Occupational Therapies Without Borders

INTEGRATING JUSTICE WITH PRACTICE

Second Edition

For Elsevier

Senior Content Strategist: Rita Demetriou-Swanwick
Senior Content Development Specialist: Nicola Lally
Project Manager: Manchu Mohan
Designer/Design Direction: Miles Hitchen
Illustration Manager: Karen Giacomucci
Illustrator: Robert Britton
Cover Photograph: Solangel Garcia-Ruiz

Occupational Therapies Without Borders

INTEGRATING JUSTICE WITH PRACTICE

Second Edition

EDITED BY

DIKAIOS SAKELLARIOU, PhD, MSc, BSc, FHEA

Senior Lecturer, School of Healthcare Sciences, Cardiff University, Cardiff, UK

NICK POLLARD, PhD, MA, MSc, DipCOT, FHEA

Senior Lecturer in Occupational Therapy, Occupational Therapy and Vocational Rehabilitation Department, Faculty of Health and Wellbeing, Sheffield Hallam University, Sheffield, UK

FOREWORDS BY

DEBBIE LALIBERTE RUDMAN, PhD, MSc, BSc

Associate Professor, Occupational Therapy, Western University, London, ON, Canada

ALEJANDRO GUAJARDO

Associate Professor, Occupational Therapy Program, Faculty of Medical Sciences, Universidad de Santiago de Chile; Member of the National Human Rights Observatory for People with Mental Disabilities, Chile

ELSEVIER   Edinburgh   London   New York   Oxford   Philadelphia   St Louis   Sydney   Toronto   2017

ELSEVIER

Previous editions © 2005 Occupational Therapy without Borders: learning from the spirit of survivors, Volume 1
© 2011 Occupational Therapies without Borders: towards an ecology of occupational-based practices, Volume 2

ISBN 978-0-7020-5920-9

Notices

Knowledge and best practice in this field are constantly changing. As new research and experience broaden our understanding, changes in research methods, professional practices, or medical treatment may become necessary.

Practitioners and researchers must always rely on their own experience and knowledge in evaluating and using any information, methods, compounds, or experiments described herein. In using such information or methods they should be mindful of their own safety and the safety of others, including parties for whom they have a professional responsibility.

With respect to any drug or pharmaceutical products identified, readers are advised to check the most current information provided (i) on procedures featured or (ii) by the manufacturer of each product to be administered, to verify the recommended dose or formula, the method and duration of administration, and contraindications. It is the responsibility of practitioners, relying on their own experience and knowledge of their patients, to make diagnoses, to determine dosages and the best treatment for each individual patient, and to take all appropriate safety precautions.

To the fullest extent of the law, neither the Publisher nor the authors, contributors, or editors, assume any liability for any injury and/or damage to persons or property as a matter of products liability, negligence or otherwise, or from any use or operation of any methods, products, instructions, or ideas contained in the material herein.

your source for books, journals and multimedia in the health sciences

www.elsevierhealth.com

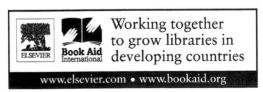

Working together to grow libraries in developing countries

www.elsevier.com • www.bookaid.org

The publisher's policy is to use paper manufactured from sustainable forests

Printed in Great Britain
Last digit is the print number: 9 8 7

CONTENTS

Section 3
THE ENACTMENT OF DIFFERENT OCCUPATIONAL THERAPIES................. 184

We would like to dedicate this book to those dear friends who through personal circumstances have been prevented from being a part of this project, and to let them know they are in our thoughts.

Y adiós
hasta más tarde
hasta más pronto
hasta que todo sea, y sea canto
Pablo Neruda (2013). Odas de todo el mundo. In I. Stavans (ed.) All the Odes. New York: Farrar, Straus and Giroux. p. 244

ACKNOWLEDGEMENTS

This book is the third volume of a joint editorial effort, which began back in the early 2000s. It started with Salvador Simó Algado and Frank Kronenberg. Nick joined the team soon after and Dikaios in 2005. We owe a big thanks to Kit Sinclair, who in her role as the president of the World Federation of Occupational Therapists brought Nick and Dikaios together back in 2004 to work on a project on Community Based Rehabilitation. Hanneke van Bruggen and Gelya Frank have offered us invaluable support over the years and we thank them both deeply.

While the composition of the editorial team has changed over the years to reflect changes in our lives, the four of us have kept on working together, in various configurations, across geographical and linguistic borders. Our personal histories have made us particularly sensitive to the need to communicate across borders and to share, acknowledge, and ultimately use knowledge from different parts of the world, grounded in a variety of paradigms and experiences. This book is the product of a happy process of experimentation.

We wish to express a special word of thanks to all contributors who generously shared their views and experiences in the chapters of this book, and who graciously responded to our feedback and engaged in a dialogical review process. The commitment and enthusiasm of everybody involved were inspirational to us. Working across geographical and linguistic borders is not always easy, but for us it is an unfailingly satisfying and enriching experience.

We also recognise that in a project involving more than 100 people, and lasting more than 2 years, life often gets in the way and things do not always go as anticipated. We are very grateful to all contributors who generously invested their time in the early phases of the book and whose work, for various reasons, has not in the end been included.

We thank our editorial team at Elsevier, and in particular Catherine Jackson for her support early on in this book series, Rita Demetriou-Swanwick for her ongoing valuable support in the continuation of the 'without borders' volumes and Manchu Mohan for seeing this book to completion. We also want to extend a special thanks and our heartfelt gratitude to Nicola Lally, the development editor for this book. Her excellent organisational skills made working with more than 100 people based all over the world a joy.

We want to express our gratitude to the Sasakawa Great Britain Foundation. A grant from this foundation made it possible for Dikaios to travel to Japan in July 2015 and work face-to-face with the authors of Chapter 56.

We have both benefitted tremendously from working and learning from many colleagues and friends, some of them also contributors to this book, from all over the world. While it is inevitable that we will not be able to mention everybody here, some of the people who offered valuable feedback, introduced us to potential contributors, or in various ways helped us during the production of this book include Hanneke van Bruggen, Sarah Kantartzis, Andrea Fabiana Albino, Mariela Nabergoi, Liliana Paganizzi, Frank Kronenberg, Sandra Galheigo, Alejandro Guajardo, Solangel Garcia-Ruiz, Salvador Simó Algado, Vagner dos Santos, and Gelya Frank. We want to extend a special thanks to Solangel Garcia-Ruiz who kindly provided the picture for the cover, beautifully illustrating the ideas of plurality and diversity that are so central in this book.

Dikaios also wishes to acknowledge the supportive environment of the School of Healthcare Sciences in Cardiff University that enabled his participation in this and numerous other projects. I have also benefitted from the hospitality and intellectual discussions in several other institutions. I would like to particularly thank the following: Pamela Block for inviting me to Stony Brook University in New York, USA; Sadako Tsubota for her unfailing support over the years and for regular invitations to Sapporo Medical University, Hokkaido Bunkyo University, and Japan Welfare University, all in Japan; and Wilson Verdugo Huenumán, and also Andrea Yupanqui Concha, Cristian Aranda Farías, Melissa Hichins Arismendi, Vanessa Vidal Castillo, and Constanza Dehays Pinochet for heartfelt hospitality at the University of Magallanes in Punta Arenas, Chile. Writing and editing are essentially solitary activities. Working with Nick meant I was working with a friend and for that I am grateful. Family and friends have always been here for me, although I have not always been able to be there for them. I thank them all deeply, and in particular the following: Julia Mpolanou, Dimitra Moustaka, Demetra Arsalidou, Erimo Okaasan, Margaret McGrath, Gareth Morgan, Dean Williams, Kazuyo Machiyama, and Elena Mounou Rotarou.

Nick would like to thank his wife, Linda, and Molly, Joshua and Daisy for their patience and support while working on this book and for holding the fort at home while I have been travelling, and also Sally, Ben, Crystal and Jack for letting me get on and work at their house at busy times. Dikaios has been a great friend and colleague and this project represents our 11th year of working together. Many thanks are due to my colleagues at Sheffield Hallam University, especially the support of those in the occupational therapy and vocational rehabilitation team. I would like to thank the students of our programmes (some represented in this volume) for their understanding and enthusiasm. I should also like to thank the staff of the occupational therapy teams at Andrés Bello National University in Santiago and Concepción in Chile for their hospitality, especially Alejandro Guajardo and Mónica Díaz Leiva. Thanks are due to Neil Carver; Moses Ikiugu; Pam Block, Devva Kasnitz and Akemi Nishida; Hetty Fransen-Jaïbi, Ines Viana Moldes, Sarah Kantartzis and Hanneke van Bruggen, who have made allowances in their work with me for some of the pressure points in this.

FOREWORD

Sakellariou and Pollard place this edition of *Occupational Therapy (Therapies) without Borders* within an 'ongoing effort to bring to the foreground of occupational therapy's consciousness the social and political context where the process of everyday living, occupation, takes place' (p. 1), and couple the aim of raising consciousness with 'what can be done' (p. 1) to work towards occupational justice. Indeed, since the 1990s, there has been a growing number of authors speaking to the transformative potential of occupation, occupation-focused scholarship, and occupation-based practice (Farias and Laliberte Rudman, 2016; Watson and Swartz, 2004). Within the current 'neoliberal world which seeks to tear asunder private troubles from public issues, and thereby social uncertainty into a personal failure that is divorced from any collective cause or remedy' (Gane and Back, 2012, p. 405), the moral imperative to mobilize consciousness of the sociopolitical shaping of occupational injustices into creative, critically informed enactments of the transformative potential of occupation urgently needs to be passionately embraced (Galheigo, 2011; Hocking and Whiteford, 2012).

Previous *Occupational Therapy (Therapies) without Borders* publications (Kronenberg et al., 2005, 2011) have been crucial igniters of awareness, dialogue and passion, particularly through creating spaces for sharing knowledges and practices generated within a diversity of contexts and through a diversity of practices. Such spaces can be hard to claim within a profession and discipline which has been dominantly 'Western', white, Anglophonic, and middle class in its 'conditions of possibility' (Kantartzis and Molineux,

2012). Continuing to break out of these foundations to promote new possibilities for thinking, being and doing in relation to occupation, this edition addresses occupational therapies; embraces varied forms of knowledges; forefronts the necessity of participatory approaches that work with those who experience inequalities; and includes contributors from wide-ranging geographical, political, and linguistic contexts. Creating such diverse spaces and dialogues is crucial to fully enacting a transformative agenda. As argued by Bonaventura de Sousa Santos (2014), there 'is no global social justice without global cognitive justice' (p. viii), and enacting social change that redresses sustained injustices in ways that avoid perpetuating forms of power that created them requires 'an intercultural dialogue and translation among different critical knowledges and practices: South-centric and North-centric, popular and scientific, religious and secular, female and male, urban and rural, and so forth' (p. 42). Embracing this book within undergraduate programmes, and as a means for practitioners and scholars to be critically reflexive regarding the assumptions that set possibilities and boundaries for their work, has the potential to further such intercultural dialogue and translation focused on issues of occupation and justice.

In line with increasing attention to the 'politics of occupation', many chapters in this book emphasize the importance of critically deconstructing and engaging with the broader context of occupation, particularly attending to how occupational injustices are shaped through political, economic and historical factors. Aligned with critical and transformative paradigms, there is a vital recognition of the need to challenge 'the status quo of an oppressive, hegemonic system in order to bring about a more equitable society' (Mertens et al., 2011, p. 231). Various authors provide means to, and examples of, critically located practices, that is, practices that attend to power; question that which has come to be taken for granted; and destabilize historically reified forms of oppression based on gender, citizenship status, race, socioeconomic status, age, and other axes of difference (Cannella and Lincoln, 2009). While such questioning and destabilizing in and of itself does not constitute social transformation, it opens up the space for possibilities (Sayer, 2009) – possibilities to reimagine different ways to 'do' realities and remobilize power relations in ways that align with occupational justice. As articulated by Holstein and Gubrium (2011):

> *Critically framed, persistent how questions remind us to bear in mind that the everyday realities of our lives ... are realities we do. Having done them, they can be undone. We can move on to dismantle and reassemble realities, producing and reproducing, time and again, the world we inhabit. Politically, this recognizes that, in the world we inhabit, we could enact alternate possibilities or alternative directions, even if common sense understandings make this seem impossible. (p. 353)*

This book forefronts key issues that require ongoing dialogue and critical reflexivity as we move forward in deploying occupation for critical and transformative purposes. There are no easy, one-size-fits-all answers to questions such as, how can occupational therapists and scientists 'turn the neoliberal themes of ownership and personal responsibility on their head' (Soss et al., 2011, p. 208), or how can we contribute to the reimagining of governance in ways that promote inclusive, just societies? However, if we accept that occupational injustice is present everywhere and that occupation is not only a means of resistance but also a site for the reproduction of inequality (Angell, 2014), occupational practices and knowledges are crucial aspects of social transformations that promote human flourishing.

DEBBIE LALIBERTE RUDMAN
Western University
January 2016, London, Ontario, Canada

REFERENCES

Angell, M.A., 2014. Occupation-centred analysis of social difference: contributions to a socially responsive occupational science. J. Occup. Sci. 21 (2), 104–116.

Cannella, G.S., Lincoln, Y.S., 2009. Deploying qualitative methods for critical social purposes. In: Denzin, N.K., Giardina, M.D. (Eds.), Qualitative Inquiry and Social Justice: Towards a Politics of Hope. Left Coast Press, Walnut Creek, CA, pp. 53–72.

de Sousa Santos, B., 2014. Epistemologies of the South. Justice against Epistemicide. Paradigm Publishers, Boulder, CO.

Farias, L., Laliberte Rudman, D., 2016. A critical interpretive synthesis of the uptake of critical perspectives in occupational science. J. Occup. Sci. 23 (1), 33–50. doi:10.1080/14427591.2014.989893.

Galheigo, S., 2011. What needs to be done? Occupational therapy responsibilities and challenges regarding human rights. Aust. Occup. Ther. J. 58 (2), 60–66.

Gane, M., Back, L., 2012. C. Wright Mills 50 years on: the promise and craft of sociology revisited. Theory Cult. Soc. 29 (7/8), 399–421.

Hocking, C., Whiteford, G.E., 2012. Introduction to critical perspectives in occupational science. In: Whiteford, G.E., Hocking, C. (Eds.), Occupational Science: Society, Inclusion, Participation. Wiley-Blackwell, Oxford, UK, pp. 3–7.

Holstein, J.A., Gubrium, J.F., 2011. The constructionist analytics of interpretive practice. In: Denzin, N.K., Lincoln, Y.S. (Eds.), The SAGE Handbook of Qualitative Research. Sage, Los Angeles, pp. 341–357.

Kantartzis, S., Molineux, M., 2012. Understanding the discursive development of occupation: historico-political perspectives. In: Whiteford, G.E., Hocking, C. (Eds.), Occupational Science: Society, Inclusion, Participation. Wiley-Blackwell, Oxford, UK, pp. 38–53.

Kronenberg, F., Pollard, N., Sakellariou, D., 2011. Occupational Therapies Without Borders: Towards an Ecology of Occupation-Based Practices, vol. 2. Elsevier Science, Edinburgh.

Kronenberg, F., Simó Algado, S., Pollard, N., 2005. Occupational Therapy Without Borders: Learning from the Spirit of Survivors. Churchill Livingstone, Oxford.

Mertens, D.M., Sullivan, M., Stace, H., 2011. Disability communities: transformative research on social justice. In: Denzin, N.K., Lincoln, Y.S. (Eds.), The SAGE Handbook of Qualitative Research. Sage, Los Angeles, pp. 227–242.

Sayer, A., 2009. Who's afraid of critical social science? Curr. Sociol. 57 (6), 767–786.

Soss, J., Fording, R.C., Schram, S.F., 2011. Disciplining the Poor: Neoliberalism Paternalism and the Persistent Power of Race. University of Chicago Press, Chicago.

Watson, R., Swartz, L., 2004. Transformation through Occupation. Whurr Publishers Ltd, London.

FOREWORD

We are witnessing a worldwide debate within occupational therapy, as its intellectual and scientific production has expanded enormously. A great part of this debate and some of the associated new developments are related to deep social changes. These changes present us with a diversity of problems, which are often at the centre of attention for public policies. To engage with these issues, occupational therapists have expanded their repertoire of expertise. Concepts such as inclusion, participation, justice, and human rights complement therapists' focus on treatment, adaptation, cure, and improvement. There has been a move from the health field to education, justice, and social development; from clinical interventions to social, justice and community programmes, and from the technical neutrality of clinical practice to political and ethical debates.

Occupational therapy is a space in dispute, of dialogues and tensions in a wide diversity of practices. It is a place of encounters and disagreements that have generated movement and fractured the notion of the profession as a stable and homogeneous concept. Discussions in occupational therapy arise from an essential need: how to produce a liberating, transformative practice, oriented to the fulfilment of people and communities, in the context of common well-being, and in recognition of diversity, of justice, dignity, and solidarity, based on common sense, daily living, and collective citizen practices. To do this, it is important to develop an occupational therapy that is firmly situated within political and historical contexts.

This book offers an account of how occupational therapists from all over the world engage with political and historical contexts to effect positive changes. In many parts of the world, human and ecological suffering has a political and historical context of poverty and misfortune through capitalism. This book offers an emancipatory transformative, political, and ethical account of how occupational therapists from all over the world can effect positive changes.

Occupational therapy is compelled to acknowledge that no single way of knowing should take priority over the others. In order to successfully address the social problems which large parts of the population across the world are facing, occupational therapy needs to draw on a variety of approaches to knowledge, both epistemologically and ontologically. This requires the complementary use of different approaches, including social, anthropological, sociological, and occupational therapy research (Avendaño et al., 2012). From this perspective, our task must be to integrate and promote self-conscious processes from community actors as central ground for social transformation.

I only see this becoming possible as theoretical and scientific production in occupational therapy adopts a radical position by rejecting reductionism while embracing holism and integrating the production of knowledge with social practices. Such a process could serve to highlight the importance of citizenship rights and respect knowledge as a social and collective production.

This is feasible in as far as occupational therapy is both not neutral and has a theoretical and scientific praxis committed to the oppressed other, rather than to an abstract notion of occupation as an object of study. Otherness is people's own relation to the world, closing up the relation between subject-object, transforming it into a subject-subject relation based upon an ethics of liberation and subject recognition, where scientific practice is founded primarily and intentionally alongside the excluded and oppressed, and is directed to their recognition and emancipation.

Knowledge production in occupational therapy must subvert the attempts of disciplinary action; there must be, in the words of Bassi (2013), improvisation, not as a fatalistic destiny, but as a process which is conscious of risks, mistakes and changes, and that manages to deal with the incompleteness of social phenomena. Such a process has no pretention of discovering the truth, but aims instead to enquire and to question. Knowledge has a plurality of actors and different social subjects. Knowledge production must be a deliberative act of freedom, one that neither reasserts new institutional professions nor legitimizes a decision-making statute. It must promote researchers' creativity and dialogue with communities and collectives. Pérez Soto (1998) calls for a league or union to defend imagination in theoretical, academic, and scientific productions.

The border between art and science in occupational therapy must be fractured. As those boundaries are diluted, usurped, and blurred, research in occupational therapy will not search for the truth, but for multiple truths. In Latin America, there is a long tradition of knowledge production that can offer guidance in collapsing the artificial boundaries between art and science: Fals Borda (Participative Action Research), Paulo Freire (Popular Education), and Enrique Dussel (Liberation Philosophy), among others. What occupational therapy needs is a plurality of epistemological traditions, drawing on social sciences, philosophy, politics, our history and region, the South, in the sense of De Sousa Santos (2012).

Emancipation and freedom, as historically situated social praxes, can be developed through human social practices; they are produced through our own subjective existence rather than through processes distanced from real life, called scientific. Giving expert knowledge a protagonist role can lead to a loss of citizens' autonomy and their right to build their future by themselves. In summary, what we need is fewer experts and more citizenship!

Occupational therapy must be based on collective rights; on people's fundamental rights under the principles of freedom, equality, and dignity. In this sense, the primary focus of our praxis must be the full self-determination of every citizen, and the freedom to make and propose personal projects aimed at achieving a dignified life and collective well-being. This involves the fulfilment of life plans, materialization of concrete actions in daily life in what is called moral autonomy (De Asís and Palacios, 2007).

Such a focus requires a strong occupational therapy that promotes action through a living culture of solidarity, from the realm of public and common sense. Such an occupational therapy can acknowledge the blurred boundaries between us and them, considering circumstances, demands, and relevant needs for everyone, and asserting common claims that may justify the existence of obligations. The lives of people and communities are not only private matters. They are primarily a citizenship and rights issue that involves us all.

ALEJANDRO GUAJARDO
Universidad de Santiago de Chile
March 2016, Santiago, Chile

REFERENCES

Avendaño, O., Canales, M., Atria, R., 2012. Sociología. Introducción a Los Clásicos. Editorial LOM, Santiago.

Bassi, J., 2013. Adios a la partitura: una defensa de los diseños flexibles en investigación social. En: Investigación Social. Lenguajes del Diseño. Editorial LOM, Santiago, p. 48.

De Asís, R., Palacios, A., 2007. Derechos Humanos y Situaciones de Dependencia. Cuadernos 'Bartolomé De Las Casas', N° 43. Editorial Dikynson, Madrid.

De Sousa Santos, B., 2012. Una Epistemología del Sur. CLACSO Ediciones, México.

Pérez Soto, C., 1998. Sobre un Concepto Histórico de Ciencia. De la Epistemología Actual a la Dialéctica. Editorial LOM, Santiago.

PREFACE

The book before you, *Occupational Therapies without Borders: Integrating Justice with Practice, Second Edition*, follows two previous volumes (which together formed the First Edition): *Occupational Therapy without Borders: learning from the spirit of survivors* (2005), of which an adapted Spanish translation was published by Editorial Médica Panamericana (2007), and *Occupational Therapies without Borders: towards an ecology of occupation-based practices* (2010). What follows is a brief account of the origins and evolution of this book series, historically situating its contents at the end of the 20th and first decades of the 21st century, a period once again characterized by global social crises (though larger and more rapidly unfolding) as those that gave birth to occupational therapy in 1917.

After exchanging a series of emails, during our first real-time meeting in Maastricht, Netherlands, in 1998 we learned to share similar concerns and interests – working with 'survivor populations' through an activist appreciation of occupational therapy, akin to the vision of some of our profession's founders. We also shared the frustrations of having to constantly defend our 'out of the box' positioning of occupational therapy against many educators and colleagues, who kept telling us that we might have chosen the wrong profession, that psychology or social work might have been more appropriate career choices. However, the pull of our personal social concerns and interests proved stronger than the pressures we experienced from within the profession. In the spirit of occupational therapy, we regarded something that 'is not' – that is, occupational therapy with marginalized populations – to mean that it was simply 'not yet', and that we may just have to get it started.

Our motivation to study occupational therapy was significantly driven by extensive travel and work experiences in different parts of the world – with immigrants, refugees (Guatemala), children survivors of war (Bosnia and Kosovo), culturally diverse people living with physical and cognitive disabilities (Pakistan, India, United States) and 'street children' (Mexico). Salvador established the *Dolphin Association* in 1997, an international internet-based initiative to attract, organize and mobilize occupational therapists to generate socially responsive practices with marginalized populations – people our profession had thus far either overlooked or neglected. In early 2002, to better capture and communicate who they were and what they were about, we renamed this initiative 'Occupational Therapists without Borders'. We then described it as an international informal network of proactive occupational therapists who share particular social concerns and who are committed to challenge and change conditions that deny or restrict access to dignified and meaningful participation in everyday life in society. Frank and Zemke (2008) first described this informal network as a movement within the international communities of occupational therapy and occupational science. The occupational therapy without borders book series can perhaps be regarded as the most tangible 'evidence' of the existence of the movement. It has also been recognized that this movement significantly influenced the generation of position papers by the World Federation of Occupational Therapists (WFOT) and also the coming about of the first ever WFOT congress in Latin America, in

Santiago de Chile in 2010, with human rights as a key theme.

During the late 1990s and early 2000s we had been sharing our intervention and research experiences with vulnerable yet resilient populations surviving adverse everyday life conditions (armed conflicts, forced displacement, living on the streets) in workshops and presentations at universities in Europe and North America. Occupational therapy students indicated a desire for reading material about the 'without borders' perspectives of occupational therapy that we presented, which provided the impetus for the original book. The students encouraged us to overcome our 'limiting perception' that books are (to be) written by native English speakers from North America, considering that the bulk of reading materials that we had been exposed to during our occupational therapy training came from there. But students were not preoccupied with this reality, pushing us with 'you write it and we will buy and read it'.

At the 2002 WFOT World Congress in Stockholm, Sweden, the late Gary Kielhofner connected us to Elsevier, which then led to an invitation to prepare and submit a proposal. We experienced this as quite a daunting task, considering that neither of us had ever been prepared for this. Through our international networks we identified and invited like-minded colleagues. Acknowledging that our education did not (and often still does not) *really* prepare us to serve people beyond those who can pay for treatment and those who present with some kind of medical diagnosis, we felt that the book ought to foreground not our profession, but those who we would have to learn from in order to become a relevant enabling resource to them. Thus the original title we proposed was *'Learning from the Spirit of Survivors'* and *'Occupational Therapy without Borders'* as the subtitle. However, the publisher urged us to reverse this order due to a concern with how books are sold nowadays (using 'occupational therapy' as the main keyword in search engines). It was our UK colleague Annie Turner who reviewed the proposal for Elsevier and who indicated that beyond its contents, she had sensed 'messages' between the lines that ought to be given a chance to get heard and published.

After the writing and editing process got under way, we realized that the project would benefit from an additional editor, someone with writing and editing experience who is a native English speaker and who would get the book's ethos. It was again through an internet-based discussion forum that Nick Pollard surfaced as the right candidate, joining the team during the course of 2003. The title and subtitle of the second volume (Kronenberg, Pollard, and Sakellariou 2010) were tweaked to posit that there is no such thing as 'occupational therapy', but instead a plurality of 'therapies' and even beyond 'occupation-based practices', including and beyond those which describe therapeutic processes to those aimed at learning, rebuilding, conflict resolution, development, etc. Having collaborated on the 2008 book *'A Political Practice of Occupational Therapy'* (Pollard, Sakellariou, and Kronenberg, 2008), Dikaios Sakellariou was invited to be the third editor of the second volume.

Considering that the first volume was 'a leap of faith' by both the authors and the publisher, the fact that a second volume came about and now a decade later a second edition – which now presents as one of the Elsevier 'Essentials' Series – is perhaps indicative of the timely and topical nature of these publications. However, it seems appropriate to exercise a point of caution regarding this achievement. We ought to remain mindful of the series' original ethos, that 'without borders' discourses and practices are to be generated from the margins of our societies and communities, to prevent falling into the trap of perpetuating the profession being positioned at the 'centre of power' instead of with the populations that our societies (tend to) push and keep at the margins.

We think that it is important to build a profession relevant to society. It is suffering, which, more than admiration, drives us to think (Boff, 2000) how to answer real contemporary challenges, respecting and acknowledging the central role of the populations we have the privilege to work with, from the perspective of empowering models. It is time to move away from grandiloquent speeches and declarations to concrete and reality-driven actions. Time to confront the situation of occupational apartheid, and develop collective occupations, including ecology in our interventions towards developing an occupational ecology approach (Simó Algado and Townsend 2015); time to develop an occupational therapy based on human rights (Guajardo and Simó Algado, 2010). Mounier (2002) pointed the need for a revolution of values that can lead to a revolution of the structures. Yes, it is time for revolution in occupational therapy! Let us create powerful interventions in order to create fairer, more inclusive and sustainable communities. We congratulate the fantastic team of editors and authors of this voluminous second edition and wish it to be widely read and engaged with.

FRANK KRONENBERG, SALVADOR SIMÓ ALGADO

REFERENCES

Boff, L., 2000. La Dignidad de la Tierra. Ecología, mundialización, espiritualidad. La emergencia de un nuevo paradigma. Trotta, Madrid.

Frank, G., Zemke, R., 2008. Occupational therapy foundations for political engagement and social transformation. In: Pollard, N., Sakellariou, D., Kronenberg, F., (Eds.), A Political Practice of Occupational Therapy. Elsevier/Churchill Livingstone, Edinburgh, pp. 111, 136.

Guajardo, A., Simó Algado, S., 2010. Una terapia ocupacional basada en los derechos humanos. Revista TOG, Galicia 7 (12), 1–25.

Kronenberg, F., Simó Algado, S., Pollard, N., (Eds.), 2005. Occupational Therapy without Borders: learning from the Spirit of Survivors. Elsevier, Oxford.

Kronenberg, F., Simó Algado, S., Pollard, N., (Eds.), 2007. Terapia Ocupacional Sin Fronteras – aprendiendo del espiritu des superivientes (2006). Panamericana, Madrid.

Kronenberg, F., Pollard, N., Sakellariou, D., (Eds.), 2010. Occupational Therapies without Borders, vol. 2. Towards an Ecology of Occupation-based Practices. Churchill Livingstone, Edinburgh.

Mounier, E., 2002. El Personalismo. Antología esencial. Ediciones Sígueme, Salamanca.

Pollard, N., Sakellariou, D., Kronenberg, F., (Eds.), 2008. A Political Practice of Occupational Therapy. Churchill Livingstone, Oxford.

Simó Algado, S., Townsend, E., 2015. Eco-social Occupational therapy. Br. J. Occup. Ther. 78 (3), 182–186.

CONTRIBUTORS LIST

ANDREA FABIANA ALBINO, PGDip, Lic
Professor, Research Methodology and Final Work
Design, School of Psychology, University of
Buenos Aires, Buenos Aires, Argentina

REBECCA M. ALDRICH, PhD, OTR/L
Assistant Professor, Occupational Science and
Occupational Therapy, Saint Louis University,
Saint Louis, MO, USA

MARION AMMERAAL, MSc
Occupational Therapist, Recovery and Rehabilitation
Research Group; Actenz, GGZ inGeest,
Amsterdam; ELSiTO member, The Netherlands

VARVARA APOSTOLOGLOU, MSc, BSc
Occupational Therapist, ELSiTO member, Athens,
Greece

CRISTIAN ARANDA FARÍAS, Mag, Lic
Occupational Therapist, PhD candidate in Cognition
and Human Evolution at University of Balearic
Islands; Associate Professor, Department of
Occupational Therapy, University of Magallanes,
Punta Arenas, Chile

ANTOINE L. BAILLIARD, PhD, OTR/L
Assistant Professor, Occupational Science and
Occupational Therapy, University of North
Carolina at Chapel Hill, Chapel Hill, NC, USA

FEDERICO BARROSO LELOUCHE, Lic
Permaculture Design Certificate, Argentine Institute
of Permaculture, Gaia Ecovillage – Navarro,
Buenos Aires, Argentina

ANGELA BERNDT, PhD, BAppSci
Lecturer, School of Health Sciences, University of
South Australia, Adelaide, SA, Australia

PAMELA BLOCK, PhD
Associate Professor, School of Health Technology and
Management, Stony Brook University, Stony
Brook, NY, USA

THEODOROS BOGEAS, BSc
Occupational Therapist, ELSiTO member, Athens,
Greece

**MARÍA MARCELA BOTTINELLI, PhD, MA,
PGDip, Lic**
Professor, Research Methodology and Final Work
Design, School of Psychology, University of
Buenos Aires and National University of Lanús,
Buenos Aires, Argentina

WENDY BRYANT, PhD, MSc, DipCOT, PGCert
Senior Lecturer, School of Health and Human
Sciences, University of Essex, Colchester, UK

OLIVE BRYANTON, MEd, BA
Project Coordinator, PEI Centre on Health and
Aging; PhD Student, Faculty of Education,
University of Prince Edward Island,
Charlottetown, PEI, Canada

HEATHER BULLEN, BSc(Hons), PGCert
Lecturer, Department of Occupational Therapy,
    University of Derby, Derby, UK

MARIJKE C. BURGER, Drs
Client Council, GGZ inGeest, Amsterdam; ELSiTO
    member, the Netherlands

PABLO A. CANTERO GARLITO, MSc, MA,
Dip(TO), Dip(Education Social)
Occupational Therapist; Social Educator; Sexologist;
    Coordinator, Occupational Therapy, Centre for
    Psychosocial Rehabilitation, Plasencia, Cáceres;
    PhD candidate; Associate Professor, Department
    of Nursing and Physiotherapy, University of
    Castile La Mancha, Toledo, Spain

MENGAN CAO, MOT, BAppScOT
Occupational Therapist, People's Republic of China

JACKIE CASEY, MSc, BSc(Hons), PGCHEP,
PGCert, FHEA
Lecturer, Occupational Therapy, School of Health
    Sciences, University of Ulster, Co. Antrim, UK

TSING-YEE (EMILY) CHAI
Undergraduate student, Community Rehabilitation
    and Disability Studies, University of Calgary, AB,
    Canada

LUIS ERNESTO CHAURA, Lic
Occupational Therapist, San Cayetano Primary
    Health Care Center; Manuel Sanguinetti External
    Area Regional Hospital, Comodoro Rivadavia,
    Argentina

SIMONE COETZEE, BSc(Hons), MSc
Lecturer, School of Health and Human Sciences,
    University of Essex, Colchester; PhD candidate,
    Brunel University, London, UK

LESLEY COLLIER, PhD, MSc, DipCOT
Senior Lecturer, Occupational Therapy, Faculty of
    Health Sciences, University of Southampton,
    Southampton, UK

JENNIFER CREEK, PhD, DipCOT
Freelance Occupational Therapist, North Yorkshire,
    UK

MIRANDA CUNNINGHAM, MSc, BA(Hons),
BSc(Hons), PGDip
Lecturer, Occupational Therapy, School of Health
    Professions, Plymouth University, Plymouth, UK

JEAN M. DALY, MSc, MSc, BA
Researcher, Cedar Foundation, Brain Injury Services,
    Belfast, Co. Antrim, UK

ALEXIS DAVIS, MSc, BSc
Pediatric Occupational Therapist/Global Health
    Project Manager, Vancouver, BC, Canada

CONSTANZA DEHAYS PINOCHET, Lic
Occupational Therapist, Adjunct Professor,
    Department of Occupational Therapy, University
    of Magallanes, Punta Arenas, Chile

JANE DIAMOND, MSc, BSc(Hons), BA(Hons)
Occupational Therapist, CWPT Partnership Trust,
    Coventry, UK

MÓNICA DÍAZ LEIVA, Mg
Magister, Occupational Therapy; Academic,
    Occupational Therapist, School of Occupational
    Therapy Andres Bello National University,
    Santiago, Chile

GUADALUPE DÏAZ USANDIVARAS, Lic
Coordinator, Tempora Psychotherapeutic Institute,
    and Association for the Development of Special
    Education and Integration (ADEEI), Buenos
    Aires, Argentina

ESTHER DOMINGUEZ VEGA, DipOT
Occupational Therapist, Consultant on International
    Cooperation, Casamance, Senegal

VAGNER DOS SANTOS, MSc, OT
PhD candidate, Assistant Professor, Occupational
    Therapy Undergraduate Program; Ceilândia
    Faculty, University of Brasília, Brazil

EVELYNE DUROCHER, PhD, MOT, BSc(Hons), RegOT
Post-doctoral Scholar, School of Occupational Therapy, Faculty of Health Sciences, Western University, London, ON, Canada

BROOKE ELLISON, PhD
Assistant Professor, School of Health Technology and Management, Stony Brook University, Stony Brook, NY, USA

DANIEL EMERIC MÉAULLE, MSc, Dip(TO)
Occupational Therapist, Care Program for the Roma Ethnic Minority in prisons, Gypsy Secretariat Foundation (NGO), Madrid V Penitentiary Center, Madrid, Spain

LENA-KARIN ERLANDSSON, RegOT
Associate Professor, Department of Occupational Therapy, Metropolitan University College, Copenhagen, Denmark

ANNE FENECH, PhD, DipCOT, MSc, MBA
Lecturer, Faculty of Health Sciences, University of Southampton, Southampton, UK

DEBORAH LEIGH FEWSTER, MPhil, BOT
PhD candidate, Lecturer, Discipline of Occupational Therapy, University of KwaZulu-Natal, Westville Campus, KwaZulu-Natal, South Africa

KRISTEN MARIE FOLEY, BAppSc
Occupational Therapist, Master of Public Health (Research) candidate, Flinders University, Adelaide, SA, Australia

GELYA FRANK, PhD, MPW, MA, BA
Professor, Mrs. T.H. Chan Division of Occupational Science and Occupational Therapy, and Department of Anthropology, University of Southern California, Los Angeles, CA, USA

HETTY FRANSEN-JAÏBI, MSc, MSc, BSc
Course Leader and Senior Lecturer, Occupational Therapy Bachelor's Program, Higher School of Health Sciences and Techniques of Tunis (ESSTST) University of Tunis El Manar, Tunis, Tunisia

ROSHAN GALVAAN, PhD, MSc, BSc
Head of Division, Division of Occupational Therapy, University of Cape Town, Cape Town, South Africa

DANIKA GALVIN, PhD, BHSc
Occupational Therapist, The Alfred; Former PhD Candidate, School of Community Health, Charles Sturt University, Albury, NSW, Australia

TRACY GARBER, MA, OTR/L
Occupational Therapist, MN, USA

SOLANGEL GARCIA-RUIZ, Specialization Degree, MA
Occupational Therapist; Coordinator of Research and Cooperation, District Secretariat of Health, Bogota; Investigator, Research group on Disability, Inclusion and Society, National University, Bogota; Member, Community Based Rehabilitation (CBR) Americas Network, Colombia

EMMA GEORGE, BAppSc, MSc, MSc
Occupational Therapist, PhD candidate, Centre for Research Excellence: Health Equity, Southgate Institute, Flinders University, Adelaide, SA, Australia

SUSAN GILBERT HUNT, MHSc, DipCOT
Senior Lecturer, School of Health Sciences, University of South Australia, Adelaide, SA, Australia

XAVIER GINESTA, PhD, Dip, BSc
Associate Professor, Department of Communications, University of Vic-Central University of Catalonia, Vic, Spain

IMOGEN GORDON, MA, DipCOT, PGDip
Senior Lecturer, Occupational Therapy and Social
   and Therapeutic Horticulture, Department of
   Health, Coventry University, Coventry, UK

PRAGASHNIE GOVENDER, PhD, MOT, BOT
Lecturer, Discipline of Occupational Therapy,
   University of KwaZulu-Natal, Westville Campus,
   KwaZulu-Natal, South Africa

**ROSEMARY JOAN GOWRAN, PhD, MSc,
BSc(Hons)**
Lecturer, Occupational Therapy, Department of
   Clinical Therapies, Faculty of Education and
   Health Sciences, University of Limerick, Limerick,
   Ireland

PAM GRETSCHEL, MS, BSc
Lecturer, Department of Health and Rehabilitation
   Sciences, Division of Occupational Therapy,
   University of Cape Town, Cape Town, Western
   Cape, PhD candidate, National Health Scholar,
   Medical Research Council, Cape Town, South
   Africa

ALEJANDRO GUAJARDO
Associate Professor, Occupational Therapy Program,
   Faculty of Medical Sciences, Universidad de
   Santiago de Chile; Member of the National
   Human Rights Observatory for People with
   Mental Disabilities, Santiago, Chile

JYOTHI GUPTA, PhD, OTR/L, FAOTA
Professor and Chair, Department of Occupational
   Therapy, Arizona School of Health Sciences, A. T.
   Still University, Mesa, AZ, USA

THAVANESI GURAYAH, MOT, BOT
PhD candidate, Lecturer, Discipline of Occupational
   Therapy, University of KwaZulu-Natal, Westville
   Campus, Kwa-Zulu Natal, South Africa

KEIICHI HASEGAWA, MSc, BSc
General Manager, Department of Rehabilitation,
   Takeda General Hospital, Fukushima, Japan

MELISSA HICHINS ARISMENDI, Lic
Occupational Therapist, Adjunct Professor,
   Department of Occupational Therapy, University
   of Magallanes, Punta Arenas, Chile

CLARE HOCKING, PhD, NZROT
Professor, Department of Occupational Science and
   Therapy, Auckland University of Technology,
   Auckland, New Zealand

MARGARET JONES, PhD, MHSc, BHSc
Lecturer, Department of Occupational Science and
   Therapy, Auckland University of Technology,
   Auckland, New Zealand

EFTYCHIA KALIMANA, BSc
Occupational Therapist, Iasis NGO Day Centre,
   Athens, Greece

SARAH KANTARTZIS, PhD, MSc, DipCOT
Senior Lecturer, Occupational Therapy, Queen
   Margaret University, Edinburgh; ELSiTO member,
   UK

MARIA KAPANADZE, MSc, BSc, BSc
Lecturer, Occupational Therapy Program; PhD
   candidate, Escola Universitària d'Infermeria i
   Teràpia Ocupacional de Terrassa/ Universitat
   Autónoma de Barcelona, Terrassa, Barcelona,
   Spain

DIMITRIOS KARAMITSOS
ELSiTO member, Athens, Greece

MARIA KARAMPETSOU, MSc
Occupational Therapist, ELSiTO member; Director
   of the Social Policy Directorate, Municipality of
   Iraklio Attikis, Athens, Greece

MARIA KATSAMAGKOU, BSc
Occupational Therapist, Chalkida, Greece

SOFIA KELEMOURIDOU, BSc
Occupational Therapist, Private Neuropsychomotor
   Rehabilitation Center for Children, Therapedia,
   Nikaia, Attica, Greece

IVANA KLEPO, BSc, OTR/L
Head of Occupational Therapy, Department of
Neurorehabilitation, Special Hospital for Medical
Rehabilitation, Krapinske Toplice; President of the
Occupational Therapy Council, Croatian
Chamber of Health Professionals, Zagreb;
Assistant, Occupational Therapy, University of
Applied Health Studies, Zagreb, Croatia

MARTHA KOKKOROU, BSc
Occupational Therapist, Central Macedonian Center
for Social Welfare, Thessaloniki, Greece

IVI KOTSINI, BSc
Occupational Therapist, Athens, Greece

MARIA KOULOUMPI, MSc
Occupational Therapist, Tutor, Department of
Occupational Therapy, School of Health and
Caring Professions, Technological Educational
Institution of Athens, Athens, Greece

HANNAH KUPER, ScD
Co-Director, International Centre for Evidence in
Disability (ICED), London School of Hygiene and
Tropical Medicine, London, UK

STEFANOS LAZOPOULOS, Dip
Accountant, ELSiTO member, Athens, Greece

THANALUTCHMY LINGAH, MBA, BOT
PhD candidate, Lecturer, Discipline of Occupational
Therapy, University of KwaZulu-Natal, Westville
Campus, KwaZulu-Natal, South Africa

ROSELI ESQUERDO LOPES, PhD
Full Professor, Department of Occupational Therapy,
Graduate Program of Occupational Therapy &
Graduate Program of Education, Member of the
Metuia Project, Federal University of São Carlos,
São Carlos, São Paulo, Brazil

DANIEL LOWRIE, MSc, BHSc
Lecturer, Occupational Therapy, James Cook
University, Townsville, QLD, Australia

JENNI MACE, DipNZOT, MSc
Senior Occupational Therapy Lecturer, Department
of Occupational Science and Therapy, Auckland
University of Technology, Auckland, New Zealand

ANA PAULA SERRATA MALFITANO, PhD
Assistant Professor, Department of Occupational
Therapy, Graduate Program of Occupational
Therapy, Member of the Metuia Project, Federal
University of São Carlos, São Carlos, São Paulo,
Brazil

MARIA MARGARI, BSc
Occupational Therapist, Sin Praxi Center for
Children with Developmental Disorders and
Learning Disabilities, Halandri, Greece

HIDENORI MATSUO, BSc, MPH
Occupational Therapist, System Science Consultants
Inc. (SSC), Tokyo, Japan

TINA MCGRATH, PhD, MA, BSc(Hons), HDip
Consultant Occupational Therapist & Independent
Scholar, Peregrine Occupational Therapy
Consultancy, Dublin, Ireland

**MARGARET MCGRATH, PhD, MSc, BSc(Hons),
PGDip**
Senior Lecturer, Discipline of Occupational Therapy,
Faculty of Health Sciences, University of Sydney,
Sydney, NSW, Australia

ANDREA VERÓNICA MEDINA, Lic
Professor, Research Methodology, School of
Psychology, University of Buenos Aires, Buenos
Aires, Argentina

KATRIEN MEERMANS, BSc
Psychiatric Nurse, Sheltered Living, Support Coach,
vzw De Hulster, Leuven; ELSiTO member,
Belgium

MARGARITA MONDACA, MSc
Lecturer & PhD candidate, Division of Occupational
Therapy, Karolinska Institutet, Stockholm, Sweden

ANNE-LE MORVILLE, PhD, MSc
Senior Lecturer, Department of Occupational
Therapy, Metropolitan University College,
Copenhagen, Denmark

MARIELA NABERGOI, PhD, PGDip, Lic
Professor, Research Methodology, Statistics and Final
Work Design, Institute of Rehabilitation and
Movement Sciences, National University of
General San Martín, Buenos Aires, Argentina

DESHINI NAIDOO, MOT, BOT
PhD candidate, Lecturer, Discipline of Occupational
Therapy, University of KwaZulu-Natal, Westville
Campus, KwaZulu Natal, South Africa

DANIELA OLIVARES, MSc
Occupational Therapist, Associate Professor, Faculty
of Medicine, Austral University of Chile, Valdivia,
Chile

MARTIN O'NEILL, PhD, BSc
Community Engagement Lead, Cardiff School of
Social Sciences, Cardiff University, Cardiff, UK

LILY OWENS, BSc(Hons), PGCert
Senior Occupational Therapist, North East London
NHS Foundation Trust, London; PhD candidate,
Department of Clinical Sciences, Brunel
University, UK

LILIANA PAGANIZZI, MSc, Lic
Professor, Public Health Institute of Rehabilitation
and Movement Sciences, National University of
General San Martín, Buenos Aires, Argentina

MÓNICA PALACIOS TOLVETT, Mg
Magister, Social Community Psychology; Academic,
Occupational Therapist, School of Occupational
Therapy, Andrés Bello National University,
Santiago, Chile

LAURA PARRAQUINI, Lic
Occupational Therapist, Permaculture Design
Certificate, Argentine Institute of Permaculture,
Gaia Ecovillage – Navarro, Buenos Aires,
Argentina

AMY PAUL-WARD, PhD, MSOT
Associate Professor, Occupational Therapy, Florida
International University, Miami, FL; Director,
Nursing PhD Program, Florida International
University, Miami, FL, USA

**ROBERT BERNARD PEREIRA, PhD, BSc(Hons),
RegOT**
Care Coordinator, Hospital Admission Risk Program,
Barwon Health, Geelong, VIC; Professional
Associate, Field of Occupational Therapy, School
of Public Health and Nutrition, Faculty of Health,
University of Canberra, Canberra, ACT, Australia

LIESL PETERS, MSc, BSc
Lecturer, Division of Occupational Therapy,
University of Cape Town, Cape Town, South
Africa

**ANNA RACHEL PETTICAN, BSc(Hons), PGCert,
MSc**
Lecturer and PhD Researcher, School of Health and
Human Sciences, University of Essex, Colchester,
UK

**LEE PRICE, PhD, MSc, BSc(Hons), DipCOT,
SFHEA**
Assistant Head, School of Health Sciences; Head,
Occupational Therapy, University of Brighton,
Eastbourne, UK

SASA RADIC, BSc, OTR/L
President, Croatian Association of Occupational
Therapists, Zagreb; Vice President, Head of
Occupational Therapy Professional Class,
Croatian Chamber for Health Professionals,
Zagreb; Assistant, Occupational Therapy,
University of Applied Health Studies, Zagreb;
Occupational Therapist, Animal Assisted Ayres
Sensory Integration Therapy, Rehabilitation
Centre Silver, Zagreb, Croatia

ELELWANI RAMUGONDO, PhD, MSc, BSc
Associate Professor, Health and Rehabilitation Sciences, University of Cape Town, Cape Town, South Africa

ELENA ROTAROU, PhD
Postdoctoral Research Fellow, Department of Economics, University of Chile, Santiago, Chile

DEBBIE LALIBERTE RUDMAN, PhD, MSc, BSc
Associate Professor, Occupational Therapy, Western University, London, ON, Canada

GAYNOR SADLO, PhD, PGDip, DipCOT
Professor, School of Health Sciences, University of Brighton, Eastbourne, UK; Visiting Professor, First Faculty of Medicine, Charles University, Prague, Czech Republic

JORDI DE SAN EUGENIO, PhD
Professor, Communication, University of Vic-Central University of Catalonia, Vic, Spain

BEN SELLAR, PhD, BSc(Hons)
Lecturer, Occupational Therapy Program, School of Health Sciences, University of South Australia, Adelaide, SA, Australia

JANE SHAMROCK, MA
PhD candidate, Graduate Centre, Faculty of Science, Health, Education and Engineering, University of the Sunshine Coast, Maroochydore, QLD, Australia

YOSHITAKA SHIINO, PhD, OT
Chief Occupational Therapist, Department of Rehabilitation, Takeda General Hospital, Fukushima, Japan

SALVADOR SIMÓ ALGADO, PhD, MBA
Lecturer and Research Coordinator, University of Vic-Central University of Catalonia, Vic, Spain

DEBORAH SIMPSON, BSc, MAEEC
Mental Health Occupational Therapist/Environmental Educator, Vancouver, BC, Canada

KIT SINCLAIR, PhD, MSc, BSc, FWFOT, FAOTA
Editor, WFOT Bulletin; Ambassador, World Federation of Occupational Therapists, Hong Kong, China

HELEN CLAIRE SMITH, MA, PGCert, DipCOT
Senior Lecturer, Occupational Therapy, Teesside University, Middlesbrough, UK

YDA SMITH, PhD, OTR/L
Assistant Professor, Director of Graduate Studies, Department of Occupational and Recreational Therapies, University of Utah, Salt Lake City, UT, USA

NATALIA SPALLATO, Lic
Professor, Research Methodology, Statistics and Final Work Design, Institute of Rehabilitation and Movement Sciences, National University of General San Martín, Buenos Aires, Argentina

MARY SQUILLACE, DOT, OTR/L
Assistant Clinical Professor, Occupational Therapy, Stony Brook University, Stony Brook, NY, USA

RICK STODDART
Adjunct Lecturer, James Cook University, Townsville, QLD, Australia

SUSAN SAYLOR STOUFFER, PhD, MS, BA
Director, The Peace Center, United University Church, Los Angeles, CA, USA

PAMELA TALERO, OTD, OTR/L
Teaching Associate, Department of Occupational Therapy, College of Health Professions, Thomas Jefferson University, PA, Philadelphia USA

KERRY THOMAS, BAppSc, GradDip
Director, International Partners in Action, Research and Training (interPART); Lecturer/Tutor, University of South Australia, Adelaide, SA, Australia

JONATHAN TIGWELL, BSc(Hons)
Research student, Life Sciences and Education,
    University of South Wales, Pontypridd, UK

LILIYA ASENOVA TODOROVA, PhD
Assistant Professor, Department of Public Health and
    Social Work, University of Ruse, Ruse, Bulgaria

ELIZABETH TOWNSEND, PhD, MAdEd, BSc,
Dip
Professor Emerita, School of Occupational Therapy,
    Dalhousie University, Halifax, NS, Coordinator,
    Graduate Studies and Adjunct Professor, Faculty
    of Education, University of Prince Edward Island,
    Charlottetown, PEI, Canada

CONCETTINA TRIMBOLI, MSc, BSc
Occupational Therapist, Bremen, Germany

VASILIKI TSONOU, MD
Laboratory Doctor, ElSiTO member, Athens, Greece

DAVID TURNBULL, BA, MA
Adjunct Lecturer, James Cook University, Townsville,
    QLD, Australia

REBECCA TWINLEY, PhD, MSc, PGCAP, BSc
Lecturer, Occupational Therapy, School of Health
    Professions, Plymouth University, Plymouth, UK

HANNEKE E. VAN BRUGGEN, DSc(Hon), BSc,
FWFOT
Director, FAPADAG (Facilitation and Participation of
    Disadvantaged Groups), Apeldoorn, The
    Netherlands; Adjunct Professor, Dalhousie
    University, Halifax, NS Canada

WILSON VERDUGO HUENUMÁN, Lic
Occupational Therapist, Assistant Professor, Director
    Department of Occupational Therapy, University
    of Magallanes, Punta Arenas, Chile.

VANESSA VIDAL CASTILLO, Lic
Occupational Therapist, Adjunct Professor,
    Department of Occupational Therapy, University
    of Magallanes, Punta Arenas, Chile

MICAELA WALDMAN, Lic
Professor, Research Methodology, School of
    Psychology, University of Buenos Aires;
    Coordinator of Laboral Association for Persons
    with Intellectual Disabilities (ALPAD); Partner in
    MiLo (Dog assisted interventions), Buenos Aires,
    Argentina

JÖRG GÜNTER WEBER, MA
Research Fellow, International Centre for Evidence in
    Disability (ICED), London School of Hygiene and
    Tropical Medicine, London, UK

GAIL WHITEFORD, PhD, MHSc, BAppSc
Principal, WHITEFORD CONSULTING;
Professor, School of Allied Health Sciences, Griffith
    University Qld; Board Member, Mid North Coast
    LHD; Chair, Occupational Therapy Australia
    Research Foundation, Australia

BEN WHITTAKER, MSc, BA
Occupational Therapy Programme Lead, Centre For
    Sustainable Healthcare, Oxford, UK

ALISON WICKS, PhD, MHSc(OT), BAppSc
Associate Professor, Discipline of Occupational
    Therapy, Faculty of Health, University of
    Canberra, Canberra, ACT, Australia

CLARE WILDING, PhD, MAppSc, BAppSc
Consultant, Knowledge Moves, Beechworth, Victoria;
    Adjunct Senior Lecturer, School of Community
    Health, Charles Sturt University, Albury, NSW,
    Australia

JESSIE WILSON, PhD, MSc, BSc
Lecturer, Occupational Therapy, James Cook
    University, Townsville, QLD, Australia

GREGOR WOLBRING, PhD
Associate Professor, Community Health Sciences;
    Program in Community Rehabilitation and
    Disability Studies, University of Calgary, Calgary,
    AB, Canada

FARZANEH YAZDANI, PhD, MSc, MA, BSc
Senior Lecturer, Health and Life Sciences, Oxford
    Brookes University, Oxford, UK

ANDREA YUPANQUI CONCHA, Mag, Lic
Occupational Therapist, PhD candidate in
    Interdisciplinary Gender Studies at University of
    Balearic Islands; Associate Professor, Department
    of Occupational Therapy, University of
    Magallanes, Punta Arenas, Chile

FEDERICO JUAN MANUEL ZORZOLI, Lic
Professor, Research Methodology, Statistics and Final
    Work Design, Institute of Rehabilitation and
    Movement Sciences, National University of
    General San Martín, Buenos Aires, Argentina

MARIA ZOUMPOPOULOU, MSc
Independent (Private) Practitioner, Paediatric
    Occupational Therapist, Lamia, Greece

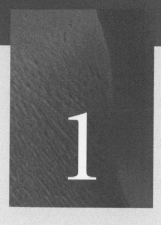

1 INTRODUCTION

DIKAIOS SAKELLARIOU ■ NICK POLLARD

INTRODUCTION

When the first edition of *Occupational Therapy without Borders* was published, some readers responded by saying that it had set out a new paradigm for the profession, a critical perspective, which looked at the wider social and political aspects of occupation and occupation-based practices. Although what that represented has been described by some people as a movement, it was already evident at the time of the first edition in 2005 that a number of writers in occupational therapy and occupational science had been working on these lines for a while. Concepts such as occupational justice and occupational deprivation had already been described in the previous decade, and our first book in this series came out almost at the same time as the late Ruth Watson and Leslie Swartz's *Transformation through Occupation* (2004) and Valerie Wright St-Clair and Gail Whiteford's *Occupation and Practice in Context* (2005). These books also contained different cultural visions of occupational therapy to the dominant ideas of the 'North' and offered political and social challenges to the profession. There have been others since, notably Lorenzo, Duncan, Buchanan and Alsop (2006), Alers and Crouch (2010), dos

Santos and Gallasi (2014) and Simo et al. (in press), while Block, Kasnitz, Nishida and Pollard (2015) have sought to engage with disability perspectives, some from political activist stances. In this introduction, we will discuss some of the context and process of the 'without borders' series and related books and our intention, and then set out an overview of this volume.

This book is part of an ongoing effort to bring to the foreground of occupational therapy's consciousness the social and political context where the process of everyday living, occupation, takes place. Our aim in this book is to highlight how access to occupation can be impeded due to structural social issues, and what can be done about this. We also want to highlight the efforts of people from all over the world to work towards a notion of occupational justice, in many different environments.

We should make it clear that the occupational therapy without borders series and the other related books that we have edited about the politics of occupational therapy and occupation-based practices, and also others in which we are involved, are not a tendency apart from other literature in the profession. Indeed, we look to and are inspired by the many

1

contributors to our edited books. With some of these authors our exchanges have continued for years, and there are now a couple of hundred people who have been involved in 'without borders' projects from the occupational therapy and occupational science archipelago. This represents a worldwide community which at the same time is very much a village.

One of the challenges we face as editors is often that of giving extensive critical feedback to people we have studied and revered. Furthermore, because this series has involved translations from other well-established traditions of professional literature, particularly in Latin America, and in this volume, Japan, we have found ourselves on a continuous journey of discovery. Over the course of editing these books our learning curves have been continuously very steep. We can admit, now, to crises of confidence in the early days about whether we could manage it. Our experience has been rather like being strapped into the seat of an academic rollercoaster for a decade – fast, very thrilling, but perhaps not as far from the ground as it might seem. We have been treated generously and with patience by our contributors, whatever their stature in the profession, institutions, or the disability organizations from which they come. All this time we have been privileged to engage in the sharing of new thinking about the potential the profession has.

It is important to mention this aspect of the experience we have had, because the process of editing and writing books is not a remote thing done by lofty people, as we once imagined, but very possible, and in many ways very ordinary. It is carried out not only in the office but in domestic spaces like kitchens, ordinary cafes and even pubs; between teaching and doing the shopping, helping with homework, family events and family tragedies.

This is hard work for our contributors as well as for us, particularly those people having to translate their work into English to make it available in the dominant lingua franca. This book, which is produced as part of the Occupational Therapy Essentials series, is aimed at undergraduates. We passionately believe that although undergraduate readers might find some of the chapters which follow challenging reading, a little difficulty will inspire them to develop their own discussion networks, practice innovations and critical accounts to be shared in the future literature. But we also hope that students will feel able to engage with the critical community of the 'occupational village'.

The suggestion that there is an occupational therapy without borders movement or paradigm shift is attractive, and perhaps it will eventually come about, but our intention has always been to develop a body of knowledge that is grounded in practices and experiences rather than being charismatic, and which reflects the different needs of different contexts while sharing practices across the world. Our intention has been to discuss *therapies*, as Alejandro Guajardo (2014) advises, rather than therapy. Our aim in this book is to highlight how access to occupation can be impeded due to structural social issues, and what can be done about this to bring about change. We want to emphasize the 'do-ability' which is inherent in occupation-based practices and the power behind it as a tool for social transformation. We also want to highlight the efforts of people from all over the world to work towards a notion of occupational justice, in many different environments.

This book and its predecessors have emphasized the need to think critically about doing things together, and not just doing, but negotiating and facilitating actions in ways that are genuinely participatory. Human experience, Jackson (1998, 2012) reminds us, is intersubjective, and occupation, being an integral part of this experiece, is also intersubjective. Rather than being independent, autonomous subjects with total control over their lives, people are linked to other people with emotional, biological, social, financial, and a multitude of other ties (Arendt, 1998). This network of human interconnections provides the foundations for human experience (Husserl, 1922/2002). Occupation happens in the spaces between people; as Hayama (2014) demonstrates, it is enabled or disabled through human networks, from the microlevel of families to the macrolevel of societies and institutions such as the legal system. In order to better understand *what* people *do*, we need to ask questions such as: *Where* does this doing take place, with *whom*, *why*, and *how*?

Occupation is inescapably connected with a political perspective of human actions. As Wilcock and Hocking (2015), for example, have set out, what people are able to do is determined by many factors such as the environment and the resources available, as well as the impact this may have on what other people can do. There has regrettably been little occupation-based literature which has focused on the historical and cultural development of human activities and occupational practices, but the review of history often shows the relationship between occupation and many other factors which influence social development. One dimension of this is the wealth of evidence about the socioeconomic determinants of health. There are pervasive inequalities in most societies that affect the health of populations all over the world (Commission on Social Determinants of Health, 2008). These inequalities are often the consequences of historical patterns such as the legacies of conflict, or colonialism, or of economic policies as well as natural events and climate change (Rushford and Thomas, 2015). Inequalities can take many different forms and affect access to healthcare, utilization of existing health services, the conditions in which people live and the occupations available, or permitted, to them. In order to address them, these inequalities cannot remain invisible. We need to explore them, trace their origins and their effects, and develop appropriate ways to address these differences and their damaging consequences, in partnership with the people affected by them.

In doing so, we want to foreground the practical, or experiential, knowledge that people possess and the ways they apply this. De Certeau (1988) argues that people implement different strategies and tactics in their efforts to 'make do' or enact everyday life. What is at stake for people is, de Certeau (1988) argues, their autonomy and power to engage in those practices that they deem to be desirable, or needed. Such practices, however, often are not valued or understood in institutions such as education and healthcare. The practical, experiential knowledge of people is often afforded a lower status compared to hegemonic scientific knowledge.

Often, needs trump desire, following a neoliberal language of cost-effectiveness, where often 'desire is of no value' (Biehl, 2007, p. 413). In this language, desires can be seen as liabilities. But, if desires are seen as liabilities, how does this language construct people who desire a good life? Questions about what a good life is, what to do when health or function cannot be restored or maintained, or when pervasive discrimination leads to people's exclusion from daily life, for example, do not have a definitive answer. Quality-of-life questions around happiness or the nature of a

good life are notoriously difficult to define because they involve so many subjective factors (Diener, 2009; Phillips, 2006). The *good* cannot be defined a priori, but only within the context of people's lives. Desire is of central importance in how people construct and lead their lives, and framing it as a liability can have repercussions on how people are enabled to live their everyday life. A recurring theme in this edition of *Occupational Therapies without Borders* concerns the rhetorics of prevailing neoliberal economic policies and their impact on health and social care practices and the experiences of people with disabilities. Over the next few years many countries will experience the consequences of a demographic shift as their populations age, and this will occur in conjunction with complex issues such as climate change, global changes in economic power, new sources of conflict and infections that are more resistant to treatments. These powerful forces determine the quality of choices that are open to many of the people that occupational therapists may work with and those of occupational therapists themselves. We hope that the discourses presented in the chapters that follow can point to some practical directions for the future.

BOOK OVERVIEW

Section 1, Key Concepts in this Book, offers a discussion on topics that are of relevance throughout this volume. Some of the concepts analysed in this section include occupational justice, the intersubjective qualities of occupation, disability, the effects of neoliberalism on health systems and the effects of austerity on public representations of people. This section also includes a discussion on the importance, and the practicalities, of monitoring and evaluation in community projects, and an overview of participatory research methods.

In Chapter 2, Evelyne Durocher provides an overview of occupational justice and injustice and firmly situates these concepts in the core of occupational therapy practice. In Chapter 3, Sarah Kantartzis discusses the collective dimension of occupation and how, rather than being an individual pursuit, occupation often happens in the spaces between people. In Chapter 4, Hannah Kuper and Jörg Günter Weber analyse a concept central to occupational therapy, disability, and trace the different dimensions and uses of it. Elena Rotarou and Daniela Olivares offer an overview of neoliberalism and its impact on health systems, using Chile as a case study, in Chapter 5. Helen Claire Smith's contribution in Chapter 6 brings to the foreground the connection between austerity and the rise of hostility toward different population groups. In Chapter 7, Kerry Thomas and Susan Gilbert Hunt discuss the importance of monitoring and evaluation in community-based practice, and offer practical advice on how to conduct it. This section concludes with Chapter 8, where Wendy Bryant and her colleagues discuss participatory research.

Section 2, Exploring Occupation and Justice, includes chapters that critically engage with the notions of occupation and justice, sometimes examining them separately and sometimes together. One of our main aims in this section is to emphasize that issues of injustice are not only relevant for practice far away from home, or for extreme situations of exclusion. Occupational injustice is present everywhere, in different forms; from clinical settings to community-based rehabilitation, occupational justice can inform occupational therapy practice.

In Chapter 9, Antoine Bailliard and Rebecca Aldrich argue that occupational justice is part of everyday practice rather than as something relevant only to some contexts. Farzaneh Yazdani in Chapter 10 offers an autoethnographical account of how one's own understanding of occupation and occupational therapy can develop, while in Chapter 11, Alejandro Guajardo and Margarita Mondaca discuss the importance of human rights for occupational therapy. Chapter 12, by Rebecca Twinley and Lee Price, brings together the notions of ageing, sexuality and occupation and explores how these can interact. Similarly, Miranda Cunningham in Chapter 13 explores the interactions between homelessness and occupation, while Anne Fenech and Lesley Collier bring together the concepts of leisure and profound disability in Chapter 14. Chapter 15, by Tina McGrath, and Chapter 16, by Jonathan Tigwell, shift the focus toward a specific diagnostic category, breast cancer, and on the effects this produces in people's everyday lives. In Chapter 17, Jyothi Gupta and Tracy Garber present the results of a systematic mapping of justice in occupational therapy. In Chapter 18, Gail Whiteford, Elizabeth Townsend

and their colleagues present the most recent version of the Participatory Occupational Justice Framework and illustrate its use through several examples. Finally, in Chapter 19, Danika Galvin and Clare Wilding discuss human rights in occupational therapy and how they can become more central in practice.

Section 3, The Enactment of Different Occupational Therapies, brings to the foreground the multiplicity of occupational therapy. Occupational therapy can assume different forms and meanings in different settings; people adapt it to their own environments to develop a practice that best suits their specific local context. Chapters in this section range in focus from the intimately personal to the broader political.

In Chapter 20, Solangel Garcia-Ruiz presents a beautiful and deeply personal account of how she developed a notion of occupational therapy relevant to her own local context while working in public policy in Bogota, Colombia. Lily Owens addresses race, an often-ignored issue, in Chapter 21, and discusses the origins and consequences of racism in occupational therapy. In Chapter 22, Vagner dos Santos explores the background and the future of the development of occupational therapy in South America. Chapter 23, by Gregor Wolbring and Emily Chai, provides readers with an ability studies lens through which to analyse occupational therapy practice. Susan Saylor Stouffer, in Chapter 24, presents her personal account of transferring and applying her occupational therapy and occupational science skills to a nontraditional setting, in Los Angeles. Chapter 25, by Clare Hocking and Jenni Fay Mace, focuses on how occupational science can inform occupational therapy practice. In Chapter 26, Jennifer Creek discusses what it means to work on the margins and presents some main characteristics of this. In Chapter 27, Roseli Esquerdo Lopes and Ana Paula Serrata Malfitano present the origins and uses of social occupational therapy, drawing on a rich tradition of relevant research and practice from Brazil. In Chapter 28, Sasa Radic and Ivana Klepo offer a detailed description of the development of occupational therapy in Croatia, clearly highlighting the social and political context and its effects. In Chapter 29, Rosemary Joan Gowran and her colleagues discuss the social and political context and how it influences wheelchair and seating provision in the island of Ireland, across two different countries. Chapter 30, by

Rick Stoddart and his colleagues, discusses the development and usefulness of an enabling occupational community, while in Chapter 31, Roshan Galvaan and Liesl Peters explore the concept of occupation-based community development. Pamela Talero, in Chapter 32, analyses the notion of culturally responsive care and presents an educational model of culturally responsive care in occupational therapy. In Chapter 33, Pam Gretschel and her colleagues discuss the different factors that can impact upon the intervention design phase, drawing on empirical data from South Africa. This section concludes with Chapter 34, by Amy Paul-Ward, discussing the importance of interdisciplinarity for addressing occupational injustice.

Section 4, The Political and Financial Context of Occupation, includes chapters that critically engage with the broader context of occupation. At the time of writing this book, between 2013 and 2015, the effects of a financial crisis were being felt in many parts of the world. The consequences are likely to continue affecting health and social care policies and availability into the next decade. Several of the chapters in this section discuss the various effects of the crisis on people's everyday life.

In Chapter 35, Debbie Laliberte Rudman offers a compelling analysis of the 'duty to age well', placing it in a broader sociopolitical context. Chapter 36, by Heather Bullen, discusses the impact of austerity on the freedoms and rights of people, drawing from examples from the United Kingdom. Chapters 37 (Greece) and 38 and 39 (both from Spain) discuss the various ways that the economic crisis (still ongoing at the time of writing in November 2015) is affecting people in two European countries. In Chapter 40, Elena Rotarou shifts the focus from the recent economic crisis to the long-standing socioeconomic exclusion of people in Easter Island (Rapa Nui) in Chile. In Chapter 41, Thavanesi Gurayah and colleagues discuss the different ways that caregiving can be enacted, drawing on data from South Africa. Chapters 42 (Denmark) and 43 (Belgium, Bulgaria, Greece, the Netherlands and Spain) discuss different ways to work towards social inclusion, for asylum seekers (Chapter 42) and people affected by the economic crisis and mental health issues (Chapter 43).

Section 5, Practices of Transformation, provides a collection of different approaches to working to enable

a notion of occupational justice. Chapters vary between small and larger scale projects, and between responding to long-term issues and addressing more urgent needs. A central element and connecting thread across all chapters is the notion of 'community' – how it is defined and how it is included in any practice of transformation.

In Chapter 44, Martin O'Neill critically discusses the notion of *community* and its centrality in community development approaches. Hanneke van Bruggen, in Chapter 45, discusses why, and how, occupational therapists can combat poverty, inequality and occupational deprivation and develop the concepts and practices necessary for an inclusive, occupationally just community. In Chapter 46, Laura Parraquini and Federico Barroso Lelouche offer an account of developing a community development project in Argentina. Yda Smith, in Chapter 47, reports on her experiences working with former refugees in the United States. In Chapter 48, María Constanza Dehays Pinochet and her colleagues present their work to address the injustices faced by mothers with learning disabilities in southern Chile. Hetty Fransen, in Chapter 49, presents a detailed discussion of disability-inclusive development, drawing on examples from Tunisia. In Chapter 50, Concettina Trimboli discusses the needs of refugee children and presents ways to explore and address them. In Chapter 51, Jane Diamond and Imogen Gordon discuss the importance of crafts in promoting a notion of community cohesion. Chapters 52, 53 and 54 discuss the position of occupational therapy in health promotion, drawing from the authors' experiences in Malawi, Senegal and Timor Leste, respectively. In Chapter 55, Margaret Jones and Clare Hocking discuss the importance of participation skills and how they can be developed. In Chapter 56, Yoshitaka Shiino and Keiichi Hasegawa present the contributions of occupational therapists in the reconstruction efforts following the Great East Japan Earthquake in Fukushima, Japan. In Chapter 57, Alexis Davis and Deborah Simpson discuss the establishment and progression of an occupational therapy-led global health project in northern India. Chapter 58, by Gaynor Sadlo and Ben Whittaker, traces the origins of sustainable occupational therapy practice and discusses its importance. Salvador Simó Algado and Maria Kapanadze, in Chapter 59, discuss the impact of ecological factors on health and well-being, as well as the potential role of occupational therapy to confront the ecological crisis. This section concludes with Chapter 60, by Pamela Block and colleagues, which presents a community programme to address some occupational issues arising from the intersections of participation, disability and need for mechanical ventilation.

Section 6, Educational Practices, includes chapters that highlight the importance and also the diversity of educational practices. Almost every chapter in this section comes from a different part of the world; there are two chapters from Argentina, and one each from Australia, Chile, China, Ireland and the United States. Educators have developed unique practices to respond to the local needs and enable the production of an occupational therapy that can remain grounded in the everyday worlds of people. Different contexts require different occupational therapies.

In Chapter 61, Margaret McGrath discusses the importance of community engagement in occupational therapy and offers practical ways this can be incorporated in educational curricula, drawing from her experiences in Ireland, Lebanon and Singapore. Susan Gilbert Hunt and colleagues, in Chapter 62, discuss in detail how to incorporate community development in an educational programme. Andrea Fabiana Albino and colleagues, in Chapter 63, reflect on the use of critical engagement with academic texts to develop new knowledge. Chapter 64, by Kit Sinclair and Mengan Cao, provides an overview of the development of occupational therapy education in China. In Chapter 65, Mónica Palacios Tolvett and Mónica Díaz Leiva address the use of *critical perspectives* in occupational therapy education. Gelya Frank, in Chapter 66, presents educational activities aimed at educating students about occupational reconstructions, that is, the ways that people can evolve and reshape their occupational identities. Finally, in Chapter 67, Liliana Paganizzi discusses the use of participatory pedagogies to enable a classroom discourse on a social and political vision of occupational therapy.

REFERENCES

Alers, V., Crouch, R., 2010. Occupational Therapy: An African Perspective. Sarah Shorten, Johannesburg.

Arendt, H., 1998. The Human Condition. Chicago University Press, Chicago.

Biehl, J., 2007. A life: between psychiatric drugs and social abandonment. In: Biehl, J., et al. (Eds.), Subjectivity: Ethnographic Investigations. University of California Press, Berkeley, CA, pp. 397–421.

Block, P., Kasnitz, D., Nishida, A., Pollard, N., 2015. Occupying Disability: Critical Approaches to Community, Justice, and Decolonizing Disability. Springer, New York.

Commission on Social Determinants of Health, 2008. Closing the Gap in a Generation: Health Equity through Action on the Social Determinants of Health. Final Report of the Commission on Social Determinants of Health. World Health Organization, Geneva.

De Certeau, M., 1988. The Practice of Everyday Life. University of California Press, Berkeley, CA.

Diener, E., 2009. The Science of Well-Being. Springer, Dordrecht, the Netherlands.

dos Santos, V., Gallasi, A.V. (Eds.), 2014. Questoes Contemporaneas da Terapia Ocupacional na America do Sul. Editora CRV, Curitiba, Brazil.

Guajardo, A., 2014. Una terapia ocupacional critica como posibilidad. In: Santos, V., Gallasi, A.V. (Eds.), Questoes Contemporaneas da Terapia Ocupacional na America do Sul. Editora CRV, Curitiba, Brazil, pp. 159–165.

Hayama, Y., 2014. Look at What You Can Do! Real Stories of Occupational Therapy in Japan. Miwo Shohen, Tokyo.

Husserl, E., 1922/2002. Ideen zu einer Reinen Phänomenologie und Phänomenologischen Philosophie (Ideas Pertaining to a Pure Phenomenology and to a Phenomenological Philosophy). Max Niemeyer Verlag, Tübingen, Germany.

Jackson, M., 1998. Minima Ethnographica: Intersubjectivity and the Anthropological Project. University of Chicago Press, Chicago.

Jackson, M., 2012. Between One and One Another. University of California Press, Berkeley, CA.

Lorenzo, T., et al. (Eds.), 2006. Practice and Service Learning in Occupational Therapy. Wiley, Chichester, UK.

Phillips, D., 2006. Quality of Life: Concept, Policy and Practice. Routledge, London.

Rushford, N., Thomas, K., 2015. Disaster, development and occupational therapy: historical perspectives and possibilities. In: Rushford, N., Thomas, K. (Eds.), Disaster and Development: An Occupational Perspective. Elsevier, Edinburgh, UK, pp. 11–20.

Simo, S., Guajardo, A., Correa, F., Galheigo, S., Garcia, S., In press. Terapias Ocupacionales Desde el Sur: Derechos Humanos, Ciudadanía y Participación. Ediciones Panamericana, Buenos Aires.

Watson, R., Swartz, L. (Eds.), 2004. Transformation through Occupation. Wiley, Chichester, UK.

Wilcock, A.A., Hocking, C., 2015. An Occupational Perspective of Health, third ed. Slack, Upper Saddle River, NJ.

Wright St-Clair, V., Whiteford, G. (Eds.), 2005. Occupation and Practice in Context. Elsevier/Churchill Livingstone, Sydney.

SECTION 1

KEY CONCEPTS IN THIS BOOK

2

OCCUPATIONAL JUSTICE: A FINE BALANCE FOR OCCUPATIONAL THERAPISTS

EVELYNE DUROCHER

CHAPTER OUTLINE

Occupational justice is based on the premise that our occupations affect our health and well-being (Christiansen and Townsend, 2010; Creek and Hughes, 2008; Stadnyk et al., 2010; Wilcock, 1998). The underlying belief is that what we do, for better and for worse, influences our health (Christiansen and Townsend, 2010); thus restrictions on opportunities for participation in meaningful occupations or the imposition of occupations that are detrimental or not meaningful can be harmful, and are therefore unjust (Stadnyk et al., 2010; Townsend and Wilcock, 2004). As occupational therapists and healthcare professionals, we directly and indirectly influence the occupations in which our clients engage. Our influence can be explicit through practice that encourages or discourages participation in particular occupations, or implicit or even unintended through aspects of practice that are

seemingly unrelated to individual occupations, but that indirectly shape opportunities for participation in occupations. Reflexive practice (Kinsella, 2000, 2001) and, more specifically, increased awareness of the potential implications of practice on participation in occupations can help us to be mindful of our role in promoting occupational justice or injustice.

In this chapter, I first provide an overview of occupational justice before reviewing forms of occupational injustice that have been presented in the literature. I then examine occupational justice and injustice in relation to clinical practice. I build this discussion by presenting a secondary analysis of data collected for a study examining discharge planning with older adults to demonstrate how current practices and processes can set up situations of occupational injustice for clients and healthcare professionals. I discuss how, as occupational therapists, we can both be instruments of occupational justice and injustice for our clients, as well as subject to occupational justice or injustice ourselves. Finally, I explore how enhanced reflexive practice and increased awareness about practice contexts can promote occupational justice for clients and healthcare professionals.

WHAT IS OCCUPATIONAL JUSTICE?

Issues of occupational justice relate to the benefits, privileges and harms associated with participation in occupations; because benefits and detriments are associated with participation in particular occupations, access to opportunities for participation in occupations becomes a matter of justice (Townsend and Wilcock, 2004). Occupational justice is based on the interrelationships between individual occupations and all aspects of health (Christiansen and Townsend, 2010). What we do undeniably affects our health. On a very basic level, active lifestyles and a nutritious diet are associated with higher levels of physical and mental health (Blair and Morris, 2009; Iqbal et al., 2008; Kesäniemi et al., 2010; Sarris et al., 2014). At the same time, an active lifestyle that includes riding a bicycle, for example, increases the risk of having a bicycle accident, which could have a negative impact on health. Occupational justice is based on the premise that *all* occupations positively and/or negatively influence various aspects of health and well-being. Occupational justice theorists argue that individuals have the right to exercise their capabilities to participate in occupations to develop and sustain their health, well-being and quality of life or the well-being of their community (Hammell, 2008; Stadnyk et al., 2010).

Theories of occupational justice portray individuals as having unique constellations of capabilities, needs, wishes and routines, set in an individual's particular context (Stadnyk et al., 2010; Townsend and Wilcock, 2004; Wilcock, 2006; Wilcock and Townsend, 2009). This unique constellation of considerations shapes the occupations in which individuals *would like* to engage, *have the opportunity* to engage, and *do* engage. Individuals may choose occupations in which they are interested, in which they find they are or would like to become skilled, and/or with which they wish to be associated. Individuals may also avoid occupations that they find tedious or at which they struggle to succeed, for example.

There is a growing body of literature about the notion that what one does shapes one's identity. Christiansen (1999, 2000, 2004) stated that 'occupations are key not just to being a person, but to being a *particular* person, and thus creating and maintaining an identity' (2000, p. 547). Values attributed to occupations and individual identities are furthermore shaped by economic, sociopolitical, and cultural determinants (Christiansen and Townsend, 2010; Phelan and Kinsella, 2009; Wilcock and Townsend, 2009). Occupations that are not valued in a particular context may not be offered in that context, or may not be offered to individuals with particular characteristics. Additionally, individuals who partake in occupations that are not valued in certain contexts may be perceived differently, and potentially in a more negative light than others. For example, in many contexts smoking is increasingly decried, and individuals who continue to smoke may be perceived as unhealthy, irresponsible or even as inconsiderate or uncaring of those around them. Conversely, there may be many opportunities for occupations that are valued in particular contexts, and there may be social recognition benefits for individuals who participate in these occupations, and even more so for those who experience success. Physical activity, and in particular participation in sports, provides an example of this idea whereby elite athletes are often glorified in the media for their achievements in their particular sports. It must be recognized, however, that success in such endeavours is not within equal reach by all given the amount of time and money required to fund training, coaching, equipment, facilities and so on.

In order to simply illustrate how individuals participate in activities that are available, expected and of interest, and how these may have positive or negative benefits, I use the example of two teenagers in school. Alia (all names in this chapter are pseudonyms) attends a school where athletics are highly valued and there are many opportunities to participate as an athlete or volunteer in various sporting activities. Alia happens to excel at sports and perceives herself as athletic. In addition to her studies, she engages in the school's sporting activities, thus experiencing physical, social, and psychological benefits. If instead Alia attended a smaller school that placed less value on athletics and had a small budget for athletics programming, she would not have as many opportunities for participation and would not experience the same benefits. Conversely, Elias is uninterested in athletics and instead prefers to participate in the photography club. Elias may feel alienated in the first school and may feel that his mandatory attendance at sport-related school events is taking time that he could spend engaging in occupations that are more meaningful to him. Thus the occupations in which individuals engage are shaped both by the context-specific opportunities and their values, as well as by individual strengths, interests and choices.

Theories of occupational justice bring attention to the interrelationships between occupation and health. Occupations are central to human existence; restrictions to participation or opportunities to participate are a matter of injustice (Townsend and Wilcock, 2004). Because of the values, potential benefits, and potential harms that are associated with participation in occupations, restrictions on participation in occupations, and on opportunities for participation, become a matter of injustice. The central tenet of occupational justice is that individuals should have the right to participate in meaningful occupations to develop and foster their own or their community's health, well-being, and quality of life (Stadnyk et al., 2010).

WHAT IS OCCUPATIONAL INJUSTICE?

The World Health Organization (WHO) was the first international organization to declare 'the enjoyment of the highest attainable standard of health as a fundamental right of every human being' (World Health Organization, 2015). WHO extends this right to comprise provision for the underlying determinants of health, in which they include not only meeting the basic necessities of life (such as food, water, shelter) but also the provision of 'healthy occupational and environmental conditions' (World Health Organization, 2013). Traditional discussions of (in)justice have been criticized as being focused on the distribution of goods and resources (such as food, water, or healthcare resources). Authors from various realms of philosophy (Gomberg, 2007; Nussbaum, 2011; Sen, 1999) have instead considered justice by focusing on capabilities,

on barriers and enablers to the development of these, and on the distribution of opportunities within society. In the field of political philosophy, for example, Gomberg (2007) presents an understanding of justice that is 'about what people are able to do, particularly how they are able to develop their abilities, give those back to society, and be respected for their contributions' (p. vi). Concepts of occupational justice and injustice (as outlined in Table 2-1) align with such formulations as these and focus not on the distribution of goods, but rather on opportunities for occupation and the subsequent benefits of such occupations for the development of capabilities, the formulation of identity, contribution to society, and the attainment of health as a human right.

TABLE 2-1
Occupational Justice and Injustice Terminology

Concepts of Occupational Justice and Injustice

Occupational justice	Individuals should have the right to exercise their capabilities to participate in occupations to develop and sustain their identity, health, well-being, and quality of life (Stadnyk et al., 2010)

Types of Occupational Injustice in the Literature

Occupational deprivation	Preclusion from participation in meaningful, health-promoting, or necessary occupations because of forces beyond one's control (Whiteford, 2000)
Occupational apartheid	Denial of or permission to participate in meaningful occupations based on personal characteristics (Kronenberg and Pollard, 2005)
Occupational marginalization	Denial or lack of opportunity for participation in occupation based on invisible societal norms or expectations (Stadnyk et al., 2010)
Occupational imbalance	Individual level: harm related to participation in one occupation at the expense of another (Stadnyk et al., 2010)
	Societal level: inequitable distribution of opportunities for participation in meaningful, beneficial, or valued occupations (Stadnyk et al., 2010)
Occupational alienation	Imposition of participation in occupations that are not meaningful (Stadnyk et al., 2010)

Occupational justice theorists argue that participation in occupations that are not meaningful, or that are even harmful, or the prevention of participation in occupations that are meaningful or beneficial to health can be detrimental to health and well-being. The imposition of participation in occupations that are harmful or not meaningful, or lack of participation in meaningful or health-contributing occupations can prevent individuals from developing their potential capabilities or from shaping their identities as they wish. Such barriers or impositions can take various explicit and implicit forms, and have been named in the literature as follows.

Occupational Deprivation

Occupational deprivation is the most often cited type of occupational injustice and refers to the 'preclusion from engagement in occupations of necessity and/or meaning due to factors that stand outside of the immediate control of the individual' (Whiteford, 2000, p. 201). External factors that impede participation in occupations can be social, political, environmental, economic, geographic, or interpersonal (Whiteford, 2000). Theorists carefully distinguish *occupational deprivation,* which has a long-term impact on individuals, from *occupational disruption,* which is temporary. Occupational deprivation was originally coined by Wilcock (1998) but was conceptually developed in more depth by Whiteford (2000), in particular in her research with prison inmates and war refugees (Whiteford, 1997, 2000). Whiteford (1997) argued that the lack of opportunities for meaningful occupation for prison inmates was detrimental to health and well-being, and impeded potential for personal growth or success in the correctional system. Another example might be encountered by occupational therapists working with clients in the community who may have decreased mobility following illness or injury. For example, older adults may be isolated and have few opportunities to participate in occupations if they cannot easily access public transportation and can no longer drive following a stroke (Patomella et al., 2009).

Occupational Apartheid

Occupational apartheid results when individuals are afforded or denied opportunities to participate in occupations based on personal characteristics such as age, gender, race, disability, nationality, or socioeconomic status (Kronenberg and Pollard, 2005). Occupational apartheid may be the result of social, political, institutional, or religious structures that systematically uphold discourses and circumstances that privilege some and exploit or deny others resources or opportunities (Kronenberg and Pollard, 2005). Many examples of this persist for women who wish to participate in amateur or professional sports. In 2013, for example, Shirin Gerami became the first woman to represent Iran in an international triathlon competition (Dehghan, 2013). Prior to this, women in Iran were not allowed to participate in overseas athletic competitions, thus barring them from achieving benefits associated with participating in international competition. A second example arises in the sport of football (soccer), in which women in many countries continue to face opposition to participating in or attending games (Isard, 2015; Nadel, 2014) and also receive much lower compensation than men for their achievements (Gibson, 2009).

Occupational Marginalization

Occupational marginalization is akin to an invisible form of deprivation and/or apartheid. Occupational marginalization occurs when individuals do not have the opportunity to make everyday choices and are excluded from participating in occupations based on *invisible* norms and expectations in the context (Stadnyk et al., 2010; Townsend and Wilcock, 2004). Occupational marginalization differs from deprivation or apartheid in that individuals are not explicitly barred from particular occupations as a result of laws or policies, but rather they are not offered opportunities for participation based on societal expectations or norms of behaviour. A child with a mobility impairment, for example, may not be explicitly excluded from participation in school activities; however, games in his physical education class may be constructed in a manner that disadvantages his abilities. He may therefore fear ridicule and choose not to engage, thus potentially experiencing marginalization.

Occupational Imbalance

Occupational imbalance can occur at two levels – individual and social. On an individual level, occupational imbalance is related to the harm that can come from participation in one occupation at the expense of others. This can be the result of a disproportionate amount of time being spent on one occupation at the expense of other occupations (Stadnyk et al., 2010), or secondary effects of participating in one occupation could negatively affect participation in other occupations (e.g., individuals working a night shift may suffer fatigue, which may affect the quality and quantity of time they are able to spend in other meaningful occupations). On a societal level, occupational imbalance occurs in situations where some individuals are offered many opportunities for occupation while others are afforded few (Stadnyk et al., 2010). In many cases, the discrepancy can result from, and be upheld by, social and political structures, in which case occupational imbalance is socially and politically constructed, and can result in situations of occupational apartheid.

Occupational Alienation

Finally, *occupational alienation* differs from the other forms of occupational injustice as it is not the omission or preclusion from participation, but rather the imposition of participation in occupations that are not meaningful or that may not promote health (Stadnyk et al., 2010). A simple example is demonstrated in a study examining mental health day programming. Users of one program reported many benefits to attending the program; however, they also reported feeling obliged to participate in activities that were not personally meaningful (Bryant et al., 2004). Given the basis of occupational justice – that participation in meaningful occupations can be beneficial to one's physical and psychological health and can contribute to the formation of individual identity – being forced to participate in occupations that are not meaningful may shape individual identity or capacities in ways one does not wish and may hinder positive individual development. Such imposition is viewed as unjust.

OCCUPATIONAL JUSTICE AND INJUSTICE IN PRACTICE

As occupational therapists, we are highly concerned with occupation and its links to health and well-being. We practise within social, political and institutional contexts consisting of discourses, norms and expectations, which undeniably assign particular values to occupations. Laliberté-Rudman (2005) introduced the concept of *occupational possibilities*, which in later work she described as 'what people take for granted as what they can and should do, and the occupations that are supported and promoted by various aspects of the broader [social and political] systems and structures' (Laliberté-Rudman, 2010, p. 55) in which they live. Contexts thus shape opportunities for participation in occupations and values associated with these. An additional aspect of contexts constitutes social, political and institutional structures that include policies to direct behaviours and practices, and determine what services and resources are available to whom. All of these shape opportunities for occupations, participation in occupations and, subsequently, the harms and benefits associated with participation in occupations, which can set up situations of occupational justice or injustice.

Clients and occupational therapists engage in occupational therapy and are subject to social, political and institutional influences inherent in practice contexts. Both the values associated with occupations and occupational therapy influence our clients and the occupations in which they engage. As occupational therapists, we can be instruments of occupational justice or injustice, or both, for our clients. Additionally, by having external influences shaping our practice, as therapists, we can also be subject to occupational justice or injustice, or both, if our occupation of being occupational therapists is somehow constrained or aspects of it that do not align with our values are imposed. In order to more concretely exemplify this, I draw on a qualitative research study in which microethnographic case study methods (Willis, 2007) were used to examine social and political influences on discharge planning from an older adult inpatient rehabilitation setting in Canada. I argue that current healthcare policies and practices are aligned in such a way that they create at least two possible situations of occupational injustice: for older adults and for healthcare professionals.

Discharge Planning Shapes Occupational Possibilities

Occupational therapists in Western countries working in clinical settings are heavily involved in processes of discharge planning (Atwal and Caldwell, 2003). Discharge planning is the process of preparing for an individual to cease use of a healthcare service. In addition to determining how an individual's personal and medical needs will be met, an important decision in discharge planning from inpatient care services is the determination of where the individual will live upon discharge. If their needs or capabilities have changed, can they manage and do they have sufficient resources to meet their needs in their previous living circumstances? If not, which type of home environment would enable them to meet all of their personal and medical needs? How might their current capabilities and anticipated home environment relate to their occupational needs and possibilities?

One's home environment shapes the social, physical and occupational aspects of one's life, which greatly influence individuals' health and well-being (McCullough et al., 1993; Moats, 2006). Circumstances of the home environment determine both occupational possibilities and requirements. If an individual lives in a house in the community, for example, she may have opportunities to engage in gardening that she may not have living in long-term care. Similarly, living alone may require one to prepare meals, whereas in many supported living environments meals would be provided and occupations of planning, shopping and meal preparation would not be required.

Durocher et al. (2016) found that discharge planning practices with older adults were strongly influenced by discourses linking ageing to inevitable declines in physical and cognitive abilities, as well as withdrawal from participation in decisions. These authors also found that the discharge planning process in this setting was heavily guided by strict adherence to a set timeline dictating a 4-week length of stay, with the discharge planning family conference being scheduled for 2 weeks into the stay (Durocher et al., in press). The discharge planning family conference is an element of the process intended to enable collaboration among older adults, their family, and healthcare professionals (Efraimsson et al., 2006; Griffith et al., 2004). Nonetheless, the results of the study suggested that practice conventions in the study setting did not encourage older adult or family contributions in discharge planning (Durocher et al., 2016). Furthermore, scheduling the family conference for 2 weeks into the inpatient rehabilitation stay meant that the first 2 weeks of the inpatient care stay were spent completing assessments to prognosticate older adults' needs upon discharge, which would then inform discharge planning recom-

mendations (Durocher et al., in press). The literature shows that it is more difficult to make an accurate prognosis early in the inpatient care stay (Wells, 1997). In conjunction, a heavy focus on the promotion of safety and discourses of ageing as a time of decline, the practice of making a prognosis early in the inpatient stay contributed to assumptions that older adults could not be safe returning to their previous home environment as they wished to do and led frequently to discharge recommendations of 24-hour care, which may not have been tailored to the individual's circumstances and would have tremendous implications for an older adult's occupational possibilities.

Occupational Injustice for Older Adults as a Result of Current Discharge Planning Processes

One of the findings in Durocher et al's (Durocher et al., 2016) study was that older adults were marginalized in a decision that had significant implications for their home circumstances and, subsequently, their health and well-being. Recommendations for 24-hour care could have significant implications for older adults and their family members, and on first glance may not seem particularly unjust. In many circumstances, the provision of 24-hour care in an older adult's preadmission living circumstances could be financially costly or could place a notable responsibility on family members or informal caregivers. The often prohibitive costs and logistical difficulties associated with providing in-home 24-hour care could lead to the sale of an older adult's home and his or her subsequent move to a long-term care setting. This move would have significant implications for older adults. Primarily, as I have argued above, the home environment shapes opportunities for occupation, which can have a significant influence on shaping individual identity (Christiansen, 1999, 2000, 2004; Phelan and Kinsella, 2009). Secondly, one's home in and of itself may hold great emotional significance and be closely related to one's identity and sense of self (Dupuis and Thorns, 1996, 1998; McCullough et al., 1993; Wise, 2000). I argue that blanket recommendations of 24-hour care have a tremendous influence on shaping older adults' occupational possibilities, as well their self-perception and identity. Such recommendations therefore set up potential situations of occupational injustice for older adults at the heart of the discharge planning process. While I acknowledge that there are options other than the provision of 24-hour care in older adults' homes and a move to long-term care, other options were rarely considered in this research setting, thus further increasing the potential for occupational injustice.

Both a move to long-term care and the provision of 24-hour care in the home would have significant implications for older adults' participation in occupations. Primarily, it is likely that in either option, they would no longer have the choice of participating in certain occupations. Individuals may be happy to give up certain occupations (I can think of many who would happily never clean their bathroom again, for example) but may no longer have opportunities to participate in long-standing meaningful occupations. Taking the examples of gardening or cooking presented above, opportunities for participating in these would be unlikely in long-term care. Alternatively they may not be deemed 'safe' for the older adult in the home environment. The older adult would thus be at risk of experiencing occupational deprivation. Secondly, with 24-hour care, older adults may be required to participate in activities in ways to which they are not accustomed, or may have to participate in occupations in which they do not wish to partake. For example, they may have to get up 1 hour later than is their habit because that is the time that the caregiver is able to accommodate, thus subjecting the older adult to spending an hour in bed waiting to get up. Similarly, in long-term care they may be expected to participate in group activities that are of little interest to them. Both of these examples suggest that older adults may be at risk of suffering occupational alienation. Finally, evidence suggests that in many situations where individuals are assumed to have decreased capabilities, paternalistic tendencies result in caregivers providing more care than is required, and thus not providing the opportunity for individuals to participate in occupations or in decisions in which they would be more than capable of participating (Sherwin and Winsby, 2010).

Occupational Injustice for Healthcare Professionals as Experienced in Their Roles in Discharge Planning

Turning our attention now to occupational therapists, there is growing attention to the idea that occupational therapists may themselves be at risk of experiencing ethical tensions and occupational injustice (Durocher, 2014; Fleming and Mattingly, 1994; Kinsella et al., 2008, 2014; Mackey, 2014). The study delineated above suggests that healthcare professionals experienced occupational alienation in their roles in discharge planning. Occupational therapists report a desire to help improve people's quality of life (Mackey, 2014). Occupational therapists' professional identity is shaped by a professional guiding tenet of taking a client-centred approach (Mackey, 2014). Client-centred approaches consist of 'a partnership between the client and the therapist that empowers the client to engage in functional performance and fulfil his or her occupational roles in a variety of environments' (Sumsion, 2000, p. 306). Client-centred practice is further qualified by an inclusion of the client in decision making and goal setting (Canadian Association of Occupational Therapists, 1997; Townsend, 1998; Townsend and Polatajko, 2013). Contemporary rehabilitation rhetoric centres on overcoming the challenges presented by illness, injury or age-related health complications in order to maximize independence and function, which aligns with professional aims of maximizing function and quality of life and professional values for client-centred approaches. When occupational therapists are not enabled to practise in manners that align with their personal and professional values, goals, and identities, they may experience moral and professional tensions (Mackey, 2014) and are therefore at risk for occupational injustice.

My colleagues and I have found that healthcare professionals experienced occupational injustice through their roles in discharge planning with older adults. The study results indicated that policies guiding shorter lengths of stay, discourses emphasizing the prioritization of safety and conventions guiding an early focus on discharge planning resulted in practice that prioritized discharge at the expense of interventions aimed at maximizing recovery and function. Furthermore, as presented above, contextual influences marginalized older adults. Such practice amounted to situations where healthcare professionals were forced to practise in ways they knew were not as client-centred as they would like because their clients were not involved in discussions and decisions, and their interventions were aimed at a discharge plan that did not align with client wishes or rehabilitation and professional aims of improving clients' function and well-being (Durocher et al., 2015; Durocher et al., 2016).

Similar experiences have been noted in other developed countries. In the United Kingdom, for example, changes in the political and economic landscapes since the early 2000s have created healthcare environments in which increasing performance expectations, growing workloads, and constrained resources shape healthcare practice towards a focus on meeting targets at the expense of client-centred practice and work–life balance (Clouston, 2014; Francis, 2013; Mackey, 2014). Mackey (2014) found that intensified pressures in the context of fiscal restraint promoted a reduced scope for occupational therapists practice centred on meeting quantifiable indicators at the expense of focusing on the client's experience and well-being. In this environment, occupational therapists were struggling to redefine their professional identity (Mackey, 2014). Similarly, the results of Clouston's (2014) study indicated that escalating demands translated into growing workloads for therapists, more intense and longer work hours, and feelings of loss of control or professional autonomy. Therapists reported that as a result of these changes, they not only had less time to spend with their families and in 'nonpaid employment' occupations, but that they also were much more exhausted after the workday, and therefore had less energy and motivation for these other aspects of their lives. In situations such as those described above, occupational therapists are themselves at risk of experiencing occupational alienation, occupational imbalance, and occupational deprivation, which can have a profound influence on how they see themselves and their role in relation to their clients, and what benefits or harms they experience from their occupation as occupational therapists.

IMPLICATIONS FOR PRACTICE: THE REFLEXIVE PATH TO BEING INSTRUMENTS OF OCCUPATIONAL JUSTICE

The purpose of this discussion is not to negate the potential value of 24-hour care discharge planning recommendations, nor is the intent to argue that occupational injustice is inevitable. Situations of occupational injustice can arise in an infinite number of living circumstances; however, the situations above demonstrate that occupational therapists may inadvertently be instruments of occupational injustice despite professional intentions to promote occupational justice (Townsend and Polatajko, 2013). Similarly, I do not suggest that institutional policies and contextual conventions are intended to coerce therapists into practising in ways that contradict personal, professional, or institutional values. I argue that the intersection of various influences can lead to practice that contradicts intended aims or values closely linked to personal and professional identity, which can have significant negative implications for occupational therapists themselves, as well as for their practice and their clients.

In the face of such forces in our practice contexts, how can we as occupational therapists align practice with personal and professional values, and not promote or be subjected to occupational injustice? Occupational therapists have moral, professional, and ethical commitments to promote justice through various aspects of practice (Townsend and Marval, 2013).

Primarily, the ever-present aim for client-centred approaches also benefits the promotion of occupational justice. Client-centred practice, as it is intended, involves taking the time to understand the client's unique intersection of needs, preferences, capabilities, resources, and contexts (Brookman et al., 2011; Gerteis et al., 1993; Townsend and Polatajko, 2013). Developing such an understanding can help occupational therapists to better understand why some options are preferable over others for their clients, and can promote recommendations and outcomes that better balance the unique situations of clients within the social and political structures, and thus promote occupational justice.

Secondly, there is a growing trend towards reflexive practice in the field of healthcare (Kinsella, 2001; Taylor, 2010; Townsend and Polatajko, 2013) that may also encourage the promotion of occupational justice. Reflexive practice involves increasing personal awareness of the varied influences and their effects on practice and outcomes (Kinsella, 2000, 2001). Within practice contexts where policies and conventions may be taken for granted, increasing reflexivity in practice may be difficult, but it can be achieved personally or through discussion with colleagues and mentors. Using frameworks for occupational justice such as the Participatory Occupational Justice Framework presented by Whiteford and Townsend (2011) or the example provided by Wolf et al. (2010) to guide reflection can help to probe reflection about practice and generate insights to guide discussion and actions to improve circumstances and promote occupational justice.

Finally, it is recognized that merely taking a client-centred approach and practising reflexively is unlikely to enable practice that undeniably promotes occupational justice. As was argued through the examples above and as may be illustrated through the use of the suggested models of occupational justice, situations of occupational injustice frequently arise through the intersection of varied influences that are beyond occupational therapists' or clients' individual control. Therefore the occupational therapists' roles as advocates (Townsend and Polatajko, 2013) for systemic change to enable practice to better meet client needs, as well as professional and institutional aims, become ever more salient. Advocacy can be done at a personal level one client at a time, can be done in the workplace, or can be achieved more broadly by addressing policy-writers and decision-makers. Change requires research to inform possible avenues to achieve better circumstances, as well as translation of this research to reach client, healthcare professional, decision-maker and general population audiences. The body of knowledge is growing, but more work needs to be done. Heightened awareness of occupational justice and the potential harms of occupational injustice can lay the foundation for more occupationally just practice to increase the well-being of all involved.

CONCLUSION

Occupational justice is an evolving concept in the fields of occupational science and occupational therapy. Based on the premise that occupations influence health, having opportunities for, and being enabled to participate in, occupations that are meaningful and contribute to health and well-being is perceived as just. Barriers to participation in such occupations or even the imposition of participation in occupations that are not meaningful, that do not contribute to health and

well-being or that even may be detrimental is considered unjust. Opportunities for occupation, however, and the liberty to participate in these opportunities, are mediated by a wide variety of factors including not only what opportunities are available and accessible in one's context, but more importantly, economic and sociocultural dimensions including social norms and expectations of who *can* and *should* be participating in which occupations, when and for what purpose. As citizens of the world acting within their varied contexts each day, and in their roles as professionals doing research, working with clients and contributing to the structure and function of healthcare systems, occupational therapists respond and contribute to the discourses that shape knowledge, behaviours, and expectations in their everyday contexts. Doing so, they can be subject to, as well as enablers of, occupational justice and injustice. While barriers remain for occupational therapists aiming to promote occupational justice (Durocher, Gibson and Rappolt, 2014; Durocher, Rappolt and Gibson, 2014; Townsend and Marval, 2013), a variety of tools and frameworks to guide the promotion of occupational justice in practice have been and continue to be developed (see for examples Chapter 18 in this book; Arthanat et al., 2012; Stadnyk et al., 2010; Townsend and Marval, 2013; Whiteford and Townsend, 2011; Wolf et al., 2010). Furthermore, the discussion is ongoing in the fields of occupational therapy, occupational science and beyond, enabling the development and evolution of ideas and theories and bringing to light novel avenues for the promotion of occupational justice. Acting together, as instruments of occupational justice, it is occupational therapists' moral and ethical obligation to contribute to orchestrating change towards a more occupationally just and inclusive world.

REFERENCES

Arthanat, S., Simmons, C.D., Favreau, M., 2012. Exploring occupational justice in consumer perspectives on assistive technology. Can. J. Occup. Ther. 79 (5), 309–319.

Atwal, A., Caldwell, K., 2003. Ethics, occupational therapy and discharge planning: four broken principles. Aust. Occup. Ther. J. 50 (4), 244–251.

Blair, S., Morris, J., 2009. Healthy hearts – and the universal benefits of being physically active: physical activity and health. Ann. Epidemiol. 19 (4), 253–256. doi:10.1016/j.annepidem.2009.01.019.

Brookman, C., Jakob, L., De Cicco, J., Bender, D., 2011. Client-Centred Care in the Canadian Home and Community Sector: A Review of Key Concepts. Saint Elizabeth, Markham, Ontario, Canada. <http://www.saintelizabeth.com/getmedia/4aba6e8e-0303-4b9c-9117-a8c22a43f8bd/Client-Centred-Care-in-the-Canadian-Home-and-Community-Sector.pdf.aspx> (accessed 15.07.15.).

Bryant, W., Craik, C., McKay, E.A., 2004. Living in a glasshouse: exploring occupational alienation. Can. J. Occup. Ther. 71 (5), 282–290.

Canadian Association of Occupational Therapists, 1997. Enabling Occupation: An Occupational Therapy Perspective. CAOT Publications ACE, Ottawa, Ontario, Canada.

Christiansen, C., 1999. Defining lives: occupation as identity: an essay on competence, coherence and the creation of meaning. Am. J. Occup. Ther. 53, 547–558.

Christiansen, C., 2000. Identity, personal projects and happiness. J. Occup. Sci. 7 (3), 98–107.

Christiansen, C., 2004. Occupation and identity: becoming who we are through what we do. In: Christiansen, C., Townsend, E. (Eds.), Introduction to Occupation: The Art and Science of Living. Prentice Hall, Upper Saddle River, NJ.

Christiansen, C., Townsend, E., 2010. An introduction to occupation. In: Christiansen, C., Townsend, E. (Eds.), Introduction to Occupation: The Art and Science of Living, second ed. Pearson Education, Upper Saddle River, NJ.

Clouston, T., 2014. Whose occupational balance is it anyway? The challenge of neoliberal capitalism and work-life imbalance. Br J. Occup. Ther. 77 (10), 507–515.

Creek, J., Hughes, A., 2008. Occupation and health: a review of selected literature. Br. J. Occup. Ther. 71 (11), 456–468.

Dehghan, S.K., 2013. Iran allows first female triathlete to compete for country. The Guardian, 12 September 2013 <http://www.theguardian.com/world/2013/sep/12/iran-first-female-triathlete-compete> (accessed 03.07.15.).

Dupuis, A., Thorns, D.C., 1996. Meanings of home for older home owners. Housing Studies 11 (4), 485–501.

Dupuis, A., Thorns, D.C., 1998. Home, home ownership and the search for ontological security. Sociol. Rev. 46 (1), 24–47.

Durocher, E., 2014. Discharge planning with older adults: The influence of social and political systems and contexts. (Doctoral dissertation). University of Toronto, Toronto, ON.

Durocher, E., Gibson, B.E., Rappolt, S., 2014. Occupational justice: a conceptual review. J. Occup. Sci. 21 (4), 418–430.

Durocher, E., Rappolt, S., Gibson, B.E., 2014. Occupational justice: future directions. J. Occup. Sci. 21 (4), 431–442.

Durocher, E., Kinsella, E.A., Ells, C., Hunt, M., 2015. Contradictions in client-centred discharge planning: through the lens of relational autonomy. Scand. J. Occup. Ther. 22 (4), 293–301.

Durocher, E., Gibson, B., Rappolt, S., 2016. Mediators of marginalization in discharge planning with older adults. Age & Soc. (First view), 1–23.

Durocher, E., Gibson, B.E., Rappolt, S., in press. Rehabilitation as "destination triage": a critical examination of discharge planning. Dis & Reh. 1–8.

Efraimsson, E., Sandman, P., Hydén, L., Rasmussen, B., 2006. 'They were talking about me' – elderly women's experiences of taking part in a discharge-planning conference. Scand. J. Caring Sci. 20, 68–78.

Fleming, M., Mattingly, C., 1994. Clinical Reasoning: Forms of Inquiry in a Therapeutic Practice. F. A. Davis Company, Philadelphia, PA.

Francis, R., 2013. Report of the Mid Staffordshire NHS Foundation Trust Public Inquiry. <http://www.midstaffspublicinquiry.com/sites/default/files/report/Executive%20summary.pdf> (accessed 15.07.15.).

Gerteis, M., Edgeman-Levitan, S., Daley, J., Delbanco, T., 1993. Introduction: medicine and health from the patient's perspective. In: Gerteis, M., et al. (Eds.), Through the Patient's Eyes. Jossey-Bass Inc, San Francisco, CA.

Gibson, O., 2009. Men's and women's football: a game of two halves. The Guardian, 8 September 2008 <http://www.theguardian.com/football/2009/sep/08/mens-football-game-two-halves> (accessed 03.07.15.).

Gomberg, P., 2007. How to Make Opportunity Equal: Race and Contributive Justice. Blackwell Publishing, Malden, MA.

Griffith, J., Brosnan, J., Lacey, K., Keeling, S., Wilkinson, T., 2004. Family meetings – a qualitative exploration of improving care planning with older people and their families. Age. Ageing 33 (6), 557–581.

Hammell, K.W., 2008. Reflections on … well-being and occupational rights. Can. J. Occup. Ther. 75 (1), 61–64.

Iqbal, R., Anand, S., Ounpuu, S., Islam, S., Zhang, X., Rangarajan, S., et al; INTERHEART Study Investigators, 2008. Dietary patterns and the risk of acute myocardial infarction in 52 countries. Epidemiology 118, 1929–1937.

Isard, R., 2015. Muslim women in sport. Soccer Politics: A Discussion Forum about the Power of Global Game. <https://sites.duke.edu/wcwp/research-projects/middle-east/muslim-women-in-sport> (accessed 03.07.15.).

Kesäniemi, A., Riddoch, C., Reeder, B., Blair, S., Sørenson, T., 2010. Advancing the future of physical activity guidelines in Canada: an independent expert panel interpretation of the evidence. Int. J. Behav. Nutr. Phys. Act. 7, 41–55.

Kinsella, E.A., 2000. Reflective Practice and Professional Development: Strategies for Learning through Professional Experience. CAOT Publication ACE, Ottawa, Ontario, Canada.

Kinsella, E.A., 2001. Reflections on reflective practice. Can. J. Occup. Ther. 68 (3), 195–198.

Kinsella, E.A., Park, A., Appiagyei, J., Chang, E., Chow, D., 2008. Through the eyes of students: ethical tensions in occupational therapy practice. Can. J. Occup. Ther. 75 (3), 176–183.

Kinsella, E.A., Phelan, S., Bossers, A., McCorquodale, L., 2014. Examining ethical tensions in occupational therapy practice: a pilot study. Canadian Association of Occupational Therapists National Conference: Reflection on Occupation: Enabling Healthy Communities, 9 May 2014.

Kronenberg, F., Pollard, N., 2005. Overcoming occupational apartheid: a preliminary exploration of the political nature of occupational therapy. In: Kronenberg, F., et al. (Eds.), Occupational Therapy without Borders: Learning from the Spirit of

Survivors. Elsevier Churchill Livingstone, Toronto, Ontario, Canada.

Laliberté-Rudman, D., 2005. Understanding political influences on occupational possibilities. J. Occup. Sci. 12 (3), 149–160.

Laliberté-Rudman, D., 2010. Occupational terminology: occupational possibilities. J. Occup. Sci. 17 (1), 55–59.

Mackey, H., 2014. Living tensions: reconstructing notions of professionalism in occupational therapy. Aust. Occup. Ther. J. 61, 168–176.

McCullough, L., Wilson, N., Teasdale, T., Kolopakchi, A., Skelly, J., 1993. Mapping personal, familial and professional values in long-term care decisions. Gerontologist 33 (3), 324–332.

Moats, G., 2006. Discharge decision making with older people: the influence of the institutional environment. Aust. Occup. Ther. J. 53, 107–116.

Nadel, J., 2014. On the precariousness of women's soccer in CON-CACAF. Soccer Politics: A Discussion Forum about the Power of the Global Game. <https://sites.duke.edu/wcwp/2014/11/08/on-the-precariousness-of-womens-soccer-in-concacaf> (accessed 03.07.15.).

Nussbaum, M., 2011. Creating Capabilities: The Human Development Approach. Harvard University Press, Boston, MA.

Patomella, A., Johansson, K., Tham, K., 2009. Lived experience of driving ability following stroke. Disabil. Rehabil. 31 (9), 726–733.

Phelan, S., Kinsella, E.A., 2009. Occupational identity: engaging socio-cultural perspectives. J. Occup. Sci. 16 (2), 85–91.

Sarris, J., O'Neil, A., Coulson, C.E., Schweitzer, I., Berk, M., 2014. Lifestyle medicine for depression. BMC Psychiatry 14 (107), 1–13.

Sen, A., 1999. Development as Freedom. Oxford University Press, Oxford, UK.

Sherwin, S., Winsby, M., 2010. A relational perspective on autonomy for older adults residing in nursing homes. Health Expect. 14, 182–190.

Stadnyk, R., Townsend, E., Wilcock, A., 2010. Occupational justice. In: Christiansen, C., Townsend, E. (Eds.), Introduction to Occupation: The Art and Science of Living, second ed. Pearson Education, Upper Saddle River, NJ.

Sumsion, T., 2000. A revised occupational therapy definition of client-centred practice. Br. J. Occup. Ther. 63 (7), 304–309.

Taylor, B., 2010. Reflective Practice for Healthcare Professionals, third ed. Open University Press, Berkshire, UK.

Townsend, E., 1998. Using Canada's 1997 guidelines for enabling occupation. Aust. Occup. Ther. J. 45, 1–6.

Townsend, E., Marval, R., 2013. Can professionals actually enable occupational justice? Caderno de Terapia Ocupacional da UFSCar 21 (2), 215–228.

Townsend, E., Polatajko, H. (Eds.), 2013. Enabling Occupation II: Advancing an occupational therapy vision for health, well-being and justice through occupation, second ed. CAOT Publications ACE, Ottawa, ON.

Townsend, E., Wilcock, A., 2004. Occupational justice and client-centered practice: a dialogue in progress. Can. J. Occup. Ther. 71 (2), 75–87.

Wells, D., 1997. A critical ethnography of the process of discharge decision making for elderly patients. Can. J. Aging 16 (4), 682–699.

Whiteford, G., 1997. Occupational deprivation and incarceration. J. Occup. Sci. 4 (3), 126–130.

Whiteford, G., 2000. Occupational deprivation: global challenge in the new millennium. Br. J. Occup. Ther. 63 (5), 200–204.

Whiteford, G., Townsend, E., 2011. Participatory Occupational Justice Framework (POJF 2010): enabling occupational participation and inclusion. In: Kronenberg, F., et al. (Eds.), Occupational Therapies without Borders, vol. 2. Towards an Ecology of Occupation-Based Practices. Elsevier, London.

Wilcock, A., 1998. An Occupational Perspective of Health. Slack, Thorofare, NJ.

Wilcock, A., 2006. An Occupational Perspective of Health, second ed. Slack, Thorofare, NJ.

Wilcock, A., Townsend, E., 2009. Occupational justice. In: Crepeau, E.B., et al. (Eds.), Willard and Spackman's Occupational Therapy, eleventh ed. Lippincott Williams and Wilkins, Philadelphia, PA.

Willis, J., 2007. Foundations of Qualitative Research: Interpretive and Critical Approaches. Sage Publications, Thousand Oaks, CA.

Wise, J., 2000. Home: territory and identity. Cult. Stud. 14 (2), 295–310.

Wolf, L., et al., 2010. Applying an occupational justice framework. Occup. Ther. Now 12 (1), 15–18.

World Health Organization, 2013. The Right to Health. <http://www.who.int/mediacentre/factsheets/fs323/en> (accessed 03.07.15.).

World Health Organization, 2015. Human Rights. <http://www.who.int/topics/human_rights/en> (accessed 03.07.15.).

3

EXPLORING OCCUPATION BEYOND THE INDIVIDUAL: FAMILY AND COLLECTIVE OCCUPATION

SARAH KANTARTZIS

CHAPTER OUTLINE

The traditional focus of occupational therapists on the individual is increasingly being challenged, with concern for the impact of societal structures on occupational possibilities (Laliberte Rudman, 2010) and occupational rights (Stadnyk et al., 2011), and concern with the 'individualizing of occupation' associated with the 'individualizing of the social' in contemporary neoliberal policies (Laliberte Rudman, 2013, p. 299). However, there also is a limited but growing discussion around a meso level of occupation, focusing on families, groups and communities. This chapter aims to contribute to the discussion problematizing an individual approach to occupation through presenting the concepts of family occupation and collective occupation. Such occupation, with different forms and offering different experiences to the occupation of the individual doing alone, was originally identified within an ethnographic study exploring occupation in the context of a Greek town (Kantartzis, 2013). In this chapter, I will present these concepts briefly as identified in the study, but primarily beyond this specific context and in relation to expanding understandings of occupation.

MOVING BEYOND AN INDIVIDUAL PERSPECTIVE

Considering family and collective occupation suggests a need to reconsider the location of the emergence, or cause, of occupation, traditionally ascribed to individual agency. A transactional perspective (Cutchin and Dickie, 2013) views occupation as the functional process emerging in the transacting relationship of all elements, and the individual's aims become temporary and flexible within the contingent elements and ever-changing nature of the situation as a whole (Dewey, 1958). This perspective supports exploration of occupation as emerging from diverse elements at multiple levels.

Discussion of family and collective occupation also addresses the relationship between the collective and the individual, originally in relation to the concept of individualistic and more collectivistic societies (Iwama, 2006). More recently, Ramugondo and Kronenberg (2015, p. 3) challenged 'the individual-collective dichotomy' in the conceptualization of occupation. They discussed the intentionality of collective occupation centred on human relations, with communities and individuals having responsibilities to each other, and collective occupations manifest on a continuum between oppressive and liberating relationships. Adam (2013) also discussed the importance of collective occupation as part of African philosophy and consciousness, identifying interconnecting elements of mutuality, connectedness and cocreating. In regards to families, studies have predominantly focused on unidirectional patterns of care (Furlong, 2001), either for an older member or for a child with a disability (Stagnitti, 2005), or on the face-to-face interaction of parents and children (Lawlor, 2003) as in co-occupations (Pierce, 2009), rather than on the family as a unit. However, Farias and Asaba (2013) focused on the family as a complex and multigenerational unit and on family-orchestrated occupations through which culture and identity are negotiated.

Fogelberg and Frauworth (2010), describing naturally occurring occupation such as national holidays, sporting events and national elections, noted that they occurred across a variety of levels including population, community, group and individual. Importantly, the authors emphasized the synergistic quality of the collective occupation, a gestalt where the whole is greater than the sum of its parts, supporting the need to develop understanding of this occupation beyond, and different from, that of the individual. In 2013, the International Society of Occupational Science (2013) furthered the discussion by hosting a web-based discussion on collective occupation.

While academic occupation-based literature on the topic may be limited, it can be argued that family and collective occupation continue to be an important element of everyday life, even in those societies considered as more individualistic. Therefore consideration of both family and collective occupation needs to be incorporated into occupational therapy practice, both in order to ensure a full consideration of the

person's occupational life and because of their importance in facilitating social interaction, development and growth (Adam, 2013).

BACKGROUND

I conducted an ethnographic study of occupation in the small market town of Melissa (a pseudonym) in central Greece between 2009 and 2011. A transactional perspective underpinned the understanding of occupation that was developed, with occupation as an ongoing and fluid process working across and between all elements of the situation, including historical, temporal, spatial, climatic and social elements. The reasons *with which* things were done were also explored, using Ricoeur's (2008, p. 188) phrase to describe the practical and ongoing reasoning that underpins the intention of action. In the town, the reasons for occupation were described as maintaining the self-in-the-world, maintaining the family, and maintaining the social fabric, and the balance between and within them (Kantartzis, 2013). Discussion here will focus on family occupation, which is important to maintaining the family, and collective occupation, which is important to maintaining the social fabric. However, all three locations of needs and purpose – self, family and social – are interrelated, and occupation worked across all three levels.

FAMILY OCCUPATION

Maintaining the family was understood to be a central element of everyday life. The perceived importance of the *oikogéneia* (family) as both ideology and practice led to occupation that aimed to uphold the household, including care of family members, and to family occupation. Family occupation was an intricate web of occupation among family members, sharing resources, sharing skills and satisfying needs. In an intricate iterative process, this ongoing occupation reconstructed on a daily basis 'the family' (Kantartzis and Molineux, 2014).

Family occupation was occupation that was not only physically with others or for their immediate needs, but was occupation that included family members in planning, discussion and doing, and that was constructed through the occupation and emotional presence of other family members both past and present. It was a network of occupation extending over time where family was a central and significant part even if not always directly involved in the moment by moment doing. Family occupation emphasizes the essentially transactional nature (Dewey, 1922/2007) of daily life in the town where people grew up within a network of family relationships, and where from day to day family occupation continually shifted and changed in order to accommodate and be responsive to the changing needs, demands and conditions of family members.

Survival, care and celebration all took place primarily with and within the family, and 'the family' can be seen as constructed and reconstructed through an elaborate orchestration of occupation and people across time. Family may be experienced and expressed through the family occupation of shared celebrations and events, for example the traditions of Christmas (Penman, 2001; Shordike and Pierce, 2005), birthday parties, christenings, weddings and funerals. However, family occupation is also the day-to-day network of doing and connectedness, of embodied memories and shared skills and knowledge, which may not always, or ever, involve doing together, but nevertheless is always present. Multiple occupations emerge with, for or because of family members: shopping, doctors' appointments, school plays, holidays, helping with house moves, telephone calls, Skype and e-mail communication, buying gifts and many more throughout the year and life span. Not only skills, knowledge and experiences of occupation are shared, but also the outcome of particular occupation influences the ongoing possibility and relevance of other family members' occupation.

It can be seen that family will be lived and can be defined in different ways by each unique family group, emerging from the ever-changing situation (Dewey and Bentley, 1949), and that fundamental to this process is family occupation. In Melissa (and, it may be suggested, throughout much of the world) family occupation is an inextricable part of what one does. However, family occupation was not the only meso-level occupation evident in the town. In addition, intertwined with this network of family occupation was occupation important for care of the self and also for maintaining the social fabric through collection occupation.

COLLECTIVE OCCUPATION

The study in Melissa identified collective occupation to be particularly important in maintaining the social fabric. The term *social fabric* incorporates a variety of elements such as social and economic institutions (from households to government), as well as more abstract concepts such as governance and social coherence (Haacker, 2004). Social relations are seen to be at its core (Huijbens, 2012) in a complex web of relations across macro, meso and micro levels. One of the primary elements supporting the social fabric is trust, and the social fabric is described as being at risk through ongoing inequality, tension and exclusionary practices, as well as damaged by civil war or extreme violence (Enander et al., 2010; Hoogenboom and Vieille, 2010). In Melissa, collective occupation predominantly contributed to the meso level of social relationships, and three types were identified: informal encounters in public spaces, local organization and associations, and celebratory and commemorative occupation.

Informal Encounters in Public Spaces

Informal daily encounters in public spaces were one form of collective occupation, with characteristics similar to family occupation, but expanding beyond the family to establish and maintain a network of occupation that provided support, information and identity across the community. In Melissa, informal encounters took place throughout the days, weeks and seasons on public streets, squares, in the *kafeneion* (coffee shops), local shops and neighbourhoods. Probably almost all communities throughout the world have some sort of shared public spaces where people meet informally (squares, streets, at the river or well), marketplaces where people shop or exchange goods, while in some countries particular meeting places have developed: the *kafeneion* in Greece, the café in France, the pub in the UK and the *bierstube* in Germany (Oldenburg, 1999), each with its own characteristics. These are where daily encounters in public space take place, a re-meeting of known people that provide the opportunity for people to learn the news and form an opinion about it, share advice and obtain practical help, discuss and do business, and move out of the intensity of the home. This is the network that someone moving to a new neighbourhood works to develop – where to buy bread and a newspaper, who is a reliable plumber or electrician, and who can provide good advice or help with the children or regarding health matters. It develops into a structure providing access to knowledge, skills, support and a sense of belonging, as the public becomes familiar (Mayol, 1998).

As with family occupation, this is not primarily the occupation of a large number of people 'doing' together, but rather is an interlinking dynamic network of occupation that takes place because of or for other people and their occupation, and resembles numerous threads that link throughout people's daily lives. This network depends on, but also enhances, trust, support and reciprocal exchange (obligations), and can be seen to have a close relationship with social capital when described as the resources embedded in one's social networks (Lin, 2006). It can also offer a sense of belonging, of being recognized by others and of being known (including one's reputation) and may encourage a sense of being part of a whole that is valued and significant. Such networks of collective occupation can facilitate the resilience of the community, offering experiences of trust, local knowledge and a commitment to act together in times of crisis (World Health Organization, 2011), facilitating the mental health and well-being of individual members (Kourkoutas and Xavier, 2010).

Networks of informal occupation are created through the ongoing coming together with others, often casually and unplanned. Occupational therapists may rarely consider these informal doings, or only incorporate them within bounded descriptions of work, self-care or leisure occupations. However, these networks of informal occupation should be considered horizontally, as numerous threads that link throughout people's daily lives, one person's occupation linked to others, and theirs to others beyond that. Therefore it is necessary to consider how such networks of informal occupation can be supported and by what they are threatened.

The importance of a place for such informal encounters has been discussed in the literature. Oldenburg (1999), for example, supported the necessity of 'third spaces' in the US, in addition to the home and workplace, for example coffee shops and pubs. He pointed out that they are important as places for relaxation, for equality of relationships removed from the intensity of the family and for developing social contacts, but also promote people to be active citizens. However, as in Melissa, informal encounters can also take place on street corners, parks, squares and any other public space. Adolescents throughout Europe hang out in their leisure time (Flammer and Schaffner, 2003), while White (2007) has discussed shopping malls as important sites of inclusion in public life for older people.

At the same time, social media, such as Facebook, would seem to be offering similar experiences of virtual belonging and the opportunity to negotiate collaborative action (discussed further in the next section), and Twitter offers the instant communication of the marketplace. However, it has been noted that they do not offer face-to-face communication, personal presence and touch, enabling the 'reading' of emotions, which is important for building trust and empathetic relationships (Olstrom, 2005; Sacks, 2011), and direct practical support and exchange of skills.

Creating places for collective engagement is the aim of many community projects working with people at risk of exclusion (e.g. ELSiTO, 2014). The quality of the place is not only in relation to the physical characteristics, but is also in relation to the interaction and engagement that it facilitates. Sharing and exchange, whether of skills, knowledge or emotions, seem to be central. Equality, respect and diversity characterize those collective occupations which facilitate a sense of belonging and identification (Ammeraal et al., 2013).

However, informal encounters in public places should not be considered as necessarily leading to a cohesive and shared vision of a common good, as the network is dynamic and fragile and challenged by a number of factors. The development of such networks is threatened by the increasing mobility of people between countries and urban areas, the closure of local shops and businesses, the increasing use of technology for everyday transactions and the unease of many at behaviour described as 'hanging out' in areas where there are concerns for safety (Panelli et al., 2002). Public meeting places such as coffee shops and pubs may be global enterprises with transient staff providing a uniform service and without the possibility for customers to make the place 'their own'. Public squares and shopping streets in many urban areas are being replaced by privately owned shopping malls, with security guards excluding those judged to be undesirable. The privatization of sports facilities and leisure activities may exclude those with lower incomes, while since industrialization there have been concerted efforts by factory owners and public officials to organize leisure time and space for the workforce towards their moral behaviour and appropriate education (Beckers and Mommaas, 1996).

Public places are also contested places where multiple voices represent conflicting groups and interests (Freeman, 2008). The possibility for voice and visibility that such public occupation potentially offers may not be available to all, with potential for discriminatory and exclusive practices (Angell, 2014). Excluded populations may experience reduced and controlled participation, limiting their experiences of trust, affiliation and belonging, while weakening the network as a whole. Such discrimination of certain groups may occur as social norms are maintained through the network of occupation, for example, reinforcing gender-appropriate behaviour and maintaining situations of occupational marginalization (Stadnyk et al., 2011). It would seem there needs to be a consciousness, a deliberate awareness of building informal encounters of collective occupation, with a particular awareness of practices that discriminate and exclude.

Collective Organization and Associations

A second form of collective occupation in Melissa was that which had developed to organize local action, particularly taking the form of local associations, for example the Farmers' Cooperative and the Athletics Association. This is the collective occupation of groups of people joining to organize, protest, debate and support. This is the form most frequently discussed in other disciplines as collective action (traditionally cited as originating with Olsen's (1985) text from economics), where the action of two or more persons relates to the pursuit of the public good, that is, some shared, nonexclusionary interest (Bimber et al., 2005). It is discussed as essential for participation in civic society and as a key component of citizenship, and is linked by some authors to social capital (e.g., Putnam,

2001), coming between the action of the individual and the institutionalized activity of macrostructures, the private and the public.

A characteristic of collective action through the centuries has been that it aimed to organize the particular form of an activity. Craftsmen in the early middle ages formed guilds in order to protect the prices and quality of their products, and to structure and regulate the learning process of their apprentices (De Moor, 2013). Trade unions and workers' councils or committees developed in various forms throughout Europe as collective actors to secure improvements in the pay, benefits and working conditions of workers (Gumbrell-McCormick and Hyman, 2013). Alongside these organizations which focus on the organization of paid work and employees, numerous other associations have emerged to support, protect, or work towards a variety of purposes depending on local needs (e.g., parent–teacher organizations, sports clubs and women's associations).

Collective action is continuing to develop in contemporary Europe. For example, grass-roots level initiatives are increasing in the political climate of the early twenty-first century with decreased government involvement and increased privatization. These include initiatives to organize collectively energy, care of the elderly and farming (De Moor, 2013). In Greece, a large number of collective organizations and actions are developing, in part, as a result of the economic crisis. These include local exchange, including time-exchange systems and producer-consumer networks, collective kitchens, social clinics and pharmacies, self-managed art spaces, seed banks and ecocommunities, and gratuitous bazaars where a large number of items may be 'bought' without payment (Institutions for Collective Action, n.d.).

There are other forms of collective occupation that work to organize, protest or support. Participation in rallies and demonstrations, civil rights marches and the nonviolent civil disobedience of Mohandas Gandhi are examples of other forms of such occupation. These demonstrate the importance of voice and visibility in the public space as discussed in Arendt's (1958) notion of 'action', particularly for those popularly identified as excluded or even illegal (Beltran, 2009). While theory of collective action was traditionally concerned with the organizational structures required to mould individual participation, recent literature and events[1] are indicating the power of technology and social media in enabling the rapid assembling of protestors and supporters, and the self-organizing powers of online groups without the traditional constraints of either individual communication or cognition, or the need for controls and hierarchy (Bimber et al., 2005).

Celebratory and Commemorative Occupation

The third form of collective occupation in Melissa was celebratory and commemorative occupation. This took place throughout the year, offering the participants opportunities for experiences beyond and different from their mundane, ongoing life, with a core characteristic of this experience being enhanced emotional expression. Such occupation included religious festivals and events, carnival celebrations, local parties and Saturday nights out, as well as national days of mourning and commemorations of historical events, events common to many communities throughout the world. Collective emotions have been part of the studies of disciplines such as sociology, psychology and philosophy (von Scheve and Salmela, 2014), but the relation of occupation to such experiences has not been addressed.

Heightened emotional experiences have been discussed as an essential component of traditional rituals and particularly the liminal phase (Turner, 1986), when unique experiences are enabled by the use of monstrous symbols, masks and costumes, for example. Such rituals may take place to mark life crises or seasonal changes, and the liminal phase is a moment of chaos, ambiguity and disorientation between the previous known structures and the expected structure still to come. Fantasy, desire and particularly the immediate subjective state are the dominating experiences. In discussing contemporary Western society, Turner (1974) suggested that many events, such as rock concerts, have the characteristics of many liminal experiences without involving a resolution to a personal crisis. Central to such liminoid experiences is the idea of a break from society and from everyday experiences, and the creation of a 'time out of space' is important

to the planning of such events regardless of the degree of intensity and their time duration (Getz, 2007).

At the same time that such collective experiences are, in some cases, deliberately planned, others emerge more spontaneously. Crowds at sporting events sing, cheer, do Mexican waves, while those watching the Olympic Games and other national and international sporting events, not only 'live' but even at home on television, become engaged in the collective experience of these events. Concerts, nightclubs and flash mobs may provide similar opportunities. The ongoing emergence of these events in nonreligious or traditional forms would suggest their importance. However, it may be questioned whether they provide the same depth of experience as those with strong historical and traditional roots, and also the importance of participation in not only the event itself but also in the preparations, as is necessary in smaller communities.

Such collective occupation may also be important in facilitating the expression of grief and mourning following natural but also socially generated crises. Collective empathy and collective compassion (Enander et al., 2010) may be expressed through commemorative services, national days of mourning and the construction of memorials.

The idea that groups of people may facilitate experiences of especial strength, particularly emotional experiences, has been recognized in mental health therapeutic settings for many years. However, less attention has been paid to these in the everyday occupation of individuals and groups, and to empowering individuals to access such experiences.

CONSIDERING A MESO LEVEL OF OCCUPATION

The preceding discussion makes it apparent that the meso level of family and collective occupation should not be considered only as characteristic of more collectivistic societies, but rather would seem to be pervasive throughout all aspects of daily life. Through people acting together, occupation is enabled beyond that possible for any one person acting alone, constructing and reconstructing both family and social fabric.

Since Aristotle the importance of 'men' acting together has been recognized, with the city described

[1]For example, the rallies held in Athens, Greece, on the days leading up to the referendum of July 5, 2015, were reported to have been largely organized through social media.

not as a physical place but as a society of men (people) acting together, and how man by his nature is a 'political animal' (Aristotle, 1998, p. 10). This idea of the potential existing in the coming together of people is also present in the writings of Arendt (1958, p. 180), and the importance of this 'sheer human togetherness' can be seen throughout the preceding discussion. The importance of the living space, the public world created by the coming together of people and the possibility for action and the associated visibility that it offers, has been noted by a number of authors (Beltran, 2009; Freeman, 2008). It may be seen how collective occupation provides opportunities not possible for the individual acting alone – whether this is occupation to organize and demonstrate, or occupation to experience alternative emotional states. It is also possible to see the power of family and collective occupation in the network of daily encounters that create a known and safe social world.

At the same time it is not possible to consider collective occupation as some kind of democratic process of like-minded people working towards some ideal of the common good. Families are also sites of tension and conflict (Kantartzis and Molineux, 2014), while collective occupation can not only provide the opportunities previously discussed but also exclude individuals and groups. For those excluded, for example, owing to the ongoing demands of labour for survival of those living in poverty, or those discriminated against by the collective, they are in effect excluded from the public world and from the possibility to fulfil their identity and their potential. It is also important to recognize that mobs, gangs and cartels are also forms of collective action (Olstrom, 2005). The public world is a contested world with struggles for recognition and dominance that may be linked to the distribution of resources.

However, it may be argued that by ignoring family and collective occupation in favour of a focus on the individual, occupational therapists are ignoring an important area of everyday life. While family and collective occupation may work against or to the disadvantage of individuals, other groups or even a whole society, such occupation also can work to support, acknowledge and provide opportunities to individuals and groups, to challenge existing processes and to work towards positive change.

It is recognized that throughout history people have engaged in multiple, overlapping and occasionally conflicting collective occupation, reconciling potentially conflicting group and individual interests (Carballo, 2013). Although the media popularly report the weakening of the social fabric, there is also evidence of increasing interest in collective occupation or action from a range of disciplines and positions, with new emerging forms being identified in some cases. These new forms are emerging in diverse ways, forms of powerful action that are responding to the needs of the local situation. For example, from the world of theatre, collective creation is discussed (Syssoyeva, 2013) as emphasizing the importance of polyphony, the harmonizing of multiple and diverse voices, instead of consensus and how this may provide a model for a better way of being together in the world. A very different form of collective action is discussed in ideas around collective intelligence or wisdom. Landemore (2012) discusses how Aristotle's idea of the wisdom of the multitude has recently resurfaced in a variety of literature referring to smart mobs, crowdsourcing and ideas around the wisdom of the crowds. New in these ideas is the possibility through technology to include millions of people, that it may not depend on any conscious deliberation or communication between the people involved, the importance of networks and the distribution of information, and that given these emerging opportunities for knowledge exchange it is increasingly likely that knowledge and solutions are more likely to emerge from bottom up amongst groups of people who are not experts rather than top down by experts. Wikipedia is an example of collective action that in a relatively short space of time has created 30 million articles and uses 287 languages. Open source is opening access, not only to software, but to a variety of product codes and designs, without restrictions of patents or licences. ThinkCycle, set up by students at Massachusetts Institute of Technology, supports distributed collaboration in design and engineering projects with individuals and groups around the world (Vallero and Brasier, 2008). Rheingold (2012) notes that the collective potential of the Internet has still not been fully utilized; the rules and processes of such collaborations are still being learnt, but they can potentially revolutionize the way people work together (again both towards and against what may be considered the common good).

Transdisciplinary approaches share a similar awareness to open source methods in recognizing the importance of moving beyond any one discipline's or combination of disciplines' knowledge in order to begin to develop solutions to the complex, 'wicked' problems facing society today (Wicks and Jamieson, 2014). At the same time as these emerging forms of collective action, the World Health Organization (2011) continues to recognize the importance of social capital including community networks, civic engagement, a sense of belonging and norms of cooperation and trust in supporting the mental health of the population.

CONCLUSION

It is important that occupational therapists recognize the meso level of family and collective occupation, beyond the traditional focus on the individual. It has been suggested that the meso level will require a distinct sphere of research (Haywood et al., 2014), while research from other disciplines on social capital, collective action and collection emotion may be usefully explored in relation to occupation.

However, I suggest that a conscious shift of focus in occupational therapy practice is also important. It is important to recognize the power of family and collective occupation in constructing both the family and the social fabric, and as providing opportunities for experiences very different from those of the individual doing alone. While pragmatically people's interrelatedness is evident throughout their everyday lives, family and collective occupation is more than recognizing the inevitable links between people and also should not be understood as an amplification of individual action. Such occupation has effects that extend beyond the intentions of any of the participating persons and therefore cannot be defined by the number of people participating, but rather by the quality of the experience and the power of the potential embedded in it. What is perhaps most important to recognize is that collective occupation is collective agency. Family occupation emerges from and reconstructs the emotional and practical connections that maintain the family both as ideology and practice. Collective

occupation contains the power to create a living space where people can access support, information and skills; where they can live safely and flourish; where they can share the collective experiences of celebration and of mourning, joy and anger; and where they can take specific action to achieve what is important in their lives.

I argue that maintaining the focus of occupational therapy practice on the micro individual level is ignoring occupation as an important process in the construction of family and public life. In doing so, occupational therapists are contributing both to an increasing individualization of daily life and to clients' exclusion from participation in the public world. Undoubtedly, further knowledge is required regarding the nature and processes of family occupation and collective occupation, not only in offering particular experiences to the individual, but also in contributing to social equality and inclusion. A conscious awareness in all areas of practice of these various forms of occupation and their importance both to the individual and to the construction of the public world will facilitate the further development of our knowledge and practice.

REFERENCES

Adam, F., 2013. Collective occupation: indigenously African. Paper presented at: Promoting Occupational Therapy in Africa. Eight OTARG Conference. 19–23 August 2013, Harare, Zimbabwe.

Ammeraal, M., et al., 2013. ELSiTO. A collaborative European initiative to foster social inclusion with persons experiencing mental illness. Occup. Ther. Int. 20, 68–77.

Angell, A.M., 2014. Occupation-centered analysis of social difference: contributions to a socially responsive occupational science. J. Occup. Sci. 21 (2), 104–116.

Arendt, H., 1958. The Human Condition, second ed. University of Chicago Press, Chicago, IL.

Aristotle, 1998. The Politics, (E. Barker, Trans.). Oxford University Press, Oxford.

Beckers, T., Mommaas, H., 1996. The international perspective in leisure research: cross-national contacts and comparisons. In: Mommaas, H., et al. (Eds.), Leisure Research in Europe. Methods and Traditions. CAB International, Wallingford, UK, pp. 209–243.

Beltran, C., 2009. Going public: Hannah Arendt, immigrant action, and the space of appearance. Polit. Theory 37 (5), 595–622.

Bimber, B., et al., 2005. Reconceptualising collective action in the contemporary media environment. Commun. Theory 15 (4), 365–388.

Carballo, D.M., 2013. Cultural and evolutionary dynamics of cooperation. In: Carballo, D.M. (Ed.), Cooperation and Collective

Action: Archeological Perspectives. University Press Colorado, Boulder, CO, pp. 3–34.

Cutchin, M.P., Dickie, V., 2013. Transactional perspectives on occupation. Springer, New York.

De Moor, T., 2013. Homo Cooperans. Institutions for Collective Action and the Compassionate Society. Inaugural lecture, 30 August 2013. Utrecht University, Faculty of Humanities, Utrecht. <http://www.collective-action.info/sites/default/files/webmaster/_PUB_Homo-cooperans_EN.pdf>.

Dewey, J., 1922/2007. Human Nature and Conduct: An Introduction to Social Psychology. Cosimo, New York.

Dewey, J., 1958. Experience and Nature, second ed. Dover, New York.

Dewey, J., Bentley, A., 1949. Knowing and the known. Beacon Preson, Boston.

ELSiTO, 2014. Empowering Learning for Social Inclusion Through Occupation (ELSiTO) (accessed 10.10.14). <www.elsito.net>.

Enander, A., et al., 2010. A tear in the social fabric: communities dealing with socially generated crises. J. Contingencies Crisis Manage. 18 (1), 39–48.

Farias, L., Asaba, E., 2013. "The family knot": Negotiating identities and cultural values through the everyday occupations of an immigrant family in Sweden. J. Occup. Sci. 20 (1), 36–47.

Flammer, A., Schaffner, B., 2003. Adolescent leisure across European nations. In: Verma, S., Larson, R. (Eds.), Examining Adolescent Leisure Time Across Cultures: Developmental Opportunities and Risks: New Directions for Child and Adolescent Development. Jossey Bass, San Francisco CA.

Fogelberg, D., Frauworth, S., 2010. A complexity science approach to occupation: moving beyond the individual. J. Occup. Sci. 17 (3), 131–139.

Freeman, J., 2008. Great, good, and divided: the politics of public space in Rio de Janeiro. J. Urban Affairs 30 (5), 529–556.

Furlong, M., 2001. Individuals live their lives within their 'tribes': accessing the practitioner's personal experience of interdependence. J Fam. Stud. 7 (2), 236–241.

Getz, D., 2007. Event studies: theory, research and policy for planned events. Butterworth-Heinemann, Burlington, MA.

Gumbrell-McCormick, R., Hyman, R., 2013. Mapping the terrain: varieties of industrial relations and trade unionism. In: Gumbrell-McCormick, R., Hyman, R. (Eds.), Trade Unions in Western Europe: Hard Times, Hard Choices. Oxford University Press, Oxford.

Haacker, M., 2004. Macro-economics of HIV/Aids. International Monetary Fund, Washington, DC.

Haywood, C., et al., 2014. Bridging the individual-collective divide: examination of 'mid-range' social analytic units. Paper presented at: Globalization & Occupational Science: Partnerships, Methods & Research. (accessed 17.10.14). <http://commons.pacificu.edu/sso_conf/2014/3/5/>.

Hoogenboom, D., Vieille, S., 2010. Rebuilding social fabric in failed states: examining transitional justice in Bosnia. Hum. Rights Rev. 11, 183–198.

Huijbens, E., 2012. Sustaining a village's social fabric? Sociol. Ruralis. 52 (3), 332–352.

Institutions for Collective Action (n.d.). Civil initiatives in Greece during crisis: social solidarity networks and co-operative organisations. <http://www.collective-action.info/sites/default/files/webmaster/_POC_CivilInitiativesGreece.pdf> (accessed 04.10.14.).

International Society of Occupational Science, 2013. On-line discussion Collective Occupations (accessed 04.10.14). <https://groups.google.com/forum/#!searchin/occupational_science_intl/collective$20occupation/occupational_science_intl/JnrwSar9cRI/hhnJbE6q-dgJ>.

Iwama, M., 2006. The Kawa Model. Culturally Relevant Occupational Therapy. Churchill Livingston Elsevier, Edinburgh, UK.

Kantartzis, S., 2013. Re-conceptualising Occupation. An Ethnographic Study of a Greek Town. Leeds Metropolitan University, Leeds, UK.

Kantartzis, S., Molineux, M., 2014. Occupation to maintain the family as ideology and practice in a Greek town. J. Occup. Sci. 21 (3), 277–295.

Kourkoutas, H., Xavier, M.R., 2010. Empowering resilience in children and adolescents with academic and psychosocial difficulties/disturbances: intervention at school (In Greek). In: Kourkoutas, H., Caldin, R. (Eds.), Families with Children with Difficulties and School Inclusion. Ellenika Grammata, Athens.

Laliberte Rudman, D., 2010. Occupational dialogue: occupational possibilities. J. Occup. Sci. 17 (1), 55–59.

Laliberte Rudman, D., 2013. Enacting the critical potential of occupational science: problematizing the 'individualization of occupation'. J. Occup. Sci. 20 (4), 298–313.

Landemore, H., 2012. Collective wisdom. In: Landemore, H., Elster, J. (Eds.), Collective Wisdom. Cambridge University Press, Cambridge, pp. 1–20.

Lawlor, M., 2003. The significance of being occupied: the social construction of childhood occupations. Am. J. Occup. Ther. 57, 424–434.

Lin, N. (Ed.), 2006. The encyclopedia of Economic Sociology. Routledge, Oxon.

Mayol, P., 1998. The neighbourhood. In: de Certeau, M., et al. (Eds.), The Practice of Everyday Life, vol. 2. Living and Cooking (T. Tomasik, Trans.). University of Minnesota Press, Minneapolis, pp. 7–14.

Oldenburg, R., 1999. The Great Good Place, second ed. Da Capo Press, Cambridge, MA.

Olstrom, E., 2005. The Complexity of Collective Action Theory. Workshop in Political Theory and Policy Analysis. 23 May 2005. Indiana University. <www.indiana.edu/-workshop/papers/ostrom_berlin.pdf>.

Panelli, R., et al., 2002. 'Hanging out': print media constructions of young people in 'public space'. Youth Stud. Aust. 21 (4), 34–48.

Penman, M., 2001. The Christmas cake. J. Occup. Sci. 9 (1), 20–24.

Pierce, D., 2009. Co-occupation: The challenges of defining concepts original to occupational science. J. Occup. Sci. 16 (3), 203–207.

Putnam, R., 2001. Bowling Along: The Collapse and Revival of American Community. Simon & Schuster, New York.

Ramugondo, E., Kronenberg, F., 2015. Explaining collective occupations from a human relations perspective: bridging the individual-collective dichotomy. J. Occup. Sci. 22 (1), 3–16.

Rheingold, H., 2012. Net Smart: How to Thrive Online. MIT Press, Cambridge, MA.

Ricoeur, P., 2008. From Text to Action (J. Blarney, K. Thompson, Trans.). Continuum, London.

Sacks, O., 2011. The Great Partnership. God, Science and the Search for Meaning. Hodder & Stoughton, London.

Shordike, A., Pierce, D., 2005. Cooking up Christmas in Kentucky: Occupation and tradition in the stream of time. J. Occup. Sci. 12 (3), 140–148.

Stadnyk, R., et al., 2011. Occupational justice. In: Christiansen, C., Townsend, E. (Eds.), Introduction to Occupation: The Art and Science of Living. Pearson, Upper Saddle River, NJ, pp. 329–358.

Stagnitti, K., 2005. The family as a unit in postmodern society: considerations for practice. In: Whiteford, G., Wright-St. Clair, V. (Eds.), Occupation and Practice in Context. Elsevier, Sydney, pp. 213–229.

Syssoyeva, K.M., 2013. Towards a new history of collective creation. In: Syssoyeva, K.M., Proudfit, S. (Eds.), A History of Collective Creation. Palgrave Macmillan, New York, pp. 1–10.

Turner, V., 1974. Liminal to liminoid in play, flow, and ritual: an essay in comparative symbology. Rice University Studies 60 (3), 53–92.

Turner, V., 1986. Dewey, Dilthey, and drama: anthropology of experience. In: Turner, V., Bruner, E. (Eds.), The Anthropology of Experience. University of Illinois, Urbana, pp. 33–44.

Vallero, D., Brasier, C., 2008. Sustainable Design: The Science of Sustainability and Green Engineering. John Wiley, Hoboken, NJ.

Von Scheve, C., Salmela, M. (Eds.), 2014. Collective Emotions. Perspectives from Psychology, Philosophy and Sociology. Oxford University Press, Oxford.

White, R., 2007. Older people hang out too. J. Occup. Sci. 14 (2), 115–118.

Wicks, A., Jamieson, M., 2014. New ways for occupational scientists to tackle 'wicked problems' impacting population health. J. Occup. Sci. 21 (1), 81–85.

World Health Organization, 2011. Impact of Economic Crises on Mental Health. WHO Regional Office Europe, Copenhagen.

4 CONCEPTUALIZING DISABILITY

HANNAH KUPER ■ JÖRG GÜNTER WEBER

WHAT IS DISABILITY?

This chapter will describe how common disability is, the effect that disability has on people's lives, and the different ways in which the impact of disability can be alleviated. An important first step is therefore to have a common understanding of what is meant by 'disability'. This is important because disability means different things to different people, and the way in which disability is conceptualized has changed over time.

To some, a disabled person is characterized as one who has something seemingly 'wrong' with them due to a medical condition. This could be someone who uses a wheelchair or someone who cannot hear. This view equates disability to the presence of bodily impairments, for instance automatically counting someone who is blind as disabled. It also assumes that someone with a lesser degree of visual impairment is not disabled. This view of disability is called the medical model and it is disputed by many people (Oliver, 1990). The primary concern is that people with the same impairment may have very different experiences as to how this impacts on their lives. A premier league footballer may be forced to retire early from a lucrative career because of a long-term ankle injury. In contrast, someone with a desk job may not experience as big an effect on their income if they failed to recover fully from a broken ankle.

Disability therefore is really about whether people can do the things that they want to do, rather than a clinical measure of function. This is also how people themselves often talk about their disability – someone who has difficulties seeing will not talk about their level of visual acuity, but whether their vision is good enough to be able to drive or recognize friends. Another problem with the medical model of disability is that it puts the responsibility for the disability on the person – a woman is disabled because of a problem in her body. This view does not appreciate the role that society plays in enabling or preventing people with impairments from enjoying a full life.

The social model is a response to the medical model (Oliver, 1990). This way of thinking views disability as being due to society's failure to respond to the needs of people with impairments. People in wheelchairs may have limited employment opportunities, not because they cannot walk, but because many offices are not set up to allow access to wheelchairs. People with schizophrenia may be marginalized in lots of different ways because they make people feel uncomfortable or nervous, and not because the illness prevents them from being able to do everyday activities. The social model is therefore important for highlighting the role that society plays in changing the experience of people with disabilities. However, some criticize this model as giving too little importance to the underlying physical impairment (Shakespeare, 2006). If someone is in pain all the time, then no amount of societal support is going to allow them to fully enjoy their life.

The human rights model of disability is a different way of approaching the concept of disability. At its core is the slogan 'nothing about us without us' (Charlton, 1998). It calls for inclusion of people with disabilities, allowing them control over their own fate. It goes beyond mere removal of barriers, as the social model would suggest, and argues that full participation is a human right that can be claimed by everybody. It goes beyond the social model and has a much more demanding character than solely pointing at barriers to participation.

The United Nations (UN) Convention on the Rights of Persons with Disabilities was constructed as a response to the human rights model of disability (UN, 2008). This is as an international human rights instrument of the UN intended to protect the rights and dignities of people with disabilities. The Convention calls upon all countries to respect and ensure the equal rights and participation of all people with disabilities (e.g., in education, healthcare, and employment). The text was adopted by the UN General Assembly in 2006 and came into force in 2008. By September 2014 it had 150 signatories and 151 parties, including the European Union. Ensuring that children with disabilities can go to school is therefore now a legal obligation for countries that have signed the Convention, rather than something that is desired for social responsibility or justice alone.

Putting all these ideas together, a common way of viewing disability today is as a bio-psycho-social model (World Health Organization, 2001). According to this model, a health condition may lead to an

impairment. For instance, polio can lead to muscle weakening and consequent physical impairment. Dementia causes cognitive impairment. The impairment may lead to reduced activities. In the previous examples, polio may lead to difficulties in walking, and dementia may lead to difficulties in communication. These limitations in activities can restrict full participation in aspects of society, for example, exclusion from employment or education, thus resulting in disability. This model therefore recognizes three levels at which disability is experienced: the body, the person, and the community.

The impact of the impairment on disability is not inevitable, but is influenced by a variety of factors. Personal factors may be important. As an example, providing additional education or training could enhance the employment prospects for a person with polio who is unable to walk. Environmental changes, such as the provision of assistive devices, adaptations to buildings, or antidiscrimination policies can also enhance participation, and thereby alleviate disability.

This view of disability is therefore an expansion beyond the limited medical view, which focuses on impairments only as the cause of disability. It also accepts the important role that impairment may play in causing disability, as a response to the social model. Figure 4-1 shows the ICF Disability and Health Conceptual Framework which illustrates this view of

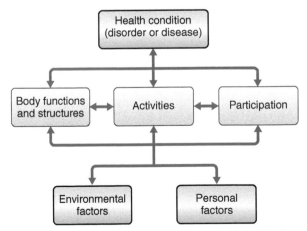

FIGURE 4-1 ■ International classification of functioning, disability and health conceptual framework. *WHO, 2011 (i.e. the World Report on Disability) Box 1.1, page 5. Available at: http://www.who.int/disabilities/world_report/2011/en/*

disability (World Health Organization, 2001). This is the model of disability that we will use for the rest of this chapter.

With this view of disability in mind, people with disabilities include those who have long-term physical, mental, intellectual, or sensory impairments which, in interaction with various barriers, may hinder their full and effective participation in society on an equal basis with others (UN, 2008). In lay terms, this means that disability arises when people cannot do the things that they want to do or are legally entitled to do because of an underlying impairment. Going to school is one example.

Disability is not a homogenous category, and people's experiences of disability are extremely varied. These experiences may be influenced by factors such as the type of disability, the age at onset, the environment in which the person lives, and their social support structure. A woman in her fifties who becomes disabled after having a stroke will not experience disability in the same way as a woman in her fifties who has had a disability all her life because of a congenital condition or a traumatic injury in childhood.

WHY ARE MODELS OF DISABILITY RELEVANT IN OCCUPATIONAL THERAPY?

These models of disability help us to develop a more differentiated view on disability. They can help us question who has a disability and who does not. Stephen Hawking has had motor neurone disease for many years, which has left him with varied and severe impairments. Yet he is able to compete at the highest levels of science while maintaining personal relationships, in no small part due to his sophisticated electronic devices and high level of education. This is not to question whether or not Professor Hawking is a person with a disability, but merely to highlight that the relationship between impairment and disability is not the same for everyone. Consider the likely living circumstances for someone with the same level of impairments, but in a low-income setting.

For occupational therapists this means that attention needs to be given not only to functional abilities, but also more broadly to whether people are able to do the things that they want to do, whether it is

travelling independently, having a job or enjoying a group sport. Another central implication is that if disability is not simply equated to impairment, then alleviation of disability can take on many forms beyond medical intervention. Occupational therapists aim to recognize these issues and to advocate for them already, and therefore do not focus just on improving physical skills, but also on supporting activities that allow inclusion in society.

WHAT IS THE MAGNITUDE AND DISTRIBUTION OF DISABILITY?

Few surveys have been conducted to estimate the prevalence of disability. This gap in knowledge means that it is hard to estimate how many people have disabilities, and this information is needed to plan services. Those studies that do exist have often used very different measures of disability. As a consequence, it is difficult for us to know overall how many people have disabilities, to gauge trends over time to see whether disability is increasing or decreasing, or to compare prevalence between different regions.

The World Report on Disability collated the best available data on disability (World Health Organization (WHO), 2011). It estimated that there are over 1 billion people with disabilities in the world, of whom 110 to 190 million experience very significant difficulties. This corresponds to about 15% of the world's population. Disability is often experienced by the whole family, rather than just the individual, so this means that a very high proportion of households in the world include a person with a disability.

The main types of disability include vision, hearing, physical or mental health. Good data are available on the prevalence of blindness. The latest WHO estimates suggest that 39 million people were blind and 285 million people were visually impaired in 2010 (Pascolini and Mariotti, 2012). Data on the prevalence of hearing impairment are more limited but suggest that there are 360 million people with disabling hearing loss around the world (WHO, 2012). There are fewer data on the overall prevalence of physical impairments or mental health conditions. However, the Global Burden of Disease Study 2010 estimated that mental and substance use disorders accounted for 7.4% of disability-adjusted life years worldwide (Whiteford et al., 2013).

The biggest determinant of disability is age (WHO, 2011). Disability is relatively rare among children and then becomes increasingly common so that more than one third of people over 60 may have some type of disability. Recent data suggest that among children, disability is more common among boys than girls (Kuper et al., 2014). Among adults disability is often more common among women than men, in part at least because women live longer on average than men (WHO, 2011). It is often stated that disability is more common among the poorer parts of the world, and this is reflected in the World Report on Disability and a recent large review (Banks and Polack, 2014; WHO, 2011).

HOW DO WE MEASURE DISABILITY?

Excellent efforts are being made to standardize the way in which disability is measured. This will allow us to produce more comparable data so that we can start to find patterns in the prevalence and cause of disability under different circumstances. There is also a growing emphasis on including measures of disability in censuses and household surveys so that we can assess whether the needs or living conditions of people with disabilities are different from the rest of the population. For instance, are people with disabilities more likely to be poor or excluded from schooling? There are two main ways in which we can assess whether a person has a disability: through self-report or through clinical assessment.

The first method is to ask the person about difficulties in functioning or if they consider themselves to have a disability. If a person is asked the question, 'Do you consider yourself to have a disability?' then few people will say yes as they do not classify themselves in this way. Instead, it is more common to ask a series of questions about difficulties in functioning and then to make a decision as to whether or not that person has a disability.

One commonly used questionnaire to measure disability is the Short Set of Questions on Disability developed by the Washington Group on Disability Statistics (Madans et al., 2011). This questionnaire asks people about whether the person experiences difficulties with seeing, hearing, walking, self-care, usual activities, and communicating. People can answer 'no difficulty', 'some difficulty', 'a lot of difficulty', or 'cannot do'. People are classified as having a disability if they answer 'some problem' in two or more domains, or 'a lot of problems'/'cannot do' in at least one domain. These questions seem simplistic, but the questionnaire will capture most of the various conditions that are considered to be disabling (e.g., dementia, severe depression, visual loss, or club foot). Assessing disability through self-report is often fairly cheap and easy, and is in line with the social model of disability. However, this method will not allow us to understand the underlying health needs of the person and plan appropriate services.

The second way to classify disability is by a clinician or a multidisciplinary team who will assess the functional capacity of a person to determine whether the person has an impairment. An occupational therapist may conduct a functional capacity evaluation to assess for a physical impairment while visual impairment can be measured through visual acuity charts. The advantage of these methods is that they identify the specific needs that a person may have for health or rehabilitation services. However, this method defines the presence of disability through impairment, which is a very limited view of disability. The missing links may include what colleagues trained in social work, speech therapy, or psychology can add to complete the assessment, such as the ability to communicate and to get along with others. Another problem is that clinical assessment relies usually on the presence of highly trained professionals, and this makes the method expensive and practically more complicated.

WHAT IS THE IMPACT OF DISABILITY?

Disability potentially has very far-reaching impacts, including on poverty, education, and employment. Disability is often viewed as both a cause and consequence of poverty. People who are poor may not have enough money to pay for services and so do not seek them until it is too late, resulting in disability. Travelling in unsafe vehicles leads to more accidents and more injuries. At the same time, people with disabilities may become poorer if they are unable to work or require care from a family member. Families may also slide into poverty because of the costs of treatments or devices needed. A recent review identified 97 studies that explored the relationship between poverty and disability in low- and middle-income countries and showed a statistically significant and positive relationship in 78 (Banks and Polack, 2014). This association may have been in part because people with disabilities were significantly less likely to be in employment in 12 of the 17 studies that assessed this relationship. In the UK, in 2012, only 46% of working-age disabled people are in employment compared to 76% of working-age nondisabled people (Department for Work and Pensions, 2014). Overall, 19% of individuals in families in the UK with at least one disabled member live in relative income poverty, on a before-housing-costs basis, compared to 15% of individuals in families with no disabled member.

Children with disabilities are also significantly less likely to attend school than their peers. A recent study found that children with disabilities across 30 countries were often 10 times less likely to attend school than their peers without disabilities (Kuper et al, 2014). Even when the disabled children were enrolled at school they were often at a lower education level. The lack of schooling of children with disabilities will ultimately reduce their earning potential when they become adults, and in the short term it limits their social interactions with other children. These barriers are also seen in high-income countries. In the UK, disabled people are around three times as likely not to hold any qualifications compared to nondisabled people, and around half as likely to hold a degree-level qualification (Department for Work and Pensions, 2014). About 19.2% of working-age disabled people do not hold any formal qualification, compared to 6.5% of working-age nondisabled people.

It is widely argued that people with disabilities have difficulties accessing preventive or curative healthcare. At the same time, they may experience higher healthcare needs, making this exclusion particularly damaging. Surprisingly, there is very little research addressing this question. One source of information on this topic is the World Health Surveys, which included data from 51 countries (WHO, 2011). These data showed that persons with disabilities were significantly more likely to seek inpatient and outpatient care, but were more likely to not receive healthcare when needed, and faced many barriers when seeking health services. Research from the UK shows that around a third of disabled people experience difficulties related to their impairment in accessing public, commercial, and leisure goods and services (Department for Work and Pensions, 2014).

There is therefore an important and negative impact of disability on inclusion in health, education and employment, and potentially in many other areas of life.

HOW CAN DISABILITY BE ALLEVIATED?

Combining all this information, we see that a focus on disability is important, because the number of people with disabilities worldwide is large and they are among the most marginalized and economically poorest people in any society. People with disabilities also have the right to be fully included in different aspects of society, in keeping with the UN Convention on the Rights of Persons with Disabilities (UN 2008). Looking again at the ICF model of disability, it is clear that there are many ways in which disability can be alleviated.

Prevention or treatment of the health condition underlying the disability is an important step. This could include preventive efforts, such as extending rubella vaccination campaigns, thereby reducing the prevalence of hearing impairment, or promoting road safety to prevent injuries. Prompt treatment of health conditions can also be effective in preventing the development of impairments. Treatment of eye conditions, such as glaucoma, can help prevent blindness. Similarly, physiotherapy can be used to alleviate functional restrictions of the motor system and help to overcome barriers to participation.

Medical treatment is also often possible once the health condition has already led to an impairment. Visual impairment due to cataract can be cured with a simple operation. Mobility can be improved after hip replacement surgery.

There is a large proportion of people, however, who have an impairment that cannot be entirely treated medically. People with spinal cord injuries, blindness due to diabetic retinopathy, cerebral palsy, Down syndrome, dementia, and more fall into this category.

Here our efforts need to focus on maximizing quality of life through enabling their full participation in society, as far as possible. There are practical means by which we can reach this lofty aim.

As every occupational therapist knows, interventions using assistive devices, training, and support can be important to maintain the independence of people living with disabilities. The effectiveness of these interventions can be assessed through randomized controlled trials, the gold standard method for assessment of impact. For instance, a systematic review of the available trial data showed that occupational therapy can help people with rheumatoid arthritis to do daily chores such as dressing, cooking, and cleaning and with less pain. In these examples, occupational therapy was offered through training, advice and counselling (Steultjens et al., 2004). Another review showed that people were more likely to maintain their ability to carry out daily activities after a stroke if they received therapy services at home, including from physiotherapists, occupational therapists, or multidisciplinary teams (Outpatient Service Trialists, 2003). These studies show that rehabilitation can maximize functioning among people with disabilities.

There is also an enormous amount that can and should be done to support participation of people with disabilities. Taking employment as an example, we need to address the physical barriers so that people can enter and engage in the workplace. The staff in the office may need support or further training in how to address the needs of people with disabilities, and similarly family members can be supported to this end. These efforts can be enshrined in law and policy, to further support the rights of people to employment, or children with disabilities to accessing education. There will be a cost for these activities, but they ultimately will be cost saving. Data from supported employment projects in Scotland suggest that every £1 spent on the programme led to a savings of £5.87 due in large part to decreased need for disability/welfare benefits and increased tax income (Durie and Wilson 2007). In the US, concerted efforts by major companies Walgreens and Verizon to employ more people with disabilities showed that this led to a 20% increase in productivity and a 67% return on investment, respectively (Houtenville and Kalargyrou, 2012; International Labour Organization, 2011).

Since disability is very common, it should be considered in all interventions and activities, to make sure that this large group of people can also enjoy the benefits of general services. This is called *mainstreaming of disability*. This could range from involving people with disabilities in the design of transport systems, provision of education, or development of health programmes, among others.

More data are needed to increase our effectiveness across all these activities. Having data on the prevalence and impact of disability will help with advocacy and planning. There is also a need for more evidence to understand what works, particularly what is cost-effective, so that these interventions can be scaled up enabling the greatest number of people to be helped within the available funds.

This discussion is highly relevant to the activities of occupational therapists. It highlights the need to look beyond treating the health condition or impairment towards considering the wider impact of the disability on the person and family. It encourages the occupational therapist to consider broader questions, such as whether social support or help accessing benefits are needed, or guidance on finding a job or improving the accessibility of a home. This does not mean that the occupational therapist needs to address all these needs, but to be aware of them and knowledgeable about different referral pathways.

DISABILITY IN LOW- AND MIDDLE-INCOME SETTINGS

The previous section demonstrated that a wide range of potential interventions exist that can enhance the participation and quality of life of people with disabilities. Comprehensive rehabilitation services may be preferred to isolated and specialized interventions, given the wide range of barriers to effective participation experienced by people with disabilities. Unfortunately, the services needed to avoid impairment and maximize participation among people with disabilities are often not available to all who need them in low- and middle-income countries.

It is still important to address disability in low- and middle-income countries, despite the many different pressing needs facing these countries. It is widely argued that the development targets cannot be achieved without the integration of disability issues since 15% of the world's population lives with disability and people with disabilities are vulnerable to poverty (Groce and Trani, 2009). Development policies therefore need to address the needs of people with disabilities and be inclusive of them. The importance of inclusive development is now acknowledged by development agencies across the world, while the Sustainable Development Goals adopted in 2015 include 11 explicit references to people with disabilities (UN, 2015). Consequently, alternative strategies to address the needs of people with disabilities must be sought in these areas.

Community-based rehabilitation (CBR) is the strategy endorsed by the WHO (2010) to address the needs of people with disabilities in low- and middle-income countries. It has become widely used since the early 1980s. The CBR matrix (Figure 4-2) provides a basic framework for the CBR strategy (WHO, 2010, p. 25). The matrix shows the need to target interventions beyond the medical aspect, focusing on other components of life such as education, livelihood, social

aspects, and empowerment. Each of the components of the matrix includes five elements where the different activities are listed. A CBR disability inclusive strategy can be formed by one or more activities in one or more of the five components. Service providers are not expected to implement every component of the CBR matrix for all people, because not all disabled people require help in all of these areas. The strategy instead is to make a range of interventions available to people with disabilities depending on their need, extending from medical (e.g., physical rehabilitation in community centres) to social (e.g., establishing family support groups). This strategy is therefore in keeping with the conceptualization of disability through the ICF model, which recognizes the range of needs of people with disabilities depending on their impairment, personal and societal circumstances. Consequently, a range of interventions can be implemented through CBR to alleviate disability and enhance quality of life.

The health component could involve provision of rehabilitation services within the community, such as

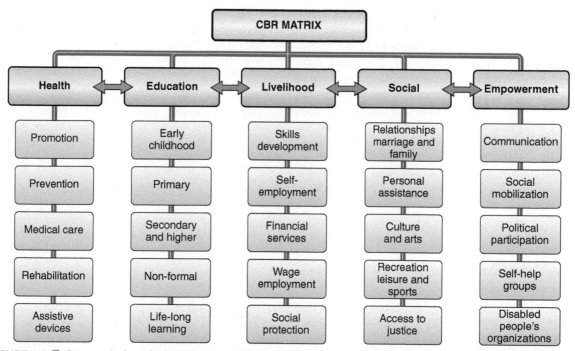

FIGURE 4-2 ■ Community-based rehabilitation (CBR) matrix. *From World Health Organization, 2010. Community-Based Rehabilitation: CBR Guidelines. World Health Organization, Geneva. Figure 1, p. 25. Available at: <http://www.who.int/disabilities/cbr/guidelines/en/> (accessed 19.07.14.).*

training family members to help with exercises for patients after stroke. The education campaign could involve training schoolteachers in how to cater to the needs of children with disabilities, or making the classroom more physically accessible. Provision of retraining to people with disabilities to increase their employment opportunities could be considered as a livelihood intervention. Providing counselling to support relationships between spouses or making public areas accessible are examples of the social component. Last, but not least, the empowerment component of the CBR matrix could include the establishment of family support groups for the parents of children with disabilities, or supporting disabled people's organizations that lobby governments for equality of rights for people with disabilities.

The characteristic feature of CBR is that it is delivered within the community using predominantly local resources. As a consequence, the interventions and activities are designed to be locally appropriate and to meet the needs of people with disabilities. This strategy also keeps the cost of the intervention low, enabling scaling up in resource-poor settings. CBR is therefore a multisectoral, 'bottom-up' strategy.

CBR is currently implemented throughout the world, but the unmet need is likely to be enormous, though exact data are lacking (Meikle, 2002). CBR therefore needs to be scaled up urgently. Strengthening the evidence base for CBR to show that it is effective, and potentially even cost-effective, would support efforts for scaling up CBR services (Finkenflugel et al., 2005; Hartley et al., 2009; WHO, 2011). Development or provision of CBR may be an excellent way by which occupational therapists working in low- and middle-income countries can best help support people with disabilities and their families.

SUMMARY

People with disabilities include those who have long-term physical, mental, intellectual, or sensory impairments which, in interaction with various barriers, may hinder their full and effective participation in society on an equal basis with others (UN, 2008). In lay terms, this means that disability arises when people cannot do the things that they want to do or are legally entitled to do because of an underlying impairment. Disability is common; there are an estimated 1 billion people with disabilities globally, and they are often poor and disadvantaged. People with disabilities face a range of exclusions, including with respect to health, employment, and education, and this can further exacerbate their poverty. There are many ways in which disability can be alleviated, ranging from treatment of the underlying impairment, provision of rehabilitation or assistive devices, or focusing on supporting inclusion in work, social life and beyond. Occupational therapists therefore have a crucial role to play in the alleviation of disability.

REFERENCES

Banks, L.M., Polack, S., 2014. Economic Costs of Exclusion and Gains of Inclusion of People with Disabilities. International Centre for Evidence in Disability, London. Accessed at: <http://disabilitycentre.lshtm.ac.uk/resources/>.

Charlton, J.I., 1998. Nothing About Us Without Us, University of California Press.

Department for Work and Pensions, Office for Disability Issues, 2014. Disability Facts and Figures. Department for Work and Pensions, Office for Disability Issues, London. Available at: <https://www.gov.uk/government/statistics/disability-facts-and-figures> (accessed 14.10.14.).

Durie, S., Wilson, L., 2007. Social Return on Investment Report. Six Mary's Place, Edinburgh.

Finkenflugel, H., Wolffers, I., Huijsman, R., 2005. The evidence base for community-based rehabilitation: a literature review. Int. J. Rehabil. Res. 28 (3), 187–201.

Groce, N.E., Trani, J.F., 2009. Millennium development goals and people with disabilities. Lancet 374 (9704), 1800–1801.

Hartley, S., Finkenflugel, H., Kuipers, P., Thomas, M., 2009. Community-based rehabilitation: opportunity and challenge. Lancet 374 (9704), 1803–1804.

Houtenville, A., Kalargyrou, V., 2012. People with disabilities employers' perspectives on recruitment practices, strategies, and challenges in leisure and hospitality. Cornell Hosp. Q. 53 (1), 40–52.

International Labour Organization, 2011. Disability in the Workplace and the ILO Global Business and Disability Network 2011. <http://www.ilo.org/wcmsp5/groups/public/@ed_emp/@emp_ent/@multi/documents/meetingdocument/wcms_159137.pdf> (accessed 14.10.14.).

Kuper, H., Monteath-van Dok, A., Wing, K., et al., 2014. The impact of disability on the lives of children; cross-sectional data including 8,900 children with disabilities and 898,834 children without disabilities across 30 countries. PLoS ONE 9 (9), e107300.

Madans, J.H., Loeb, M.E., Altman, B.M., 2011. Measuring disability and monitoring the UN Convention on the Rights of Persons with Disabilities: the work of the Washington Group on Disability Statistics. BMC Public Health 11 (Suppl. 4), S4.

Meikle, L., 2002. Disability, poverty and development. World Hosp. Health Serv. 38 (1), 21–33.

Oliver, M., 1990. The Politics of Disablement. Macmillan and St Martin's Press, Basingstoke, UK.

Outpatient Service Trialists, 2003. Therapy-based rehabilitation services for stroke patients at home. Cochrane Database Syst. Rev. (1), CD002925.

Pascolini, D., Mariotti, S.P., 2012. Global estimates of visual impairment: 2010. Br. J. Ophthalmol. 96 (5), 614–618.

Shakespeare, T., 2006. Disability Rights and Wrongs. Taylor and Francis, Abingdon, UK.

Steultjens, E.M., Dekker, J., Bouter, L.M., et al., 2004. Occupational therapy for rheumatoid arthritis. Cochrane Database Syst. Rev. (1), CD003114.

United Nations (UN), 2008. UN Convention on the Rights of Persons with Disabilities. United Nations, New York. Available at: <http://www.un.org/disabilities/documents/convention/convoptprot-e.pdf> (accessed 19.07.14.).

United Nations (UN), 2015. Sustainable Development Goals. <https://sustainabledevelopment.un.org/> (accessed 14.04.16.).

Whiteford, H.A., Degenhardt, L., Rehm, J., et al., 2013. Global burden of disease attributable to mental and substance use disorders: findings from the Global Burden of Disease Study 2010. Lancet 382 (9904), 1575–1586.

WHO Global Estimates on Prevalence of Hearing Loss. 2012. World Health Organization, Geneva. Available at: <http://www.who.int/pbd/deafness/estimates> (accessed 25.11.13.).

World Health Organization, 2001. International Classification of Functioning Disability and Health (ICF). World Health Organization, Geneva.

World Health Organization, 2010. Community-Based Rehabilitation: CBR Guidelines. World Health Organization, Geneva. Available at: <http://www.who.int/disabilities/cbr/guidelines/en/> (accessed 19.07.14.).

World Health Organization, World Bank, 2011. World Report on Disability. World Health Organization, Geneva. Available at: <http://www.who.int/disabilities/world_report/2011/en/> (accessed 19.07.14.).

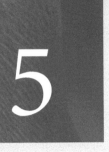

THE IMPACT OF NEOLIBERALISM ON HEALTH AND THE HEALTH SYSTEM: THE CASE OF CHILE

ELENA ROTAROU ▪ DANIELA OLIVARES

Neoliberalism is the term often used to describe the existing global economic regime. Neoliberal economic theory promotes free market or laissez-faire economics; as a political ideology, it argues that the role of national governments is to provide regulatory frameworks that enable markets to function successfully (Scholte, 2005). Private institutions are deemed as more capable and effective at delivering social services, including health and education. This has resulted in slashing of government welfare spending in many parts of the world, a fact that has often led to an increase in poverty and inequality rates.

Since the 1970s, the world's economies have experienced a wide-ranging transformation from a state-centric to a neoliberal form, as a more 'monetarist' approach to the economy – inspired by the theories and work of Milton Friedman – started to take hold (Sewell, 2005). By the 1990s, many countries had proceeded to lifting capital controls, massive and unregulated privatization of state enterprises, and limiting social welfare, often under the guideline of international institutions, such as the International Monetary Fund and the World Bank. The neoliberal measures adopted included a reduction in health spending, introduction of private health providers and the notion of 'health consumer' (McGregor, 2001).

Chile is regarded as the first country where neoliberal economic reforms started taking place in 1975, under the government of General Augusto Pinochet. While the neoliberal 'shock therapy' and structural adjustment programmes that were adopted by many developing countries led to instability and poor growth, this was not the case with Chile. Despite serious human rights abuses during Pinochet's government, Chile is viewed as an economic miracle by neoliberal advocates and strong critics of neoliberalism alike. Nevertheless, neoliberal policies in Chile have had a negative impact on welfare provision, especially concerning health and education systems. Although great improvements have been made during the last few decades, particularly regarding poverty, the country still suffers from high inequality levels.

The aim of this chapter is to present neoliberalism, its main characteristics and its impacts on health and health systems. Chile is taken as a clear example of a country that applied neoliberal measures to its economy, with both positive and negative socioeconomic impacts. It is argued that neoliberalism – with its focus on free markets, individualism, liberalization, and deregulation – does not include in its agenda the welfare of people, communities, and societies. Neoliberal policies applied to the health system have led to greater inequality and dehumanization of healthcare.

NEOLIBERALISM AND HEALTH

The relationship between neoliberalism and health has been characterized by a rather turbulent history, considering that neoliberal economic theory advocates for the minimization of the welfare state – that sees health and education as a right for all its citizens – and the promotion of an entrepreneurial and individualistic 'homo economicus.' Before proceeding to the relationship between neoliberalism and the health system, it would be useful to first define these two sides of the equation.

Neoliberalism

Neoliberalism rests on the 'beliefs in the efficacy of the free market and the adoption of policies that prioritise deregulation, foreign debt reduction, privatisation of the public sector…and a (new) orthodoxy of individual responsibility and the "emergency" safety net - thus replacing collective provision through a more residualist welfare state' (Hancock, 1999, p. 5).

The 1980s were for most countries a period of economic stagnation, widespread strife and confusion, persistent inflation and disillusionment with the role of the state in activating the economy. It was at this point that neoliberal economic and political ideology emerged in the public and political debate, with economists Friedrich Hayek and Milton Friedman on one hand, and the election of neoliberals Margaret Thatcher in the UK and Ronald Reagan in the US on the other (Evans and Sewell, 2013).

During the late 1980s and early 1990s, the 'Washington Consensus' – a set of 10 economic policy prescriptions for developing countries under crisis – was introduced. However, despite the confidence in neoliberal policies to invigorate the world economy, this did not happen. In the 1990s, the 'Washington Consensus' was being criticized worldwide; the East Asia financial crisis, the chaos surrounding liberalization in Russia and the worldwide failure of neoliberal policies had started to discredit the growth paradigm used by the International Monetary Fund and the World Bank (Maddison, 2008).

Current debates on the consequences of neoliberalism are divided between those that see only benefits and others that see only harms; in reality, the results are more mixed. Nevertheless, it is usually the case that more emphasis is placed on the negative impacts of neoliberalism. This is not to undermine the fact that neoliberalism has led to improvements in productivity, consumer choice and material welfare as a result of carefully designed and implemented processes of privatization, liberalization, and deregulation. Also, it is unfair to blame solely neoliberal policies for negative outcomes since there are a number of other forces that are at play in a globalized world: demographic challenges, institutional factors, preexisting macroeconomic conditions, and natural disasters (Scholte, 2005).

On the other hand, it can be argued that neoliberalism, as an economic model, has lost its human dimension since it focuses on concepts such as individualism, efficiency, competition and profits. Exactly the opposite is the concept of the economy suggested by Manfred Max-Neef (see Box 5-1).

Neoliberalism has been heavily criticized for a range of social harms: increase in socioeconomic inequality and poverty, concentration of wealth, and reduction in social security. Neoliberal labour policies have failed to provide enough waged work for the world's labour force; instead, they have often worsened working conditions through reduction of job guarantees, union protection, and other labour rights. The insecurity and increased competitiveness in the market have also encouraged greater violence, criminality, and family breakdown (Scholte, 2005). Furthermore, neoliberal ideology rejects the notion of providing policy interventions – such as redistributive mechanisms in taxes or health – in order to reduce gaps.

A clear example is the US: at the beginning of the twentieth century, the top 1% income share in the US concentrated 17% to 18% of total income. This dropped to about 8% at the end of 1970s, but with the introduction of neoliberal policies, the top 1% income share has since been increasing and reached 17.5% in 2013; that is, it regressed to the same level as a century

BOX 5-1
THE ALTERNATIVE ANSWER FROM A CHILEAN BAREFOOT ECONOMIST

In the 1980s, while the neoliberal system was gradually established as the sole global economic system, a Chilean economist, Manfred Max-Neef, raised the concept of 'barefoot economy', which bore direct reference to his experience living in rural and remote areas where nothing of what he had learned in relation to how the world should work was useful. He focused on the *invisible* people who do not fit into an economic theory based on a mechanistic paradigm, which does not assign value, for example, to house chores or to the most basic subsistence activities, thus excluding the poorest groups and most women. Max-Neef (1992) explains that 'economics, originally the offspring of moral philosophy, lost a good deal of its human dimension, to see it replaced by fancy theories and technical trivialities that are incomprehensible to most and useful to none, except to their authors who sometimes win prizes with them' (p. 20). Therefore he decided to transform himself from a 'pure economist' to a 'barefoot economist', whose subsequent work led to the Human Scale Development.

The economy as such has always fulfilled the function of supporting a class structure, with the help of the existing law system. In the West, with the rise of the modern era and the middle class, the difference between rich and poor, which until then was considered natural as if by divine causes, had to be justified from an intellectual viewpoint. Since the Renaissance, the indisputable fact that some are born with natural rights to property and others are not began to fracture, revealing a conflict that persists today, one that is characterized by simplistic approaches that ignore social complexity (Max-Neef et al., 1991). In this manner, and with the aim of maintaining social order, a 'new economy' is born, which is no longer based on the art of household management (*oikonomia*), but on the art of acquisition (*krémastique*) (Smith and Max-Neef, 2011).

The neoliberal system is the ultimate expression of a capitalist model that supports the current industrial civilization. Max-Neef (2014) explains:

> [T]he foundations of mainstream economics are composed of three dangerous principles. First, the growth obsession, with exponential increases in consumerism. Second, the assumption of externalities which expunge all negative side effects from the responsibility of the economic process. Third, the macroeconomic aberration of accounting loss of patrimony as increase of income. While each of these can generate negative effects, the three together can be devastating for both Nature and Society. (p. 1)

Max-Neef suggests considering the economy as capable of committing crimes against humanity, according to the categories provided by the Rome Statute of the International Criminal Court Explanatory Memorandum.

In order to find a solution to the problems planted here, according to the Human Scale Development, we can start by changing the notion of human capital into human

capacity. Under the human capital notion, human beings are taken as mere productive tools for wealth generation, such as machinery and raw materials. In contrast, the second notion relates to the possibility of real development, where people possess the freedom to choose their own forms of existence. To accomplish this, it is necessary to modify both the economic and the political structure, allowing the generation of a bottom-up approach, and integrating macro and micro levels, without the first ones coopting or instrumentalizing the second (Smith and Max-Neef, 2011).

Consequently, 'the most important contribution of a human-scale economics is that it may allow for the transition from a paradigm based on greed, competition and accumulation to one based on solidarity, cooperation and compassion' (Smith and Max-Neef, 2011, p. 136), with the aim of overcoming inequality and restoring the social fabric disintegrated by the current dominant system. While no economic model has been sufficiently developed to replace the existing one, it is necessary that any possible alternatives should consider the following five principles and the principle of fundamental value (Smith and Max-Neef, 2011):

Postulate 1. The economy is to serve the people, not the people to serve the economy.

Postulate 2. Development is about people, not about the objects.

Postulate 3. Growth is not the same as development, and development does not necessarily require growth.

Postulate 4. No economy is possible in the absence of ecosystem services.

Postulate 5. The economy is a sub-system of a larger and finite system, the biosphere; hence permanent growth is impossible.

Value principle. No economic interest, under any circumstance, can be above the reverence for life. (p. 137)

According to Smith and Max-Neef (2011):

> [T]he parameters for human-scale economics could include... the use of local currencies...the production of goods and services as locally and regionally as possible...the protection of local economies...local cooperation in order to avoid monopolies...ecological taxes on energy, pollution and other negatives...a greater democratic commitment to insure effectiveness and equity in the transition towards local economies. (p. 136)

Thus, fundamental human needs can be resolved through synergic satisfiers that are directed to the development of individuals and communities; this would result in the actual elimination of all types of poverty, not only of income poverty, since every unmet need generates impoverishment in some aspect of life and leads to all kinds of social pathologies, including exclusion, violence, and social segregation.

ago. In contrast, in Sweden – a welfare state – the top 1% income share concentrated 27% of total income in 1903; by 2013, this had dropped to 7.2%, a fact which makes Sweden a much more equal society than the US (Alvaredo et al., 2015).

Health and Health Systems

There are many definitions available of what *health* is; however, many of these definitions have been criticized as incomplete, idealistic, vague, or unattainable. One of the most used definitions is the one provided by the World Health Organization (WHO), which states that 'health is a state of complete physical, mental, and social well-being and not merely the absence of disease or infirmity' (WHO, 1946, cited in WHO, 2015). This definition, though, does not include other dimensions of health, including sexual, emotional, and spiritual (Ewles and Simnett, 2003). Other definitions stress the importance of various factors that can enable us to understand health, such as quality of life (Lee and McCormick, 2004), health as a commodity (Aggleton,

1990), health as self-actualization, achievement, and empowerment (Acton and Malathum, 2008; Seedhouse, 2001), and health as a resource (WHO, 1984, 1986). Overall, as Downie and Macnaughton (2001, cited in Warwick-Booth et al., 2012, p. 11) argue, 'health does not have a clear identity of its own'; therefore, we are faced with a defying task in trying to define what it is.

A health system can be described as a series of institutional measures and programmes that are constructed in order to satisfy the health needs of a population or community (Feo, 2008). The main aims of a well-functioning health system are presented in Figure 5-1.

Health financing can be achieved through the following means: (a) public provision through taxation, (b) social insurance through a percentage of an individual's wages, (c) reliance on market mechanisms and private providers through private insurance companies, (d) out-of-pocket payments through direct payment for services, and (e) donations or community

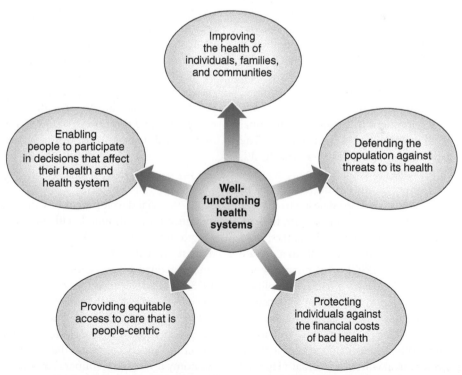

FIGURE 5-1 ■ Aims of well-functioning health systems. *(Based on data from WHO 2010).*

health insurance (Association of Faculties of Medicine of Canada, 2013). More and more countries, however, rely on a mixture of public provision and market mechanisms regarding health service provision (Organization for Economic Co-operation and Development, 2010). In any case, even in market-based countries, the government usually provides a safety net for vulnerable people.

Health systems are evaluated in terms of quality, efficiency, acceptability, and equity (Duckett, 2004). Health indicators are often used to understand or compare health quality and the effectiveness of the health system, for example mortality rates (such as infant mortality per 1000 births), health aspects (including practicing physicians per 1000 people), and health expenditure (such as public expenditure as a percentage of the total expenditure on health).

Neoliberalism and Its Impact on the Health System

Before the mid-1970s, the concepts used for the reorganization of health systems envisioned health as a public good and responsibility of states. However, due to global recession and domination of finance capital in the world economic system, the role of the state was redefined, since the state itself was viewed as inefficient and the cause of the crisis (Iriart et al., 2000). As a result, in the late 1980s and 1990s, Latin American countries were forced to accept the policies promoted by multilateral lending organizations (World Bank, Inter-American Development Bank, and International Monetary Fund) in order to access finance loans. The structural adjustment plans extended to the health sector as an area that needed restructuring.

The elaboration of regulations in the area of health and the deterioration of the welfare state led to the loss of the notion that health was a universal right; instead, it became a market commodity that individuals should acquire, thus transforming it from a public to a private good (Laurell, 1995; Testa, 1997). This phenomenon of the *health consumer* reveals the interest of neoliberalism in the possession of goods at the expense of people's well-being. In a society focused on the acquisition of wealth, consumerism, and power, 'the *health consumer* label effectively discriminates against a group whose spending power is, at worst, ineffectual' (Horton, 2007, p. 5); the term itself fails to underline the

inequalities between various social groups because patients, unlike consumers, do not have much power in making decisions regarding healthcare. Overall, the neoliberal philosophy regarding health assigns responsibility to the individual; that is, it fails to distinguish between people's roles as consumers and citizens (Horton, 2007). Figure 5-2 presents the main ideas behind the neoliberal approach to health and neoliberal restructuring of the health system.

Neoliberalism also had a great impact on the training of healthcare professionals, through the imposition of education as an individual consumer good that is to be acquired in the free market. Numerous private schools and private courses arose that were often 'excessively theoretical, elitist, exclusive, removed from reality, and marked by foreign concepts' (Feo, 2008, p. 228). The result was the production of health professionals for the private sector, who even though they did their training in public clinics with public funding, focused merely on the disease rather than on a more holistic conception of health (Feo, 2008).

While there are differences between countries, the neoliberal restructuring of health systems shares common patterns. Some of these patterns include the creation and/or strengthening of the market as a regulator of prices and quality, dedication of the state to standardization and regulation, introduction of different health packages subject to the risk associated with the individual (depending on age, sex or pathology), purchase of local health providers by multinational companies, and promotion of flexibility of labour relations of public health workers (Iriart et al., 2000).

NEOLIBERAL POLICIES IN CHILE

By 1970, social development in Chile – including level of education, national health system, school meals programmes, and unionized workers – was among the highest in Latin America. Neoliberal policies first emerged during the Pinochet government after the 1973 coup that toppled the socialist President Salvador Allende. To recover the embattled Chilean economy – suffering from chronic inflation, falling gross domestic product (GDP), and lack of foreign reserves – General Pinochet began the reorientation of the economy towards a neoliberal model, by adopting the free market economic policies advocated by Milton

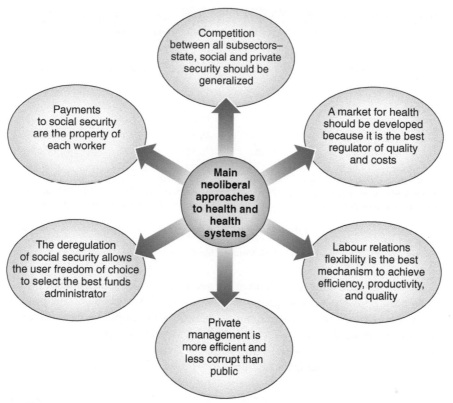

FIGURE 5-2 ■ Main neoliberal approaches to health and health systems. *(Based on data from Iriart et al. 2000.)*

Friedman and the 'Chicago boys'[1]. The economic reforms that transformed the Chilean economic landscape were aimed at:

- Minimizing the role of the state in the economy through privatization of state-owned companies and deregulation;
- Opening the economy to external competition;
- Liberalizing financial markets;
- Suppressing most labour union rights;
- Proceeding to tax reform, which sharply reduced the share of direct and more progressive taxes; and

- Reducing public spending on education, health and housing (Bräuchle, 2010; Centro de Estudios Miguel Enríquez, 2010; Ffrench-Davis, 2005).

The first round of the reforms, 1974 to 1983, was characterized by mass unemployment, purchasing power losses, extreme inequalities in income distribution and severe socioeconomic damage (Wittelsbürger and von Hoff, 2004). As discontent with the socioeconomic condition increased, the Pinochet government was forced to revise some of its neoliberal strategies. After 1984, this change resulted in a high GDP growth and lower unemployment and inflation. However, the government was still biased in favour of upper-income sectors and various business interests; the consequence was a further deterioration in income distribution and increase in poverty (Ffrench-Davis, 2005).

The measures of social assistance implemented by the Pinochet government aimed at addressing only the basic needs of the poorest people. These measures,

---

[1]'Chicago boys' is the term used to refer to a group of mostly male Chilean economists who were trained during the 1970s at the University of Chicago by Milton Friedman and Arnold Harberger. Upon their return to Latin America, they gained high positions in the government as economic advisors, where they advocated and implemented free market neoliberal policies.

TABLE 5-1							
Various Indicators for Chile: 1960–2014							
Variable	1960–1970	Allende 1971–1973	Pinochet 1974–1989	1990–1999	2000–2009	2013	2014
GDP growth (%)	3.9	1.2	2.9	5.1	3.7	4.3	1.9
Inflation rate (%)	26.5	293.8	79.9	7.0	3.4	1.8	4.4
Unemployment rate (%)	5.6	4.7	18.1	8.7	9.7	6.0	6.3
Poverty rate (%)[a]	–	–	45.1	28.8	16.0	7.8	–
GINI index[b]	0.489	0.466	0.547	0.523	0.521	0.509	–
Income distribution (Q5/Q1)	12.9	12.8	17.7	15.7	14.9	–	–

[a]Previous studies have indicated that poverty in 1970 was 17% (Fazio, 1996) or 20% (Ffrench-Davis, 2014). Although the poverty rate might have been underestimated, it is considered that it was much lower than in the Pinochet period. Poverty for the period 1974–1989 is the 1987 available figure.
[b]The Gini index assesses the income distribution of a nation and is the most common measurement of inequality. It ranges from 0 (perfect equality) to 1 (perfect inequality).
Some data from Banco Central de Chile (2015), Ffrench-Davis (2014), Ministry of Social Development (2014), and University of Chile (2015).

however, did not include any investments in human capital or capacity building for the poor to generate income[2]. On the other hand, whilst these programmes increased the provision of basic services to society's poorest, the government reduced public social assistance to the rest of the population, including the middle and working class.

While some social indicators continued to improve during the Pinochet era[3] – such as literacy rates, life expectancy, and general and infant mortality – the economic policies adopted are often regarded as an attempt to dismantle the social security system, which had been substantially expanded during the government of Eduardo Frei Montalva (1964–1970) and Salvador Allende (1970–1973) (Centro de Estudios Miguel Enríquez, 2010). Table 5-1 provides some indicators to compare the pre-, during, and post-Pinochet Chile.

A tangible example of the neoliberal economic model employed in Chile was the delivery of public goods through concessions to private companies, whose final aim was economic profitability over social benefit. For example, with regards to education, Matear (2007) explains that:

Inspired by economic neoliberalism and the New Public Management model, the reforms fostered competition between schools for students and resources with the aim of increasing choice, promoting efficiency and improving standards. They centred on several core initiatives including the decentralisation of the education administration to local government, and the financing of schools based on a voucher system to cover operational and capital costs, as calculated on average monthly student attendance. (pp. 103–104)

Furthermore, in the 1990s, road construction was conceded to private firms; although infrastructure improved, tolls rose considerably (Fundación Paz Ciudadana and Interamerican Bank of Development, 2013). Prison infrastructure and administration were also conceded; today, Chile has one of the highest incarceration rates in Latin America, overcrowding still remains and social reintegration is very low (Interamerican Bank of Development, 2013).

The regressive trends in the Chilean society were reversed by the socioeconomic policies implemented by the succeeding democratic governments, which, however, sustained the neoliberal economic model,

---

[2]The main idea of focusing social assistance on the poorest formed part of the Chicago boys' philosophy. They considered poverty as the result of rigidities in the social structure and market distortions; their aim was to identify these groups of extreme poverty and provide them with the goods and services to maintain their standard of living, without trying to solve the problem (CEME, 2010).

[3]The improvements in many health indicators – including maternal mortality and child malnutrition – were the results of policies implemented by previous governments.

albeit with a more social focus. Thus there was an increased emphasis on social spending, favouring growth with equity, reducing unemployment, safeguarding macroeconomic stability, and improving the standard of living of the middle class and the poorest (Centro de Estudios Miguel Enríquez, 2010). These measures managed to decrease poverty significantly, although with regards to redistribution they were less successful.

Despite the vast improvements experienced by the country in the last 20 years, Chile is still regarded as one of the worst countries in terms of income distribution. Out of Chile's approximately 17.5 million inhabitants and an active population of a little over 8 million, 74% earn less than 400 000 Chilean pesos a month and out of these, more than 1 million receive only the statutory minimum wage (241 000 pesos). Also, only 15% of working women receive a wage above 500 000 pesos, and 75% of pensioners receive less than 185 000 pesos. In short, 50% of Chileans live on less than 5000 pesos per day (exchange rate US $1 = 650 pesos, average July 2015) (Fundación SOL, 2015a,b,c,d,e).

As a result, economic inequality in Chile has gradually become profound social inequality, where territorial segregation has been changing the relationship between different social groups. There are schools, healthcare centres, and universities for the poor and the rich, leaving a middle class whose aim is to move away from the marginalized groups and integrate with the privileged groups rather than fight for the construction of a more just country, a middle class which is impregnated with a social imaginary characterized by individualism and consumerism, and fuelled by the media and advertising (Smith and Max-Neef, 2011).

NEOLIBERALISM AND THE CHILEAN HEALTH SYSTEM

The first neoliberal policies in the health system were applied in Chile during the Pinochet government and began with the abolition of the Unified Health Service, which provided free public healthcare for the entire population. Decentralization was also implemented through several initiatives, which included the municipalization of primary health centres and the creation of the National Health Fund (FONASA, in Spanish).

The two major milestones of privatization were the creation of Pension Fund Administrators (AFPs, in Spanish) in 1980 and private health insurance institutions (ISAPRE, in Spanish) in 1981.

Between 1974 and 1989, the goal of reducing the role of the state in the health system was partly accomplished: fiscal contributions dropped from 67.7% to 34.8%, contributions for insurance increased from 15.6% to 45.3%, and participation of the private health system increased to reach half of services in the health system by 1989 (Labra, 1995, reported in Hernández-Álvarez, 2003)[4].

The separation of the health system in Chile into mainly FONASA and ISAPRE constituted a 'regressive form of targeting and it helped to deepen the crisis in the public health system' (Ffrench-Davis, 2005, p. 202). The contract premium for ISAPRE is determined by sex, age and risk; therefore women of fertile age, the elderly, or the young are often excluded. The provision of health services by FONASA and ISAPRE led to the stratification of access to health: (a) the higher socioeconomic classes pay for private health insurance available in the market (ISAPRE); (b) the middle-income classes access public health insurance, with variable copayments depending on their income (FONASA); and (c) the lower socioeconomic classes and the poor access the public health system for free or paying an amount depending on their income (Labra, 2002).

The goals of the health reform initiated in 2000 were to increase equity in health access, financing, and equitable service provision. The reform provides a strong strengthening and extension of the health social protection (especially for the most vulnerable groups), the establishment of explicit guarantees for people in a group of prioritized pathologies independent of their ability to pay for health services and treatment, and new models for the attention and management in health (Kuncar Fritz, 2013). As a result, total spending on health as a percentage of GDP has increased from

---

[4]Although basic health indicators improved during the Pinochet era, morbidity indicators worsened, especially with regards to mental disorders caused by the high unemployment, as well as childhood diseases resulting from poverty, all of which could have been avoided if adequate health services were available (Medina, 1989, cited in Labra, 2002).

5.15% in 1995 to 7.4% in 2013 (Organization for Economic Co-operation and Development, 2015).

FINAL REMARKS

Neoliberalism can be more accurately defined as 'the ideology and practice of the dominant classes of the developed and developing worlds alike' (Navarro, 2007, p. 53), which usually results in aggravating poverty and increasing inequality. According to Evans and Sewell (2013), '[N]eoliberalism has actually been more successful as a means of shifting the balance of class political power than as an instrument for reinvigorating capitalist growth' (p. 47). Due to its growing conceptual ambiguity, neoliberalism is now widely seen as a controversial, omnipresent, oft-invoked, and confusing term (Clarke, 2008; Mudge, 2008; Turner, 2008).

Neoliberal policies were first introduced in Chile during the Pinochet government in the 1970s, thus turning the country into a neoliberal laboratory, a test for policies to be reproduced worldwide. While many economists talk of 'the miracle of Chile' and juxtapose the country against other Latin America states, others see the low growth, high inflation and unemployment, and increased poverty as an indication of the actual failure of neoliberal policies, especially during the 'pure monetarist experiment' of 1973 to 1981 (Drèze and Sen, 1989). However, the 'Chilean miracle' is far from being a miracle: the country's economy is a clear result of an economic model forged during the military government and inherited during democracy, a model defended by institutions of global order, such as the International Monetary Fund, World Bank, and World Trade Organization (Smith and Max-Neef, 2011).

Neoliberal policies are still being dictated by these international institutions to a number of developing countries or countries in crisis, despite the wide evidence that the strict application of such measures does not guarantee economic growth and development for all (Stiglitz, 2008). In most cases, especially when good institutions are not in place, these policies fail at producing results, and instead create more instability and inequality, while serving only the interests of certain groups.

In the case of healthcare, the introduction of neoliberal policies and private actors in service delivery and management has led to an increase in the price of healthcare and inequality of access (Huber and Solt, 2004). One of the main principles of neoliberal policies in the health system is the promotion of the *health consumer,* a notion according to which individuals are responsible for their own healthcare. On the other hand, the continuous budget-cutting in health, the increase in the number of private healthcare providers and the decline of the welfare state have turned health into a market commodity that not all people can access: from being a universal right, it has become a private good that excludes disadvantaged people.

In order to promote equal access to quality healthcare – and ensure sustainable growth, stability, and society's well-being alongside – it is necessary to proceed to larger investment in education, healthcare and nutrition, housing, social security, and sanitation. A combination of carefully thought-out economic reforms and the building of strong institutions accompanied by social policies based on a people-first philosophy can be a much more promising alternative to the unregulated free market measures championed by neoliberalism.

REFERENCES

Acton, G.J., Malathum, P., 2008. Basic need status and health promoting self-care behavior in adults. West. J. Nurs. Res. 22, 796–811.

Aggleton, P., 1990. Health. Routledge, London.

Alvaredo, F., et al., 2015. The World Top Incomes Database. <http://topincomes.g-mond.parisschoolofeconomics.eu> (accessed 22.06.15.).

Association of Faculties of Medicine of Canada, 2013. Primer on population health: a virtual textbook on public health concepts for clinicians. <http://phprimer.afmc.ca/Part1-TheoryThinking AboutHealth> (accessed 17.06.15.).

Banco Central de Chile, 2015. Base de datos estadísticos. <http://si3.bcentral.cl/Siete/secure/cuadros/home.aspx> (accessed 01.07.15.).

Bräuchle, M., 2010. Applied theory: the reforms in Chile. <http://www.powershow.com/view1/1dbbe8-ZDc1Z/Applied_Theory _The_Reforms_in_Chile_powerpoint_ppt_presentation> (accessed 23.06.15.).

Centro de Estudios Miguel Enríquez, 2010. Análisis económico de los gobiernos chilenos 1964–2000. Centro de Estudios Miguel Enríquez. <http://www.archivochile.com/Gobiernos/varios_otros _gob/GOBotros0010.pdf> (accessed 23.06.15.).

Clarke, J., 2008. Living with/in and without neo-liberalism. Focaal 2008 (51), 135–147.

Drèze, J., Sen, A., 1989. Hunger and Public Action. Oxford University Press, Oxford.

Duckett, S.J., 2004. The Australian Health Care System, second ed. Oxford University Press, South Melbourne, VIC, Australia.

Evans, P., Sewell, W.H. Jr., 2013. Neoliberalism: policy regimes, international regimes, and social effects. In: Hall, P., Lamont, M. (Eds.), Social Resilience in the Neoliberal Era. Cambridge University Press, Cambridge, pp. 35–69.

Ewles, L., Simnett, I., 2003. Promoting Health: A Practical Guide, fifth ed. Ballière Tindall, Edinburgh, UK.

Fazio, H., 1996. El Programa Abandonado. Balance Económico del Gobierno de Aylwin. ARCIS-CENDA, Santiago de Chile.

Feo, O., 2008. Neoliberal policies and their impact on public health education: observations on the Venezuelan experience. Soc. Med. 3 (4), 223–231.

Ffrench-Davis, R., 2005. Economic reforms in Chile: from dictatorship to democracy. University of Michigan Press, Ann Arbor, MI.

Ffrench-Davis, R., 2014. Sáez, J.C. (Ed.), Chile entre el neoliberalismo y el crecimiento con equidad, fifth ed. SpA, Santiago, Chile.

Fundación Paz Ciudadana and Interamerican Bank for Development, 2013. Evaluación del Sistema Concesionado versus el Sistema Tradicional en la Reducción de la Reinsidencia Delictual. <http://www.pazciudadana.cl/wp-content/uploads2013/07/2013-07-02_Evaluaci%C3%83%C2%B3n-del-sistema-concesionado-versus-el-sistema-tradicional-en-la-reducci%C3%83%C2%B3n-de-la-reincidencia-delictual.pdf> (accessed 16.06.15).

Fundación, S.O.L., 2015a. Distibución de trabajadores que ganan el sueldo mínimo según tamaño de la empresa. Fundación SOL. <http://www.fundacionsol.cl/graficos/distribucion-de-trabajadores-que-ganan-el-sm-o-menos-segun-tamano-de-empresa-panel-1-distribucion-porcentual-panel-2-porcentaje-relativo-ra-su-propia-categoria> (accessed 16.06.15.).

Fundación, S.O.L., 2015b. Distribución general de los ingresos de la ocupación principal nesi 2013. Fundación SOL. <http://www.fundacionsol.cl/graficos/distribucion-general-de-los-ingresos-de-la-ocupacion-principal-nesi-2013> (accessed 13.06.15.).

Fundación, S.O.L., 2015c. Los verdaderos sueldos en Chile. Fundación SOL. <http://www.fundacionsol.cl/estudios/los-verdaderos-sueldos-en-chile> (accessed 13.06.15.).

Fundación, S.O.L., 2015d. Mujeres trabajando, una exploración al valor del trabajo y la calidad del empleo en Chile. Fundación SOL. <http://www.fundacionsol.cl/estudios/mujeres-trabajando-una-exploracion-al-valor-del-trabajo-y-la-calidad-del-empleo-en-chile> (accessed 13.06.15.).

Fundación, S.O.L., 2015e. Radiografía al salario mínimo de más de un millon de chilenos. Fundación SOL. <http://www.fundacionsol.cl/2015/07/radiografia-al-salario-minimo-mas-de-un-millon-de-chilenos-recibe-esta-remuneracion-o-menos> (accessed 13.06.15.).

Hancock, L., 1999. Women, Public Policy and the State. Macmillan, Melbourne.

Hernández-Álvarez, M., 2003. Neoliberalismo en salud: desarrollos, supuestos y alternativas. In: Restrepo Botero, D.I. (Ed.), La Falacia Neoliberal: Crítica y Alternativas. Universidad Nacional de Colombia, Bogotá, Colombia, pp. 347–355.

Horton, E.S., 2007. Neoliberalism and the Australian healthcare system (factory). In: Proceedings 2007 Conference of the Philosophy of Education Society of Australasia, Wellington, New Zealand.

Huber, E., Solt, F., 2004. Successes and failures of neoliberalism. Latin Am. Res. Rev. 39 (3), 150–164.

Interamerican Bank for Development, 2013. Evaluación del Sistema Concesionado versus el Sistema Tradicional en la Reducción de la Reinsidencia Delictual. Interamerican Bank for Development.

Iriart, C., Merhy, E.E., Aitzkin, H., 2000. Managed care in Latin America: transnationalisation of the health sector in a context of reform. Caderno Saúde Pública 16 (1), 95–105.

Kuncar Fritz, E.U.C., 2013. Sistema de Salud en Chile. Universidad San Sebastián, Santiago, Chile.

Labra, M.E., 2002. La reinvención neoliberal de la inequidad en Chile. El caso de la salud. Cad. Saúde Pública 18 (4), 1041–1052.

Laurell, A.C., 1995. La salud: de derecho social a mercancía. In: Laurell, A.C. (Coord.), Nuevas Tendencias y Alternativas en el Sector Salud. Ed. Universidad Autónoma Metropolitana Unidad Xochimilco/Ed. Representación en México de la Fundación Friedrich Ebert, Mexico, pp. 9–31.

Lee, Y., McCormick, B.P., 2004. Subjective well-being of people with spinal cord injury: does leisure contribute? J. Rehabil. 70 (3), 5–12.

Maddison, A., 2008. Shares of the rich and the rest in the world economy: income divergence between nations, 1820-2030. Asian Econ. Policy Rev. 3 (1), 67–82.

Matear, A., 2007. Equity in education in Chile: the tensions between policy and practice. Int. J. Educ. Dev. 27 (1), 101–113.

Max-Neef, M., 1992. From the Outside Looking in. Experiences in 'Barefoot Economics'. Zed Books, London.

Max-Neef, M., 2014. The good is the bad that we don't do. Economic crimes against humanity: a proposal. Ecol. Econ. 104, 152–154.

Max-Neef, M., Elizalde, A., Hopenhayn, M., 1991. Human Scale Development. Apex Press, New York.

McGregor, S.L.T., 2001. Neoliberalism and health care. Int. J. Consum. Stud. 25 (2), 84.

Ministry of Public Works, 2003. Sistema de Concesiones en Chile 1990–2003. Ministry of Public Works, Santiago, Chile.

Ministry of Social Development, 2014. CASEN 2013: Situación de la Pobreza en Chile. Ministry of Social Development, Santiago, Chile.

Mudge, S., 2008. What is neo-liberalism? Socioecon. Rev. 6 (4), 703–731.

Navarro, V., 2007. Neoliberalism as a class ideology; or, the political causes of the growth of inequalities. Int. J. Health Serv. 37 (1), 47–62.

Organization for Economic Co-operation and Development, 2010. Health care systems: getting more value for money. OECD Economics Department Policy Notes, No. 2. OECD publishing, Paris.

Organization for Economic Co-operation and Development, 2015. OECD health data: health expenditure and financing: health expenditure indicators. <https://data.oecd.org/healthres/health-spending.htm> (accessed 17.06.15.).

Scholte, J.A., 2005. The Sources of Neoliberal Globalisation. Over-arching Concerns Programme Paper, No. 8. United Nations Research Institute for Social Development, Geneva.

Seedhouse, D., 2001. Health: The Foundations for Achievement, second ed. John Wiley & Sons Ltd, West Sussex, UK.

Sewell, W.H. Jr., 2005. From state-centrism to neoliberalism: macro-historical contexts of population health since World War II. In: Hall, P., Lamont, M. (Eds.), Successful Societies: Institutions, Cultural Repertoires, and Health. Cambridge University Press, Cambridge, pp. 254–287.

Smith, P., Max-Neef, M., 2011. Economics Unmasked. From the Power and Greed to Compassion and the Common Good. Green Books, London.

Stiglitz, J., 2008. The end of neoliberalism? Project Syndicate. <https://www.project-syndicate.org/commentary/the-end-of-neo-liberalism> (accessed 30.06.15.).

Testa, M., 1997. Saber en Salud. La Construcción del Conocimiento. Lugar Editorial, Buenos Aires.

Turner, R., 2008. Neo-liberal Ideology. Edinburgh University Press, Edinburgh, UK.

University of Chile, 2015. Encuesta de ocupación y desocupación – Documentos: Informe ingresos. University of Chile, Faculty of Economy and Business, Department of Micro-data, Santiago, Chile. <http://www.empleo.microdatos.cl/encuesta_ocupacion/encuesta-ocupacion-documentos.php?op=4> (accessed 01.07.15.).

Warwick-Booth, L., Cross, R., Lowcock, D., 2012. Contemporary Health Studies: An Introduction. Polity Press, Cambridge.

Wittelsbürger, H., von Hoff, A., 2004. Chiles Wegzur Sozialen Marktwirtschaft. Auslandsinfo 01/04, Konrad Adenauer Foundation. <http://www.kas.de/wf/doc/kas_4084-544-1-30.pdf?040415182627> (accessed 23.06.15.).

World Health Organization, 1984. A discussion document on the concepts and principles of health promotion. Copenhagen, 9–13 July 1984. WHO publishing, Copenhagen.

World Health Organization, 1986. The Ottawa charter for health promotion. First International Conference on Health Promotion. Ottawa, 17–21 November 1986. WHO publishing, Copenhagen.

World Health Organization, 2010. Key components of a well functioning health system. <http://www.who.int/healthsystems/EN_HSSkeycomponents.pdf> (accessed 17.06.15.).

World Health Organization, 2015. Glossary of globalisation, trade and health terms: health. <http://www.who.int/trade/glossary/story046/en> (accessed 17.06.15.).

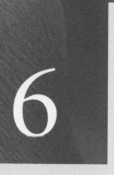

6

AUSTERITY AND THE RISE OF HOSTILITY TOWARDS MARGINALIZED GROUPS

HELEN CLAIRE SMITH

CHAPTER OUTLINE

At times of economic hardship, occupational therapists are aware of the challenge of managing precious resources in overstretched health and social care services. It is important, however, that the reasoning and judgements underpinning the provision of occupational therapy are fair. Therapy does not occur in a vacuum, and occupational therapists are not immune to political and social opinions, which often convey ideas about the needs, rights and opportunities of groups and individuals within society. There is a growing recognition of a link between economic hardship and changing attitudes towards marginalized groups, with influences from politics and the media steering public opinion (Briant et al., 2013; Philo et al., 2013).

Whilst occupational therapists are required to provide services without prejudice, they are still susceptible to socially constructed messages about the needs, or even the worthiness, of clients. In this chapter, I use a mixture of literature, theory, and student opinions to encourage critical awareness of what shapes people's opinions and how this might impact upon the services occupational therapists provide.

In preparation for this chapter, and to better understand the learning needs of my students, I undertook a stand-alone project with volunteers from the BSc and MSc Occupational Therapy programmes at Teesside University, discussing the impact of media on perceptions of marginalized groups. Below, I explore the interplay among austerity, marginalization, politics and media to understand their impact on attitudes towards individuals.

THE IMPACT OF AUSTERITY

Austerity is the process by which difficult policy measures are introduced to manage national economic crises. Austerity measures have become a major feature of the contemporary sociopolitical landscape, with varied but substantial impact across nations and across groups (Holthuis, 2013). Although many of the

49

examples used here are from the UK, similar debates occur across Europe and beyond (Ciobanu, 2012; Holthuis, 2013; Karanikolos et al., 2013).

Whilst some assert that austerity measures are essential to redress existing financial difficulties (Winder, 2015), the need for austerity measures is contentious (Blyth, 2015). The approaches taken to austerity are widely criticized as unnecessarily draconian as they are associated with economic hardship and reduced social spending (Blyth, 2015). These measures create a 'cold climate' of reduced income and opportunity, particularly for those most reliant on statutory support (Joseph Rowntree Foundation, 2014).

Austerity is seen as magnifying disadvantage, as individuals experience unemployment, job insecurity, income reduction, soaring living costs, welfare cuts and reduced access to services (Butler, 2012; Ifanti et al., 2013; O'Hara, 2014a). These circumstances have significant implications for health and social well-being, as there is an important relationship between a prosperous economy and the health of the population (Hudson, 2013). The correlation between poor health and unemployment, debt and financial insecurity is well established and incontrovertible (Wind-Cowie, 2013), with some of the most negatively affected groups experiencing the most significant health implications (Duffy, 2013; Elliott, 2014; Karanikolos et al., 2013).

In addition to the impact directly on health and well-being, austerity measures have implications for service provision, with service reforms and spending cuts leading to lower statutory provision and greater reliance on voluntary organizations (Holthuis, 2013; Ifanti et al., 2013; O'Hara, 2014b). There is also inefficiency and inequality in the manner in which available funding is used, with waste still a major issue and questions raised about the equanimity of spending (Duffy, 2013; Molloy, 2014). The British National Health Service has become an increasingly and unsustainably costly service (National Audit Office, 2012), and major efforts are being undertaken to review all services to make huge efficiencies (Department of Health, 2015). The necessity to reduce waste is widely accepted; however, savings made at the current rate are potentially unsustainable, and it is not yet possible to measure the impact of savings on patient care (National Audit Office, 2012). There are also concerns

raised by public health strategists about the focused prioritization of services, where expensive showcase treatments are made available because they appear to have public support, without any analysis of how the funds could be spent on other priorities (Potter and Knight, 2011).

In the UK, austerity measures require a 10.8% reduction in public expenditure; however, 50% of these cuts occur within local government, whose primary function is the provision of social care (Duffy, 2013). This creates a disproportionate burden, particularly for those most vulnerable, such as people with disabilities, those with mental health problems, and immigrants (Ciobanu, 2012; Duffy, 2013; Elliott, 2014; Heap, 2013; Valentine, 2014).

Vulnerable groups often experience multiple layers of disadvantage, and the impact of austerity measures can be cumulative, due to the combined effects of regressive taxation and cuts across social care, benefits, and housing (Duffy, 2013). In considering this cumulative impact, Duffy (2013) asserts that the burden for people in poverty is 5 times that of the rest of the population, for people with disabilities it is 9 times that of the rest of the population, and for people experiencing the most severe disabilities it is 19 times that of the rest of the population.

Cumulative cuts may add to existing challenges, which are part of an ongoing fight for equality (Equality and Human Rights Commission, 2010), such as higher than average living costs for people with disabilities (Zaidi and Burchardt, 2005) or labour market exclusion for migrants (Kingston et al., 2015). Additionally, policies around austerity are rarely responsive enough to the kind of complex lives and interlocking challenges experienced by people in need, so the limited social protection provided often compounds difficulties by being inflexible and unresponsive (Perry et al., 2014).

As a result, people with existing needs, already facing inequalities, experience a range of circumstances made more challenging by austerity. They experience more frequent and less manageable personal crises and become less able to participate in their communities. They rely more heavily on families, and health and social care services, which are increasingly providing limited services due to budgetary constraints (Duffy, 2013). In addition to this increased need, there are features of increased marginalization for the groups highlighted as most vulnerable, adding an extra element of complexity to both their need and the likelihood of getting their needs met (Joseph Rowntree Foundation, 2014; Valentine and Harris, 2014).

MARGINALIZED GROUPS

Having become concerned about what I saw as increasingly troubling attitudes towards marginalized groups in wider society, I decided to explore the perspectives of occupational therapy students, in order to gauge their learning needs. I undertook a project with nine volunteer students, where they were asked to consider the nature of marginalization and some of the possible influences and outcomes. This was undertaken in two parts, via e-mail. The students were given a series of open questions, followed separately by a number of examples of media coverage of a particular group, to explore how marginalization may be fostered.

When the students were asked, 'Who would you imagine might be "marginalized" in the United Kingdom?' they identified a diverse range of people, but most commonly immigrants and benefit recipients. There was an appreciation that people may become marginalized as a result of age, ability, ethnicity, faith, origins, health, need, culture, opportunity, appearance, or lifestyle choices. This highlights the complexity of the issue, where so many groups can be identified as marginalized, perhaps with multiple layers of exclusion, and where factors may vary by location and over the course of time (Cohen, 2011).

The process of marginalization can often develop through a combination of the dynamics of three processes: 'othering', perceived deservedness and moralizing, which are discussed below. These processes allow people to be seen and treated as separate, distant and disconnected from wider communities and can impact upon their health and well-being (Grove and Zwi, 2006).

Othering

Othering involves the creation and use of labels to define and characterize groups, objectifying them, and establishing them as subordinate (Grove and Zwi, 2006; Shapiro, 2008).

Many stereotypes exist regarding marginalized groups, taking the form of 'tropes' (overused images, words, and representations) (Fahnestock, 2011) from the repeated use of words such as *swamped* and *bogus* in relation to immigration (Chakrabortty, 2013) to the representation of people with disabilities as either sinister or pitiful (Haller, 2010). Such representations have the potential to create lasting impressions about, for example, disability and mental ill health (Coyle and Craig, 2012; O'Hara, 2014a), engendering sympathy or pity, or hostility and ridicule, neither of which leaves room for progressive opportunity and fulfilled potential (O'Hara, 2014a).

Othering creates an environment where individual identity ceases to be recognized. Individuals are not simply devalued, but also denied status, and considered unworthy of respect (Fraser, 2000). Fraser (2000) describes how the battle for recognition is at the heart of issues around identity, multiculturalism, and human rights. As people balance their need for a shared humanity with the desire to maintain cultural and personal distinctiveness, group identities can be drastically simplified, increasing the sense of separation and generating intolerance (Danermark and Gellerstedt, 2004; Fraser, 2000).

There has been a marked decline in empathy and understanding for some of the most disadvantaged groups in our society, corroding compassion for those most in need and having a negative impact on social cohesion (Valentine, 2014; Valentine and Harris, 2014). Large-scale studies by the Equality Commission (Northern Ireland) (2011) and the British Social Attitudes Survey (2014) noted an increased hardening of attitudes and growing social division, suggestive of a shift in public opinion. When people were asked to reflect on their views on various groups of people, imagining them as a work colleague, neighbour, relative, or friend, there was less compassion and greater prejudice than in previous surveys, with the most negative attitudes expressed about travellers, transgender people, Eastern European migrant workers, and people experiencing mental health problems (Equality Commission, 2011). Researchers found that negativity had particularly increased towards welfare recipients and immigrants, but they also found diminishing compassion for groups such as disabled or retired people, previously considered the deserving poor (British Social Attitudes Survey, 2014).

Deservedness

The concepts of the deserving and undeserving poor have long been an aspect of attitudes towards people in need. Since medieval times there have been efforts, including public floggings, branding, and hanging, used to dissuade 'idleness' in the poor. British legislation from 1563, and the Elizabethan Poor Law of 1601, offered categorizations of poverty: the deserving poor were those who were poor through no fault of their own, either too young, old, or ill to work, or those who would work but could not find work (Alchin, 2012). The undeserving poor were those who could work but would not, and consequently they were considered as the idle poor, and they were to be publicly castigated (Bloy, 2002). There was no recognition of external factors which created hardship at these times, which were beyond the control of the poor, such as the excesses of the ruling classes, rapid inflation, and decreased charitable support due to the dissolution of the monasteries (Boyer, 1990). In the intervening years, attitudes towards deservedness have continued to dominate perceptions of individuals who require help and support, with the current period of austerity facilitating the reemergence of traditional distinctions between the 'deserving' and 'undeserving' poor (Pennington, 2011; Valentine, 2014). Currently (i.e., as of September 2015), much of the debate on deservedness centres on welfare and benefits with powerful messages regarding the place and value individuals hold in society (Bowlby, 2010; Clarey, 2012; Johnes, 2012).

Moralizing

The debate around the needs of some groups often takes on a moral dimension, with divisions fostered by 'moral panic', a theory characterized by a disproportionate perception of the threat of a particular group on society, with a resultant growth of hostility (Cohen, 2011; Goode and Ben-Yehuda, 2009). Moral panic occurs when people are provided with information, from a source they perceive as credible, which presents behaviour in terms of some form of moral violation (Goodwin et al., 2001). This defines a target group as a threat to societal values and interests, vilifying them and increasing the likelihood of them becoming marginalized.

Groups begin to be portrayed as 'folk devils', with extreme negative portrayals and perspectives circulated by press and public opinion (Cohen, 2011).

Ideas of deservedness are propagated by the media and politicians, but also resonate with the experiences of ordinary citizens in their everyday lives, meaning that they now attribute issues such as unemployment and poverty to the failings of individuals (Valentine, 2014). This focus on the moral or cultural worth of others demonizes people in need, obscuring other causes of inequality and socioeconomic exclusion and eroding care, compassion, and social responsibility (Valentine, 2014; Valentine and Harris, 2014).

AUSTERITY AND MARGINALIZATION

This link among attitudes, marginalization, and austerity is a phenomenon which has been repeated a number of times throughout history, when economic pressures have eroded compassion and social cohesion (Ponticelli and Voth, 2011).

Just as Tudor hardships fostered hostility towards the 'undeserving' poor, the Great Depression of the 1930s fuelled the rise of German National Socialism (the Nazi Party). When, in the 1930s and 1940s, the Nazi Party ran media campaigns attacking groups they perceived as undeserving, few would have anticipated the implications.

The process began with the exploitation of the vulnerability of people with disabilities and major illness. They utilized propaganda describing people with disabilities as 'useless eaters', bemoaning the cost to the hardworking German of maintaining their 'unworthy lives' (Mostert, 2002). See Fig. 6-1.

From this, the German people experienced reduced empathy and a heightened sense of burden, enabling people with disability and ill health to become the first victims of the holocaust, with vast numbers of children and adults exterminated and experimented upon as part of the Action T4 programme.[1]

---

[1]Action T4 was a programme of forced euthanasia, in wartime Nazi Germany, which officially ran between 1939 and 1941, and unofficially until 1945. Physicians were directed to judge patients 'incurably sick, by critical medical examination' and then administer to these patients a 'mercy death'. A total of 70 273 children and adults with disabilities and ill health were killed during the official period, and a further 200 000 later on (Action T4, 2014).

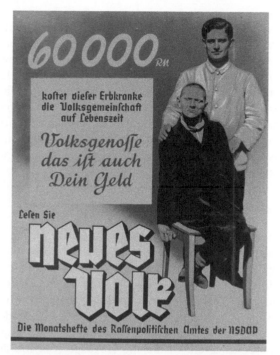

FIGURE 6-1 ■ 'This hereditarily ill person will cost our national community 60,000 Reichmarks over the course of his lifetime. Citizen, this is your money.' *(Reproduced courtesy of the Deutsches Historisches Museum.)*

Whilst we may reflect on such events as historical aberrations, they are repeated with enough frequency to create an association among economic challenges, attitudes toward marginalized groups and horrific outcomes (Mostert, 2002; Seymour, 2014).

Changing perspectives of particular groups, driven by othering, deservedness, and moralizing, could indeed be the beginnings of the kind of demonization we have seen in the past and continue to see across the present-day world (Disability Rights UK, 2012; Ponticelli and Voth, 2012). At the very least such demonization presents a major additional challenge to people as they become vulnerable to negative public judgement (Bambra and Smith, 2010; British Social Attitudes Survey, 2014). The example of National Socialism and the 'useless eaters' also shows the connection among politics, media, propaganda, and attitudes which, then as now, play a role in shaping public opinion (Mostert, 2002).

POLITICS AND ATTITUDES

Governments have the potential to influence social attitudes through policies that set out government priorities, establishing who and what is 'worthy' of benefitting from public money (Collingwood, 2015). As successive governments in the UK have sought to reduce the substantial costs of welfare and social support, there has been an increased use of stereotyping about specific groups, leading to individuals being negatively portrayed (Garthwaite, 2011). Just as previous generations have perceived generosity as benefitting the idle poor (Pennington, 2011), there continues to be an assertion that social support rewards fecklessness and irresponsibility (Bowlby, 2010; Clarey, 2012), and there have been calls to remoralize services around the principle of deservedness (Bowlby, 2010; Clarey, 2012).

The language of deservedness and the language of policy have become entwined in what Duffy (2013) describes as falsehoods, distortions, and ugly rhetoric. The UK government approach to unemployment benefit fraud, for example, changed some years ago to routinely use the terms *cheats* and *thieves*; yet, their own evidence shows that only 0.7% of benefit overpayments are due to fraud (Department for Work and Pensions, 2014). Similarly, over recent years social security provision in the UK has been reframed as 'welfare', which Parliament members assert conveys a shift from entitlement towards stigma (Baumberg et al., 2011). Language changes such as this are not insignificant and may be part of a process of dehumanizing benefit recipients; as Williams (2013) says, 'We never used to talk about welfare in terms of humans, but the word has been in everyday UK usage, for as long as I can remember, to describe animals' (p. 1).

The debate regarding benefit payments for individuals out of work has become framed in the rhetoric of 'skivers versus strivers' following a number of high-profile speeches by political figures (Bambra and Smith, 2010; Heap, 2013; O'Hara, 2014a). The suggestion is that some individuals are worthy recipients of support and others not, generating what Williams calls a 'fictional feckless bogeyman' (2013, p. 1), an individual viewed as having little to contribute and being at the root of societal ills. The dehumanizing of people receiving benefits allows difficult economic decisions, such as extensive budget cuts, to be justified (Bambra and Smith, 2010; Heap, 2013; O'Hara, 2014a), with little or no acknowledgement of wider socioeconomic causes that may contribute to individual difficulties (Chauhan and Foster, 2013).

During the current period of austerity, as in the past, there is evidence of movement towards the far right. Increases in far right politics and activism can be seen in many countries, ranging from increased support for political parties such as Front National in France and Golden Dawn in Greece, to single-issue groups such as Germany's anti-Islamic Pegida and Russia's homophobic Occupy Paedophilia. Despite differences of activity between these groups and parties, they all hold strong conservative views associated with authoritarianism, resistance to change, dislike of uncertainty, and fear of the 'other' (Jost et al., 2003; Leone and Chirumbolo, 2008). These features of right wing thinking are often heightened at times of economic uncertainty, and people who are naturally more fearful and uncertain are more likely to be supportive of policies that provide them with a sense of surety and security (Blinder et al., 2013; Hatemi et al., 2013).

Messages that appear to be attuned to these conservative fears are often popular (Robin, 2004), and organizations, political groups and media agencies which utilize these are believed to strengthen their standing by exploiting public anxieties (Hatemi et al., 2013). There is often a disproportionate focus on marginalized groups, intensifying the focus on differences and minimizing awareness of needs. Consider how often mental ill health is linked with violence, homosexuality with paedophilia, or immigration with terrorism. This negative attention is not grounded in evidence, but captures people's imagination and heightens their paranoia (Furedi, 2006; Gardner, 2009).

Such messages promote separateness, widening the gap between 'them and us' (Hatemi et al., 2013). In addition to generating distance between groups, these attitudes foster an appealing sense of group solidarity, with the desire to stand together and exclude others a natural and seductive response to economic hardship (Vasilopoulou et al., 2014; Goodwin et al., 2001; Karyotis and Rudig, 2013). By grouping people

together, and demonizing minorities, the majority feel a greater sense of togetherness and personal value (Vasilopoulou et al., 2014). Indeed, it has been suggested that in Greece, the European nation most profoundly affected by austerity (Ifanti et al., 2013), hardship has led individuals who identify themselves as native Greeks to feel a sense of entitlement in comparison to immigrant populations, providing a focus for blame and allowing them to channel their anger as an antidote to their own economic hardship (Carastathis, 2015).

MEDIA AND ATTITUDES

Intertwined with political influences, various forms of media take an important role in shaping public opinion, with television, print and social media providing a backdrop of hostile commentary. Tabloid newspaper articles often adopt a deliberately provocative tone, written to shock, anger and disgust readers (Briant et al., 2013; Philo et al., 2013), using divisive, irresponsible and damaging language (Clayton and Vickers, 2014; Vickers et al., 2013) and focusing on individuals whose extreme and polarized lifestyles reflect little of the majority experience.

Briant et al. (2013) and Philo et al. (2013) reported a clear increase in negative reporting on issues such as disability and immigration, with the use of pejorative language and a focus on economic burden. They explored the views of members of the public to the needs of benefit claimants, refugees and people with disabilities, finding that attitudes were harsh and based on distorted facts that people justified because they had read about them in the popular press (Briant et al., 2013; Philo et al., 2013).

By way of example, in November 2013, the *Daily Mail* newspaper ran the headline 'Taxpayers' £10,000 bill to teach failed asylum seeker to fly.' It tells the tale of brothers Yonas and Abiy Kebede who, after coming to the UK from Ethiopia as children, were abandoned and entered the care system. On leaving care, Yonas, aged 21, planned to take flying lessons prior to a university place to train as a pilot, and Abiy, aged 20, planned to start a degree. The *Daily Mail* expresses shock at their entitlement and the cost of this decision, which is based on the council's legal obligation to help meet training costs for care leavers. The opinion of the author is clear as they express their outrage at the 'enormous sums' provided to support the professional qualifications of the two men (Harding, 2013, p. 1). The article uses quotations describing 'farcical decisions', 'free rides' and 'blank cheques' and focuses on the 'deeply unfair' impact on taxpayers, with an emphasis on the worthy hardworking people who 'scrimp and save' to provide their children higher education (Harding, 2013).

This portrayal is typical of such tales of the undeserving (Coyle and Craig, 2012; Vickers et al., 2013). The article, like many of its kind, shows the use of othering, deservedness, and moralizing, representing the reported problems as an unacceptable responsibility for the rest of society (Chauhan and Foster, 2013).

Another example began around 2007, through e-mail and social media messages, stating that people entering a nation illegally get a job, driver's license, pension card, welfare, credit cards, subsidized rent or a loan to buy a house, free education, and free healthcare. The messages also suggested that illegal immigrants were entitled to financial assistance worth up to £29 900 per year, in contrast to pensioners who received only £6000 a year in benefits (Kennedy, 2015). The messages circulated in many nations, including America, Australia, Canada, and India, and the content was altered to reflect the specifics of the intended nation. Various national governments and refugee agencies have investigated the original source, which is unknown, raising concerns about the inaccurate content and its intention to create resentment towards refugees (Refugee Council of Australia, 2010). The clear juxtaposition of illegal immigrants and pensioners not only raises an issue of cost, but also reflects the principles of othering and deservedness.

In order to raise awareness on the role of the media, a group of volunteer occupational therapy students in Teesside University in the UK were asked to share their perspectives on marginalization. Opinions were elicited in two phases, first exploring ideas about marginalization in general and secondly focusing on media portrayals. The students were provided with a series of tabloid newspaper articles relating to the payment of Incapacity Benefit. The students highlighted how complex issues were explored through unqualified facts, statistics and pseudoevidence such as 'official

tests show', with sound bites from influential characters, all of which made the content more compelling and harder to challenge. The material was constructed to be personal, with the use of individual stories and examples providing a target for the readers' anger. Images were carefully selected and language used to paint a powerful picture, condemning individuals with words such as idleness, festering, and waste, which carry the subliminal associations of disgust. They noted how individuals are caricatured to exaggerate themes, while their needs and circumstances are rarely considered and greatly simplified. Each article focused on groups less likely to evoke empathy and individuals who are rarely typical, including those whose issues are hidden or harder to define. The students were concerned that accessing only one source of information left the reader with a greatly simplified and unchallenged message.

The students acknowledged that the evidence they gained was often limited and skewed, containing distorted facts and failing to fully reflect the underpinning sociopolitical factors that may have created or contributed to the hardship faced by individuals. They recognized that much of the information they received had an emotional element that focused on blame and burden, and suggestions that the actions of a few can be taken as a reflection of the behaviour of the masses. In many instances, marginalized individuals, because they did not follow the majority, were seen as morally, religiously or financially corrupting, with television, print, and social media sensationalizing stories, making entertainment out of negative stereotypes and fostering fears.

The students described these various sources of information as propaganda, recognizing it as the selective use of partial facts, from narrow sources, to reinforce a particular message (Shah, 2005). Fiske and Taylor (1991) described people as 'cognitive misers', keen to simplify their approach to information and therefore drawn to clear and direct messages rather than complex ones. Powerfully persuasive, information presented in this way provides a simplified message, attractive in the context of a volume-heavy information age (Johnston, 2013).

Often, the primary media or political messages are not received firsthand, and the student group identified that they are often accessed second- or third-hand from the opinions of family, friends, or colleagues. This reflects the two-step flow theory (Katz and Lazarsfeld, 1955), which suggests that information from the mass media is processed and disseminated by opinion leaders at a local level, who add personal influence to the message. We rely on the integrity of these leaders to ensure the appropriateness of the message, but with increasing streams of media, particularly accessible online, our messages may become increasingly simplified and come from multiple, unreliable sources.

With the rise of social media, people are bombarded with information, processed by a range of opinion leaders of various levels of credibility, providing swathes of information we cannot meaningfully process. The ease with which we can 'like' a sentiment or an idea, without critically considering the quality of it, can be seductive, turning social media into a modern propaganda channel (Johnston, 2013).

THE IMPACT OF AUSTERITY AND MARGINALIZATION

There are multiple features at play in the process and continuation of marginalization (Fig. 6-2). There is a cyclical process by which austerity increases the need for prioritization of services and support (Duffy, 2013), and as the public is required to accept or support these priorities, the planned cuts are linked to deservedness (Bambra and Smith, 2010; Valentine, 2014). To promote this message, the media and politicians convey messages using fear and the distortion of facts to promote othering (Briant et al., 2013; Philo et al., 2013). Support is diminished for those people labelled 'undeserving', with reduced public empathy leading to increased marginalization (Valentine, 2014). From there, further exclusion becomes easier, as the individuals have less support and their needs are less well acknowledged (Duffy, 2013).

As a result of austerity and changing attitudes, individuals may find themselves facing increased economic hardship combined with the impact of negative attitudes. Their everyday hardship is reduced to a purely economic issue, debated, often without compassion, with assumptions and generalizations eroding public sympathies. This has the potential to worsen personal

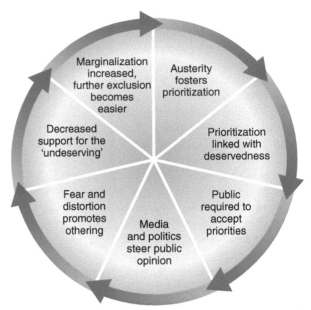

FIGURE 6-2 ■ The process and continuation of marginalization.

outcomes by feeding myths and fostering exploitation, reversing the efforts made over recent decades to give recognition to individuals as fully equitable members of society (Crawford, 2013; Wolbring, 2012).

Through the process of 'othering', normal moral rules can be broken, allowing society to care less and act more punitively (Clarey, 2012; Coyle and Craig, 2012; Eyben, 2004). Hate crimes, though severely underreported, have shown an increase of 18% in 2014–2015 alone, with the rise affecting all hate crime strands (race, religion, sexual orientation, disability, and transgender identity) (Corcoran et al., 2015). Ninety-one percent of respondents to a survey by Disability Rights UK (2012) identified rising negative press portrayals as fostering hostility and hate crime, having little doubt that the deteriorating situation is being driven by 'benefit scrounger' abuse, with media attitude legitimizing bullying (Philo, 2013).

The dynamics of marginalization not only alter public opinion, but shape opportunities and access to services through a process called *bordering* where boundaries develop which prevent people from equitable opportunities (Eyben, 2004). There is a significant human cost to this, as individuals experience increased isolation, loneliness, heightened stigma and shame, increased psychological pressure, and physical and mental ill health (Grove and Zwi, 2006; Heap, 2013; O'Hara, 2014b). Alongside this lies the perceived lack of empathy from others, including those administering the welfare system, and a lack of self-esteem fuelled by media and political rhetoric (O'Hara, 2014b).

Exclusion and deprivation occur in multiple layers; people are left to face the impact of daily hardships, the challenges of austerity, reduced access to services, and hardened attitudes and discrimination (Elliott, 2014; Philo et al., 2013). These interconnected issues can foster exclusion, reduce outcomes and opportunities for recovery, increase carer burden, and further widen already problematic gaps in opportunity (Butler, 2012; Elliott, 2014; Purton, 2014). The multilayered and pervasive impact creates 'durable inequality', entrenched, and extremely hard to escape.

FORGING BETTER OUTCOMES

Austerity undeniably presents a challenge to effective service provision, but creativity and energy can present opportunities where stretched services may otherwise feel unable to help (Wind-Cowie, 2013). O'Hara (2014a) and Butler (2012) encountered what they described as extraordinary support where individuals and organizations improvised 'grassroots' solutions to everyday hardship. These projects often ran with minimal funding, showing the resilience and ingenuity of individuals and organizations. Their examples included parents taking over a support group for families of children with a learning disability, and people on a housing estate coming together to pool resources and advice to help with day-to-day solutions. They provided practical and emotional support, built networks for inclusion and integration, focused on solutions, and helped one another to manage crises (Butler, 2012; Grove and Zwi, 2006; O'Hara, 2014a).

Occupational therapists often demonstrate the kind of creative, solution focused, and sustainable practice suited to meeting needs in austere times (Pollard and Kronenberg, 2008). Traditionally, services have focused on downstream 'repairing' following crises, but a focus

on 'preparing' upstream can develop individual and community capacity, resilience and control (Holthuis, 2013).

Occupational therapists have the opportunity to use positive attitudes, advocacy, and creative problem solving to make a difference to this process of marginalization. The principles of occupational therapy acknowledge the value and uniqueness of the individual, encouraging a person-centred, possibilities-driven approach to meeting needs and exploring solutions.

In order to retain values in tune with occupational therapy's guiding principles, it is important to reflect on the processes that influence their perceptions of others around them. A busy working world and a barrage of negative impressions may erode empathy and make the maintenance of a person-centred mindset more difficult to achieve (Shapiro, 2008). It is sometimes easier to maintain a distance from need and vulnerability in others; however, empathy is the foundation of meeting challenges and honouring difference (Shapiro, 2008). A genuinely person-centred approach safeguards human dignity and appropriate moral values (Ifanti et al., 2013), countering the cynicism of the agenda of marginalization to foster what Kronenberg et al. (2010) call 'possibilities based practice' (p. 11).

Lane and Tribe (2010) describe the client as the most valuable knowledge resource, so instead of attending to the misused and distorted narratives presented by others, occupational therapists can maintain awareness of their clients' needs and unique experiences through their firsthand narrative. This can be augmented by sound evidence, from varied and reliable sources, explored with an open and critical mind.

Within practice, occupational therapists have a responsibility to challenge and, where possible, address the occupational injustices that form part of marginalized lives (World Federation of Occupational Therapists, 2006). By seeing the impact of policy and media on public attitude and acknowledging its implications in the lives of others, it is possible to advocate for better access to services and opportunities, and address prevailing harsh attitudes.

Occupational therapists can adopt the role of 'opinion leader' to educate and raise awareness, challenging stereotypes or poor-quality evidence shared by others. By sharing balanced, research-informed evidence (such as the short animated film *All in This Together: Are Benefits Ever a Lifestyle Choice?* by Dole Animators (2014)), it is possible to raise awareness of the realities of marginalization in a meaningful and accessible way.

The power of a single contradictory message should not be underestimated. Consider, for example, the impact of the photographs of Aylan Kurdi, the Syrian child who drowned off the coast of Turkey in the summer of 2015. The image followed prolonged and almost exclusively negative coverage of migrants to the UK, yet it not only challenged the opinions of many members of the public, but also influenced media reporting and political rhetoric and mobilized increased aid (Barnard and Shoumali, 2015).

CONCLUSION

At times of hardship the need for service prioritization is a reality; however, the question remains whether professionals are being persuaded by insidious messages that one client deserves services more than the next? Occupational therapy has great potential to focus on the most meaningful possible outcomes for an individual, to take account of their context and circumstances, and to use ingenuity to find low-cost solutions to occupational issues. However, if we do not see need fairly and equitably across client populations, we are failing to uphold our values.

Similarly, if we silently ignore the rising hostilities around us, we are failing to challenge injustices which impact widely on occupational choice and opportunity. As Holocaust survivor Elie Wiesel said in his Nobel acceptance speech, '[W]e must always take sides. Neutrality helps the oppressor, never the victim. Silence encourages the tormentor, never the tormented' (1986, p. 1).

The tale of the Kebede brothers, presented earlier in this chapter, is an example of how political and media message can devalue individuals and add to their marginalization. It is also an example of two young men whose determination and aspiration has allowed them to rise above those barriers.

By seeing the capacity and potential of the individual, and challenging the rhetoric of demonization, occupational therapists can work with individuals who have been impacted by the interplay of hardship and negative attitudes. After all, what is occupational therapy if not an opportunity for all people to learn to fly?

Acknowledgements

I wish to express my gratitude to the following students from Teesside University BSc and MSc Occupational Therapy courses for giving their time and opinions in the preparation of this chapter: Chris Britton, Richie Brown, Vicky Field, Natalie Greenwell, Clare Johnson, Amanda Peach, Rachael Ward, Hayley Watson and Rachel Wetherall.

REFERENCES

Action T4, 2014. Remembering Action T4. <http://www.actiont4.com> (accessed 15.07.15.).

Alchin, L.K., 2012. Elizabethan Era:1563 Act for the Relief of the Poor. <www.elizabethan-era.org.uk> (accessed 25.10.14.).

Bambra, C., Smith, K., 2010. 'No longer deserving'? Sickness benefit reform and the politics of (ill) health in the UK. Crit. Publ. Health 20 (1), 71–83.

Barnard, A., Shoumali, K., 2015. Image of Drowned Syrian, Aylan Kurdi, 3, Brings Migrant Crisis into Focus. <http://www.nytimes.com/2015/09/04/world/europe/syria-boy-drowning.html> (accessed 03.10.15.).

Baumberg, B., Bell K., Gaffney, D., 2011. Benefit Stigma In Britain. Turn2us. Available at: <https://www.turn2us.org.uk/T2UWebsite/media/Documents/Benefits-Stigma-in-Britain.pdf>.

Blinder, S., Ford, R., Ivarsflaten, E., 2013. The better angels of our nature: how the antiprejudice norm affects policy and party preferences in Great Britain and Germany. Am. J. Polit. Sci. 57 (4), 841–857.

Bloy, M., 2002. The 1601 Elizabethan Poor Law. <http://www.victorianweb.org/history/poorlaw/elizpl.html> (accessed 25.10.14.).

Blyth, M., 2015. Austerity: the history of a dangerous idea. Open University Press, Maidenhead, UK.

Bowlby, C., 2010. Who deserves welfare? BBC. <http://www.bbc.co.uk/news/magazine-11778284> (accessed 25.10.14.).

Boyer, G.R., 1990. An Economic History of the English Poor Law, 1750–1850. Cambridge University Press, Cambridge.

Briant, E., Watson, N., Philo, G., 2013. Reporting disability in the age of austerity: the changing face of media representation of disability and disabled people in the UK and the creation of new 'folk devils'. Disabil. Society 28 (6), 874–889.

British Social Attitudes Survey, 2014. <http://www.natcen.ac.uk/our-research/research/british-social-attitudes/> (accessed 15.07.15.).

Butler, P., 2012. The 'despair' and 'loneliness' of austerity Britain. The Guardian, 17 July 2012. Available at: <http://www.theguardian.com/society/2012/jul/17/despair-loneliness-austerity-britain> (accessed 25.10.14.).

Carastathis, A., 2015. The politics of austerity and the affective economy of hostility: racialised gendered violence and crises of belonging in Greece. Fem. Rev. 109, 73–95.

Chakrabortty, A., 2013. Press freedom: is that the right to make up stories about asylum seekers? The Guardian, 7 October 2013. Available at: <http://www.theguardian.com/commentisfree/2013/oct/07/press-freedom-asylum-seekers-ed-miliband> (accessed 25.10.14.).

Chauhan, A., Foster, J., 2013. Representations of poverty in British newspapers: a case of 'othering' the threat? J. Commun. Appl. Soc. Psychol. 24, 390–405.

Ciobanu, C., 2012. European Refugees Meet Austerity-Era Hostility. <http://www.ipsnews.net/2012/04/european-refugees-meet-austerity-era-hostility/> (accessed 25.10.14.).

Clarey, E., 2012. Welfare. Are tough times affecting attitudes to welfare? British Social Attitudes. Available at: <http://www.bsa-29.natcen.ac.uk/read-thereport/welfare/introduction.aspx> (accessed 25.10.14.).

Clayton, J., Vickers, T., 2014. Black, male, care leaver, seeking asylum: access to higher education in Britain. Open Democracy. Available at: <http://www.opendemocracy.net/5050/john-clayton-and-tom-vickers/black-male-careleaver-seeking-asylum-access-to-higher-education-i> (accessed 25.10.14.).

Cohen, S., 2011. Folk Devils and Moral Panics. Taylor & Francis, Abingdon, UK.

Collingwood, A., 2015. Who has gained and lost most since 2010? The Joseph Rowntree Foundation, York.

Corcoran, H., Lader, D., Smith, K., 2015. Hate Crime, England and Wales, 2014/15. Statistical Bulletin 05/15. Home Office. <http://www.report-it.org.uk/files/ho_hate_crime_statistics_201415.pdf> (accessed 02.11.15.).

Coyle, N., Craig, K., 2012. Press portrayal of disabled people: a rise in hostility fuelled by austerity? Disability Rights UK. <http://www.disabilityrightsuk.org/press-portrayaldisabled-people-rise-hostility-fuelled-austerity> (accessed 25.10.14.).

Crawford, R., 2013. The Immigration Bill: hostility won't tackle austerity. Migration Pulse 18. October 2013. <http://www.migrantsrights.org.uk/migration-pulse/2013/immigration-bill-hostility-won-t-tackle-austerity> (accessed 25.10.14.).

Danermark, B., Gellerstedt, L.C., 2004. Social justice: redistribution and recognition—a non-reductionist perspective on disability. Disabil. Society 19 (4), 339–353.

Department of Health, 2015. Review of Operational Productivity in NHS providers: An independent report for the Department of Health. Online: <https://www.gov.uk/government/uploads/system/uploads/attachment_data/file/434202/carter-interim-report.pdf>.

Department for Work and Pensions, 2014. Press release: new benefit fraud and error campaign: 'Benefits. Are you doing the right thing?' <https://www.gov.uk/government/news/new-benefit-fraud-anderror-campaign-benefits-are-you-doing-the-right-thing> (accessed 25.10.14.).

Disability Rights UK, 2012. Press portrayal of disabled people: a rise in hostility fuelled by austerity? <http://www.disabilityrightsuk.org/press-portrayal-disabled-people-rise-hostility-fuelled-austerity> (accessed 25.10.14.).

Duffy, S., 2013. A fair society? How the cuts target disabled people. Centre for Welfare Reform, Sheffield.

Elliott, J., 2014. Austerity is making life unbearable for those with mental health conditions. <http://www.newstatesman.com/politics/2014/09/austerity-making-life-unbearable-those-mental-health-conditions> (accessed 25.10.14.).

Equality and Human Rights Commission, 2010. Triennial Review 2010, How Fair is Britain? The First Triennial Review. Available at: <www.equalityhumanrights.com/uploaded_files/triennial_review/how_fair_is_britain_ch6.pdf> (accessed 04.07.15.).

Equality Commission NI, 2011. Do you mean me? <http://www.hscbusiness.hscni.net/pdf/ECNI_Equality_Awareness_Survey_2011.pdf> (accessed 25.10.14.).

Eyben, R., 2004. Inequality as process and experience. In: Eyben, R., Lovett, J. (Eds.), Political and Social Inequality: A Review. IDS Development Bibliography 20, Institute of Development Studies, Brighton, UK.

Fahnestock, J., 2011. Rhetorical Style: The Uses of Language in Persuasion. Oxford University Press, Oxford.

Fiske, S.T., Taylor, S.E., 1991. Social Cognition, second ed. McGraw-Hill, Philadelphia, PA.

Fraser, N., 2000. Rethinking recognition. New Left Review 3. Available at: <http://newleftreview.org/II/3/nancy-fraser-rethinking-recognition> (accessed 15.07.15.).

Furedi, F., 2006. The Politics of Fear; Beyond Left and Right. Continuum Press, London.

Gardner, D., 2009. Risk: The Science and Politics of Fear. Virgin Books, London.

Garthwaite, K., 2011. The language of shirkers and scroungers?' Talking about illness, disability and coalition welfare reform. Disabil. Society 26 (3), 369–372.

Goode, E., Ben-Yehuda, N., 2009. Moral Panics: The Social Construction of Deviance, second ed. Wiley-Blackwell, Chichester, UK.

Goodwin, J., Jasper, J.M., Polletta, F., 2001. Passionate Politics; Emotions and Social Movements. University of Chicago Press, Chicago.

Grove, N.J., Zwi, A.B., 2006. Our health and theirs: forced migration, othering, and public health. Soc. Sci. Med. 62 (8), 1931–1942.

Harding, E., 2013, Taxpayers £10,000 bill to teach failed asylum seeker to fly. Daily Mail. Available at: <http://www.dailymail.co.uk/news/article-2487444/Taxpayers-10-000-teach-failedasylum-seeker-fly.html#ixzz2twfLQHaR> (accessed 25.10.14.).

Hatemi, P.K., McDermott, R., Eaves, L.J., Kendler, K.S., Neale, M.C., 2013. Fear as a disposition and an emotional state: a genetic and environmental approach to out-group political preferences. Am. J. Polit. Sci. 57 (2), 279–293.

Heap, D., 2013. Shame, stigma and benefit cuts: a symposium. SPA Conference, 27 February 2013. <http://danheap.wordpress.com/2013/02/27/spa-conference-2013/> (accessed 25.10.14.).

Holthuis, E., 2013. Social protection and health as a means to invest in people. European Commission Sixth European Public Health Conference, 14 November 2013. <https://eupha.org/repository/conference/2013/Brussels_2013_summary_report.pdf> (Last accessed 21.09.15.).

Hudson, R., 2013. Conclusion: divided kingdom? Health, the regions and austerity economics. In: Wood, C. (Ed.), The NHS at 65 Is Facing a Triple-Pinch of Recession. Austerity and Demographic Change, pp. 65–72. <http://www.demos.co.uk/files/DEMOS_Health_in_Austerity_-_web.pdf?1379898927> (accessed 12.7.15.). DEMOS, London.

Ifanti, A.A., Argyriou, A.A., Kalofonou, F.H., Kalofonos, H.P., 2013. Financial crisis and austerity measures in Greece: their impact on health promotion policies and public health care. Health Policy (New York) 113 (1–2), 8–12.

Johnes, C., 2012. Has David Cameron opened a new front on welfare? Oxfam. <http://policy-practice.oxfam.org.uk/camerons-front-on-welfare> (accessed 25.10.14.).

Johnston, P., 2013. The Internet, social media and propaganda: the final frontier? <http://britishlibrary.typepad.co.uk/socialscience/2013/08/the-internet-social-media-and-propaganda-the-final-frontier.html#sthash.YKqy1pgD.dpuf> (accessed 12.5.15.).

Joseph Rowntree Foundation., 2014. Austerity in the UK. <http://www.jrf.org.uk/topic/austerity?gclid=CNTUo6_6xMACFfSWtAodpSAAnQ> (accessed 25.10.14.).

Jost, J.T., 2003. Political conservatism as motivated social cognition. Psychol. Bull. 129 (3), 339–375.

Karanikolos, M., Mladovsky, P., Cylus, J., Thomson, S., Basu, S., Stuckle, D., 2013. Financial crisis, austerity, and health in Europe. Lancet 381 (9874), 1323–1331.

Karyotis, G., Rudig, W., 2013. Blame and punishment? The electoral politics of extreme austerity in Greece. Pol. Stud. 63 (1), 2–24. Available at: <http://onlinelibrary.wiley.com/doi/10.1111/1467-9248.12076/full> (accessed 25.10.14.).

Katz, E., Lazarsfeld, P.F., 1955. Personal Influence. Free Press, New York.

Kennedy, S., 2015. Viral emails protesting about financial assistance for 'illegal immigrants/refugees living in Britain'. House of Commons Social Policy Section, House of Commons Library, London.

Kingston, G., McGinnity, F., O'Connell, P.J., 2015. Discrimination in the labour market: nationality, ethnicity and the recession. Work Employ. Soc. 29 (2), 213–232.

Kronenberg, F., Pollard, N., Sakellariou, D., 2010. Occupational Therapies without Borders, vol. 2. Towards an Ecology of Occupation Based Practices. Churchill Livingstone, London.

Lane, P., Tribe, R., 2010. Following NICE 2008: a practical guide for health professionals: community engagement with local black and minority ethnic (BME) community groups. Divers. Health Care (Don Mills) 7 (2), 105–114.

Leone, L., Chirumbolo, A., 2008. Conservatism as motivated avoidance of affect: need for affect scales predict conservatism measures. J. Res. Personal. 42 (3), 755–762.

Molloy, C., 2014 The billions of wasted NHS cash no-one wants to mention. <https://www.opendemocracy.net/ournhs/caroline-molloy/billions-of-wasted-nhs-cash-noone-wants-to-mention> (accessed 09.10.15.).

Mostert, M.P., 2002. Useless eaters: disability as genocidal marker in Nazi Germany. Catholic Culture. Available at: <https://www.catholicculture.org/culture/library/view.cfm?recnum=7019> (accessed 25.10.14.).

National Audit Office, 2012. Progress in making NHS efficiency savings. Report By The Comptroller And Auditor General London. The Stationary Office.

O'Hara, M., 2014a. Austerity Bites: Journey to the sharp end of the cuts. Policy Press, Bristol.

O'Hara, M., 2014b. Deprivation, depression and demonisation part of daily struggle. Joseph Rowntree Foundation. Available at: <http://www.jrf.org.uk/austerity-birmingham> (accessed 25.10.14.).

Pennington, J., 2011. Beneath the surface: a country of two nations. <http://www.bbc.co.uk/history/british/victorians/bsurface_01.shtml> (accessed 25.10.14.).

Perry, J., Williams, M., Sefton, T., Haddad, M., 2014. Emergency Use Only: Understanding and Reducing the Use of Food Banks in the UK. Child Poverty Action Group, Church of England, Oxfam GB and The Trussell Trust, The Trussell Trust, Salisbury.

Philo, G., Briant, E., Donald, P., 2013. Bad News for Refugees. Pluto, London.

Pollard, N., Kronenberg, F., 2008. Working with people on the margins. In: Creek, J., Lougher, L. (Eds.), Occupational Therapy and Mental Health. Churchill Livingstone, London.

Ponticelli, J., Voth, J.H., 2011. Austerity and Anarchy: Budget Cuts and Social Unrest in Europe, 1919–2008. <http://crei.cat/people/voth/voth_austerity_anarchy.pdf> (accessed 25.10.14.).

Potter, A., Knight, A., 2011. The Cancer Drugs Fund. <http://ukpolicymatters.thelancet.com/policy-summary-the-cancer-drugs-fund/> (accessed 09.10.15.).

Purton, P., 2014. Mental health at work and austerity. Working life. <tuc.org.uk/equality-issues/disability-issues/disabled-people-fighting-austerity> (accessed 25.10.14.).

Refugee Council of Australia, 2010. Response to outlandish claims about benefits to refugees: update. <http://www.refugeecouncil.org.au/docs/releases/2010/100309%20Updated%20Response%20to%20email%20on%20Centrelink%20benefits.pdf> (accessed on 25.10.14.).

Robin, C., 2004. Fear: The History of a Political Idea. Oxford University Press, New York.

Seymour, R., 2014. Against austerity. <https://ceasefiremagazine.co.uk/austerity-uk-ideology-public-opinion/> (accessed 09.10.15.).

Shapiro, J., 2008. Walking a mile in their patients' shoes: empathy and othering in medical students' education. Philos. Ethics Humanit. Med. 3, 10.

Valentine, G., 2014. Inequality and class prejudice in an age of austerity. Sheffield Political Economy Research Institute, Sheffield.

Valentine, G., Harris, C., 2014. Strivers vs skivers: class prejudice and the demonisation of dependency in everyday life. Geoforum 53, 84–92.

Vasilopoulou, S., Halikiopoulou, D., Exadaktylos, T., 2014. Greece in crisis: austerity, populism and the politics of blame. J. Common Mark. Stud. 52 (2), 388–402.

Vickers, T., et al., 2013. Right judgment. Times Higher Education. Available at: <https://www.timeshighereducation.com/comment/letters/right-judgment/2008984.article> (accessed 25.10.14.).

Wiesel, E., 1986. Nobel acceptance speech, delivered in Oslo on 10 December 1986. <http://www.pbs.org/eliewiesel/nobel/index.html> (accessed 12.07.15.).

World Federation of Occupational Therapists, 2006. Position statement on human rights. <http://www.wfot.org/ResourceCentre.aspx> (accessed 02.06.15.).

Williams, Z., 2013. Skivers v strivers: the argument that pollutes people's minds. The Guardian. 9 January 13. Available at: <http://www.theguardian.com/politics/2013/jan/09/skivers-v-strivers-argument-pollutes> (accessed 12.5.15.).

Wind-Cowie, M., 2013. Health and innovation in a time of austerity. In: Wood, C. (Ed.), Health in Austerity. Demos, London. <http://www.demos.co.uk/files/DEMOS_Health_in_Austerity_-_web.pdf?1379898927> (accessed 25.10.14.).

Winder, E., 2015. Austerity is essential if Britain wants to reduce inequality – why can't the left-wingers who march against it realise this? <http://www.independent.co.uk/voices/comment/austerity-is-essential-if-britain-wants-to-reduce-inequality-in-the-future-why-cant-the-left-wingers-10339081.html> (accessed 02.10.15.).

Wolbring, G., 2012. Societies 2 (3), 75–83.

Zaidi, A., Burchadt, T., 2005. Comparing incomes when needs differ: equivalization for the extra costs of disability in the UK. Rev. Income Wealth 51 (1), 89–114.

7

ARE WE REALLY MAKING A DIFFERENCE? MONITORING AND EVALUATION IN COMMUNITY-BASED PRACTICE

KERRY THOMAS ■ SUSAN GILBERT HUNT

CHAPTER OUTLINE

Health professionals are increasingly required to demonstrate that what they do really makes a difference, articulating how their efforts make a difference to the health and well-being of the people and communities with whom they work. In community-based practice, the focus is on working in partnership with the community to address health inequalities through the development of high-quality relevant programmes that take account of social and economic factors (Labonte, 2005). Evaluation needs to identify the extent to which the programme has developed the community's capacity to sustain programme benefits and adapt to the changing (policy, funding, climatic and socioeconomic) conditions that are characterizing global, national and local contexts. Demonstrating such impact is not only important for professional and personal identity and credibility, but it is also an essential requirement of managers and funders of programmes. This is especially so where occupational therapists are working with vulnerable communities in cross-disciplinary programme areas such as community-based rehabilitation. Moreover, the task is magnified in cross-cultural contexts.

This chapter aims to contribute to the ongoing dialogue regarding how occupational therapists determine effectiveness and account for their effort in community-based practice, particularly with disadvantaged communities and in low-resource settings. Reflection on years of experience in designing and undertaking small-scale, community-based programme evaluation in contexts where evaluation capacity and culture is still evolving has informed the dialogue.

We begin with an overview of monitoring and evaluation (M&E), reviewing its purpose and associated tensions and challenges in getting started. This is a foundation from which to consider practical strategies in navigating the complexities inherent in designing and implementing effective evaluation of community-based programmes. Within this we share some insights into developing a moral stance to M&E practice for professionals. In considering approaches to evaluation practice, it is not our intention to promote one methodology over another; rather, we introduce 'Making MERI' (monitoring, evaluation, reporting/communication and improvement), a framework that has potential to integrate relevant, ethical, evidence-based programme, and professional 'monitoring, evaluation, reporting and improvement' strategies. The discussion in this chapter applies equally to programmes and projects, but for ease of reading we primarily use the term *project*.

EVALUATION

Over time there has been a shift in the focus of project evaluation. In the 1950s, the focus was on simple measurement of predetermined categories using simple counting and aggregation to explain before and after effects with a focus on cost–benefit analysis (Mayoux and Chambers, 2005). However, such approaches do not necessarily produce sustained benefits for the community, as this requires participatory and empowering strategies to develop the capacity of communities to effect their own change. Moreover, improving practice through the learning afforded by effective participatory evaluation has gained prominence in order to encourage and sustain the time and resources required to undertake the evaluation (Mayoux and Chambers, 2005). Evaluation is now a complex process of collecting a portfolio of evidence to describe the impact of the project.

UNDERSTANDING THE ROLE OF MONITORING AND EVALUATION

Although the terms *monitoring* and *evaluation* are often used synonymously, or together, it is important to understand how they differ from each other. At its simplest level, M&E is about gathering and analysing information to track progress, modify actions and assess the results (Estrella, 2000). As human beings, we do this almost intuitively as part of everyday living. However, in community-based practice, it is not only important to determine the extent to which the project results have enabled the community to develop the capacity to better address existing needs, but also to adapt to ongoing change in policy, funding and socio-economic conditions.

The two components of M&E have different purposes and only together can they provide evidence of a project's effectiveness. *Monitoring* involves collecting, analysing and using information about progress and performance as a programme or project goes along; it allows activities and processes to be modified to accommodate changing contexts and enhance appropriateness and effectiveness across the project cycle (Figure 7-1). *Evaluation* is distinguished from monitoring by being a periodic, critical appraisal of overall performance and results (Estrella, 2000). Evaluation focuses on the extent to which project aims and objectives have been achieved including the effectiveness and efficiency of effort and the relevance of chosen strategies to deliver and sustain desired outcomes. Thus monitoring generates data on inputs, outputs and shorter-term outcomes that contribute to a portfolio of 'so what' evaluative information and evidence from which overall performance can be judged and lessons learned.

As can be seen in Figure 7-1, M&E are critical elements of the project cycle, and as Talbot and Verrinder (2014) explain, '[I]n practice, effective and efficient

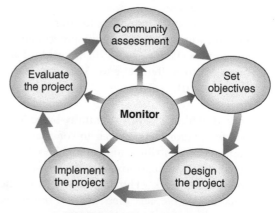

FIGURE 7-1 The project cycle.

[health promotion] is guided by a recurring process of assessing, planning, acting, implementing and evaluating, followed by reassessing, replanning, reacting...in a continuous cycle of reflection and action' (p. 204).

In order to achieve and evidence the desired outcomes, M&E is an integral component of a project plan and should be planned at the outset. Indeed, many funding bodies now require it as a condition of funding release. Once all key stakeholders agree on the overarching purpose of evaluation, M&E needs to follow a systematic process to ensure all key aspects are effectively addressed. In doing so, the role of M&E in community-based practice can meet its multiple and quite diverse purposes, which include:

- monitoring of performance against plans, baselines and agreed criteria;
- assessing progress towards achieving intended aims, objectives and outcomes;
- coordinating, rationalizing and managing data collection and analysis;
- demonstrating contribution of project actions towards capacity building, change and ultimately community health and well-being;
- providing information to inform strategic planning, future investment, management and improvement functions that address effectiveness, efficiency, appropriateness and sustainability;
- being accountable to community stakeholders, managers and funders;
- enabling effective and appropriate contributions to reporting and communication processes, and supporting ongoing engagement, learning and development; *and*
- reflecting on and accounting for our own performance as stakeholders in the process and as practitioners (Patton, 2002, 2008; Rushford and Thomas, 2015; Talbot and Verrinder, 2014; Thomas, 2010).

This practical blueprint of community-based M&E provides a foundation upon which to consider some of the features that contribute to forming the substantive character and moral landscape of humanitarian and development work (Hunt, 2011; Pollard and Sakellariou, 2009). We can then use the normative guidelines and approaches relevant for this work,

against which performance in 'making a difference' can be evaluated. The Making MERI framework presented later in the chapter provides a scaffold within which to consider these, but first an exploration of some of the challenges is presented.

COMMON CHALLENGES IN GETTING STARTED

There is a range of intersecting tensions and challenges associated with M&E, some of which relate to the perceptions associated with M&E, others reflect the political landscape, and then those that simply reflect the complexity of the task (Newell and Graham, 2012). Evaluation is a value-laden process (Guttman, 2000; Patton, 2008); therefore it is important to understand how potential tensions can present significant challenges for practitioners who may themselves be developing their skills and competencies in this area.

Challenges Related to Perceptions of Monitoring and Evaluation

Often the first challenge is to overcome negative perceptions of M&E as a necessary evil to appease bureaucrats and accountants. As a result, M&E suffers from a poor reputation and has in the past been a neglected component in programme planning and management, with respect to the consideration and emphasis it is given (Newell and Graham, 2012). Fostering an understanding of how M&E can contribute to recognition and shared learning regarding strategies that work in specific contexts is important. Moreover, dissemination of this knowledge and experience is critical for the development of improved practice. Thus in planning for M&E, it is necessary to consider how best it can be promoted as opportunity for engagement, learning and development within the project while still accommodating upwards and outwards accountability requirements.

Limitations in M&E skills and the inherent suspicions outlined above create a tendency for it to be tacked on at the end of the project rather than be an instrumental and integrated component of the project's work (Talbot and Verrinder, 2014). It is necessary to facilitate the integration of M&E across all the work in an interesting, empowering and effective way that inherently contributes to the project's aim and objectives.

Challenges Related to the Complexity of Monitoring and Evaluation

The context within which M&E occurs is dynamic and characterized by a variety of interacting factors. Every situation is unique, negating a prescriptive approach. Practitioners need to understand many variables, including the cultural and historical background of the community, as well as the demographics and individual, group and power dynamics. There is a need to give consideration to what the M&E process will require, including counterpart availability and capacities, and to determine if the requisite time, skills and resources are available. Given that these factors are finite and evaluation capacities may still be emerging, designing the M&E process to capture data necessary to evidence outcomes involves determining the limits of information that can be reasonably collected, absorbed and effectively used (Estrella, 2000; Feuerstein, 1986).

Effective M&E is an inclusive process requiring the involvement of a broad stakeholder group that can include beneficiaries and community people, political leaders, programme staff and managers, funders, and policymakers. The diversity of people and organisations that have a connection with even small projects can be extensive. This diversity creates a significant challenge when there are competing needs, interests and expectations (Newell and Graham, 2012). Understanding the potential agendas of different groups and ensuring a focus on the project and the key people is critical to managing these dynamics in the M&E process.

Furthermore, the M&E process needs to account for the project inputs (money provided, personnel involved, resources used), project outputs (activities undertaken, people reached), project outcomes (results of activities, changes in capacity including understanding and behaviour) and project impact (long-term effect on the well-being of people or situations) (Oakley et al., 1998; Thomas, 2010; Woodhill and Robins, 1998). Systems and processes to gather and review data in relation to project inputs and outputs are more straightforward and frequently involve quantitative data collection. However, outcome assessment is more complex as it requires the disaggregation and/or attribution of project effort and activity to project outcomes. For example, how can you evidence that participation in a workshop on child development and play using low-cost household items resulted in increased play opportunities for the children with disabilities who took part in it? Moreover, what provisions can be made to secure postproject impact evaluation, which often occurs 12 to 24 months after a project's completion?

If the core task of the M&E process is to evidence the effectiveness, efficiency, appropriateness and sustainability of a project, it is necessary to determine how these will be defined and by whom, and by what criteria they will be measured. While quantitative data may contribute to the empirical evidence-based analysis that is particularly sought by some stakeholders, applying dialogue and other participatory qualitative methods in M&E of development aid and programme performance to deliver progress against longer-term community outcomes is increasingly being pursued (Newell and Graham, 2012; Oakley et al., 1998; Roughley, 2009).

This leads to a further complexity challenge, that of generating credible evidence that is robust, relevant and responsive to evaluation and serves the community's interest, while also meeting professional guidelines and standards, including community and cultural considerations. This is particularly challenging when the desired project outcomes relate to value-laden social changes such as inclusion, democratic participation and capacity building for leadership and advocacy (Kotvojs and Hurworth, 2011; Marsden et al., 1994; Newell and Graham, 2012). Not only do these defy quantitative measures, but they can also ignite internal conflict, for example when advocacy by empowered people begins to annoy funders or threaten political stakeholders.

Challenges Related to Political Tensions Associated with Monitoring and Evaluation

In addition to managing the political dynamics that exist between stakeholders at local levels, M&E is impacted by shifts in international and community development policies and funding arrangements, which themselves are a response to various geopolitical, economic, social, environmental and health trends.

While the rhetoric of democratic politics and development policies promotes participatory and empowerment approaches, in practice the pendulum is currently shifting back towards an overarching requirement for externally facilitated evaluation with prescribed reporting that allows the aggregation and manipulation of quantitative data (Greenaway, 2013). This is generating increasing tension between funders and programmes with respect to whose needs are being privileged (see, e.g., Newell and Graham, 2012). The situation is exacerbated by shorter-term and politicized policies and interventions (e.g., Berry 2014). How can M&E be designed in ways that leverage community participation and influence whilst servicing wider political needs and accommodating midprogramme policy changes?

Challenges in Aligning Community-Based Programmes and Monitoring and Evaluation Approaches

To develop a credible M&E approach, it is important to ensure that it is aligned with the underlying philosophy, sociocultural context, goals and programmatic approach with which the partner organization and community are working. This too is a value-laden, politically sensitive endeavour. However, a lack of congruency with the underlying principles upon which the programme or project is based risks measuring wrong or inappropriate outcomes, things the initiative never aimed to achieve. The integrity of findings can also be impacted by application of M&E methods that are inconsistent with programme values and approaches. For example, projects in disability and development, indigenous health and other disadvantaged community sectors are invariably underpinned, explicitly or unconsciously, by empowerment and rights-based approaches (Newell and Graham, 2012; Johnson, 2004; Scougall, 2006). Such programmes have an emphasis on participatory and capacity-building processes and activities that endeavour to enhance inclusion and equity in access to services and resources. While a range of evaluation approaches has emerged that reflect and incorporate similar principles and embrace analogous practices, identifying and assessing their fit with planned and/or operating programme approaches can be challenging (Kotvojs and Hurworth, 2013). In this regard, it can be helpful to refer to evaluation approaches that elaborate clear rationales together with practical operating principles, such as Fetterman and Wandersman (2005) and Lentz et al. (2005) on empowerment evaluation and its 10 principles.

Concomitantly, development interventions often need to address the more immediate, practical needs of vulnerable people, such as food, water, shelter, security and income before they can physically engage in the health and advocacy initiatives about which local organizations, policymakers and donors seek data and information to service their needs. In tandem with capacity constraints that characterize smaller-scale programmes in disadvantaged communities, such situations may call for realist review (Pawson et al., 2005) and utilization-focused evaluation (Patton, 2008) approaches.

Collaborative approaches and carefully considered methodological flexibility have proved to be particularly appropriate and useful in designing and conducting M&E with vulnerable and disadvantaged communities (Pollard and Sakellariou, 2009; Rushford and Thomas, 2015; Scougall, 2006). Such approaches focus on what is meaningful to key stakeholders, build ownership, reduce the potential for harm, utilize local assets, increase efficiencies and inherently strengthen M&E participation, capacity, engagement and sustainability (Estrella, 2000; Newell and Graham, 2012; Thomas, 2010). Of course, in practice the task is a little more problematic.

Challenges in Managing Professional Motives and Community Needs

Community practice professionals are often 'outsiders' to the community they are working with (Pollard and Sakellariou, 2009), particularly in humanitarian contexts and where external project and/or evaluative expertise is sought. Personally and professionally, there is a drive to 'do good' and to 'deliver', respectively, but 'these motives do not always meet community needs and good intentions do not necessarily transpire into sustainable, culturally appropriate action' (Pollard and Sakellariou, 2009, p. 3); these challenges apply equally to project facilitation and evaluation roles. As Mayhew and Kennedy (2005) elaborate, virtue in humanitarian action can have many dark and detrimental effects that require conscious attention. Constraints related to workloads, geographical coverage, logistical arrangements, fragile data management systems, limited resources, finite contract timelines and sociocultural differences are common and may be exacerbated by language challenges. Managing the competing tensions that exist between professional motives and community needs brings practical as well as moral and ethical challenges (Clarinval and Biller-Andorno, 2014; Hunt et al., 2014; Kaplan, 2002; Pollard and Sakellariou, 2009). How to be compassionate yet professional? Whose interests are being supported, subsumed or subjugated?

Examining one's own motivations is imperative (Kaplan, 2002; Pande and Dalal, 2004). Reflective practice strategies are powerful tools in helping manage the task but can be difficult to apply in the midst of an intensive evaluation process. Similarly, safeguards such as those related to recruitment, police clearance checks and the handling of complaints are important but not sufficient. Demonstrating compliance with humanitarian, professional and evaluation mandates and codes of conduct is now commonly sought (e.g., Australian Evaluation Society, 2013; International Federation of Red Cross, 1994), and even accreditation processes are being implemented. However, it is the active involvement of the community that is critical to ensuring that M&E remains accountable and relevant to community needs and takes precedence over any personal and professional motivations (Hillhort, 2002; Hunt et al., 2014; Pollard and Sakellariou, 2009).

MAKING MERI: A FRAMEWORK TO GUIDE COMMUNITY-BASED EVALUATION

Making MERI represents an integrated, flexible, evidence-based approach for community-based evaluation that endeavours to respond to the realities, needs, lessons and challenges outlined above. As the acronym suggests, it integrates and makes explicit the communication ('reporting') and utilization of information arising from M&E, which are particularly poorly addressed in M&E practice and budgets, and signals that M&E can be enjoyable and energizing.

Having already defined *monitoring* and *evaluation,* it is now pertinent to define what is meant by *reporting* and *improvement.* Reporting embraces the dissemination, communication and sharing of project results, learning and outcomes (Roughley, 2009; Thomas, 2010); in the context of MERI, the tendency of reporting as a one-way, formal, upwards accountability process is expanded to include a wide range of mediums that promote two-way communication, discussion and engagement. Improvement shifts the focus from judgement to learning and promotes reflective practice on both successes and failures in order to adapt, refine and improve performance (Roughley, 2009; Thomas 2010). It is a lot more than reviewing data and information; it is about collectively generating meaning, knowledge and even wisdom, and applying this to problem solving, decision making and ongoing development (Thomas, 2010; Woodhill and Robins, 1998).

The Making MERI framework outlined here has emerged from work undertaken by the lead author in collaboration with a wide range of colleagues and organizational partners (including Roughley and Dart). It combines, builds on and adapts concepts, practice and research from across various sectors including natural resource management (Roughley, 2009; Roughley and Dart, 2009), community health, and international aid and development (Thomas, 2010), and with reference to contemporary trends and debates in evaluation discourse. As a dynamic framework, it has been continually evolving through experience extending over a decade and across a considerable range of programmes, projects, communities, cultures and sectors. Figure 7-2 portrays its use with a local nongovernmental organization working with children and youth with disabilities and their families in Cambodia. Experience through such partnerships and review of MERI application (which is largely documented in grey literature including consultancy and donor reports and training materials) has been distilled to crystallize core principles, elements and processes; these are reflected in the MERI framework outlined below, and are intended as a guide to assist practitioners navigate through and develop effective evaluation.

Making MERI is a framework that comprises two main elements: firstly, it elaborates a series of steps and considerations in planning for MERI, which in turn inform the structure for the design and implementation of performance story reporting (PSR) (Mayne,

2003; McLaughlin and Jordan, 1999; Roughley, 2009). PSR is a highly participatory process used to generate information, analyse data, compile findings and critique results (Davies and Dart, 2005; Roughley and Dart, 2009; Thomas, 2010).

Neither of the two elements is prescriptive; rather, they provide a guiding process and format that is responsive to different contexts, allowing the mixing-and-matching of different methodological approaches and tools whilst supporting the generation of robust

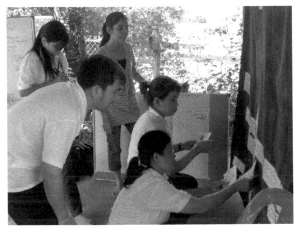

FIGURE 7-2 Participatory development of a MERI framework. A rural team from the Komar Pikar Foundation in Cambodia codeveloping a 'programme logic' describing the foundations and expected inputs, activities, short- and longer-term outcomes to achieve goals related to provision of community-based rehabilitation services for children with disabilities and their families. Logic models from each team were integrated to form an overarching organizational diagrammatic summary depicting the strategic plan and providing the structure for the Komar Pikar Foundation MERI Framework (Komar Pikar Foundation, 2013). This has proved valuable in guiding planning and evaluation with community stakeholders, as well as donors and the government, and has supported ongoing learning and capacity building within the organization.

evidence that promotes utilization of findings. On its own it does not compel the critical reflection and analysis that is necessary to genuinely determine if and how we are making a difference; rather, as a process, it creates opportunities, nurtures potential and enables positive engagement in M&E, and has the capability to scale up its sophistication and complexity as experience, interest and situations develop. For example, the Murdi Paaki Drug and Alcohol Network MERI Framework (2012) designed and implemented over 5 years with several independent Aboriginal health services in New South Wales in Australia, in collaboration with state and national government authorities, allowed for individual services to select evaluation questions and indicators from a common pool and add to these annually. It also enabled frontline Aboriginal workers, community elders and people to contribute equally to MERI activities with tertiary qualified professionals and administrators, deepening and expanding the range of measures and methods they utilized, as confidence, meaning and value built. With varying success, it serviced community and service needs, partnerships and network programme development, and mandatory government and project reporting (Thomas et al., 2012, 2013, 2015).

Underpinning the MERI framework are principles and values that guide sustainable development, and humanitarian action and public health ethics more generally. Beyond identifying substantive core values, as an integrated planning and evaluation framework it also includes a seven-step process (Figure 7-3) that promotes a transparent and clear decision-making process across the project cycle, improves the M&E of project interventions and performance, and promotes an appropriate culture of learning and improvement reflective of the context or situation. Giving attention to the principles as listed in Box 7-1, all of which reflect general good practice in M&E, supports this effort.

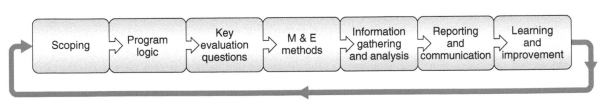

FIGURE 7-3 The seven steps in developing a MERI plan.

BOX 7-1
PRINCIPLES FOR EFFECTIVE MERI

- Planned at the outset
- Meaningful and relevant to project goals and community interests
- Focused in scope, scale, priorities and outcomes
- Feasible and practical in relation to available resources
- Considerate of capacity within the community
- Participatory
- Promotes learning, understanding and continuous improvement
- Contributes, through process and results, to ongoing adaptive and transformative capacity

---

Making MERI: Developing a Plan

There are seven steps in Making MERI planning (Figure 7-3). This suggests a simple linearity that belies a dynamic and cyclical process. Developing a MERI plan entails significant iteration, juggling and aligning of a range of variables and considerations at each of the seven steps.

Scoping involves clarifying the purpose of a project and the community, policy and programmatic context within which it will be or is already operating. It includes determining who the key stakeholders are, what information they need and why. For example, is evaluative information required to inform policy, address regulatory implications, influence advocacy initiatives or refine operational strategies? It is important at this stage to build common understandings and expectations about MERI and ensure that there is alignment with the project approach and principles. In considering the context of the project and evaluation, it is important to be mindful of transcultural considerations and any potential conflict that may arise due to personalities or differences in perspectives. Being realistic about constraints, such as available resources including time, money and skills, helps to determine the capacity and identify potential risk factors. Undertaking a risk analysis and determining mitigation strategies helps to minimize the 'foul-up factors'. This step is essentially about agreeing on the MERI purpose and parameters, and determining what is enough.

Programme logic is a diagrammatic map developed with key stakeholders depicting the proposed pathways by which project actions are intended to

deliver desired shorter- and longer-term outcomes and so collectively achieve the aim and objectives. It is based on the project's theory of change; if we do this, then X and Y will happen. Its participatory development allows everyone an opportunity to develop a shared understanding of how all aspects of the project can work together to effect change, and in the process of collaborative development allows key assumptions to be unpacked and addressed. It encourages smart, integrated thinking by illustrating how actions and processes can simultaneously contribute to achieving multiple outcomes; this results in a 'noodle' pathway diagram rather than linear or 'pillared' approach. There should be a mix of outcomes reflecting client/community needs, advocacy and networking initiatives and organizational requirements.

Key evaluation questions and measures of success need to be focused and limited to collectively determine the most important things the community and stakeholders want to know about the project's performance. While keeping key agreed project outcomes in mind, as set out in the programme logic, it is useful to develop a set of generic questions that everyone can use to capture and assess the project experience, such as:

- What has been happening? Who has been doing what, with whom and how?
- What has worked well and why?
- What have been the challenges and how have they been managed?
- 'So what' has changed? What has been the most significant change and why? Any unexpected changes?
- What has been learnt?
- How will learning be applied in the future? How will we know if this has occurred?

These questions can then be supplemented with targeted and/or technical questions about specific elements of the project's design, implementation and management. In more sophisticated evaluations, a range of questions will be developed that address each element in the programme logic.

It is important to agree upon the measures or indicators to be used. In community-based work, a combination of quantitative, qualitative and process indicators is generally required to capture the information needed to generate meaningful evidence-based responses to key evaluation questions. These are best formulated by asking stakeholders, 'What will change look like?'

M&E methods also need to be focused and limited to make best use of the resources available and ensure that they can answer the key evaluation questions in a way that helps build a portfolio of evidence. In selecting an appropriate mix of methods, collectively they should:

- Employ participatory methods and processes that are meaningful to the project community and key stakeholders.
- Align programme and evaluation principles and approaches.
- Consider how collectively the same methods can serve formative, baseline and summative evaluation purposes.
- Build on existing data and processes.
- Take account of local capacity, including skills, time, language and resources for people to engage as coevaluators and participants.
- Utilize techniques such as thematic analysis and triangulation to enhance rigour.

There is an enormous range of participatory M&E methods available to choose from. Commonly, community projects will use a combination of methods, such as data review, semistructured interviews or conversations, focus groups, site visits, stories of significant change, and creative activities that enable stakeholders of different ages, abilities and experiences to engage equitably in M&E processes, including children and people with disabilities. Surveys are rarely used but can be valuable to canvass feedback from widely spread populations particularly where online options exist.

Information gathering and analysis occurs as a rolling process during information gathering, as well as a distinct step to formulate results and recommendations. These activities must be supported by strategies to ensure appropriate and effective systems for data and information recording, collection, collation, storage and retrieval. Respect must be given for different types of knowledge, as well as intellectual property requirements. Strategies for maintaining confidential-

ity are essential. Where possible, train local people to assist in gathering information and provide opportunities for stakeholders to review and critique emerging findings and codevelop results and recommendations. It is best to collect less and use more; consider how the information being gathered can serve multiple functions including reports, media, advocacy, education and publicity.

Reporting and communicating results to key internal and external stakeholders addresses accountability requirements. Give consideration to who needs what information and in what form; while governments and donors expect written documents, community people may prefer information to be disseminated and discussed through forums and social media. Literacy and disability impairments may influence how reporting and communication occurs. Engage key project participants in sharing their experience with stakeholders.

Learning and improvement is core to the MERI process and requires project facilitators to develop embedded processes for reflection, learning and improvement across the project cycle with stakeholders. This can include utilizing existing monitoring, review and performance management strategies, staff development and mentoring activities, and community forums. Structuring these into project design and implementation processes at the outset demonstrates a commitment to learning and continual improvement, supports problem solving and promotes capacity building, sustainability and transformation. It is important to monitor and evaluate the MERI plan itself; this is an important task to include in the overall MERI process.

Making MERI: Performance Story Reporting

PSR provides a structure and participatory process to systematically consolidate, manage and present information arising from implementation of the MERI plan. In addition to assessing the extent to which a project aim and objectives have been met, it explicitly addresses the 'so what' questions related to the change in knowledge, behaviour and health conditions or services. The PSR process does this by building multiple lines of evidence, empirical and experiential, quantitative and qualitative, against the hierarchy of outcomes as set out in the programme logic. This

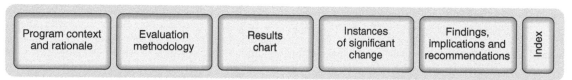

FIGURE 7-4 Performance story report structure.

portfolio of evidence assists stakeholders in assessing project performance, including through peer review or expert panels and participatory summit workshops as appropriate.

The process concludes with the production of a performance story report. This is a succinct document that balances completeness with conciseness; it can be as short as 10 to 15 pages. Figure 7-4 outlines the content and structure of a performance story report.

The programme context and rationale includes background information about the project and the context within which it operates, its location, objectives, structure and funding sources. It also includes the programme logic or project's theory of change.

The evaluation methodology briefly describes the approach and process used in undertaking the evaluation.

The results chart is a table containing the most relevant and rigorous evidence against the outcomes in the programme logic hierarchy. This is often provided as dot points, linked to sources listed in the index. Notes can be added to identify or explain unusual or skewed data or gaps in evidence.

Instances of significant change are carefully crafted stories of experience, often including reasons for significance as identified by participants at a PSR summit workshop. These stories contain insights and nuanced information that is unmeasurable but often catalytic in project processes and outcomes.

Findings, implications and recommendations comprise discussion framed by the evaluation questions, progress towards expected outcomes, unintended outcomes, contribution to the project aim, as well as key learning and implications, and recommendations for the future.

The index is a list of sources of evidence considered in the evaluation (including, e.g., documents reviewed, people interviewed, focus groups held) and any other references used in compiling findings and analysing results.

Together, MERI planning and PSR evaluation provide practitioners and stakeholders with a means to honour the way in which project activities are undertaken, as well as to systematically account for progress against desired outcomes, and to do so in a rigorous and ethical manner.

CONCLUSION

Community-based work and evaluation is complex and evolving. The demands on occupational therapists engaged in project work to evidence practice and change continue to grow. While acknowledging that no single approach will work in every context, this chapter has introduced a range of key professional and ethical considerations while advancing some practical strategies for tackling the challenges in undertaking effective project monitoring, evaluation, reporting and improvement.

REFERENCES

Australasian Evaluation Society (AES), 2013. Guidelines for the ethical conduct of evaluations. <www.aes.asn.au> (accessed 15.04.16.).

Berry, N., 2014. Did we do good? NGOs, conflicts of interest and the evaluation of short-term medical missions in Sololá, Guatemala. Soc. Sci. Med. 120, 344–351.

Clarinval, C., Biller-Andorno, N., 2014. Challenging operations: an ethical framework to assist humanitarian aid workers in their decision-making processes. PLoS Currents 6, 1–14.

Davies, R., Dart, J., 2005. The 'most significant change' technique. A guide to its use. <http://www.mande.co.uk/docs/MSCGuide .pdf> (accessed 15.04.16.).

Estrella, M. (Ed.), 2000. Learning from Change. Issues and Experiences in Participatory Monitoring and Evaluation. Intermediate Technology Publications and the International Development Research Centre, London and Ottawa.

Fetterman, D., Wandersman, A. (Eds.), 2005. Empowerment Evaluation: Principles in Practice. Guildford Press, New York.

Feuerstein, M.T., 1986. Partners in Evaluation. Evaluating Development and Community Programmes with Participants. Macmillan Publishers, London.

Greenaway, L., 2013. 'Evaluation that Empowers'. A model for generating evaluation-minded organisations. Eval. J. Austral. 13 (2), 3–8.

Guttman, N., 2000. Public Health Communication Interventions: Values and Ethical Dilemmas. Sage Publications, Thousand Oaks, CA.

Hillhort, D., 2002. Being Good at Doing Good? Quality and Accountability of Humanitarian NGOs. Disasters 26, 193–212.

Hunt, M., 2011. Establishing moral bearings: ethics and expatriate health care professionals in humanitarian work. Disasters 35 (3), 606–622.

Hunt, M., Schwartz, L., Sinding, C., Elit, L., 2014. The ethics of engaged presence: a framework for health professionals in humanitarian assistance and development work. Dev. World Bioeth. 14, 47–55.

International Federation of Red Cross (IFRC) and Red Crescent Societies, 1994. Code of Conduct for the International Red Cross and Red Crescent Movement and NGOs in Disaster Relief. IFRC, Geneva. <http://www.ifrc.org/Docs/idrl/I259EN.pdf> (accessed 15.04.16.).

Johnson, A., 2004. Engaging Queenslanders – Evaluating Community Engagement. Queensland Government Department of Communities, Brisbane, Australia.

Kaplan, A., 2002. Development Practitioners and Social Process. Artists of the Invisible. Pluto Press, London.

Komar Pikar Foundation, 2013. KPF MERI Framework. Developed in collaboration with K. Thomas, interPART. Komar Pikar Foundation, Phnom Penh, Cambodia.

Kotvojs, F., Hurworth, R., 2011. Making evaluations of capacity development programs more influential. Paper presented at the Australasian Evaluation Society International Conference, Sydney, Australia, 29 August – 2 September 2011. <http://www.aes.asn.au/previous-conferences/189-2011-aes-international-conference-sydney-presentations.html> (accessed 15.04.16.).

Kotvojs, F., Hurworth, R., 2013. Evaluating capacity development: what do we really want to know? Eval. J. Australas. 13 (1), 4–14.

Labonte, R., 2005. The future of health promotion. Health Promot. J. Austr. 16, 172–176.

Lentz, B., Imm, P., Yost, J., Johnson, N., Barron, C., Lindberg, M., et al., 2005. Empowerment evaluation and organizational learning: a case study of a community coalition designed to prevent child abuse and neglect'. In: Fetterman, D., Wandersman, A. (Eds.), Empowerment Evaluation: Principles in Practice. Guildford Press, New York.

Marsden, D., Oakley, P., Pratt, B., 1994. Measuring the Process: Guidelines for Evaluating Social Development. INTRAC, Oxford.

Mayhew, D., Kennedy, D., 2005. The Dark Sides of Virtue: Reassessing International Humanitarianism. Princeton University Press, Princeton, NJ.

Mayne, J., 2003. Reporting on outcomes: setting performance expectations and telling performance stories. Office of the Auditor General of Canada, Ottawa.

Mayoux, L., Chambers, R., 2005. Reversing the paradigm: quantification, participatory methods and pro-poor impact assessment. J. Int. Dev. 17 (2), 271–298.

McLaughlin, J., Jordan, G., 1999. Logic models: a tool for telling your program's performance story. Eval. Program. Plan. 22, 65–72.

Murdi Paaki Drug and Alcohol Network, 2012. MPDAN MERI Framework. Developed in collaboration with interPART. MPDAN, Orange, NSW, Australia.

Newell Sand Graham, A., 2012. Using an empowerment evaluation approach with community-based programs. Reflections from the front line. Eval. J. Australasia 12 (2), 15–27.

Oakley, P., Pratt, B., Clayton, A., 1998. Outcomes and Impact: Evaluating Change in Social Development. INTRAC, Oxford.

Pande, N., Dalal, A.K., 2004. In reflection: making sense of achievements and failures of a CBR initiative. Asia Pac. Disabil. Rehabil. J. 15, 95–105.

Patton, M.Q., 2002. Qualitative Research and Evaluation Methods, third ed. Sage Publications, London.

Patton, M.Q., 2008. Utilization-Focused Evaluation, fourth ed. Sage Publications, London.

Pawson, R., Greenhalgh, T., Harvey, G., Walshe, K., 2005. Realist review – a new method of systematic review designed for complex policy interventions. J. Health Serv. Res. Policy 10 (Suppl. 1), 21–34.

Pollard, N., Sakellariou, D., 2009. Is doing good 'good': professional motives vs. community need. Asia Pac. Disabil. Rehabil. J. 20 (2), 3–16.

Roughley, A., 2009. Developing and Using Program Logic in Natural Resource Management. User Guide. Commonwealth of Australia, Canberra, Australia.

Roughley, A., Dart, J., 2009. Developing a Performance Story Report. User Guide. Commonwealth of Australia, Canberra, Australia.

Rushford, N., Thomas, K., 2015. Disaster and Development. An Occupational Perspective. Elsevier, Oxford.

Scougall, J., 2006. Reconciling tensions between principles and practice in indigenous evaluation. Eval. J. Australas. 6 (2), 49–55.

Talbot, L., Verrinder, G., 2014. Promoting Health. The Primary Health Care Approach, fifth ed. Elsevier/Churchill Livingstone, Oxford.

Thomas, K., 2010. MERI Training Resource Materials. interPART, with reference to various sources including the Australian Government. Unpublished documents available from International Partners in Action, Research and Training. Macclesfield, South Australia.

Thomas, K., Allen, J., Biven, A., Lincoln, B., O'Donnell, K., 2012. Formative, Summative and Impact evaluations of the Murdi Paaki Drug and Alcohol Network MERI Framework. MPDAN and interPART, Orange, NSW, Australia.

Thomas, K., Allen, J., Biven, A., Lincoln, B., O'Donnell, K., 2013. Formative, Summative and Impact evaluations of the Murdi Paaki Drug and Alcohol Network MERI Framework. MPDAN and interPART, Orange, NSW, Australia.

Thomas, K., Allen, J., Biven, A., Lincoln, B., O'Donnell, K., 2015. Formative, Summative and Impact evaluations of the Murdi Paaki Drug and Alcohol Network MERI Framework. MPDAN and interPART, Orange, NSW, Australia.

Woodhill, J., Robins, L., 1998. Participatory evaluation for landcare and catchment groups. A guide for facilitators. Greening Australia, Canberra, Australia.

8

DESIGNING PARTICIPATORY ACTION RESEARCH TO RELOCATE MARGINS, BORDERS AND CENTRES

WENDY BRYANT ■ ANNA RACHEL PETTICAN ■ SIMONE COETZEE

CHAPTER OUTLINE

P articipatory action research methods are sometimes used to explore experiences of community projects. This approach to research can be enhanced by a critical and analytical grasp of the theory of occupational injustice and in particular occupational alienation, considering who is included in what, where and how. This chapter is illustrated by two participatory action research projects in London, UK: first, an organizational case study of a market garden, and second, a participatory action research project involving members of a football club. These projects were led by occupational therapy researchers who were experts in using occupation to promote and enable participation of relevant groups, including people often marginalized from research because of their learning disabilities or mental health problems. As researchers, we used our expertise, based on practical skills and advanced understanding of participation, to overcome real and imagined barriers. This enabled diverse voices to be heard within discourses about how vulnerable people can achieve social inclusion through community projects.

This expertise could translate into research activity, drawing on professional occupational therapy prac-

tice. The skill of analysing activities and adapting them can be applied to doing collaborative research. Knowledge about the impact of health problems on human function can be used for research design, anticipating and resolving possible problems. Reflection in action and reasoning skills can be used to create opportunities and shape experiences at all stages. The central focus on occupation gives particular value to doing things with people in real-world settings. Thus it has to be questioned why so much occupational therapy research is based on controlled and contrived measuring (Gillen, 2013), or encounters with disabled people that are restricted to verbal exchanges of experiences and opinions. It has been suggested that there are limitations to the randomized controlled trial or qualitative studies based on interviews (Greenhalgh et al., 2014). Yet, a growing number of occupational therapists and many others recognize the potential of engaging people in participatory action research to understand experiences of disability and the impact of health problems (Jagosh et al., 2012).

This chapter offers analysis and reflection on how participatory action research design can create opportunities for the people involved to experience a sense of belonging and shared ownership of research outcomes and products, overcoming occupational alienation.

PARTICIPATORY ACTION RESEARCH DEFINED AND DISCUSSED

By definition, research involving human subjects requires participation. Participatory action research aims to actively involve people in the research process, drawing on their expertise, knowledge, skills and experiences to give the research findings authenticity (Jagosh et al., 2012). The essential use of 'participant' information sheets to ensure people are able to consent in an informed way illustrates the focus on participation in the ethical review process. Generally in research ethics approval it is assumed that participants will be subject to one or more procedures, defined and stated clearly to guarantee that no harm will be done (INVOLVE, 2012). This approach of subjecting people to defined procedures, reflects a scientific worldview which seeks to see participants as human subjects responding to an identified independent variable. Alternatively, participants can be seen as having a relevant experience or knowledge which can be extracted using interviews. Either view gives narrow recognition of what participants can contribute to healthcare research.

Participatory action research is an approach to research or a methodology, rather than a single method, valuing combinations of methods which involve people as active participants. Therefore, methods such as interviewing and measuring can still be used. Multiple methods can be used to build a detailed data set, analysed and interpreted to elicit new knowledge and understandings of human experience, especially from people who are often excluded from research, because of perceived difficulties associated with disability, communication and/or acute ill health. This exclusion means that participatory action research often has an emancipatory purpose, giving a voice to people who would otherwise not be heard (Faulkner, 2004).

This focus on including people who are marginalized for various and often multiple reasons resonates with occupational therapists who work to promote occupational justice. Wilcock (2006) proposed that participatory approaches are fundamentally important for highlighting how occupational injustices are

---

BOX 8-1

DEFINITION OF OCCUPATIONAL ALIENATION

Occupational alienation is indicated when a person is doing something he or she is not engaging with (Bryant, 2014). This is indicated in lay terms such as 'going through the motions' or 'her heart wasn't in it'. Repeatedly experiencing occupational alienation has adverse consequences for health, associated with prolonged exposure to the physiological and psychological stress response. A person may feel they are not themselves, suggesting an intrapersonal, or internal, sense of alienation which in extreme situations would be dissociation. The person may also be socially alienated from others. It is useful to distinguish among occupational, intrapersonal and social alienation.

---

experienced. There can be a simultaneous focus on investigating occupational injustices as research topics and at the same time designing research to minimize occupational injustices, such as occupational alienation, being experienced by participants during the study.

OCCUPATIONAL ALIENATION

Researchers can engage with the challenges of participatory action research in a practical way, using the idea of occupational alienation, which is defined in Box 8-1. It is closely related to other forms of occupational injustice and can be addressed by attending to several factors. One is the occupational form or way in which a person is doing something; this can be adapted or changed to be more engaging, satisfying or meaningful. Involving the person in this process of adaptation gives them more control of the occupation, or what they are doing, so that they feel a greater sense of ownership. The occupation can then be considered to belong to them, being part of their occupational identity. These elements are core to therapeutic practice and should be equally valued in participatory action research (Bryant, 2014). Participatory action research offers an opportunity to understand alienation and demonstrate within the research process how to address it, through inclusive and collaborative projects. However, there can be concern about how researchers prepare people for the inevitable end of the project. Occupational therapists have skills and knowledge of how to manage the therapeutic process, so that the people they work with are aware of the ending and prepared for it. This knowledge can be used in participatory action research: recognizing that endings are important for a sense of achievement. This apparent limitation of participatory action research – that it comes to an end which might distress participants – should not be seen as a reason not to do the project at all, but represents a call to focus on the ethical aspects of enabling and supporting participation in an honest and fair way. Allied to this, and evident in our examples, is the idea that participation can be transitory and situated at any point on a participation continuum, such as the one proposed by Bradbury and Huang (2010). This continuum suggests involvement can vary from being a key person in shaping and implementing research to making a one-off response. People can vary their own involvement over time, giving them flexibility as a human resource for the project and making the best use of their individual capacities. The process of deciding the nature of involvement is an ongoing part of collaboration, with times when possibilities have to be explored and negotiated which might leave people feeling alienated. Openly valuing diverse activities and occupations can prevent occupational and social alienation, or at least enable participants to be aware that the situation could be transitory and renegotiated. Occupational alienation is a risk factor for occupational injustice, so in the long term people can explore how they are alienated as an issue of injustice and institute changes from the findings.

In this chapter, we focus on processes rather than outcomes of research, seeing occupational alienation as an issue of belonging and ownership, rather than focusing on negative feelings which have been emphasized in previous definitions (Wilcock 2006). Being actively involved overcomes marginalization and strengthens evidence, influencing future service structures and approaches. Participatory action research is much more than people becoming participants. The examples in this chapter seek to illustrate the opportunities, challenges, benefits and tensions in detail.

CASE 8-1

'Seeing Myself Doing': *An Organizational Case Study Involving People with Learning Disabilities, Exploring Inclusion and Occupation in a Market Garden*

This research project was based with a social enterprise run by a cooperative. The cooperative had established themselves initially in an allotment space as a small community gardening project, which grew into a larger organization on the outskirts of London. The social enterprise now has several branches to it: a 12-acre market garden, a community café and many small 'outreach' gardens in previously unused spaces. There is a core of dedicated volunteers and paid workers involved in each branch. The cooperative is committed to running the organization according to permaculture philosophy. This philosophy encourages a creative design process in which relationships and knowledge learned from the natural world are used to build sustainable, resilient and ecologically mindful growing spaces, services and communities, grounded on three ethics (Holmgren,

2011). The three ethics are 'earth care, people care and fair shares', demonstrating the broad scope of the permaculture philosophy and its application to health and social care and community development. These ethics, together with 12 guiding principles of permaculture design (Holmgren, 2011) such as 'value the marginal' and 'integrate rather than segregate', arguably encourage a naturally inclusive culture.

A volunteer in the organization, Simone was interested in whether the permaculture approach created a space of less judgement, where people with differing abilities felt able to participate within their individual capacities. The cooperative members and the garden participants were interested in understanding this, too, and evaluating whether changes could be made within their practice to enable further

Continued on following page

'Seeing Myself Doing': *An Organizational Case Study Involving People with Learning Disabilities, Exploring Inclusion and Occupation in a Market Garden (Continued)*

inclusion of people with different abilities within their gardening community. Simone proposed a research design that would fit with the ethos of the cooperative. Participatory action research met this aim, being based on collaborative enquiry and focused on community empowerment (Denzin and Lincoln, 2011), both characteristics that reflected the cooperative's own values.

As a social enterprise, the market garden cooperative aimed to share knowledge and skills about food growing and self-sufficiency, providing a space for people to participate in outdoor activity in a social environment. They had a specific outreach focus for people with learning disabilities or mental health problems who, due to their disability, experienced both occupational alienation (due to limited work and leisure opportunities) and social alienation, due to a reduction in local services. Cooperative members, Simone and garden volunteers, wanting to understand the organization's specific contribution to local services and to individual participants with disabilities more clearly, aimed to explore the social and occupational experiences of participants in the market garden. The research aimed to include everyone willing to participate, with and without a declared disability. Consideration was given to making research information and methods as accessible as possible, and personal assistants were included in the research group to enable participation. Here, the participatory action research group with people with learning disabilities is discussed, as it highlighted the most important issues raised with regards to social and occupational alienation.

This group involved a mix of some new and some repeat participants in a 10-week programme that normally focused only on basic gardening skills. In this case, basic gardening skills were covered, alongside additional research activities aiming to capture the gardening experience as it happened. This involved Simone co-facilitating the group as researcher and facilitator in the gardening space alongside another garden worker, doing food growing,

mapping and other garden maintenance tasks while exploring how the experience contributed to a sense of ownership and belonging.

The group's communication skills varied widely, some participants being vocal and others having no verbal communication at all, although all had a variety of ways to communicate needs, wants and dislikes. Simone considered this when choosing the methods of data gathering, along with the issue of the group not knowing each other and consequently lacking in social confidence. Activity participation was more successful in engaging the group than traditional group discussions were. For Simone, this highlighted the difference between social and occupational perspectives: facilitating occupational engagement would lead to a greater sense of social inclusion due to acknowledgement from cooperative members and other volunteers of their coparticipation in and contribution to the garden in multiple ways. This is supported by findings from Fieldhouse (2003) and Sempik et al. (2005).

'IN THE MOMENT' ENGAGEMENT: THE BUILDING BLOCKS TO LONGER-TERM ENGAGEMENT

The group was captivated by novel occupations, including gardening and maintenance activities on the site and, in particular, the main activity of growing vegetables. These occupations were novel to them, because elsewhere gardens were inaccessible and sometimes hostile environments, for them and for other disabled people. Occupational alienation is evident when people cannot participate in a meaningful way and have to observe or undertake very limited tasks. This organization, however, held that all gardening tasks should make a contribution to the site or food production to prevent tokenistic participation. One participant, Leo (all names are pseudonyms), felt that he did not enjoy all the tasks, but the advantage of being on such a big growing site was that there was always something that was engaging to do. Being given the opportunity to try out different tasks was one of the most important

'Seeing Myself Doing': *An Organizational Case Study Involving People with Learning Disabilities, Exploring Inclusion and Occupation in a Market Garden (Continued)*

things to him: 'I mean, if you don't like it they give you a chance to say but at least you had the chance to do it. Which is really good'.

Early on in the research project, Simone observed that the group members with learning disabilities sometimes had difficulty remembering activities or information from week to week, resulting in the loss of connection with place and occupation and suggesting a problem with ownership. So, she adapted the research design to incorporate activities such as taking photographs of each other doing tasks in the garden, capturing parts of the site they liked and being photographed doing activities they liked by other group members. The analysis of these photographs as a group enabled the participants to:

1. See themselves making a contribution towards the wider garden community's aim of production and distribution of fresh fruit and vegetables;
2. Reflect on the physical and sensory experiences of the activities, their meaning and the environment, and evaluate their positive or negative experiences; and
3. See themselves as part of a consistent group of gardeners who could recall shared weekly events and position these within seasonal growing calendars.

The use of photography became key in facilitating a sense of ownership and belonging. Another activity that contributed to a sense of belonging was constructing a wall-sized map of the garden. The participants attached photographs of themselves as individuals in places they liked most and drew or attached other artefacts to it to represent activities they had done. Figure 8-1 is an example of this. The map was a reflective tool, and like the photographs, it contributed to a growing confidence in what they were doing both as individuals and as a group.

TIME AND FAMILIARITY EMBED OWNERSHIP

The occupation of gardening together, including the embodied sensory and visual involvement, enabled

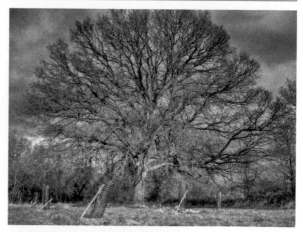

FIGURE 8-1 ■ The mapping task: the group identified an ancient tree they all admired as a landmark. They eventually referred to it as 'Big Tree' as it developed more meaning for them. *(Photograph taken by research participant.)*

participants to develop a greater sense of familiarity with each other and of being 'in place'. They felt part of a larger food growing community, identifying their own contribution to production for the vegetable box scheme, pest and soil management and seasonal growing tasks, as well as expanding on activities for the following term. Two members considered the option of joining the permanent volunteer team as they felt they wanted a more regular involvement in the garden. Others committed to return on a termly basis for supported sessions.

They reflected on all of this in the group meetings. As the familiarity grew, the sense of ownership within the group also developed. Members took on the responsibility to bring shared food for break times and when reflecting on the photographs, the group members started to relate and refer to each other, not just themselves. Issues of occupational alienation, including participating in research that lacks meaning to the individual, can be addressed by using inclusive research methods. The participatory action research group experienced 'in the moment' or transient engagement in the tasks. This

Continued on following page

CASE 8-1

'Seeing Myself Doing': *An Organizational Case Study Involving People with Learning Disabilities, Exploring Inclusion and Occupation in a Market Garden (Continued)*

engagement was consolidated each week to embed ownership of the tasks and the place and a familiarity with each other. Time to engage with places within the site and being acknowledged through photographs as 'doing' were key aspects of building a sense of meaning into occupations, a sense of ownership of the outcomes produced and a sense of belonging to and within a space or organization. The philosophy of the organization, engendering an inclusive, nontokenistic attitude, could reduce occupational alienation for people with learning disabilities.

BY SIMONE COETZEE

CASE 8-2

Ways of Being Involved: *Participatory Action Research with members of a community-based football club*

Our second example is participatory action research with the Positive Mental Attitude (PMA) Sports Academy. It particularly illustrates how an occupational justice perspective can shape and inform the participatory action research process over time. The PMA is a registered charity in the UK and has been operating academies in London and Yorkshire that utilize sport, mainly football, as a therapeutic activity to support the lives of people living with mental health problems. Mental health service users become players within a community-based football team, which ultimately forms part of a PMA league. The research study sought to explore the experience of participating in the PMA from the perspective of those who take part. Through structured discussion with the PMA players, two aspects of their participation in the PMA were identified as important: the nature of participation in the organization and the value derived from taking part. Throughout the PMA, research study has been focused on access to meaningful occupation as a matter of justice (Durocher et al., 2014), and therefore there has been a fundamental concern with offering multiple and inclusive ways of being involved. A research steering group was convened, with Anna initially engaging players and gaining perspectives by fitting into existing PMA structures and activities, such as training sessions and team meetings. Unusually, the research impetus came from the organization itself, which was looking for a researcher to evaluate and explore the work it was doing. Therefore a collaborative partnership was relatively easy to establish between Anna and the members of the research steering group. The level of involvement of the steering group members was openly discussed and debated whenever necessary in order to avoid any misinterpretation about where on the participation continuum the research expectations and activities were occurring at any given time (Bradbury Huang, 2010). However, active involvement in all stages of the research study was sought, rather than one-off consultation.

Porter et al. (2006) discussed the practical challenges that can make or break efforts to establish such a steering group. With the PMA, efforts were continuously made to reduce the practical disruption that might potentially occur from participating. For example, the research steering group meetings were scheduled to take place immediately after a football training session, so that no additional travel was necessary, while the location of meeting was negotiated and flexible, with numerous meetings taking place within a preferred local community café setting. Participants were able to attend such meetings accompanied by a support worker, leave for periods of time to manage difficult or distressing thoughts, and help themselves to refreshments. The value of creating space (in terms of both physical space and time) has been indicated in other participatory action research projects, such as the project by the Researching Psychosis Together group (2012; Bryant et al.,

Ways of Being Involved: *Participatory Action Research with members of a community-based football club (Continued)*

2012). For the PMA study, the temporal structure of the football season[1] was useful in framing a cycle of planning, action and reflection.

Furthermore, data collection was planned in the form of related strands, to offer diverse ways of being involved and with the open acknowledgement that data collection methods are not culturally neutral (Rose, 2014). Instead, data collection methods were chosen and planned with the aim of reflecting the PMA's cultural processes of knowledge production and with the intention of enabling expression and communication. For example, the first strand of data collection consisted of a series of open participation research world café events (Brown and Issacs, 2005), which sought to replicate the familiar and accessible environment of the community cafés regularly accessed by the players after training sessions and matches. The world cafés involved structuring group discussions within a café-like environment, with refreshments and paper tablecloths, where participants could write or draw their responses to research questions and topics. Through the PMA research steering group meetings it had been observed that community café spaces provided players with an important place for discussion, reflection, match analysis and team planning. The world café was therefore agreed as a method that would be accessible and inclusive to those involved. The café events engaged people in collaborative discussions and players were free to move around the tables in their own time, responding to each of the table questions and recording their discussion on the paper tablecloths on each table. The café environment, the refreshments available and the rituals and activities involved provided focus for conversations, associations and collaboration. The series of café events also offered the opportunity for players to observe participation before deciding whether or not to take part. Similarly to previous activity-orientated data collection (Redwood et al., 2012), this method avoided the direct style of questioning associated with conventional qualitative interviewing and sought to provide a sensitive and familiar (to the players) way of facilitating expression.

The work of the PMA research steering group and the resulting methods of data collection can be linked with the concept of occupational marginalization, which is explained as arising from situations where individuals or groups may not have been afforded the choice to participate in valued occupations, and may be relegated to those that are less prestigious or allow little choice, control or opportunity for decision making (Stadnyk et al., 2010; Townsend and Wilcock, 2004). This concept is relevant to the PMA research study because established power relations were fundamentally challenged by the involvement of mental health service users in the entire research process, rather than a more conventional and narrow involvement as research participant. The aim is that such active participation contributes towards meaningful social change (Beresford, 2005, 2013). Additionally, the strands of data collection provided dynamic and alternative methods of engaging PMA players in diverse and culturally meaningful ways, with the intention of increasing participation amongst a frequently excluded group of individuals (Department of Health, 2010).

The second data collection strand involved players participating in a walking interview (Evans and Jones, 2011), as the nature of participation in the PMA is synonymous with being outdoors and frequenting specific places and spaces (such as football training pitches, local community cafés and the league clubhouse). Walking (Evans and Jones, 2011) or 'go-along' (Carpiano, 2009) interviews involve a researcher walking with a participant, and it is argued that richer data are generated because participants are prompted by meanings and connections to the surrounding environment (Carpiano, 2009). Similarly to the first strand, this method of data collection sought to enhance data elicitation by avoiding a direct style of questioning. Instead, topics were introduced in a conversational style and through the environmental prompts of places visited and seen. The topics introduced were based on findings from the first strand. This did not mean that only players who had participated in the first strand

Continued on following page

could take part in the second strand, as the PMA study's data collection took place over a period of 3 years. A further third strand involved repeating the walking interviews with some players. This data collection occurred after the London PMA project had ceased and a group of players had decided to continue the football teams as an informal service user-led community project. Throughout the study transitory involvement was very much accommodated and valued, due to unavoidable fluctuations in health, interest and personal circumstances. The method was flexible enough to enable players to construct meaning for themselves. For example,

some players chose to complete the walking interview individually so that it provided a private, confidential space, whilst others completed it as a paired experience because they felt this was representative of their participation in the PMA. Additionally, some used the walking interview as an opportunity to complete other tasks, such as buying food and holding conversations. This method of data collection can therefore be linked back to the earlier outline of addressing occupational alienation, in terms of involving participants in the process of adapting an occupation in order to promote belonging and ownership.

[1]The length and time of year of a football season varies around the world, but typically the season comprises a single period within the year in which league competition is contested alongside any cup competitions. The typical English football season occurs August through May.

BY ANNA PETTICAN

CONCLUSIONS

Research methods can provide a platform through which different understandings and experiences can be captured, to address gaps in knowledge that result from exclusion. The two research studies presented in this chapter focused on access to meaningful occupation and participation as a matter of justice. It is important to be creative and culturally sensitive, particularly when researching with often excluded and seldom heard groups and individuals. In theory, applying the principles of occupational justice to the research process and topic should be straightforward for occupational therapists, who use occupation as a means and ends for transformation (Creek, 2009). In practice, there are challenges. This could be due to a dominant mechanistic metaphor for practice and research, where toolkits and skills are emphasized. Even the metaphors of pathways and flowcharts control the direction of collaborative work, with little consideration of what to do when the tools fail and the pathways are blocked. It has to be recognized that people will define their own way of participating, in negotiation with others. Sometimes it is necessary to be on the margins of group activity and collaboration,

and other times to be in the centre. The cycles of action and reflection, common to all action research, can be essential to enable researchers and participants to negotiate their participation and avoid enduring occupational and social alienation (Reason and Bradbury, 2008). As participants become more familiar with each other and the research process, the cycle can become a valued structure to support the development of new understandings. This suggests an evolving, organic, living process (Mancini, 2011).

In this chapter, we have explored how concepts such as occupational alienation and occupational marginalization can be used to inform research practice when participatory approaches are used. Occupational therapists are urged to consider what participatory action research could bring to their own enquiries, as a means of enabling occupational justice and engaging with marginalized populations.

REFERENCES

Beresford, P., 2005. Developing the theoretical basis for service user/survivor-led research and equal involvement in research. Epidemiol. Psichiatr. Soc. 14 (1), 4–9.

Beresford, P., 2013. From 'other' to involved: user involvement in research: an emerging paradigm. Nordic Social Work Res. 1–10

Available at: <www.tandfonline.com/doi/full/10.1080/2156857X.2013.835138> (accessed 25.09.13.).

Bradbury Huang, H., 2010. What is good action research? Why the resurgent interest? Action Res. 8 (1), 93–109.

Brown, J., Issacs, D., 2005. The World Café: Shaping Our Future through Conversations that Matter. Berrett-Koehler Publishers Inc, San Francisco.

Bryant, W., 2014. A definition of occupational alienation. <https://drwendy08.wordpress.com/2014/11/21/defining-occupational-alienation/> (accessed 18.04.16.).

Bryant, W., Parsonage, J., Tibbs, A., Andrews, C., Clark, J., Franco, L., 2012. Meeting in the mist: key considerations in a collaborative research partnership with people with mental health issues. Work 43 (1), 23–31.

Carpiano, R.M., 2009. Come take a walk with me: the 'go-along' interview as a novel method for studying the implications of place for health and well-being. Health Place 15, 263–272.

Creek, J., 2009. Something lost and something gained. Ment. Health Occup. Ther. 14 (2), 45–51.

Denzin, N.K., Lincoln, Y.S., 2011. The SAGE Handbook of Qualitative Research, fourth ed. Sage Publications, Inc: London.

Department of Health, 2010. High Quality Care for All; Inclusion Health: Improving Primary Care for Socially Excluded People. DH, London.

Durocher, E., Gibson, B.E., Rappolt, S., 2014. Occupational justice: a conceptual review. J. Occup. Sci. 21 (4), 418–430.

Evans, J., Jones, P., 2011. The walking interview: methodology, mobility and place. Appl. Geogr. 31 (2), 849–858.

Faulkner, A., 2004. The Ethics of Survivor Research. Guidelines for the Ethical Conduct of Research Carried out by Mental Health Users and Survivors. The Policy Press, Bristol, UK.

Fieldhouse, J., 2003. The impact of an allotment group on mental health clients' health, wellbeing and social networking. Br. J. Occup. Ther. 66 (7), 286–296.

Gillen, G., 2013. A fork in the road: an occupational hazard? (Eleanor Clarke Slagle Lecture). Am. J. Occup. Ther. 67, 641–652.

Greenhalgh, T.J., Howick, N., Maskrey, N., et al., 2014. Evidence based medicine: a movement in crisis? Br. Med. J. 348 (4), g3725–g3725.

Holmgren, D., 2011. Permaculture: Principles and Pathways Beyond Sustainability. Permanent Publications, Hampshire, UK.

INVOLVE, 2012. Public Involvement in Research: Impact on Ethical Aspects of Research. INVOLVE, Eastleigh, UK.

Jagosh, J., Macaulay, A., Pluye, P., Salsberg, J., Bush, P., Henderson, J., 2012. Uncovering the benefits of participatory research: implications of a realist review for health research and practice. Milbank Q. 90 (2), 311–346.

Mancini, M., 2011. Understanding change in community mental health practices through critical discourse analysis. Br. J. Social Work 41, 645–667.

Porter, J., Parsons, S., Robertson, C., 2006. Time for review: supporting the work of an advisory group. J. Res. Spec. Educ. Needs 6 (1), 11–16.

Reason, P., Bradbury, H. (Eds.), 2008. The Sage Handbook of Action Research. Participative Inquiry and Practice, second ed. Sage Publications, Los Angeles.

Redwood, S., Gale, N., Greenfield, S., 2012. 'You give us rangoli, we give you talk': using an art-based activity to elicit data from a seldom heard group. BMC Med. Res. Methodol. 12, 7.

Researching Psychosis Together. 2012. Living with Psychosis. Report for Hillingdon Mind and CNWL Mental Health NHS Foundation Trust. <http://bura.brunel.ac.uk/handle/2438/7462> (accessed 18.04.16.).

Rose, G., 2014. On the relation between 'visual research methods' and contemporary visual culture. Soc. Rev. 62 (1), 24–46.

Sempik, J., Aldridge, J., Becker, S. (Eds.), 2005. Health, Well-being and Social Inclusion – Therapeutic Horticulture in the UK. Policy Press, University of Bristol, in association with Thrive, Bristol, UK.

Stadnyk, R.L., Townsend, E.A., Wilcock, A.A., 2010. Occupational justice. In: Christiansen, C.H., Townsend, E.A. (Eds.), Introduction to Occupation: The Art and Science of Living, second ed. Prentice Hall, Englewood Cliffs, NJ, pp. 329–358.

Townsend, E., Wilcock, A., 2004. Occupational justice and client-centred practice: a dialogue in progress. Can. J. Occup. Ther. 71 (2), 75–87.

Wilcock, A., 2006. An Occupational Perspective of Health, second ed. Slack Inc, Thorofare, NJ.

SECTION 2

EXPLORING OCCUPATION AND JUSTICE

9

OCCUPATIONAL JUSTICE IN EVERYDAY OCCUPATIONAL THERAPY PRACTICE

ANTOINE L. BAILLIARD ■ REBECCA M. ALDRICH

CHAPTER OUTLINE

Since the 1990s, occupational scientists and occupational therapists have sought to develop and clarify the concepts of occupational justice and injustice. Durocher, Rappolt and Gibson (2014) state that 'occupational justice is oriented to promoting fairness, equity, and empowerment to enable opportunities for participation in occupations for the purposes of health and quality of life' (pp. 431–432). Occupational injustice implies the inverse of occupational justice, referring to situations in which people are unable to access or participate in meaningful occupations due to factors beyond their control. Ideas about occupational justice have been translated from academic discourses into frameworks (Whiteford and Townsend, 2011) and questionnaires (Wilcock and Townsend, 2014) that aim to identify and ameliorate occupational injustices.

The shift from theoretical development to application may seem to suggest consensus regarding the concepts of occupational justice and injustice; however, continued debate indicates that the conversation is still evolving.

One facet of the dialogue about occupational justice deserves particular attention: scholars and practitioners question whether or not occupational therapists can seek justice through everyday practices. Prior to addressing this question, we would like to identify aspects of the dialogue that we will not include in this chapter. Wilcock and Hocking (2015) proposed that 'discussions of occupational justice are underpinned by a growing awareness that odious and health-depleting occupations are unfairly apportioned across different groups in society and that some groups are excluded from beneficial occupations that support and enhance health' (p. 392). This statement suggests that some occupations are 'good' and that others are 'bad'. Although we recognize that social and cultural values can make some occupations seem beneficial and others harmful, we will not address the inherent value of particular occupations in relation to occupational justice. In line with other elements of Wilcock and Hocking's argument, however, we *will* focus on how to develop a better understanding of the circumstances that give people particular possibilities (Laliberte Rudman, 2010) to engage in occupations. In addition, Whiteford et al. (2016) set up a dichotomous view of occupational therapy, suggesting that 'critical occupational therapy practice [that takes up issues of occupational justice] diverges from general occupational therapy through an explicit focus on disadvantaged and oppressed populations, and on processes that bring critical awareness to, and target change in, broad environmental forces' (p. 9). We agree that applying a critical perspective can change the scope of occupational therapy practice; however, we believe that setting critical occupational therapy apart from 'general' practice only serves to make occupational justice appear further removed from everyday life and occupational therapy. Therefore our discussion focuses on how a critical awareness of social and political circumstances can be brought into all occupational therapy practices.

Although occupational science and occupational therapy's 'awakening to occupational injustice' (Townsend and Marval, 2013, p. 216) has foregrounded the pursuit of justice via everyday interventions, it seems that the idea of occupational injustice tends to be associated with 'extreme' life situations that hinder occupational performance. As explained in the coming pages, by 'extreme' situations, we refer to circumstances that tend to lie outside the dominant or middle-class socioeconomic experience. We believe that the social positioning of many occupational therapists fosters 'extreme' connotations of occupational injustice. Systemic barriers that limit equitable access to education, combined with the need for advanced education to practice occupational therapy, make it common for occupational therapists to occupy socioeconomic positions that are not marginalized or disadvantaged. If a majority of occupational therapists belong to 'agent' social groups (Harro, 1999) that possess more relative power in society, they may not

regularly experience injustices and consequently may feel that seeking occupational justice is not a part of their practices (Galvin et al., 2011). In this chapter, we propose ways to reframe the conversation about occupational injustice to better illuminate how promoting justice falls under the purview of everyday occupational therapy practices.

Throughout our discussion, the phrase *everyday occupational therapy practice* will refer to practice settings and client populations that are considered 'traditional' in Western and Northern parts of the world. Such a focus does not aim to diminish the importance of other practice situations or disregard how the conversation about occupational justice has developed outside Western and Northern domains; rather, the purpose of this reference point is to break down potential 'extreme/everyday' dichotomies and encourage *all* occupational therapists to view their practices as justice-promoting efforts. In the coming pages, we reinforce the belief that occupational injustices arise when *any* person experiences *any* situation that prevents access to meaningful occupations. As Wilcock and Hocking (2015) note, occupational injustices are much more than instances of unhappiness: they arise when everyday realities squander human potential and foster social strife. In line with that perspective, we aim to demonstrate how everyday occupational therapy practices already acknowledge potentials for injustice and constitute the active pursuit of justice.

We will begin by reviewing the conceptual development of occupational justice and discussing theoretical underpinnings that support occupational therapy as a justice-focused practice. We will also offer examples of practice frameworks and educational approaches that underscore the link between everyday occupational therapy practices and occupational justice. We will end by discussing the implications of orienting occupational therapy practice more broadly to the pursuit of justice.

BACKGROUND

Imbalanced Connotations of Occupational Justice

Evelyne Durocher, Gibson, and Rappolt (2014) undertook a scoping review to clarify the conceptual development of occupational justice in the occupational science and occupational therapy literature. Their review yielded four articles and nine book chapters that substantively addressed occupational justice and injustice, all of which have informed our position in this chapter. Table 9-1 sorts examples of occupational injustice in scholarly literature based on our analytic distinction between 'everyday' and 'extreme' situations, where everyday situations represent those more familiar to people who occupy a dominant social position. For instance, although homelessness is becoming more common and is experienced as an everyday situation for people who do not have stable shelter, it is not a situation that dominant social groups will typically experience and it is not directly addressed in traditional occupational therapy practice settings. Accordingly, for the purposes of this chapter, we have classified homelessness as a situation that might be perceived as extreme, and therefore outside the arena of everyday occupational therapy practice. As Table 9-1 illustrates, published literature about occupational injustices references more than twice as many everyday situations than extreme situations. Given the prevalence of everyday examples of occupational injustice in existing scholarship, why might occupational injustice continue to be primarily associated with extreme situations? We suggest two factors to explain this phenomenon: (a) occupational therapists' typical social positioning shapes their perception of everyday versus extreme forms of injustice, and (b) extreme examples are easier to understand and remember than everyday examples because they seem to represent more urgent needs. Although Townsend and Wilcock (2004) assert that 'justice is an implicit, invisible foundation' of occupational therapy in general (p. 77), repeated references to situations of slavery, refugeeism and incarceration in the literature overshadow the idea of justice in relation to everyday practice. This may illuminate Galvin et al.'s (2011) finding that occupational therapists do not see occupational justice as relevant to their traditional practices: If therapists in traditional settings tend to associate occupational justice with extreme situations, then that association may override the connection between occupational justice and everyday practice.

Durocher, Gibson and Rappolt's (2014) scoping review found that the concept of occupational justice: (a) assumes that humans have a right to use their unique set of capacities to achieve well-being within their circumstances (Stadnyk, Townsend and Wilcock, 2010), but (b) is fraught with 'the lack of conceptual clarity regarding how to determine which occupations should be prevented or compelled for which individuals' (Durocher, Gibson and Rappolt, 2014, p. 423). This second finding highlights an important consideration for locating justice within everyday occupational therapy practice: how can practitioners determine what *is* and *is not* a situation of occupational injustice, and *who* ought to address identified injustices? Or, as Wilcock and Hocking (2015) phrased it, how can practitioners employ an 'occupational justice approach to health' (p. 404)?

Political Awareness: The Key to Determining Situations of Injustice

Determining what constitutes a situation of occupational injustice requires understanding that everyday occupation is political. A 'political' orientation entails recognizing that occupations are shaped by decisions and power relations that overtly and covertly structure society (Pollard et al., 2008). Everyday occupation is political because its performance is inextricably linked to an actor's sociocultural position. In a given society, the dominant group is portrayed as the standard to which all other groups are compared; accordingly, the meaningful occupations of dominant groups are praised and valued while ways of being or behaving that vary from the dominant standard are labelled as deviant aberrations (Young, 1990). Power dynamics such as these implicitly manifest in a person's everyday occupational behaviour and are unavoidably evoked when occupational performance is inhibited. Recognizing that such power dynamics affect occupation represents a political orientation.

By extension, we argue that the act of helping people engage in occupations is also political. Believing that people have the right to engage in occupation is a political position, and believing otherwise is also a political position; therefore people who choose to become occupational therapists take up a particular political position. Some therapists may hesitate to call their daily practices 'political,' but in our experience, that hesitation stems primarily from equating the word *political* with a particular ideology or governmental party. However, recognizing the existence of

TABLE 9-1

Examples of Factors that Promote Occupational Injustice in Occupational Science and Occupational Therapy Literature

Reference	Example(s) of Occupational Injustice	Everyday Situation	Extreme Situation
Whiteford's (2000) article on occupational deprivation	Refugeeism		X
	Minority group status	X	
	Imprisonment		X
	Chronic unemployment	X	
Townsend and Wilcock's (2004) article on occupational justice and client-centred practice	Slavery		X
	Refugeeism		X
	Oppressive industrial policies	X	X
	Disability status	X	
	Ageism	X	
	Unemployment	X	
	Geographical isolation		X
	War		X
	Mass relocation		X
	Long-term institutionalization		X
	Unsatisfactory employment conditions	X	
	Incarceration		X
	Sex-role stereotyping	X	
	Racism	X	
Kronenberg and Pollard's (2005) chapter on occupational apartheid	Homelessness		X
	Minority group status	X	
	Disability status	X	
Wilcock's (2006) book on the occupational perspective of health	War		X
	Homelessness		X
Hammell's (2008) article on well-being and occupational rights	Inequitable access to employment	X	
	Segregation		X
	Confinement		X
	Political apartheid		X
	Lack of affordable/accessible transportation	X	
Stadnyk's (2008) chapter on occupational justice for older adults	Confinement to skilled nursing/assisted living facilities	X	
	Ageism	X	
Wilcock and Townsend's (2009) chapter on occupational justice	Lack of housing	X	
	Inadequate employment	X	
	Lack of financial resources	X	
Stadnyk et al.'s (2010) chapter on occupational justice	Being over/under-occupied	X	
	Poverty	X	
	Imprisonment		X
	Discrimination	X	
	Lack of occupational choice/variety	X	
Whiteford's (2010) chapter on occupational deprivation	Geographic isolation	X	
	Unemployment/underemployment/overemployment	X	
	Imprisonment		X
	Refugeeism		X
	Sex-role stereotyping	X	

<table>

TABLE 9-1
Examples of Factors that Promote Occupational Injustice in Occupational Science and Occupational Therapy Literature *(Continued)*

</table>

Reference	Example(s) of Occupational Injustice	Everyday Situation	Extreme Situation
Whiteford and Townsend's (2011) chapter on the Participatory Occupational Justice Framework	Lack of safe learning and playing contexts	X	
	Lack of meaningful employment	X	
	Lack of occupational choice	X	
	Living with HIV/AIDS		X
	Surviving war		X
Thibeault's chapter (2013) on occupational justice's intents and impacts	Beneficent acts that create injustices		X
	Living with HIV/AIDS/leprosy		X
	War		X
	The presence of landmines		X
	Extreme violence		X
	Gender inequality	X	
	Posttraumatic stress disorder		X
	Being an ex-child soldier		X
	Disability status	X	

power relations does not equate to casting a vote for a particular governmental party – it means acknowledging that occupational therapists and their clients operate within webs of power that govern society. For example, in addition to helping clients optimize their functional capacities, many occupational therapists also teach their clients strategies for coping with stigma against disability. Activities that raise clients' awareness of stigma exist because people with disabilities are marginalized due to dominant social expectations. Some therapists may choose to ignore the power relations that perpetuate stigma against people with disabilities, but many therapists act in ways that challenge such power relations. The act of helping clients engage in occupations and educating against stigma represents a political decision, be it implicit or explicit, to protect clients' rights and redress the naivety that may threaten those rights.

Understanding everyday occupational therapy practices as pursuits of justice extends beyond viewing occupational engagement as a human right; it also requires shifting occupational therapists' perspective of what represents an infringement upon a person's rights. According to Galvin, Wilding and Whiteford (2011), Western nations tend to frame 'human rights

along civil and political lines rather than as social, economic and cultural issues', and this stance 'serves to diminish the significance of everyday occupational problems' (p. 381). Conceptualizing human rights in civil and political terms restricts the idea of injustice to situations involving discrimination (e.g., by race, gender, religion) or procedural unfairness (e.g., due process, participation in politics, right to vote). Apart from discrimination against people with disabilities, a civil/political approach to justice may not seem directly applicable to occupational therapists' everyday practices. Yet, the social, economic and cultural factors that afford or constrain occupational engagement are basic elements of experience that undergird civil and political injustices, as well as occupational therapy practice. Whiteford and Townsend (2011) remind us that 'occupational justice is occupational therapy's implied social vision when the consequences of *not* providing occupational therapy are restricted participation and social exclusion' (p. 69). If occupational therapists ascribe to the social vision that all people should be able to engage in meaningful occupations, then occupational therapists must acknowledge that they are taking an inherently political position that seeks justice beyond civil and political equity.

THEORETICAL UNDERPINNINGS FOR JUSTICE-ORIENTED EVERYDAY PRACTICES

The previous section demonstrates that situations of occupational injustice are those in which power relations infringe upon rights and yield negative effects on occupational participation. In this section, we discuss the related topic of *who* should address occupational injustices. Drawing from the Framework for Occupational Justice (FOJ) (Stadnyk et al., 2010), the Capabilities Approach (Nussbaum, 2000; Sen, 2009; Venkatapuram, 2011) and the American Occupational Therapy Association (AOTA) Practice Framework (2014), we argue not only that occupational therapists *can* ameliorate occupational injustices, but that most occupational therapists already *do* address injustices given the theoretical underpinnings that guide their practices.

Framework for Occupational Justice

Stadnyk et al.'s (2010) FOJ is the major and most frequently cited conceptualization of occupational justice within current literature (Durocher, Rappolt and Gibson, 2014), and one of its primary concerns is the 'enablement of occupational potential' (Stadnyk, Townsend and Wilcock, 2010, p. 345). Although practitioners do not typically recognize their interventions within the purview of justice, we argue that many typical occupational therapy practices address the FOJ's concerns. When coupled with the lens of the multidisciplinary Capabilities Approach to social justice (Nussbaum, 2000; Sen, 2009; Venkatapuram, 2011), the FOJ illustrates that enabling occupational participation clearly constitutes a justice-focused endeavour. The Capabilities Approach eschews traditional views of distributive justice (Nussbaum, 2000; Sen, 2009; Venkatapuram, 2011) and posits that the primary metric of justice is the extent to which a society supports individuals' and groups' capabilities to achieve desired functionings – in other words, whether individuals can *be* and *do* what they value (Nussbaum, 2000; Sen, 2009; Venkatapuram, 2011). Accordingly, the Capabilities Approach asserts that efforts to promote justice should focus on enhancing capabilities. Thus occupational therapists' efforts to rehabilitate their clients' skills (capabilities) to partici-

pate in occupation (functionings) can be framed as works of justice using a Capabilities Approach. In support of this perspective, Mousavi et al. (2015) found that a cohort of occupational therapists in mental health practice, when presented with the Capabilities Approach, saw 'themselves as playing a role in enhancing the capabilities of people with mental illness' (p. 1).

The philosophical synergy between the FOJ and the Capabilities Approach has been referenced in occupational science (Bailliard, 2013, 2014; Pereira, 2013; Stadnyk et al., 2010; Townsend, 2012; Townsend and Marval, 2013; Whiteford and Pereira, 2012), and its application via occupational therapy is important. Occupational therapy interventions focus on enhancing occupational participation, the vehicle through which humans integrate with their social, cultural and physical environments (Cutchin et al., 2008). Efforts to enhance clients' participation in occupation can therefore be seen as efforts to enhance clients' integration with sociocultural and physical environments. The FOJ asserts that occupational justice facilitates 'the enablement of diverse participation in society' (Stadnyk et al., 2010, p. 331) through the enhancement of occupational capabilities. Therefore typical occupational therapy interventions that support social inclusion and participation may be framed as pursuits of justice. However, only interventions that both aim to enhance participation *and* adhere to other core standards of the profession constitute pursuits of justice.

Client-Centred Therapy

The application of core professional values to help clients function and integrate with environments is essential to using everyday occupational therapy as a vehicle for justice. The value of client-centredness is integral to occupational therapy and involves empowering clients to actively shape the direction and mode of the therapeutic process, including codetermining the goals of therapy (AOTA, 2014). For Townsend and Wilcock (2004), client-centred therapy provides an explicit link between everyday occupational therapy practices and occupational justice by promoting social inclusion through client enablement. Whereas Townsend and Wilcock's view of justice and client-centred therapy focuses on advocacy at a broader systems level, we maintain that microlevel client-centred therapy in everyday practice can also constitute an act of justice. Client-centred therapy respects clients' personal conceptions of the good and avoids forcing them into predetermined modes of functioning. According to Nussbaum (2000), it is important for therapists to avoid prescribing particular modes of functioning to prevent imposing their specific conceptualization of the good on those they aim to help. Therapy that assumes a one-size-fits-all approach or coerces clients into particular ways of being is itself a form of injustice (Nussbaum, 2000) that reifies problematic power differentials in society. Such therapy becomes a political act of oppression and a form of cultural imperialism (Young, 1990), which reinforces normative standards and ignores diversity. As with the recognition of power dynamics, many occupational therapists already strive to 'promote [clients'] *capacity for occupational participation* and not a particular *form of occupational participation*' (emphasis in original, Bailliard, 2013, p. 352). Being client-centred thus exemplifies one small-scale pursuit of justice that already occurs in everyday occupational therapy practice. By providing clients with the freedom of choice to determine who they are and how they perform their occupations, occupational therapists help ensure that those individuals retain power over their capability to function.

Respect for Pluralism

Genuine client-centred therapy necessarily entails respecting a plurality of worldviews and ways of being. The acceptance of pluralism requires that therapists go beyond measuring clients against normative standards, instead viewing clients as inseparably embedded within complex situations. Respect for pluralism is something that many therapists already strive to achieve, and the language of justice fits well with that endeavour. Stadnyk et al. (2010) note that 'the concept of occupational justice rests on the idea that individuals are different and have different needs' (p. 334) that are expressed through occupation. This view of occupational justice echoes the Capabilities Approach and illustrates how pluralism can frame client-centred interventions as justice-focused interventions. If clients from heterogeneous backgrounds with different values and desires are empowered to actively shape

the direction and mode of their therapy, then the resulting therapeutic processes will necessarily foster diverse participation in society. Beyond accepting the heterogeneity of clients via respect for pluralism, occupational therapists welcome, support and advocate for diverse manifestations of human beings and doings.

Empathic Understandings

Acknowledging and respecting pluralism through genuine client-centred care requires that therapists try to see the world through clients' eyes. Empathic care is core to occupational therapy and 'one of the basic ingredients responsible for changes that occur during intervention' (Abreu, 2011, p. 623). Most occupational therapists strive to be empathetic in their everyday practices. Empathy requires 'being sensitive, respectful of differences, and fully present to the other person' (p. 624), and it reinforces therapists' commitment to protecting the dignity and worth of each person (AOTA, 1993). Promoting justice involves treating each individual as a worthy moral end that deserves to experience dignity through participation in valued occupations (Nussbaum, 2000; Sen, 2009; Venkatapuram, 2011, 2013). Occupational therapists use empathy in everyday practices to try to understand clients' self-perceived dignity and the ways in which clients' occupations are or are not deemed dignified; such empathic understandings reflect a professional position that treats clients as worthy moral ends, thus facilitating the promotion of justice.

WHAT DO THESE THEORETICAL UNDERPINNINGS MEAN FOR EVERYDAY OCCUPATIONAL THERAPY PRACTICES?

The above paragraphs demonstrate that basic aspects of occupational therapy practice, including client-centredness, respect for pluralism and empathy, align with multidisciplinary assertions about the promotion of justice. Enhancing people's participation in occupation with the goal of promoting dignity and social inclusion undeniably constitutes a pursuit of justice – the challenge is to help occupational therapists become aware of it. We recognize that many occupational therapists see themselves as health professionals who have not been trained to understand how societal power structures manifest in everyday living. However, we believe that occupational therapists can quickly become aware of social structures and power dynamics because they routinely experience such structures and dynamics in their everyday lives and practices. Given that occupational therapists have the experience, tools and 'responsibility to advance understanding of occupational injustices, to educate others, and to effect change' (Wilcock and Townsend, 2014, p. 547), we offer two suggestions about how they can come to understand everyday practices as acts of justice.

Modifying Practice Frameworks

Wolf et al. suggest (2010) that 'adopting an occupational justice framework requires occupational therapists to adjust the way they view issues that prevent a client's occupational engagement. To frame an issue in occupational justice terms means to identify the environmental and systems barriers that prevent the client from engaging in occupations that promote health and quality of life' (p. 15).

While we agree that focusing on environmental and systemic barriers is important, we believe that encouraging occupational therapists to view their practices as pursuits of justice can occur through other mechanisms as well. For instance, occupational therapy practice frameworks can be modified to frame everyday occupational therapy as acts of justice. The World Federation of Occupational Therapists' Statement on Occupational Therapy (2011) alluded to justice in declaring that occupational therapists can work with clients 'who are socially excluded owing to their membership of social or cultural minority groups' (p. 1); however, the statement stopped short of identifying such work as an act of justice and did not frame traditional practice in terms of justice. Likewise, the Canadian Framework for Ethical Occupational Therapy Practice (Canadian Association of Occupational Therapists, 2006) portrayed practitioners as moral agents who must consider the moral dimensions of their everyday practice, but it failed to label such considerations in terms of justice. The AOTA's (2014) Practice Framework explicitly cited occupational justice within its scope of practice 'as both an aspect of contexts and environments and an outcome of intervention' (p. S9). Although the AOTA Practice Framework makes justice more explicit than the World Federation of Occupa-

tional Therapists' statement or the Canadian Framework, it still keeps occupational justice somewhat separate from everyday occupational therapy practices because it describes occupational injustice relative to physical or environmental limitations but does not address power relations. Moreover, although the AOTA Practice Framework links occupational justice to a specific type of practice – advocacy – it falls short in situating power relations as contextual factors that affect all areas of practice. These frameworks seem to illustrate the dichotomization of 'genera' and 'critical' occupational therapy practice that Whiteford et al. (2016) describe in this book. However, we believe that such a dichotomization is unnecessary given the foundations for justice which we have outlined. We believe that current practice frameworks and statements from around the world have inadequately portrayed the embedment of human occupation in sociopolitical forces. Articulating the impact of those forces on everyday occupations across practice areas and global frameworks would constitute a great stride towards framing everyday occupational therapy practice as an act of justice. We recognize that occupational therapy associations must carefully and strategically navigate such a move because acknowledging a political orientation (as we have defined it here) may challenge and subvert the very systems through which occupational therapists operate.

As practice frameworks develop, they can assume a more explicit focus on rights with the understanding that rights are incommensurable and must be equitably addressed. Hammell (2008) has proclaimed 'the profession's commitment to the occupational rights of all people and not solely those people who are defined as disabled' (p. 61). The World Federation of Occupational Therapists (2006) has also issued a statement that challenges occupational therapists to 'identify and address occupational injustices' (p. 2) based on the promotion of human rights. While occupational therapists embrace their responsibility to empower and enhance the quality of life of individuals with disabilities, many therapists may worry that promoting 'rights' will ensnare them in political ideological debates and distract them from the true aim of their work (i.e., helping clients). However, as mentioned above, occupation and occupational therapy are both unavoidably political, and donning a political orientation necessarily entails a focus on rights and justice. Highlighting rights in practice frameworks offers helpful language for underscoring the justice work that already occurs in everyday occupational therapy practice: by helping clients access and engage in occupations, occupational therapists are assuring clients' rights to live healthy, fulfilling lives as occupational beings.

Enhancing Educational Courses and Curricula

Although modifying practice frameworks can help occupational therapists envision their practices as justice-seeking efforts, changes to educational curricula might also allow future occupational therapists to more easily see their practices in relation to occupational justice. To illustrate, we offer examples of how contemporary educational efforts aim to associate everyday occupational therapy practices and justice. By helping students make these associations before they formally enter the world of practice, we believe that educators can help students to more easily see practice as a justice-seeking endeavour.

Example 1: A Justice-Focused Undergraduate Occupational Science Course

Saint Louis University's (SLU's) Bachelor of Science in Occupational Science programme is underpinned by a university-wide focus on justice; an undergraduate occupational science course focused on occupational justice therefore aligns with most students' previous educational experiences. The course is structured around experiential learning activities that expose students to local and global occupational injustices and occupational therapy practices (Aldrich, 2015). Course discussions between SLU students and students at the Karolinska Institute in Stockholm, Sweden, focus on the connections between the political practice of occupational therapy and occupational justice. For those discussions, students begin by answering a series of questions, including: (a) What do you think of when you hear the word *political*? (b) In what ways do you see engagement in occupation as a 'political' phenomenon? (c) Should the practice of occupational therapy be 'political'? and (d) In what ways do you see your future occupational therapy practices as being 'political' or pursuing occupational justice? Students from both institutions deliberate and discuss these

questions, knowing that their understandings are provisional and will evolve as they progress through their education and into their practices. Although the SLU students are generally reluctant to say that occupational therapy is a political practice, the Karolinska Institute students tend to communicate a broader view of politics that supports the power-based perspective we have described in this chapter. Through discussions with the Karolinska Institute students, the SLU students learn how to talk about the political practice of occupational therapy and to consider how the pursuit of occupational justice intersects with politically oriented practice. SLU students also share examples of occupational injustices based on their experiential learning in the Saint Louis community, helping their Karolinska Institute peers understand the range of everyday circumstances, including poverty and minority status, that are enveloped by the concept of occupational justice. These discussions all happen in year-long context of reframing the notion of 'being critical' as a positive trait that all professionals can and should take up (Marterella and Aldrich, 2015).

For this course, SLU students also complete two culminating projects that provide opportunities to: (a) apply knowledge about occupational injustice, and (b) begin conceptualizing future occupational therapy practices as political or justice-seeking efforts. The first project is linked to another occupational science course that requires student groups to develop a wellness programme in collaboration with a community partner. As a prelude to this wellness project, student groups use the Occupational Justice and Health Questionnaire (Wilcock and Townsend, 2014) to identify occupational injustices that may threaten their community partners. Using the Participatory Occupational Justice Framework (Whiteford and Townsend, 2011), the students then propose ways to address identified occupational injustices through enablement skills. For the second project, students create individual 5-minute videos that convey who they are, what they have learned, and whether they see their future practices embodying a political practice of occupational therapy or engaging with the pursuit of occupational justice. Taken together, these two culminating projects give SLU students space and time to explicitly consider the political and justice-related dimensions of occupational therapy. Upon graduating from their occupational therapy programme, SLU students are already primed to consider occupational therapy practice as involving the pursuit of justice, giving them a more solid basis for seeing everyday practice through a lens of occupational justice.

Example 2: Justice-Focused Occupational Therapy Curricular Streams

The University of North Carolina at Chapel Hill's Division of Occupational Science and Occupational Therapy embraces 'ethics, justice, and care' as one of its core curriculum themes. 'Justice' is framed as working towards the protection of human rights and equitable access to occupational participation. The faculty believes in moving beyond the use of didactic teaching methods to provide basic exposure to justice principles. To habituate students to embody considerations of justice and care in every aspect of their reasoning, deliberations about justice are infused into seminars, assignments and extracurricular activities through which students repeatedly and critically analyse situations using a justice lens. Through experiential and peer problem-based learning, students learn how to build a professional community culture that supports ethical deliberations and creates a structure for voicing justice-related concerns in everyday practice. For instance, students from the University of North Carolina at Chapel Hill and Boston University participated in a joint research project to observe older adults' occupational participation in different environments through the lens of occupational justice (Berger et al., 2012). Students were encouraged to identify structural and systemic conditions that facilitated or impeded the occupational participation of their participants. Informed by readings and discussions, students from both institutions collaboratively analysed their observations to identify themes related to occupational justice. This experience facilitated students' habits of analysing situations through an occupational justice perspective. The interinstitutional collaboration cemented students' appreciation of occupational injustices as everyday phenomena that occur through different environments.

In addition, students at University of North Carolina at Chapel Hill are trained to view occupational participation using a transactional perspective. The transactional perspective on occupation is a relational theory that conceptualizes humans and the environments through which they operate as codefining and coconstitutive (Cutchin and Dickie, 2012). This perspective broadens students' views of how various forces come to bear on participation in occupation and encourages them to consider occupation as inherently affected by power relationships. These considerations are woven throughout the curriculum and assignments such that students are accustomed to analysing occupation as inextricably embedded in and affected by sociocultural and political forces.

Similarly, the faculty of the Department of Occupational Therapy at the University of the Western Cape transformed their occupational therapy curriculum to nurture the political consciousness of their students (de Jongh et al., 2012). To begin the transformation, the faculty engaged in reflective activities and workshops that fostered a critical awareness of the social and political contexts of South Africa, including occupational therapy's broad role within those contexts. Their goal was to encourage students 'to critically examine their attitude and to broaden their understanding of their political role as occupational therapy practitioners' (p. 17). The faculty revised their mission statement to highlight their goal of producing 'politically conscious, graduates [who] will understand the dynamics of power and their role as advocates as being central to addressing occupational injustices and human needs' (p. 19). To achieve that goal, they incorporated learning strategies that fostered the exercise of political reasoning and purposefully sought marginalized and underresourced fieldwork placements for their students. De Jongh et al. (2012) emphasized that transforming the curriculum content was necessary but insufficient to achieve their goal. It also required that the faculty internalize political consciousness in their everyday doings and teaching.

FUTURE DIRECTIONS AND CONSIDERATIONS

As the profession becomes increasingly attuned to the power relations that influence everyday occupational therapy practice, it will become more important to continuously critique occupational therapy's role in the advancement of justice. In addition to promoting justice in everyday situations, occupational therapists will need to consider how their practices may perpetuate or transform the societal power relations that lead to experiences of injustice. Occupational therapists will need to consider the appropriateness of their involvement in extreme situations of injustice. Durocher, Gibson and Rappolt (2014) wrote, '[C]ertainly situations of slavery, war, poverty, abuse, displacement, and countless other circumstances may indicate the need for a response to injustice, but whether or not these and other injustices indicate the need for intervention against *occupational* injustices requires deliberation' (emphasis added, p. 423). The dialogue about occupational injustice must continue to evolve to guide therapists in recognizing when occupational justice interventions are warranted. In addition, that dialogue must address the potential for collateral harm in occupational justice interventions; that is, occupational therapists must ensure that their efforts to help one client or group do not yield an experience of injustice for other individuals or groups (Bailliard, 2014).

CONCLUSIONS AND IMPLICATIONS

Throughout this chapter we have argued that occupational injustices arise in any situation that prevents a person's access to meaningful occupations. Participation in everyday occupation is inherently political because it is unavoidably affected by power dynamics and social norms, and occupational therapists must view their practices as political by extension. Through client-centred therapy, respect for pluralism and empathic understandings, everyday occupational therapy interventions already constitute acts of justice as outlined in the Capabilities Approach and FOJ. Portraying everyday occupational therapy practice using justice terms in frameworks and curricula can mobilize students and practitioners to explicitly attend to the political and justice-focused dimensions of occupation. We believe that embodying these understandings in everyday practices will encourage students and practitioners to recognize their important role in global efforts to establish a just world where all individuals have an equitable opportunity to participate in meaningful and valued occupations.

REFERENCES

Abreu, B.C., 2011. Accentuate the positive: reflections on empathic interpersonal interactions (Eleanor Clarke Slagle Lecture). Am. J. Occup. Ther. 65 (6), 623–634. doi:10.5014/ajot.2011/656002.

Aldrich, R., 2015. The importance of experiential learning spaces and an occupational science foundation for global occupational therapy education. South Afr. J. Occup. Ther. 45 (1), 56–62. doi:10.17159/2310-3833/2015/v45no1a10.

American Occupational Therapy Association (AOTA), 1993. Core values and attitudes of occupational therapy practice. Am. J. Occup. Ther. 47 (12), 1085–1086. doi:10.5014/ajot.47.12.1085.

American Occupational Therapy Association (AOTA), 2014. Occupational therapy practice framework: doman and process (3rd ed.). Am. J. Occup. Ther. 68 (Suppl. 1), S1–S48. Available at:: <http://dx.doi.org/10.5014/ajot.2014.682006>.

Bailliard, A., 2013. Laying low: fear and injustice for Latino immigrants to Smalltown, USA. J. Occup. Sci. 20 (4), 342–356. doi: 10.1080/14427591.2013.799114.

Bailliard, A., 2016. Justice, difference, and the capability to function. J. Occup. Sci. 23 (1), 3–16. doi:10.1080/14427591.2014.957886.

Berger, S., et al., 2012. Occupational justice for older adults. AOTA Gerontology Special Interest Section Newsletter, 35 (1), 1–4.

Canadian Association of Occupational Therapists, 2006. The Canadian Framework for Ethical Occupational Therapy Practice. Available at: <http://www.caot.ca/pdfs/EthicalFrameworkJuly 2006.pdf>.

Cutchin, M.P., Dickie, V.A., 2012. Transactionalism: occupational science and the pragmatic attitude. In: Whiteford, G., Hocking, C. (Eds.), Occupational Science: Society, Inclusion, Participation. Wiley, London.

Cutchin, M.P., Aldrich, R.M., Bailliard, A.L., Coppola, S., 2008. Action theories for occupational science: the contributions of Dewey and Bourdieu. J. Occup. Sci. 15 (3), 157–165. doi:10.1080 /14427591.2008.9686625.

de Jongh, J., Hess-April, L., Wegner, L., 2012. Curriculum transformation: a proposed route to reflect a political consciousness in occupational therapy education. South Afr. J. Occup. Ther. 42 (1), 16–20.

Durocher, E., et al., 2014. Occupational justice: a conceptual review. J. Occup. Sci. 21 (4), 418–430. doi:10.1080/14427591.2013.775692.

Durocher, E., Gibson, B.E., Rappolt, S., 2014. Occupational justice: future directions. J. Occup. Sci. 21 (4), 431–442. doi:10.1080 /14427591.2013.775693.

Galvin, D., Wilding, C., Whiteford, G., 2011. Utopian visions/dystopian realities: exploring practice and taking action to enable human rights and occupational justice in a hospital context. Austr. Occup. Ther. J. 58 (5), 378–385. doi:10.1111/j.1440-1630.2011.00967.x.

Hammell, K.W., 2008. Reflections on ... wellbeing and occupational rights. Can. J. Occup. Ther. 75 (1), 61–64. doi:10.2182/cjot.07007.

Harro, R.L., 1999. The cycle of socialization. In: Adams, M., et al. (Eds.), Readings for Diversity and Social Justice. Routledge, London, pp. 15–21.

Kronenberg, F., Pollard, N., 2005. Overcoming occupational apartheid: a preliminary exploration of the political nature of occupational therapy. In: Kronenberg, F., et al. (Eds.), Occupational Therapy Without Borders: Learning From the Spirit of Survivors. Churchill Livingstone Elsevier, Toronto, ON.

Laliberte Rudman, D., 2010. Occupational terminology: occupational possibilities. J. Occup. Sci. 17 (1), 55–59. doi:10.1080/14427591.2010.9686673.

Marterella, A., Aldrich, R., 2015. Developing occupational therapy students' practice habits via qualitative inquiry education. Can. J. Occup. Ther. 82 (2), 119–128. doi:10.1177/0008417414562955.

Mousavi, T., Forwell, S., Dharamsi, S., Dean, E., 2015. Occupational therapists' views of Nussbaum's practice reason and affiliation capabilities. Occup. Ther. Ment. Health. 31 (1), 1–18. doi:10.1080/0164212X.2014.1003265.

Nussbaum, M.C., 2000. Women and Human Development. Cambridge University Press, New York.

Pereira, R.B., 2013. The Politics of Participation: A Critical Occupational Science Analysis of Social Inclusion Policy and Entrenched Disadvantage. Unpublished doctoral dissertation. Macquarie University, Sydney, Australia.

Pollard, N., Sakellariou, D., Kronenberg, F., 2008. A Political Practice of Occupational Therapy. Churchill Livingstone Elsevier, New York.

Sen, A., 2009. The Idea of Justice. Harvard University Press, Cambridge, MA.

Stadnyk, R., 2008. Occupational justice for older adults. In: Coppola, S., et al. (Eds.), Strategies to Advance Gerontology Excellence. AOTA Press, Bethesda, MD.

Stadnyk, R.L., Townsend, E.A., Wilcock, A.A., 2010. Occupational justice. In: Christiansen, C.H., Townsend, E.A. (Eds.), Introduction to Occupation: The Art and Science of Living, second ed. Pearson, Upper Saddle River, NJ.

Thibeault, R., 2013. Occupational justice's intents and impacts: from personal choices to community consequences. In: Cutchin, M.P., Dickie, V.A. (Eds.), Transactional Perspectives on Occupation. Wiley, Hoboken, NJ.

Townsend, E.A., 2012. Boundaries and bridges to adult mental health: critical occupational and capabilities perspectives of justice. J. Occup. Sci. 19 (1), 8–24. doi:10.1080/14427591.2011.639723.

Townsend, E.A., Marval, R., 2013. Can professionals actually enable occupational justice? Cadernos de Terapia Ocupacional da UFSCar 21 (2), 215–228. doi:10.4322/cto.2013.025.

Townsend, E.A., Wilcock, A.A., 2004. Occupational justice and client-centred practice: a dialogue in progress. Can. J. Occup. Ther. 71 (2), 75–87. doi:10.1177/000841740407100203.

Whiteford, G., 2000. Occupational deprivation: global challenge in the new millennium. Br. J. Occup. Ther. 63 (5), 200–204. doi:10.1177/030802260006300503.

Whiteford, G., 2010. Occupational deprivation: understanding limited participation. In: Christiansen, C., Townsend, E. (Eds.), Introduction to Occupation the Art and Science of Living, second ed. Pearson Education Inc, Cranbury, NJ.

Whiteford, G., Pereira, R.B., 2012. Occupation, inclusion and participation. In: Whiteford, G., Hocking, C. (Eds.), Occupational Science: Society, Inclusion, Participation. Blackwell Publishing, Hoboken, NJ.

Whiteford, G., Townsend, E., 2011. Participatory occupational justice framework (POTJ): enabling occupational participation and inclusion. In: Kronenberg, F., et al. (Eds.), Occupational Therapies without Borders. Churchill Livingstone Elsevier, New York.

Whiteford, G., Townsend, E., Bryanton, O., Wicks, A., Pereira, R., 2016. The Participatory Occupational Justice Framework: salience across contexts. In: Pollard, N., Sakellariou, D. (Eds.), Occupational Therapies without Borders. Churchill Livingstone Elsevier, Oxford.

Wilcock, A.A., 2006. An Occupational Perspective of Health, second ed. Slack, Thorofare, NJ.

Wilcock, A.A., Hocking, C., 2015. An Occupational Perspective of Health, third ed. Slack, Thorofare, NJ.

Wilcock, A., Townsend, E., 2009. Occupational justice. In: Crepeau, E.B., et al. (Eds.), Willard and Spackman's Occupational Therapy, eleventh ed. Lippincott Williams & Wilkins, Philadelphia, pp. 192–199.

Wilcock, A.A., Townsend, E., 2014. Occupational justice. In: Crepeau, E.B., et al. (Eds.), Willard and Spackman's Occupational Therapy, twelfth ed. Lippincott Williams & Wilkins, Philadelphia.

Wolf, L., Ripat, J., Davis, E., Becker, P., MacSwiggan, J., 2010. Applying an occupational justice framework. Occup. Ther. Now. 12, 15–18.

World Federation of Occupational Therapists, 2006. Statement on Human Rights. <http://www.wfot.org/ResourceCentre.aspx> (accessed 15.09.14.).

World Federation of Occupational Therapists, 2011. Statement on Occupational Therapy. <http://www.wfot.org/Portals/0/PDF/STATEMENT%20ON%20OCCUPATIONAL%20THERAPY%20300811.pdf> (accessed 20.10.14.).

Venkatapuram, S., 2011. Health Justice: An Argument from the Capabilities Approach. Polity Press, Cambridge.

Venkatapuram, S., 2013. Health, vital goals, and central human capabilities. Bioethics 27 (5), 271–279. doi:10.1111/j.1467-8519.2011.01953.x.

Young, I.M., 1990. Justice and the Politics of Difference. Princeton University Press, Princeton, NJ.

10

OWNING OCCUPATIONAL THERAPY THEORIES AND CONCEPTS: WEARING YOUR OWN COAT!

FARZANEH YAZDANI

CHAPTER OUTLINE

I have worked for many years as an occupational therapist and educator with diverse groups of clients and students from a variety of backgrounds and in different contexts. At times I have mainly noticed the similarities between people; at other times the differences are more apparent. Understanding and valuing diversity is a process that comes with time, exposure to learning and willingness to learn. So, in this chapter, I illustrate some of the experiences in my professional journey that have moulded my identity as a therapist and an educator who has tried to tailor the theory and practice of occupational therapy to suit whoever would wear it.

I hope my experience helps others to see occupational therapy in different international contexts and be more critical about the fundamental concepts of occupational therapy and their application.

CONTEXTUALIZING THE AUTHOR'S NARRATIVE

I am a child of the revolution (1979) and war (1980–1989) in Iran, both of which events have clearly influenced my choice of occupational therapy as a career. My memories of the Iranian Revolution begin at age 8; I could see both fear and hope in the eyes of the adults around me. So many whispers I did not understand. I can remember the highly charged atmosphere – a flow of energy in school, in the streets and even at home. Soon after the revolution the war between Iran and Iraq began. I was 10 then and lived the next 8 years of my life surrounded by new friends who had moved away from the front line to my city. My childhood and teenage years were full of stories of sorrow of people displaced from cities under rocket fire and bombings. The war ended when I was 18 years old, the year I had to choose my university major. Inevitably my experiences of war shaped my decision. So many people had been left with physical and mental trauma, and I needed to find a future career that would reflect my desire to help my country: occupational therapy. The following lines from the description of occupational therapy in the university prospectus are embedded in my mind and guided my choice of future career:

The war between Iran and Iraq has left us
with many victims who deserve to live with
their full capacity and occupational therapy
is a profession that can help these people to
achieve this and live their life with the dignity
that they deserve. (Ministry of Higher
Education, 1989)

And, yes, that was it. I went for it. In those days (1990s) at university, occupational therapy was considered to be the use of occupation as intervention. Carpentry, ceramics, weaving and fine art were used as therapeutic media. The understanding of occupational therapy did not extend beyond the use of activity as a therapeutic tool, based on what Iranian occupational therapists had learnt from a World Health Organization training course (1971) held in Iran. This first generation of occupational therapists also emphasized activities of daily living and environmental adaptation to facilitate patients' performance (Mehraban et al., 2008). The emphasis was on purposeful rather than meaningful activities. Concepts such as occupational participation and engagement were not emphasized in education or practice.

Worldwide, the emphasis on improving function and performance had led to a departure from occupation-centred practice, and this later led to a paradigm shift in occupational therapy to return to occupation centredness (Kielhofner, 2009). Kielhofner (2009) considers rethinking the use of self as a therapeutic tool as another paradigm shift in occupational therapy.

There were some pioneers who greatly influenced occupational therapy education and practice, and aimed to facilitate this paradigm shift in Iran. They guided my philosophical thinking about occupational therapy. Shafaroodi (1993) taught me that occupational therapy is not only about improving performance but also about quality of life. Her work helped me make sense of the humanistic philosophy of occupational therapy that informs client-centred practice. Another key figure was Rassafiani, whose application of theory to the field of occupational therapy with children and their parents opened the gates to another world for me, enhancing my sense of professional identity (Dalvand et al., 2014).

In 2000 I was invited to establish an occupational therapy department in the Faculty of Medicine at the University of Jordan. Jordan is a relatively young country (it gained full independence in 1946) in the Middle East, which at that time was making a rapid transition towards becoming a more open and modern society. Its population at the time was about 6 million, including a large population of people of Palestinian origin who had emigrated or were exiled. Most Palestinians were fully integrated with the inhabitants of Jordanian origin. It was clear that the people all had a sense of pride about their national and cultural identity as members of a modern Arab society.

I grew to appreciate both cultural differences and similarities with Iran, and to establish my status as a young Iranian professional woman. I needed to work hard to be taken seriously as I felt that my age, gender and nationality counted against me, and people's perceptions, particularly the younger generation, had been influenced by negative media portrayals of Iran.

I had to start from scratch and develop a course that would meet both local needs and international standards of occupational therapy. On my daily trips to town using public transport, I started to communicate with local people. This was not difficult because Jordanians were used to tourists visiting their country and were very sociable and welcoming, though I must have appeared different from the usual Western visitors. They were also mostly fluent in English, which was helpful in conversations as I did not know colloquial Arabic then.

I developed an understanding of the Arab world through my students who were from Jordan, Palestine, Egypt, Iraq, Bahrein, Oman, Kuwait, Saudi Arabia, the Emirates and Syria. I learnt about the similarities and differences between them and Iran. I reflected on my own previous learning and experiences, reviewing theories of occupational therapy in relation to the new context of Jordan.

DAY-TO-DAY OCCUPATION

As an outsider, I needed to make sense of what people were doing, based on my then understanding of occupation as work, leisure and activities of daily living. Even the simplest day-to-day activities appeared to be different from what I was familiar with and had taken for granted. The first day at work I waited for someone to come and ask me if I wanted tea, unaware that this was not the custom at work. Most people would start their working day with a small strong coffee which they made themselves. So I had to learn to make my morning tea/coffee or buy it from the canteen. On my first day at a meeting with the university president, a man came to me with a flask of Arabic coffee and a series of small cups which were stacked on top of each other and offered me coffee. There was a small amount of coffee at the bottom of the cup. He stood over me until I had finished it, then put it under the other cups and repeated this with the next person. This ritual happened mostly in the office of senior staff as a gesture of hospitality and respect. Although it was not easy for me to drink that very bitter coffee, with the thought that someone else might have just drunk from the same cup, later I developed a taste for it and realized that each cup was used only once.

As I mentioned before, not only were some 'doings' different in Jordan, but also the way they were conducted differed from what I was used to in Iran. Greetings are similar in many different cultures. However, I was interested to see male students and colleagues kiss each other as part of their greeting – one or two kisses on each cheek. In Iran, males would usually only shake hands as a greeting. As I became more familiar with these simple day-to-day customs it made me think about how easily the 'strange' turns into 'normal' if we keep an open mind. These day-to-day behaviours have a meaning and not knowing them could lead to misunderstandings. The challenge for me was making sense of these cultural rituals and transferring my 'textbook' learning about communication and relationships into this new professional context. For example, it was normal practice to assign female therapists or nurses to clients of the same gender if possible.

In Iran, this had not been standard practice before the Islamic revolution; it was later introduced by the Islamic government. For me it was strange to see a practice the Islamic government of Iran had introduced, in the face of some resistance from Iranians, as normal and well-established practice in Jordan. This underlined for me the significance of culture, religion and politics in occupational patterns.

I went through a journey of recognizing both cultural differences and similarities, often at a deeper level. I can draw a comparison with Wikan's (2015) ethnographic analysis of working within Arab cultures. She discusses how we as people can live together in the world and understand one another with cultural differences. However, the journey was more complicated for me as I needed to understand how the Western concept of occupational therapy interacted with Jordanian culture.

Islam is the most practiced religion in both Iran and Jordan. Moving to Jordan made me think about how Islam is interpreted in these two countries. As a Muslim Iranian woman, I realized that many things which were interpreted as an Islamic lifestyle in Iran were aspects of Arab culture, an interrelationship emphasized by Khalaf and Khalaf (2009). To me, it was clear that Islam has developed in interaction with local culture: from a sociological perspective, Ansari (2006) has identified how Islam has influenced Iran's social transformation, whilst also reflecting traditional Iranian culture. One example of the interaction of religion and culture could be seen in the interpretation of *spirituality.* I was teaching models of practice, using the Canadian model of occupational performance and engagement, and we needed to discuss patients' spirituality. Interestingly, most students were referring to religion as spirituality while my previous experience of teaching and applying the same concept in Iran was different. In Iran, students thought that spirituality is different from religion. In Iran, religion was considered as a form of belief that could shape one's spirituality. There was less emphasis on rituals of religion to represent spirituality while in Jordan, rituals of Islam were used to describe one's spirituality.

Another discovery for me was how the meaning of what is considered as work, leisure or activity of daily living was interpreted differently. For example, at times I would sit at my desk in the evening after work reading a scientific article and drinking coffee. Colleagues would see this as work, perhaps even labelling me as a workaholic, but to me it was a relaxing time when I could read an article about a subject I am passionate about. It was productive because it enhanced my knowledge, but productivity was not the aim. Choosing what I wanted, not needed, to read helped me to feel connected to my global professional family and gave me a sense of personal fulfilment. For me, this was recreation, not work. Although this was not necessarily 'normal' in Iran or Jordan, my colleagues' critical words made me realize that occupation cannot be understood outside its specific, even individual, context. In Iran, particularly after the revolution and war, being a hard worker and even a workaholic was not seen as a bad thing but gave value to one's identity. So it was prestigious to work late, look tired and be busy. In Jordan, almost no one I knew took work home. The approach to work was different, and keeping the balance between home and work life was much more significant.

On reflection, these differences in attitudes to work could apply to any context and not just Jordan or Iran. As well as differences between countries, individuals are also different in the way they attribute meaning to different doings (Hammell, 2014). This was apparent between different generations. For instance, in Jordan, long visits to relatives reinforced a sense of belonging for the older generation, but for younger people it was often seen as time consuming and burdensome to a modern lifestyle (Yazdani, 2011). The more I was exposed to Jordanian culture, the more I reflected on the fundamental concepts of occupational therapy. What would grandchildren do to make their grandmother happy, bringing tea, taking care of them, and would they see this as a burden? What would these things mean to the grandmother: their right, their duty? Many things are done to reinforce connectedness with loved ones. Iwama (2006) addresses this in Japanese culture as a fundamental motivation for initiating occupation. However, the nature of this belonging appeared to be different in Iran compared to Jordan. Activity reinforcing belonging is important in all cultures, though who or what people feel affiliated with is different for every person (Ghazimoradi, 2012; Khalaf and Khalaf, 2009; Wikan, 1992; Yazdani, 2011). Apart from individual differences, there were patterns

that were more common in Jordan and these are illustrated in the next section.

OCCUPATION IN A GROUP-ORIENTED COMMUNITY

The first thing that attracted my attention was the way Jordanians did a lot of things together. Even in supermarkets you would see families doing their shopping together, sometimes including their grandmother. In Amman, particularly in richer areas, a babysitter was mostly within this group too. Soon I realized the importance of family life during the weekend. You could not find anyone using mobile phones as they were all switched off to allow family-related activities. Later, during group activities with students, it became apparent to me that almost all students had large and lengthy gatherings at weekends with grandparents. This was interesting because in Iranian towns and villages people still had this type of lifestyle, but not in the big cities. Complicated lifestyles, traffic congestion and a competitive job market made this incompatible with life in urban Iran in 2000. In a piece of research I conducted later about the subjective well-being of students (Yazdani, 2011), my participants expressed dissatisfaction and stress about their transition into student life alongside time-consuming family commitments. Arab families are mostly big and extended which means that gatherings need a real commitment of time and energy which could conflict with the demands of university life. This is particularly true for female students, who have more family responsibilities. That was one of my very first lessons about the social environment of my students and their clients.

The issue of being part of a bigger group did not end here. The dynamics of extended families and even their tribe[1] was very complicated and hard to understand for a newcomer like me. I remember the day one of my students came to me and said the notion of client centredness did not work in Jordan. She said:

I had prescribed an assistive tool for a child to help him to hold his spoon. I worked with the child to motivate him to use it and he was excited about it.

---

[1]Tribe in this text is used as equivalent of clan which is a group of people united by actual or perceived kinship and descent.

His mother was hesitant to tell me her opinion and said she would think about it. At the next session she brought the aid back and said that she could not use it for her child, reluctantly explaining that her mother-in-law did not like the idea of her grandson wearing something that looked stupid!

I began to consider who the client was in this context, the child, mother, grandmother or all three? Who else might be involved and how should this be managed? How about the client's choice and autonomy as emphasized in the textbooks? It felt like the extended family and relationships among members could not be ignored in any decision making. Hunt and Ells (2011) discuss the issue of independence, choice and autonomy for patients, presenting the concept of partnership towards autonomy in healthcare. They discuss the concept of relational autonomy that bridges the gap between the very individualized autonomy usually found in Western countries and the more interdependent and relational social modes found in Asia. Relational autonomy is based on understanding individuals as interconnected and situated and not isolated decision-makers. Therefore the social and cultural context of the client should be considered when addressing autonomy and choice.

THE CONCEPT OF SELF

As in most occupational therapy programmes worldwide, in Iran, we had learnt to apply the 'therapeutic use of self' based on psychotherapy models – for example, making use of the transference between therapist and client based on a psychodynamic approach, or unconditional positive regard based on person-centred therapy (Kielhofner, 2009). These techniques had mostly translated to occupational therapy in mental health and in developing therapeutic relationships (Kielhofner, 2009). As a novice therapist, it had not been possible for me to apply these yet into occupational therapy practice. I still hoped to be able to develop this aspect of my practice when I went to Jordan. For me, this was a part of my aim of establishing a holistic approach in occupational therapy practice. I planned to educate students in the therapeutic use of self in all areas of occupational therapy: mental health, physical, adults or children. But how could I

design classroom activities that supported students' learning about therapeutic use of self? My journey involved further reading about self, listening to therapists' narratives and reflecting on my own practice as a therapist. I applied my learning in developing a module called 'self'. The students and I went through three main pathways together: knowing who we are, what the occupational therapy profession requires and how they are married together. Classroom discussions made it clear to me that culture, politics, religion and community groups had an impact on the way students presented who they were and these were significant elements in shaping who they wished to be as occupational therapists (Ikiugu et al., 2003; Yazdani, 2014). In the process of developing their professional self they needed to understand how who they were at the beginning of the course and how they could integrate this into occupational therapy practice.

This 'self' needed to be used therapeutically in relation to their clients. They needed to learn how to translate warmth, empathy and caring, for example, into a language that could be shared with clients from their own community and within the same sociopolitical context, in a way which was congruent with their being a Jordanian therapist (Yazdani, 2014). My students would call an elderly client Haj or Hajje, meaning someone who has been to Mecca; this is an expression of respect, a title that is linked with spirituality and religious status. On the other hand, a mother of a child with a disability calling a female therapist 'auntie' would not be considered as crossing a boundary, but would indicate that the therapist was considered warm and approachable by her client.

I also realized that there was a great family, tribal and community group presence in the individual self. I needed to be aware of this and support students in reflection on how this presence determined decision-making at a personal and professional level, and in developing a self-awareness about who they were and how their self could be used therapeutically. For example, students needed to be fair and provide equal services to their clients regardless of their family connections, but this was hard in practice given the strong family loyalties. Having a parent of a student calling his daughter or son and asking her or him to give a certain type of service to a particular client was not unusual. There is a concept of 'wasta' which means someone who has power and works between the service giver and service user to facilitate better service. Many students did not like to follow this tradition and within the complex social system it could be very difficult to manage, requiring experience and wisdom. In other words, dealing with the issue of 'wasta' and managing that within the legal and professional requirements of the profession was not at the novice level and needed some cultural expertise.

As a foreigner, I did not have the same social sensitivities. It took me some time to understand the politics surrounding this issue. In Iran, it was more likely for there to be an expectation of preferential treatment based on political allegiance. In Jordan, in common with other Arab countries, this was linked more to tribal groups, which in turn could have an impact on the politics of the country (Al-Omari, 2008). Similar things probably happen in different ways in different countries throughout the world. It took me some time after I moved to the UK to understand what it meant when my seniors asked to 'have a word' with me in order to 'swing' something based on the politics of the system. Having some understanding of local culture helps to manage these pressures within the professional code of conduct.

THE SIGNIFICANCE OF TRANSITION

As an occupational therapist whose thinking is based on systems theories, considering change within societies and their impact on people's lives is not new to me. The speed of change varies in different parts of the world, but change is happening every moment, everywhere. There are various ways that people respond to and manage change and transition in their lives. I began to realize this when I started travelling and observing this phenomenon in Jordan and how it was similar and also different from Iran. Jordan, as a country with a young and developing identity, appeared to me as a country in rapid transition, and at times struggling to cope with change. Occupational therapists are in close contact with clients and their environment, and I had to educate a young generation of occupational therapists to develop within this transitory context. A strong Arab culture which is largely inseparable from Islam had shaped people's thinking and lifestyles (Khalaf and Khalaf, 2009). On the other hand, the open door towards modernity and Western culture, admired by the new generation in particular, could also influence occupational therapy practice.

Theories and models represented in textbooks were mostly based on Western concepts, and my role was helping students to translate this into the Jordanian context. For example, using the model of human occupation, we had groups for students to start understanding the concepts of the model by applying them to themselves. According to the model of human occupation, occupation is motivated by internal factors consisting of interests, personal causation and values in interaction with the environment (Kielhofner, 2008).

As a young generation who had easy access to media, students made choices and developed a variety of interests within a global online community. However, there were limited opportunities to experience these within the social context of Jordan. Also, sometimes their interests clashed with the community's values, in a society where community approval is highly significant. Community values and their influence have strong significance in the lives of people living in countries like Iran (Yazdani, 2012) and Jordan (Yazdani, 2011). This can present real challenges to young people trying to manage their lives in a period of social change.

The experience of one of my students illustrates this. She liked salsa dancing but attending a class required having a dance partner who might not be a brother, father or husband, which is not acceptable within traditional Islamic values. The student was Muslim and even though she was happy to bend the rules and go, she could not face the admonishment of the community for such inappropriate behaviour. This issue could also happen in Iran, where politics (i.e. the application of Islamic principles by force of law) has a strong impact on lifestyles. Within the classroom, students discussed how these dilemmas could be understood from a theoretical perspective, helping students to think about their application in practice. Students needed to practise this in order to develop skills in handling complicated situations that clients would also face.

A big part of my learning about Jordan was through my little daughter. She was almost 4 when she came to Jordan and had to learn and adjust to her new world.

She needed to make a link between our family norms, values and lifestyle and what she was confronting daily in school and the playground outside our building. Through her I learned how children's occupational life and the value of different 'doings' were forming. My experience of living in Jordan guided me to constantly think critically and reflect on what occupational therapy is and how I could train my students to apply it effectively in their own contexts. This experience felt like tailoring an occupational therapy coat that was as stylish as the international ones that pioneers of the profession would wear, but was suitable for the size, shape and taste of Jordanians – a fashionable coat with a new style that was made from Jordanian fabric. I learnt that we need to *own* our coat.

CONCLUSION

To have a good grasp of diversity, whether it is related to religion, ethnicity, language or sociopolitical factors, for example, occupational therapists should have an understanding of themselves. In translating ideas, knowledge and skills across different cultures, similarities are as important as differences. Similarities are often seen in people's common humanity while differences appear more in the diverse manifestations of this humanity. The basic concepts of human occupation need to be understood in terms of these diverse but global experiences of occupation across the world. Through developing this understanding, occupational therapists can make sure that they not only have considered diverse groups of people and environments, but also the interaction between the two. It is within this complex interaction that the diversity of occupation emerges.

REFERENCES

Al-Omari, J., 2008. Understanding the Arab culture: A Practical Cross-Cultural Guide to Working in the Arab World (working with other cultures), second ed. How To Books Ltd, Oxford.

Ansari, A., 2006. Iran, Islam and Democracy: The Politics of Managing Change. Chatham House, London.

Dalvand, M., Rassafiani, M., Bagheri, H., 2014. Family centred approach: a literature review. Novin J. Sci. Res. 8 (1), 2–8.

Ghazimoradi, H., 2012. Work and Leisure of Iranians. A'amme Ketab, Tehran, Iran.

Hammell, K.W., 2014. Belonging, occupation, and human wellbeing: an exploration. Can. J. Occup. Ther. 81 (1), 39–50. doi:10.1177/0008417413520489.

Hunt, M.R., Ells, C., 2011. Partners towards autonomy: risky choices and relational autonomy in rehabilitation care. Disabil. Rehabil. 33 (11), 961–967.

Ikiugu, M.N., Rosso, H.M., 2003. Facilitating professional identity in occupational therapy students. Occup. Ther. Int. 10 (3), 206–225.

Iwama, M.K., 2006. The Kawa Model, Culturally Relevant Occupational Therapy. Churchill Livingstone Elsevier, Philadelphia.

Kielhofner, G., 2008. Model of Human Occupation: Theory and Application. Lippincott Williams & Wilkins, Chicago.

Kielhofner, G., 2009. Conceptual Foundations of Occupational Therapy, third ed. F.A. Davis, Philadelphia.

Khalaf, S., Khalaf, R., 2009. Arab Society and Culture: An Essential Guide. SAQI, London.

Mehraban, A., Azad, A., Akbarfahimi, N., 2008. The History of Occupational therapy in Iran. The Sixteenth Iran National Congress of Occupational Therapy, Iran Medical University Press, Tehran, Iran.

Ministry of Higher Education, 1989. Guide to Choose University Courses. Higher Education Press, Tehran, Iran.

Shafaroodi, N., 1993. Occupational Therapy History. The First Occupational Therapy Congress, Tehran, Iran.

Wikan, U., 1992. Beyond the words: the power of resonance. Am Ethnol. 19, 460–482.

Wikan, U., 2012. Resonance: Beyond the Words. The University of Chicago Press, London.

Yazdani, F., 2011. How students with low level subjective wellbeing perceive the impact of the environment on occupational behaviour. Int. J. Ther. Rehabil. 18 (8), 462–470.

Yazdani, F., 2012. The dynamic nature of attributing meaning and value to occupation in Iran. J. Occup. Sci. 19 (4), 371–375.

Yazdani, F., 2014. The triad of community group, politics and religion in forming the 'professional self'. Philos. Pract. 9 (1), 1336–1343.

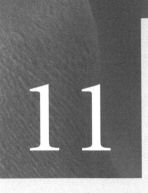

11

HUMAN RIGHTS, OCCUPATIONAL THERAPY AND THE CENTRALITY OF SOCIAL PRACTICES

ALEJANDRO GUAJARDO ■ MARGARITA MONDACA

Our aim in this chapter is to explore some of the dominant epistemologies in occupational therapy and present some alternative ones. We argue that a human rights and ethical perspective needs to be a central component of an understanding of humans as occupational beings.

HOW TO UNDERSTAND THE NOTION THAT WE ARE OCCUPATIONAL BEINGS

The assumption that humans are occupational beings has been examined extensively by Wilcock (2006) in her study on the relationship between occupation and health. Despite an apparent consensus in occupational therapy regarding this assumption, it is necessary to problematize both *being* and *occupational*. From an occupational therapy perspective, occupation is often seen as an attribute, a quality of the living being. The original foundation of occupational therapy relies on a naturalistic understanding of what *being* means, grounded primarily in the understanding of being as

biological. Occupation is then a quality, an effect of the living being which is grounded in biological roots. This has an inevitable consequence: in order to explore and know the being, we need to explore its attributes, one of which is occupation. Thus there is a living being, which is characterized as an individual, and there is an object called *occupation*. This naturalistic understanding philosophically explains the origin of reality centred in biological laws but disregards the influence of sociohistorical processes. The premise that the being is equivalent to the subject and the subject is equivalent to the person underpins this understanding (Pérez, 1998).

This Darwinian naturalistic understanding of the being, grounded in the natural sciences, medicine and in the health sciences, has dominated occupational therapy. Within this framework the individual is understood in isolation, as an atom relates to other atoms, or in its relationship with the environment. This understanding is a result of historical conditions which constitute modern reason, that is, what Hegel (1770–1831) called the constants of modern scientific rationality: rationalism, realism, atomism, reductionism, freedom defined by the fact of being individual and the idea of human nature (Pérez, 1998). This understanding develops through a rupture with the previously theocentric understanding of the world. The individual, rather than a divine entity, is put at the centre of the world and into a situation where humans will no longer depends on a superior entity. Instead, will is dependent on a dyadic and external relationship with the subject itself. This new will is none other than the human reason that would illuminate the darkness of consciousness, but its reasoning limits any possibility of freedom. Freedom is deposited in each individual as a political act (liberalism), under the preeminence of the natural sciences (mathematics/physics), industrialization and the new form of social production, capitalism. In this line of reasoning, it is only possible to be free, to the extent that the external reality called nature is known (Pérez, 2008). This ontological foundation has led to the development of a specific kind of epistemology in occupational therapy whereby occupational beings are natural beings. Natural beings are living beings, involving biological, individual structures and processes; so reality is internal, intrinsic and phenomenally knowable only through an externally observable object: occupation.

The possibility of understanding occupation from any other angle, such as the social, remains anchored to this discursive means. Thus the possibility of the social will be understood as interaction between individuals rather than in a wider community context. This explains, in part, the individually focused methodologies often used in occupational therapy (Hammell, 2009). Thus occupation is based ultimately on a biological rather than a social understanding. A good example of this is the notion of intrinsic motivation. There is a tendency in the literature to unpack occupation from a positivist perspective, as an observable object, which is disaggregated in parts: occupation, performance, ability, skills, the neurological, the anatomical, and so forth. This anatomical dissection is the basis from which occupational therapy has been organized. In this account, the social does not fit; instead, the discipline is concerned with a realization of the liberal vision of the subject as the individual par excellence, and so gives ideological support to the current neoliberal order (Von Hayek, 2005).

This positivistic tendency to see occupation as being open to disaggregation is also evident in, for example, Nelson's (1988) description of occupational performance and occupational form, where performance is referred to as the process of doing something, and occupational forms are described as the circumstances that elicit, guide and structure that performance. Occupational form then is separated as a distinct entity, observable and not intertwined with human aspects as a whole. We argue that this individualized understanding of occupation is present in other influential theoretical models such as Kielfhofner's model of human occupation (Kielhofner, 2008). With the intention of addressing the complexity of human occupation, the model of human occupation dissects aspects of human occupation that are inseparable. This understanding of human occupation can lead to the reification, naturalization and dehumanization of the human subject, affecting occupational therapy practice. There is no space for an ethical or political positioning in this naturalistic foundation of the profession. The biological is ultimately independent of the human will and operates with its own laws, being a natural element of reality. The ethical and the political dimensions are not fundamental aspects of occupational therapy, but a sociohistorical interpellation or calling of the suffering and pain experienced by large groups with which the occupational therapist is in contact. Therefore it can be argued that occupational therapy acts as one kind of ideological apparatus through which pain and suffering can be directed and addressed: for some people who experience pain and suffering, an intervention is socially necessary, and occupational therapy is a social and historical construction developed to meet some of these needs. The knowledge of nature (in an aseptic or abstract form) is one thing, and what people make of that knowledge (as a response to nature through ethics, e.g., through genetic modification) is another; similarly, knowledge of occupation is different to the kinds of knowledge we generate about it and from it.

In the dominant epistemology of occupational therapy, human occupation is understood as the subjects' manifestation of an attribute, as exteriority, an external process through which humans can mediate the social environment. This view has gradually been overcome by a more subjective and situated understanding of the person, where the focus becomes the meanings of occupations in particular sociocultural contexts; with regard to narratives, the situatedness of narratives becomes a particular focal point of interest (Laliberte Rudman and Huot, 2013; Prodinger et al., 2013; Stoetzler and Yuval-Davis, 2002). These shifts in focus are important steps to overcoming the criticism of the ontological individualism prevalent in occupational therapy (Hammell, 2009). Gradually, a different epistemology of occupational therapy, grounded in social and political dimensions, has started to emerge. A clear example of this is the Participatory Occupational Justice Framework developed by Whiteford and Townsend (2011). Another sign of this change is the growing literature about the limitations to understanding human occupation, qualifying the predominant discourses of it as Western biased, culturally specific, contestable and lacking of supporting evidence (see, e.g., Hammell, 2009).

OCCUPATION AS SOCIAL PRAXIS

From an ontological perspective, we propose that within occupational therapy the object of study is not an object but instead a subject that thinks, acts, decides and is historically situated in the process of being. From this perspective, the subject can be understood constitutively, that is, as a conscious being, as a being able to transform, act upon and produce reality. The subject is understood as being embedded, acting and produced within the sociohistorical context. The subject is understood as a reflecting and active part of the social praxis framework. This praxis is nothing other than the activities that precede the subject, which progressively becomes instituted and recognizable in the act of being occupied. Thus the subject is understood not as a form of individuality but as a social relationship determined through action (Guajardo, 2014); that is, it is not separate from the reality in which it exists. We differentiate between the terms *individual* and *subject* by stating that the former is an outcome of an individualization process that results in each person being unique, different and singular. However, this process has a generic common base, where persons are cognizant. The subject will be then the confluence of the more stable dimensions, with the constantly unfolding social relationships, the struggle

to become individualized, able to transform the reality through occupation (Pérez, 2014; Rubio and Sanabria, 2011). This field of subjectivity produces our experiences of ourselves as singularities composed of our interactions to construct the inner reality that we have about the world and ourselves (Pérez, 2014). The dominant modern subject in occupational therapy, by contrast, is the Cartesian, rational, homogeneous, intrinsically busy, instrumental, pragmatic and individual subject. We propose that social relations are the foundation of the subject: at the same time, other people embody our personal subjectivities, our personal identities. We produce ourselves as beings, and at the same time we constitute our personal identity. This is only possible in the context of social relations, in the context of occupational praxis (Rubio and Sanabria, 2011).

Why is it important to talk about the subject as a conceptual entity, through which the phenomenon of occupation is revealed? Which relationship can we establish between subject and subjectivity-subjectivation? We propose that it is important to explore human occupation not as if it is separated from the subject, but through understanding the subject as *being in human occupation*. Therefore, we argue that we are not occupational beings, but occupational *subjects* in the act of being. We argue for an understanding of 'the occupational' in the Hegelian sense, as a totality (Pérez, 2008; Hegel, 2011). That is, there are no subjects who 'occupy themselves' or subjects who 'acquire subjectivity', in the psychological sense, through 'the act of being occupied'. Instead, there is a field of social relations that produces reality and subjects as two entities *in the same* space. This field is historical, situated, cultural and concrete. This field as a *totality* is human occupation, where occupation as a field produces both occupied subjects and their occupational relationships, and thus oneself as subject is produced by occupations. This view is only possible through taking a dialectical perspective of how we are constituted as human beings, that is, that we are organized through a constant transformational process which is never complete, constantly unfolding, a process of being in the making (Ricoeur, 1992). To summarize our argument, we argue that occupations are social practices and relationships, and within themselves constitute and produce subjects. There is no occupation that exists by itself. All singularization (the process by which singular characteristics become visible) is actually the manifestation in a subject of an occupational field of a relational character. No occupation can be understood then as separate from its relationships with others. Every occupation exemplifies culture, meaning and relationships. Occupation is the expression of collective occupations, the practice of social relations that have been historically produced, incarnated, embodied and materialized in the singularities. Practices are social acts, and therefore no practice is individual, not even when a single person carries it out independently. All human occupation makes reference to a context, to a personal sense and to a process of cultural appropriation. All that can be called individual is the singular materialization of a collective occupational field.

A HUMAN RIGHTS PERSPECTIVE

Occupational therapy has started to recognize and acknowledge the precariousness of modern life, the emptiness of the subject, inequities, violence, poverty and exclusion. Human rights violations have been very evident in the historical development of Latin America (Galeano, 1985) and Africa. The more recent experiences of social and economic degradation and structural violence in the southern hemisphere through neoliberal capitalism have also extended to the developed countries in the past two decades. Migration, ethical or morally 'just' wars (such as United Nations missions engaged in by the powerful in the world order to preserve the status quo), and poverty are found in countries all over the world, including some of the world's richest economics such as the US, UK and Sweden, with severe political, cultural, social and economic effects (Dirkx, 2014). As de Certeau (1988) foresaw, marginality is no longer limited to minority groups, but, rather, is massive and pervasive, becoming a universal silent majority. Occupational therapy cannot be grounded in any foundation other than an ethical and political approach. Its centrality relies in the recovery of life's projects, the recognition of others and inclusion. The whole range of occupational therapy practices have the obligation to embrace a human rights perspective, from those working in sociopolitical practices to those in clinical settings.

Everything that is related to people, their well-being, quality of life, justice and participation in an unequal, structurally segregated and violent world is an issue for occupational therapy. The profession has to say something about these issues and be part of transformative actions aimed at changing them. Indifference is not an option.

There are two dimensions of interest to occupational therapy with regards to adopting a human rights approach. The first dimension has to do with maintaining a reflexive practice. The second dimension relates to the recognition of the *other*. For Galheigo (2011), one of the most damaging effects of neoliberalism has been the invisibility of human needs and social issues produced by the dominance of economic and political interests, by cultural differences and ethnic conflicts, and by the lack of political will to address social issues and by approaching human affairs in a reductionist manner. This invisibility extends to the marginalization of needs and rights which the neoliberal agenda considers to be unproductive. This effect of neoliberal political and economic strategy effectively denies people's rights and their opportunities to have active roles in managing their daily struggles. Inequalities in access to human rights and full participation in social life is a huge social problem that occupational therapists should not overlook. Social vulnerability can be amplified by political invisibility, rendering marginalized people voiceless, and denying them the possibility of participating as citizens. Their influence in policymaking, regulations and perspectives is practically absent from the dominant discourses. Their difficulties in obtaining access and influence for social, civil and political rights is reproduced everywhere in society. The neoliberal economic model has globally increased vulnerability and worsened living conditions across countries, producing new patterns and forms of social exclusion (Kallen, 2004). These issues are no longer limited to the Southern Hemisphere developing countries, or to severely impoverished countries. However, as the latter suffer the major burden, efforts are needed to address promptly the structural causes of the problems. We are in agreement with Galheigo (2011) that there are particular groups of people who are in urgent need of attention. The poor, migrants, displaced groups, ethnical minorities, women and people with disabilities or mental health problems have experienced the effects of social exclusion most. Galheigo (2011) claims that the current debate on human rights is central to the future of occupational therapy.

Occupational therapy practice is not only obliged to be a political practice (Kronenberg and Pollard, 2006; Pollard et al., 2008), but needs to *actively engage* in social and political issues. Occupational therapy is a political praxis because it deals with a concrete world, within a particular society. It relates to the kind of subjects that are produced by our actions in a neoliberal society, and how these relations between actions and society are primarily expressed in everyday life practices. Occupational therapy can play a major role in maintaining the status quo or influencing the stability of social systems. Therefore our actions *as practitioners* do not escape the ethical and political, as they reproduce or transform various forms of practices through our interventions and their effect in producing different ways of constructing social life and negotiating actions between people. A human rights perspective is often understood in terms of legal frameworks, organized under a legal corpus (Guajardo and Galheigo, 2015). However, we argue that human rights are essentially relational, produced in historical contexts where the tangible everyday life of the subjects is produced, through social projects and the specific power relationships associated with these. Occupational therapy practices within the human rights framework are not about rehabilitating capacities as a pragmatic exercise of the right thing to do, but to promote and embrace rights as producers of capacities and capabilities (Bloodworth, 2006; Nussbaum, 2011). In the terms proposed by Arendt (1998), human rights are only possible to the extent that they support the existence of a political community. It is in this political community that the recognition of the other is constituted and translated into citizenship. Human rights are recognized in their relationship to the existence of citizenship. That is, rights are the effect of the citizens' participation in everyday life through being part of a political community. Therefore a critical practice of occupational therapy should promote the transformation of the conditions of subjects and the transformation of alienating everyday practices. Occupational therapy should focus on the deprivatization of human suffering and oppose the dominant individualistic methodologies in the analysis of intervention processes. A critical practice of occupational therapy should be based on human rights, in the recognition of the otherness, advocating a full practice of citizenship.

CHALLENGES WITHIN OCCUPATIONAL THERAPY PRAXIS

Which is the everyday life that occupational therapy promotes? To which future of everyday life should occupational therapy contribute? We live in a particular historical period, characterized by dynamic and rapid changes, accelerated development of technology and the productive forces – a period characterized by migration, remarkable advances, great contradictions and social injustices. It is a time marked by globalization, neoliberalism and the market economy, that generates a tension between the significant increase in the supply of goods and services and growing disparities; many groups of people and communities are excluded from these symbolic exchanges and materials. In this social, political, economic and cultural context, great human suffering emerges, through the violation of human rights or the absence of them. Poverty, social exclusion, the weakening of affective and social ties, lack of access to education, health and housing are common conditions. The loss of social welfare and quality of life of large sectors of populations involves psychosocial damage and creates detrimental changes in the health–disease process. Violence, substance misuse, increases in the prevalence of mental health problems and the absence of dignified and respectful conditions for occupational participation are the most critical expressions of the exclusion of groups and individuals in many societies (Bauman, 2005). It is in these realms that occupational therapy is being called to act. Occupational therapy is not, neither can it ever become, a homogeneous and standardized discipline; it is determined through historical processes, and it is imprinted by the socioeconomic, political and historical contexts where it develops. Therefore there are many occupational *therapies*. Occupational therapy is not, then, an abstract, ahistorical or metaphysical entelechy or vital principle. It exists because there is a concrete world that has produced it, a social world that deemed the presence of this profession and discipline necessary. It has been produced to operate on social problems. The social conditions of a particular historical period are the ones that define the existence and status of occupational therapy (da Rocha Medeiros, 2008).

From this perspective, the reflection of the cultural and social must be grounded within the occupational therapy profession itself. Occupational therapy knowledge is grounded in the practices of human occupations themselves, within and not outside of them, and thus is grounded and informed by occupational experiences. Human occupations are not something external to the subject, a phenomenological expression of the interiority of persons, a method by which one can achieve the essence of being human through this phenomenon called *human occupation*. If human occupations are social practices, relationships, in which subjects are constituted and produced, then occupational therapy knowledge is not something beyond that. Occupational knowledge resides in the subjects themselves, in many places, in many actors. Occupational therapy is just another way of understanding and knowing these forms of knowledge. A substantive knowledge for the profession emerges through critical reflection, a problematizing of the actors themselves, a questioning of common sense. At the same time, we must also problematize the assumptions that underlie all scientific knowledge.

CONCLUSIONS

When this problematization is at the centre, what would then be occupational therapy identities, knowledge and practices? What positions do these hold? It would not be an occupational therapy that intends to promote the adaptation of people to the dominant social system, that adapts people who are vulnerable and excluded to the system that excludes them, that focuses on the development of skills and know-hows, so that the subjects become integrated into the context without the possibility of transformation. Instead, what is required is an occupational therapy that transforms and promotes other forms of social relations and alternative forms of living, of everyday practices. Every occupational therapy practice should be an exercise of democratization, freedom validation as collective production, a claim and promotion of human rights as free and conscious occupations, focusing

on the subject, but grounded in a particular community. The variety of professional practices should validate the differences and skills that allow a democratic exercise of the difference, where knowledge is in all places and experiences. Occupational therapy practices should recognize and engage in dialogue with diverse worldviews, to imagine and build other possible worlds, other subjects, other ways of life.

REFERENCES

Arendt, H., 1998. Los Orígenes del Totalitarismo. Taurus, Madrid, Spain.

Bauman, Z., 2005. Vidas Desperdiciadas: La Modernidad y Sus Parias. Paidos Ibérica, Barcelona, Spain.

Bloodworth, A., 2006. Nussbaum's 'capabilites approach'. Nurs. Philos. 7 (1), 58–60. doi:10.1111/j.1466-769X.2006.00240.x.

da Rocha Medeiros, M., 2008. Terapia Ocupacional. Un Enfoque Epistemológico y Social. (Occupational Therapy. An Epistemological and Social Approach). Universidad Santa Fé, Universidad Nacional del Litoral, Buenos Aires, Argentina.

de Certeau, M., 1988. The Practice of Everyday Life. University of California Press, Berkeley, CA.

Dirkx, P., 2014. Estado europeos desmembrados. Le Monde Diplomatique XV, 14–16.

Galeano, E., 1985. Las Venas Abiertas de América Latina. Editorial siglo XXI, Madrid, Spain.

Galheigo, S., 2011. What needs to be done? Occupational therapy responsibilities and challenges regarding human rights. Austr. Occup. Ther. J. 58 (2), 60–66. doi:10.1111/j.1440-1630.2011.00922.x.

Guajardo, A., 2014. Una terapia ocupacional critica como posibilidad. In: dos Santos, V., Gallassi, A.D. (Eds.), En Cuestiones Contemporáneas de la Terapia Ocupacional en América del Sur. Edit CRV, Brazil.

Guajardo, A., Galheigo, S., 2015. Los Derechos Humanos y la Terapia Ocupacional Crítica: Construyendo una Perspectiva Contra Hegemónica desde América Latina. [Human Rights and Critical Occupational Therapy: Building an Antihegemonic Perspective from Latin-America]. WFOT Bulletin, volume 71, pages 73–80.

Hammell, K.W., 2009. Sacred texts: a sceptical exploration of the assumptions underpinning theories of occupation. Can. J. Occup. Ther. 76 (1), 6–13. Available at:: <http://cjo.sagepub.com/content/76/1/6.abstractN2>.

Hegel, G., 2011. Ciencia de la Lógica, vol. I. Lógica Objetiva. Ediciones Solar S. A., Madrid, Spain.

Kallen, E., 2004. Social Inequality and Social Injustice. A Human Rights Perspective. Palgrave Macmillan, New York.

Kielhofner, G., 2008. A Model of Human Occupation, fourth ed. Lippincott Williams & Wilkins, Philadelphia.

Kronenberg, F., Pollard, N., 2006. Political dimensions of occupation and the roles of occupational therapy. Am. J. Occup. Ther. 60 (6), 617–625. Available at: <http://ajot.aota.org/data/Journals/AJOT/930159/617.pdf>.

Laliberte Rudman, D., Huot, S., 2013. Conceptual insights for expanding thinking regarding the situated nature of occupation. In: Cutchin, M.P., Dickie, V.A. (Eds.), Transactional Perspectives on Occupation. Springer, London, pp. 51–63.

Nelson, D.L., 1988. Occupation: form and performance. Am. J. Occup. Ther. 42 (10), 633–641.

Nussbaum, M., 2011. Creating Capabilities. The Human Development Approach. Belknap Press of Harvard University Press, Cambridge, MA.

Pérez, C., 1998. Sobre un Concepto Histórico de Ciencias. De la Epistemología a la Dialéctica [About an Historical Concept of Science. From Epistemology to Dialectic]. Editorial LOM, Santiago, Chile.

Pérez, C., 2008. Desde Hegel. Para una Crítica Radical de las Ciencias Sociales (From Hegel. For a Radical Critique of Social Sciences). (Itaca Ed.) LOM, Mexico.

Pérez, C., 2014. Sobre la Condición Social de la Psicología. Editorial LOM, Santiago, Chile.

Pollard, N., et al., 2008. A Political Practice of Occupational Therapy. Churchill Livingstone-Elsevier, Oxford.

Prodinger, B., et al., 2013. Institutional ethnography: studying the situated nature of human occupation. J. Occup. Sci. 22 (1), 71–81. doi:10.1080/14427591.2013.813429.

Ricoeur, P., 1992. Onself as Another. University of Chicago Press, Chicago.

Rubio, S., Sanabria, L., 2011. Occupación como proceso subjetivante [Occupation as a subjetivant process]. In: Claudia, R., Humana, G.D. (Eds.), Occupación: sentido, realización y realidad. Dialogos occupacionales en torno al sujeto, la sociedad y el medio ambiente [Occupation: meaning,realization and reality. Occupational dialogues about the subject, society and the environment]. Editorial Universidad de Colombia, Bogotá, Colombia.

Stoetzler, M., Yuval-Davis, N., 2002. Standpoint theory, situated knowledge and the situated imagination. Fem. Theory 3 (3), 315–333. Available at:: <http://fty.sagepub.com/content/3/3/315.abstractN2>.

Von Hayek, F.A., 2005. Camino de la Servidumbre. Alianza editorial, Madrid.

Whiteford, G., Townsend, E., 2011. Participatory Occupational Justice Framework (POJF 2010): enabling occupational participation and inclusion. In: Kronenberg, F., et al. (Eds.), Occupational Therapies Without Borders, vol. 2: Towards an Ecology of Occupation-Based Practices. Churchill Livingstone, London, pp. 65–84.

Wilcock, A.A., 2006. An Occupational Perspective of Health, second ed. Slack, Thorofare, NJ.

12

APPRECIATING THE LIVED EXPERIENCE OF SOME OLDER GAY PEOPLE: CONSIDERATIONS FOR CONTEMPORARY OCCUPATIONAL THERAPY PRACTICE

REBECCA TWINLEY ■ LEE PRICE

Ageing populations are presenting ever-increasing societal challenges globally. With the number of older people and the length of life expectancy increasing throughout the world, occupational therapy practice needs to respond to the needs of this ageing population. Some older people will experience longer periods of good health, social engagement and productivity; others will be socially isolated, living with multiple chronic health problems and disabilities (Department of Health, 2010). In many countries, including the UK, US, Australia, Canada and New Zealand, the health and care needs of these older people are receiving much attention from their respective health and care systems. However, thus far, there has been a limited consideration of the needs and experiences of older gay people. It is our contention that the discrimination and marginalization gay people have experienced, and may continue to experience, due to their sexual orientation, in addition to any other demographic factors, warrants understanding if their occupational and health needs are to be met; indeed, the importance of gaining an accurate life history is necessary if occupational therapists are to appreciate the subjective experience of occupation for people.

The aim of this chapter is to advocate for inclusive, occupation-focused occupational therapy practice with older gay people. To do so, we: (a) highlight the key issues for ageing gay people identified from a literature review, and (b) discuss the key themes from a thematic analysis of the opinions of student and qualified occupational therapists who engaged in an online discussion. The participants discussed issues related to the provision and use of health and care services for older gay people.

We have written this chapter from our own auto/biographical positions, acknowledging the significance of what we individually brought to this project. The forward slash between *auto* and *biography* is intentional because – as an approach to research – auto/biography allows for the study of other people's lives which is grounded in the researchers' own social context and experience. As Bagnoli (2004, no page) explains:

> [J]ust as the selves under study are considered within their network of significant others, and not in isolation from their context, so too the researcher's subjectivity is present throughout the research, and resonates of the themes raised in the inquiry (Stanley, 1993). The adoption of such a reflexive approach in research may thus ultimately result in personal growth for the researched and researcher alike.

As auto/biographical researchers we are, therefore, explicit about our insider status and our positionality within this work (Letherby et al., 2013). Rebecca's position is as a self-identified gay woman who was born and grew up in the UK, and Lee's position is as a self-identified gay man, born and still living in the UK. It is from these auto/biographical positions that we have written about gay women and men. We do not seek to exclude people who self-identify with other sexual and gender identities (e.g., bisexual, lesbian, and trans), and we acknowledge that some of the content of discussion may relate to a variety of people's lived experiences.

SEXUAL ORIENTATION AND SEXUALITY AS IDENTITY

A person's sexual orientation is the general attraction they feel towards others (Equality and Human Rights Commission, 2009), and might therefore be characterized by who they love, desire or are attracted to. A person's sexuality is expressed through how and what they desire, or what they do, sexually and intimately. Hence sexual orientation and sexuality are intrinsically linked to what people do and their sense of self; it is one aspect of each person that makes them different from others and, therefore, unique. However, scholars such as Whalley Hammell (2011) have argued that, similar to mainstream feminist theories regarding women's experience, theories of occupation have been based upon authors' own perspectives and assumptions. Consequently, key contributors have ignored difference of experience (e.g., regarding meaningful or purposeful occupation) that is attributed to demo-

graphic factors, including sexual orientation and sexuality (Sakellariou and Pollard, 2008).

Harrison's (2001) early work regarding the invisibility of older gay people in aged care highlighted the importance of sexual orientation and sexuality as part of a person's identity. Harrison (2001, p. 145) concludes that considering sexuality as private is a 'potentially dangerous cop out and a serious obstacle to people realising their human potential with their sexual identities as integral'. As Harrison (2001) explains, this issue is not about advocating for everyone to disclose their sexual orientation; rather, it is each individual occupational therapist's duty to ensure people experience them – their therapist – and the therapy environment as open, accepting, nondiscriminatory, and nonassuming. Occupational therapists and all other health and care professionals can do so by the language they use, their approach to practice and by eliminating signs of heterosexism in the environments within which they work.

THE EXPERIENCES OF OLDER GAY PEOPLE

Everyone has the right to social and occupational justice, regardless of various personal and contextual factors, such as older age and sexual orientation. With the public concerns about how to respond to an ageing society (Scrutton et al., 2014), current healthcare environments have entered an era where the highest numbers of older people need to use services. Indeed, the majority of older people face issues related to ageing and ageism (Blaine, 2013). Of those who identify as gay, there are likely to be additional challenges related to the inclusivity of health and social care services, particularly if the promotion of social and occupational justice is to be achieved.

The lived experience of many older gay people is known to be characterized by social exclusion, injustice and discrimination, encountered because of their sexual orientation (Hammack and Cohler, 2011). It is pertinent to remember the sociopolitical context when exploring the lives of older gay people in the UK as occupational beings and their experience of occupational justice. Historically, their experience of equality has been poor and fraught with constant barriers and challenges, which may well impact upon their current health, care and occupational needs. Many older gay people are from a generation of activists, that is, they grew up resisting and often fighting against a backdrop of overt homophobia and discrimination. They came of age in the pre-Stonewall era[1] when homophobia and discrimination were far more overtly prevalent and acceptable than they are today. It is understood that this is because homosexuality was criminalized and pathologized significantly during this era (Knauer, 2009). This experience is expressed by people such as William, a 73-year-old gay man quoted in a Stonewall report (Guasp, 2011, p. 8), who observed: 'In my younger days I paid taxes to be hounded and criminalised by the police'.

Indeed, many older gay people in the UK experienced unique social struggles caused by these abuses against their human rights; abuses which some gay people are still being subjected to in many countries across the world (Amnesty International, 2012). The implications of being marginalized as members of the communities and societies in which they live are multiple and include, amongst other inequalities, the experience of health disparities (Institute of Medicine, 2011). Post-Stonewall, many important legislative changes have occurred that have led to increased equality for gay people currently living in Western societies. However, there are still issues related to inclusivity of services. For instance, a UK-based survey involving 1036 gay people over the age of 55 found that 60% were not confident that social care and support services would be able to understand and, therefore, meet their needs (Guasp, 2011).

The joint paper by AGE Platform Europe and the European Region of the International Lesbian, Gay, Bisexual, Trans and Intersex Association (ILGA-Europe, 2012) outlines three key challenges older gay people experience throughout their lives: (a) the lack of recognition of same-sex relationships; (b) ongoing stigmatization in the realm of health and care; and (c)

---

[1]In 1969, the Stonewall Inn (in Greenwich Village, New York City, where being gay in public was prohibited) was raided by police. Police raids on gay establishments were a regular occurrence, but on 29 June the patrons fought back and a riot ensued. This event is understood to have led to the uprising of the gay liberation movement in the United States, and inspired gay people in other countries to join the gay rights movement.

> ### BOX 12-1
>
> 'For many gay and lesbian elders, the invisibility and isolation that they face in their later years are, unfortunately, familiar territory. As members of the pre-Stonewall generation, gay and lesbian elders are well acquainted with the themes of estrangement, alienation, and secrecy'. (Knauer, 2011, p. 11)

social exclusion and invisibility, which can include a lack of or no family support. With particular regard to the latter, as people age they become more likely to live alone, particularly women (Rutherford, 2012); gay people are known to be at an increased risk of living in isolation (Guasp, 2011). This can be either purposeful isolation or isolation as a consequence of being rejected and alienated from biological family and friends which, in turn, leads to lack of connectedness, or sense of belonging as illustrated in text Box 12-1.

As people enter the later stages of their lives, it is not uncommon to reflect upon their past – upon the choices they made and the way they spent their time – as a form of life review (Cohler and Galatzer-Levy, 2000). Unfortunately, such self-reflections can yield memories of feeling or experiencing any combination of homophobia, stigma, shame, heterosexism, heteronormativity and issues of family and social support. We discuss the significance of each in turn below.

Homophobia

Homophobia is 'the irrational hatred, intolerance, and fear of lesbian, gay and bisexual (LGB) people' (Stonewall, 2014, no page). Homophobia can be experienced on four levels: cultural, institutional, interpersonal and personal (internalized). Cultural homophobia is expressed through societal standards and norms that are based upon the combination of negative feelings, attitudes and stereotypes held towards a person, and discrimination against a person, because of their gay identity. Institutional homophobia sees these negative attitudes manifest as direct discrimination against gay people (through, e.g., policies) in institutions such as businesses and governmental organizations. A key example of institutional homophobia experienced by many older gay people can be found amongst those who served in the military; today's older gay adult served in the military at a time when gay people were banned. It was not until 2000 that gay people were allowed to openly serve in the UK military service.

Interpersonal homophobia is expressed through the speech and actions of a person towards another person they perceive to be gay. Experiences of interpersonal homophobia and discrimination occur amongst people in health and care services. Fear of experiencing this discrimination as they age impacts upon older gay people's health and well-being (Jackson et al., 2008). Conceivably, this fear can make it difficult for older gay people to proactively look after their health.

Internalized homophobia occurs when the individual internalizes negative societal depictions, attitudes and beliefs about gay people. This can lead to feelings of self-hatred and low self-esteem, and can explain the higher rates of depression amongst gay people, due to its effects upon their mental health (Kimmel, 2014). On the individual level, such negative views of self, and of their sexual orientation, can impact upon the sense of who the person feels they are, and what they wish to become, as an occupational being (i.e., their occupational identity).

Stigma

Hicks (2011) argues that when working with older gay people an awareness of the role sexuality has played in shaping peoples' lives is necessary. The experience of 'coming out' and the possible associated effects of sexual orientation-related stigma could be an example. Indeed, gay people who have experienced a lifetime of stigma may face unique barriers to accessing healthcare sensitive to their needs as they age. There are reports of individuals living in residential homes or in the community who hide their sexuality through fear of stigma and prejudice (Hicks, 2011). Hatzenbuehler and Link (2014) explored structural stigma, 'societal-level conditions, cultural norms, and institutional policies that constrain the opportunities, resources, and well-being of the stigmatized' (p. 2), highlighting the effect these factors can have on the individual. They found that structural stigma had adverse impacts upon the morbidity and mortality of lesbian, gay and bisexual people living in the US. Those living in communities where there is a high level of structural stigma were found to be at a higher mortality risk

than lesbian, gay and bisexual people living in less prejudiced communities. Sexual orientation-related stigma and discrimination have negative effects on the health of gay people (Pan American Health Organization, 2013). Work seeking to explore the experience of older gay people from an occupational perspective must recognize the negative and powerful effects stigma has upon people's physical and mental health.

The Politics of 'Shame'

Stigma is associated with identity, and for gay women and men can fuel what Warner (2000) described as the 'politics of shame'. This involves deliberately attempting to shame a person or group of people in relation to sexual activity. Warner (2000) argues that most people can easily be made to feel embarrassed about sex; this is a product of the societies in which people live, and the way that people are exposed to dominant beliefs and values. Yet some people are at greater risk of sexual shame than others. Sexual shame for gay women and men is brought about by political and legal stigma of homosexuality and the prohibition of sexual activity considered to be outside the norm and morals of a society. Sexual politics ministered through the law have described homosexuality as obscene, offensive, lewd, lascivious, abominable and unnatural to the norm of heterosexuality (Warner, 2000). It is therefore little wonder that researchers found older gay people who are isolated and who experience inequalities and restricted access to predominately heteronormative public health and social care services (Beauchamp et al., 2003; Brotman et al., 2003; Clark et al., 2001; Jackson et al., 2008).

The shame society places on sexual activity and the stigma of homosexuality appear to be inextricably linked. The indignity of sexual shame, derived from stigma, can be humiliating and destructive to the individual's concept of self (Warner, 2000). For these reasons, some people may conceal their sexuality from others, making inclusive service provision challenging (Knochel et al., 2010). Longhofer (2013), in his commentary on shame in clinical encounters with gay clients, challenges health and social care practitioners to be sensitive to shame and its social and psychodynamic manifestations. He argues that in order to provide inclusive care, practitioners must be cognisant of the factors which may influence and affect how gay women and men communicate with service providers and make use of what are heteronormative services.

Heteronormativity and Heterosexism

Health and care services in the UK are often described as heteronormative (Hayman et al., 2013), that is, predominantly heterosexual orientated, owing to the belief that heterosexual sexual orientation is the norm. Heteronormativity informs the policies and discourses related to the needs of older people, which according to Heaphy and Yip (2006) limits social inclusion and the services and supports for older gay people. Heterosexism is the belief, or assumption, that everyone is, should be or wants to be heterosexual. However, being heterosexist does not necessarily incorporate homophobia, particularly in instances where gay people are unconsciously excluded by individuals, institutions or their wider communities. Nevertheless, privileging and assuming heterosexuality can reduce the possibility for accurate and important information sharing (Mercier et al., 2013) which, in itself, is an immense barrier to gay people having their needs met. By assuming heterosexuality, people who identify as gay are faced with the dilemma of whether to disclose their sexual orientation or to hide it. NHS Education for Scotland (2007, p. 4) provides an example of how engrained heterosexism is in today's society by providing an extract from a real conversation between two nurses, Tracy and Julie. In text Box 12-2, Tracy assumes Julie is heterosexual.

BOX 12-2

Tracy: 'I've got nothing against gay people, but I don't understand why they feel they need to come out and tell people about it. I mean, I'm heterosexual and I don't go on about that'.

Julie: 'I am a lesbian and the reason I am coming out and telling you is because you assumed I am heterosexual. I would also like to point out that just last week you brought your wedding photos in to show everyone…you wear a wedding ring every day and talk openly about your husband. I can assure you that you are very out and proud about your heterosexuality and you do "go on about it" all the time.'

For older gay people living in residential (retirement, care or nursing) homes, institutional heterosexism is experienced through nonaffirmative policies and practices based upon heterosexual norms. For such reasons, the fear of eventually living in such an environment has been found to be common amongst older gay people (Taylor, 2012). Indeed, Morrison and Dinkel (2012), in their concept analysis of heterosexism in healthcare, inform us that people do not have to be homophobic to alienate gay people, but by working in heteronormative services practitioners may inadvertently do this.

So how do occupational therapists work to overcome this phenomenon? Wilton (2000) warns that attempting to treat everyone the same way does not guarantee equality. She argues practitioners should strive to offer the same standard of care, treating people equally and recognizing cultural differences. She invites people to consider what would happen if heterosexual people were treated as if they were gay. Wilton (2000) highlighted the importance of sexuality in people's lives for their sense of self, that is, who they are. Similarly, Twinley (2014) asserts that working towards occupational justice necessitates the understanding that 'working to uphold principles of equality does not always mean we should treat everyone the same; it is about recognizing and respecting diversity and difference of experience' (p. 624).

Family of Choice

Dewaele et al. (2011) discussed 'family of choice' as a phrase used by some gay people to identify friends who take the place of their biological family. Gay women and men can be isolated from their biological family due to indifference or negativity of the family because of the individual's sexuality (Shippy et al., 2004). One example of a gay man's experience of this is presented in a Stonewall report about gay people in their older adult lives: 'My family rejected me a long time ago hence no contact or support – no children and my partner of 43 years died from cancer as soon as we retired' (Neil, age 67, North West England; Guasp, 2011, p. 8).

Friends who constitute a 'family of choice' offer support, role modelling and a sense of unity often lacking from the person's biological family (Elizur and Ziv, 2001; Heaphy and Yip, 2003; Pugh, 2002). As people age, they generally find the need for increased social support. Although gay men, for instance, appear no more socially isolated than heterosexual men, they differ in tending to rely on friendship networks for support rather than biological family (Doffman et al., 1995; Grossman et al., 2000).

Shippy et al. (2004) investigated the social networks of 223 gay men aged between 50 and 82 years who lived in New York. Contrary to previous studies, most of their participants were not estranged from their biological families. Nevertheless, social networks of friends remained vital for physical and emotional support. They also discovered that 'families of choice' were sometimes unable to provide sufficient support because these individuals were also growing older and frail.

UNIQUE CONSIDERATIONS FOR GAY WOMEN AND MEN

As the authors of this chapter, we share the lived experience of being gay and growing up gay. However, we wanted to highlight unique considerations for gay women and men, as informed by our auto/biographical positions. These are presented in Boxes 12-3 and 12-4.

OCCUPATIONAL THERAPY WORK WITH OLDER GAY PEOPLE: YOUR STORIES

Using the online Twitter (microblogging) forum,[2] the #OTalk team facilitate weekly discussions about occupational therapy and occupational science (#OTalk, 2014). As a guest host, Rebecca facilitated one of these weekly discussions. Anyone with a Twitter account could participate in the discussion. The participants were predominantly qualified occupational therapists and occupational therapy students who discussed the experience of older gay people, health and care provision, and issues for occupational therapists and other

---

[2]See #OTalk 8 July 2014 titled 'Appreciating the Experience of Using Health and Care Services for Some Older Gay People' (http://otalk.co.uk/2014/06/26/otalk-8th-july-appreciating-the-experience-of-using-health-and-care-services-for-some-older-gay-people/).

BOX 12-3
GAY WOMEN

On explaining the need to write a book about lesbian health, Wilton (1997, p. ix) suggested there are 'major flaws in most health handbooks for "women". On the whole, they are really health handbooks for heterosexual women (although they fail to acknowledge this), since they generally neglect to recognize that lesbians exist.' Herein lies the most significant barrier to recognizing the social, occupational, health and care needs of gay women: their invisibility. Living in a society where some people hate you is not good for your health or well-being (Lesbian and Gay Foundation, 2013); living in a society in which you, or your needs, are largely invisible is an altogether different challenge.

Gay women are considerably more likely to experience a range of health inequalities, in comparison to heterosexual women (Conron et al., 2010; McNair, 2003). Fish and Bewley (2010) suggest that analysing the difference of experience amongst gay women from a health and human rights perspective would facilitate recognition that the social inequalities and discrimination they experience have a direct impact upon their health. Research exploring the health inequalities of gay women confirms that the facilitation of disclosure of sexual orientation is socially and clinically relevant (McNair et al., 2012), and so may well have therapeutic significance. Mercier et al. (2013) found that disclosure focused the relevance of the interaction between gay women and healthcare professionals. Facilitation of disclosure is a complex process, particularly when gay women choose to remain silent about their sexual orientation. Although, for older gay women this choice is understandable when the sociopolitical and historical context is considered and understood (Hooyman and Kiyak, 2011). The repercussion of this silence can render them invisible because health and care professionals can overlook the possibility that some of their ageing female clients are gay (Brotman et al., 2003).

---

healthcare professionals. Lee performed thematic analysis of the transcript from this online discussion; this revealed four themes, as illustrated in Table 12-1.

CONCLUSION

Thankfully, sociocultural and political attitudes and beliefs have changed during the course of older gay people's lives. However, the very people who lived through these changes are now amongst the general population of older people in society. While research

BOX 12-4
GAY MEN

Much of Western health and social care research literature and services tend to focus on young gay men. It often relates to safer sex, mental health and HIV, yet these issues are equally important for middle-aged and older gay men. Thanks to effective antiretroviral therapy, HIV has become a chronic health condition resulting in increased numbers of HIV-positive adults living into old age (Martin et al., 2008). Many Western gay men in their mid and late adulthood who are HIV-positive are the first generation living with HIV as a long-term condition (Lyons et al., 2010). This has the potential to impact on their human occupation in its widest conception; there is a paucity of occupational therapy literature related to this population. Generally, current health and social care research does not explore the experiences and expectations older gay men have of their health and social care.

Price (2014) explored the views of gay men over 60 years of age from the UK concerning their health and social care needs. His study yielded a range of issues related to communicating needs, sociocultural issues and issues of perceived heteronormativity. These men talked about the difficulty of being 'out' sexually with healthcare providers and not with their biological family. They discussed wanting to be accepted as individuals and not seen in stereotypical terms with assumptions made about their lives. In particular, they rejected the notion that they had a 'gay lifestyle'; they lived individual lives with particular cultural characteristics arising from belonging to a minority group in a predominately heterosexual society.

The UK's current generation of gay men aged over 60 is the first sizeable generation of 'gay rights activists'. Many have lived through early, mid and late adulthood fighting for sociopolitical change, with expectations and a drive for change that is now on the health and social care providers' threshold. They envisaged requiring intimate health and social care as they aged, potentially exposing them to dependency and vulnerability in an environment which they perceived to be based on heteronormative assumptions and perceptions. This is the very ideology they have struggled against for 40 years. These perceptions caused them to question how they will be treated when they are alone – an isolated minority without 'family of choice' to support and advocate for them.

TABLE 12-1
Themes Identified From Thematic Analysis of #OTalk Transcript

Theme	Issues
Asking, not stereotyping: Participants thought occupational therapists were not doing enough to recognize older gay people and may be making assumptions and stereotyping.	Older gay people were invisible to them as professionals and, therefore, to services. Speculated that occupational therapists are not asking the 'right' questions, although types of questions were not elaborated. Occupational therapists should ask about a person's sexuality as part of initial assessment.
Heteronormativity: Those participating thought that the prevailing assumption about a person's sexuality in British health and social care services was of heteronormativity.	Suggested to counteract these assumptions people should consider each other as diverse individuals. Occupational therapists who worked in healthcare services with regular contact with gay service users stated they were used to 'being aware' of difference.
Stigma and shame: Participants believed that there is stigma in being gay in British society which may impact on the disclosure of sexual orientation.	Participants discussed stigma as linked to the act of sex between gay (same-sex) couples, although there was discussion that sexuality is about self-identity and should not simply be linked to sexual intercourse.
Our limited understanding: Contributors said that occupational therapists do not know enough about the influence sexual orientation and sexuality have on human occupation.	Participants believed not enough focus is given to human sexuality in occupational therapy education. They posited that more occupational therapy-focused research is needed if occupational therapists are to understand and embrace diversity in their practice.

has started to focus on the health and care needs of older gay people, there is a need to transform the findings into public policy. Moreover, government policy and practice must focus on equalizing the experience of health and access for all people. It is only in doing

so that healthcare and social care professionals can understand the relevance of sexual identity throughout people's lives. This requires recognition that a number of health and care service users are gay and may have needs that will go unmet unless they feel able to disclose their sexual identity. The potential for disclosure can be facilitated by providing opportunities for the people occupational therapists work with to feel comfortable that they can self-disclose, without fear of a negative or judgemental reaction. This might require an adjustment in the focus of an occupational therapist's preliminary work with people. For example, a shift away from an emphasis on ascertaining a person's strengths and needs, to more attention in identifying and exploring their subjective and unique life experiences, could, equally, still reveal what has caused their current health status, and their associated occupational strengths and needs.

Occupational therapy practitioners, educators and researchers should consider the impact of intrapersonal, interpersonal and contextual factors upon the health and well-being outcomes of older gay people. Occupational therapists can be advocates for the health issues and occupational needs of marginalized populations in the society in which they live. To do so, they need to be able to recognize and articulate the health and occupational impact of, for example, the social inequalities and discrimination that older gay people have experienced. Experiences of stigma, heterosexism, homophobia, stereotypes, internalized negative feelings, inequality, exclusion and isolation, real and perceived barriers, are complex and unique to each individual. Sexual orientation is one of many demographic factors that can impact upon an individual's experience of occupational justice. Our focus here has primarily been upon sexual orientation and age. Occupational therapists should be working towards achieving an equality of occupational opportunities for the people they work with; this will be evident when people have equal rights, responsibilities and opportunities. Equality does not mean sameness, and so occupational therapists should not be taking the approach in their work that they will treat each person the same; people's uniqueness as occupational and human beings demands that they be treated accordingly.

REFERENCES

AGE Platform Europe and the European Region of the International Lesbian, Gay, Bisexual, Trans and Intersex Association (ILGA-Europe). 2012. Equality for older lesbian, gay, bisexual, trans and intersex people in Europe. <http://www.age-platform.eu/images/stories/Combating_discrimination_on_the_grounds_of_age_and_SOGI_final.pdf> (accessed 01.08.14.).

Amnesty International, 2012. Amnesty International Report 2012: The State of the World's Human Rights. Amnesty International Ltd, London.

Bagnoli, A., 2004. Researching identities with multi-method autobiographies. Sociol. Res. Online 9 (2), Available at: <http://www.socresonline.org.uk/9/2/bagnoli.html> (accessed 10.03.15.).

Beauchamp, D., Skinner, J., Wiggins, P., 2003. LGBT Persons in Chicago: Growing Older – A Survey of Needs and Perceptions. Chicago Task Force on LGBT Aging, Chicago.

Blaine, B.E., 2013. Understanding the Psychology of Diversity, second ed. SAGE Publications Ltd, London.

Brotman, S., Ryan, B., Cormier, R., 2003. The health and social services needs of gay and lesbian elders and their families in Canada. Gerontologist 43, 192–201.

Clark, M., Landers, S., Linde, R., Sperber, J., 2001. The GLBT health access project: a state-funded effort to improve access to care. Am. J. Public Health 91, 895–896.

Cohler, B.J., Galatzer-Levy, R.M., 2000. The Course of Gay and Lesbian Lives: Social and Psychoanalytic Perspectives. University of Chicago Press, London.

Conron, K.J., Mimiaga, M.J., Landers, S.J., 2010. A population-based study of sexual orientation identity and gender differences in adult health. Am. J. Public Health 100 (10), 1953–1960.

Department of Health, 2010. Healthy Lives, Healthy People: Our Strategy for Public Health in England. <https://www.gov.uk/government/uploads/system/uploads/attachment_data/file/216096/dh_127424.pdf> (accessed 23.01.15.).

Dewaele, A., Cox, N., Van den Berghe, W., Vincke, J., 2011. Families of Choice? Exploring the supportive networks of lesbians, gay men, and bisexuals. J. Appl. Soc. Psychol. 41, 312–331.

Doffman, R., Walters, K., Burke, P., Hardin, L., Karanik, T., 1995. Old, sad and alone: the myth of the aging homosexual. J. Gerontol. Soc. Work 24 (1/2), 29–44.

Elizur, Y., Ziv, M., 2001. Family support and acceptance, gay male identity formation, and psychological adjustment: a path model. Fam. Process 40, 125–144.

Equality and Human Rights Commission, 2009. What does sexual orientation mean? <http://www.equalityhumanrights.com/your-rights/equal-rights/sexual-orientation/what-does-sexual-orientation-mean> (accessed 23.01.15.).

Fish, J., Bewley, S., 2010. Using human rights-based approaches to conceptualise lesbian and bisexual women's health inequalities. Health Soc. Care Community 18 (4), 355–362.

Grossman, A.H., D'Augelli, A.R., Hershberger, S.L., 2000. Social support networks of lesbian, gay and bisexual adults 60 years of age and older. J. Gerontol. Psychol. Sci. 55B (3), 171–179.

Guasp, A., 2011. Lesbian, Gay and Bisexual People in Later Life. Stonewall, London.

Hammack, P.L., Cohler, B.J., 2011. Narrative, identity, and the politics of exclusion: social change and the gay and lesbian life course. Sex. Res. Social Policy 8 (3), 162–182.

Harrison, J., 2001. Viewpoint: 'it's none of my business': gay and lesbian invisibility in aged care. Aust. Occup. Ther. J. 48, 142–145.

Hatzenbuehler, M.L., Link, B.G., 2014. Introduction to special issue on structural stigma and health. Soc. Sci. Med. 103, 1–6.

Hayman, B., Wilkes, L., Halcomb, E., Jackson, D., 2013. Marginalised mothers: lesbian women negotiating heteronormative healthcare services. Contemp. Nurse 44 (1), 120–127.

Heaphy, B., Yip, A.K., 2003. Uneven possibilities: understanding non-heterosexual ageing and the implications of social change. Sociol. Res. Online 8 (4), Available at: <http://www.socresonline .org.uk/8/4/heaphy.html> (accessed 03.08.14.).

Heaphy, B., Yip, A.K., 2006. Policy implications of ageing sexualities. Soc. Policy Society. 5 (4), 443–451.

Hicks, D.W., 2011. Case discussion of treatment of an 83-year-old gay white male. J. Gay Lesbian Ment. Health 15 (4), 392–400.

Hooyman, N.R., Kiyak, H.A., 2011. Social Gerontology: A Multidisciplinary Perspective, ninth ed. Pearson, Upper Saddle River, NJ.

Institute of Medicine (of the National Archives), 2011. The Health of Lesbian, Gay, Bisexual, and Transgender People: Building a Foundation for Better Understanding. <http://www.ncbi.nlm .nih.gov/books/NBK64806/pdf/TOC.pdf> (accessed 09.03.15.).

Jackson, N.C., Johnson, M.J., Roberts, R., 2008. The potential impact of discrimination fears of older gays, lesbians, bisexuals and transgender individuals living in small to moderate-sized cities on long-term health care. J. Homosex. 54 (3), 325–339.

Kimmel, D., 2014. Lesbian, gay, bisexual, and transgender aging concerns. Clin. Gerontol. 37 (1), 49–63.

Knauer, N.J., 2009. LGBT elder law: toward equity in aging. Harvard J. Law Gender 32, 1–58, Temple University Legal Studies Research Paper No. 2009-9. <http://ssrn.com/abstract=1309182> (accessed 10.03.15.).

Knauer, N.J., 2011. Gay and lesbian elders: history, law, and identity politics in the United States. Ashgate Publishing Limited, Surrey, UK.

Knochel, K.A., Quam, J.K., Croghan, C.F., 2010. Are old lesbian and gay people well served? Understanding the perceptions, preparation and experiences of aging service providers. J. Appl. Gerontol. 30 (3), 370–389.

Lesbian and Gay Foundation, 2013. Mental Health and Wellbeing: A Guide for Lesbian, Gay and Bisexual People. Lesbian and Gay Foundation, Manchester.

Letherby, G., Scott, J., Williams, M., 2013. Objectivity and Subjectivity in Social Research. SAGE Publications Ltd, London.

Longhofer, J.L., 2013. Shame in the clinical process with LGBTQ clients. Clin. Soc. Work J. 41, 297–301.

Lyons, A., Pitts, M., Grierson, J., Thorpe, R., Power, J., 2010. Ageing with HIV: health and psychosocial well-being of older gay men. AIDS Care 22 (10), 1236–1244.

McNair, R.P., 2003. Lesbian health inequalities: a cultural minority issue for health professionals. Med. J. Aust. 178 (16), 643–645.

McNair, R.P., Hegarty, K., Taft, A., 2012. From silence to sensitivity: a new Identity Disclosure model to facilitate disclosure for same-sex attracted women in general practice consultations. Soc. Sci. Med. 75, 208–216.

Martin, C.P., Fain, M.J., Klotz, S.A., 2008. The older HIV-positive adult: a critical review of the medical literature. Am. J. Med. 121, 1032–1037.

Mercier, L.R., Harold, R.D., Dimond, M., Berlin, S., 2013. Lesbian health care: women's experiences and the role for social work. J. Soc. Serv. Res. 39 (1), 16–37.

Morrison, S., Dinkel, S., 2012. Heterosexism and health care: a concept analysis. Nurs. Forum 47 (2), 123–130.

NHS Education for Scotland, 2007. Addressing LGBT health inequalities: an educational resource: heterosexism notes for trainers. <http://webcache.googleusercontent.com/search?q=cache :zR4PVEgzrl4J:www.lgbt-healthinequalities.scot.nhs.uk/ documents/6%2520Training_activities_resources/3%2520 Barriers_to_LGBT_equality/Resources/Heterosexism_notes.doc +&cd=3&hl=en&ct=clnk&gl=uk> (accessed 31.07.14.).

#OTalk, 2014. About #OTalk. <http://otalk.co.uk/about-2/> (accessed 20.02.15.).

Pan American Health Organization, 2013. Stigma and discrimination jeopardize the health of lesbians, gays, bisexuals, and transgender people. <http://www.paho.org/hq/index.php?option =com_content&view=article&id=8670%3Astigma-and -discrimination-jeopardize-the-health-of-lesbians-gays-bisexuals -and-transgender-people&catid=740%3Anews-press-rele> (accessed 29.07.14.).

Price, L., 2014. Queering older gay male lives: academic theory and real-life research. In: Zeeman, L., et al. (Eds.), Queering Health: Critical Challenges to Normative Health and Healthcare. PCCS Books, Ross-on-Wye, UK.

Pugh, S., 2002. The forgotten: a community without a generation-older lesbians and gay men. In: Richardson, D., Seidman, S. (Eds.), Handbook of Lesbian and Gay Studies. Sage, Thousand Oaks, CA, pp. 81–104.

Rutherford, T., 2012. Population ageing: statistics. <http://www .parliament.uk/business/publications/research/briefing-papers/ SN03228/population-ageing-statistics> (accessed 22.01.15.).

Sakellariou, D., Pollard, N., 2008. Three sites of conflict and cooperation: class, gender and sexuality. In: Pollard, N., et al. (Eds.), A Political Practice of Occupational Therapy. Churchill Livingstone Elsevier, Edinburgh, UK, pp. 69–90.

Scrutton, J., Sinclair, D., Watson, J., Hawkins, M., Chong, A., 2014. Public health responses to an ageing society: opportunities and challenges. ILC-UK, London.

Shippy, R.A., Cantor, M.H., Brennan, M., 2004. Social networks of aging gay men. J. Mens Stud. 13 (1), 107–120, <http://search.pro quest.com/printviewfile?accountid=9727> (accessed 03.08.14.).

Stonewall, 2014. What is homophobia? <http://www.stonewall .org.uk/at_home/sexual_orientation_faqs/2697.asp> (accessed 30.07.14.).

Taylor, J., 2012. Working with Older Lesbian, Gay and Bisexual People: A Guide for Care and Support Services. Stonewall, London.

Twinley, R., 2014. Sexual orientation and occupation: some issues to consider when working with older gay people to meet their occupational needs. Br. J. Occup. Ther. 77 (12), 623–625.

Warner, M., 2000. The Trouble with Normal: Sex, Politics, and the Ethics of Queer Life. Harvard University Press, Cambridge, MA.

Whalley Hammell, K., 2011. Resisting theoretical imperialism in the disciplines of occupational science and occupational therapy. Br. J. Occup. Ther. 74 (1), 27–33.

Wilton, T., 1997. Good for You: A Handbook on Lesbian Health and Wellbeing. Cassell, London.

Wilton, T., 2000. Sexualities in Health and Social Care: A Textbook. Open University Press, Buckingham, UK.

13

BROADENING UNDERSTANDINGS OF OCCUPATIONAL IDENTITY: ILLUSTRATIONS FROM A RESEARCH STUDY OF HOMELESS ADULTS

MIRANDA CUNNINGHAM

Occupational identity is an emerging construct that is relatively unexplored in occupational science and occupational therapy literature. It has been described as a broad and value-laden concept (Wiseman and Whiteford, 2007) that is often discussed without clarification of the theory that underlies it (Phelan and Kinsella, 2009). Laliberte-Rudman and Dennhardt (2008) have suggested that the evolution of occupational identity has been limited due to the prevalence of Western cultural norms held amongst theorists developing the concept. Therefore they argue that the focus of occupational identity is on 'emphasising a future orientation, achievement-based doing, individual choice, and mastery of individuals over nature' (Laliberte-Rudman and Dennhardt, 2008, p. 153). It is important for the credibility of the occupational therapy profession, and the usability of occupation-based concepts, that the theoretical underpinnings of occupational therapy practice encompass the diversity of human experience.

The aim of this chapter is to broaden understandings of the concept of occupational identity. This will be achieved by firstly exploring key concepts from the wider literature on identity theory. Secondly, the concept of occupational identity will be examined from its historical beginnings to current occupational science conceptualizations. Finally, findings from a British study of homeless people are used to explore links between occupation and identity. This will provide a basis on which to broaden current thinking around occupational identity.

THE CONCEPT OF IDENTITY

Within the social sciences, there is a significant body of literature pertaining to the concept of identity (Vignoles et al., 2011). This literature is complex and diverse, emanating from disciplines including psychology, anthropology, sociology, education, and criminology, among others. It should be noted that within psychology there is a division of this work which

118

includes a dimension called *occupational identity,* which refers to 'the conscious awareness of oneself as a worker' (Skorikov and Vondracek, 2011, p. 693).

Examining the breadth of social science identity theory could be illuminating for occupational science because the literature considers identity from many more parameters than have previously been explored in relation to occupational identity. For example, identity scholars debate two different but equally significant aspects of identity: the content of identity and identity processes. The content of identity could include such diverse subjects as self-esteem, or a person's role (e.g., spouse) or a nationality (e.g., British). Identity processes are concerned with how identity is formed, maintained or changed (Vignoles et al., 2011).

Scholars from diverse theoretical backgrounds tend to explore different levels of identity content and processes. For example, those who adopt a psychological approach may focus on identity at the personal or individual level. In this approach, the content of the identity might be a personal goal or belief, and the process is the self-agency through which a person works towards a set of goals. Those from a sociological background consider relational identity and argue that an identity can only be established if it is recognized socially within a relational group (Swann, 2005). There is also recognition of wider social influences. For example, collective identity is related to associations with groups, such as ethnic and religious groups, and the beliefs or behaviours that occur as a consequence of identifying with them (Vignoles et al., 2011).

Additionally, there is debate in the identity literature about whether identity remains stable or whether it changes. Erikson's (1968) seminal theory on identity proposed that adolescence was the time when identity was developed and that it remained comparatively fixed once it was. Vignoles et al. (2011, p. 10) argue that 'developmental psychological approaches continue to view identity as relatively stable once it has been formed'. In contrast, other social perspectives suggest that context can influence conceptions of the self (English and Chen, 2007) and that identity is more dynamic, albeit in relation to short-term changes. As an example, being made redundant may cause a person to reconsider their previous identity as a worker.

It is clear from this brief overview that the construct of identity is multifaceted and layered. It is seen by some scholars in the field to be problematic because it is difficult to develop a clearly defined and demarcated body of work due to this complexity (Rattansi and Phoenix, 2005). This may have implications if scholars from occupational science wish to further develop the concept of occupational identity by drawing from existing identity theory. The following section considers how the concept of occupational identity has been developed within occupational science to date.

DEVELOPMENT OF THE CONCEPT OF OCCUPATIONAL IDENTITY WITHIN OCCUPATIONAL SCIENCE

In occupational science, occupational identity was first addressed by Christiansen (1999), who suggested that occupation was the primary vehicle through which a person would communicate their personal identity. He suggested that personal identity is shaped by relationships with others, is tied to what people do, provides coherence and meaning through life, and is an essential element in promoting well-being (Christiansen, 1999). From an occupational perspective, Christiansen suggested that identity construction might be considered as 'becoming who we are through what we do' (2004, p. 121). However, Christiansen (1999) also stated that his ideas were speculative and required further research to determine their appropriateness. A number of writers have taken up this challenge, and there is a small but growing literature base within occupational science that considers the links between occupation and identity.

Writing shortly after Christiansen, Kielhofner brought the words *occupation* and *identity* together to coin the phrase *occupational identity*. He described occupational identity as 'a composite sense of who one is and wishes to become as an occupational being generated from one's history of occupational participation' (Kielhofner, 2002, p. 119). He elaborated further on this, suggesting occupational identity was linked to volition, habituation and performance, which are systems within the model of human occupation (Kielhofner, 2008). Some of the subsequent literature used constructs (or assessments) from the model of human occupation to explore occupational identity (see, e.g., Braveman et al., 2006; Cotton, 2012; Howie et al., 2004; Martin et al., 2011).

Further examination of the occupational science literature reveals that there is a lack of clarity around the usage of some terms in relation to identity. For example, the terms *self-identity* and *occupational identity* are used interchangeably. This is significant given the complex nature of the construct of identity described previously. Some authors suggest that occupational identity is a specific element within the wider construct of identity (Laliberte-Rudman and Dennhart, 2008). Bryson-Campbell et al. (2013) explore this further by distinguishing self-identity as a broad concept whilst occupational identity is more specific (Bryson-Campbell et al., 2013). They argue that they can infer relevant information from literature on occupational identity because it is part of self-identity. However, the focus of their discussion is on the self and neglects aspects of social or collective identity.

Taking a solely individualistic view of occupational identity limits the potential for understanding the links between occupation and identity from a collective or culturally informed standpoint, particularly as there is growing recognition that occupation is seldom purely the domain of the individual (Hammell, 2011). Occupation is after all connected to locations, history, culture, community, politics and economics (Dickie et al., 2006; Kantartzis and Molineux, 2011), meaning that the development of occupational identity is likely to be influenced by these aspects too.

Taylor and Kay (2013) recently undertook research to identify how engaging in 'serious leisure occupations' led to the construction of identity amongst a group of people in the UK. Serious leisure occupations were defined as those that were particularly significant to participants, where engagement was intense and often involved being part of an occupational community, specialist skills were developed and positive meanings for individuals were derived. Their study concluded with the development of an empirically based 'conceptualization of the occupied self' which included three dimensions: the located self, the active self and the changing self (Taylor and Kay, 2013, p. 12). The located self refers to the influence of cultural expectations, group membership and positive or negative aspects of social image, and as such provides a framework that broadens current conceptualizations of occupational identity because it

acknowledges not only the self, but also relational and collective influences on identity developed through occupation.

In Taylor and Kay's (2013) study, the sample population was leisure enthusiasts, some of whom were in employment and some retired, with the majority being educated to at least degree level. The profile of participants reflects criticism of the construct of occupational identity in that it has been developed in the affluent West where personal choice is valued. The social class of the participants may have also influenced their ability to engage in rewarding occupations that were personally meaningful to them and valued by wider society. Identity formation developed through engaging in intensely enjoyable and meaningful occupations is likely to be positive. One might therefore question what happens to identity when people engage in occupations that they experience as alienating, or society perceives to be negative? What happens to your occupational identity if you experience stigma because of what you do, or if you are excluded from society? How do you construct an occupational identity if you are deprived of engaging in meaningful occupations because of the environment you live in, for example, on the streets or in a homeless hostel? How do you construct an occupational identity without a place to occupy? These questions and others like them sparked a personal interest in finding out more about occupational identity from the perspective of homeless people. The following section explores this in more depth.

THE LIVED EXPERIENCE OF HOMELESSNESS AND THE IMPACT ON IDENTITY: PRESENTING THE STUDY

I used a phenomenological approach with the aim to understand homeless peoples' subjective experience of their occupations and how this contributed to their identity construction. Five men, aged from 18 to 61, took part in the study. The participants were residing in a homeless hostel in the south of England. They were asked to describe their day-to-day activities by completing a photographic diary of their daily occupations. A subsequent semistructured interview was undertaken with each participant and this included questions about how the person felt about themselves in relation to their occupations. The analysis was guided by interpretative phenomenological analysis (Smith et al., 2009). The following section discusses the study findings.

Knowing Who I Am Through Occupation, Fixed or Sustained Identity

Participants were able to articulate aspects of their identity in terms of who they were through what they did. For example, Sean (all names used are pseudonyms) viewed himself as a butcher: 'I mean I'm a butcher by trade'.

It is apparent that this aspect of Sean's identity was relatively stable, as he talked about being a butcher in the present tense, despite not being employed at the time of the research. Mark, who participated in football games whilst at the hostel, identified himself as a goal keeper: 'So I've been playing in goal like, and I'm a good goal keeper like, believe it or not'.

These examples allude to ideas from social science theory on identity content and processes, where the occupations Sean will have engaged in to become a butcher (training, work experience) were part of the identity creation process. His role as a butcher is formally recognized as a qualification. Playing football would have been the process through which Mark developed his identity as a footballer, and this could have been achieved either informally or formally. The content of people's identity is the role they assume; for Sean this is being a butcher and for Mark it is being a good goal keeper. Knowing that you are good at something suggests content identity at the personal level, but being good at goal keeping relies on others to play football with you, which resonates with the relational level of content identity and also the interconnectedness of occupations.

There is a sense of participating in occupations over time that has led to these beliefs, or understandings of the self. This fits with Kielhofner's (2002) original conceptualization of occupational identity as being 'generated from one's history of occupational participation' (p. 119). There are other aspects of identity that were sustained and came from past experiences of occupations. For example, Mark's identity as a football fan was particularly meaningful to him. One of his few possessions was an Arsenal (English football team) poster, and his photo diary included a photograph of the poster in his room in the hostel. Mark described his long-term occupation as a football fan:

Well, I've always been an Arsenal fan. I used to go up to, when it was Highbury [area in London], used to go to every home game for about four years I used to go. Every home game, I was a junior gunner as they say. I went when it used to cost two pound a ticket.

Being a junior gunner suggests belonging to a group and having a collective or social identity that was achieved through the process of going to home games. Holding on to this valued identity may have served to counter the negative impact of homelessness. One could surmise that the devastating losses of homelessness that Mark experienced, including becoming estranged from his young sons, would have a significant impact on his well-being. Perhaps having a consistent sense of self, as an Arsenal fan, supported his well-being and provided continuity when the rest of his life was disrupted. Howie et al. (2004) studied older people's engagement in lifelong craft occupations and found a beneficial effect of sustaining engagement on identity and sense of self over time.

Occupational Engagement and Fluid Identities

There is a growing consensus in the occupational science literature that occupational identities might not be static (Asaba and Jackson, 2011; Howie et al., 2004; Taylor and Kay, 2013; Vrkljan and Miller-Polgar, 2007). In social psychology, short-term changes in identity are also recognized (Vignoles et al., 2011). This is contradictory to the idea of a stable identity discussed previously. However, Vignoles et al. (2011, p. 11) explain this as 'difference of emphasis rather than a difference in the nature of the phenomena', suggesting that there is a possible middle ground between stable and changing identity.

Participants in the study described aspects of their identity that had obviously changed as a result of the experience of homelessness and engaging in certain antisocial occupations. This engagement created a negative identity, as Neil and Mark describe:

Neil: Picking up dog ends, going through bins…it's not who I am.

Mark: I'm not happy with myself, no. Not happy with myself at all. That's what I mean like, obviously when I'm in court, I've done a lot of bad things last, you know, over the last year, you know just theft wise and stealing and whatever.

There is a hint of *spoiled identities* in these accounts, a term that was first used by Goffman (1963) to describe an identity that causes a person to experience stigma. However, at the time, Neil was able to override his personal standards and engage in activities like going through bins to ensure his survival. Spoiled identity was felt personally by individuals, and the stigma of a homeless identity resulted in abusive behaviour from the public:

Neil: I've had, erm, when I was at the soup run, I've been walking back home, so and so has thrown a water bomb at me, I've been called names, walking up you know, yeah it's just cruel, like.

A stigmatized occupational identity has also been found in other populations following disruption including people with brain injury (Bryson-Campbell et al., 2013) and HIV (Braveman et al., 2006). When Sean was asked about his identity, his focus was on past occupations, perhaps because his current identity would be spoilt by links to negative occupations.

Miranda: From the things that you do day to day, does that give you a sense of who you are? Is your personal identity linked to what you do?
Sean: No, I don't think so. Erm, my personal identity, is linked to what I've done in the past, what I've, what I've achieved in my life.

Although Sean links his identity to doing, he does not describe an identity for himself now, based on homelessness and the occupations he engages in at present. He has a stable identity as a butcher that he is prepared to reveal, but his changed identity in relation to being homeless is not one that he chooses to share in the same way. Neil stated that he would only disclose his homeless experience to others when he felt his life was back on track, for example, when he had money and a car. This illustrates how context affects identity, something also illustrated in English and Chen's (2007) study on the stability of the self-concept of East Asian and European Americans across contexts. Notably,

they argue for an 'if-then' profile where 'if' relates to a situation and 'then' is the response to it (English and Chen, 2007). In Neil's case, *if* he is able to get his life back on track, *then* he will disclose his homeless experiences to his relatives.

Despite these stigmatized aspects to identity, there were positive elements and hope for a changed identity in the future. Alex expressed how his homeless experience had contributed to changing who he wanted to become as a person:

No, 'cos when I was younger I wanted to be a care worker, I wanted to work for the elderly, so it's a total career path change, it's just what I've been through, just changed me totally.

Neil explained how his previous identity related to his girlfriend and his employment. Here he describes his previous role as a skilled programmer, which he refers to as 'C and C':

And that's why I kind of stuck with the C and C for so long, 'cos she was like, you know that's a good job, she would tell people like, oh you know my chap works in C and C, so yeah to keep her happy, keep her impressed, you know and it was like, and now I get a job, I do what I want to do.

Neil remained in this occupation that he did not particularly enjoy because his girlfriend valued it. This aspect of his identity was about what somebody else 'wants you to be through what you do' and illustrates the potential powerful influence of relationships on occupational identity. However, the loss of his relationship with his girlfriend and his experiences of homelessness allowed him to consider pursuing a new career path of his own choosing. He later alludes to his decision to pursue a career as a personal trainer that he developed since living in the hostel.

Rowles (2008, p. 129) suggests people are 'defined by a particular location and a particular time'. However, both Neil and Sean resist definitions of themselves based on homelessness – that is, Neil's difficulty in accepting a view of himself as a person who goes through bins and Sean's suggestion that his identity is linked to what he has achieved previously. In Sean's experience, place and occupation are undeniably powerful in influencing his sense of self, as the discussion about his experience of hostel living illustrates:

Every now and again something happens, and I get a sense of who I am, and I, I kind of think, I am still there, I am still me, it's just I need to get, I need to move forward a bit further than and be a bit more happier. But I think that's not going to happen until I'm in my own place, you know a remote control for my TV, you know, put on what I want to watch, put the kettle on, eat what I want to eat, do what I want to do, and then I'll get a sense of who I am [laughs].

Exploring Theoretical Assumptions of Occupational Identity From the Lived Experience of Homelessness

Critics of the construct of occupational identity suggest that there are certain assumptions that underpin it (Laliberte-Rudman and Dennhardt, 2008; Phelan and Kinsella, 2009). These include: '(a) the individual at the core of identity formation, (b) choice, (c) productivity and (d) social dimensions' (Phelan and Kinsella, 2009, p. 86). To examine the associations between homelessness and occupational identity further, data were analysed against these theoretical assumptions.

This research into the lived experience of homelessness challenges the idea that individuals have control over their identity, as demonstrated by the emergence of spoiled identities. The reaction of the public, such as Neil being called names when rough sleeping, suggests that identities are not just shaped by the self (Dickie et al., 2006) and this is also evident in literature on homelessness (Rayburn and Guittar, 2013; Skosireva et al., 2014). Furthermore, participants in this study experienced occupational deprivation which impacted on their ability to make choices about occupations, both when sleeping rough and whilst living in the hostel. For example, Mark valued and enjoyed cooking, and regularly participated in a cooking group run by a volunteer at the hostel. The majority of his photographs were of dishes he had cooked, suggesting some correlation between this occupation and a positive sense of self, or identity. However, he was not able to make choices about what to eat or when to cook. He stated: 'Yeah, I like cooking, yeah. But obviously here, you know, this [the cooking group] is on a Thursday'.

This illustrates how both agency (the self) and structure (society/culture) influence identity (Huot and Laliberte-Rudman, 2010). Mark was committed to cooking and demonstrated personal agency in respect of this; however, there were structural barriers to his participation because he was only able to access the kitchen when the volunteer ran the cooking group.

Productivity is also an element that is emphasized in occupational identity theory (Phelan and Kinsella, 2009). The participants were embedded in a Western culture and were subject to society's values. The norm for males of a working age is to be in employment. This socially constructed aspect to occupational identity influenced the men in the study, and it is therefore unsurprising that all of the participants articulated aspirations in relation to a productive role. Arguably, achieving that aim might be more problematic for them because of the social discourse surrounding homelessness and prevailing negative attitudes that influence the occupational choices of homeless people. Moreover, some of the participants acquired criminal records as a result of engaging in illegal occupations, and they commented on how this engagement impacted on them:

Alex: To be honest, being in that situation [living on the streets] you get in rocky roads, and where I got in got in rocky roads, I used to go and steal, just to have funds and get somewhere in life, and look at me now, it's caught up with me and I've got burglary charges, I'm on bail so, not good.

The influence of society on identity formation has been acknowledged in the literature (Phelan and Kinsella, 2009). For Neil, his previous occupation as a computer programmer carried status in society and influenced his identity in a positive way (Christiansen, 2004). However, thinking has extended beyond the idea of socially approved occupations to suggest that society can actually 'form, shape or even produce identities' (Phelan and Kinsella, 2009, p. 89). This was the case where negative identities were formed due to stigma and discrimination. Participants did not wish to belong to the homeless population and sought ways to distance themselves from other homeless people, as the following quote illustrates:

Neil: I think, I think, that people saw that I wasn't a criminal, a proper homeless person, erm, but I think everyone, everyone, staff wise, saw the potential in me you know.

This illustrates the power of sociocultural influences on identity (Kantartzis and Molineux, 2011). In a similar way, people with disabilities often reject labels given to them. A study by Asaba and Jackson (2011) that explored disability, identities and occupation discussed the case of Sam, a wheelchair-user with a recent spinal cord injury who did 'not consider himself as disabled' (Asaba and Jackson, 2011, p. 142) because of the negative social discourse around disability. The participants in this study disassociated themselves from negative connotations of homelessness which they achieved through describing identity in terms of either previous achievements (Sean) or future aspirations (Neil and Alex).

CONCLUSION

This chapter has added to the occupational identity literature by examining both existing identity theory *and* occupational identity theory whilst relating these to the lived experience of a group of homeless people in the UK.

Identity scholars discuss both identity *content* and *process*. It does appear that engaging in occupations is one of the main *processes* through which identity is formed, and this was Christiansen's original premise (1999). Being able to call yourself a footballer would necessitate engaging in playing football. It is interesting that for Sean, the content of his identity as a butcher remained long after he stopped engaging in the occupations that were part of the process of forming that identity. His memory and the narrative he constructs allow him to integrate his memories with his present experiences, which supports his connection to others. Kielhofner (2002) alluded to both content and process in his original definition of occupational identity. This was in terms of who one is and wishes to become (content) generated from one's history of occupational participation (process). Generally, however, the distinction between identity content and process has not been elaborated upon in the occupational science literature, and this may be a useful area of future research, particularly as both aspects can impact on sense of self and well-being.

This chapter has shown that identity content and processes can be experienced as humiliating or alienating by people; the spoiled identities discussed illustrate this (e.g., going through bins and picking up cigarette ends, and being labelled as homeless by others). However, Kielhofner's (2002) original definition does not allude to these more negative aspects. To understand humans as occupational beings, occupational science needs to be inclusive of the full range of human occupational experience. It is important to understand that structural factors can impede personal agency and choice in respect of engaging in meaningful occupations (e.g. Mark and his cooking) and make the development of a positive identity challenging. Working therapeutically with others, one might therefore need to consider the impact on identity of 'who you are unable to become because of what you are excluded from doing' and 'who you do not want to be through what you have done' (e.g., Mark and his criminal record).

The idea that a person's previous and ongoing positive identities (e.g., football fan, Sean's previous achievements) might provide protection against adversity is useful because these aspects of a person's occupational history may provide a base against which other new positive identities can be formed. It was clear from this research that participants had aspirations to change their future occupational identity. Whilst in a time of crisis, for example, homelessness, identity might become damaged. Opportunities to experience the self in a positive way, such as through engaging in new, more constructive occupations, could support changes in identity and consequently wellbeing. Finally there is the collective or social aspect of identity that might be described as 'who you are perceived to be by others through what you do'. The participants in this study were motivated to take part and described future occupational aspirations. They also disassociated themselves from wider society's negative connotations of homeless people by mentally distancing themselves from fellow residents. This raises questions as to how a person might experience belonging when they are within a socially excluded section of society. These aspects merit further research.

The study presented in this chapter has shown that understanding occupational identity as 'who we are through what we do' is far too simplistic. A number of other valid permutations of this simple definition have been suggested, for example, 'who you don't want to be through what you've done'. There are doubtless many other permutations, which suggest a simple definition of occupational identity is not realistic. What is useful from a therapeutic perspective is to continue to take an occupational lens to considering issues of identity, as this links to a person's or community's self-esteem and well-being. Occupational therapists need to consider how occupations support identity construction, maintenance and change; this should continue from a multilayered approach in relation not only to the individual, but also their relationships, taking into account the wider societal perspective.

REFERENCES

Asaba, E., Jackson, J., 2011. Social ideologies embedded in everyday life: a narrative analysis about disability, identities, and occupation. J. Occup. Sci. 18 (2), 139–152.

Braveman, B., Kielhofner, G., Albrecht, G., Helfrich, C., 2006. Occupational identity, occupational competence and occupational settings (environment): influences on return to work in men living with HIV/AIDS. Work 27, 267–276.

Bryson-Campbell, M., Shaw, L., O'Brien, J., Holmes, J., Magalhaes, L., 2013. A scoping review on occupational and self-identity after a brain injury. Work 44, 57–67.

Christiansen, C.H., 1999. Defining lives: occupation as identity: an essay on competence, coherence, and the creation of meaning. Am. J. Occup. Ther. 53 (6), 547–558.

Christiansen, C.H., 2004. Occupation and identity: becoming who we are through what we do. In: Christiansen, C.H., Townsend, E.A. (Eds.), Introduction to Occupation: The Art and Science of Living. Prentice Hall, Upper Saddle River, NJ, pp. 121–139.

Cotton, G., 2012. Occupational identity disruption after traumatic brain injury: an approach to occupational therapy evaluation and treatment. Occup. Ther. Health Care 26 (4), 270–282.

Dickie, V., Cutchin, M.P., Humphry, R., 2006. Occupation as transactional experience: a critique of individualism in occupational science. J. Occup. Sci. 13 (1), 83–93.

English, T., Chen, S., 2007. Culture and self-concept stability: consistency across and within contexts among Asian Americans and European Americans. J. Pers. Soc. Psychol. 93 (3), 478–490.

Erikson, E.H., 1968. Identity, Youth and Crisis. W.W. Norton and Company, New York.

Goffman, E., 1963. Stigma: Notes on the Management of Spoiled Identity. Prentice-Hall, New Jersey.

Hammell, K.W., 2011. Resisting theoretical imperialism in the disciplines of occupational science and occupational therapy. Br. J. Occup. Ther. 74 (1), 27–33.

Howie, L., Coulter, M., Feldman, S., 2004. Crafting the self: older persons' narratives of occupational identity. Am. J. Occup. Ther. 54 (4), 446–454.

Huot, S., Laliberte-Rudman, D., 2010. The performances and places of identity: conceptualising intersections of occupation, identity and place in the process of migration. J. Occup. Sci. 17 (2), 68–77.

Kantartzis, S., Molineux, M., 2011. The influence of Western society's construction of a healthy daily life on the conceptualisation of occupation. J. Occup. Sci. 18 (1), 62–80.

Kielhofner, G., 2002. Model of Human Occupation: Theory and Application, third ed. Lippincott Williams & Wilkins, Philadelphia.

Kielhofner, G., 2008. Model of Human Occupation: Theory and Application, fourth ed. Lippincott Williams & Wilkins, Philadelphia.

Laliberte-Rudman, D., Dennhardt, S., 2008. Shaping knowledge regarding occupation: examining the cultural underpinnings of the evolving concept of occupational identity. Aust. J. Occup. Ther. 55, 153–162.

Martin, L.M., Smith, M., Rogers, J., Wallen, T., Boisvert, R., 2011. Mothers in recovery: an occupational perspective. Occup. Ther. Int. 18, 152–161.

Phelan, S., Kinsella, E.A., 2009. Occupational identity: engaging socio-cultural perspectives. J. Occup. Sci. 16 (2), 85–91.

Rattansi, R., Phoenix, A., 2005. Rethinking you identities: modernist and postmodernist frameworks. Identity Int. J. Theory Res. 5 (2), 97–123.

Rayburn, R.L., Guittar, N.A., 2013. This is where you are supposed to be: how homeless individuals cope with stigma. Sociol. Spectr. 33, 159–174.

Rowles, G.D., 2008. Place in occupational science: a life course perspective on the role of environmental context in the quest for meaning. J. Occup. Sci. 15 (3), 127–135.

Skorikov, V.B., Vondracek, F.W., 2011. Occupational identity. In: Schwartz, S.J., et al. (Eds.), Handbook of Identity Theory and Research, vol. 2: Domains and Categories. Springer, New York, pp. 693–714.

Skosireva, A., O'Campo, P., Zerger, S., Chambers, C., Gapka, S., Stergiopoulos, V., 2014. Different faces of discrimination: perceived discrimination among homeless adults with mental illness in health care settings. BMC Health Serv. Res. 14, 376.

Smith, J.A., Flowers, P., Larkin, P., 2009. Interpretative Phenomenological Analysis: Theory, Method and Research. Sage, London.

Swann, W.B. Jr., 2005. The self and identity negotiation. Interact. Stud. 6, 69–83.

Taylor, J., Kay, S., 2013. The construction of identities in narratives about serious leisure occupations. J. Occup. Sci. 1–17. doi:10.1080/14427591.2013.803298.

Vignoles, V.L., Schwartz, S.J., Luyckx, K., 2011. Introduction: toward an integrative view of identity. In: Schwartz, S.J., et al. (Eds.), Handbook of Identity Theory and Research, vol. 1. Springer, New York, pp. 1–27.

Vrkljan, B.H., Miller-Polgar, J., 2007. Linking occupational participation and occupational identity: an exploratory study of the transition from driving to driving cessation in older adulthood. J. Occup. Sci. 14 (1), 30–39.

Wiseman, L.M., Whiteford, G., 2007. Life history as a tool for understanding occupation, identity and context. J. Occup. Sci. 14 (2), 108–114.

14

LEISURE AS A ROUTE TO SOCIAL AND OCCUPATIONAL JUSTICE FOR INDIVIDUALS WITH PROFOUND LEVELS OF DISABILITY

ANNE FENECH ■ LESLEY COLLIER

Meaningful occupations enhance people's sense of self and facilitate occupational engagement (Perruzza and Kinsella, 2010). During rehabilitation the priority tends to be on self-care, leaving many people struggling to reestablish new or existing leisure occupations. However, meaningful leisure may predict well-being (Krishnagiri and Southam, 2013). This chapter promotes a notion of social justice by arguing that individuals with neuropalliative conditions (NPCs) have the right to engage in leisure occupations of their choice. This chapter emphasizes consideration of the leisure occupation itself, the contextual factors surrounding it, and the participants' preferences and abilities. It highlights the increasing incidence of NPCs, and the influences on occupational engagement, before exploring meaningful leisure and some of the barriers to leisure engagement faced by individuals living with NPCs, prior to considering some of

the factors that could contribute to an engaging occupation as defined by Jonsson (2014). Finally, this chapter presents a case study about engaging leisure occupations.

BACKGROUND

Increasing Incidence of Neuropalliative Conditions

The subspecialties in neurology include, among others, specialist neurology, rehabilitation and neurological palliative (neuropalliative) services. Palliative care involves the prevention and reduction of suffering by means of preemptive assessment and treatment, without curing (Robinson and Barrett, 2014). A condition becomes neuropalliative at the point where improvement in terms of health, autonomy or independence is no longer probable, and rehabilitation ceases. The expectation becomes one of compensation for limitations through modification of the built, social and physical environment surrounding the occupation, to empower the individual as much as possible. NPCs include neurological conditions such as locked-in syndrome, multiple sclerosis or Huntington disease (British Society of Rehabilitation Medicine, 2010), which result in profound and complex levels of disability (British Society of Rehabilitation Medicine, 2010). Increases in survival rates and longevity mean that their incidence is increasing (Neurological Alliance, 2014). Consequently, individuals with disabilities are living longer, with greater impairments and fewer occupational choices (Monti et al., 2010). Accordingly, leisure engagement is the goal of many individuals who cannot return to past employment (Fenech and Shaw-Fisher, 2012). Many individuals with NPCs have permanent and profound disabilities that lead to reliance on others for their self-care, productivity and leisure (Fenech, 2013, 2015). Leisure participation may focus on passive roles, living life through others, and therefore increasing the risk of passive occupational engagement or even occupational deprivation (Fenech, 2013, 2015).

Influences on Occupational Engagement

Providing engaging and meaningful leisure opportunities is challenging. Only the individual can decide the categorization of an occupation and whether it is an engaging pursuit (Jonsson, 2014). Self-determination of leisure for people with NPCs is problematic as biopsychosocial factors and the sensory environment influence occupational performance (Jonsson, 2014). Indeed, Galvaan (2014) suggests that leisure engagement is not simply a matter of individual choice. Accessibility, for example, may influence engagement, leading carers to impose activities that are easy to provide. The level of support received and a desire for carers to prevent boredom may influence engagement, leading to resentment if interventions are not appreciated by the person with the NPC. In order to achieve optimal engagement, leisure activity needs to be of suitable length to maintain interest and arousal. Another influencing factor could be the individual's sense of contributing to their community or social circle, or their level of interest, and their sense of occupational balance. Other factors include the novelty and complexity of an occupation, and the individual's

occupational capacity, as well as the occupational role actually experienced. Jonsson (2014) suggested that occupational engagement may be influenced by internal motivations and external demands, for example, the depletion or enrichment of the participants' physical and psychological resources through their occupational engagement.

Definitions of Meaningful Leisure

Many publications have discussed meaningfulness, engagement worthiness, and how imposed, nonmeaningful, 'time-filler' occupations may result in stagnation and a sense of emptiness (Fenech, 2013). Jonsson (2014) described how a single occupation can have different meanings for each participant. This idea was supported by Pollard and Sakellariou (2012), who suggested that occupation contains multiple meanings for the individual depending on the reasons for doing it, the sensory experience, temporality and context. This suggests that meaning could be defined from an individual's perspective, and that of fellow participants, and the sense of well-being experienced. Participation in a range of occupations was also associated with ageing well, breaking patterns of isolation and increasing social engagement (Wright-St Clair, 2012).

Occupations gain meaning within the multiple contexts in which they take place. This meaning is shaped by a dynamic interplay among what people choose to engage in given cultural expectations, others who are part of the activity, past experiences, and influences and expectations for the future (Reed et al., 2010). This interplay changes over the lifespan, presenting choices to alter the meaning of an occupation. Jonsson (2014) suggested that the meaning derived could be positive or negative which would possibly resonate with the experience of individuals with NPCs. The meaningfulness of occupations contributes to providing a meaningful social world for the participant. The challenges, new skills learned and goals achieved may all contribute to a sense of accomplishment and a raison d'être. The meaning of occupational engagement can therefore be understood from different theoretical and philosophical angles, such as the social and cultural perspectives of meaning and the experience of the individual (Jonsson, 2014). These will be explored in more depth in relation to individuals with NPCs.

LEISURE AND 'OCCUPATIONAL CHOICE' FOR INDIVIDUALS LIVING WITH NEUROPALLIATIVE CONDITIONS

Throughout life, impediments to occupational engagement may arise, requiring new patterns of occupation (Perruzza and Kinsella, 2010). For instance, individuals with physical and cognitive disabilities experience reduced leisure participation compared with those without (Sharp et al., 2011). Fenech (2013) observed that passive engagement was the experience of profoundly disabled individuals who were expected to do or be part of just any occupation, or whatever came their way, suggesting that this was less engaging than active participation. Studies exploring the use of leisure by individuals with disabilities have been quite prescriptive about what activities are perceived as leisure and also the activities to be studied. This prescriptiveness runs counter to the concept of leisure as self-determined, but may resonate with the experience of individuals whose leisure choices are selected from a menu (Wright-St Claire, 2012). As such, determining the value of occupations that clearly do not match the features of meaningful activity is problematic. Fenech and Shaw-Fisher's (2012) study revealed the importance of leisure for health, well-being, sense of being capable, reduced boredom, increased self-expression and creativity, a sense of belonging and self-identity. Opportunities to experience challenge, links with past self, individual growth and life satisfaction were also mentioned, as were a sense of life's rhythm, goal orientation, a sense of self-efficacy and adjustment to disability. Arguably, individuals who do not have many opportunities for engagement in productivity/work or self-care may engage in leisure in order to gain a sense of meaning and self-determination.

Krishnagiri and Southam (2013) suggest that individuals choose leisure occupations that they enjoy. Therefore only the individual can determine whether an occupation is leisure, enjoyable and of interest. Leisure is defined as being free from commitments (Dattilo and Rusch, 2012), freely chosen, meaningful and done for its own sake (Fenech, 2013). Leisure occupations can offer roles such as being actively involved or being a passive onlooker, for example, playing or watching a sport (Dahan-Oliel et al., 2012).

Roy et al. (2013) defined active leisure as doing and passive leisure as watching, listening and being. A link may exist between individuals with NPCs and passive leisure, changed leisure patterns or a lack of leisure activities, for example, having more free time than self-care or productivity opportunities, and reduced morale in the absence of occupational balance (Fenech, 2013).

Facilitating active leisure occupations requires occupational analysis in order to match the abilities of the individual with the demands of the task. Without choice about whether to engage, a leisure occupation becomes an imposed experience. This is relevant because therapeutic interventions may include adapting leisure occupations or the occupational environment, assisting an individual to develop new leisure interests and using recreational occupations as a therapeutic medium. Cuenca et al. (2014) suggested that individuals with NPCs may need to redefine their sense of self, their roles and goals. This might focus on self-care and productivity, because adapting them is difficult (Krishnagiri and Southam, 2013).

Profound disability results in a 'catastrophic reaction' (Martelli et al., 2008, p. 18), exacerbating the limitations experienced, leading to a steep decline in the individual's well-being, self-identity and valued roles. Besides the reduced ability to participate, leisure opportunities may be limited because formal and informal supporters may view them as unearned or unsuitable (Fenech, 2013). However, leisure is of particular importance to individuals whose lifestyle does not include employment (Eriksson et al., 2009).

The aim of the occupation differentiates leisure from recreation. Defining leisure as freely chosen may be problematic because prescribing leisure occupations changes the focus to that of a therapeutic regime, requiring facilitation. It is therefore no longer freely chosen leisure but becomes recreation (Aitchison, 2009). Additionally, what is leisure to one individual could be work to another, and so it is the reasons why and the participation method which determine the categorization of an occupation (Jonsson, 2014). The disability itself may reduce the number, frequency and duration of leisure opportunities, increasing the amount of support required (Wise et al. 2010). Because of this, individuals with disabilities may predominantly participate in physically passive, solitary, home-based, casual leisure occupations which enable independence, rather than requiring assistance to engage in active leisure. Physical difficulties may have less influence on well-being than the cognitive, perceptual, communication and sensory sequelae of an NPC (Bateman et al., 2005). There needs to be a cohesive relationship between these features, taking into account both the demands of the activity and the coregulation of those interacting with the individual with an NPC, particularly when the activity provides a high sensory challenge. Indeed, overarousal can be easily caused by an overenthusiastic carer who is unable to pick up on the nonverbal cues. Positioning an individual in a busy, noisy environment also places excess demand on attention and modulation. These challenges make it increasingly difficult for the individual to discriminate and appraise stimuli, which in turn leads to disorganization in motor and cognitive output. This concludes with failure to engage that, in time, can lead to occupational deprivation.

Given these challenges and the increasing incidence of NPCs globally, increasing numbers of individuals could be at risk of occupational deprivation. This is important, given that leisure may provide an experience of competence and self-determination, promoting self-efficacy and well-being, and combating the catastrophic reaction and occupational deprivation resulting from NPCs (Fenech and Shaw-Fisher, 2012). Leisure-based relationships reduce stress, enabling adjustment to life role changes and enhancing social identity, social interaction skills and the expression of creativity (Fenech and Shaw-Fisher, 2012).

Leisure choices reflect ability and the cultural value judgements of the participant and those about them (Fenech and Shaw-Fisher, 2012). An inability to maintain previous leisure occupations could reinforce uncertainty about the future (Cuenca et al., 2014). Consequently, leisure satisfaction may be associated with adjustment to disability (Cuenca et al., 2014). Additionally, leisure engagement may enhance coping with stress, self-identity and occupational balance, influencing hope and optimism (Sellar and Stanley, 2010; Wise et al., 2010).

Knowing that individuals with NPCs have more 'free' time, consideration of the occupations engaged in and why, and the individual, cultural and historical context of an individual is required. Free time and leisure are different. Imposed free time, without the means to fill it, is oppressive and unsatisfying (Stebbins, 2014). Therefore boredom or occupations imposed to fill free time do not equate to leisure (Stebbins, 2014).

Enabling engagement for individuals with NPCs is challenging. Therefore the organization of leisure and interaction opportunities is a core skill for carers (Fenech, 2013). A 'just right' occupational challenge encourages self-actualization, through the provision of opportunities and choice, rather than prescriptions or a menu of set activities. Self-determination of leisure for individuals with NPC can be challenging because the sensory and biopsychosocial environment influences occupational performance, as do an individual's preferences (Jonsson, 2014) and abilities. Therefore engagement may be influenced by accessibility, turning a leisure occupation into an imposed, arbitrary or easy option to provide. Other factors could include the novelty of an occupation, the complexity of the occupation as well as the occupational role offered. Fenech (2013) suggested that fewer individuals with NPCs engage in serious leisure than casual leisure occupations, with highly dependent individuals tending to prefer a spectator role. This tendency to engage in inactive or solitary leisure pursuits could be due to the effort required to engage in more physically active leisure occupations, which could lead to high satisfaction rates, influencing well-being (Fenech, 2013).

THE BORDERS BETWEEN LEISURE ENGAGEMENT AND INDIVIDUALS LIVING WITH NEUROPALLIATIVE CONDITIONS

Arguably, individuals with NPCs experience many of the external conditions of occupational deprivation. These include isolation, restraint, displacement, lack of transportation, poverty and homelessness (Fenech, 2013). Particular restraints experienced by individuals with NPC could include:

- Displacement from normal routines and roles to live with atrophied occupational capacities;
- Being restricted by immobility, or disability;

■ Being isolated from others by cognitive, perceptual or communication difficulties which influence reciprocal understanding;

■ Being unoccupied because of a lack of opportunities available; or

■ Being stigmatized by others' beliefs about capacity and suitability.

A disparity exists between wished for and experienced leisure (Wise et al., 2010), due to constraints such as lack of interest, facilities and environmental obstacles (Bier et al., 2009). In addition, reduced concentration, memory, initiative, practical transport or compensatory strategies may constrain leisure engagement for individuals with NPCs (Wise et al., 2010).

The meaningfulness of occupations may change following impairment or illness (Perruzza and Kinsella, 2010). Many environmental, physical and psychological barriers influence leisure participation such as transport issues, accessibility, loss of energy and stamina, inadequate finances, lack of interest, feelings of uncertainty and fear of harm (Fenech, 2013). Other barriers to engagement could include a lack of opportunities to take risks or experience challenge, differences in perceptions about leisure and the individual's role preference versus the role offered by leisure supporters (Fenech, 2013). Fenech (2013) reported a sense of constraint, a lack of imagination on the part of leisure supporters and a lack of self-determination. Perceptions also influenced a desire to do something more physically active versus ability (Fenech, 2013).

The occupational context for each individual within a group of individuals with NPCs requires consideration. This consideration should include the ease of accessibility and the role and the level of support required. The timing, the participant's sense of contributing to their community or social circle, as well as the meaning of the occupation and the sense of experiencing occupational balance might all influence engagement. Individual interest could motivate occupational engagement, especially if occupations are a compromise between what is desired and what is convenient. The level and skill of facilitation and collaboration from carers may also influence the engagingness of an occupation, as could the sensory attributes offered versus preferred.

The right time for engagement may also be a factor, making the most of limited ability to complete an occupation (given their sitting tolerance, for example); therefore the challenge to finish or achieve occupational balance may also be influential (Aegler and Satink, 2009). Additionally, novelty, requiring a higher level of perceptive processing (Larson and Von Eye, 2010), may encourage time to pass more quickly. Conversely, overly challenging occupations could overwhelm the individual, making time seem to pass slowly. The relative merits of familiarity with the occupation, that is, a comparison between nonroutine and routine occupations, may influence engagement. Arguably, routine occupations could be familiar, safe and engaging, or overfamiliar, boring and nonengaging. Fenech (2013) suggested that leisure choices should include deciding between either watching or doing, across the whole range of occupational and sensory experiences.

Sensory experiences and sensory activity have been underused by care staff for individuals with NPCs as they may be perceived as 'childish' (Collier and Truman, 2008), but matching the sensory ability of the individual to the sensory demand of the task can facilitate engagement on a number of levels. For example, increasing arousal has the potential to influence temperament and awareness, whilst influencing sensory processing; attention not only influences motor control, but contributes to the sense of flow and socially mediated attention. Achieving an appropriate sensory balance mediates stress and anxiety, hence contributing to a sense of wellness (Engel-Yeger and Dunn, 2011) and promoting emotional engagement.

Building on existing knowledge about the meaning of occupation and considering the influence of contextual factors may remove borders that traditionally have reduced opportunities for occupational engagement. Reed et al. (2010) described interconnectedness in the meaning of occupation. This contributes towards turning an occupation from a basic or necessary one into an engaging one (Jonsson, 2014).

FACTORS THAT COULD ENHANCE AN ENGAGING OCCUPATION

Three interrelated facets (Figure 14-1) have the potential to either enable or constrain engagement in

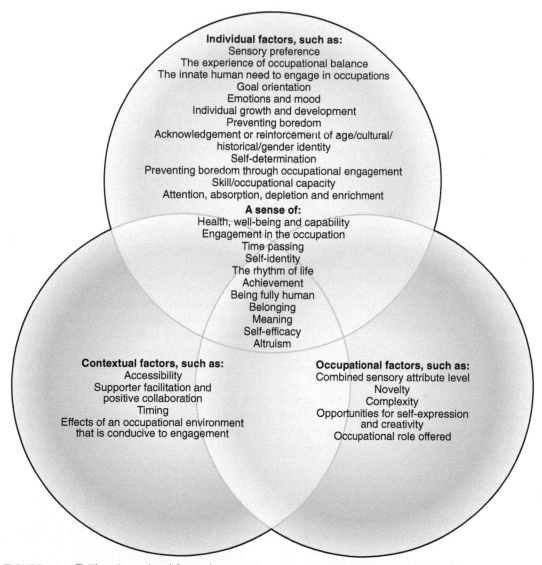

FIGURE 14-1 ■ Three interrelated facets that contribute to an engaging occupation. *(Adapted from Fenech, 2013)*

general (Fenech, 2013). The three interrelated facets pertain to the individual, to the occupation and to the environment, thus mirroring the Canadian Model of Occupational Performance and Engagement (Polatajko, et al., 2013) as influencing occupational performance. Using the three interrelated facets, Case Study 14-1 illustrates how leisure occupations may be modified to facilitate engagement for someone with an NPC.

CONCLUSIONS

Meaningful leisure occupations enhance one's sense of self; however, NPCs leave many people struggling to reestablish new or existing leisure occupations. Facilitating active leisure occupations requires occupational analysis in order to match the abilities of the individual with the demands of the task, but also choice. Impediments to occupational engagement may result in new

CASE 14-1

Environmental and Contextual Factors

Amanda (a pseudonym) has locked-in syndrome and had previously enjoyed printing cards, and using her computer for e-mail and information sourcing. Nowadays, supporting Amanda involves positioning resources so that she can connect them to her head pointer, for painting and printing of greetings cards. Her cousin acts as a helper and design advisor. Amanda enjoyed making spare cards for when family members were unable to make them themselves. Therefore Amanda makes a positive contribution to the family's card-making culture. Potentially, locked-in syndrome could be very isolating; however, Amanda's card making enables her not only to stay in touch with her friends and family but to play an important role within her social environment. As a result, Amanda became the go-to individual for card-making advice and spares.

THE OCCUPATION

Using her head pointer offers Amanda vestibular stimulation. Auditory stimulation comes from her quiet, calming music. Olfactory stimulation comes from the resources used, especially the paints and glues. As she became more proficient, an additional attachment had to be made for her head pointer to allow her to stick cut-out items onto them. Amanda is physically and actively engaged in her card making. Not having her head pointer to use one day facilitated the exploration of different way of making cards, using an eye gaze input device to access her computer. She is able to search for images on the Internet, as well as paint using the software and type using different fonts. This extended the range of her card making, as has discovering how to print them on different textured paper or altering the images in many ways.

THE INDIVIDUAL

Amanda does not like loud or sudden noises, bitter or artificial smells, or flashing lights. Her cards are a source of achievement and satisfaction, which reinforce her links with her family and friends, some of whom admired her tenacity at keeping up with this family tradition. Amanda is keen to be 'doing' because her paralysis and limited head movements limit what she can do. The card making gives Amanda the chance to reminisce with her cousin about making cards as children, with other relatives and about precious memories.

---

patterns of occupation. Individuals with NPCs experience many of the external conditions of occupational deprivation, further limiting the individual's opportunities to engage.

Building on existing knowledge about the meaning of occupation and considering the influence of contextual factors have the potential to either enable or constrain occupational engagement. The contextual factors which may influence meaning pertain to the individual, to the occupation and to the environment, as illustrated in the case study of Amanda.

REFERENCES

Aegler, B., Satink, T., 2009. Performing occupations under pain the experience of persons with chronic pain. Scand. J. Occup. Ther. 16, 49–56.

Aitchison, C., 2009. Exclusive discourses leisure studies and disability. Leisure Stud. 28 (4), 375–386.

Bateman, A., et al., 2005. Outcomes of intensive neuropsychological rehabilitation: the relationship between the Dysexecutive Questionnaire (Dex) and European Brain Injury Questionnaire (Ebiq) and smart goals attainment. Brain Impair. 6, 132.

Bier, N., Dutil, E., Couture, M., 2009. Factors affecting leisure participation after a traumatic brain injury an exploratory study. J. Head Trauma Rehabil. 24 (3), 187.

British Society of Rehabilitation Medicine, 2010. Specialist neurorehabilitation services: providing for patients with complex rehabilitation needs. British Society of Rehabilitation Medicine, London.

Collier, L., Truman, J., 2008. Exploring the multi-sensory environment as a leisure resource for people with complex neurological disabilities. Neurorehabilitation 23, 361–367.

Cuenca, J., Kleiber, D., Monteagudo, M.J., Linde, B.D., Jaumot-Pascual, N., 2014. The influence of meaningful leisure on the subjective well-being of older adults in the Basque Country of Northern Spain. World Leisure J. 56 (2), 120–129.

Dahan-Oliel, N., Shikako-Thomas, K., Majnemer, A., 2012. Quality of life and leisure participation in children with neurodevelopmental disabilities: a thematic analysis of the literature. Qual. Life Res. 21 (3), 427–439.

Dattilo, J., Rusch, F., 2012. Teaching problem solving to promote self-determined leisure engagement. J. Phys. Act. Health XLVI (2), 91–105.

Engel-Yeger, B., Dunn, W., 2011. Exploring the relationship between affect and sensory processing patterns in adults. Br. J. Occup. Ther. 74 (10), 456–464.

Eriksson, G., Kottorp, A., Borg, J., Tham, K., 2009. Relationship between occupational gaps in everyday life, depressive mood and life satisfaction after acquired neuropalliative condition. J. Rehabil. Med. 41 (3), 187–194.

Fenech, A., 2013. A study of engagement in casual leisure occupations by individuals who are living with neuropalliative conditions. Unpublished doctoral thesis, University of Southampton, Faculty of Health Sciences. Available at: <http://eprints.soton.ac.uk/361588/> (accessed 05.02.14.).

Fenech, A., 2015. A study of engagement in active and passive roles in casual leisure occupations. Open J. Occup. Ther. 3 (2).

Fenech, A., Shaw-Fisher, K., 2012. Lifelong leisure and therapeutic recreation. In: Zasler, N.D., et al. (Eds.), Brain Injury Medicine Principles and Practice, second ed. Demos Medical Publishing, New York.

Galvaan, R., 2014. The contextually situated nature of occupational choice: marginalised young adolescents' experiences in South Africa. J. Occup. Sci. 21 (4), 532–547.

Jonsson, H., 2014. Towards an experience-based categorisation of occupation. <http://commons.pacificu.edu/sso_conf/2014/4/64/> (accessed 22.01.15.).

Krishnagiri, S., Southam, M., 2013. Leisure occupations. In: McHugh Pendleton, H., Schultz-Krohn, W. (Eds.), Pedretti's Occupational Therapy: Practice Skills for Physical Dysfunction. Mosby, St Louis, MO, pp. 412–426.

Larson, E., Von Eye, A., 2010. Beyond flow temporality and participation in everyday activities. Am. J. Occup. Ther. 64, 152.

Martelli, M., Nicholson, K., Zasler, N., 2008. Skill reacquisition after acquired brain injury a holistic habit retraining model of neurorehabilitation. Neurorehabilitation 23 (2), 115–126.

Monti, M.M., Vanhaudenhuyse, A., Coleman, M.R., Boly, M., Pickard, J.D., Tshibanda, L., 2010. Willful modulation of brain activity in disorders of consciousness. N. Engl. J. Med. 362 (7), 579–589.

Neurological Alliance, 2014. Neuro numbers: a brief review of the numbers of people in the UK with a neurological condition. Neurological Alliance, London.

Perruzza, N., Kinsella, E.A., 2010. Creative arts occupations in therapeutic practice: a review of the literature. Br. J. Occup. Ther. 73 (6), 261–268.

Polatajko, H.J., Townsend, E.A., Craik, J., 2013. The Canadian Model of Occupational Performance and Engagement (CMOP-E). In: Townsend, E.A., Polatajko, H.J. (Eds.), Enabling Occupation II: Advancing an Occupational Therapy Vision for Health, Wellbeing, and Justice through Occupation, rev. ed. CAOT Publications ACE, Ottawa, ON, p. 23.

Pollard, N., Sakellariou, D., 2012. Towards a transformational grammar of occupation. In: Pollard, N., Sakellariou, D. (Eds.), Politics of Occupation-Centred Practice: Reflections on Occupational Engagement across Cultures. Wiley-Blackwell, Hoboken, NJ.

Reed, K., Hocking, C., Smythe, L., 2010. The interconnected meaning of occupation: the call, being-with, possibilities. J. Occup. Sci. 17 (3), 140–149.

Robinson, M.T., Barrett, K.M., 2014. Emerging subspecialties in neurology: neuropalliative care. Neurology 82 (21), e180–e182.

Roy, L., Rousseau, J., Fortier, P., Mottard, J.-P., 2013. Patterns of daily time-use of young adults with or without first-episode psychosis. Occup. Ther. Ment. Health 29, 232–245.

Sellar, B., Stanley, M., 2010. Leisure. In: Curtin, M., et al. (Eds.), Occupational Therapy and Physical Dysfunction Enabling Occupation, sixth ed. Elsevier, Oxford.

Sharp, E.H., Coffman, D.L., Caldwell, L.L., Smith, E.A., Wegner, L., Vergnani, T., 2011. Predicting substance use behavior among South African adolescents: the role of leisure experiences across time. Int. J. Behav. Dev. 35 (4), 343–351.

Stebbins, R.A., 2014. Leisure, happiness, and positive lifestyle. In: Elkington, S., Gammon, S.J. (Eds.), Contemporary Perspectives in Leisure: Meanings, Motives, and Lifelong Learning. Routledge, New York, pp. 28–38.

Wise, E.K., Mathews-Dalton, C., Dikmen, S., Temkin, N., Machamer, J., Bell, K., 2010. Impact of traumatic neuropalliative condition on participation in leisure activities. Arch. Phys. Med. Rehabil. 91 (9), 1357–1362.

Wright-St Clair, V.A., 2012. Being occupied with what matters in advanced age. J. Occup. Sci. 19 (1), 44–53.

15

IN OUR OWN HANDS AND IN THE EYES OF OTHERS: THE EMANCIPATORY IMPERATIVE OF OCCUPATIONAL WITNESSING FOR BELONGING AND BECOMING

TINA MCGRATH

CHAPTER OUTLINE

This chapter explores the subjective and intersubjective nature of human occupation and argues that belonging and becoming are not neutral or passive aspects of occupational being, but rather are complexly negotiated within individual and collective sociocultural and temporal contexts. I develop the concept of an *occupational subject* who actively builds a personal occupational identity both with and for others. I then apply this construct to examine the political nature of belonging and becoming.

Informed by feminist critical theory and derived from existential phenomenological exploration of embodied experience, the lived category of gender is used as an exemplar to demonstrate the political nature of human occupation as lived through the meanings and purposes which are brought to women's sociocultrally sanctioned occupations in particular times and places. I introduce the notion of *breasted occupation* to explore how gendered subjectivity influences the negotiation of female occupational identity in Western heteronormative culture. This examination challenges a unified and stable notion of femininity, revealing multiple and splintered femininities lived differently at different times and in different places both individually and collectively through occupation by women. The implications of these understandings are revealed in the cocreated personal occupational narratives of a group of Irish women living with breast cancer.

I propose *occupational witnessing* as a clinical reasoning mechanism that can validate the mutual subjectivity and intersubjectivity in the occupational therapy encounter, enabling a practice without and beyond borders. Occupational witnessing provides a framework for the urgent and necessary interrogation of the political nature of human occupation, making an important contribution to the emancipatory agenda of occupational justice.

BREAST LOSS AND OCCUPATIONAL LOSS

How does the loss of the female breast result in feelings of being 'half a woman', 'ugly' and 'unattractive'? How does this breast loss result in neglect of self-care, a dread of dressing and an active aversion to viewing one's reflection? Why, in the sickness and tiredness of the lived breast cancer experience, do women ignore bodily cues in order to privilege the performance of established routines and roles? Why does the resultant compromised function result in a painful and frustrating loss of satisfaction with occupational performance that leads women to feel that they are no longer themselves?

These were some of the questions that arose during my doctoral research into the occupational lives of Irish women as they lived with and through female breast cancer (McGrath, 2013a). These took me far beyond the boundaries of traditional theories of occupation, challenging me to redraw the borders of my own established understandings in order to appreciate the women's personal occupational narratives of living out their deeply felt losses.

The study was undertaken in Dublin, Ireland, and examined the lived experience of female breast cancer from an occupational perspective through the collaborative generation of occupational biographies of life before, during and after breast cancer (McGrath, 2013a). Purposive sampling at a city-centre cancer support centre was used to recruit 10 women who had a diagnosis of breast cancer. Every woman chose her own pseudonym. Three semistructured interviews were conducted over a period of 3 years, with seven women completing all interviews. Each was collated into one longitudinal transcript. Data were analysed using interpretative phenomenological analysis (Smith et al., 2009). This chapter is focused on my interpretations of our preliminary coconstructed occupational narratives in the immediate aftermath of breast cancer treatment and my subsequent theorizations of how these women negotiated their occupational identities.

All 10 women described the aftermath of surgery and treatment as having made significant changes to bodily areas associated with breast cancer, as well as to their bodies in general, describing an altered relationship with their bodily selves. Most disclosed that the appearance of their bodies initially postsurgery was a source of distress and upset for them. Participants described a sense of separation from bodily self with some going so far as to express strong disaffection with and distancing from their postoperative bodies. This alienation was focused primarily on the female body as a sexual entity, manifesting in a variety of ways, varying from disassociation from the body to dissatisfaction with bodily appearance to active dislike of the body's reflection in a mirror. Miranda described being 'mentally detached' from her 'mutilated' postsurgical body which 'revolted' her, stating that she would 'not have cared for' her body as much. This resulted in her neglect of her personal hygiene and self-care and in changes to how the body was privately managed. Aoife said that she now 'hated' her body and the sight of it, no longer feeling attractive, with subsequent alterations to her public management of her body. For example, when clothes shopping, Aoife avoided communal dressing rooms and reluctantly chose loose garments that hid her shape.

The women strove, at great personal cost, to maintain premorbid levels of occupational engagement (McGrath, 2013b). They refused to accept the functional changes brought about by treatment and continued to try to force the body to perform as they believed it should have, resulting in frustration with occupational performance. Norah described herself as 'wired' for the period when she was taking steroids during her chemotherapy treatment. She used the sense of energy they provided to get 'somewhere cleaned' or 'something done'. She would 'calm down' as the drug effects wore off, and felt 'so what' if the housework tired her out completely.

The women were particularly distressed by their limitations in regards to household tasks and the expression of roles relating to relationships. Ruth felt that she could no longer enjoy her homemaking, stating that everything in 'day-to-day life' was very stressful and that even preparing meals left her feeing unable 'to cope', with 'the least little things' annoying her. Ruth spoke of 'trying to catch up on the house stuff' and feeling that she could 'not deal with it'. She pushed herself to keep going until she was forced to rest and reported feeling constantly tired. At one point, she had considered asking her husband to move out for a little while to alleviate her stress.

For the women in this study, their occupational natures had become problematic. Personal activities of daily living brought sadness. Instrumental activities of daily living created frustration. Valued roles were emptied of their fulfilment, and functional limitations resulted in loss of satisfaction with familiar occupations. It was apparent that beyond altered occupational performance, their occupational identities were challenged and that these difficulties had to do with their bodies. The prevailing androgynous and disembodied nature of the concept of occupation lacked explanatory power to account for the gendered nature of the findings (McGrath, 2013a). This necessitated deeper interrogation of how being in, and doing with, a body relates to the belonging and becoming that assemble the female occupational being.

HUMAN OCCUPATION: A FEMINIST CRITICAL THEORETICAL PERSPECTIVE

Occupational therapists are familiar with Reilly's seminal hypothesis that our health and well-being is in our own hands (Reilly, 1962), learning that the Latin root of the term *occupation* implies an active seizing or holding of time and space (Christiansen and Townsend, 2011). As the theory of occupation has evolved and the practice of occupational therapy has developed, understandings of human occupation have deepened sufficiently for mature questioning of the profession's principles and core tenets (Pollard and Sakellariou, 2012). This allows the creation of an important rhetorical platform where the philosophy and practice of occupational therapy can be explored, questioned, contested and problematized (Hammell, 2009). The current move towards critical theory[1] brings with it a constructive sceptical stance that

destabilizes established traditional ways of thinking (Hammell, 2013). Critical theory brings an important political dimension to understandings of the relationship between occupation, health and well-being at both individual and population levels, exposing to scrutiny the multiple structures that offer and deny opportunities for exploration of and engagement in occupations.

If roles are a function of sociocultural convention, then the personal formulation of one's occupational identity is a reflection of this (Pollard and Sakellariou, 2012). Human occupation is understood as simultaneously an individual and collectively shared phenomenon. Membership of a given community, society and culture in a given time and place is formative, in that it shapes what occupations are normal and expected (Christiansen and Townsend, 2011). Belonging and becoming extend from this contextualized being and doing, creating the individual and collective conditions that determine what is occupationally possible (Laliberte-Rudman, 2010). For example, Kantartzis and Molineux (2011) examine how the concept of human occupation is strongly informed by Western and Anglophone constructions of good and healthy living which emphasize individualism, productivity and self-actualization. Iwama (2005) problematizes such Western perspectives, calling for appreciation of differing worldviews in order to better understand our own and others' ways of relating to each other and the world.

The occupational is inherently political; thus, as well as being in our own hands, occupational identity dwells in the eyes of others. Politics refers to the making of a shared public realm that creates the structures within which people live out their lives (Young, 2005). Such contexts appear to change little over time, creating a perceived sense of stable and collective continuity. The ways that people are positioned in relation to these structures (e.g., institutions such as rules, regulations, distribution of resources, physical access, power and status) are made up of how persons position themselves and how they are positioned by others.

BREASTED OCCUPATION

Gender can be seen as a form of such relative social positioning, and living out the category of 'woman'

---

[1]Critical theories attempt to examine the multiple contexts of people's lives such as the sociocultural, historical and structural in order to challenge the often hidden and taken-for-granted ideologies, assumptions and theories that make up the circumstances within which people strive to build personhood and identity. The notion of 'critical' also encompasses a commitment to confront inequity, inequality, power imbalances, exclusion and oppression in order to manifest a more just society (adapted from Hammell and Iwama, 2012).

within this positioning is influenced by the mix of individual factors and constituent structural factors (Young, 2005). Using female embodiment in Western heteronormative culture as an exemplar, I introduce the notion of *breasted occupation* (McGrath, 2013a, 2014).

Being and doing in a female body means learning to live with a particular anatomy and physiology and requires accommodating its form, feelings and capacities into the performance of occupations. This allows an individual to appreciate her own body's intrinsic potential (Grosz, 1994). However, to live with female breasts in Western culture is to live in many respects without secure borders. The human body can be seen as a collection or assemblage of body parts where bodily components associated with reproductive function attract increased political significance in the structuring of political and social relations (Woodward, 2008). Breasts are a woman's most visible signal of femininity and most potent symbol of sexuality in Western culture and are subject to socioculturally sanctioned notions of the 'normal' breast. These integrate with a woman's body image and her notion of self as she internalizes and conforms to the customs of heteronormative appraisal (Young, 2005).

The breasted occupational being reflects the expected traditions and values of her culture in a given time through her occupations. I define the term *breasted occupation* as 'both the implied notion and actual performance of occupations associated with women as a result of anatomical structure, biological processes and functional capacities in the context of socio-cultural and historical norms' (McGrath, 2014, p. 51). For example, female motility, comportment, grooming and dressing are often subject to sociocultural sanction (Young, 2005). Breasted occupation refers to the tacit socioculturally sanctioned normativity of female occupations in Western culture. For instance, implicit assumptions associated with the category of 'woman' promote women's roles as carers, mothers and homemakers with consequences for education, work roles, career progression and subsequent financial security and independence. Such presuppositions can foreclose occupational opportunities and impoverish the process of building an occupational identity.

THE OCCUPATIONAL SUBJECT

Subjectivity refers to the ongoing process of building a personal selfhood that encompasses both a sense of place in the world and the nature of connections to others in the world. Our valourised ideas about purpose, meaning, our own becoming and our deepest desires for belonging, what in philosophical terms are called our 'projects', are contextually bound in a sociocultural context (Finlay, 2011).

If the premise of human occupation is founded on the notion of subjectively sanctioned purpose and meaning, then it is imperative in theory and in practice to explore and advance occupational understandings of subjectivity and, thus, to acknowledge the existence of the *occupational subject* (McGrath, 2013a). The concept of the occupational subject that I develop is derived from existential and phenomenological exploration of the lived experience of embodiment. Existential philosophy addresses the complexity and challenges of the concrete human condition such as living, dying, temporality, and personal and communal identity (Wartenberg, 2008). Phenomenology focuses on the meaning and sense-making that is attached to living in and with a body through time (Finlay, 2011).

Human occupation must be considered in the light of active agency and in contest to the reduction of subjectivity to passive bodies. Occupation can be seen as a practical form of subjectivity, where people 'do' identity through purposeful and meaningful interactions with the world. The notion of an occupational subject privileges the fact that occupations are bodily lived. Such consideration must then acknowledge lived occupational experience and the formative and transformative properties of historical and sociocultural contexts as they influence subjectivity.

GENDERED SUBJECTIVITY

By lending a feminist approach to a critical theoretical perspective, the frequently hidden complexity of human occupation is exposed in the lived every day for women in Western culture. The relations between lived bodies are structured by the material environment, as well as the established historical and sociocultural institutions within which occupations are facilitated or constrained. Sakellariou and Pollard (2009) discuss 'engendered occupation' and identify gender as a cultural identity and a powerful regulator of behavioural patterns (p. 77). Gender can be understood as a structure that positions people in a societal hierarchy, with implications for both women and men, where the dominant group exerts power and privilege over another through social interaction, everyday activities and occupational opportunities.

A fixed construct of gender identity cannot be extracted from the dynamic interactions of given identities in the historical and sociocultural milieu. Indeed, any era can be immediately recognized by such things as the customs and fashions of that time. When engaged critically with the notions of womanhood and of femininity within an occupational perspective, these concepts quickly rupture. It is not possible to speak of a singular notion of femininity, because how it is defined will always vary depending on the circumstances that it attempts to describe. This is because occupational beings are perspectival, with permeable boundaries that traverse the many specifics of being embodied and embedded in time and place. The material fact of a particular biological body is but one contribution to the constitution of the feminine self and to the sort of woman that a person strives to become. Being, doing, belonging and becoming manifest femininity differently within differing contexts and are the result of the dynamic intersection of other features of identity such as age, sexuality, class, religion, health status, economic status, ethnicity, geographic specificity and sociocultural context.

Hegemonic gender relations become embedded in particular contexts and can be seen to alter across time and culture in their contemporaneous reflections of the dominant fixed ideals of 'natural' or 'normal' femininity. This demands consideration of the existence of multiple and splintered femininities across time and place, rather than regard femininity as an essential single stable category. I emphasize the plural notion of femininities, which I define as the constellations of structures and circumstances that formulate the customary situations and expressions of womanhood in given temporal and sociocultural contexts, as well as the embodied living out of these situations through occupation (de Beauvoir, 1949/ 2011; Young, 2005). Of significance here is the slow sedimentation of femininities that occurs within the female body itself over time and through lived interpreted experience, its insidious assimilation into everyday occupational performance. This process is captured in de Beauvoir's (1949/2011) celebrated observation that a woman is not born, but is what one becomes. Pierce (2003) acknowledges that the construction of gender exerts a formative influence on occupational patterning. Bodily form is managed in space and across time through comportment, gestures and activities that represent thematic repetitions of socially normative feminine occupations. These become the ordinary ways that womanhood and femininity are lived out for a given female in a particular time and place.

Belonging and becoming are politically problematic as women live out the construction and contestation of femininities within the confines of the categories that they inhabit. This occurs particularly through the interiorization of the male gaze where generalized norms and expectations become reflected in self-awareness and self-appraisal. A sense emerges of the self as object-like with the resultant experience of shame. In de Beauvoir's account (1949/2011), shame is fundamental to women's everyday activities, as women's circumstances are deeply gendered.

Young (2005) advocates a focus on the lived body through which gendered structures are daily lived out in experiences of 'facticity', where people find themselves passively placed within particular structural categories that are historically and socioculturally given in ways that precondition the consciousness and action of individuals. Facticity refers to the hard facts of existence – the concrete realities of human embodiment in the world such as biological body, physical environment and sociocultural context. However, the occupational being has agency and can choose how to interpret and assemble the self in response to this facticity, a capacity described in philosophical terms as 'freedom' (Moi, 1999).

De Beauvoir (1949/2011) sees subjectivity as the focus of a freedom that is constrained within a dialectical perspective on embodiment, in which the female body is lived as a 'situation' that combines the biological and sociohistorical, with the projects, both individual and shared with others, through which a woman reaches for her belonging and becoming.

Situation refers to the complex interplay of facticity and projects, and how they are interpreted through the lived body (Young, 2005). Gendered structures are a component of individual situation; from how to look, to what to wear, to how a home is maintained, to what you are permitted to hope for (Moi, 1999).

Freedom refers to the ability to take up freely chosen projects and express one's subjectivity. There exists an ontological freedom to choose how to interpret the context of one's situation (de Beauvoir, 1949/2011). This is linked with the lifelong occupational projects of becoming – where individual potential is recognized and reached for – and belonging – where the intersubjective necessity of living in relation to, and in relationship with, others is expressed (Wilcock, 2006). There concurrently exists a practical freedom which functions in the presence of historical, sociocultural, economic and political circumstances to either enable or constrain this ontological freedom (de Beauvoir, 1949/2011). Practical freedom is about the factors that impact on the fullest expression of the subjective self. It encompasses the enablers and barriers that must be considered when attempting to negotiate occupational identity.

I argue that human occupation is premised on an individual's ontological freedom to make choices within the constraints of the practical freedoms available to each person. This leads to an occupational friction between an individual's ontological and practical freedoms, marked by a struggle between what is potentially possible and what is practically possible, as the occupational being strives to construct an occupational identity. This is illustrated poignantly in Deirdre's account of her situation and demonstrates the occupational friction between her ontological freedom which envisages a life beyond her mothering and homemaking, and the practical freedoms that place her as primary caregiver, economically dependent and tied to the domestic sphere.

Deirdre was a highly qualified health professional with international work experience and had put her career on hold to support her husband and children full time at home. Deirdre chose to struggle with debilitating treatment side effects, extreme tiredness and low mood to ensure that the family were 'not put out' by her cancer treatment. Deirdre, despite choosing her family over her career, yearned 'to get out of the house' and would have liked a 'small little job' to focus on herself and yearned 'to do something life-changing' after her cancer experience. However, Deirdre felt that this was not possible, as her children were still too young, and summarized her situation with the words: *I can't*.

OCCUPATIONAL WITNESSING

Human occupation is intricately entwined with the sense-making capacities of persons that confer and express subjectivity. Our subjectivity may be in our own hands, but it is also in the eyes of others. We perform our occupations to express our occupational selfhoods for ourselves and also for others. Our becomings require that we are seen and we need others in order to belong.

Subjectivity, as constituted intersubjectively, is dialogical, relational and dependent. This requires new ethical understandings of the occupational subject beyond the process of recognition. Oliver (2001) sees the demand for recognition as symptomatic of the pathological nature of oppression where the very need to be recognized by the oppressors both reinforces and replicates the conditions of the oppression itself. The mechanisms of oppression result in an objectification that assaults the structure and, thus, the agency and voice necessary for subjectivity (Oliver, 2004). In this process, the occupational subject is both diminished and silenced.

The occupational subject needs to be an active and communicating subject in order to belong and become. Oliver (2001) argues for a model of subjectivity that involves an address-response structure composed of the ability to address oneself to the other and to be addressed, and the ability to respond to self and the other. Implicit in this model is the ethical consideration of subject position, identified as one's personal placement in sociohistorical context and immersion in politics, and of subjectivity, which is envisaged as the agentic and communicative self in continuous open encounter with the vastness of otherness. Oliver (2004) identifies the inherent tension between subject position and subjectivity as the internalized experience of the self, and terms this process 'witnessing'.

Following Oliver, I have developed a concept of *occupational witnessing* as an ethical model of subjectivity and intersubjectivity where through human occupation, occupational beings can both address and respond to each other (McGrath, 2013a; Oliver, 2001;2004). Such an address-response configuration envisages the occupational subject as able to address others and be responded to through the medium of human occupation. This brings ethical obligations in terms of ensuring an openness that facilitates the ongoing possibility of address and response so that the agency and voice needed to experience selfhood and express subjectivity are present (Oliver, 2004).

When the women in this study were appreciated as occupational subjects, I could make occupational sense of their narratives. All expressed values that were part of their upbringings in a very conservative era. A pervasive traditional patriarchal culture of sexual repression and strong gender role stereotyping remains evident in Ireland as part of the legacy of the dominance of the Roman Catholic Church in Irish society (Share, Corcoran and Conway, 2012). Rattigan (2012) describes the infiltration of this influence into private morality within an extremely conservative heteronormative viewpoint. The notion of Irishness itself is a gender-biased concept which exerts strong influence on the normative female occupations of homemaking and motherhood (Lentin, 1998). This reflects the dominant gendered construction of the Irish notion of 'home' and demonstrates how hegemonic interpretations of femininity solidify the idea of home as a naturalized feminine location (Laurie et al., 1999; Lentin, 1998). These attitudes are beginning to change with Irish exposure to globalization (Inglis, 2008).

I identified the essence of the women's lived occupational experiences with breast cancer surgery and treatments characterized by two levels of distress, with the first associated with living the difference of a non-conforming female body, and the second associated with the occupational losses brought about by the compromise of previous function due to the iatrogenic complications of medical intervention (McGrath, 2014). These were found to be strongly gendered through the women's internalizations of mid-twentieth-century Irish sociocultural heterosexual normativities of the female body, female roles, and thus female occupations.

APPLICATION OF OCCUPATIONAL WITNESSING TO CLINICAL REASONING

The traditional dual axis of occupational therapy where a reductive and functional biomedical view is blended with attention to the phenomenological aspects of human occupational nature requires careful and sensitive practice (Mattingly, 1991). For the occupational therapist, such a stance requires critical vigilance to ensure that methodologies, technologies and evaluations do not replicate dominant or oppressive structures that objectify the occupational subject and diminish her ontological status to 'other' or different. No occupational subject is self-sufficient as subjectivity is built with and through each other.

Occupational therapists can, through reciprocity, recognize another occupational subject through her occupations (Hammell, 2004). This opens occupational therapy practice to the possibility of political change through conscious challenging of the structures that create otherness and impair a fair vision of another subject. This results in reciprocal acknowledgement of the other's status as an occupational subject and provides a platform from where the other can express their own subjectivity and explore occupational identity. This reveals the interdependency of subjectivities in the client-centred clinical encounter, encouraging a stance of 'being with' another occupational subject.

In the endeavour to witness the active agency of other occupational subjects as they negotiate their subjectivities within given structures and practices, occupational therapists can understand better the meanings and purposes that drive occupational performance. In deepening understandings of the situation of the occupational subject, the occupational therapist can work towards expansion of freedoms and the extension of possibilities. Operation of occupational therapy clinical reasoning at the level of occupational witnessing requires that the occupational perspectives of doing, being, belonging and becoming must be interpreted in totality as the unified expression of another occupational subject beyond difference.

Occupational therapists can work towards the emancipation of other occupational subjects using the core skill of enablement. This can take various forms such as striving to end oppressive institutions, supporting people to overcome the barriers to their participation, using occupation to assist people to examine and expand their occupational subjectivities and exploring resistant occupational engagement for emancipatory potential. In all cases, the process of occupational witnessing can work to repair and build subjectivity through thoughtful advancement of occupational opportunities that enable the expression of agency and voice that are fundamental to the structure of occupational subjectivity itself.

CONCLUSION

The location of the body simultaneously in nature and culture has profound implications for the ways occupation is understood, particularly as an instrument of therapeutic intervention. This chapter has explored how belonging and becoming contribute to the subjective and intersubjective nature of human occupation, advancing the concept of an occupational subject.

The gendered subjectivity of women in Western culture was explored through the notion of breasted occupation and examination of women's experiences of breast cancer, in order to demonstrate the often hidden political aspects of occupation in place and across time. Occupational witnessing was introduced as a political lens through which the mutual subjective and intersubjective nature of occupational being can be appreciated. This can be harnessed in the occupational therapy encounter to uncover and lessen the structural influences on client-centred practice where the occupational therapist endeavours to realize the freedoms that hold out for the possibility of political and personal liberatory change for all occupational subjects.

Acknowledgements

This work is developed from the author's doctoral thesis which was supervised by Professor Susan Ryan and Professor Gill Chard, Department of Occupational Science and Occupational Therapy, University College Cork, and Dr. Kathy Glavanis-Grantham, Department of Sociology, University College Cork. University ethical approval was granted for this research.

As always, thanks to my coresearchers, the women who lived to tell the tale of their occupational lives with breast cancer. Our occupational witnessing has expanded my freedoms.

REFERENCES

Christiansen, C.H., Townsend, E.A., 2011. Introduction to Occupation: The Art and Science of Living, second ed. Pearson, Upper Saddle River, NJ.

de Beauvoir, S., 2011. The Second Sex (Borde, C., Malovany-Chevallier, S., Trans.). Vintage, London. (Original work published 1949.)

Finlay, L., 2011. Phenomenology for Therapists: Researching the Lived World. Wiley-Blackwell, West Sussex, UK.

Grosz, E., 1994. Volatile Bodies: Toward a Corporeal Feminism. Indiana University Press, Bloomington, IN.

Hammell, K.W., 2004. Dimensions of meaning in the occupations of daily life. Can. J. Occup. Ther. 71 (5), 296–305.

Hammell, K.W., 2009. Sacred texts: a sceptical exploration of the assumptions underpinning theories of occupation. Can. J. Occup. Ther. 76 (1), 6–13.

Hammell, R.K.W., 2013. Client-centred practice in occupational therapy: critical reflections. Scand. J. Occup. Ther. 20 (3), 174–181.

Hammell, R.K.W., Iwama, M.K., 2012. Well-being and occupational rights: an imperative for critical occupational therapy. Scand. J. Occup. Ther. 19 (5), 385–394.

Inglis, T., 2008. Global Ireland: Same Difference. Routledge, London.

Iwama, M.K., 2005. Situated meaning: an issue of culture, inclusion and occupational therapy. In: Kronenberg, F., et al. (Eds.), Occupational Therapy without Borders: Learning from the Spirit of Survivors. Elsevier Churchill Livingstone, Edinburgh, pp. 127–139.

Kantartzis, S., Molineux, M., 2011. The influence of western society's construction of a healthy daily life on the conceptualisation of occupation. J. Occup. Sci. 18 (1), 62–80.

Laliberte-Rudman, D., 2010. Occupational Terminology: Occupational possibilities. J. Occup. Sci. 17 (1), 55–59.

Laurie, N., Dwyer, C., Holloway, S., Smith, F., 1999. Geographies of New Femininities. Pearson Education Limited, New York.

Lentin, R., 1998. 'Irishness', the 1937 Constitution, and citizenship: a gender and ethnicity view. Irish J. Sociol. 8, 5–24.

McGrath, T., 2013a. Living to Tell the Tale: Narratives of Occupational Engagement, Creativity and Living with Breast Cancer. Unpublished thesis. University College Cork, Cork, Ireland.

McGrath, T., 2013b. Irish insights into the lived experience of breast cancer related lymphoedema: implications for occupation focused practice. WFOT Bulletin 68, 44–50.

McGrath, T., 2014. Occupational therapy news: PhD conferring: living to tell the tale: narratives of occupational engagement, creativity and living with breast cancer. Irish J. Occup. Ther. 42 (1), 51–52.

Mattingly, C., 1991. What is clinical reasoning? Am. J. Occup. Ther. 45 (11), 979–986.

Moi, T., 1999. What Is a Woman? And Other Essays. Oxford University Press, Oxford.

Oliver, K., 2001. Witnessing: Beyond Recognition. University of Minnesota Press, Minneapolis, MN.

Oliver, K., 2004. Witnessing and testimony. Parallax 10 (1), 79–88.

Pierce, D., 2003. Occupation by Design: Building Therapeutic Power. F.A. Davis, Philadelphia.

Pollard, N., Sakellariou, D., 2012. Politics of Occupation-Centred Practice: Reflections on Occupational Engagement across Cultures. Wiley-Blackwell, West Sussex, UK.

Rattigan, C., 2012. What else could I do? Single mothers and infanticide, Ireland 1900-1950. Irish Academic Press, Dublin.

Reilly, M., 1962. Occupational therapy can be one of the great ideas of 20th century medicine. Am. J. Occup. Ther. 26, 1–9.

Sakellariou, D., Pollard, N., 2009. Three sites of conflict and cooperation: class, gender and sexuality. In: Pollard, N., et al. (Eds.), A Political Practice of Occupational Therapy. Churchill Livingstone Elsevier, Edinburgh, pp. 69–90.

Share, P., Tovey, H., Corcoran, M.P., 2012. A Sociology of Ireland, 4th ed. Gill and MacMillan, Dublin.

Smith, J., Flowers, P., Larkin, M., 2009. Interpretative Phenomenological Analysis: Theory, Method and Research. SAGE Publications, London.

Wartenberg, T.E., 2008. Existentialism: A Beginner's Guide. Oneworld Publications, London.

Wilcock, A.A., 2006. An Occupational Perspective of Health, second ed. Slack Inc, Thorofare, NJ.

Woodward, K., 2008. Gendered bodies: gendered lives. In: Richardson, D., Robinson, V. (Eds.), Introducing Gender and Women's Studies, third ed. Palgrave MacMillan, Hampshire, UK, pp. 75–90.

Young, I.M., 2005. On Female Body Experience: 'Throwing Like a Girl' and Other Essays. Oxford University Press, Oxford.

16

RETURN TO WORK SUPPORT FOR BREAST CANCER SURVIVORS: A RECENTLY QUALIFIED OCCUPATIONAL THERAPIST'S JOURNEY INTO RESEARCH

JONATHAN TIGWELL

■ ■ ■ ■ ■ ■ ■ ■ ■ ■ ■ ■ ■ ■ ■ ■ ■ ■ ■

CHAPTER OUTLINE

The practice of occupational therapy, as with any specialist discipline, requires the ability to operate within multiple worldviews simultaneously. There is the worldview which is developed through individual lived experience and the more recently acquired view of the world gained from the experiences of occupational therapy training and practice (Hooper, 1997). It is the linking of these two worldviews that is essential in order to provide effective occupational therapy in a healthcare environment that is increasingly challenging. Without a link between the occupational therapy world and the wider context in which it operates, occupational therapy runs the risk of becoming a marginalized entity, potentially leading to an entire profession being subject to the occupational injustices and deprivations that its raison d'être was intended to alleviate (Pettican and Bryant, 2007). This chapter will attempt to communicate the parallels between the challenges in the occupational therapy world and the opportunities for improvement within breast cancer survivor support. To illustrate these parallels, examples will be provided from a research study with users of breast cancer support services in the UK who often experience a dissonance between the ideal service as promoted by policymakers and the reality of the services delivered (Gupta et al., 2014; National Cancer Survivorship Initiative, 2013). The central argument of this chapter is to communicate the importance of aligning the multiple worldviews to create a harmonious alliance; to not only ensure the survival of the profession, but to guarantee that service users receive the interventions that they have a right to access and that can greatly improve their quality of life. In order to prevent the perpetuation of the occupational injustices discussed in several chapters in this book, there must be a renewed emphasis on engagement with and application of research. The chapter will proceed with a personal narrative of the author's experience of engaging with clinically applicable research and how this demonstrated the need and utility of discovering person-centred solutions to improve services.

MY PERSONAL JOURNEY INTO RESEARCH: THE DOORSTEP MILE

When I began my training, I was immersed in a whole new way of viewing the world, enabling me to become aware of how everyday activities I had previously taken for granted had such a positive effect on health and well-being. As my training developed I saw so many examples of the restorative power of meaningful occupations. From the use of adaptive technology to enable someone with a spinal injury to attend and succeed at university, to the use of purposeful, chosen activities to control and improve the symptoms of people with severe mental health conditions, occupational therapy was not only enhancing people's lives, it was reducing a mutually negative dependence on services. These and innumerable other examples inspired a new awareness of the potential for people to adapt to their challenging situations in a positive way. Occupational therapy provided a new approach to rehabilitation and health maintenance that was seen to create significant, positive and sustainable change for its participants. However, what was missing in all the settings I worked in was the lack of measurement of these achievements. The improvements being made were substantial and observable, but were unreported and unrecorded by service users, staff or managers. Indeed, a significant and sometimes disproportionate amount of time was dedicated to documenting the process of the interventions but not the outcomes.

During my first appointments after graduation I attempted to apply the theoretical principles of my training to the complex, real-world setting and find ways of measuring and recording the therapeutic gains being made. I soon came to realize that the aligning of the academic and clinical worlds was a difficult and often frustrating endeavour. The rapidly changing health and social care system in which I was working and the progressive and expanding occupational therapy theoretical base seemed to exist in two separate parallel worlds. There seemed to be a discord between the academic ideals and the practical everyday clinical setting. The challenges I experienced trying to apply the principles of occupational therapy and evidence-based improvement led me to look further into engagement with research and how this could be applied to clinical practice. This resulted in researching outcome measures to apply to an occupational therapy service within a community mental health team. It was my aim to capture the positive improvement I was seeing, display the improvements being made, but also identify service users who were not moving forward and goals that were not being achieved. I felt this form of measurement was especially needed, as at the time occupational therapists were moving towards a more generic care coordination role and away from their core therapeutic role.

Firstly, I reviewed the literature on outcome measures and mental health and matched this with the practicalities of the setting. I decided that the Canadian Occupational Performance Measure (COPM) provided a standardized format that could quickly and unobtrusively be applied best to this particular service user group in a culturally appropriate way (Law et al., 2005). The COPM would provide a list of service-user led goals on which numerical benchmarks and subsequent outcomes could be measured. I applied the COPM to appropriate service users over a 9-month rotational post within the community mental health team in which I was working. The recorded outcomes were positive on many levels. Firstly, the majority of the results showed a clinically significant improvement in the service user's occupational performance and satisfaction levels (Rehab Measures, 2014). This provided a real sense of achievement for myself and the service users, and was also a useful communication tool for other healthcare professionals within and outside of the multidisciplinary team. Secondly, the results highlighted where service users were not achieving their goals. This can be a difficult area to broach within a mental health setting, and the COPM provided a useful prompt to help the service user and practitioner to constructively redirect their efforts to address the areas of deficit. Thirdly, the collation of the results data provided a better understanding of the types of problems experienced and the frequency at which they occurred. These data could then be used for making the case for occupational therapy to remain or even be expanded within the setting. This experience gave me a renewed enthusiasm for getting involved with the assessment and measurement of interventions and services. In Norway, the phrase 'the doorstep mile' is used to describe the first step of a long journey, with the implication that it is the most difficult one to take (Allen, 2013). I feel this is especially true of becoming involved with research, and yet once this first step is taken, a new world of opportunities presents itself. Also, by overcoming this first step, I realized the relative ease with which occupational therapists can become engaged in the first stages of service improvement and the assertive advocacy needed to build evidence to ensure service users receive the correct service. As my knowledge grew I became increasingly aware that there were many threats to the provision of holistic occupational therapy and that building the evidence for its efficacy through accurate research was essential to defend it. The following section will briefly highlight some specific threats to occupational therapy, which will then be linked with the opportunities to improve breast cancer survivor support.

THE WIDER CONTEXT AND THREATS TO OCCUPATIONAL THERAPY

There is currently an international push for occupational therapists to become engaged with evidence-based practice and clinically led research in order to confirm to the service user and commissioning authorities the efficacy and efficiency of the service (Pighills et al., 2013; Swedlove and Etcheverry, 2012). Over the next decade and on into the longer term, healthcare services will be put under further strain from increasing demands from growing patient populations and the after-effects of the global financial crisis of 2008 (Appleby, 2011; Karanikolos et al., 2013). The financial, demographic and political drivers affecting the future of healthcare may precipitate the depletion or even deletion of services such as occupational therapy (Lambert et al., 2014). Any occupational therapist would undoubtedly define their service as essential; however, without the evidence to support it, how might they persuade a healthcare commissioner or policymaker – with perhaps no previous experience of occupational therapy – that the service is essential, best value and worthy of investment (Nancarrow and Borthwick, 2005). The imperative for both newly qualified and established occupational therapists must be to challenge the status quo and to advance and improve the services for the good of the service user and to ensure the continuation of an outcome-improving

occupational therapy service. A contention of this chapter is that as occupational therapy faces threats from many different directions, it is imperative for occupational therapists to make these difficult choices and to confront institutionalized and redundant practices in order to maintain a truly holistic and person-centred occupational therapy.

With the increasingly complex daily occupations associated with contemporary living and escalating consumption of digital media content, there can often be an overload of information that can lead to an increased focus on the immediate discipline-specific environment. This can lead to professional silos, or isolated disciplines that can produce barriers to effective teamwork and patient care (Margalit et al., 2009). An example of this could be seen with the dichotomy between the progressive and horizon-expanding influence of the educational and research establishment and the pragmatic and focused necessities of frontline practice (Lyons et al., 2011). For example, during training in the UK, it is part of the requirements for students to maintain a thorough review of the current occupational therapy literature. However, once an occupational therapist is qualified, this practice may be eroded as work demands take up all available energies and time (Clouston, 2014; Cooper, 2012). There is also an increasing trend in the UK towards occupational therapists assuming a narrowed role of discharge liaison or care coordinator and moving away from a holistic therapeutic role. If this trend continues and occupational therapists change from being therapists – that is, someone who facilitates the improvement of health and well-being of a person – to someone who is primarily focused on getting people discharged from care services as soon as is practicably safe, it would surely represent a threat to their professional integrity (College of Occupational Therapists, 2010). If occupational therapists are increasingly less therapeutic and more logistical and administrative, executive managers might make the decision to replace occupational therapists for non-occupational therapist discharge planners. It would seem that in some settings in the UK this has already occurred and represents a reduction of service standards and quality.

The imperative and underlying element that underpins any attempt to ameliorate any of these threats is to produce a robust evidence base (Upton et al., 2014). To achieve an evidence base, there needs to be research conducted by occupational therapists and for occupational therapists to engage with this research (Finlay, 2004). For the research to become meaningful and applicable to practice there must be a grassroots change in the approach, utilization and dissemination of research that becomes not only accessible to all occupational therapists, but also to other disciplines and policymakers (Bannigan, 2007). In an analogy to the ongoing global climate and environmental crisis, there have been innumerable historical warnings and repeated calls to action, and we have been slow in addressing the problem that threatens us all; however, it does not mean it is too late to become engaged and make a difference.

The remainder of the chapter will contain the details of a study that provides an example of how occupational therapists can become engaged with research and how they could expand, rather than contract, their role to meet the needs of service users. It will illustrate an example of engaging in interdisciplinary research and the positive outcomes that this has produced.

THE EXPERIENCE OF RETURNING TO WORK FOR BREAST CANCER SURVIVORS

Throughout the world there is a steadily increasing cohort of women diagnosed with breast cancer. Each year around 1.7 million new cases of breast cancer are diagnosed around the world, and nearly 50,000 women are diagnosed with breast cancer every year in the UK alone (Ferlay et al., 2010; World Cancer Research Fund International, 2012). Survival rates are also increasing: around 85% of those diagnosed will complete treatment and not have a recurrence of cancer for at least 5 years (Cancer Research UK, 2014). There are now estimated to be around 570,000 women living currently in the UK who have been diagnosed with breast cancer and can be classed as cancer survivors (Breast Cancer Campaign, 2014). A cancer survivor[1] is defined

---

[1]The term *survivor* is not universally accepted within the academic and service user community but currently serves as the generally accepted term (Kaiser, 2008).

by Feunerstein (2007a) as an adult cancer patient following medical treatment until the end of life. A large number of breast cancer survivors will have been in paid employment when diagnosed and will either need, or want, to return to work during or after treatment. These statistics indicate a significant cohort of people affected by the condition and represent an opportunity for healthcare professionals to support the service user's efforts to achieve their desired level of recovery and improve their outcomes (Fantoni et al., 2010; Tamminga et al., 2012). There are also widespread calls within the academic, healthcare and service user association literature to increase understanding in this area (Banning, 2011; Desiron, 2013; Hoving et al., 2009; Macmillan Cancer Care, 2008).

The recommendations from government, healthcare and tertiary sources highlight the importance of gaining service user perspectives when creating and adapting services and interventions (Amir et al., 2008; Welsh Government, 2012). If the experiences of the patient group are not investigated and analysed, then the health professionals responsible for creating and adapting services will be less informed, potentially leading to less effective services and poorer outcomes for the service users. If the service users then do not return to work at the optimum time, this will represent a significant social and financial burden on society and can lead to further negative implications for the service user (Feunerstein, 2007b). The argument for effective intervention with this cohort is further verified by a significant and increasing evidence base supporting the link between meaningful employment and improved physical and mental health (Eva et al., 2012; Waddell et al., 2013). Therefore there is an impetus for healthcare, government and support services to consider appropriate interventions concerning helping breast cancer survivors back to work at the optimum time (Macmillan Cancer Care, 2008). As with many areas involving complex problems, the core principles of occupational therapy align well with the needs of breast cancer survivors as described in the literature and the ideal service provision advocated by the healthcare authorities (Department of Health, 2011; Macmillan Cancer Care, 2015). The findings of the study will show evidence to support the argument that occupational therapists have a potentially larger role to play in the rehabilitation of breast cancer survivors.

The study aimed to build on the existing research by investigating the personal insights of breast cancer survivors to gain an in-depth understanding of their lived experience of the post-treatment period and what elements helped and hindered in their rehabilitation and return to work. The study was guided by phenomenology, and data were collected through the use of semistructured interviews. Phenomenology seeks to understand phenomena that are perceived or experienced, and the use of phenomenology encourages participants to extensively describe their experiences in their own words from their own perspective (Flood, 2010). The researcher then attempts to explore the phenomenon in further detail with the participants to find why such perceptions exist (Laverty, 2003). Through this exploration, new insights can emerge, which can inform participants, researchers and service providers. It can also provide the opportunity to highlight challenges to the previous assumptions of the phenomena and indicate further areas requiring additional study.

FINDINGS

Each of the 15 participants' single interviews were recorded and later transcribed verbatim. The transcripts were then analysed using thematic analysis, which is a structured process designed to rigorously and reliably identify patterns, or themes, within the data (Vaismoradi et al., 2013). As analysis progressed, many themes emerged from the interviews. Four of these themes have been chosen to highlight particularly important issues that were raised. These themes will be explained, with quotes from the transcripts used to illustrate the themes. These themes will then be linked to the previous contentions regarding occupational therapy threats and opportunities.

A Sudden Drop in Support

Amongst all the participants there was a unanimous opinion that the treatment and service they received from the cancer services and charities were excellent and exceeded their expectations. Each participant repeatedly praised the professional and caring role of healthcare and charity staff. However, there was a majority of participants reporting a sudden 'drop' in support after treatment that significantly affected their psychological state and in some cases was felt to have affected their rehabilitation and subsequent return to work. This phenomenon was best described by Paula, who explained the psychological impact of the abrupt ending of treatment:

> I think it would have been nice to have contact after I finished my treatment, just like follow-ups, I guess. Because you are so, kind of, like, mollycoddled through it all, you do have a lot of support, and it's amazing, but once you've finished your last treatment: nothing. And that's quite, you feel vulnerable.

A Change in Identity

All the participants described the importance of work to their lives. From the fundamental need to remain financially secure, to genuine enjoyment of the working environment, there were many different motivations to return to work. Many participants talked about how work to them was part of their identity and that by not working this affected them negatively. This was also the case with independence in general. Nadia described the positive effect of regaining her independence:

> I've always been quite independent so to have someone doing everything for me is quite annoying to a certain extent. So being able to just do my things, organize my life, do my own thing again, it was awesome I have to say.

The other change in identity that was expressed by a number of participants involved the feeling that they were no longer the same as they were before the treatment. This was reflected by negative reactions at work and difficulties with family members. Nia described the change as follows:

> It's not about getting back to normality because normality is not the same as it was because I'm a different kind of person. I look at things slightly differently but I feel I want to move on now. I want to start to rebuild my future if you like.

The Negative and Positive Effects of Treatment

The treatment schedule for breast cancer is dependent on a variety of factors and can differ for each person. The participants of the study had a combination of four different types of treatment: surgery, radiotherapy, chemotherapy and hormone therapy. The interviews presented startling differences in their reactions to treatment. There were the predicted and well-known experiences of side effects such as fatigue, nausea and low mood, but there were also more complex effects such as cognitive impairment and disabling fears of the return of cancer. Also, the participant sample represented a broad spectrum of treatment effects, from mild symptoms that lasted only hours, to continual debilitating effects that would last for months. However, in amongst the long list of negative symptoms, there were also positive effects. One example was that many participants expressed an actual reduction in anxieties that they had before the diagnosis. They described acquiring a new, liberating perspective on their lives. This was explained by Adrienne and Trisha:

> **Adrienne:** I was scared, very, very scared. Scared but…I suddenly thought it's quite liberating, because I thought, well actually I'd gone through all this treatment, I'd come out the other side and it will always be with me. And so, why am I frightened of anything?

> **Trisha:** I don't think I'm any worse from the experience, in fact it most probably made me a whole lot better person. I think it makes you appreciate everything in life, you look at everything differently.

The Importance of Occupation

Throughout the data the importance of occupation was significant. Participants described the debilitating and occupationally depriving effect of the treatment which fostered a renewed appreciation of the occupations that they previously valued. Once the participants resumed their meaningful occupations this significantly improved their well-being. The following excerpt illustrates the diversity of occupations that were beneficial to one participant:

> **Interviewer:** Was there anything else that helped during that [post-treatment] period?
> **Laura:** Well, being occupied, doing things, yeah.
> **Interviewer:** Can you tell me a bit more about that?
> **Laura:** Well, you know, being able to do some work and, you know, I sing in a choir so I kept going to the choir…and do things that really made me happy, and travelling you know, being able to plan for things. Well, you know, little short term objectives, practical things you know, life, looking after my family, my daughter, having little projects, travels, treats.

There was also the frequent theme of realizing that the participants needed to remain active and engaged with meaningful activities:

> **Trisha:** I just kept busy, because I wasn't working, I kept busy. We were always doing something because I think if you don't do anything, you're just going to sit and wallow in it and it's ten times worse, I thought, 'Right, I've got to do it!' I went to skittles, I carried on skittling, in fact I didn't miss a match all the way through my treatment, none of it!

Many participants described the positive effects of activities that were held to be therapeutic such as spa days and relaxation sessions, but they also described the positive effects that occurred as a result in engaging in a broad range of stimulating everyday occupations such as volunteering, genealogy research, child care and dog walking. These examples provide a welcome illustration of occupational therapy theory in action, in the fundamental sense that the engagement in meaningful occupations was described as resulting in better health and well-being outcomes. The question arises of how much more could the rehabilitation of breast cancer survivors be improved by the implementation of holistic occupational therapy and how might an increase in occupational therapy interventions improve the rehabilitation and return to work of breast cancer survivors, especially in light of the 'drop' in support described by the participants.

These four themes represent an introductory insight into a complex, changing and varied phenomenon. The full findings could be used by health professionals to gain a more in-depth understanding of the area and be able to address the needs of cancer survivors more effectively. The broader themes, such as the importance of occupations in rehabilitation, could be usefully applied to all settings. These four themes highlight unmet needs for the participants which might represent an opportunity for occupational therapists to expand their role in this area. With its holistic, occupation-focused ethos and wide knowledge base in health and social care, occupational therapy is very well placed to deliver a comprehensive service that can ensure that rehabilitation and return to work of breast cancer survivors is both effective and efficient.

The current provision of occupational therapy in cancer services could be seen as a real-world example of occupational therapy being in prime location for delivering a high-quality service but not expanding their role to optimally fulfilling the holistic needs of the service user. The main findings from the study indicate a need for an expanded role in dealing with breast cancer survivors who have finished their medical treatment and want to return to work. It perhaps represents an opportunity for occupational therapy managers to reassess the prospect of developing occupational therapy services in this and other areas. Following on from the previously stated threats to occupational therapy, this adds to the argument for occupational therapists to expand rather than contract their roles and use their fundamental professional expertise to provide a service that best fits the needs of service users within the limitations of resources available.

CONCLUSION

The uniting of multiple worldviews is a complex and difficult endeavour. However, a stronger link between the theoretical and clinical world is needed in order for occupational therapists to provide appropriate and effective services. Occupational therapists must become more engaged in research and service evaluation to provide the evidence of the value of their service and to mitigate the many threats to the profession. This chapter has offered an example of gaining new perspectives from breast cancer survivors on their experience of rehabilitation and returning to work,

and presented the viewpoint from a recently qualified occupational therapist concerned for the future of the profession. The presentation of the threats and potential solutions are admittedly limited by the provisional knowledge of an inexperienced practitioner; however, it is hoped that these examples may offer some inspiration to both newly qualified and experienced occupational therapists to become more engaged in building evidence to counter the threats to this valuable life-enhancing profession. There remains the call to action for all occupational therapists to provide evidence for their interventions and the imperative that this occurs before financial, political or managerial factors take the options out of our hands.

Acknowledgements

The author would like to acknowledge the Research Capacity Building Collaboration Wales and Tenovus Cancer Care for their support with the study, and the guidance of Dr. Paul Gill, Dr. Gina Dolan, Dr. Rachel Iredale, and Dr. Allyson Lipp during its production. All participant names in this chapter have been changed to preserve anonymity.

REFERENCES

Allen, T., 2013. Janapar. Janapar Media, London.

Amir, Z., Neary, D., Luker, K., 2008. Cancer survivors' views of work 3 years post diagnosis: a UK perspective. Eur. J. Oncol. Nurs. (12), 190–197.

Appleby, J., 2011. Can we afford the NHS in future? Br. Med. J. (343), 4321.

Bannigan, K., 2007. Making sense of research utilisation. In: Creek, J., Lawson-Porter, A. (Eds.), Contemporary Issues in Occupational Therapy: Reasoning and Reflection. John Wiley, Chichester, UK.

Banning, M., 2011. Employment and breast cancer: a meta-ethnography. Eur. J. Cancer Care. 20 (6), 708–719.

Breast Cancer Campaign, 2014. Breast cancer statistics. <http://www.breastcancercampaign.org/about-breast-cancer/breast-cancer-statistics> (accessed 06.06.14.).

Cancer Research UK, 2014. How we deliver our research. <http://www.cancerresearchuk.org/science/research/how-we-deliver-our-research/> (accessed 31.09.14.).

Clouston, T., 2014. Whose occupation is it anyway? The challenge of neoliberal capitalism and work life balance. Br. J. Occup. Ther. 77 (10), P507–P515.

College of Occupational Therapists (COT), 2010. Code of Ethics and Professional Conduct. COT, London.

Cooper, J.E., 2012. Reflections on the professionalization of occupational therapy: time to put down the looking glass. Can. J. Occup. Ther. 79 (4), 199–210.

Department of Health, 2011. Improving Outcomes: A Strategy for Cancer. Department of Health, London.

Desiron, H., 2013. A conceptual-practice model for occupational therapy to facilitate return to work in breast cancer patients. J. Occup. Rehabil. 23 (4), 516.

Eva, G., Playford, D., Sach, T., Radford, K., Burton, C., 2012. Thinking Positively about Work. Macmillan, London.

Fantoni, S., et al., 2010. Factors related to return to work by women with breast cancer in Northern France. J. Occup. Rehabil. (20), 49–58.

Ferlay, J., Peugniez, C., Duhamel, A., Skrzypczak, J., Frimat, P., Leroyer, A., 2010. Global burden of breast cancer. Breast Cancer Epidemiol. (8), 1–19.

Feunerstein, M., 2007a. Defining cancer survivorship. J. Cancer Surviv. (1), 5–7.

Feunerstein, M., 2007b. Handbook of Cancer Survivorship. Springer, New York.

Finlay, L., 2004. The Practice of Psychosocial Occupational Therapy, third ed. Nelson Thornes, Cheltenham, UK.

Flood, A., 2010. Understanding phenomenology. Nurse Res. (17), 2–15.

Gupta, D., Rodeghier, M., Lis, C., 2014. Patient satisfaction with service quality as a predictor of survival outcomes in breast cancer. Support. Care Cancer 22 (1), 129–134.

Hooper, B., 1997. The relationship between pretheoretical assumptions and clinical reasoning. Am. J. Occup. Ther. 51 (5), 328–338.

Hoving, J.L., Broekhuizen, M.L., Frings-Dresen, M.H., 2009. Return to work of breast cancer survivors: a systematic review of intervention studies. BMC Cancer 9 (117), 1471–2407.

Kaiser, K., 2008. The meaning of the survivor identity for women with breast cancer. Soc. Sci. Med. 67 (1), 79–87.

Karanikolos, M., Mladovsky, P., Cylus, J., Thomson, S., Basu, S., Stuckler, D., et al., 2013. Financial crisis, austerity, and health in Europe. Lancet (381), 1323–1331.

Lambert, R., Radford, K., Smyth, G., Morley, M., Ahmed-Landeryou, M., Rastrick, S., 2014. Occupational therapy can flourish in the 21st century – a case for professional engagement with health economics. Br. J. Occup. Ther. 77 (5), 260–263.

Laverty, M., 2003. Hermenuetic phenomenology and phenomenology: a comparison of historical and methodological considerations. Int. J. Qual. Methods 2 (3), 21–35.

Law, M., Baptiste, S., Carswell, A., McColl, M., Polatajko, H.J., Pollock, N., 2005. COPM Canadian Occupational Performance Measure, fourth ed. CAOT Publications ACE, Ottawa.

Lyons, C., Brown, T., Tseng, M., Casey, J., McDonald, R., 2011. Evidence-based practice and research utilisation: perceived research knowledge, attitudes, practices and barriers among Australian paediatric occupational therapists. Aust. Occup. Ther. J. 58 (3), 178–186.

Macmillan Cancer Care, 2008. Returning to Work: Cancer and Vocational Rehabilitation. <http://www.macmillan.org.uk/ Documents/GetInvolved/Campaigns/Campaigns/working_ through_cancer.pdf> (accessed 04.08.14.).

Macmillan Cancer Care, 2015. Macmillan's 'Nine Outcomes': what matters most to people with cancer. <http://www.macmillan .org.uk/Aboutus/WhatWeDo/Nineoutcomes/NineOutcomes .aspx> (accessed 09.03.15.).

Margalit, R., Thompson, S., Visovsky, C., Geske, J., Collier, D., Birk, T., et al., 2009. From professional silos to interprofessional education: campus wide focus on quality of care. Qual. Manag. Health Care 18 (3), 165–173.

Nancarrow, S., Borthwick, A., 2005. Dynamic professional boundaries in the healthcare workforce. Sociol. Health Illness. (27), 897–919.

National Cancer Survivorship Initiative, 2013. The Recovery Package. <http://www.ncsi.org.uk/what-we-are-doing/the-recovery -package/> (accessed 21.03.15.).

Pettican, A., Bryant, W., 2007. Sustaining a focus on occupation in community mental health practice. Br. J. Occup. Ther. 70 (4), 140–146.

Pighills, A., Plummer, C., Harvey, D., Pain, T., 2013. Positioning occupational therapy as a discipline on the research continuum: results of a cross-sectional survey of research experience. Aust. Occup. Ther. J. 60 (4), 241–251.

Rehab Measures, 2014. Rehab Measures: Canadian Occupational Performance Measures. <http://www.rehabmeasures.org/Lists/ RehabMeasures/DispForm.aspx?ID=928> (accessed 20.02.15.).

Swedlove, F., Etcheverry, E., 2012. Occupational therapists' perceptions of the value of research. New Zealand J. Occup. Ther. 59 (1), 5–12.

Tamminga, S.J., De Boer, A.G., Verbeek, J.H., Frings-Dresen, H.W., 2012. Breast cancer survivors' views of factors that influence the return-to-work process – a qualitative study. Scand. J. Work Environ. Health 38 (2), 144–154.

Upton, D., Stephens, D., Williams, B., Scurlock-Evans, L., 2014. Occupational therapists' attitudes, knowledge, and implementation of evidence-based practice: a systematic review of published research. Br. J. Occup. Ther. 77 (1), 24–38.

Vaismoradi, M., Turunen, H., Bondas, T., 2013. Content analysis and thematic analysis: implications for conducting a qualitative descriptive study. Nurs. Health Sci. 15, 398–405.

Waddell, G., Burton, K., Kendall, N., 2013. Vocational rehabilitation: what works, for whom, and when? <https://www.gov.uk/ government/publications/vocational-rehabilitation-scientific- evidence-review> (accessed 06.06.14.).

Welsh Government, 2012. Together For Health – Cancer Delivery Plan. A Delivery Plan up to 2016 for NHS Wales and Its Partners. <http://wales.gov.uk/docs/dhss/publications/ z120613cancerplanen.pdf> (accessed 22.10.14.).

World Cancer Research Fund International, 2012. Breast cancer statistics. <http://www.wcrf.org/int/cancer-facts-figures/data -specific-cancers/breast-cancer-statistics> (accessed 22.09.14.).

SYSTEMATIC MAPPING REVIEW OF NOTIONS OF JUSTICE IN OCCUPATIONAL THERAPY

JYOTHI GUPTA ▪ TRACY GARBER

CHAPTER OUTLINE

The genesis of the profession of occupational therapy is historically linked to the moral treatment era that moved through France, England and North America during the eighteenth and nineteenth centuries (Gordon, 2009; Peters, 2011). The intention of moral treatment was 'to replace brutality with kindness and idleness with occupation' (Gordon, 2009, p. 203). The central role of occupation in the human experience is *the* core tenet of occupational therapy. This original belief of occupational engagement as a requisite for health and well-being has endured the maturing of the profession and the emergence of the discipline of occupational science (Yerxa et al., 1989). Ideas of justice that have grounded the profession in implicit ways have been brought to the foreground

with the coining of *occupational justice* (OJ) and its associated terminology (Townsend and Wilcock, 2004). The belief that humans are occupational beings that require occupation for survival and life itself was the impetus to identify different forms of injustices such as occupational deprivation, imbalance, alienation, marginalization and apartheid (Kronenberg and Pollard, 2005; Townsend and Wilcock, 2004). Therefore, by depriving or restricting people from occupational engagement, one is essentially denying them access to their humanity. Justice has been and remains intricately woven into the profession's philosophy and conceptual models.

The aim of this chapter is a synthesis and examination of a broad exploration of how justice-based values of the profession are articulated within the occupational therapy and occupational science literature to determine whether or not they are present in modern practice contexts. The chapter begins with a brief description of the methodology to illustrate the systematic diligence of the mapping review process. Next, a discussion of the findings organized as justice-related themes from the literature is presented. The remaining two sections offer a critique on the current state of justice ideas in occupational science and occupational therapy and the practice of occupational therapy in the US.

MAPPING 'JUSTICE' IN THE PROFESSION'S DISCOURSE

The Process of Mapping

As the aim of the study was to generate a topographic map of 'justice', two broad research questions were asked: (a) How has justice been presented in the profession's discourse? and (b) Is justice operationalized (or not) in clinical practice? A broad and inclusive systematic mapping review process was used (Hooper et al., 2013) to search PubMed, CINAHL, Medline, SocINDEX and OT Search databases from 1980 to 2014. Through multiple iterative reviews, the search yielded a final count of 120 articles. The framework analysis (Ritchie and Spencer 2004) guided the content analysis process and included the following steps: (a) familiarization (articles read and reviewed multiple times); (b) identification of framework-(International Classification of Functioning, Disability and Health [ICF] (World Health Organization, 2001) and Person-Environment-Occupation Model (Law et al., 1996)); (c) indexing (categorization, coding and thematic analysis); (d) charting (synthesis of data); and (e) mapping and interpretation (identification of key concepts and themes).

JUSTICE IS EVIDENT IN BOTH IMPLICIT AND EXPLICIT WAYS IN THE LITERATURE

The systematic mapping review process helped identify the topics and contexts that have been linked to ideas of justice. Overall, ideas of justice were more implied in occupational therapy literature and far more explicit in the occupational science literature.

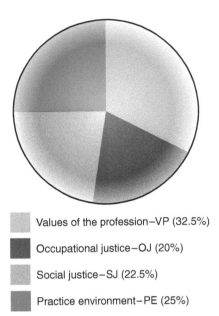

Values of the profession–VP (32.5%)

Occupational justice–OJ (20%)

Social justice–SJ (22.5%)

Practice environment–PE (25%)

FIGURE 17-1 ■ Distribution of articles by primary categories: values of the profession (VP), practice environment (PE), occupational justice (OJ) and social justice (SJ).

The four major categories for the articles are shown in Figure 17-1. Nearly 32.5% of the articles categorized as *values of the profession* represented the largest group, followed by practice environment (25%), social justice (SJ; 22.5%), and OJ (20%). Each article was assigned one primary subcategory code (Figure 17-2) and two secondary codes (Figure 17-3).

The quantitative results highlight the following key points:

■ OJ was represented by 36% of the articles (n = 43) as a secondary topic.
■ OJ articles were dominated by occupational deprivation subcategory (46%).
■ SJ was present in 63% of the articles (n = 76) as a secondary topic.
■ SJ was not explicitly labelled as such, but was clearly evident as an undercurrent.
■ Nearly 78% of articles (n = 93) discussed the environment, indicating that context matters to occupational therapy and occupational science.

The qualitative content analysis of the literature revealed the following four overarching themes:

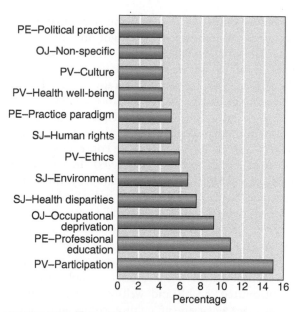

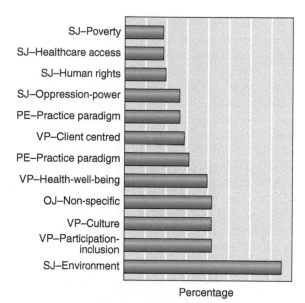

FIGURE 17-2 ■ Top 12 primary code subcategories of articles. Values of the profession (VP) was dominated by the subcategory participation. Occupational justice (OJ) category had articles on occupational deprivation as the most represented subcategory. Health disparities was the main subcategory under social justice (SJ). Professional education dominated the practice environment (PE) category.

FIGURE 17-3 ■ Top 12 secondary subcategories of articles. This figure shows the representation of occupational therapy's values of inclusion, client-centred practice, health and well-being, culture, justice and the influences of the environment in doing justice in the literature. OJ, occupational justice; PE, practice environment; SJ, social justice; VP, values of the profession.

- Occupational therapy practitioners are called to be true to the profession's heritage and values.
- The dominant group controls the contextual and social conditions.
- Socially constructed barriers to participation are risk factors for occupational injustices and poor health.
- Dissonance in practice contexts and espoused values ensues as crisis in professional identity.

While the following discussion of the themes is based on the complete review (n = 120 articles), only key references will be cited as exemplars of themes.

Occupational Therapy Practitioners are Called to be True to the Profession's Heritage and Values

Occupational therapy is a profession with a heritage in justice, activism and advocacy (Cage, 2007). Historically, occupation was used as the vehicle to promote

the health and well-being of *disadvantaged* individuals through enabling participation in activities they found meaningful (Gordon, 2009). The early political activism and reformist tendencies of occupational therapy were lost in 1917 with the recognition of occupational therapy as a profession in the US, at which point the profession allied itself with biomedicine (Frank and Zemke, 2008). Regardless of this departure from social concerns, notions of justice were evident in the literature. Justice was associated with the vulnerable and oppressed populations such as refugees, unemployed (Burchett and Matheson, 2010; Jakobsen, 2009), prisoners of war (Cockburn, 2005), the mentally ill (Farrell and Bryant, 2009; Magasi and Hammel, 2009), older adults (Holthe et al., 2007; Rudman and Molke, 2008), foster children (Paul-Ward, 2009), those with disabilities (Gossett et al., 2009; Magasi and Hammel, 2009), indigenous peoples (Thomas et al., 2011), women (Cage, 2007) and those living in poverty (Thew, 2008). These populations also experience inequities in access to the goods of the society, and social exclusion based on attributes such as race, disability and socioeconomic status. The profession was born out of the conviction that all individuals are of worth regardless of differences, and that through occupation, health and well-being could be achieved for all. This belief has been revitalized with the emergence of the discipline of occupational science (Yerxa et al., 1989), which puts occupation at the forefront as a health determinant, and occupational enablement as the goal of occupational therapy. It is understood that by enabling all individuals or groups to participate in meaningful, productive and self-chosen activities it will not only benefit their health and well-being, but help them fulfil roles and responsibilities and make a contribution to society. Furthermore, everyday occupations are powerful tools for promoting justice and change at both the individual and the societal level; participation in occupation promotes action and reflection in the real world (Townsend 1993, p. 178).

In order to be effective and to honour the profession's core values, occupational therapists must demonstrate solidarity with those who are restricted or barred from participation in health-promoting activities due to issues of power and privilege. The profession's orientation and values can help guide practitioners to use occupation to empower participation for individuals and groups experiencing social exclusion or marginalization. Justice is inherently political, and espoused values in justice demand politically competent practitioners who are socially conscious, justice-oriented and prepared to tackle system-level issues. Sakellariou et al. (2008) state that because occupation is at the centre of the profession, practitioners have a responsibility to advocate for the right to engage in occupation. Political competency can involve various strategies including writing letters to the editors of local newspapers and publications, participating in community-based rehabilitation, meeting with policy-makers, committing to a client-centred practice, using therapeutic rather than simulated occupation and working with populations outside the traditional scope of modern practice (Braveman and Bass-Haugen, 2009; Cage, 2007; Kronenberg, 2003; Rebeiro-Gruhl, 2009; Townsend, 1993). 'In recognizing and working for the right to do, be, become, and belong, occupational therapists have a role in safeguarding equitable

access to occupation and ensuring that situations of occupational injustice are brought to the surface' (Sakellariou et al., 2008, p. 359). This viewpoint was implicit in the nature of the work being done during the early years of occupational therapy practice and has remained unchanged within the profession's values for nearly a century. Although principles of justice are woven into the professional documents, many practitioners struggle to integrate these concepts into daily practice (Riegel and Eglseder, 2009). In Chapter 9, Bailliard and Aldrich discuss some ways by which therapists can be justice oriented with individual clients in their everyday practice. Townsend (1993) identified the core of occupational therapy philosophy as the use of everyday occupations to enable participation. When discussing occupational therapy's core values, the professional lexicon includes terminology such as client-centred, health and well-being, participation, enablement, engagement, cultural competence, advocacy, inclusion and nondiscrimination. These are the values that guided the early stages of the profession's development nearly 100 years ago and are still present in the profession's guiding texts and literature.

The profession is hence called upon to honour its legacy of activism by advocating for those who are vulnerable or marginalized, including victims of domestic violence, individuals with learning disabilities and children with special needs (Cage, 2007). More recently, Frank and Murithi (2015) have proposed the occupational reconstruction theory that may serve as a framework for bridging justice-oriented occupations and social transformation at the level of the individual, community and social policy. This framework links occupational injustices, SJ, political activism and critical theories to occupational science and occupational therapy. The profession's political involvement in the US has largely focused on maintaining or broadening the scope of occupational therapy practice and advocating for more occupational therapy services, particularly for the Medicare entitlement programme[1]. While

---

[1]Medicare is the federal government-administered health insurance for US citizens and residents over 65 years and those less than 65 years with certain disabilities and end-stage renal disease. It is funded through Medicare tax that is paid half by employees through payroll deductions and half by the employer (Centres for Medicare and Medicaid Services, 2014).

this is perhaps a justified goal for the professional association, the American Association of Occupational Therapy (AOTA), it is essentially self-serving. It falls short of advocating for the social change needed to address the impoverished contexts of daily living, and the gross inequities in access and opportunities to a diverse range of occupations for many vulnerable clients.

The Dominant Group Controls the Contextual and Social Conditions

In all societies, '[T]he dominant culture defines who is valued and who is marginalized and determines a hierarchy of valued occupations (for example, paid employment is 'more valuable' than volunteerism or the care of others)' (Hammell, 2008, pp. 62–63). Those with power, privilege and socioeconomic means influence social institutions, and it is in their self-interest to maintain the status quo. In most societies, political and economic power is with the wealthy who, by virtue of their socioeconomic status, have the capacity to determine how others will live (Thew, 2008). The dominant view is often a white, Western cultural perspective that is deemed as 'normal' and informs the values that are promoted within the society (Kantartzis and Molineux, 2011; Nelson, 2009). Occupational therapy is value-laden and is influenced by dominant ways of knowing and doing; these values are then transposed onto 'others' through practice (Molke and Rudman, 2009; Nelson, 2009). The dominant professional perspective can also be transmitted through professional documents, funding guidelines and institutional policies that define and govern the practice of occupational therapy (Molke and Rudman, 2009; Nelson, 2009; Townsend et al., 2003). Power and justice are at the heart of the dissonance that therapists and clients experience in society. The profession of occupational therapy itself lacks power due to its subordinate status to medicine and the health systems (Townsend et al., 2003). In its early years, occupational therapy was less dominated by medicine; sponsorship of the American Medical Association during the early 1930s brought visibility and recognition at the cost of professional autonomy (Reed and Peters, 2006). However, during 1950 to 1980, when occupational therapy was being transformed into a profession, there were tensions that still persist 'between those therapists embracing an objective, and arguably male, science and those supporting a characteristically feminine caring philosophical base' (Peters, 2011).

OJ implies that all individuals are ensured adequate access to occupational opportunities (Braveman and Suarez-Balcazar, 2009). Yet marginalized groups are perceived as having less social, cultural, political and economic value than the dominant group, resulting in conditions of occupational marginalization, occupational alienation, occupational deprivation, occupational imbalance and occupational apartheid. Within a framework of OJ, power and oppression contribute to injustices. Power is based on concepts of participation, equality and empowerment, the latter being defined as 'the giving of power to another' (Smith and Hilton, 2008, p. 170). Oppression is a risk factor for poor health (Gupta and Walloch, 2006), social invisibility and health disparities (Flowers, 2006). Oppression is rooted in the politics of identity manifested as cultural imperialism, marginalization and exploitation (Hammell, 2008; Young, 1990). The dual influences of power and oppression, both implicit and explicit, have been used as a means to disable certain subgroups within the dominant culture through deprivation, segregation, marginalization, control and alienation. Systems of oppressing power were identified as government, medical establishments, corporate entities, Western culture, ableist thinking and social attitudes (Blakeney and Marshall, 2009; Gupta and Walloch, 2006; Magasi and Hammel, 2009; Nelson, 2009; Paul-Ward, 2009).

Socially Constructed Barriers to Participation are Risk Factors for Occupational Injustices and Poor Health

Social determinants of health that impact health and produce inequities in health (Marmot and Wilkinsen, 2006) also restrict access and opportunities to occupations in context that create inequities in participation. The environment can be empowering or disabling for individuals and groups (Sakellariou, 2006), and factors such as social attitudes, policies, technology and civil unrest create unjust conditions (Whiteford and Townsend, 2011). Inequalities in health and quality of life are more often a result of contextual aspects of the environment owing to unequal access to resources and issues of social injustice (Padilla et al., 2004). The US

Centers for Disease Control and Prevention identified the following social determinants of health: socioeconomic conditions, culture, social support, social norms and attitudes, community resources to support health lifestyles including recreational opportunities, access to education, economic and employment opportunities, and transportation (Centers for Disease Control and Prevention, 2012). Sakellariou et al. (2008) point out the preventable nature of contextual factors that restrict access to occupation and their 'pervasive impact on the resources and opportunities available, presenting a potential violation of the right to occupation' (p. 359). Since occupation is a health determinant, being restricted from participation by factors that exist outside the individual's control is a matter of justice (Gupta and Walloch, 2006).

Systemic barriers, such as government and public policies, exert power over certain populations. Paul-Ward (2009) identified that those that have 'unequal access to education, political participation, basic healthcare, and economic security are victims of structural violence' (p. 82). Magasi and Hammel (2009) explored institutional power and barriers to community living for women with disabilities in nursing homes. These women experienced social isolation and loss of control that significantly impacted their health and well-being. Environmental impacts of surface mining practices and water pollution restricted availability of clean water that led to occupational deprivation and alienation for residents of a poor, coal-mining community (Blakeney and Marshall, 2009). Children in foster care reported many environmental barriers including the inability to acquire independent living skills, limited access to transportation, poor communication within the system and placement instability (Paul-Ward, 2009).

Since the theoretical models propose the *transactional* relationship between the person, occupation and the environment (Dickie et al., 2006; Law et al., 1996), occupational therapists have a professional responsibility to identify and address environmental barriers to occupational participation, at the individual and the macro level (Gupta and Walloch, 2006). For individuals with disabilities, environmental barriers can result in the inability to access housing, limited recreational or employment opportunities, social isolation, the inability to access transportation and

decreased political power. These barriers in essence create the disabling conditions (Magasi and Hammel, 2009; Sakellariou, 2006).

Dissonance in Practice Contexts and Espoused Values Ensues as Crisis in Professional Identity

The literature revealed a discrepancy between the current context of practice in biomedical settings and the profession's espoused values and theories. This is not new as even the first generation of therapists struggled 'to create a concise body of knowledge, authority, and identity in the early twentieth century's evolving culture of professionalism and medical hierarchy' (Quiroga, 1995, p. 14). Concern over occupational therapy losing its focus on occupation and its holistic view of health has been acknowledged within the profession (Pettican and Bryant, 2007). The reductionist approach in biomedical settings is more relevant to professions that focus on impairments such as medicine and physical therapy. Occupational therapy's focus is on occupational behaviour in natural contexts that are far more nebulous and difficult to quantify using the metrics of biomedicine. Hence decontextualized, impairment-focused practice that is incongruent with the profession's beliefs about occupation, health and conceptual models of practice creates dissonance between belief and action (Gupta and Taff, 2015). As noted by Carlsson (2009), 'we still have far to go to articulate our professional identity, as we continue to break free of the biomedical shackles that practice seemingly remains embedded [in]' (p. 6). Relevant to practice in the US is the corporatization of healthcare and the power wielded by the health insurance industry (Gupta and Taff, 2015). The profession not only needs to claim its identity with confidence, but more importantly evaluate objectively its presence in biomedical institutions, which are clearly not the contexts for everyday occupations.

An OJ perspective takes a stance that all people have a right to participate in occupations for meaning, purpose, development, health and social inclusion and to contribute to their communities and society. In any society, daily life is experienced within complex and nested social arrangements with differential power. Occupational therapists are also embedded in power relations within the healthcare industrial complex, and a majority of therapists in the US (66%) practice in environments that are driven by reimbursement practices (AOTA, 2015). In such environments, the profession's discourse on occupation and client-centred practice are muted by the more powerful discourses of medicine and the healthcare industry (Mackey, 2014). This socialization is insidious and happens gradually over time such that therapists, acculturated into the dominant culture of medicine and business practices, are distanced from their professional socialization. The profession of occupational therapy that began in mental health today has a fraction (2.4%) of therapists in the US who work in this practice area (AOTA, 2015). Many therapists are relegated to the position of generic workers within healthcare teams, causing some to express concern that occupational therapists may lose core skills and, inevitably, professional identity (Pettican and Bryant, 2007). Similarly, therapists in medical settings pondered whether a generic transprofessional skill set was a better fit for job security (Mackey, 2014).

The corporatization of healthcare with its high demands for productivity, rigorous documentation for reimbursement, and focus on impairment and function add further challenges to enact the profession's values (Gupta and Taff, 2015). For example, in medical settings it was difficult to maintain a client-centred, value-driven focus due to the constraints of daily practice (Mackey, 2014). The profession's identity is further challenged, as other professions are unable to differentiate occupational therapy from the other therapies. This is inevitable when practice is impairment focused and distal from the core of the profession—occupation paradigm (Letts, 2011). Hammell (2008) asks, '[I]f occupational therapists believe that engagement in occupation influences human well-being, why are occupational therapists so preoccupied with people who have impairments and not more concerned about the well-being of all people?' (p. 62). Authentic occupational therapy practice is client-centred, has occupation at its core and occurs in the natural context of everyday living (Gupta and Taff, 2015). It is worth remembering that although occupational therapy was associated with medical institutions, such as hospitals and sanitariums in its early years, the focus of practice was activity and occupation, not impairment reduction or remediation. Our identity is at its strongest when practice is grounded in core values, beliefs and occupation-based practice in the context of everyday living.

A CRITIQUE OF THE EVOLVING JUSTICE NOTIONS

More recently, with the emergence of occupational science, significant changes within the vocabulary of the profession have spawned new ways of thinking about occupation and justice: OJ, occupational deprivation, occupational possibilities, occupational apartheid and occupational balance, to mention a few. These terms have made the concepts of occupation and justice more explicit within the lexicon of occupational science and occupational therapy. Durocher et al. (2014) question whether the abundance of nuanced forms of OJ causes more confusion in understanding the basic concept of OJ, which itself is yet to be consistently defined. Clark and Lawlor (2009) state that defining professional terminology can help to identify the most significant aspects of a discipline and offer insights into the perspective of the profession. These evolving notions of justice have been instrumental in enhancing how injustices that prevent people from engaging in necessary, meaningful and required occupations can negatively impact their health and well-being. This in turn impacts the health of the society they live in. Our study is in agreement with the conclusions of Durocher et al. (2014) that further conceptual clarity is required for OJ to be operationalized in practice. One discrepancy noted is that, although occupational therapy professes the importance of context and environment, it is given only cursory importance in OJ literature.

OJ has been described as the 'implied social vision' of occupational therapy (Whiteford and Townsend, 2011, p. 69). Just as occupations do not occur in a vacuum, OJ cannot exist in one. The larger context of human occupation, the macro-level social influences, must be factored in the conceptualization of OJ. This essentially means that OJ cannot be achieved without social change – in other words, policy and legislation based on principles of SJ. The profession has also taken a very narrow view of SJ as one of distributive justice, and distinguishes OJ from SJ as justice of difference (Townsend and Wilcock, 2004). One cannot alleviate occupational injustices without adequate resources, and redistribution is one way most government bodies address inequities. Furthermore, justice of difference that originated in identity politics falls under the category of recognition justice. Young (1990) and Fraser (1996), prominent scholars in this area, acknowledge that neither distribution nor recognition is sufficient on its own. They favour an integrative approach that is based on redistribution *and* recognition for social inclusion and parity in participation. Social participation is essentially membership to society or citizenship that entails the rights and responsibility to participate in the social, cultural and economic life of civil society and its political process (Fransen et al., 2013). When certain groups are denied their rights to participate in social life, they are excluded from social membership or citizenship, which is an injustice.

The term *occupational* is best understood by those associated with occupational science or occupational therapy, and this perhaps isolates this emerging discourse of OJ from the justice discourses occurring in other disciplines. OJ needs to be conceptualized and situated in broader justice theories. Moreover, while not intended, the authors believe the way OJ is presented further perpetuates the focus on the person and puts the context in the background. As most barriers to participation are socially constructed, promoting individual occupational rights will not go far without understanding OJ in the context of social systems. For instance, Stadnyk et al. (2010), in their framework for OJ, describe that OJ differs from SJ as it perceives humans as occupational beings and is concerned with individual differences. This is an artificial demarcation as humans are occupational *and* social beings who exist in transactional relationships within multiple, nested contexts that contribute to their multifaceted identity. Even in individualistic societies such as the US, social organization necessitates a certain degree of collective thinking. The difference is that societies differ in the relative degree of individualism versus collectivism that is best seen as a continuum. Language of shared advantage, interdependence, contextual factors and quality of life was used in discussing OJ. These terms are *social* in nature and speak of social cohesion and collectives; moreover, participation in life happens in the life-world that includes both the individual and their social world. Other authors also note the cursory attention to SJ in the conceptualization of OJ

(Durocher et al. 2014). The inadequacy of capturing the complex relationships by the simplistic and mechanistic conceptualization of occupational injustices and their systemic root causes has been put forth (Bailliard, 2014). The causal pathways to injustices are complex, intersecting, and are based on historical, economic and social arrangements that inequitably distribute power, privilege and access to resources.

Peloquin (2005) describes a professional ethos as a tapestry of sentiment, value and thought that serves as a touchstone and is used to convey a profession's character, demonstrate its unique genius and embody its spirit. The profession is challenged to think about occupation, participation, the environment and client-centred practice in ways that enact our beliefs in authentic practice (Gupta and Taff, 2015).

IMPLICATIONS FOR PRACTICE – 'WALK OUR TALK'

Occupational science has made explicit the importance of occupation to meaning, health and quality of life. The viability and vitality of the profession calls for practice to be guided by its espoused values, theories, conceptual models and belief in the power of occupation as a health determinant for the benefit of individuals, communities and societies.

The importance of context to occupation is captured in all the conceptual models of practice (e.g., Law et al., 1996). Occupational science has elaborated on the transactional relationship of the person, occupation and context (Dickie et al., 2006), and recognized that context creates meaning and identity (Hasselkus, 2002; Huot and Rudman, 2010). Yet these precepts are not applied sufficiently to professional practice that largely occurs in decontextualized environs. Occupational lives are enacted in communities and within their specific milieu the members of the community are the experts of their lives and their context. Would community not be a far better contextual fit for client-centred, occupation-based practice? Therapists recognize that biomedical practice settings are not compatible for occupation-based practice, yet practice continues in this suboptimal context at the risk of eroding the core identity of the profession.

While clinical practice is a valuable and necessary domain for the profession, the authors believe that occupational therapists' absence in communities is a lost opportunity for the profession and its clients. As long as occupational therapy remains predominantly in medical establishments, practice will remain distanced from occupational engagement. In acute and rehabilitation settings, reimbursement-driven practice is focused on getting clients discharged as quickly as possible, and hence emphasis is on safety and function of very basic activities of daily living – those tasks that are concerned with taking care of one's own body (Gupta and Taff, 2015). This also impacts how others perceive the profession – that perhaps this type of therapy can be done by anyone (Mackey, 2014).

If occupational therapy in the US is to honour its commitment to the health and well-being of society, to realize its potential and to remain relevant, the profession must expand the context of practice into community practice. With rising costs of healthcare and shifting attention to prevention and primary care, the timing is right to liberate the profession from a context that has constrained the flourishing of occupational therapy. For instance, even if occupational therapy is tied to healthcare reimbursement, perhaps more of the therapy ought to occur in client's homes and in the community rather than in hospitals and rehabilitation settings.

Issues of social inequities are of concern to occupational therapy as they are the root cause of inequities in opportunities and resources that create barriers for some individuals and groups to realize their occupational potential. Health determinants and occupational determinants are contextual and shaped by dominant group politics and societal attitudes towards others. Kantartzis and Molineaux (2011) proposed that social institutions and professions such as occupational therapy are social constructions that reflect an expected way to live that is seen as 'normal' and desirable. This worldview works to disempower those with different values, abilities, or lifestyles, and also restricts access and opportunities. These injustices invisibly construct impediments to participation for less valued members of society and silently exert power and oppression to maintain privilege over those that society has deemed not worthy of equal access to certain goods and services. The result of being denied occupational participation contributes to these disparities in health for minority or devalued groups.

Health is an asset and a resource for 'everyday life' that is essential to human development (Hofrichter, 2003; World Health Organization, 1986, p. 1). In the US, health and healthcare are not considered as basic rights. Healthcare is a commodity in the free market that is dominated by market justice rooted in individualism, personal responsibility, self-interest and voluntary behaviour (Bundetti, 2008). Research has demonstrated that among those who are most likely to suffer from health disparities are individuals who are poor and belong to racial/ethnic minority groups (Blanchard, 2009; Cahill and Suarez-Balcazar, 2009). Results further indicate other marginalized groups such as those with mental health issues, disabilities and victims of domestic abuse are also at risk for health disparities as these groups experience occupational deprivation, marginalization and social exclusion. Many social issues are prevalent in the US, a country that has the largest income disparities among industrialized Western nations (Organization for Economic Cooperation and Development, 2014). It has the highest rates of incarceration (The Sentencing Project, 2013) and teen pregnancy (Kearney and Levine, 2012), and one in five of all children (22%) live in families below the poverty level (National Center for Children in Poverty, 2014). These findings are directly relevant to justice-oriented occupational therapy practice that can enable occupational engagement to these groups that experience grave occupational injustices.

As a profession concerned with enabling occupation, occupational therapists have a social responsibility to raise awareness of the importance of occupation to health and quality of life, how environmental barriers prevent participation and the ensuing cost to society. Practice that addressed barriers to participation for marginalized populations is what spawned the profession of occupational therapy and guided its development and evolution, yet in the US this type of practice has been largely replaced by reimbursement-driven biomedical practice. The 'Centennial Vision' to commemorate the 100th anniversary of the national professional association in the US asserts: 'We envision that occupational therapy is a powerful, widely recognized, science-driven, and evidence-based profession with a globally connected and diverse workforce meeting society's occupational needs'

(AOTA, 2006, p. 626). If we are to meet society's occupational needs, we must be visible in communities where people live their daily lives. As the link between health and social determinants becomes more evident, occupational therapists must step forward and form allegiances with other disciplines, such as public health, to address systemic issues or risk becoming irrelevant and obsolete. For 'if we fail to serve society's need for action, we will most assuredly die out as a health profession…another group similarly purposed and similarly organized and prepared would have to be invented' (Reilly, 1961, p. 84).

CONCLUSION

Occupational therapy has tremendous potential to make a positive contribution to the health and well-being of individuals, communities and society. In order to realize this potential, the profession must not abandon its rich, historical legacy and commitment to justice. To bring occupational therapy into the next century, professional values will need to be used as the touchstone to guide occupational therapy education, research and practice. To remain relevant and to drive the evolution of healthcare, occupational therapy needs to be grounded in its core values and beliefs, and promote occupation-based practice. If the profession does not make explicit its unique contribution and put meaningful occupation back at the centre of occupational therapy and practice in contexts where occupations happen, occupational therapists risk losing their professional identity and relevance to society.

REFERENCES

American Occupational Therapy Association (AOTA), 2006. The Road to the Centennial Vision. <www.aota.org/en/AboutAOTA/Centennial-Vision.aspx> (accessed 02.10.14.).

American Occupational Therapy Association (AOTA), 2015. Occupational Therapy Salary and Workforce Survey. http://www.aota.org/-/media/corporate/files/secure/educations-careers/salary-survey/2015-aota-workforce-salary-survey-high-res.pdf> (accessed 04.07.15.).

Bailliard, A., 2014. Justice, difference, and the capability to function. J. Occup. Sci. 1–14. doi:10.1080/14427591.2014.957886.

Blakeney, A.B., Marshall, A., 2009. Water quality, health, and human occupations. Am. J. Occup. Ther. 63 (1), 46–57.

Blanchard, S., 2009. Variables associated with obesity among African-American women in Omaha. Am. J. Occup. Ther. 63 (1), 58–68.

Braveman, B., Bass-Haugen, J., 2009. Social justice and health disparities: an evolving discourse in occupational therapy research and intervention. Am. J. Occup. Ther. 63 (1), 7–12.

Braveman, B., Suarez-Balcazar, Y., 2009. Social justice and resource utilization in a community-based organization: a case illustration of the role of the occupational therapist. Am. J. Occup. Ther. 63 (1), 13–23.

Bundetti, P.P., 2008. Market justice and US health care. J. Am. Med. Assoc. 299 (1), 92–94.

Burchett, N., Matheson, R., 2010. The need for belonging: the impact of restrictions on working on the well-being of an asylum seeker. J. Occup. Sci. 17 (2), 85–91.

Cage, A., 2007. Occupational therapy with women and children survivors of domestic violence: are we fulfilling our activist heritage? A review of the literature. Br. J. Occup. Ther. 70 (5), 192–198.

Cahill, S., Suarez-Balcazar, Y., 2009. Promoting children's nutrition and fitness in the urban context. Am. J. Occup. Ther. 63 (1), 113–116.

Carlsson, C., 2009. The 2008 Frances Rutherford Lecture: taking a stand for inclusion: seeing beyond impairment! New Zealand J. Occup. Ther. 56 (1), 4–11.

Centers for Disease Control and Prevention, 2012. Social Determinants of Health. <http://www.cdc.gov/socialdeterminants/FAQ.html#a> (accessed 04.10.14.).

Centers for Medicare and Medicaid Services, 2014. Medicare Program – General Information. Available at: <https://www.cms.gov/Medicare/Medicare-General-Information/MedicareGenInfo/index.html> (accessed 04.18.15.).

Clark, F., Lawlor, M., 2009. The making and mattering of occupational science. In: Crepeau, E., et al. (Eds.), Willard and Spackman's Occupational Therapy. Lippincott Williams & Wilkins, Philadelphia, pp. 2–14.

Cockburn, L., 2005. Reflections on … Canadian occupational therapists' contributions to prisoners of war in World War II. Can. J. Occup. Ther. 72 (3), 183–188.

Dickie, V., Cutchin, M.P., Humphry, R., 2006. Occupation as transactional experience: a critique of individualism in occupational science. J. Occup. Sci. 13 (1), 83–93.

Durocher, E., Gibson, B., Rappolt, S., 2014. Occupational justice: a conceptual review. J. Occup. Sci. 21 (4), 418–430.

Farrell, C., Bryant, W., 2009. Voluntary work for adults with mental health problems: a route to inclusion? A review of the literature. Br. J. Occup. Ther. 72 (4), 163–173.

Flowers, K., 2006. Empowering clients to participate: a report of AOTA's workshop on health disparities and social justice. Adv. Occup. Ther. Pract. 22 (18), 64–65.

Frank, G., Murithi, B., 2015. Theorizing social transformation in occupational science: the American civil rights movement and South African struggle against apartheid as 'occupational reconstructions'. South Afr. J. Occup. Ther. 45 (1), 11–19. Available from: <http://www.scielo.org.za/pdf/sajot/v45n1/03.pdf> (accessed 04.07.15.).

Frank, G., Zemke, R., 2008. Occupational therapy foundations for political engagement and social transformation. In: Pollard, N., Sakellariou, D., et al. (Eds.), A Political Practice of Occupational

Therapy. Elsevier Health Sciences, Philadelphia, PA, pp. 111–135.

Fransen, H., Kantartzis, S., Pollard, N., Viana-Moldes, I., 2013. Citizenship: Exploring the Contribution of Occupational Therapy <http://www.enothe.eu/activities/meet/ac13/CITIZENSHIP_STATEMENT_ENGLISH.pdf> (accessed 09.01.15.).

Fraser, N., 1996. Social Justice in the Age of Identity Politics: Redistribution, Recognition, and Participation. The Tanner Lectures on Human Values. Stanford University, 30 April–2 May 1996. <http://tannerlectures.utah.edu/_documents/a-to-z/f/Fraser98.pdf> (accessed 15.09.15.).

Gordon, D., 2009. The history of occupational therapy. In: Crepeau, E., Cohn, E., et al. (Eds.), Willard and Spackman's Occupational Therapy. Lippincott Williams and Wilkins, Philadelphia, pp. 202–215.

Gossett, A., Mirza, M., Barnds, A.K., Feidt, D., 2009. Beyond access: a case study on the intersection between accessibility, sustainability, and universal design. Disabil. Rehabil. Assist. Technol. 4 (6), 439–450.

Gupta, J., Taff, D.W., 2015. The illusion of client-centred practice. Scand. J. Occup. Ther. 22 (4), 244–251.

Gupta, J., Walloch, C., 2006. Process of infusing social justice into the Practice Framework: a case study. OT Pract. 11 (15), CE1–CE8.

Hammell, K., 2008. Reflections on … well-being and occupational rights. Can. J. Occup. Ther. 75 (1), 61–64.

Hasselkus, B.R., 2002. The Meaning of Everyday Occupation. SLACK, Thorofare, NJ.

Hofrichter, R. (Ed.), 2003. Health and Social Justice: Politics, Ideology, and Inequity in the Distribution of Disease. Jossey Bass, San Francisco, CA, pp. xvii–xxi. (preface).

Holthe, T., Thorsen, K., Josephsson, S., 2007. Occupational patterns of people with dementia in residential care: an ethnographic study. Scand. J. Occup. Ther. 14 (2), 96–107.

Hooper, B., King, R., Wood, W., Billics, A., Gupta, J., 2013. An international systematic mapping review of educational approaches and teaching methods in occupational therapy. Br. J. Occup. Ther. 7 (1), 9–22.

Huot, S., Rudman, D.L., 2010. The performances and places of identity: conceptualizing intersections of occupation, identity and place in the process of migration. J. Occup. Sci. 17 (2), 68–77.

Jakobsen, K., 2009. The right to work: experiences of employees with rheumatism. J. Occup. Sci. 16 (2), 120–127.

Kantartzis, S., Molineux, M., 2011. The influence of western society's construction of a healthy daily life on the conceptualisation of occupation. J. Occup. Sci. 18 (1), 62–80.

Kearney, M.S., Levine, P.B., 2012. Why is the teen birth rate in the United States so high and why does it matter? J. Econ. Perspect. 26 (2), 141–166.

Kronenberg, F., 2003. The WFOT position paper on community-based rehabilitation: a call upon the profession to engage with people affected by occupational apartheid. World Fed. Occup. Therapists Bull. 51, 5–13.

Kronenbereg, F., Pollard, N., 2005. Overcoming occupational apartheid. A preliminary exploration of the political nature of occupational therapy. In: Kronenberg, F., et al. (Eds.), Occupational

Therapy without Borders: Learning from the Spirit of Survivors. Elsevier, Edinburgh, pp. 58–86.

Law, M., Cooper, B., Strong, S., Stewart, D., Rigby, P., Letts, L., 1996. The Person-Environment-Occupation model: a transactive approach to occupational performance. Can. J. Occup. Ther. 63 (1), 9–23.

Letts, L., 2011. Optimal positioning of occupational therapy. Can. J. Occup. Ther. 78 (8), 209–217.

Mackey, H., 2014. Living tensions: reconstructing notions of professionalism in occupational therapy. Aust. Occup. Ther. J. 61 (3), 168–176.

Magasi, S., Hammel, J., 2009. Women with disabilities' experiences in long-term care: a case for social justice. Am. J. Occup. Ther. 63 (1), 35–45.

Marmot, M., Wilkinsen, R.J., 2006. Social Health Determinants, second ed. University Press, Oxford.

Molke, D.K., Rudman, D.L., 2009. Governing the majority world? Critical reflections on the role of occupation technology in international contexts. Aust. Occup. Ther. J. 56 (4), 239–248.

National Center for Children in Poverty, 2014. Child poverty. <http://www.nccp.org/topics/childpoverty.html> (accessed 20.12.14.).

Nelson, A., 2009. Learning from the past, looking to the future: exploring our place with indigenous Australians. Aust. Occup. Ther. J. 56 (2), 97–102.

Organization for Economic Cooperation and Development, 2014. Society at a Glance 2014: OECD Social Indicators. OECD Publishing. <http://dx.doi.org/10.1787/soc_glance-2014-en> (accessed 05.01.14.).

Padilla, R., Gupta, J., Liotta-Kleinfeld, L., 2004. Occupational therapy and social justice: a school-based example. OT Pract. 9 (16), CE-1–CE-8.

Paul-Ward, A., 2009. Social and occupational justice barriers in the transition from foster care to independent adulthood. Am. J. Occup. Ther. 63 (1), 81–88.

Peloquin, S.M., 2005. The 2005 Eleanor Clarke Slagle Lecture: embracing our ethos, reclaiming our heart. Am. J. Occup. Ther. 59 (6), 611–625.

Peters, C.O., 2011. Powerful occupational therapists: a community of professionals, 1950–1980. Occup. Ther. Ment. Health. 27 (3–4), 199–410.

Pettican, A., Bryant, W., 2007. Sustaining a focus on occupation in community mental health practice. Br. J. Occup. Ther. 70 (4), 140–146.

Quiroga, V.A.M., 1995. Occupational therapy: the first 30 years 1900-1930. AOTA Press, Bethesda, MD.

Rebeiro-Gruhl, K., 2009. The politics of practice: strategies to secure our occupational claim and to address occupational injustice. New Zealand J. Occup. Ther. 56 (1), 19–26.

Reed, K., Peters, C., 2006. Occupational therapy: values and beliefs, Part II. OT Pract. 18 (22), 17–22.

Reilly, M., 1961. Occupational therapy can be one of the great ideas of 20th century medicine. Am. J. Occup. Ther. 16, 1–9.

Riegel, S.K., Eglseder, K., 2009. Occupational justice as a quality indicator for occupational therapy services. Occup. Ther. Health Care. 23 (4), 288–301.

Ritchie, J., Spencer, L., 2004. Qualitative data analysis for applied policy research. In: Bryman, A., Burgess, R.G. (Eds.), Analyzing Qualitative Data. Routledge, London, pp. 173–194.

Rudman, D., Molke, D., 2008. Forever productive: the discursive shaping of later life workers in contemporary Canadian newspapers. Work 32, 377–389.

Sakellariou, D., 2006. The disabler, the disablee and their context: a tripartite view of disability. Br. J. Occup. Ther. 69 (2), 49–57.

Sakellariou, D., Pollard, N., Kronenberg, F., 2008. Time to get political. Br. J. Occup. Ther. 71 (9), 359.

Smith, D., Hilton, C., 2008. An occupational justice perspective of domestic violence against women with disabilities. J. Occup. Sci. 15 (3), 166–172.

Stadnyk, R., Townsend, E., Wilcock, A., 2010. Occupational justice. In: Christiansen, C., Townsend, E. (Eds.), Introduction to Occupation: The Art and Science of Living. Pearson Education, Upper Saddle River, NJ, pp. 329–358.

The Sentencing Project, 2013. Report of the sentencing project to the United Nations Human Rights Commission. <http://sentencingproject.org/doc/publications/rd_ICCPR%20Race%20and%20Justice%20Shadow%20Report.pdf> (accessed 04.02.15.).

Thew, M., 2008. Occupational profile: an interview with professor Gary Craig. J. Occup. Sci. 15 (3), 181–185.

Thomas, Y., Gray, M., McGinty, S., 2011. Occupational therapy at the 'cultural interface': lessons from research with Aboriginal and Torres Strait Islander Australians. Aust. Occup. Ther. J. 58 (1), 11–16.

Townsend, E., 1993. Muriel Driver lecture: occupational therapy's social vision. Can. J. Occup. Ther. 60 (4), 174–184.

Townsend, E., Galipeault, J.P., Gliddon, K., Little, S., Moore, C., Klein, B.S., 2003. Reflections on power and justice in enabling occupation. Can. J. Occup. Ther. 70 (2), 74–87.

Townsend, E., Wilcock, A.A., 2004. Occupational justice and client-centred practice: a dialogue in progress. Can. J. Occup. Ther. 71 (2), 75–87.

Whiteford, G., Townsend, E., 2011. Participatory occupational justice framework (POJF): enabling occupational participation and inclusion. In: Kronenberg, F., et al. (Eds.), Occupational Therapy without Borders, vol. 2: Towards an Ecology of Occupation-Based Practice. Elsevier Churchill Livingstone, Toronto, pp. 65–84.

World Health Organization, 1986. The Ottawa Charter for Health Promotion, <http://www.who.int/healthpromotion/conferences/previous/ottawa/en/> (accessed 04.18.15.).

World Health Organization, 2001. International Classification of Functioning, Disability and Health. <http://www.who.int/classifications/icf/en/> (accessed 11.10.15.).

Yerxa, E.J., Clark, F., Frank, G., Jackson, J., Parham, D., Pierce, D., 1989. Occupational science: the foundation for new models of practice. Occup. Ther. Health Care. 6 (4), 1–17.

Young, I.M., 1990. Justice and the Politics of Difference. Princeton University Press, Princeton, NJ.

18

THE PARTICIPATORY OCCUPATIONAL JUSTICE FRAMEWORK: SALIENCE ACROSS CONTEXTS

GAIL ELIZABETH WHITEFORD ■ ELIZABETH TOWNSEND ■ OLIVE BRYANTON ■ ALISON WICKS ■ ROBERT PEREIRA

CHAPTER OUTLINE

The Participatory Occupational Justice Framework (POJF) was first developed and published in 2005 as a scholarly collaboration between Townsend and Whiteford (2005). It was based on their experiences of working with different populations of people in differing sociopolitical contexts, and their hope was that the framework would be a useful tool for occupational therapists working with groups of people facing occupational injustices. It was also their intention at the time that the framework – and its grounding within a critical occupational therapy – would have theoretical utility. In this chapter, we represent an expanded group of authors able to further develop the narrative of the POJF and its salience in practice and in research. In this regard it is our intention to continue the dialogue with therapists internationally through reflections on the extent to which the POJF can be used in different contexts as a basis for doing justice in everyday life.

The first section of the chapter presents the three conceptual foundations of the POJF: occupation, enablement and justice. In this section we also discuss the philosophical underpinnings of the POJF in the form of critical occupational therapy. Here we present the articles of such a critical practice and within them an acknowledgement of the centrality of human rights. We then move on to consider the theoretical utility of the POJF through a case study-based discussion of Pereira's use of it in a research project focused on poverty and disability and, because of its inherent orientation towards acknowledgement of power relations in society, its complementarity with a discourse analysis approach. The next sections discuss, through a case study approach, how the POJF was used in two communities in initiatives generated, respectively, by Wicks and then Townsend and Bryanton aimed at tackling situated occupational injustices. In conclusion, we reflect on how the POJF may be utilized by occupational therapists and their community partners to achieve transformative and sustainable change.

FOUNDATIONS OF THE PARTICIPATORY OCCUPATIONAL JUSTICE FRAMEWORK

The POJF draws on the Western historical development of occupational therapy and occupational science

and the ideas, values and beliefs underpinning three related concepts: occupation, enablement and justice. To profile WHAT interests occupational therapists in using the POJF, we focus on occupational therapists' domain of concern: participation in the *occupations* of daily life. To explain HOW occupational therapists may work with populations using the POJF, we integrate approaches for *enabling* social change, notably change to transform social structures and power relations that are determinants of occupational participation. In exploring WHY occupational therapists are concerned with social inclusion, we emphasize occupational therapists' concern for a *justice of difference* (see Table 18-1) to promote inclusive occupational participation.

With justice as a distinguishing feature, we emphasize that use of the POJF requires critical reflexivity, collaborative negotiation of power relations, a focus on the environment, notably the policy, funding and legal context. Finally, we address the WHERE – that is, the rich contexts in which occupations are enacted. We emphasize that all occupations are situated and can neither be fully understood nor addressed without due

	TABLE 18-1			
	Concepts of Justice			
	Social Justice			**Occupational Justice**
	Procedural	*Distributive*	*Restorative*	*Participatory*
Concerns	Processes of dispute resolution	Having or acquisition	Repair or renewal	Meaningful engagement in valued occupations
Contested terrain	Equality of voice, unequal human and fiscal resources	Measurement and comparison of assets and deficiencies of social groups	Credibility of perpetrators and victims, measurement of damage and fair compensation	Occupational classification: social versus economic value of occupations, competing needs for opportunities and resources
Aims	Equal voice and procedural rights	Equal rights to and equal responsibility for goods, services and privileges	Restoration of perpetrators, restitution to victims	Enablement of different opportunities and resources, taking differences into account in social structures
Issues of power	Individual defendants and prosecutors to be heard without bias	All social groups to have equal advantages for participation in daily life	Individual defendants to be exonerated, individual or class victims to be compensated	Different opportunities and resources to enable full citizen participation by all individuals, families and social groups
Actions for justice	Equal procedural processes	Equal distribution or allocation	Confession of guilt, compensation to victims	Enablement of difference for social inclusion

TABLE 18-2			
Four Pillars of Occupational Therapy Knowledge			
WHAT	HOW	WHY	WHERE
is core knowledge?	do occupational therapists practice?	enable occupation?	do occupational therapists engage with others?
Occupations: participation in necessary, obligatory and voluntary occupations	Enabling: Collaborative and person centred with individuals, families, communities and populations	Social change: Reducing everyday injustices/ advancing occupational justice	Context: Occupations are situated – physically, historically, socioculturally and politically. Occupational therapists actively address this whatever specific setting they work in
= Everyday life	= Empowerment	= Social inclusion	= Relevance

consideration of physical, cultural, political and historical forces that shape their form and shared meaning (Table 18-2).

WHAT – Occupation: Our Domain of Concern

Given the occupational therapy core domain of concern in occupation, everyday practice engages people in negotiated processes to enable contextually meaningful modes of occupational participation. This will, and should, look and be experienced differently depending on the site, setting and specific sociocultural and political milieu. Consistent with a stance of critical reflexivity on difference and inclusion, we emphasize here the complex and interconnected weave of structural factors in society that enable and preclude participation in occupations of meaning, necessity and obligation. Clearly, the POJF guides practice that extends beyond enabling individual occupational performance components, a focus we argue has hitherto delimited the social contribution of occupational therapy (Townsend, 1998). Indeed, it can be argued that a historical biomedical emphasis and focus on functionality has truncated occupational therapists' ability to understand and address the social determinants of occupational participation (Pereira and Whiteford, 2013). We acknowledge the inherent pluralism and diversity of occupations and forms of occupations in society and of diverse languages and cultures, not just those in narrowly defined economic categories (Christiansen and Townsend, 2004; Jarman, 2004; Kielhofner, 2002; Wilcock, 2002). Similarly, we interpret occupational participation as being about

active engagement in all the occupations central to daily life, not just the occupation of paid employment. We note, however, that equity of access to appropriately paid, sustainable employment remains a significant issue around the globe for many people living in poverty.

HOW – Enabling: How We Work with People

Given a core competency in enabling (also known as enablement), everyday practice consistent with the POJF is distinguished by culturally appropriate collaborative enabling approaches. Occupational therapists' enabling perspective predicates participatory, empowerment-oriented approaches – what the profession has described for 25 years as client-centred (collaborative) practice contrasted with profession–expert prescriptive practice (Canadian Association of Occupational Therapists, 1993). There are, however, many complex issues with respect to the power relations of enabling change in client-centred practice (Townsend and Landry, 2004). The linguistic standpoint is challenging in that the term *client* is not universally applicable (especially cross-culturally), tends to guide individualized rather than community or other collective practices, and has a commercial orientation. Given the problematic nature of the term and its associated connotations, we refer hereafter in this chapter to *people* or *persons*, communities or populations consistent with the philosophy underpinning critical occupational therapy and the POJF (see next section).

Enabling approaches are recognized in occupational therapy as being on a continuum. Ineffective enablement that reinforces addictive or codependent behaviour, including dependence on professionals, is at the opposite end of the spectrum to enablement approaches that are directed towards empowerment and transformative change. With ineffective enablement, good intentions may be derailed or actually be detrimental if well-meaning practitioners take over where collaborative planning, decision making and evaluation should prevail. Ineffective enablement is evident when practitioners presume to know best without consultation with those involved, or prescribe solutions without listening to and learning about what will work in a particular sociocultural context with a particular population. With effective enablement, individuals, communities or populations are full partners in enabling occupational justice.

The POJF directs practice that is grounded in what people need and want to do. Occupational justice practice stretches beyond technical or instrumental goals (e.g., developing skills, improving body function, using technical supports) to address the local, national or international restrictions that limit possibilities for some populations or communities to participate fully in the areas of society that others take for granted, such as schools or the workplace. Enabling occupational justice includes a range of active strategies aimed at changing or reforming the policy and legislative environment to enhance the rights of citizens to participate in valued, meaningful occupations. An occupational justice practice would address the diversity of capacity and resources globally and acknowledge important differences between groups in a range of contexts rather than attempting to standardize and universalize what people do across the life course (Dunst and Trivette, 1989).

WHY – Addressing Injustice and Focusing on Inclusion

The centrepiece of the POJF that stretches beyond typical occupational therapy process frameworks is the overt attention to inequities and pursuit of what has been described as the appropriate ends of occupational therapy: social inclusion (Pereira and Whiteford, 2013). A practitioner would explicitly identify and name occupational issues of inequity, and explicate the sociocultural, political and economic determinants that limit participation in different countries

and communities. In describing the POJF, we emphasize a population approach, occupational participation and, inter alia, a constant vigilance to inequity in everyday life.

Clearly, one of the most significant outcomes in working towards occupational justice would be the achievement of greater levels of equity in occupational engagement: a justice of empowerment, inclusion and participation for all regardless of differences in ability, age, gender and other characteristics. Importantly, at the level of internationally accepted nomenclature, this framing or construction of occupational injustice is congruent with the International Classification of Function (World Health Organization, 2001) concept of *participation restrictions*. In naming occupational justice as a pillar of occupational therapy knowledge, the profession extends the International Classification of Function meaning of participation restriction to *rights for all to participate in the occupations they define as necessary and meaningful in their context*. Occupational injustices exist when, for example, participation is barred, confined, segregated, prohibited, undeveloped, disrupted, alienated, marginalized, exploited or otherwise devalued for some more than others.

WHERE – Being and Doing in Place: Culture and Context

Whilst it is beyond the scope of this chapter to present an in-depth discussion of the situated nature of occupations (see Whiteford, 2010), as authors we felt that it was important to emphasize that enablement is always within a particular context and that to ignore this can lead to irrelevant or, worse, oppressive practices. Occupational therapists need to go beyond 'taken for grantedness' and make no assumptions about the attendant meaning of a given occupation, but seek to understand it from the existential standpoint of the persons with whom they are interacting. What is required in this regard is a reflexive standpoint which is not unlike that of narrative enquiry, that is, one in which the starting point is an understanding of self as a gendered, culturally constructed being with a particular worldview and attendant biases (Iwama, 2003). Only from this place can occupational therapists approach some understanding of the lived experience of specific occupations in specific locations.

A CRITICAL OCCUPATIONAL THERAPY: UNDERSTANDING POWER RELATIONS AS A BASIS FOR UTILIZING THE PARTICIPATORY OCCUPATIONAL JUSTICE FRAMEWORK

Whilst noting in the discussion of the pillars of occupational therapy knowledge above that practice is predicated by a reflexive stance, we wish to develop this perspective more fully through discussing reflexivity as an essential element of a critical occupational therapy. A critical stance is one in which the structural arrangements and attendant power relations in society are foregrounded in the enactment of everyday practice. First named by Townsend and Whiteford in 2005 and subsequently used by authors including, for example, Laliberte Rudman (2010) and Hammell and Iwama (2012), we promote a *critical occupational therapy* defined by six key features, which we present here as articles:

Article I: Occupational therapists strive to engage in critical reflexivity to constantly challenge gaps between specific occupational therapy philosophy and theories and everyday practice, as well as between universal principles of human rights and institutional policies, practices and environmental conditions.

Article II: Occupational therapists aim to be collaborative and participatory in all stages of decision making and throughout all decision-making processes.

Article III: Occupational therapy objectives ideally address the means and ends of social inclusion for the people with whom they work who are, or may be at risk of becoming, marginalized, disadvantaged or oppressed.

Article IV: Occupational therapy approaches and methods are those which seek to engage people as individuals, as families and as communities in obligatory, necessary and voluntary occupations which are deemed culturally appropriate by those persons, individually or collectively.

Article V: Occupational therapy collaborative objectives are those ideally aimed at ensuring more equitable opportunities and resources are available for people to exert optimal levels of control and choice in everyday occupations.

Article VI: Occupational therapists strive to work with others in pursuit of the ideal of occupational justice irrespective of attendant political and economic challenges and current environmental limitations. Hope, and a vision of possibility, underpins their efforts.

Critical occupational therapy requires a conscious foregrounding of power relations, not just with respect to the individuals, families, groups or other people occupational therapists work with, but also with other professionals, funders, administrators, and others. Accordingly, when professionals structure programmes and implement and evaluate them, particular attention must be paid as to 'the who and how' of power in negotiations. We note that occupational therapists' conception of occupational justice – a justice of empowerment and inclusion regardless of difference – is necessarily aligned with postmodern interests in multiple perspectives, distributed and collaborative power (see Table 18-1), diversity and critiques of universal theories (Rolfe, 2001). Although these may seem familiar to many occupational therapists, a critical occupational therapy practice diverges from general occupational therapy through an explicit focus on disadvantaged and oppressed populations, and on processes that bring critical awareness to, and target change in, broad environmental forces, such as regional, national and global policies, laws and economic structures. Whilst disadvantage and oppression will be experienced very differently in different national contexts, the central concern is the impact of restrictions in occupational participation over time and how this can be tackled through a range of means.

USING THE PARTICIPATORY OCCUPATIONAL JUSTICE FRAMEWORK: PROCESSES AND STRATEGIES

Having presented the conceptual and philosophical underpinnings of the POJF, we discuss here its key features. One of these, indeed one which distinguishes it from other frameworks utilized in occupational

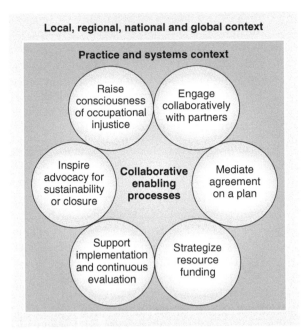

FIGURE 18-1 ■ Participatory Occupational Justice Framework.

therapy, is its *nonlinear nature*; for this reason, the POJF is portrayed as a circle of interconnected processes (see Figure 18-1). The circle of collaborative and enabling processes is embedded and interconnected within a practice and systems context that may include (but not be limited to): availability of resources – fiscal and human; professional frames of reference; scope of practice; professional regulation; workloads; labour unions; codes of ethics; protocols; policies and liabilities. These processes are in turn embedded within a local, regional, national and global context that may include, but not be limited to, for example: economic policies, public and private control of education, health and social network supports, telecommunications and transportation, primary resource policies and industry standards.

Although we emphasize that the processes are nonlinear, the typical starting process for an occupational therapist is to raise consciousness in others of occupational injustice. A typical closing process completes the agreement based on evaluation from all partner perspectives on the partnership, processes of engagement, resources and outcomes. The end-point evaluation may trigger another agreement. Ideally, the evaluation

signals longer-term sustainability and the use of context-appropriate resources to continue towards justice *without* professional involvement. Each process is grounded in issues of injustice, is participatory and focuses on the environment with an emphasis on population approaches to structural changes in society. It is worth noting that the processes may be repeated or adjusted depending on specific contextual forces and events.

Table 18-3 provides a series of stimulus questions that are linked to each process and are intended to assist a practitioner to focus in a reflexive way on the what, how and who of each process within the specific context in which the collaborative action is occurring. Ultimately, the POJF is about enabling change *in* everyday occupations *through* engagement in everyday occupations. Programmes guided by the POJF would be monitored and modified through continuous evaluation with all participants and partners of all facets of the relationship and the actions taken within successive process cycles.

Before going on to present some case studies which detail how these processes were used in two different contexts, the next section speaks to the utility of the POJF in research. Below, Pereira presents his narrative account of why and how he adopted the POJF.

From Theoretical Salience to Practical Application: Pereira's Account of Using the Participatory Occupational Justice Framework to Critically Analyse Policy

Commencing doctoral research for me, as for many students undertaking their Ph.D., meant a beginning point of reading widely. The purpose of the reading was to consider the conceptual terrain in which my topic was grounded. As I was interested in exploring critical occupational science research into occupational justice issues manifested by policy, I wanted to explore how the POJF could be used as an analytic tool for 'doing justice' (Whiteford and Townsend, 2011, p. 65) by using it in conjunction with a critical discursive approach (Pereira, 2013, 2014).

Additionally, the POJF provided a platform to acknowledge and reflect on my participants' stories of everyday participation, inclusion and social exclusion – adults living with a range of disabling conditions in one of Australia's most disadvantaged urban areas.

TABLE 18-3	
Participatory Occupational Justice Framework Processes and Guiding Questions for Reflexive Practice	
Processes – Nonlinear Sequence	**Guiding Questions/Foci**
Raise consciousness of occupational injustices	■ Is a particular community or population inequitably excluded from participation in typical occupations? ■ What forms of consciousness raising are culturally appropriate and relevant? ■ What forms of collaboration are contextually appropriate? ■ How is social exclusion experienced as an everyday, embodied injustice? ■ What documentation is being created to illustrate and make publicly explicit injustices for a given population? ■ What is the knowledge exchange strategy and how will narratives and other data be accessible to others – for example, through social media?
Engage collaboratively with partners	■ How ready are partners to participate and how resilient are they? ■ What cultural beliefs, values and power issues that may be problematic need attention? ■ What education, mediation or negotiations will be enacted to show respect for the dignity, worth and rights of all involved? ■ How will partners participate, for example, verbally, through storytelling, focus groups or nonverbally through visual/creative expressive means? ■ What records are being generated, and how will the agreed justice frameworks be documented?
Mediate agreement on a plan	■ What goals, objectives and outcomes are mutually desirable? ■ What occupationally based programmes and services would have the greatest collective impact to reduce the occupational injustice for the given group? ■ How will the design be participatory? ■ What types of documentation will communicate the plan to interested stakeholders? ■ What are the knowledge generation and capture strategies in the plan?
Strategize resource finding	■ Who will advocate for human and financial resources, and what are the funding options? ■ What are the primary occupational issues for the given population and what collective resources/social capital do they have to address perceived injustices? ■ How will the occupational therapist coordinate efforts between agencies involved and the given group? ■ What is the communication strategy to inform others about the resource issues involved?
Support implementation and continuous evaluation of the plan	■ How are the partners enabling change through occupational engagement? ■ How is the learning through doing philosophy explicitly being used and understood by all partners? ■ How will the impact of the service/programme/initiative be monitored throughout from population, professional, management and other perspectives? ■ What formative and summative evaluation processes and strategies are feasible and appropriate to context? ■ How will data and documentation of it be utilized in proving programme effectiveness or otherwise?
Inspire advocacy for sustainability or closure	■ How might advocacy for and with partners be best achieved in the setting? ■ What decisions would guide advocacy for sustainability or closure? ■ What is the perception of success and lessons learned for each partner? ■ What empowerment strategies may be employed to positively conclude the professional relationship? ■ What conditions might warrant termination or renegotiation of professional involvement? ■ In what form will the documented legacy of the initiative be and how will it be communicated across relevant platforms?

A key feature of the POJF (Whiteford and Townsend, 2011) is its overt attention to power relations among individuals, communities, agencies and other stakeholders. What emerged from my analysis of social inclusion policy discourses was the utility and usefulness of the POJF to explore matters of occupational justice and injustice within and practiced at the political level. Because it was developed within an 'ethics of care' ethos (Townsend, 1998) to support marginalized groups (such as citizens living with entrenched disadvantage characterized by poverty, disability and other social issues), the foregrounding of occupational justice within policy provided a natural fit to expose political accountabilities, rationalities and areas of concern. The POJF provided further analytic support in favour of marginalized citizens through its application of critical occupational therapy (Townsend and Whiteford, 2005; Whiteford and Townsend, 2011), which has been discussed earlier in the chapter.

Through adopting the POJF (Whiteford and Townsend, 2011) as a complementary analytic tool to Bacchi's (2009) 'What's the problem represented to be?' approach (Pereira, 2014), the predominant finding from my research suggested that social inclusion – as it was presented and discussed with a number of government documents over several years – suggested an ideologically driven, *selective* occupational justice practice. The policies reflected in the material pointed to a tacit participation hierarchy (Pereira, 2013) and an extremely narrow, neoliberal framing of participation (Gidley et al., 2010), evidenced by an overt emphasis on productivity, rather than on occupational choice (Galvaan, 2012). Using the critical lens of the POJF enabled me to examine this focus on work and productivity within the discursive material and consider whether it represented constrained occupational possibilities (Laliberte Rudman, 2010) for citizens. Ultimately, my analysis pointed to the reality that employing a participation hierarchy (through prioritizing and politically recognizing paid work above all other forms of participation, e.g., volunteering) brings about what I have termed 'occupational misrecognition'. Based on my research, I define this as 'the act of promoting, recognizing and legitimizing certain types of occupations (i.e. paid employment) over others in the interests of hegemonic practices' (Pereira, 2013, p. 1). Inherent in this conceptualization is the influence of political or organizational power on occupational choice and control leading to both limited opportunities to do and be, as well as restricted occupational outcomes. Participants in my research spoke to this as it impacted on their daily lives, in stories which highlighted that occupations such as caring for others, engaging in social support networks or creative leisure pursuits were considered institutionally invalid. Alongside the experiential accounts, I also drew upon theoretical influences in development of the term; namely, theories of recognition and misrecognition originating from the fields of moral and political philosophy (e.g., Honneth, 1995; Thompson and Yar, 2011).

In summary, then, employing the POJF enabled me to analyse policy through illuminating hidden discourses of occupational injustice within a seemingly positive and 'inclusive' policy agenda. This enabled me to identify the disturbing phenomenon in which, despite an apparently inclusive orientation, the national discourse and its interpretation through policy and operationalization at a service level, did the opposite: potential was truncated and choice and control delimited through attendant power inequities within the institutional cultures and the processes utilized within them.

Using the POJF in research of a critical nature, as described in Pereira's account, is an approach that the authors are hopeful may be adopted by others given the indications that it was valuable in this contextual application. Next, we present Wicks's description of how the POJF was utilized in the development of a community garden project in an aged care facility in Australia.

Utilizing the Participatory Occupational Justice Framework in an Institutional Context: An Aquaponics Garden Project

Good fortune led to my involvement in the aquaponics garden project at the Basin View Masonic Village, a residential aged care facility on the south coast of New South Wales, Australia. The project's vision is that the village is a vibrant place to live and an interesting place to visit. Initially, specific aims were to address a perceived lack of social cohesion within the village and increase engagement with the local community. From an occupational perspective, the project promotes individual and community well-being by creating opportunities for village residents, families and local people to participate in meaningful occupations such as growing, tending and harvesting flowers, vegetables and fish.

The village is home for about 80 elderly residents. Approximately 30 residents live independently in self-care villas while the others require varying levels of care and support. The dementia support unit caters for about 20 residents. Most residents previously lived in the local area, a popular haven for retirees attracted to the relaxed rural lifestyle and ready access to the national marine park. Gardening and fishing were popular occupations for many residents prior to their move to the village.

Occupational justice per se has never been an explicit focus of the project, yet it is inherent in many aspects of the project. For example, the brief was to establish a garden which was accessible to all, easy to maintain, low cost, environmentally friendly, containing every feature requested by residents, and a pleasant place for spending time, doing meaningful and enjoyable things. Moreover, when I reflect on the various processes that have evolved, serendipitously, since the project began in July 2011, the processes described in the POJF are clearly evident, highlighting the salience of the POJF.

Engaging Collaboratively with Partners

This ongoing project is transdisciplinary, fostering imagination (Brown et al., 2010), fusing multiple disciplinary perspectives (Lawrence, 2004) and incorporating and acknowledging the expertise of laypersons as well as experts (Thompson Klein, 2004). The eclectic team includes residents, their families, village staff, a retired teacher, an informatics expert, a marine ecologist, a structural engineer, local schoolchildren, service club members and community organizations.

Mediating Agreement on a Plan

The village owners agreed to fund and support the project after the structural engineer, an aquaponics expert, gave a passionate presentation on the benefits and technology of aquaponics. Meetings with residents provided 'wish lists' of what they wanted to grow and what the garden should look like. Each item on the wish list, such as wheelchair access, raised garden beds with easy-to-dig soil, water and artistic features was incorporated into the garden design.

Strategizing Resource Funding

In-kind support and donations of materials are continuously sought from the community. Volunteers help with garden maintenance and harvesting the organically grown vegetables which are used in the village kitchen and shared among residents. The garden is a unique, attractive venue for community events, such as Australia's Biggest Morning Tea, which raise public awareness of the garden project and lead to additional community support.

Supporting Implementation and Evaluating Continuously

Team members regularly take photographs to create a pictorial garden history. Informal focus groups (Mackay, 2012) with residents, their family and staff have been used to capture feedback and attain new ideas for the garden. Some comments overheard opportunistically demonstrate the positive effect of the garden on some residents. One day while feeding the fish, Mary, who has late-stage dementia said, 'It is so peaceful here. It [the garden] makes me feel so calm.' Super granny Edna, 102 years old and living with minimal support, was inspecting some of the huge spinach crop when she said, 'Coming up here, I feel I am free, that I am alive again.' Local schoolchildren have assisted with the monitoring of the water quality and fish growth, undertaken every 4 months.

Inspiring Advocacy for Sustainability

Gaining a High Commendation in the salutogenic category in the 2013 International Academy of Design and Health awards certainly cemented the project's sustainability. The village owners, ecstatic with this outcome, subsequently confirmed ongoing support and development of the garden. A new playground and a remodeled barbecue area are being planned for the garden.

Raising Consciousness of Occupational Injustices

Proactively sharing the story and images of the aquaponics garden project through print and social media, oral and poster presentations at conferences, publications in lay and academic literature, and YouTube videos has influenced people's perceptions of the occupational opportunities that an aged care facility can offer residents. National and international interest has been significant, and similar projects are being developed in other aged care facilities.

All people, at any stage in the life course, have a right, indeed a need, to participate in meaningful everyday occupations. Therefore, when people move into a residential aged care facility, they should not be deprived of their occupational rights and needs. Projects such as the Basin View aquaponics garden focus on what people can and want to do and on keeping people well.

The final case study presented here that highlights the retrospective use of the POJF in framing, planning and actively tackling an extant occupational injustice within a given community is from Prince Edward Island (PEI), Canada's smallest province. Townsend, also known as Liz, and Bryanton, also known as Olive, conjointly tell the story that highlights key features of POJF processes, especially the mobilization of resources.

The Participatory Occupational Justice Framework in Community: Olive and Liz's Story

Liz and Olive met through Olive's University of PEI admission to the Ph.D. in Educational Studies programme in 2012. They are seniors (over 60 years of age) and as Olive says, 'Loving it'. Olive is a long-time community activist most recently researching transportation systems for older women, particularly in rural and small communities (Bryanton et al., 2010). Liz is also a long-time community activist who also spent more than 30 years linking occupational therapy practice with theory, recently in the POJF with Gail Whiteford and a film on activist occupational therapy (Townsend and Sandiford, 2012). In Liz and Olive's story, Liz asked Olive about starting the Seniors Active Living Centre in Charlottetown, the provincial capital city of PEI. The story illustrates how the POJF is not individualized and can be used in community activism to critically reflect on actions already taken.

Raising Consciousness of Occupational Injustices

Although the starting place in using the POJF can be at any point, we started by talking about raising awareness of the injustice for a population of community-dwelling older adults who were being alienated, deprived and ultimately marginalized within their homes without city and provincial support for a seniors activity programme and transportation to get out and around the community.

Liz: When did you become interested in developing the Seniors Active Living Centre and how did you get started?

Olive: It was in the late 1990s … I worked well with the President of the Seniors Federation of PEI and we were aware that many people were not members. There were many small seniors clubs in PEI villages, but Charlottetown had nothing. At a conference called Yes We Can, many people raised awareness that PEI had no 'seniors centre'.

Engage Collaboratively with Partners and Mediate Agreement on a Plan

Liz: How did you get people together to start and reach agreement to go ahead?

Olive: A few of us decided on a pilot project for seniors to get together and have fun. Previous attempts by other groups had not been successful. This time I wrote a proposal to New Horizons [a Federal fund for seniors' projects] because I was working for the Seniors Federation. We got the funding. We brought out different points of view and planning issues, and we sought consensus. Majority rules!

Strategize Resource Funding

Liz: How did you use your limited resources?

Olive: We had to find a place to meet, but we could not use our funds to renovate an empty space with a rent we could pay. Our funding did not cover renovations, but we agreed with the owner of a local mall to pay back the costs after we made some money. We found the money for curtains informally.

Support Implementation and Continuous Evaluation

Liz: How did you fund the programme?

Olive: We charged a bit for activities every week. One of the activities of interest was a card game called 'Auction', so we asked one of the men who loved cards to head up the card games. Although the activists were women to start, when the men joined we made a lot of money on card games. We reached out to people with volunteers to organize bingo, catering and social events. People took organizing very seriously. We get feedback by people coming back. And we always survey what people want to do.

Inspire Advocacy for Sustainability

Liz: One of the challenges for groups is to go from enthusiasm to sustainability. How did you keep the centre going?

Olive: We took advantage of the talents of local seniors, for instance, we hired an artist to run painting classes, and he also provided paintings for sale to raise funds. We had to reapply for funding after the first year, after we had already become an official organization with bylaws, a constitution, and so forth. We kept applying for yearly funding, and looked for donations – chairs, materials, you name it. Finally, we approached the city for support and received $10,000 [CAD] for the year. The city also offered us space in a new sports centre at the University of Prince Edward Island where we are today for $1.00 [CAD] per year with the annual $10,000 [CAD] grant from the city. We have many fund-raising events and have raised a huge amount in partnership with local business people. We are working toward our second 10-year plan.

Liz: Any advice for a group wanting to start something or make a change?

Olive: If you want something you have to just make it happen. You want to team up with positive people. The naysayers are not helpful. We had to suggest to one naysaying person that he was not enjoying the board when he repeatedly expressed concerns that older persons are not worthy of getting out and around. Ageism is still very much alive but we took charge to make things happen.

Critical Reflection

Reflecting on the empowerment of a group of older women, Olive highlights success *with* seniors where attempts to start similar programmes *for* seniors had failed. They involved persons in authority, sought funds through a grant for seniors' programming, and legitimized the Seniors Active Living Centre with local leaders who knew how resources could be found and put together, succeeding against the odds.

THE FUTURE: THE PARTICIPATORY OCCUPATIONAL JUSTICE FRAMEWORK AND SUSTAINABLE CHANGE

In this chapter we have presented the POJF and its conceptual and theoretical underpinnings, and reinforced that its enactment is grounded in a critical occupational therapy in which human rights are foregrounded. The three case studies speak respectively to the theoretical utility of the framework and its use in research, and to the salience of the POJF in two differing contexts in which its adoption guided social change for persons at risk of (further) marginalization. The reasons for presenting these case studies, especially in narrative form, is to encourage others to use the POJF in the spirit in which it is intended: experimentally, collaboratively and with the ends of empowerment, social inclusion and participatory citizenship as guiding ideals.

What we hope is that through engaging with the case studies, occupational therapists in diverse settings and national and local contexts will be able to get a sense of how the six processes are a *practical* means of identifying injustices, not through rhetoric, but by determining what people need and want to do, then acting *with them*. Ultimately, the success of the POJF will be realized when the input of an occupational therapist is time limited and their role, which starts out as facilitatory, becomes redundant as the people they work with are mobilized, empowered and self-directed in the achievement of greater levels of inclusion and participation.

We face a future with many uncertainties, including high levels of civic unrest, environmental degradation, economic instability and human displacement. In the title of this chapter and throughout, we have attempted to demonstrate salience with respect to the POJF, but the real test of its salience will be how it may be used in actively addressing these uncertainties and in the mitigation of heightened levels of alienation, displacement and marginalization that are often corollary to such conditions. At least, the face of occupational therapy practice will need to transform and, in some settings and contexts, radically if such salience is indeed to be realized.

REFERENCES

Bacchi, C., 2009. Analysing Policy: What is the Problem Represented to Be? Pearson, Frenchs Forest, Sydney.

Brown, V., Harris, J., Russell, J., 2010. Tackling Wicked Problems through Transdisciplinary Imagination. Earthscan, London.

Bryanton, O., Weeks, L.E., Lees, J.M., 2010. Supporting older women in the transition to driving cessation. Acti. Adapt. Aging 34 (3), 181–195. doi:10.1080/01924788.2010.501483.

Canadian Association of Occupational Therapists, 1993. Occupational Therapy Guidelines for Client Centred Mental Health Practice. CAOT Publications ACE, Toronto.

Christiansen, C., Townsend, E., 2004. Introduction to Occupation: The Art and Science of Everyday Living. Prentice Hall, Upper Saddle River, NJ.

Dunst, C.J., Trivette, C., 1989. An enablement and empowerment of case management. Topics Early Child. Spec. Educ. 8, 87–102.

Galvaan, R., 2012. Occupational choice: the significance of socio-economic and political factors. In: Whiteford, G.E., Hocking, C. (Eds.), Occupational Science: Society, Inclusion, Participation. Blackwell Publishing Ltd, Chichester, West Sussex, UK, pp. 152–162.

Gidley, J.M., Hampson, G.P., Wheeler, L., Bereded-Samuel, E., 2010. From access to success: an integrated approach to quality higher education informed by social inclusion theory and practice. Higher Educ. Policy 23, 123–147. doi:10.1057/hep.2009.24.

Hammell, K.W.R., Iwama, M.K., 2012. Wellbeing and occupational rights: an imperative for critical occupational therapy. Scand. J. Occup. Ther. 19 (5), 385–394.

Honneth, A., 1995. Struggle for Recognition: The Moral Grammar of Social Conflicts (Anderson, J., Trans.). Polity Press, Cambridge, UK.

Iwama, M., 2003. The issue is … toward culturally relevant epistemologies in occupational therapy. Am. J. Occup. Ther. 57 (5), 217–223. doi:10.5014/ajot.57.5.582.

Jarman, J., 2004. What is occupation: interdisciplinary perspectives on defining and classifying human activity. In: Christiansen, C., Townsend, E. (Eds.), Introduction to Occupation: The Art and Science of Living. Prentice Hall, Upper Saddle River, NJ, pp. 47–62.

Kielhofner, G., 2002. Model of Human Occupation. Slack, Thorofare, NJ.

Laliberte Rudman, D., 2010. Occupational terminology: occupational possibilities. J. Occup. Sci. 17 (1), 55–59. doi:10.1080/14427591.2010.9686673.

Lawrence, R., 2004. Housing and health: from interdisciplinary principles to transdisciplinary research and practice. Futures 36 (4), 487–502.

Mackay, H., 2012. The 'unfocused' group discussion technique. Australas. J. Market Soc. Res. 20 (2), 47–58.

Pereira, R.B., 2013. The politics of participation: a critical occupational science analysis of social inclusion policy and entrenched disadvantage. Unpublished doctoral dissertation. Macquarie University, Sydney, Australia. <http://hdl.handle.net/1959.14/282427> (accessed 25.10.14.).

Pereira, R.B., 2014. Using critical policy analysis in occupational science research: exploring Bacchi's methodology. J. Occup. Sci. 21 (4), 389–402. doi:10.1080/14427591.2013.806207.

Pereira, R.B., Whiteford, G.E., 2013. Understanding social inclusion as an international discourse: implications for enabling participation. Br. J. Occup. Ther. 76 (2), 112–115. doi:10.4276/030802213X13603244419392.

Rolfe, G., 2001. Postmodernism for healthcare workers. Nurse Educ. Today 21 (1), 38–47.

Thompson, S., Yar, M. (Eds.), 2011. The Politics of Misrecognition: Rethinking Political and International Theory. Ashgate Publishing Limited, Farnham, Surrey, UK.

Thompson Klein, J., 2004. Prospects for transdisciplinarity. Futures 36 (4), 515–526. doi:10.1016/j.futures.2003.10.007.

Townsend, E., 1998. Good Intentions Overruled: A Critique of Empowerment in the Routine Organization of Mental Health Services. University of Toronto Press, Toronto.

Townsend, E., Landry, J., 2004. Enabling participation in occupations. In: Christiansen, C., Townsend, E. (Eds.), Introduction to Occupation: The Art and Science of Living. Prentice Hall, Upper Saddle River, NJ.

Townsend, E.A., Sandiford, M., 2012. Reaching Out: Today's Activist Occupational Therapy. Beachwalker Films, Inc. Full version available at: <http://youtu.be/LIcfyQ3RwT0>. Short version available at: <http://youtu.be/_RXL4V505Bw>. Youtube video (accessed 21.04.16.).

Townsend, E., Whiteford, G., 2005. A participatory occupational justice framework: population-based processes of practice. In: Kronenberg, F., Simó Algado, S., et al. (Eds.), Occupational Therapy without Borders: Learning from the Spirit of Survivors. Elsevier Limited, London, pp. 110–126.

Whiteford, G., 2010. Occupation in context. In: Curtin, M., Molineux, M., et al. (Eds.), Occupational Therapy and Physical Dysfunction, Enabling Occupation. Churchill Livingstone, London, pp. 135–149.

Whiteford, G., Townsend, E., 2011. Participatory Occupational Justice Framework (POJF 2010): enabling occupational participation and inclusion. In: Kronenberg, F., Pollard, N., et al. (Eds.), Occupational Therapies without Borders, vol. 2: Towards an Ecology of Occupation-Based Practices. Elsevier, London, pp. 65–84.

Wilcock, A., 2002. A Journey from Prescription to Self Health, vol. 2. British Association of Occupational Therapists, London.

World Health Organization, 2001. International Classification of Functioning, Disability and Health (ICF). <http://www.who.int/classifications/icf/en/> (accessed 25.09.14.).

19

CULTIVATING A HUMAN RIGHTS CULTURE FOR OCCUPATIONAL THERAPY

DANIKA GALVIN ■ CLARE WILDING

CHAPTER OUTLINE

In recent years, occupational therapists have increasingly been engaged in critical thinking and dialogue about the need to consider how issues of power and justice are embedded in society and occupational therapy practice (Whiteford et al., 2000). This contemplation has helped to make the relationship of justice to core occupational therapy concepts of occupation and enablement more explicit (Townsend and Polatajko, 2007; Townsend and Wilcock, 2004). For example, Pollard et al. (2008) argued that occupational therapists have a role and a responsibility to enable the perspectives of their clients' experiences of exclusion and injustice to be heard and to work out meaningful solutions for these issues. In addition, occupational scientists have raised moral and political questions that are of relevance to occupational therapy and that support the development of occupationally just societies (Frank, 2012).

In this chapter, we use a broad and simple definition of 'occupational justice' as the right of all people to participate in occupations of their choosing. This is similar to Whiteford and Townsend's (2011) description of this concept as 'a vision of society in which all populations have the opportunities, resources, privilege and rights to participate to their potential in their desired occupations' (p. 66). Taking an occupationally just approach includes fostering awareness of injustices that arise for people individually and collectively, and for how professional practices, laws, policies, regulations, funding, attitudes and so on govern opportunities for occupational participation (Whiteford and Townsend, 2011). When occupational therapists consider the impacts of these issues on occupational participation, they may have increased understanding of the ways in which particular occupations become 'possible, ideal and ethical' for some people, and yet are marked by various authorities as 'not possible, nonideal and unethical' for others (Rudman, 2012, p. 110).

In this chapter, we propose that it is possible for occupational justice concepts to exert influence upon occupational therapists' practice through the use of discursive practices. To provide some context for readers, the chapter begins with a brief overview about why occupational justice concepts do not currently routinely inform occupational therapy practice. We then discuss human rights theory and philosophy, especially as they pertain to Australia. This Australian viewpoint is highlighted because we are Australian therapists and we formed our ideas from a study that was conducted in Australia. Next, we describe some challenges and opportunities in understanding and applying human rights and occupational justice in occupational therapy practice, drawing upon an action research study that was undertaken by the first author (Galvin, 2013). Finally, we will argue that when occupational therapists engage in local, contextualized dialogue about human rights and occupational justice, it is possible for them to generate solutions about how to make their practice more occupationally just.

BACKGROUND: THE UNREALIZED POTENTIAL OF OCCUPATIONAL JUSTICE

There are several factors that have created challenges to occupational therapists' use of occupational justice concepts in their practice. For example, misunderstanding and complexity in the theory of occupational justice can make the application of ideas difficult. The concept of occupational rights has arisen from the theory of occupational justice and the meanings of these two ideas are similar; for example, Hammell (2008) proposed that there ought to be one all-inclusive occupational right for 'all people to engage in meaningful occupations that contribute positively to their own well-being and the well-being of their communities' (p. 75). Concepts of justice are concerned with what people *have* (such as their materials and resources); however, Hammell and Iwama (2012, p. 386) argued that concepts of rights refer to whether there is an 'opportunity to act'. Because of this focus on action rather than having, Hammell and Iwama (2012) contended that occupational therapy ought to be aligned with occupational rights rather than occupational justice since occupational therapy is a profession that is concerned with people's opportunities to *do*. Although there is a distinction, we use occupational rights and occupational justice interchangeably.

This is because these concepts can describe both processes and outcomes depending upon how these expressions are used. That is, an approach of occupational justice is necessary to achieve one's occupational rights, and the claiming or experience of one's occupational rights is necessary for an experience of occupational justice.

Additionally, although there have been significant advances in theorizing about occupational justice, there are some gaps in understanding about how occupational justice is practised. Lack of action may stem from a lack of theoretical clarity about the emergent concepts of occupational justice and occupational rights (Durocher, Gibson, and Rappolt, 2013; Hammell, 2008). A further barrier to the practice of occupational justice may be that the dominant theories of occupational therapy have been largely shaped through the contributions of Western occupational therapists in developed nations, and therefore oppressive conditions such as poverty, discrimination and social exclusion have not traditionally been central concerns (Hammell and Iwama, 2012).

The occupational therapy profession appears to have been slow in addressing issues of occupational injustice due to alignment with the medical model (Durocher, Rappolt, and Gibson, 2013). Frank and Zemke (2008) contended that the alliance of occupational therapy with the medical profession during the founding of occupational therapy has narrowed the focus of occupational therapy to the client's presenting clinical diagnosis, rather than to other issues such as those of the prevention of illness or addressing problematic social concerns (such as poverty, lack of employment and inclusivity). Furthermore, with the exception of research in community development, there is a limited amount of research to help occupational therapists understand how to *do* occupational justice, particularly in medical practice contexts (Galvin et al., 2011).

Long-standing patterns of hegemony may also pose a challenge to occupational therapists in addressing issues of occupational injustice in their practice (Kronenberg et al., 2011; Wilding, 2011). Hegemony refers to the ways in which a dominant group exerts control over others through systematically fostering ideologies that promote their own interests and in turn, people who are subordinate come to accept these ideas without question (Gesler, 1992). For example, during an action research in the UK, Atwal and Caldwell (2003) found that in response to fiscal pressures, occupational therapists tended to engage in thinking about the organization's needs rather than the needs and rights of the people with whom they were working. In South Africa, Dayal (2010) found that national health service policy reforms towards a rights-based framework were in conflict with the institutional imperatives of a metropolitan rehabilitation service. Therefore it was difficult to shift practitioners away from individualized biomedical approaches (Dayal, 2010). The issue of hegemony, by its very nature, is an entrenched problem, especially because others (such as employers) have a vested interest in maintaining the status quo. Indeed, this hegemony is terrifyingly successful precisely because of the way in which health services are governed and structured at their very cores.

HUMAN RIGHTS: THEORY AND PHILOSOPHY

Although human rights ideas have been recorded in earlier ages, as understood in contemporary society they originated from Enlightenment era (1695–1800) perspectives about *natural rights* (Griffin, 2008). According to a viewpoint that considers natural law and natural rights, human beings have inherent rights because they are creatures with a particular capability to reason (Winston, 1989). Thus in this view, all people are born free and equal, and therefore all people naturally acquire human rights.

During the course of the Enlightenment, the protection of rights came to be understood as the responsibility of government (Griffin, 2008). Nations listed 'human rights' in key declarations or bills of rights as an expression of their political and moral values and their governing principles (Griffin, 2008). Over time, however, views about the role of the state in governing natural rights became politicized. For example, feminist philosopher Mary Wollstonecraft (1759–1797) and revolutionary Karl Marx (1813–1883) argued that listings of rights contained exclusions based upon issues of economics, gender and cultural distinctions (Winston, 1989). Thus injustice is created when all people do not have their claims to fundamental human

rights upheld because they are not recognized as deserving citizens by the governing organization.

Human rights were advanced in response to the Holocaust and other atrocities of the Second World War. Arising from a desire to set a moral standard that all peoples and nations should strive to respect and observe, in 1948, the newly formed United Nations agreed upon the Universal Declaration of Human Rights (UDHR) (Griffin, 2008). The UDHR is a set of entitlements that are universal and that belong equally to all people as a condition of being human (United Nations, 1948). Therefore everyone is entitled to human rights without distinction; there ought to be no discrimination, whether according to place, culture, gender, religion, or so forth (Winston, 1989). It is this statement of human rights that remains most well-known in contemporary society.

Wilcock (2006) described the UDHR as inherently occupational due to its emphasis on human rights related to participation in occupations such as work, cultural life, leisure, education and so on. Although similar, human rights and occupational rights are distinct ideas. Statements of human rights are universally accepted as the kinds of rights that ought to apply to all humans. In contrast, there has been no such dialogue and debate about occupational rights; a dialogue about occupational rights would present occupational therapists with the opportunity to promote occupational rights as vitally important for achieving health and well-being and, therefore, along with human rights, as valuable human entitlements.

The UDHR was the first international conceptualization of human rights in a way that accommodated different political, cultural and economic beliefs and systems (Winston, 1989). However, it has been criticized for its creation in a forum that was dominated by Western political leadership and the championing of individual rights while devaluing collective understandings of human rights, which are more prominent in other cultural, religious and philosophical traditions (Ife, 2012). A philosopher of the Dinka people in Sudan, Francis Deng (2009) argued that dominant Western conceptualizations of human rights provide a powerful starting point for dialogue about human rights, but that every culture has humanitarian ideals or principles to which it can add and contribute to the redefinition of universal standards of human rights.

Therefore, although the UDHR is an important reference point for enacting human rights globally, the importance of local cultures and local circumstances is also highly relevant. Thus, it would appear that for occupational therapists to enact human rights and occupational justice, they ought to realize that these concepts and practices are necessarily both global and local in nature.

THE AUSTRALIAN HUMAN RIGHTS CONTEXT: CHALLENGES AND OPPORTUNITIES

Australia is a signatory to the UDHR and to legally enforceable United Nations treaties enacted in 1966: the International Covenant on Civil and Political Rights and the International Covenant on Economic, Social and Cultural Rights (United Nations, 1966a, 1966b). Australia has also agreed to uphold and respect additional conventions enacted through the United Nations to protect the rights of minority groups, such as the Convention on the Rights of Persons with Disabilities (United Nations, 2006).

Even though Australia has a strong record of ratification of United Nations covenants and treaties, it does not have a dedicated national system of human rights protections. Unlike other nations across the European Union, and in South Africa, Canada and New Zealand, Australia is the only liberal democracy that does not provide constitutional guarantee for human rights (Grover, 2009). This situation limits citizen access to remedies for human rights breaches (Australian Human Rights Commission, 2010).

When Australia first became a federated nation in 1901, human rights protections were not embedded in the constitution (Chappell et al., 2009). The Australian parliamentary founders believed that the legislature and a strong parliament were sufficient protectors of freedoms. Furthermore, they were concerned that a constitution that was dense with limitations would restrict the ability of government to effectively respond to the changing needs and desires of Australian citizens (Chappell et al., 2009).

There is a lack of a well-developed human rights culture in Australia; in the country's first Universal Periodic Review at the United Nations Human Rights Council in 2011, member states highlighted their concerns for particular vulnerable groups, including the marked disadvantage experienced by First Australians, issues of gender equality and domestic violence against women, and the ongoing use of mandatory immigration detention and transfer of asylum seekers to third countries (Australian Human Rights Commission, 2012). The National Human Rights Consultation Committee (2009) found that citizens know little about the constitution of human rights, including what they are, where they come from, and how they ought to be protected. The committee's report also highlighted that there was significant support among Australian community organizations and citizens for the introduction of a national Human Rights Act (National Human Rights Consultation Committee, 2009); however, the Australian Government declined to create such an act.

Rather than embracing liberalism and its associated constitutional protections for human rights, an Australian polity has tended to be governed by a utilitarian mentality and this has sometimes led to Australian governments ignoring the human rights of minorities in order to achieve objectives considered to be good for the majority (Byrnes et al., 2008). According to utilitarian ethical theory, founded by Jeremy Bentham, the sum total of individual *utility* or happiness must be considered when deciding what should be done (Sen, 2009). A direct interpretation of utilitarianism (such as that espoused by Bentham) is in conflict with ideas of human rights (and occupational justice) because although the needs of the majority are met, the rights of some individuals may be overlooked. In contrast, a human rights perspective is that all people have rights that ought to be met; no one ought to be obliged to relinquish his or her rights (Sen, 2009).

Australian political culture is strongly imbued with egalitarian notions of social justice (Chappell et al., 2009). Thus, Australian citizens consider that legislative and democratic electoral processes will naturally work to uphold human rights in accordance with cultural values of equality and the ethics of a 'fair go' (Victorian Equal Opportunity and Human Rights Commission, 2011). A fair go reflects a widely shared and contemporary Australian view that all people are equal in worth and ought to be afforded an equal chance, despite their differing life circumstances (Burnside, 2007).

Despite the limitations that have been described, Australia has made progress in enhancing protections of human rights. The Australian Government adopted Australia's Human Rights Framework, which outlines a commitment to education and enhanced legislative review, and consolidates federal antidiscrimination laws into a single act (Australian Government, 2010). Some Australian states and territories have also strengthened their human rights protections. For example, the Victorian Charter of Human Rights and Responsibilities Act 2006 (Victorian Charter) enacts into law some civil and political rights drawn from the International Covenant on Civil and Political Rights (Byrnes et al., 2008). The Victorian Charter makes a human rights framework for governance explicit: all public authorities and professionals in the state of Victoria are legally responsible for upholding the human rights in the charter (Victorian Equal Opportunity and Human Rights Commission, 2012). Consequently, it would appear that occupational therapists working in Victoria, Australia, have a legal and ethical imperative to uphold human rights in their practice.

CONSIDERING HUMAN RIGHTS IN OCCUPATIONAL THERAPY PRACTICE

One area in which occupational therapists in Australia are confronted by occupational justice issues is when managing their waiting lists and prioritizing who should receive services, in a context of scarcity. This challenge arose for a group of occupational therapists who were part of an action research study that explored the therapists' understanding and practice of occupational justice at a metropolitan hospital in Melbourne, Australia (Galvin, 2013). In Galvin's (2013) study, nine occupational therapists participated in monthly focus groups and in three rounds of individual interviews over the course of 10 months. Data were collected by audio-recording the group discussions and interviews and transcribing them verbatim. The transcripts were inductively analysed using coding, categorization and theme building.

Utilizing action research, Galvin (2013) assisted the occupational therapists to participate in discussions about human rights. In the monthly meetings, the therapists engaged in the steps of reflecting, planning, acting and evaluating. Initially, the therapists reflected

upon the themes of occupation, enablement, enabling occupation and occupational rights. They shared stories of their practice with each other and considered questions such as, 'What are the rights issues in this story? What duties go with those rights? Who is responsible for meeting these rights?'

The therapists were assisted in learning more about occupationally just practice by reading chapters from *Enabling Occupation II: Advancing an Occupational Therapy Vision for Health, Well-Being and Justice Through Occupation* (Townsend and Polatajko, 2007) and a range of international occupational science and occupational therapy publications (e.g., Mji, 2008; Van Niekerk, 2008; Wilcock, 2001; World Federation of Occupational Therapists, 2006). Next, they engaged more explicitly in planning for change by considering questions such as, 'What kinds of rights issues evoke my interest, and how will I make a difference? What supports will help me?'

The therapists put their plans into action and afterwards reflected on the questions, 'What worked well and what could I have done differently? What do I plan to do next?' Thus the action research approach enabled the occupational therapists to develop their understanding of human rights and occupational justice and work towards developing a practice that was more occupationally just.

Occupational Justice and Priority Setting

The therapists in Galvin's (2013) study did not have sufficient resources to meet all of the needs of their clients; therefore, they had to make judgements about who should be prioritized to receive a service. For example, older people who were admitted from residential care were generally not given priority for occupational therapy unless their discharge was in jeopardy or they had significant need for rehabilitation. A service was not offered even though in many instances these clients would have likely benefitted from occupational therapy. Not offering services to this particular group of people is contrary to ideas about occupational justice. In an occupationally just society, all people have the opportunity to develop their capabilities through engagement in occupation (Wilcock, 2006). However, the therapists had to make difficult ethical choices because they did not have the ability to provide a service to all possible recipients.

The therapists used utilitarian decision making to solve their ethical dilemma. When using a utilitarian framework, a person considers the consequences of action on others and aims to bring about the best outcome for the majority of people (Ife, 2012). One of the participating occupational therapists, Harry (a pseudonym), allocated his time and resources according to utilitarian principles:

If I spent a lot of time trying to get someone who is at high level care to be able to transfer easier and spend two to three hours doing that, that means that two to three other people that also need intervention don't get it. So it is deciding which one you are going to provide that intervention to. And then in terms of human rights, well how do you weigh that up, of almost who has got more of a right between being able to transfer versus being able to go home. (Galvin, 2013, p. 153)

When a solely utilitarian framework for decision making is used, the needs of individuals may be overlooked. For example, Nussbaum (2001) argues that when a person considers utilitarianism, one 'tends to think of the social total, or average, as an aggregate, neglecting the salience of the boundaries between individual lives' (pp. 218–219). Indeed, not only might opportunities for enabling occupational justice with some individuals be missed, occupational injustice may be created for others, if in providing a service to more people an ineffective or poor quality of occupational therapy results. In Galvin's (2013) study, the therapists' judgements of what was fair may have contributed to create injustice, even as they strove to achieve occupational justice for all.

Using Discursive Processes to Cultivate a Rights Culture

Galvin (2013) found that when the occupational therapists participated in discussion about human rights and occupational justice they were better able to solve moral dilemmas about how to spend limited resources and also to promote a just and inclusive approach to providing occupational therapy. Thus, learning about human rights provided the therapists with an additional way of making of practice decisions. When a human rights perspective is considered, the human

rights of all people, as well as the breadth of a person's human rights, are taken into account (Ife, 2012); that is, the therapists thought about their responsibility to work not only for the right to health, but also for rights to housing, employment, and so on. The therapists' thinking was enriched through the use of different ethical theories, which is consistent with Chappell et al.'s (2009) view that Australian citizens would benefit from finding a way of understanding the concepts of utility and rights as complementary to, rather than rivalling, one another.

By engaging in discursive processes, the therapists in Galvin's (2013) study found ways to make their practice more inclusive of a range of clients. For example, prior to her participation in the study, Sophie (a pseudonym) had tended to limit the scope of her practice to that of undertaking initial assessments and helping her clients in using the toilet, bathing or dressing independently. However, the dialogue and debate with her colleagues enabled Sophie to see the ways that she had potentially contributed to occupational injustice through her system of prioritizing clients:

I've thought a lot about human rights and occupational justice when I think about developing nations and Indigenous communities, but I've never brought it back to us in comfortable Melbourne society. I'd never really sat back and thought about what are the injustices and the human rights issues about my aged care population? It's been quite evident there are quite a lot, especially with who I see on the ward, like the ones from low-level care who are much less a priority than the ones from home alone; and naturally I enforce that sort of injustice. (Galvin, 2013, p. 176)

After she reflected on and discussed issues of occupational justice and injustice with her colleagues, Sophie began to recognize her clients' needs for engagement in social and leisure occupations; Sophie sought opportunities to assist her clients to participate in this broader range of meaningful occupations. This recognition of individual difference and diversity is an important aspect of practising in an occupationally just way.

A discursive approach can assist occupational therapists to understand clients' perspectives and experiences about rights and justice issues. This is because discursive processes encourage talking about what it might mean to be human, rather than directly focusing on statements of rights per se (Ife, 2012). An understanding of human rights is achieved through using an inductive approach that is grounded in practitioners' discussions of stories from practice with real people. In addition to Ife (2012), several scholars have argued that taking a discursive approach may develop and deepen understanding of human rights and justice issues. Osler and Zhu (2011) recommended that telling the 'untold stories' of marginalized individuals or groups may deepen practitioners' learning about the various forms of oppression and injustice in society and help to 'fill the blind spots' in dominant discourses. Similarly, the philosopher Upendra Baxi (2009) considered that traditional forms of human rights discourse tend to tell large global stories or metanarratives, and therefore they become disconnected from local people and communities who are struggling. Therefore Baxi (2009, p. 184) argues that the task for discourse about human rights is that of 'humanising human rights' by sharing stories about concrete ways in which people have experienced oppression or human suffering.

Opportunities for dialogue and shared learning enabled the therapists in Galvin's (2013) study to better understand local issues of human suffering and injustice. Joshua (a pseudonym) considered that thinking and talking about occupational justice with his peers enhanced his leadership in a collaborative project that he was undertaking with occupational therapy students; the project was about exploring employment opportunities for people with mental illness:

That particular project I didn't have very much time to dedicate to, but whenever I came to the study it would re-invigorate my ideas about occupational justice, and so therefore it would help me refine some of the questions I was already thinking about the project. Therefore, I think I was probably a better supervisor to the students and was able to advocate more strongly for that ... So keeping it [occupational justice] in my mind is one [change] and because I can keep it in my mind, I can act on any opportunities that I see through that lens, whereas it might not have been as alive to

me if I hadn't participated in the study. (Galvin, 2013, p. 175)

The group discussions enabled the therapists to better see the issues of power and inequity that shaped people's everyday occupations and lives. Freire (2000) proposed that acting and reflecting together allow people to develop a growing consciousness or insight into an oppressive situation, and to learn about their capacities to transform those unfair power arrangements in society.

CONCLUSION: ADVANCING OCCUPATIONAL JUSTICE

It may be argued that occupational therapists have a responsibility to enable the right of all people to participate in meaningful occupations that contribute to their health and well-being. However, a reality of everyday occupational therapy practice is that it may not always be possible to achieve clients' needs and rights due to a range of contextual issues, including competing claims on occupational therapists' time and resources. When making these difficult decisions about who to prioritize, therapists need to be able to justify that their choices are based on sound reasoning (Barnitt et al., 1998).

We propose that occupational therapists' ethical decision making may be enhanced when they join with their colleagues in dialogue about human rights and occupational justice. Discussions about occupational justice can assist in bringing to light issues affecting marginalized and neglected individuals and groups. These conversations can also help in generating insights about the relevant actions that therapists could take to enable human rights and occupational justice in practice.

The public nature of the discussions is important. Sen (2009) argues that some rights are not recognized and therefore are better promoted through public discussions. When a claim to a human right is debated openly and endures arguments from well-informed critics, it can be presumed as relevant within that particular culture or context (Sen, 2009). Therefore, it would appear to be important for occupational therapists to engage in dialogue about occupational rights, and what it might mean to incorporate occupational rights into their everyday practice. We propose that a discursive approach is a way of building collective understandings of shared values about occupational rights, thereby assisting occupational therapists to see ways of challenging dominant ideas and practice hegemonies.

Although we have emphasized human rights and occupational justice in an Australian context, we propose that the use of a discursive approach to developing a culture of occupational justice amongst occupational therapists is also relevant elsewhere. Taking a discursive approach enables people's understandings and practices of rights and justice to be shaped by their culture and particular context. For the profession of occupational therapy to advance an agenda of promoting occupational justice, we recommend that all occupational therapists, worldwide, engage in discussion and debate about what occupational justice is and how they have enacted it within local and global contexts.

REFERENCES

Atwal, A., Caldwell, K., 2003. Ethics, occupational therapy and discharge planning: four broken principles. Aust. Occup. Ther. J. 50, 244–251.

Australian Government, 2010. Australian Human Rights Framework. Commonwealth of Australia, Canberra, Australia. <http://www.ag.gov.au/Consultations/Documents/Publicsubmissionsonthedraftbaselinestudy/AustraliasHumanRightsFramework.pdf> (accessed 17.04.16.).

Australian Human Rights Commission, 2010. Taking stock of Australia's human rights record. Australian Human Right Commission, Sydney, Australia. <http://www.humanrights.gov.au/sites/default/files/content/upr/AHRC_UPR_guide.pdf> (accessed 17.04.16.).

Australian Human Rights Commission, 2012. Australia's Universal Periodic Review: progress report prepared by the Australian Human Rights Commission on behalf of the Australian Council of Human Rights Agencies 2012. Australian Human Rights Commission, Sydney, Australia. <http://www.humanrights.gov.au/sites/default/files/document/publication/ACHRA_UPR_Progress_Report_2012.pdf> (accessed 17.04.16.).

Barnitt, R., Warbey, J., Rawlins, S., 1998. Two case discussions of ethics: editing the truth and the right to resources. Br. J. Occup. Ther. 61 (2), 52–56.

Baxi, U., 2009. Voices of suffering and the future of human rights. In: Twining, W. (Ed.), Human Rights, Southern Voices. Cambridge University Press, Cambridge, pp. 162–204. (Original work published 1998.)

Burnside, J., 2007. Australian values. Austr. Q. 79 (3), 15–20.

Byrnes, A., Charlesworth, H., McKinnon, G., 2008. Bills of Rights in Australia: History, Politics and Law. University of NSW Press, Sydney, Australia.

Chappell, L., Chesterman, J., Hill, L., 2009. The Politics of Human Rights in Australia. Cambridge University Press, Melbourne, Australia.

Dayal, H., 2010. Provision of rehabilitation services within the District Health System: the experiences of rehabilitation managers in facilitating this right for people with disabilities. South Afr. J. Occup. Ther. 40 (1), 22–26. Available at:: <http://www.sajot.co.za/index.php/sajot>.

Deng, F., 2009. A cultural approach to human rights among the Dinka. In: Twining, W. (Ed.), Human Rights, Southern Voices. Cambridge University Press, Cambridge, UK, pp. 44–52. (Original work published 1998.)

Durocher, E., et al., 2013. Occupational justice: a conceptual review. J. Occup. Sci. 21 (4), 418–430. doi:10.1080/14427591.2013.775692.

Durocher, E., Rappolt, S., Gibson, B., 2013. Occupational justice: future directions. J. Occup. Sci. 21 (4), 431–442. doi:10.1080/14427591.2013.775693.

Frank, G., 2012. The 2010 Ruth Zemke Lecture in Occupational Science – Occupational therapy/ occupational science/ occupational justice: moral commitments and global assemblages. J. Occup. Sci. 19 (1), 25–35. doi:10.1080/14427591.2011.607792.

Frank, G., Zemke, R., 2008. Occupational therapy foundations for political engagement and social transformation. In: Pollard, N., et al. (Eds.), A Political Practice of Occupational Therapy. Elsevier, Edinburgh, UK, pp. 111–136.

Freire, P., 2000. Pedagogy of the Oppressed: 30th Anniversary Edition, 30th Anniversary ed. Continuum, New York. (Original work published 1970.)

Galvin, D., 2013. Exploring practice and taking action to enable human rights and occupational justice in an Australian hospital context: an action research study. Unpublished doctoral thesis, Charles Sturt University, Albury, Australia.

Galvin, D., Wilding, C., Whiteford, G., 2011. Utopian visions/dystopian realities: exploring practice and taking action to enable human rights and occupational justice in a hospital context. Aust. Occup. Ther. J. 58, 378–385. doi:10.1111/j.1440-1630.2011.00967.x.

Gesler, W., 1992. Therapeutic landscapes: medical issues in light of the new cultural geography. Soc. Sci. Med. 34 (7), 735–746.

Griffin, J., 2008. On Human Rights. Oxford University Press, Oxford.

Grover, A., 2009. United Nations Special Rapporteur on the right of everyone to the enjoyment of the highest attainable standard of physical and mental health: preliminary observations and recommendations. 4 December 2009, Canberra, Australia. <http://www.hr-dp.org/files/2013/09/22/UN_Statement_-_Intervention_-_4Dec09.pdf> (accessed 17.04.16.).

Hammell, K.W., 2008. Reflections on … well-being and occupational rights. Can. J. Occup. Ther. 75 (1), 61–64. doi:10.2182/cjot.07.007.

Hammell, K.W., Iwama, M., 2012. Well-being and occupational rights: an imperative for critical occupational therapy. Scand. J. Occup. Ther. 19, 385–394. doi:10.3109/11038128.2011.611821.

Ife, J., 2012. Human Rights and Social Work: Towards Rights-Based Practice, third ed. Cambridge University Press, Cambridge.

Kronenberg, F., Pollard, N., Ramugondo, E., 2011. Introduction: courage to dance politics. In: Kronenberg, F., et al. (Eds.), Occupational Therapies without Borders: Towards an Ecology of Occupation-Based Practices, vol. 2. Churchill Livingstone Elsevier, Edinburgh, UK, pp. 1–16.

Mji, G., 2008. The use of the confessional tale as a tool to enter the critical tale and become an advocate for those at the margins – a researcher's journey and reflection. South Afr. J. Occup. Ther. 38 (1), 3–8.

National Human Rights Consultation Committee, 2009. Human Rights Consultation Committee Report. Commonwealth of Australia, Canberra, Australia. <https://www.humanrights.gov.au/sites/default/files/content/legal/submissions/2009/200906_NHRC_complete.pdf> (accessed 17.04.16.).

Nussbaum, M., 2001. Capabilities and human rights. In: Hayden, P. (Ed.), The Philosophy of Human Rights. Paragon House, St. Paul, MN, pp. 212–235.

Osler, A., Zhu, J., 2011. Narratives in teaching and research for justice and human rights. Educ. Citizsh. Soc. Justice 6, 223–235. doi:10.1177/1746197911417414.

Pollard, N., Kronenberg, F., Sakellariou, D., 2008. A political practice of occupational therapy. In: Pollard, N., et al. (Eds.), A Political Practice of Occupational Therapy. Elsevier, Edinburgh, UK, pp. 3–19.

Rudman, D.L., 2012. Governing through occupation: shaping expectations and possibilities. In: Whiteford, G., Hocking, C. (Eds.), Occupational Science: Society, Inclusion, Participation. Blackwell Publishing, Oxford, pp. 100–116.

Sen, A., 2009. The Idea of Justice. Allen Lane, London.

Townsend, E., Polatajko, H. (Eds.), 2007. Enabling Occupation II: Advancing an Occupational Therapy Vision for Health, Well-Being and Justice through Occupation. Canadian Association of Occupational Therapists, Ottawa.

Townsend, E., Wilcock, A., 2004. Occupational justice and client-centred practice: a dialogue in progress. Can. J. Occup. Ther. 71 (2), 75–87.

United Nations, 1948. Universal Declaration of Human Rights. <http://www.ohchr.org/EN/UDHR/Documents/UDHR_Translations/eng.pdf> (accessed 17.04.16.).

United Nations, 1966a. International Covenant on Civil and Political Rights. <http://www.ohchr.org/en/professionalinterest/pages/ccpr.aspx> (accessed 17.04.16.).

United Nations, 1966b. International Covenant on Economic, Social and Cultural Rights. United Nations. <http://www.ohchr.org/Documents/ProfessionalInterest/cescr.pdf> (accessed 17.04.16.).

United Nations, 2006. Convention on the Rights of Persons with Disabilities. United Nations. <http://www.un.org/esa/socdev/enable/rights/convtexte.htm> (accessed 17.04.16.).

Van Niekerk, L., 2008. Participation in work: a human rights issue for people with psychiatric disabilities. South Afr. J. Occup. Ther. 38 (1), 9–15. Available at:: <http://www.sajot.co.za/index.php/sajot>.

Victorian Equal Opportunity and Human Rights Commission, 2011. Talking rights: consulting with Victorians about economic, social and cultural rights and the Charter. State of Victoria, Melbourne, Australia. <http://www.humanrightscommission.vic.gov.au/index.php/our-resources-and-publications/charter-reports/item/158-talking-rights-consulting-with-victorians-about-economic-social-and-cultural-rights-and-the-charter-mar-2011>.

Victorian Equal Opportunity and Human Rights Commission, 2012. Rights in focus: 2011 report on the operation of the Charter of Human Rights and Responsibilities. State of Victoria, Melbourne, Australia. <http://www.humanrightscommission.vic.gov.au/index.php/our-resources-and-publications/charter-reports/item/152-rights-in-focus-2011-report-on-the-operation-of-the-charter-of-human-rights-and-responsibilities-jun-2012>.

Whiteford, G., Townsend, E., 2011. Participatory Occupational Justice Framework 2010: enabling occupational participation and inclusion. In: Kronenberg, F., et al. (Eds.), Occupational Therapies without Borders: Towards an Ecology of Occupation-Based Practices, vol. 2. Churchill Livingstone Elsevier, Edinburgh, UK, pp. 65–84.

Whiteford, G., Townsend, E., Hocking, C., 2000. Reflections on a renaissance of occupation. Can. J. Occup. Ther. 67 (1), 61–69.

Wilcock, A., 2001. Occupational utopias: back to the future. J. Occup. Sci. 1 (1), 5–12.

Wilcock, A., 2006. An Occupational Perspective of Health, second ed. SLACK Incorporated, Thorofare, NJ.

Wilding, C., 2011. Raising awareness of hegemony in occupational therapy: the value of action research for improving practice. Aust. Occup. Ther. J. 58 (4), 293–299. doi:10.1111/j.1440-1630.2010.00910.x.

Winston, M., 1989. Introduction: understanding human rights. In: Winston, M. (Ed.), The Philosophy of Human Rights. Wadsorth Publishing Company, Belmont, CA.

World Federation of Occupational Therapists, 2006. Position Statement on Human Rights. World Federation of Occupational Therapists. <http://www.wfot.org/ResourceCentre.aspx> (accessed 17.04.16.).

20 OCCUPATIONAL THERAPY IN A GLOCALIZED[1] WORLD

SOLANGEL GARCIA-RUIZ

'Describe your village, and you will describe the world'.
Leo Tolstoy, cited in Treat Whittier (1988, p. 6)

CHAPTER OUTLINE

My purpose in this chapter is to share my experiences and reflections on my practice of occupational therapy. I will do this by addressing my different identities as a woman, as a Colombian and Latin American, and as a professional. I have worked as a manager of public policy (in the area of disability), as an advisor for public health policies, leading the Community-Based Rehabilitation programme in Bogotá (Colombia), and as a consultant for Community-Based Rehabilitation in Latin America, as well as a researcher and manager of the Health Research Department in Bogotá.

For a long time, I thought that what I was doing was not exactly occupational therapy. What I knew about occupational therapy was related to direct patient care. I was not working directly with patients, but instead with people and organizations aspiring to participate in the construction of a city, of a better common life. After sharing my points of view with colleagues across Latin America – from Colombia, Chile, Costa Rica, Argentina and Peru – I came to understand that what I am currently doing is thinking about the duty of an occupational therapist that is less to do with academia and traditional, or clinical, intervention models, and very close to the political practice and policy in a specific urban context.

In this path, I have identified issues related to history, geography, populations, ecology and the environment, and I have begun to explore some of the intersections between these matters and occupational therapy. A different colour and shade of occupational therapy has emerged, as well as the nuances of the place where I live, the South. A South in the process of

---

[1]Thinking globally, acting locally.

progressive construction of social responses to the real needs of individuals and groups, responses to disasters and conflicts, or simply, responses to help the day-to-day local affairs of life, in the context of a global world. All this has led me to recognize myself as a political subject and to act in politics and research. It is in the midst of this trajectory where my occupational therapy emerges; mine is an occupational therapy that happens outside of clinics and hospitals and close to where people live. I am a policymaker. This is the journey I want to discuss in this chapter.

THE WORLD OF TODAY AND THE WORLD OF TOMORROW

What is the world of today like? What are its features? What kind of world do we currently inhabit? What kind of world are we building for tomorrow? I usually see the world from the windows of my apartment: a world full of trees, birds singing at dawn, kids and dogs playing during the day. I also observe the world from the window of my office: the eastern hills of Bogotá with picturesque Monserrate mountain in the background, the dirty neighbourhood full of factories, the pollution of the city, TransMilenio buses and some white clouds shaping figures on the blue sky. I close my eyes to activate the windows of my soul and spirit, and I give a glance to my emotions, dreams and beliefs.

We are in the twenty-first century, walking in the postmodern era, trying to overcome modernity where technology plays the central role, where life (human, animal, natural) is often in conflict with a focus on money and where the economy seems to have assumed centre stage. I talk about modernity as a historical process originating in Europe, where formal and expert knowledge prevails, where everyday life is governed by the institutional and the regulated, where professions such as occupational therapy are normalized, supported by laws and standards defined in some places in the world and exerted in other places. Meanwhile, postmodernism is a form of rebellion to this situation. Lyotard says that postmodernism is a form of emancipation of reason; it is the liberation from the discourses which homogenize and eliminate diversity and plurality (Lyotard cited in Vásquez Roca, 2011).

We live in times of focusing to overcome poverty of the most while the wealth of the few is growing stronger. Libertad (a character from the Argentinean comic strip *Mafalda*), said it very well (Quino, 2004a):

For me, what is wrong is that a few have much, many have little, and some have nothing
If those few who have nothing had something of the little that the many that have little had
And, if the many who have a little had a bit of the much that the few who have much had,
there would be less trouble
But nobody does anything to improve something as simple.

While all this happens, in some parts of the world, in Colombia, for instance, conflicts are a part of everyday life; global warming results in seasons of endless rain and lands of infernal heat, while earthquakes happen worldwide. We have recently experienced earthquakes (Chile, 2010), floods (Bogotá, 2011) and droughts. These issues can have a major impact on the lives of people.

Meanwhile, during the economic crisis that began in 2008 and was still affecting many countries at the time this book went to press, people in Latin America were not sure of the motivations of some European governments in reaching out to the South: did they want to come to fund projects for our development, or to access financial resources for themselves? International aid asks for many requirements for uncertain small rewards. Asia, in turn, has, in China and Japan, some of the world's biggest economic powers; therefore its influence is beginning to affect political and social decisions. Africa is considered to be a continent blighted by poverty, where there are proposals for social developments. Meanwhile, Latin America lives in the third wave of democracy and the Washington Consensus (Martínez Rangel and Soto Reyes Garmendia, 2012). That is, the state adapted to market requirements, which was characterized by elections, economic openness and changes in the state structure (Gómez Buendía et al., 2010).

In this context, conditions emerge that may generate inequities and injustices, occasioned by conditions such as migration, displacement, disability and gender. Also, many new locations emerge, where individuals are in search of their own dreams and well-being, while facing challenges caused by the environmental crisis, as proposed by Simó Algado (2012). In the late 1990s, I started working, whilst with the Health Department of Bogotá, on the policy of inclusion of people with disabilities in the city. This work consisted of the analysis of the situation of the population in the city in order to formulate policy, in partnership with disabled people, universities and local government. One of our aims was to understand the context of social policies, and in particular how the disability policy arose as part of the targeting process in the context of the Washington Consensus of economic reforms then being applied to Colombia.

RECOVERING HISTORY

'How have we become what we are today, and what forms have allowed us to think in this way or in a different way?' (Melgarejo and del Pilar, 2000, p. 35). Occupational therapy was born in a specific context and place, and it has since transformed itself, in different ways, according to needs and places. It is influenced by the history of each country, each city and place. For example, for Colombians, our history is a mix of situations involving armed conflict, political, economic, and financial international interests, and colonial interests, among others. Our history includes migration, disability, the story of our lives and of the lives of our families, the story of each of the people and places.

It is important to understand history beyond the mere account of events; we need to explore the meanings associated with each event, and how all these together make up history. Through research on the historical analysis of the political category of disability in Colombia, we understood how power relations are alive in Colombian history. Colombia is a country with a history of a centrist State that changed after the 1991 Constitution. Citizens are just beginning to identify themselves as political subjects (Cruz-Velandia et al., 2015).

The first historical features of Latin America are concerned with the story inherited from the Mayans, the Incas and the Aztecs. The Mayans, who inhabited what is now Mexico and Central America, left us a legacy which is still visible in architecture, mathematics and astronomy. The Aztecs left us their military organization and the construction of ceremonial cities, while the Incas, from the Andes, left us major

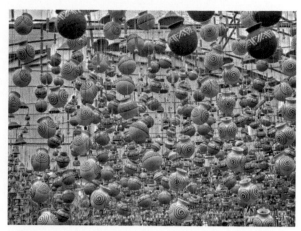

FIGURE 20-1 ■ Reproductions of Muiscas artefacts. *(Solangel Garcia-Ruiz.)*

engineering, agriculture and weaving works. From the Muiscas, who lived in the region where I grew up, Facatativá (Cundinamarca), which was immortalized in the legend of El Dorado, the greatest legacy is the military–political organization, the worship of the sun and the moon. The Muiscas still tell us their histories and traditions through thousands of objects made of gold (Figure 20-1).

Traces of colonialism are still visible in Latin America, especially the legacies of the Spanish and Portuguese, and to a lesser extent of the Dutch, French and English, who in the past had territorial and economic control of the continent. Although the independence wars put an end to this outside control, we still preserve forms and attitudes from this historical period; we are faced with the effects of postcolonialism (Gareis, 2005). The past is also an *other,* and in the case of South America, the colonial past has a special condition of otherness, although in recent years the de-colonial process has increasingly been incorporated and developed (Gareis, 2005).

The traces of colonialism can be clearly seen in a conversation between Mafalda and Libertad in Quino's comic strip. As Libertad is putting a world map upside down on the wall, she comments:

Upside down of what? The Earth is in space, and space does not have up or down. The fact that the Northern hemisphere is on the top is a psychological trick invented by those who believe they are on the top, so that we, who think we are down, will keep thinking we are down. The problem is that if we keep on thinking that we are down, we will remain staying down. But from now on…it's over!

(Quino, 2004b)

There are many stories that make history, rather than a single story; thus in the field as an occupational therapist, understanding social relationships, cultural policies, environment and places means to understand that making decisions is a political act that makes part of the history. We began to study, in 2014, occupational therapy histories in Colombia to mark the anniversary of 50 years of practice in the country. The purpose of this research was to understand, from a historical perspective, the occupational therapy discourses and practices in the country. See Box 20-1.

AWARENESS OF GEOGRAPHY

Geography is more than rivers and mountains; it is about being aware of the geography of thoughts, of positions, interests, powers, and relationships. Geography also has to do with 'the territorial practices of social movements, territorial conflicts associated with political ecology, as well as the counter-hegemonic alternatives of land use that incorporate novel forms of representation of the territory and rights claims through critical social cartography and participatory

geographical information systems' (Barrera Lopbaton, 2009, p. 9).

This means that talking about the territory (e.g.. discussions about water in the Amazon, or oil on the Plains, both in Colombia) cannot be done without talking about the power over land and power relations that are built around it. This means recognizing the social spaces and relations of power in spaces: in the perceived space (material), in the conceived space (mental) and in the lived space (experiences) (Barrera Lopbaton, 2009). Institutional geography is not the only version; it is just one of them. There are other geographies, like the social and political geographies, which have to do with everyday existence and with the geographies that each one of us, individually and collectively, is building. See Box 20-2.

Following Michel de Certeau et al. (1999), the geographies of places are built and histories are made in the places of everyday life such as the neighbourhood or the kitchen. Those places are inhabited by people. They nurture people as they weave stories holding olfactory memories like the smell of the neighbourhood bakery when we were kids or like the smell of marijuana when we attended the university campus.

KEEPING GENERATIONS IN MIND

Usually policies, programmes and services in the field of health and social services are organized around phenomena such as pathologies. For instance, people often talk about programmes for people with spinal cord injury, chronic illness or autism. An alternative way to address this issue is by considering the stages of the life cycle or life course, understood as the passage

---

BOX 20-1

In 2014, Rosario University and the Health Secretariat concluded a study entitled 'Historical Analysis of the Political Construction of the Disability Category in Colombia (1985–2012)'. We identified international, national and local scenarios and three time periods: (a) 1986 to 1990, about biomedical hegemony, dependence and the lack of political subjects; (b) 1991 to 2001, on the crisis of the institutions working on disability, and the genesis of the Colombian political subjects; and (c) 2002 to 2012, paradigmatic rupture of the concept of disability with the emergence of new political subjects and development of territorial social action. This historical study allowed us to understand the development of a disability policy coming from the economic and social development at a national and international historical context (Cruz et al., 2015).

BOX 20-2

Mauricio Fuentes Vallejo (2010), in his master's research in public health, invited some people with different disabilities living in the Fontibón area of Bogota to produce maps of their most frequented places. Persons with disabilities made maps identifying places that were accessible and easy to navigate, as well as places that were impossible and became barriers. Therefore other maps were constructed of places seen through the eyes of those who could not see, with the steps of those who could not walk, in the words of those who could not speak. See Figure 20-2.

Barreras y facilitadores identificados y caracterizados en la zona central de Fontibón

CATEGORÍA: INFRAESTRUCTURA URBANA

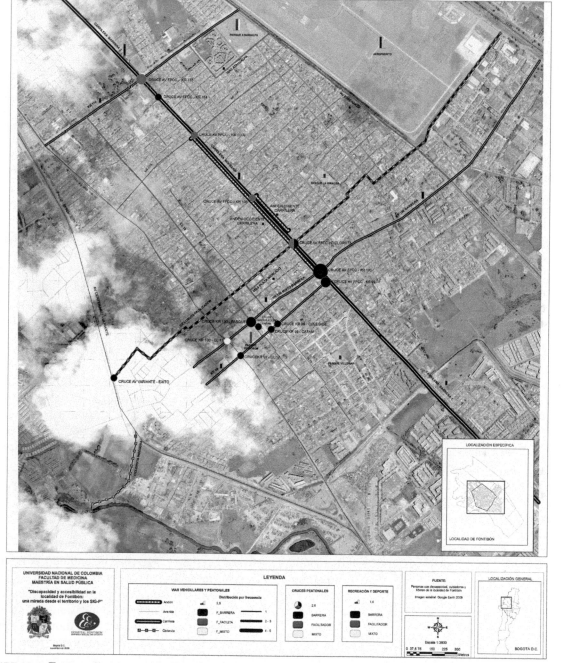

FIGURE 20-2 ■ Map of barriers and facilities for disabled people and their carers in Fontibón, Bogotá. *(Mauricio Fuentes Vallejo.)*

through life, from conception to death, as a continuous development in a complex process that can be studied from the physical, cognitive, emotional and social development (García-Ruíz et al., 2010), which refers to childhood, youth, adulthood and old age, stages defined by modernity.

Beyond the lifecycle, we find the concept of generation. I go on trying to find answers to my inquiries: What is a generation? Generation is the accumulated cultural heritage that suggests multiple aspects related to demography, economy, political ideologies and aesthetic constructions of groups of people living in specific times and places. Some authors classify generations according to national and international policies or events (milestones) that occur throughout people's lives.

The term *generation* allows us to think about and understand the actions, speeches, worldviews, feelings and ways of life of people at a time of life, in specific historical contexts, taking into account their collective, accumulated experiences. This calls for a comprehensive domain that challenges a logical, linear understanding of historical processes, because each generation appropriates the transformations that preceded it and reconstructs them in order to incorporate them into the present moment. This process can characterize each generation by a series of particularities in relation to roles, status, communicative expressions, with differential nominations, common attributes, set of possibilities and constraints imposed by the previous generations. The relationship between the generations is intergenerational, which has to do with interdependence, solidarity and reciprocity for the transformation and reconstruction of roles and status that facilitate learning, and with the recognition and exchange of knowledge that are of mutual benefit (García-Ruíz et al., 2010, 2012). Thus the understanding of the generations invites us to take into account the history, past and future of each person and group we have in front of us. See Box 20-3.

LIVING DIVERSITY

Diversity (from the Latin word *diversitas*) refers to the difference, variety, abundance of different things, dissimilarities, nonhomogeneity or heterogeneity. Diversity implies recognition of the particular within the

---

BOX 20-3

Traditionally, public health policies have as a reference the stages of life cycle to define actions for people during childhood, youth, adulthood and old age. These stages are defined by the evolutionary process of people, characterized by physical, physiological and psychological changes. However, this frame of reference has its limitations. The formulation and implementation of policies require an understanding of the social, historical and political contexts. For example, policies for young people today cannot be the same as the ones made when our parents were young, as they belong to a different generation. Issues such as the use of technology mark a new way of acting and relating to each other.

---

universal, of how such particularities are constructed and lived, as a result of collective interactions.

Social policy in Colombia is designed with a focus on meeting the needs of specific groups of the population, generally the poor and most vulnerable (Departamento Nacional de Planeación, 2007). Thus every minority group which is considered to have been excluded is now the focus for a specific public policy. Thus there are public policies for children, for victims, for women, for disabled persons, among others. The problem is that these public policies end up addressing the needs of minorities, but not the needs of a wider society, and the perspective of a wider consensus is thus lost. The proposal here is to recognize diversity: diversity in gods, skin colours, faces, origins, sexual orientation, life choices, and to design inclusive public policies based on social justice.

UNDERSTANDING INTERSECTIONALITIES

Intersectionality refers to a process derived from black activists. Creshaw (1991, cited in Jaramillo, 2012), used this term to analyse discriminations of class, gender and employment in the US. The word also refers to the 'relationship among multiple dimensions and modalities of social relations and the formation of people as subjects' (McCall, 2005, p. 1771). It is a term that is widely accepted in political processes worldwide and has been used since the 1990s.

In Colombia people talk about a differential approach to public policy, which means seeing each person from his or her difference in order to develop programmes according to the specific situation. This can have the effect of focusing on actions that can contribute to the construction of stereotyping and ghettoization of people and their experiences. In contrast, the concepts of diversity and intersectionality can be useful in understanding populations from multiple, intersecting categories of gender, disability, displacement, among others, where there is evidence of discrimination and inequality. However, in some forms of states, especially when they are based on neoliberalism, as Jaramillo (2012) says, it is easier to work on additive models than on creating intersectional policies. It is easier to focus action on targeting specific groups of people within those societies, such as the unemployed or people with disabilities, than on a strategy for the implementation of policies. See Box 20-4.

LET'S NOT FORGET ETHICS

It is not possible to talk about policies without discussing the ethical and philosophical principles that form the basis of daily living. The ethical discussion should be a natural part of the discussions in occupational therapy and should go beyond the mere existence of codes of professional ethics endorsed by professional associations. In fact, one of the issues that sometimes goes unnoticed has to do with the ethical and moral principles that drive people to act one way or another. These principles have their roots in philosophy and culture, and relate to the concepts of respect, dignity, autonomy and freedom. We should not only know and define in words ethical processes, but we should incorporate them in all activities of our daily life.

These inconsistencies and tensions are shown in simple cases such as when institutions promote the rights of people and their performance focuses on economic sustainability or in the individual and personal interests of a few. Vélez Correa and Maya Mejía (n.d.) argue:

> [T]he effort today is focused on building a civil or civic ethics that can be shared by all, whatever the worldview may be. It involves an agreement on the minimum to live in society in a dignified and humane manner. It is constituted by the acceptance of shared rationality and the rejection of any exclusionary intransigence, being a basic element on which a collective vision of society can be built, facilitating the personal growth of each person. (p. 166)

OCCUPATIONAL THERAPY IN A GLOCALIZED CONTEXT

I understand occupational therapy as the relationship among doing, occupation and happiness, that is, trying to be happy with what we do and encouraging people to be happy with what they do. Day-to-day work and the conceptual developments in occupational therapy have changed as much as the world. Professional requirements and actions are transformed in response to conflicts and post conflicts and their aftermath, to dictatorships, to natural disasters and to climate change, in the era of public policies, of construction of democracy, decentralization and local development. It is in these circumstances where we act locally in a globalized way, that is, with global thinking and local action – this is glocalization (Cruz and Bodnar, 2008; de Sousa Santos, 2009). It is as if the life-world requires, by chance or by knowledge, the creation of conceptual developments as the model of human occupation, occupational behaviour, occupational science and more.

What all this may mean is that through practice, or in order to understand these processes, occupational therapy has seen the need to respond to social, political, economic and even environmental issues of individuals and groups, and many times has had to learn by doing – sometimes by generating distances between theory and practice, and sometimes with a practice that is faster than the theory, with the risk that the actors involved become *doers without reflection*.

THE OCCUPATIONAL THERAPIST AS A RESEARCHER, AS A POLITICIAN AND IN THE POLICIES

Research is a natural act of life and it has to do with what is done aseptically in the laboratory, as well as with what happens at any stage of life. The research, action and participation, and systematization of knowledge have become natural in political and community processes, hence the possibility of turning practice into a research exercise, converting practice into reflection (Fals Borda et al., 1986).

Guajardo and Simo Algado (2010) invite us to reflect on occupational therapy from an ethical and political perspective of human rights, quality of life and psychosocial well-being. From the point of view of social cohesion and governance, occupational therapy plays a role of stability of social systems, often acting from the periphery for social transformation. Sandra Galheigo (2014), in her closing speech at the World Federation of Occupational Therapists congress in Chile in 2010, invited occupational therapists from Latin America to speak more often of professional identity in the South, to differentiate themselves (ourselves!) from identities imported from the North. She placed special emphasis on the richness of our context and on discussions on gender and employment. Simó Algado (2009), in his proposal of El Jardín de Martí in Spain, shows us the possibility of occupational justice from gardening, mixed with poetry, passion and love in the performance of the activity, which results in the transformation of persons with mental illness into political subjects through action, research and participation. Kronenberg and Pollard (2006) introduced the concept of occupational apartheid, emphasizing that some people have a value and a social and economic status different from others. Fernández (2011) invites us to make a political-ethical reflection from recognition as a category for social justice, while Pollard and Sakellariou (2014) refer to occupational therapy as a political and transformational act. My experiences have led me to recognize myself as a political subject in interaction with other political actors in a local action, within a global context, and interpreted from the different disciplines that nurture my work.

This is how occupational therapies transform and are being transformed, how they are globally contextualized and localized, departing from the simplicity

of life, working for happiness, well-being, justice and fairness. That is how we become political subjects and transformers of local realities and lives. For Foucault (2007), political subjects are recognized as autonomous beings, free, sovereign and with awareness, that is, empowered. If so, occupational therapists are political subjects who are actors who can transform and help in transforming the lives of those with whom they interact. Hence capabilities can be generated at individual and collective levels, leading to participation in decision making. These practices and reflections are part of the renewal of knowledge in occupational therapy, where research plays a central role.

CONCLUSIONS

We can talk about many kinds of occupational therapies, those of the South, the North, the West and the East; therapies that invite us to act locally and think globally, which are critical and recognized as a social practice, which invite the development of professionals with skills to lead and organize individual and collective engagements.

The world does not only require occupational therapists to work in projects, in nongovernmental organizations or in institutions solely dedicated to theory development. It rather needs professionals who can develop ideas and ideals, and help in the transformation and improvement through decision making. What I mean is that occupational therapy must strategically place leaders inside decision-making organizations, ministries, and national and international institutions.

In this chapter I shared a story, my story, from *below,* from the South, from the South of the Americas, from the local level, from my womanhood and from being a Latin American, a policymaker. It is from this positionality and through my practice as an occupational therapist that I have learned to understand occupational therapy as a practice emerging from history, from geography, from the generations, from diversity and from ethical and political reflections. It is there that I find local value understood within a global world.

Acknowledgements

Initially, this paper was prepared for the Chilean meeting of students of occupational therapy, Chile

(2012), and subsequently presented to the Colombian meeting of students of occupational therapy, Colombia (2013). I want to thank Dikaios Sakellariou and Nicholas Pollard for the affectionate dedication and professional commitment that helped me to clearly introduce my ideas in this writing. I want to also say thank you to Teresa Santos Rojas, for the translation and looking after intercultural accuracy in the way my ideas are written.

REFERENCES

Barrera Lopbaton, S., 2009. Reflexiones sobre el Sistema de Información Geográfica Participativo (SIGP) y cartografía social. Geography Notebooks. Colomb. Geo. J. 18, 9–23.

Cruz, J., et al., 2015. Historias de las Terapias Ocupacionales en Colombia (Colombian occupational therapy histories). Universidad Nacional de Colombia & Universidad del Valle, Bogota. unpublished.

Cruz, P.M., Bodnar, Z., 2008. Pensar globalmente y actuar localmente: el estado transnacional ambiental em Ulrich Beck. 5 (2), 13–25, July-December 2008. Jurid, Manizales, Colombia.

Cruz-Velandia, I., García-Ruíz, S., Rodríguez-Prieto, I., Rojas-Cárdenas, A., Chaves-Ortiz, A., 2015. Configuración política de la categoría discapacidad en Colombia: relación Estado y ciudadanía. Revista de la Facultad de Medicina 63 (Suppl. 3), 25–32. Available at: <http://revistas.unal.edu.co/index.php/revfacmed/article/view/49350/53062> (accessed 01.11.15.).

de Certeau, M., Giard, L., Mayol, P., 1999. La invención de lo cotidiano 2 Habitar y cocinar. Universidad Iberoamericna & Instituto Tecnológico de Estudios Superiores de Occidente. México.

de Sousa Santos, B., 2009. Una epistemologia del Sur. Clacso Editories. México.

Departamento Nacional de Planeación, 2007. Mecanismos de focalización cuatro estudios de caso. Sistema de indicadores sociodemográficos para Colombia. SISD 32, Bogotá. Colombia.

Fals-Borda, O., Brandão, C.R., Cetrulo, R., 1986. Investigación Participativa. Instituto del Hombre, Montevideo, Uruguay.

Fernández, A., 2011. Jóvenes con discapacidades: sujetos de reconocimiento. Thesis doctoral. Centro de estudios avanzados en niñez y juventud. Manizales, Universidad de Manizales – Cinde, Colombia.

Foucault, M., 2007. Nacimiento de la Biopolítica. Fondo de Cultura Económica, Ciudad de Mexico, México.

Fuentes Vallejo, M., 2010. Discapacidad y accesibilidad en la localidad de Fontibón: una mirada desde el territorio y los sistemas de información geográfica participativos. Work submitted for the Master's Degree in Public Health. National University of Colombia, School of Medicine, Institute of Public Health, Bogotá, Columbia. <http://www.coloquiodiscapacidad.com/investigaciones/phocadownload/participacion-social-y-vida-en-comunidad/fuentes_2010.pdf> (accessed 14.10.14.).

Galheigo, S.M., 2014. O cotidiano na terapia ocupacional: cultura, subjetividade e contexto histórico-social. Occup. Ther. J. Univ. São Paulo Brazil 14 (3), 104–109.

García-Ruíz, S., Ruíz, E., Díaz, T., Rozo, P., Espinosa, G., 2010. El enfoque poblacional: las personas como centro de las políticas. J. Res. Soc. Security Health 12, 129–142.

García-Ruíz, S., Ruíz, E., Díaz, T., Rozo, P., 2012. Reflexiones Sobre el Enfoque Poblacional. District Department of Health of Bogotá, Bogotá, Colombia.

Gareis, I., 2005. Identidades latinoamericanas frente al colonialismo, una apreciación histórico-antropológica: introducción al dossier. INDIANA 22, 9–18.

Gómez Buendía, H., Arciniegas, E., Hernández, A., Maríani, R., 2010. De las transiciones a los desafíos actuales de la democracia. Virtual School, UNDP, Bogotá, Colombia.

Guajardo, A., Simo Algado, S., 2010. Una terapia ocupacional basada en los derechos humanos. TOG (A Coruña). Consultada Julio de 2015 7 (12), 1–25. Available at: <www.revistatog.com/num12/pdfs/maestros.pdf>.

Jaramillo, P., 2012. El enfoque poblacional desde una perspectiva de interseccionalidad cultural. In: García-Ruíz, S., et al. (Eds.), Reflections on the Population Approach. [Reflexiones sobre el enfoque poblacional]. Bogotá, Colombia, District Department of Health of Bogotá.

Kronenberg, F., Pollard, N., 2006. Superar el apartheid ocupacional. Exploración preliminary de la naturaleza política de la terapia ocupacional. En terapia ocupacional sin fronteras. Aprendiendo del espíritu de supervivientes. Editorial Medica Panamericana, Buenos Aires, Madrid.

McCall, L., 2005. The Complexity of Intersectionality. Signs (Chic) 3 (3), 1771.

Martínez Rangel, R., Soto Reyes Garmendia, E., 2012. El Consenso de Washington: la instauración de las políticas neoliberales en América Latina. Política y Cultura 35–64.

Melgarejo, A., del Pilar, M., 2000. Historical thinking as genealogy: interpretive act and construction of subjectivity [El pensar histórico como genealogía: acto ierpretativo y construcción de la subjetividad]. Fronteras de la Justicia 5, 35–50.

Pollard, N., Sakellariou, D., 2014. The occupational therapist as a political being. Cadernos de Terapia Ocupacional da UFSCar 22 (3), 643–652.

Quino, J.S., 2004a. Mafalda, 8. Editorial Lumen, Barcelona.

Quino, J.S., 2004b. Mafalda, 10. Editorial Lumen, Barcelona.

Simó Algado, S., 2009. Desafíos contemporáneos para la educacion y la ciencia de la ocupación: la ecología, la ética y la justicia ocupacional. TOG (A. Coruña) 6 (Suppl. 5), Available at: <www.revistatog.com>.

Simó Algado, S., 2012. Terapia Ocupacional eco-social: hacia una ecología ocupacional/Eco-social. Cad. Ter. Ocup. UFSCar, São Carlos 20 (1), 7–16. <http://dx.doi.org/10.4322/cto.2012.001>.

Treat Whittier, J., 1988. Polls of water, pillars of fire: the literature of Ibuse Masuji. University of Washington Press, Seattle, WA.

Vásquez Roca, A., 2011. La posmodernidad. Nuevo régimen de verdad, violencia metafísica y fin de los metarrelatos. Nómadas. Revista Crítica de Ciencias Sociales y Jurídicas 29 (2011.1).

Vélez Correa, L.A., Maya Mejía, J.M., n.d. ética y salud pública. Ethics Public Health 14, 166–176.

21

OUR PROFESSIONAL EXISTENCE *IS* POLITICAL: CRITICAL REFLECTIONS ON 'SEEING WHITE' IN OCCUPATIONAL THERAPY

LILY OWENS

SETTING THE SCENE

The implications of 'seeing white'[1] in occupational therapy theory, academia and practice are potentially devastating in regards to its *relevance* to the 'other' and may thus arguably impact on the very survival of our profession in an increasingly globalized world. Furthermore, systematic underrepresentation of the 'other' within all remits of occupational therapy concerns not only issues of relevance and irrelevance, but also of access to social and occupational justice, equality and ultimately of power and control. Importantly, 'seeing white' in this sense does not refer to skin colour, but to a form of ethnocentrism (see Table 21-1) in which Western or Eurocentric ways of knowing, thinking and experiencing the world ultimately become taken-for-granted assumptions (Quijano, 2007). Indeed, 'whiteness' as a social construction in this context arguably 'forms the invisible absolute vertical by which all else is defined and judged' (de Beauvoir, 1989,

p. xxi), whilst the 'other' in this sense refers to the less powerful: those who may not subscribe to this propagated and dominant Eurocentric way of seeing the world (Iwama, 2006).

Rather problematically, recognizing 'whiteness' necessitates acute awareness of deeply imbedded assumptions so engrained epistemologically and ontologically that they are invisible to those who not only harbour them (Walter et al., 2011), but give them life. Fundamentally, it is this status quo which systematically informs occupational therapy and sends out a powerful political message to key 'other' stakeholders, including clients, students, practitioners, communities, organizations and society, whether such has been consciously intended or not. Arguably, claiming ignorance of such inadvertent political messages should no longer be a permissible option if occupational therapists are to fulfil their role as change agents at the forefront of social justice and human rights agendas. Indeed, the profession's frequent self-affirmation based on idealized subscriptions to human rights and social justice ideals without critical awareness of

---

[1]Term adopted from Nelson (2007).

TABLE 21-1
Defining Ethnocentrism, Theoretical Imperialism and Hegemony

Ethnocentrism	Encompasses a belief that one's own culture demands superiority over that of others and represents a standard by which others ought to be measured or judged (Leavitt, 1999).
Theoretical imperialism	Broadly thought to refer to the development and perpetuation of theories by therapists, privileging their own perspectives, whilst the perspectives of others are overlooked, ignored or simply silenced (Mann, 1995).
Hegemony	Refers to the dominant vision of reality being postulated as universal and valid for all groups (Gramsci, 1971).

capacity for injustices in its own backyard is deeply concerning. To avoid complacency, it is important to investigate whether adopted ideals can genuinely be sustained or kept alive by conditions within occupational therapy. In other words, one must investigate whether the profession itself truly enables social justice and holism ideals or whether good intentions, coupled with a systematic lack of critical awareness, actually support injustice and the continued propagation of dominant ways of knowing, valuing, learning and doing.

This chapter aims to critically reflect on 'whiteness' within occupational therapy theory, incorporating possible political and social implications of this monocultural status quo. Such reflection will hopefully contribute to speaking justice to power by offering an alternative critical view on deeply rooted Western philosophical assumptions that underpin all remits of occupational therapy, with far-reaching consequences. Notably, such consequences may be particularly devastating if 'white ways of knowing' (Nelson, 2007, p. 242) are not zealously made visible. Critical race theory will lend understanding to emerging themes, whilst urgent calls are made for interventions beyond external training in 'cultural safety' and 'cultural competence' to that of systematically working to change the 'whiteness' of occupational therapy from within.

My Voice ...

[Colonel Maynadier] was surprised to see tears well up in Spotted Tail's eyes; he did not know that an Indian could weep.

(Bury My Heart at Wounded Knee, Brown, 1987, p. 146)

In recognition of the self as political and the belief that my individual positioning has a bearing on the content of this chapter, it is morally important that my own voice is situated transparently within this work. I was born into a household of contradictory world views (Western/non-Western), deeply impacted by burdensome histories on both sides. Ideas of normalcy or ways of knowing therefore had little opportunity to become taken-for-granted assumptions. Such perceived assumptions, however, in regards to the 'other' have routinely been encountered in both academia and clinical practice and have, in light of life experiences and my own 'other' ethnic and cultural background, not sat comfortably with me. Grappling with such tensions has led to increased sensitivity, as 'by struggling I [have] become conscious/aware' (Freire, 1989, p. 46).

Formal documentation ordinarily categorizes me as 'mixed other' ethnically, a social construct that tells me that I have become 'other' on account of my mother's devoted love and marriage to a person outside of the dominant group. I tend to consider such a 'mixed other' vantage point not solely a meaningful opportunity but more so a profound responsibility to explore perceived issues of inclusivity, justice and power within my chosen profession.

I am considered an ethnic 'minority' occupational therapist because I am underrepresented amongst represented occupational therapist colleagues. As an occupational therapy student, I was an ethnic 'minority' occupational therapy student because I was underrepresented amongst represented students, lecturers and placement educators, particularly aesthetically. As an occupational therapy student and practitioner, I was and am underrepresented within some of the theories and assumptions that underpin occupational therapy practice.

I have personally grappled with belonging at times, despite encounters with the most kind and dedicated occupational therapist colleagues and the profession's wider stance on participation and inclusion. I have experienced particular frustration (and hurt) at encountering a systematic lack of deeper critical awareness from well-meaning therapists and the profession itself around the wider contextual impact of structural inequalities, discrimination, injustice and human rights. This has been coupled with a seemingly deafening silence around the fallibility of occupational therapy in contributing to such inequalities. Within the working context of inner-city London and some of the most economically deprived and richly diverse communities, such encounters have led to a realization that immense danger exists when one's practitioner focal lens is directed solely at the individual 'minority' client, student and/or practitioner at ground level without acute critical awareness of the immense wider structural inequalities that may have and still do weigh heavily on persons and their communities.

I have wondered whether it is fair or realistic to look for fault or solutions purely at the level of individual occupational therapists working within organizations, without holding the relevant professional bodies to account: this is especially important in regards to addressing and tackling these issues systematically and honestly within all remits of occupational therapy, inclusive of the need to decolonise our discourses of knowledge, our pedagogy. Occupational therapists need to become critically aware of the dangers of their wishful, but uncritical, idealism and advocate for genuine emancipation from the status quo, thereby enabling social action (Freire, 1985). They need to critically steer away from the practice of solely allowing the 'other' to sit at their table, but only to eat in the way that they do. This would not only be required for the sake of the survival of occupational therapy, but also is essential to justifying the profession's moral and ethical conduct subscriptions and mantras of holism. Naturally, immediate action is also dictated by continued evident health inequalities and occupational therapy's arguable contribution to such inequity in this present day.

History teaches us that complicity to violations does not necessarily require active (obvious) participation but may amount to silent hand-holding and walking with the violator. Our actions and inactions are political and moral, whether we systematically and critically allow for such recognition or not.

'SEEING WHITE' AND OCCUPATIONAL THERAPY

Perhaps some of the lack of engagement with issues of racism and inequality in occupational therapy discourse was due to poor representation of the oppressed in the profession. Those who were tasked with generating knowledge for the profession may have seen little value in entertaining such discourse ... what was included as important ... depended on the knowledge generators.

(Ramugondo, 2000, p. 9)

During the Seventeenth Meeting of the European Network of Occupational Therapy in Higher Education Conference, Jennifer Creek's speech 'In Praise of Diversity' rather poignantly asked:

Our remit is to work with people who are occupationally disadvantaged by impairment, disability, poverty, displacement or exclusion but how many occupational therapists have experienced and overcome such disadvantages in their own lives ... how willing are we to change the status quo of our profession?

(Creek, 2011)

However, the incorporation and retention of a diverse workforce has been difficult, with some arguing:

[S]tudents of different migrant or ethnic minority backgrounds often feel excluded by teachers and fellow students and not attracted to occupational therapy programmes. Furthermore, there is a high drop-out rate ... it is quite difficult to find good practice about successfully implemented diversity policy in occupational therapy practice and education.

(van Bruggen, 2009, p. xv)

Beagan and Chakala (2012) argue that the occupational therapy literature has greatly disregarded the experiences of therapists who are from culturally and ethnically diverse backgrounds. It should also be questioned whether 'their absence [has] thus become normalised' (Richards, 2003, p. 296) within occupational therapy and what impact this political message has fundamentally on those who do not form the dominant group. Similarly damning US studies from other disciplines have pointed to 'minority' therapist experiences of marginalization, 'racial battle fatigue' and racial microaggressions to name a few (see, e.g., Solorzano et al., 2000). Indeed, in their critical exposé entitled 'Racial Microaggressions in Everyday Life, Implications for Clinical Practice,' Sue et al. (2007) from Columbia University, New York, asserted that ideals of cultural competence by helping professionals would not be realized when 'white clinicians fail to understand how issues of race influence the therapy process and how racism potentially infects the delivery of services' (Sue et al., 2007, p. 271)[2].

These authors further called for research to be conducted of 'ethnic minority' therapist and student experiences in relation to racial microaggressions. Notably, a subsequent US small-scale study of this kind, which addressed the experiences of ethnic minority students and practitioners within the psychological realm, discovered themes akin to 'assumptions of inferior status' (Sue et al., 2008, p. 333), the 'assumed superiority of white cultural values/communication styles' (Sue et al., 2008, p. 334), feeling like an 'alien in one's own land' (Sue et al., 2007, p.75), 'denial of [participant] racial realities' (Sue et al., 2007, p.76) and 'invisibility' (Sue et al., 2007, p. 77), with further contentions that some students were forced to 'confront unrelenting oppression and discrimination as part of their everyday college experiences at historically white institutions' (Smith et al., 2007, p. 552).

The limited focus on recruiting a diverse workforce, without commitment to critical awareness of structural societal discriminatory processes that have compounded the exclusion of particular groups historically, has been criticized (Willie and Sanford, 1995). Indeed, Smith (2010) has pointed to some Freirean perspectives to aid understanding of such arguably superficial efforts:

I have already mentioned the kind of 'help' that Freire described as false generosity, which is assistance offered by people with privilege, to the oppressed in the absence of any acknowledgement of the context of oppression. (p. 134)

---

[2]See also Suman Fernando (2000) for a UK perspective.

EXPLORING 'WHITENESS'

Who are better prepared than the oppressed to understand the terrible significance of an oppressive society?

(Freire, 1972, p. 26)

It has become apparent over the years that occupational therapy is situated within white, middle-class norms and values (see, e.g., Hammell, 2009). Indeed, despite occupational therapy's inclusive stance of occupational engagement and participation, Hammell (2011) has argued that 'it is difficult to avoid the impression that theories of occupation *belong* to white, middle-class, English-speaking Western theorists' (p. 31).

According to critical race theorists, Western society ordinarily presents whiteness as constituting the 'norm', and the 'other' is categorized in accordance with this norm (Ladson-Billings, 1999). What constitutes 'white' in this sense refers to taken-for-granted assumptions in the way one views the world, which are ordinarily and inherently adopted by those forming the dominant sociocultural group (Moreton-Robinson, 2000). Importantly, such assumptions of thinking and knowing are often taken for granted, becoming invisible to those constituting the dominant majority (Hammell, 2009). Occupational therapists and occupational scientists form major bearers of such invisibility within 'white' culture, impacting on clients from all cultural backgrounds (Iwama, 2006) and arguably contributing to disparities in health (Andrulis, 2005).

The social theorist Foucault (1980) argues that the domination of a particular theoretical stance concerns not issues of superiority but of knowledge and power, which in lack of alternative theories arising would ensure 'power not truth determ[ining] which version of reality w[ould] prevail' (Riger, 1992, p. 736). Iwama (2006) has pointed to inherent power implications when the ways of knowing, valuing and being of a profession are fundamentally grounded on the ideas of knowing, valuing and being as deemed 'normal' by a specific cultural group. Indeed, there is increased interest in the way 'disciplinary power and control may take place within the realm of occupational therapy practice' (Galheigo, 2012, p. 1).

Kantartzis and Molineux (2011) argue that occupational therapists and occupational scientists hold power in the maintenance (or not) and the imposition (or not) of their perceived reality in relation to the way occupation and a 'normal' daily life is construed in practice (p. 74). Some have therefore deemed it necessary to address the exposition of such theories of normalcy in colonial and imperialistic domination terms (see, e.g., Hammell, 2011). Furthermore, several authors argue that the peddling of unquestioned assumptions in occupational therapy and the actions of deeming such to be universally applicable could amount to not merely inadequately informed theories, but ethnocentrism (Iwama, 2006), theoretical imperialism (Hammell, 2011) and even cultural or 'white' hegemony (Magalhaes, 2012) (see Table 21-1). Clients unable or unwilling to conform to such preconceived ideas of normalcy during practice encounters could be categorized as being deviant and even marginalized by means of silencing or disregarding of alternative viewpoints, leading one to consider 'whose reality counts' (Fernando, 2009). Contextually, of course, it is noteworthy that claims of imperialism extend beyond occupational therapy[3].

THE OCCUPATIONAL THERAPIST AS AN ETHICAL, MORAL AND POLITICAL ADVOCATE

After Apartheid, the question of complicity is unavoidable – not simply because it is necessary to know whose resources gave apartheid life, nourished and defended it, but also because apartheid, by its very nature, occasions a questioning of and thinking about complicity itself.

(Sanders, 2002, p. 1)

Increasingly, research evidence points to a link between valued diverse workforces and good patient care (see, e.g., West et al., 2012). Despite this, a damning research report has recently highlighted a major gap between workforce diversity and the diversity found within local populations served by the National Health Service (NHS) (Kline, 2014). Furthermore, it was found that executives from Black Minority Ethnic (BME) backgrounds were 'entirely absent' (Kline, 2014, p. 4), whilst ethnicity and diversity data were scarcely being monitored by most NHS organizations in England. Indeed, the highly critical report drew associations with the Francis Report (Francis, 2013)[4], pointing to the need for 'radical change of culture and leadership style' (p. 4). It further argued:

Now would seem a good time to apply that approach to the treatment of the most undervalued and least rewarded section of the NHS workforce – its BME (black and minority) staff – not least since the evidence is that their treatment is a good predictor of the quality of patient care. At a time when there appears consensus on the benefits of diversity for all those receiving health services there can be no better time to change, once and for all, the 'snowy peaks' of the NHS.

(Kline, 2014, pp. 4–5)

Kline went further, suggesting that the lack of action against racial discrimination within the NHS could arguably be compared to the institutional racism defined in relation to the London Metropolitan Police (Macpherson Report, 1999)[5] a decade earlier (Kline, 2014, p. 21).

Occupational therapy deems itself to be highly committed to the ethical, moral and political cause of promoting an equitable society (Canadian Association of Occupational Therapists, 2014), fundamentally

---

[3]It has previously been argued, for example, that 'imperialism carried over from slavery and colonialism is now manifested through psychiatry' (Fernando, 2000, p. 84), whilst in social work, antioppressive discourse has emerged as a means of addressing practices of power in relation to difference, inclusivity and diversity (Brown, 2012).

[4]The Francis Report (led by Robert Francis QC) was published in 2013 as a result of a public enquiry which sought to examine the causes of systemic failings in care at Mid Staffordshire NHS Foundation Trust between 2005 and 2009, during which mortality rates significantly increased and standards of care were 'unacceptable' (Francis, 2013, p. 7).

[5]The Macpherson Report (led by William Macpherson) was published in 1999 as a result of a public enquiry which sought to examine the murder of black teenager Stephen Lawrence in an unprovoked racist attack in London and allegations of a systematic failure by the police to investigate the murder as they should have.

rooted in human rights and social justice agendas and actively working towards health equity (World Federation of Occupational Therapists, 2006). Professional responsibilities bespeak notions of ethically fair, just and moral conduct as seemingly deeply engrained within the healthcare system. The enterprise then as healthcare professionals essentially appears to be a 'moral' endeavour, prescribing to moral obligations that are deeply rooted in philosophical frameworks which ascribe infinite value and dignity to human beings. The rights to dignity and respect are further reinforced by human rights legislation and reflected within human rights position statements guiding the various healthcare professions, including occupational therapy (World Federation of Occupational Therapists, 2006). In professional practices, these rights are often demonstrated by requirements to uphold the right to autonomy and informed consent as far as is possible. Such obligatory responsibilities seek to safeguard the best interests of the most vulnerable and perhaps retain the practitioner's place as moral agent. The World Federation of Occupational Therapists (2006) acknowledges such a responsibility and calls for practitioners to recognize their role as agents of social change, placing fundamental onus on enabling a wider whole of advocacy and social reform, and in essence on human rights and participation. Such sentiments were supported by Law (2011), who at the 2011 College of Occupational Therapy Conference in Brighton asserted that 'participation in occupation is a human right' and is vitally important to both health and well-being.

It is arguably the case that the profession's fundamental focus on maximizing health and well-being affirms not only an occupational perspective, but political and moral stances on rights of access to health and well-being for all, affirming responsibilities to advocate on behalf of the most vulnerable in keeping with wider social and political roles as change agents (World Federation of Occupational Therapists, 2006).

The US Department of Health (2004) was spurred into action by way of publications standardizing cultural competence within healthcare, following concerns about health disparities (Pole et al., 2008)[6]. Cul-

tural competence constitutes the 'dominant approach' within occupational therapy (Canadian Association of Occupational Therapists, 2014) and has broadly been described as the ability of practitioners to both understand and practice within the culturally specific contexts of their clients. It further requires practitioners to critically examine their own biases towards clients from differing cultural backgrounds, whilst recognizing their own privileged standing socially and existing power imbalances in practitioner–client encounters. Others (e.g., Tervalon and Murray-Garcia, 1998) have argued that it encompasses cultural humility and a life-long self-reflective commitment.

Diverse communities cannot be assumed or expected to subscribe to a Western worldview. Rather, traditional practices and belief systems are likely to be actively maintained, heavily underpinned by gender, ethnic origin and religious practices. Studies show that generally, ethnic minority communities living in the UK perceive their ethnic and racial background to heavily influence their identity (Department for Communities and Local Government, 2009). Daily discrimination and resultant isolation on grounds of race and ethnicity is a reality for many people (e.g., Bhui, 2002; Karlson and Nazroo, 2002).

CONSIDERING REFLEXIVITY

Educating physicians skilled at addressing the healthcare needs of a diverse society involves not the fulfilment of a competency, as some sort of educational nirvana, but the development of an orientation – a critical consciousness.
(Kumagai and Lypson, 2009, p. 782)

Occupational therapists are encouraged to 'engage the whole person – their body, mind and soul – either on an individual basis or as a group' (Polgar and Landy, 2004, p. 199). Such a stance would recognize that effective and ethically sound occupational therapy provision must also include genuine understanding of client needs within their particular contexts and that for certain individuals, for example, the prospect of becoming 'independent' amounts to a notion of disdain or even amusement (Geurts, 2002). Indeed, many cultures represented within the Asian and African communities in Europe and North America

---

[6]For example, minority groups underusing services or terminating treatment early and the quality of healthcare differing significantly between minority/nonminority groups (Pole et al., 2008).

share beliefs which place emphasis on belonging to others and thereby reflect a worldview that does not separate the individual from their community (Ogbonnaya, 1994). This requires that all aspects of the person work collectively and interdependently without losing the uniqueness of each aspect or self; in essence, the person is community as the two are inseparable and inextricably linked (Ogbonnaya, 1994, p. 82). Mikhize (2008) points to Zulu teachings from South Africa, depicting the person as intertwined with their community, their families, God and the universe, suggesting that such harmony constituted a balanced life. The greeting 'sawubona' (literally translated as 'I see you', originating from the wisdom of the Bantu peoples of Africa) exemplifies this notion that 'my humanity is caught up, is inextricably bound up, in yours'; it is the spirit of Ubuntu (Covey, 2011, p. 34)[7].

Krog (2008) pointed to the potentiality of discriminatory practices and ethically problematic interpretations by practitioners of narratives told from non-Western perspectives. She called on individuals to 'interpret the narrative via its embeddedness in an indigenous world view' (Krog, 2008, p. 231); only then could the understanding of such narratives be deemed to be ethical and fair, even logical.

Only through practicing reflexivity as an outsider looking in[8] is the practitioner able to be ethically and morally responsive, accepting or declining practices of normalcy (Mackey, 2007, p. 98). Indeed, the basis on which ethical engagement occurs is firmly situated in the practitioner's obligation to the other (Mackey, 2007, p. 99). Such obligation may arguably include the 'moral act of listening' (Frank, 1995, p. 25). A recognition of critical disability studies literature and its intervention calls for practitioners to address sociocultural and sociopolitical levels, focusing heavily on social justice (Galheigo, 2005), advocacy (Kubina, 2000) and experiences of discrimination/racism. Essentially, critical reflexivity intends to avert, as much as possible, the replication of 'oppressive social relations in practice' (Healy, 2005, p. 80).

---

[7]Ubuntu is difficult to translate, but it has been likened to 'personhood' and more than this – that a person depends on other persons to be a person (Covey, 2011, p. 34).

[8]Or as the theoretical self (see Mackey, 2007, p. 98).

CONCLUDING THOUGHTS

True compassion is more than flinging a coin to a beggar. It comes to see that an edifice which produces beggars needs restructuring. (Martin Luther King Speech, Beyond Vietnam: A Time to Break Silence, 1967)

Feminist authors have for some time contended that the personal *is* political and so engagement in permitting the 'subordinate' voice to be heard fundamentally affects social change (Wilkinson and Kitzinger, 1996). Similarly, since the era of the civil rights movement, critical race theory has been fundamentally concerned with dismantling power differentials by encouraging the reconstruction of dominant 'white' narratives in favour of naming racist injury and identifying its origins using counterstories. Such counterstories are intended to 'cast doubt on the validity of accepted premises or myths, especially ones held by the majority' (Delgado and Stefancic, 2001, p. 144), and invite questioning around who has the power to define reality and who does not.

'Diverse voices' remain systematically absent within occupational therapy and there is a tendency to accord primacy to dominant group experiences with 'diverse' subjects over 'diverse' voices themselves. Furthermore, silence pertaining to issues of racism and inequality may be attributable to a systematic underrepresentation of 'minorities' in the profession, leaving a concerning vacuum of unheard perspectives and potentially valuable insight.

The rhetoric of client-centredness, inclusion, participation, holism and advocacy has no meaning to the person whose suitcase you have not offered to weigh and whose burdens you cannot see. Underrepresented voices can 'sharpen … moral conscience to a point where personal responsibility is [never again] abdicated' (Sanders, 2002, p. 133). Indeed, such voices have the ability to challenge our circles of certainty (Freire, 1972), a necessary contribution to an orientation of critical consciousness in a spirit of dialogue, curiosity and humility.

Freire (1972) suggests that we must reexamine ourselves constantly if we are to be authentically committed to the people we are working with. Such a re-examination may remind us of Adorno (1978), who believed that the highest form of morality is not to feel at home in one's own home, or Heywood (1994), who saw knowledge itself as a social construct which served to legitimize social structures. True change from the status quo in occupational therapy, then, necessitates not romanticized subscriptions to cultural 'competence' ideals which can contribute to a lulling into complacency and self-adulation, but a radical shift of consciousness. Let us begin with decolonizing occupational therapy's 'knowledge'; decolonize the curriculum and thereby the mind![9]

[9]For further reading on this topic, see also Nandy (1983).

REFERENCES

Adorno, T., 1978. Minima Moralia: Reflections from Damaged Life. Surkamp Verlag, Frankfurt, Germany.

Andrulis, D.P., 2005. Moving beyond the status quo in reducing racial and ethnic disparities in children's health. Public Health Rep. 120, 370–377.

Beagan, B.L., Chakala, A., 2012. Culture and diversity among occupational therapists in Ireland: when the therapist is the diverse one. Br. J. Occup. Ther. 75 (3), 144–151.

Bhui, K., 2002. Racism and Mental Health. Jessica Kingsley Publishers, London.

Brown, D., 1987. Bury My Heart at Wounded Knee: An Indian history of the American West. Vintage, London.

Brown, C.G., 2012. Anti-oppression through a postmodern lens: dismantling the masters conceptual tools in discursive social work practice. Crit. Soc. Work 13 (1), 34–65.

Canadian Association of Occupational Therapists, 2014. Position statement: diversity. <http://www.caot.ca> (accessed 15.10.15.).

Covey, S., 2011. The 3rd Alternative: Solving Life's Most Difficult Problems. Simon & Schuster, Inc., New York.

Creek, J., 2011. In praise of diversity. European Network of Occupational Therapists in Higher Education Conference, ENOTHE, Belgium. <http://www.enothe.eu>.

de Beauvoir, S., 1989. The Second Sex. Vintage, New York.

Delgado, R., Stefanic, J., 2001. Critical Race Theory: in introduction. New York University Press, New York.

Department for Communities and Local Government, 2009. Tackling race inequalities: a discussion document. Communities and Local Government Publications, London, UK. <http://www.communities.gov.uk> (accessed 14.10.15).

Fernando, S., 2000. Imperialism, racism and psychiatry. In: Barker, P., Stevenson, C. (Eds.), The Construction of Power and Authority in Psychiatry. Butterworth Publishers, Oxford.

Fernando, S., 2009. Whose reality counts? Open Mind 155, 21.

Foucault, M., 1980. Power/Knowledge: Selected Interviews and Other Writings, 1972–1977. Knopf Doubleday Publishing Group, London.

Francis, R., 2013. Report of the Mid Staffordshire NHS Foundation Trust Public Inquiry. <http://www.midstaffspublicinquiry.com/report> (accessed 15.10.15.).

Frank, A.W., 1995. The wounded storyteller: body, illness and ethics. The University of Chicago press, Chicago.

Freire, P., 1972. Pedagogy of the Oppressed. Continuum, New York.

Freire, P., 1985. Education for Critical Consciousness. Continuum, New York.

Freire, P., 1989. Education for the Critical Consciousness. Continuum, New York.

Galheigo, S.M., 2005. Occupational therapy and the social field: clarifying concepts and ideas. In: Kronenberg, F., Simo Algado, S., Pollard, N. (Eds.), Occupational therapy without borders. Elsevier; Churchill Livingstone, Oxford, pp. 87–98.

Galheigo, S., 2012. Editorial board member profiles: Sandra Galheigo. J. Occup. Sci. 19 (1), 1–2.

Geurts, K.L., 2002. Culture and the Senses: Bodily Ways of Knowing in an African Community. University of California Press, Ltd, Berkeley, CA.

Gramsci, A., 1971. Selections from the Prison Notebooks of Antonio Gramsci. International Publishers, New York.

Hammell, K.W., 2009. Sacred texts: a sceptical exploration of the assumptions underpinning theories of occupation. Can. J. Occup. Ther. 76 (1), 6–22.

Hammell, K.W., 2011. Resisting theoretical imperialism in the disciplines of occupational science and occupational therapy. Br. J. Occup. Ther. 74 (1), 27–33.

Healy, K., 2005. Social Work Theories in Context: Creating Frameworks for Practice. Palgrave MacMillan, New York.

Heywood, A., 1994. Political Ideas and Concepts: An Introduction. Macmillan Publishers, London.

Iwama, M.K., 2006. The Kawa Model: Culturally Relevant Occupational Therapy. Elsevier Churchill Livingstone, Toronto.

Kantartzis, S., Molineux, M., 2011. The influence of Western society's construction of a healthy daily life on the conceptualisation of occupation. J. Occup. Sci. 18 (1), 62–80.

Karlson, S., Nazroo, J.Y., 2002. The relationship between racial discrimination, social class and health among ethnic minority groups. Am. J. Public Health 92 (4), 624–631.

Kline, R., 2014. The 'snowy white peaks' of the NHS: a survey of discrimination in governance and leadership and the potential impact on patient care in London & England. Middlesex University Research Repository, Middlesex, England. <http://eprints.mdx.ac.uk>.

Krog, A., 2008. My heart is on my tongue: the untranslated self in a translated world. J. Anal. Psychol. 53 (2), 225–239.

Kubina, L.A., 2000. Assertive community treatment: Risk, challenge and opportunity. Occup. Ther. Now 2 (5), 7–9.

Kumagai, A.K., Lypson, M.L., 2009. Beyond cultural competence: critical consciousness, social justice, and multicultural education. Acad. Med. 84 (6), 782–787.

Ladson-Billings, G., 1999. Just what is critical race theory, and what's it doing in a nice field like education? In: Parker, L., et al. (Eds.), Race Is Race Isn't: Critical Race Theory and Qualitative Studies in Education. Westview Press, Boulder, CO, pp. 7–30.

Law, M., 2011. Occupation, evidence and outcomes: the future of our profession. College of Occupational Therapists (COT) Conference, Brighton, UK.

Leavitt, R.L., 1999. Moving rehabilitation professionals towards cultural competence: strategies for change. In: Leavitt, R.L. (Ed.), Cross-Cultural Rehabilitation: An International Perspective. WB Saunders, London, pp. 375–385.

Mackey, H., 2007. 'Do not ask me to remain the same': Foucault and the professional identities of occupational therapists. Aust. Occup. Ther. J. 54 (2), 95–102.

Macpherson, W., 1999. The Stephen Lawrence Inquiry. The Macpherson Report. London. <https://www.gov.uk/government/publications/the-stephen-lawrence-inquiry> (accessed 15.10.15.).

Magalhaes, L., 2012. What would Paolo Freire think of occupational science? In: Whiteford, G.E., Hocking, C. (Eds.), Occupational Science: Society, Inclusion and Participation. Blackwell Publishing, Chichester, UK, pp. 8–19.

Mann, H.S., 1995. Women's rights versus feminism? Postcolonial perspectives. In: Rajan, G., Mohabram, R. (Eds.), Postcolonial Discourse and Changing Cultural Contexts: Theory and Criticism. Greenwood Press, Westport, CT, pp. 69–88.

Mikhize, N., 2008. Ubuntu and harmony: an African approach to morality and ethics. In: Nicolson, R. (Ed.), Persons in Community: African Ethics in a Global Culture. University of KwaZulu-Natal Press, Scottsville, South Africa, pp. 35–43.

Moreton-Robinson, A., 2000. Talkin' up to the white woman: Aboriginal women and feminism. University of Queensland Press, Brisbane, Australia.

Nandy, A., 1983. The Intimate Enemy: Loss and Recovery of the Self under Colonialism. Oxford University Press, Delhi.

Nelson, A., 2007. Seeing white: a critical exploration of occupational therapy with indigenous Australian people. Occup. Ther. Int. 14 (4), 237–255.

Ogbonnaya, A.O., 1994. Person as community: an African understanding of the person as an intra-psychic community. J. Black Psychol. 20 (1), 75–87.

Pole, N., Gone, J.P., Kulkarni, M., 2008. Posttraumatic stress disorder among ethno-racial minorities in the United States. Clin. Psychol. Sci. Pract. 15 (1), 35–61.

Polgar, J., Landy, J.E., 2004. Occupations as a means for individual and group participation of life. In: Christiansen, C.H., Townsend, E.A. (Eds.), Introduction to occupation: The art and science of living. Pearson Education, Upper Saddle River, New Jersey.

Quijano, A., 2007. Coloniality and modernity/rationality. Cult. Stud. 21 (3), 168–178.

Ramugondo, E., 2000. The experience of being an occupational therapy student with an underrepresented ethnic and cultural background. University of Cape Town, South Africa. Available at: <http://uctscholar.uct.ac.za/PDF/112716_Ramugondo_E.pdf> (accessed 15.10.15.).

Richards, G., 2003. Race, Racism and Psychology: Towards a Reflexive History. Routledge Publishers, London, UK.

Riger, S., 1992. Epistemological debates, feminist voices: science, social values and the study of women. Am. Psychol. 47 (6), 730–740.

Sanders, M., 2002. Complicities: The Intellectual and Apartheid. Duke University Press, Durham, NC.

Smith, L., 2010. Psychology, Poverty, and the End of Social Exclusion: Putting Our Practice to Work. Columbia University, New York.

Smith, W.A., Allen, W.R., Danley, L.L., 2007. Assume the position… you fit the description': psychosocial experiences and racial battle fatigue among African American male college students. Am. Behav. Sci. 51, 551–578.

Solorzano, D., Ceja, M., Yosso, T., 2000. Critical race theory, racial microaggressions and campus racial climate: the experiences of African American college students. J. Negro Educ. 69 (1/2), 60–73.

Sue, D.W., Bucceri, J., Lin, A.I., Nadal, K.L., Torino, G.C., 2007. Racial microaggressions and the Asian American experience. Cult. Divers. Ethnic Minor. Psychol. 13 (1), 271–281.

Sue, D.W., Capodilupo, C.M., Torino, K.L., Gina, C., 2008. Racial microaggressions and the power to define reality. Am. Psychol. 63 (4), 277–279.

Tervalon, M., Murray-Garcia, J., 1998. Cultural humility versus cultural competence: a critical distinction in defining physician training outcomes in multicultural education. J. Health Care Poor Underserved 9 (2), 117–125.

US Department of Health, 2004. Setting the Agenda of Cultural Competence in Health Care. US Department of Health & Human Services, Rockville, MD.

van Bruggen, H., 2009. Foreword. In: Pollard, N., et al. (Eds.), A Political Practice of Occupational Therapy. Elsevier Churchill Livingstone, Edinburgh, UK, pp. xiii–xv.

Walter, M., Taylor, S., Habibis, D., 2011. How white is social work in Australia. Aust. Soc. Work 64 (1), 6–19.

West, M., Dawson, J., Admasachew, L., Topakas, A., 2012. NHS Staff Management and Health Service Quality Results from the NHS Staff Survey and Related Data. Lancaster University Management School and the Work Foundation Aston Business School. <https://www.gov.uk/government/uploads/system/uploads/attachment_data/file/215455/dh_129656.pdf> (accessed 16.10.15.).

Wilkinson, S., Kitzinger, C., 1996. Theorizing representing the other. In: Wilksinon, S., Kitzinger, C. (Eds.), Representing the Other: A Feminism and Psychology Reader. Sage Publications, London.

Willie, C.V., Sanford, J.S., 1995. Turbulence on the college campus and the frustration-aggression hypothesis. In: Willie, C.V., et al. (Eds.), Mental Health, Racism and Sexism. University of Pittsburgh Press, Pittsburgh, PA, pp. 253–276.

World Federation of Occupational Therapists, 2006. Human Rights Position Statement. <http://www.wfot.org/office_files/Human%20Rights%20Position%20Statement> (accessed 14.10.15.).

OCCUPATIONAL THERAPY ACROSS SOUTH AMERICA: AN OVERVIEW OF ITS BACKGROUNDS, CURRENT SITUATION AND SOME CONTEMPORARY ISSUES

VAGNER DOS SANTOS

■ ■

CHAPTER OUTLINE

My aim in this chapter is to highlight a wide range of elements and the ways in which they became issues for South American occupational therapists. These issues pertain to professional training, practice, advocacy and knowledge production. In this chapter I will explore some of the following questions: How is South American occupational therapy distinguished from that of other regions? Have we, South American occupational therapists, established our own independent academic and practice agendas? Do we have a regional identity and common framework that crosses our borders? In bringing a variety of issues together, I do not aim to offer definitive answers, but rather to shed some light on the discussion. I will not defend the idea of a consolidated and unified South American occupational therapy. Neither will I argue that there is a lack of it. In my perspective, there are tensions between the universalized occupational therapy values, prac-

tices, theories and local and regional perspectives. These contemporary issues are both a product and a producer of our professional identity that have spatial/geographical and historical roots. I argue that it is within these tensions that we are defining our self-concept as South American occupational therapists. Since these spatial/geographical and historical backgrounds are the layout of our present status, in the first section of this chapter I will briefly explore these two points.

SOUTH AMERICA

With nearly 390 million inhabitants (World Bank, 2015), South America is a subregion of the American continent. The 12 countries that constitute South America are characterized by a wide diversity of cultures, ecosystems and demographic and epidemiological profiles. From small, rural villages to some of the world's largest megacities, there is a large scope of languages, religions, traditions and social organizations within, and between, our countries.

These realities are also shaped by large disparities and inequalities regarding social and economic opportunities along with historically rooted racism and violence. However, what seems to define a region of diversity and differentiation also represents a rather common socioeconomic and political history. Indeed, the countries in the region share a similar history when it comes to colonization process, dictatorial regimes and, more recently, political shifts and economic ideology.

During the second half of the twentieth century, South America endured a process of social change characterized by strong economic instability, inequality, military dictatorships, restoration of democracy and deployment of neoliberal values followed by the pink tide, that is, the newest wave of leftist governments. The social turn of some governments towards redistributive and social policies have made relative advances in integrating the region and reducing disparities. However, there are common and prevailing challenges in most of our countries, such as political corruption, social violence, inequality, drug production/traffic and abuse, lack of a strong environmental agenda and economic vulnerability, to name only a few.

THE EXPANSION OF MAINSTREAM OCCUPATIONAL THERAPY IN SOUTH AMERICA

Occupational therapy was expanded to South America from the Global North by international agencies in the second half of the twentieth century. The international rehabilitation movement promoted this expansion through agencies such as the World Health Organization, International Labour Organization and United Nations. These agencies found a national interest in implementing these 'new' forms of assistance and training programmes in several countries across the region. Internal factors such as the interest of local governments to reduce treatment costs and tackle the poliomyelitis epidemic supported the process (Testa, 2012, 2013).

During these first decades, occupational therapy in South America was characterized by heavy interna-

tional influence, especially from the United States. It was mainly implemented and practised within strong hierarchical institutions, such as general and psychiatric hospitals, and rehabilitation centres. There was not much space to reflect upon the discipline through our own reality nor to define a self-concept distinguished from the mainstream of occupational therapy, that is, a female majority, health-allied profession subordinated to medicine and based on white, middle-class values.

For instance, in 1956, the United Nations in cooperation with the Hospital of the Medical School at the University of São Paulo created the Instituto Nacional de Reabilitação (do Prado de Carlo and Bartalotti, 2001). The first of its kind in Brazil, it aimed to provide both assistance and training. The training programme in rehabilitation included occupational therapy courses for the hospital staff. International cooperation together with national institutions provided assistance and training in occupational therapy during the 1950s. This was true not only for Brazil, but also for Argentina and Venezuela, followed by Chile and Colombia in the 1960s and Peru in the 1970s (do Prado de Carlo and Bartalotti, 2001; Moreno, 2012; Rodríguez and Blanco, 2014; Testa, 2012). It was from these thematic courses that occupational therapy progressively became an undergraduate programme at universities within the region.

During the following decades practitioners and scholars incipiently developed a professional identity and started to accumulate an increasing body of original and critical thought (see, e.g., Galheigo, 1988; Guajardo, 2014; Moreno and Ruiz, 2014; Paganizzi, 2014). During the dictatorships[1] it is possible to recognize a turning point towards more local and national engaged occupational therapy. I argue that a second turning point is a shift towards South American assemblages within occupational therapy.

---

[1] Several authoritarian regimes ruled South America during the second half of the last century. Military dictatorships were established in several countries (e.g., Uruguay, 1973–1985; Brazil, 1964–1985; Argentina, 1976–1983; Chile, 1973–1990) supported by the United States of America due to its political and economic interest in the region. This was one of the US Cold War policies to depose and prevent leftist governments within the region. 'The United States also cultivated Latin American armed forces by providing training, financing, and equipment' (Dávila, 2013, p. 13).

TURNING POINTS: LOCAL/NATIONAL RUPTURES FROM THE MAINSTREAM OCCUPATIONAL THERAPY TO REGIONAL ASSEMBLAGES

I mentioned previously that occupational therapy in South America has been characterized by a strong influence of northern frameworks. However, throughout political and economic transitions, some occupational therapists were neither mere spectators nor passive actors. I argue that, to some extent, political and social change has produced ruptures within the discipline across the region. Much of the questioning of mainstream occupational therapy began during the 1980s. It was a relative side effect of social movements against the military dictatorships in several countries and it had different results in each country.

Despite the expansion and institutionalization of occupational therapy under military regimes – as in the cases of Brazil, Chile and Argentina – many occupational therapists, together with grassroots movements, favoured the restoration of democracy. Along with this also came other engagements such as political, health and social reforms. This shifted the agenda of occupational therapy towards a critical position regarding globalization, political freedom, and economic and social issues. More recently, this combination of local and national perspectives started to be shared and discussed within the region. It has mobilized occupational therapists to pursue common interests and has established regional professional identities.

In this scenario of similitudes and differences, contemporary issues in occupational therapy within the region can be perceived and presented in a number of ways. The elements and discussion presented in the next section are the result of my engagement and experience as a South American occupational therapist. My perspective is one of many different perspectives of what is a contemporary issue in occupational therapy, relevant and significant in South America.

CONTEMPORARY ISSUES

A key contemporary issue is whether it would be possible to consolidate regional assemblages by valorizing common pasts, respecting diversity and looking for a shared future. Firstly, advocacy, agency and practice have characterized our political actions. Secondly, meetings and congresses have become a key element in defining commons agendas. Thirdly, education at different levels remains a challenge and is a central issue at both the national and the regional level.

Hay que Participar y Negociar [We Must Engage and Negotiate]

The pink tide governments (newest wave of leftist governments) during the first decade of the twenty-first century have increased investments in health and welfare. Social change has been acknowledged as an element that has also influenced occupational therapy (e.g., Blanco and Rodríguez, 2012). To some extent, the region has moved towards social inclusion guided by policies in different sectors, such as education, health, culture, social security, environment and labour.

Agency and advocacy have been new fields of interaction for occupational therapists in the region. There are examples of how occupational therapists have contributed to the development and implementation of these policies. For instance, Chaura and Zorzoli (2014) argue that professional actions have to assure social inclusion and participation based on the principles of human rights. They articulated the involvement of several social groups to assure both cultural representativeness and a range of technical elements of accessibility within the Argentinian telecommunication system (Chaura and Zorzoli, 2014).

Cultural accessibility has also been an element of interest for occupational therapy in Brazil. Dorneles (2014) has discussed cultural accessibility and the implications of occupational therapy's political action. She indicates that political reforms in Brazil have modified policies regarding culture. Consequently, there has been an incentive to decentralize resources and invest in different forms of cultural expressions in the country. Dorneles (2014) exceeded the individual and technical dimension of occupational therapy, and began to influence the political agenda around culture accessibility at the federal level.

It is also important to note that the frameworks and responsibilities of practice have broadened. For instance, mental healthcare is an ongoing challenge in South America. Espinosa and Toro (2014), presenting the *Comunidad Terapeutica de Peñalolén* (Peñalolén Therapeutic Community) in Chile, explain how they articulated different axes of care and social inclusion in practice. They combined intersectoral work, based on the principles of autonomy, citizenship and participation. This centre remarkably breaks away from hierarchical forms of organization, meaning that those who use the service are involved in institutional decision making (Espinosa and Toro, 2014). In the same way, Furtado et al. (2013) also indicate a need to improve theoretical frameworks within our practice. In their project they aimed to offer educational inclusion for people with mental suffering in Brazil, using Paulo Freire's[2] perspective to implement an educational inclusive programme. Here, the intervention intended both to provide formal education for people with mental suffering and to reposition students' and teachers' knowledge within the classroom.

There is some interest towards environmental issues. New fields of action are emerging, such as the intervention of occupational therapy after natural disasters. One example is the efforts of a group of colleagues to build an occupational-oriented intervention for the community after the flood in Santa Fé, Argentina, in 2003 (Ariño et al., 2014). They also supported the development of policies regarding this issue along with local government.

These examples illustrate how occupational therapy can integrate political action and new frameworks. Despite the positive examples mentioned above, there are still plenty of challenges to tackle. Institutions still lack structure and resources that tend to generate socially excluded groups. Furthermore, in times when an 'economic crisis' is affecting South Americans, several countries are reducing social investments and several pink tide governments are redefining their expenditure based on austerity and economic adjustments. Thus social inclusion and integrative care remain a concern of our practice and advocacy.

---

[2]Paulo Freire (1921–1997) was a Brazilian intellectual. He developed an ethics-, critic- and political-oriented comprehension of education. The basis of his theory is the notion of dialogue to overcome and change social, economic and political injustices. His work has had a growing interest among occupational therapists (see, e.g., Magalhães, 2012).

Hay que Compartir y Colaborar [We Must Share and Collaborate]

Much of the regional articulation has been organized through the *Confederação Latinoamericana de Terapia Ocupacional* (CLATO), along with collaborative initiatives. Created in 1997, CLATO aims to develop the profession, strengthening its professional identity and expanding its field of action, as well as increasing international cooperation in the region (Jorge, 2013). Along with national associations CLATO has organized and promoted several congresses.

Many national, regional and international events have been held during the past decade, which have seen an increase in audience and participation. The region gained international attention in 2010, when the World Federation of Occupational Therapists World Congress, traditionally held in the Global North, was hosted for the first time in the Global South, in Chile. To some extent, the congress positioned South American occupational therapy in the global arena and supported regional interaction. Thus, nowadays, many national events reflect a strong interest in promoting cross-national discussion and regional interaction. For instance, the Argentinian Congress held in Paraná, Entre Rios (September 2015) included invited guests from Brazil, Chile, Uruguay and Colombia. It is also worth mentioning the effort in producing complementary documents that systematize and analyse information across the region (see, e.g., Lopes et al., 2012; Moreno, 2012; Oliver et al., 2011; del Carmen Muñoz Palm et al., 2012).

There is still a lack of literature produced within the region. The existing literature has been mainly translated into Portuguese and Spanish from English. Meanwhile, most of the local and regional productions have been limited to some articles (Moreno, 2012). However, there is a growing interest in collective work, especially around collaborative books. Such a book was published in 2014, aiming to explore and analyse contemporary issues in occupational therapy in South America (Dos Santos and Gallassi, 2014). It included contributions from more than 30 occupational therapists from Argentina, Brazil, Chile, Colombia, Peru and Venezuela. Previous books have shared to some extent the same international collaborative interest (Boaretto et al., 2007; Guajardo, 2011).

A forthcoming collaborative publication is another example of this effort and shows the growing interest in discussing Southern occupational therapy. Edited by Alejandro Guajardo, Fátima Correa, Sandra Galheigo, Solángel Garcia and Salvador Simó, colleagues from Chile, Brazil, Colombia, Venezuela and Argentina, along with Spain, explore what they refer to as 'occupational therapies from the south' (Simó et al., forthcoming).

I argue that we still need to critically reflect on and discuss the symbolic and territorial limits of 'the south', since social and historical contexts in South America can be distinguished from other 'southern' perspectives, such as the South of Europe. A traditional definition would include Spain within the Global North (Aulette, 2012). However, it must be acknowledged that occupational therapy in Spain has faced some similar challenges to the profession in South America[3].

Finally, a key element regarding this issue is studies developed through a cross-national comparative perspective. Some projects have already gained this cross-national comparative form; for instance, the ongoing project of Pamela Cristina Bianchi in which she explores the outreach of Brazilian Social Occupational Therapy within education programmes across the region (Bianchi, 2014).

Hay que Enseñar y Aprender [We Must Teach and Learn]

Some countries, such as Brazil and Chile, have had a steady expansion of undergraduate programmes. In Chile, the number of undergraduate students in occupational therapy increased from 2330 in 2009 to 6927 in 2014 across 18 institutions (Colegio de Terapeutas Ocupacionales de Chile, COLTO, 2014). In Brazil, there has also been a remarkable increase. Nowadays, the country has about 70 undergraduate programmes, which is a great step forward when compared to fewer than 20 in the early 1990s. However, there has been a massive concentration of educational programmes in metropolitan regions in both countries. More than half of the programmes are to be found in Santiago de Chile and the Southeast region in Brazil. Meanwhile,

some countries, such as Uruguay, still have challenges in establishing and maintaining new university programmes.

Despite these challenges, the growth of occupational therapy within the region is a reality. Lopes et al. (2008) have acknowledged the need to prioritize critical reflection based on our realities and the way this is discussed in professional practices. However, there is still an element of deep concern about how to promote critical thinking inside the classroom, and there exist contradictions in relation to the education provided within undergraduate programmes. In her study on the expansion of undergraduate programmes in Brazil, Celegati Pan (2014) indicates that most academics had only recently graduated and had limited clinical and research experience. As a consequence, there is a massive reproduction of institutional discourses along with a lack of critical reflection for future actions (Celegati Pan, 2014). There is also an excessive, or even almost exclusive, healthcare focus within the undergraduate programmes, with limited education and training to intervention and work in other fields, such as the social field.

Recognizing that the expansion of education in occupational therapy has not been fully accompanied by a reflexive process or critical thinking, there have been two kinds of responses. One is related to noninstitutional collaborative actions and the other is related to the improvement of institutional presence through graduate programmes and scientific production.

In general, science in academia has increased its strength and resources within the region. The number of doctorates is a clear indication of regional growth, along with other investments (Catanzaro et al., 2014). Graduate programmes in occupational therapy have become an element for concern across the region, especially in Brazil, Chile and Colombia (Oliver et al., 2011). For instance, in Brazil, the improvement of the institutional presence is illustrated by the doctoral and master's programmes in occupational therapy at the Universidade Federal de São Carlos (http://ppgto.ufscar.br/). The programmes are organized in two axes of research, dealing with:

1. The promotion of human development in the context of everyday life, and
2. Social networks and vulnerability (Malfitano et al., 2014).

---

[3]In this sense, comparative and collaborative work to deepen this reflection has been necessary. An example may be a collaborative project among the *Escola Universitària d'Infermeria i Teràpia Ocupacional de Terrassa* (Spain) and the *Universidade de Brasília* (Brazil) (Dos Santos and Sanz, 2015).

This programme is not an isolated event but reflects a long and sustained effort to consolidate a more relevant scholarship within Brazil and in the region. It acquires such relevance not only because it will consolidate our profession (attracting occupational therapists and graduate students from other disciplines), but because it will support a growth regarding research and scientific knowledge, specifically in the two axes of research.

Despite the advances in the institutional level, there have been demands for complementary actions. Regarding noninstitutional education actions, there are some cases that have articulated knowledge with the reality and everyday life of students, scholars and practitioners. Furtado (2014) argues that for students there has been a disconnection between institutional training and personal experience. To fulfil this gap, she created the *Grupo de Estudos sobre a Atividade Humana* (Group for Studies on Human Activity). Recognizing the abilities of her students to reposition themselves, she focused on revisiting the discipline through a more ethically, politically and socially engaged posture in occupational therapy. This experience is a result of her long experience in practice, teaching and researching (Furtado, 2014). Similarly, recognizing that critical reflection, creativity and interdisciplinary knowledge contribute to consolidating professional identity, de Lourdes Feriotti (2014) developed a group outside the institutional bureaucracy called *Grupo de Estudo Interdisciplinar em Terapia Ocupacional* (Group for Interdisciplinary Studies in Occupational Therapy) (de Lourdes Feriotti, 2014).

Both study groups in Brazil have aimed to define an identity sharing the everyday challenges of being an occupational therapist. But even if the reach of these actions is limited to its participants, they are valuable because they facilitate the production of a professional identity.

CONCLUSION

My aim in this chapter was to explore some contemporary issues in occupational therapy across South America. These points are obviously moving targets, never static or fixed. The development of occupational therapy in our region is moving fast, and with it comes a necessity to pursue our discussion and our reflexivity over the possibilities of regional assemblages. I have brought into the discussion some elements that will slowly but surely be replaced by new elements that will need both scientific scrutiny and political engagement – in other words, fresh, new contemporary issues.

Frank and Zemke (2008, p. 115) argued that there is 'a need for a comparative and critical history of the occupational therapy profession in various countries, regions and linguistic-cultural spheres'. In this sense, occupational therapy across South America is experiencing a movement towards more interactions, developments and agreements. Our challenge is to consolidate this movement of regional assemblages, while respecting national and local realities.

Occupational therapy has the capacity to expand its borders across national frontiers. South American occupational therapy identity has been built from the tensions between dominant occupational therapy paradigms and local and national realities and frameworks. These tensions could lead to a fully engaged body of occupational therapists, working to define regional assemblages. I believe that it is only by looking back into our past, understanding where we come from, and acknowledging our challenges that we can draw a clear path towards a common future.

Acknowledgements

I would like to thank my wife, Sara Leon, a social anthropologist, who kindly addressed questions that helped to build and shape this chapter. I am also very thankful to Eliana dos Anjos Furtado, who sparked my interest for occupational therapy, for her unconditional support.

REFERENCES

Ariño, R., Bofelli, M., Chiapessoni, D., Boggio, C., Demichelis, M., Demiry, M., et al., 2014. Terapia Ocupacional en situaciones de desastres. La construción de nuevos territórios. In: Dos Santos, V., Gallassi, A. (Eds.), Questões Contemporâneas Da Terapia Ocupacional Na América Do Sul. CRV, Curitiba, Brazil, pp. 205–218.

Aulette, J., 2012. North-South. In: Ritezer, G. (Ed.), Wiley-Blackwell Encyclopedia of Globalization. Wiley-Blackwell, Hoboken, NJ.

Bianchi, P., 2014. A formação da Terapia Ocupacional na América Latina sob a perspectiva da Terapia Ocupacional Social Brasileira. (Master Project). Universidade Federal de São Carlos, São Carlos.

Blanco, G., Rodríguez, V., 2012. Cambios sociales y Terapia Ocupacional. Rol del terapeuta ocupacional en el contexto contemporáneo. Rev. Ter. Ocupacional Galicia 9, 190–325.

Boaretto, R., Galvani, D., Barros, D., Lopes, R., Reis, T., 2007. Terapéutica Ocupacional en el Campo Social: construyendo caminos y rescatando proyectos con adultos que viven en calles. In: Paganizzi, L. (Ed.), Terapia Ocupacional Psicosocial: Escenarios Clínicos y Comunitarios. Polemos, Buenos Aires, pp. 203–208.

Catanzaro, M., Miranda, G., Palmer, L., Bajak, A., 2014. South American science: big players. Nature 510, 204–206. doi:10.1038/510204a.

Celegati Pan, L., 2014. Políticas de ensino superior, graduação em Terapia Ocupacional e o ensino de Terapia Ocupacional Social no Brasil. Master's dissertation. Universidade Federal de São Carlos, São Carlos.

Chaura, L.E., Zorzoli, F.J.M., 2014. Televisón Digital. Desafíos el processo en Argentina. Comunicación, Participación social y Derechos Humanos. In: Dos Santos, V., Gallassi, A. (Eds.), Questões Contemporâneas Da Terapia Ocupacional Na América Do Sul. CRV, Curitiba, Brazil, pp. 185–204.

COLTO, 2014. Antecedentes sobre la formación Universitaria de Terapeutas Ocupacionales en Chile. Colegio de Terapeutas Ocupacionales de Chile, Santiago, Chile.

Dávila, J., 2013. Dictatorship in South America. John Wiley & Sons, Hoboken, NJ.

de Lourdes Feriotti, M., 2014. Educação fora da sala de aula. In: Dos Santos, V., Gallassi, A. (Eds.), Questões Contemporâneas Da Terapia Ocupacional Na América Do Sul. CRV, Curitiba, Brazil, pp. 103–112.

del Carmen Muñoz Palm, R., Navas, A., Puche, A.R., Mengelberg, E.G., Salas, E.N., Bolaños, M.C., 2012. Catálogo Latinoamericano de libros y revistas de Terapia Ocupacional. <http://www.scribd.com/doc/145985868/Catalogo-latinoamericano-de-livros-e-revistas-de-terapia-ocupacional#scribd> Published 6 June 2013.

do Prado de Carlo, M.M.R., Bartalotti, C.C., 2001. Terapia ocupacional no Brasil: fundamentos e perspectivas. Plexus Editora, São Paulo.

Dorneles, P., 2014. Acessibilidade Cultural. Uma nova atuação dos Terapeutas Ocupacionais. In: Dos Santos, V., Gallassi, A. (Eds.), Questões Contemporâneas Da Terapia Ocupacional Na América Do Sul. CRV, Curitiba, Brazil, pp. 151–158.

Dos Santos, V., Gallassi, A., 2014. Questões Contemporâneas da Terapia Ocupacional na América do Sul. CRV, Curitiba, Brazil.

Dos Santos, V., Sanz, S., 2015. Terapia Ocupacional en España y Brasil. Un estudio critico de las realidades. Universidade de Brasília/Fundação de Apoio à Pesquisa do Distrito Federal, Brasília.

Espinosa, G.S., Toro, A.M., 2014. Salud Mental en Chile. Lo cotidiano, Generación de redes y Lazo. In: Dos Santos, V., Gallassi, A. (Eds.), Questões Contemporâneas Da Terapia Ocupacional Na América Do Sul. CRV, Curitiba, Brazil, pp. 169–184.

Frank, G., Zemke, R., 2008. Occupational Therapy fondations for political engagement and social transformation. In: Pollard, N., et al. (Eds.), A Political Practice of Occupational Therapy. Elsevier Health Sciences, Edinburgh.

Furtado, E., 2014. Um novo processo educativo para a formação de Terapeutas Ocupacionais. In: Dos Santos, V., Donatti, A. (Eds.), Questões Contemporâneas Da Terapia Ocupacional Na América Do Sul. CRV, Curitiba, Brazil, pp. 93–102.

Furtado, E., Alves, G., Dos Santos, V., Marin, P., Chrempach, E., Nobre, C., et al., 2013. Relato de experiência inclusiva. In: Danesi, M., Timm, E. (Eds.), Caminhos Para Educação Inclusiva. EDiPUCRS, Porto Alegre, Brazil, pp. 31–40.

Galheigo, S.M., 1988. Terapia Ocupacional: a produção do conhecimento e o cotidiano da prática sob o poder disciplinar – em busca de um depoimento coletivo. Master's dissertation. Universidade de Campinas, Campinas, Brazil.

Guajardo, A., 2011. Prólogo. In: Rojas, C. (Ed.), Ocupación: Sentido, Realización y Libertad. Diálogos Ocupacionales En Torno Al Sujeto, La Sociedad y El Medio Ambiente. Universidad Nacional de Colombia, Bogotá.

Guajardo, A., 2014. Una Terapia Ocupacional crítica como posibilidad. In: Dos Santos, V., Gallassi, A. (Eds.), Questões Contemporâneas Da Terapia Ocupacional Na América Do Sul. CRV, Curitiba, Brazil, pp. 159–165.

Jorge, Z.S., 2013. Terapia Ocupacional de Latinoamérica para el Mundo. Rev. Ter. Ocupacional Galicia 10, 1–8.

Lopes, R.E., Oliver, F.C., Malfitano, A.P.S., Galheigo, S.M., de Almeida, M.C., 2008. XI Encontro Nacional de Docentes de Terapia Ocupacional: refletindo sobre os processos de formação acadêmica e profissional. Rev. Ter. Ocupacional Universidade São Paulo 19, 159–166. doi:10.11606/issn.2238-6149.v19i3.

Lopes, R.E., de Oliveira Borba, P.L., Silva, C.R., Malfitano, A.P.S., 2012. Terapia Ocupacional no campo social no Brasil e na América Latina: panorama, tensões e reflexões a partir de práticas profissionais. Cad. Ter. Ocupacional Ufscar 20 (1).

Magalhães, L., 2012. What would Paulo Freire think of occupational science? In: Whiteford, G.E., Hocking, C. (Eds.), Occupational Science. Wiley-Blackwell, Chichester, West Sussex, pp. 8–19.

Malfitano, A.P.S., Matsukura, T., Martinez, C., Emmel, M.L., Lopes, R.E., 2014. Pós-Gradução em Terapia Ocupacional: primeiro programa de mestrado acadêmico na América do Sul. In: Dos Santos, V., Gallassi, A. (Eds.), Questões Contemporâneas Da Terapia Ocupacional Na América do Sul. CRV, Curitiba, Brazil, pp. 113–122.

Moreno, A.F., 2012. Publicações periódicas da terapia ocupacional na América Latina. Cad. Ter. Ocupacional Ufscar 20 (2).

Moreno, A., Ruiz, S., 2014. Fundamentos conceituales reflexiones sobre el abandono e Institucionalización Y la Terapia Ocupacional. In: Dos Santos, V., Gallassi, A. (Eds.), Questões Contemporâneas Da Terapia Ocupacional Na América Do Sul. CRV, Curitiba, Brazil, pp. 141–158.

Oliver, F.C., Almeida, M.C., Toldrá, R.C., Galheigo, S.M., Lancman, S., Lopes, R.E., et al., 2011. Desafios da educação em Terapia Ocupacional na América Latina para a próxima década. Rev. Ter. Ocupacional Universidade São Paulo 22, 298–307. doi:10.11606/issn.2238-6149.v22i3.

Paganizzi, L., 2014. Sobre la Emergencia de los Fundamentos sociales: notas sobre las prácticas comunitarias en Argentina 1980-2010. In: Dos Santos, V., Gallassi, A. (Eds.), Questões

Contemporâneas Da Terapia Ocupacional Na América Do Sul. CRV, Curitiba, Brazil, pp. 123–140.

Rodríguez, V., Blanco, G., 2014. Venezuela. Contextualización, História y Cultura de la Terapia Ocupacional. In: Dos Santos, V., Donatti, A. (Eds.), Questões Contemporâneas Da Terapia Ocupacional Na América Do Sul. CRV, Curitiba, Brazil, pp. 81–90.

Simó, S., et al. (Eds.), In press. Terapias Ocupacionales desde el Sur. Derechos humanos, ciudadanía y participación. Ediciones Panamericana, Buenos Aires.

Testa, D., 2012. Aportes para el debate sobre los inicios de la profesionalización de la terapia ocupacional en Argentina. Rev. Chil. Ter. Ocupacional 12, 72.

Testa, D.E., 2013. Curing by doing: la poliomielitis y el surgimiento de la terapia ocupacional en Argentina, 1956–1959. Hist Ciênc Saúde-Manguinhos 20, 1571–1584.

World Bank, 2015. <http://data.worldbank.org> (accessed 09.12.15.).

23

INVESTIGATING OCCUPATIONAL THERAPY: FROM DISABILITY STUDIES TO ABILITY STUDIES

GREGOR WOLBRING ■ TSING-YEE (EMILY) CHAI

Occupational therapy was formed in the context of historical events that created its purpose and aim, with its origins traced back to providing services to war veterans and those institutionalized in mental hospitals, tuberculosis sanatoriums, and community workshops (Friedland et al., 2000). In the 1980s, occupational therapists were challenged to advocate on behalf of people living with chronic illness and disability and to take a global interest in the social issues that affect the lives of the people they serve (Trentham, 2001). Since then, occupational therapy has added promotion of well-being, enablement, person-centred services, evidence-based practice and community-based practices with new roles in companies, greater government relations and greater access to information and communication technology to its focus (Green et al., 2001). Occupational therapy is a profession that is seen as being crucial to the development of society and to addressing societal issues of the present and future (Freeman et al., 2014). Occupational therapy research has started to investigate societal issues such as the ecological sustainability of occupations (Wagman, 2014). In 2014, the Canadian Association of Occupational Therapists (CAOT) identified the following trends as being important to the redirection of the occupational therapy field: an ageing population, increased survival in events of accidents and injuries, increased awareness of disability, job stress, greater promotion of well-being and prevention, greater numbers of mental problems, and a more informed audience about health and health concerns (CAOT, 2014a). In 2014, CAOT also outlined the values and beliefs (Box 23-1) that should guide occupational therapists (CAOT, 2014b).

BOX 23-1
BELIEFS OF THE CANADIAN ASSOCIATION OF OCCUPATIONAL THERAPISTS

About occupation, we believe that:
- Occupation gives meaning to life;
- Occupation is an important determinant of health, well-being, and justice;
- Occupation organizes behaviour;
- Occupation develops and changes over a lifetime;
- Occupation shapes and is shaped by environments;
- Occupation has therapeutic potential.

About the person, we believe that:
- Humans are occupational beings;
- Every person is unique;
- Every person has intrinsic dignity and worth;
- Every person has the right to make choices about life;
- Every person has the right to self-determination;
- People have some ability to participate in occupations;
- People have some potential to change;
- People are social and spiritual beings;
- People have diverse abilities for participating in occupations;
- People shape and are shaped by their environments.

About the environment, we believe that:
- The environment includes cultural, institutional, physical, and social components;
- The environment influences choice, organization, performance, and satisfaction in occupations.

About health, well-being, and justice, we believe that:
- Health is more than the absence of disease;
- Health is strongly influenced by having choice and control in everyday occupations;
- Health has personal dimensions associated with spiritual meaning and satisfaction in occupations, and it has social dimensions associated with fairness and equitable opportunity in occupations;
- Well-being extends beyond health to quality of life;
- Justice concerns are for meaningful choice and social inclusion, so that all people may participate as fully as possible in society.

Source: Canadian Association of Occupational Therapists (2014b).

According to Service Canada statistics, the average annual growth rate for occupational therapist jobs from 2012 to 2016 is 3.2%, compared to 0.7% for all occupations (Service Canada, 2013), with the trend expected to grow sharply. As such, a foresight and broad education of occupational therapy students becomes ever-increasingly essential. We contribute two lenses to the endeavour that will sharpen students' engagement with the social aspects of occupational therapy. One is the disability studies lens, which is an academic field that investigates the social disablement experienced by people labelled as impaired or ability deficient. The second is the lens of ability studies, which investigates ability expectation hierarchies, preferences and their impact (Wolbring, 2008, 2012). Engaging with these two lenses allows occupational therapy students to engage with an ever-changing landscape of challenges occupational therapists face in a foresight fashion and to engage with the trends, values and beliefs identified.

WHAT IS DISABILITY STUDIES?

Disability studies is an academic field that investigates the social disablement experienced by people labelled as impaired or ability deficient. Its scholars question the narrative that claims that the disablism (the problems faced by people labelled as physical, mental, neuro or cognitive ability impaired) originates from a body that does not fulfil species-typical physical, mental, neuro, and cognitive abilities (medical model of disablement). Instead, disability studies scholars posit that the problems originate from the societal environment that expects certain physical, mental, neuro or cognitive abilities (social model of disablement). Disability studies scholars question the labelling of someone as impaired if one does not have species-typical abilities. Deaf culture and the discourse around neurodiversity question the species-typical normatization of body-linked abilities. Indeed, 'many disabled people perceive themselves in a cultural identity war with the so called non-disabled people where their self-identity understanding of being ability diverse and ability variant, as being a culture and not being ability deviant and ability deficient is rejected by many' (Wolbring, 2013a, p. 189).

DISABILITY STUDIES AND OCCUPATIONAL THERAPY

Engaging with disability studies allows occupational therapists to critically engage with the characterization and identifications of disablements, the characterization of the body of their client and the characterization of the assistive devices used by their clients, to name just three areas. The following CAOT statements can be found in Box 23-1: every person is unique, every person has intrinsic dignity and worth, every person has the right to make choices about their life; and every person has the right to self-determination. If occupational therapy, as a field, truly believes in the right to self-determination, this would have to include the right to self-identification. This means that occupational therapy and its students, researchers, and practitioners have to use factual language, thus leaving it up to the person to self-identify. For example, to say that person X cannot walk is a factual statement but to say person X is 'walking impaired' assumes that one has to walk and reproduces the cultural construction of the normativity of walking. To give another example, based on the genetic make-up of the human species, humans do not have the ability to fly and must rely on planes or other assistive devices to achieve this ability; however, humans do not refer to this lack of ability as a 'flying impairment'. However, if one looks at the section 'Practice Settings' on the CAOT web page <https://www.caot.ca/default.asp?pageid=3824>. (CAOT, 2014c), the use of medical and not factual language is evident, denying people their right to self-determination of their identity.

The characterization of an assistive device is another example of self-determination. A hierarchy of worthiness of assistive devices is evident in the general literature. The term *wheelchair bound* is used to sell bionic legs as the liberator from such confinement (Panesar and Wolbring, 2014) and ignores that the wheelchair is for many a tool of liberation and that humans are more confined to their legs than most wheelchair users are confined to their wheelchair (Wolbring, 2003). On 9 October, 2014, a search of the CAOT website for the term *wheelchair bound* resulted in 23 hits, indicating a rather biased approach to at least one assistive device.

As to the overall medical labelling of the person, this is a long-standing criticism of occupational therapy (Townsend, 1993). Chacala et al. (2014) state:

Occupational therapy's view of disability has traditionally drawn on a medical model, in which disability means impairment, limitation, inferiority, deviance from the norm, warranting discomfort,

pity, charity, or concern. Despite theoretical attention to environment and social inclusion in occupational therapy, disability still tends to be seen as an individual deficit requiring remediation. The emphasis remains on disability as undesirable, while rehabilitation reinscribes notions of normal and abnormal ways of doing things. (p. 108)

At the same time, the dominance of biased, judgemental language around ability-diverse people seems to be puzzling given the claim that 'occupational therapy's language, ideas and practice are similar to civil rights, feminist, ethnic, gay and lesbian, disability and other social justice movements' (Townsend, 1993, p. 176).

It has been proposed that occupational therapists should increase their engagement with disability studies and disability theory, which is so far seen as lacking, because it would 'raise important questions about many of occupational therapy's central issues, and critique professional power and privilege and the systemic oppression of disabled people with which rehabilitation professionals are perceived to collude' (Hammell, 2007, p. 366). Engaging with disability studies is seen as a way for occupational therapists to 'become more aware and reflexive practitioners with respect to the disability experience and their roles as advocates' (Phelan, 2011, p. 170). Hamilton (2013) states:

Occupational therapists are natural helpers, but our helping can contribute to oppression of people with disabilities rather than enablement of participation by them. We believe that introducing occupational therapy students to disability studies specifically and to critical thinking generally may decrease the frequency with which occupational therapy is oppressive. (p. 80)

The 2005 September/October open access issue of the *American Journal of Occupational Therapy* has various articles highlighting the utility of disability studies for occupational therapy (e.g., Kielhofner, 2005).

However, the utility for occupational therapists to engage with disability studies is not only about obtaining a different view on people labelled as impaired. Engaging with disability studies will expose occupational therapy educators, students, researchers and practitioners to the cultural dynamic of ability expectations (want stage) and ableism (need stage). The disabled people rights movement coined the term *ableism* in the 1970s to highlight the negative societal consequences people can experience if they perform below species-typical physical, mental, neuro or cognitive ability expectations (Wolbring, 2012). However, the cultural reality of ability expectations and ableism goes far beyond how it is used in disability studies and is of importance to engage with by the occupational therapy field, as we will show in the remaining sections of this chapter.

ABILITY EXPECTATIONS AND ABLEISM BEYOND DISABILITY STUDIES

Every individual, household, community, group, sector, region and country cherishes and promotes some abilities and finds others nonessential; for example, some individuals see the ability to buy a given product as essential, while others do not; some perceive living in an equitable society as important, others do not. Countries make comparisons between themselves and others based on whether they have certain abilities (e.g., provision of good education or high employment, or being competitive) (Wolbring, 2008, 2012). Although ability expectations can be applied in positive ways, they are often used to justify negative treatments of others whereby one powerful group decides that a certain ability is essential and that another group lacks this 'essential' ability (Wolbring, 2008). To provide one example not covered by the disability studies field, the power structure controlled by men has constructed a narrative that values rationality as an essential cognitive ability and men ultimately had (in many places still have) the power to control the narrative around who were, and who were not, deemed rational beings. In the UK in the last century, the issue of irrationality played itself out around the suffragette's fight for women's right to vote, whereby the dominant narrative was that women were irrational beings and therefore could not vote (Buechler, 1990; Van Helmond, 1992). The claim that women are irrational beings is still used (Daily, 2014).

Ability expectations constantly change. Changes in ability expectations are often triggered by scientific research and technological developments. At the same time, ability expectations also influence the direction of scientific research and technological developments. The *Deus Ex: Invisible War* computer game dialogue between Alex D and Paul Denton, the two main protagonists in the game from 2003, captures many ability expectation and ableism dynamics:

Conversation between Alex D and Paul Denton

Paul Denton: If you want to even out the social order, you have to change the nature of power itself. Right? And what creates power? Wealth, physical strength, legislation – maybe – but none of those is the root principle of power.

Alex D: I'm listening.

Paul Denton: Ability is the ideal that drives the modern state. It's a synonym for one's worth, one's social reach, one's 'election', in the Biblical sense, and it's the ideal that needs to be changed if people are to begin living as equals.

Alex D: And you think you can equalize humanity with biomodification?

Paul Denton: The commodification of ability – tuition, of course, but, increasingly, genetic treatments, cybernetic protocols, now biomods – has had the side effect of creating a self-perpetuating aristocracy in all advanced societies. When ability becomes a public resource, what will distinguish people will be what they do with it. Intention. Dedication. Integrity. The qualities we would choose as the bedrock of the social order. (Wikiquote)

Ability expectations do not only influence how humans relate to each other; the ways humans interact with nature are also characterized by ability expectations with, for example, anthropocentrism and bio/eco-centrism exhibiting different ability expectations of what nature provides to humans (Wolbring, 2011a, 2013b, 2014).

ECO-ABILITY EXPECTATIONS AND ECO-ABLEISM

Ecology is about the interrelationship of organisms and their environment. According to Aoyama et al. (2012), Wilcock was the first to make explicit links between occupation and ecological sustainability. They acknowledge that research in this area is still sparse (Aoyama et al., 2012). Wagman investigated in 2014 'what has recently been written about how occupational therapy/therapists/science can contribute to ecological sustainability and the prevention of more severe climate change' (p. 161). Aoyama et al. (2012) state:

> *With a concern for the ecosystem and sustainable resources, occupational therapists could become advocates for, and advisers of, the occupations suited to individuals to meet their needs yet to sustain resources and the ecology. The way forward is to be part of the economic and ecological debate, with the occupation for health needs at the forefront of the agenda. It is a different role, but it is the practice of occupational therapy at the global level. (p. 217)*

They further state that 'occupations can certainly support human well-being, but many human occupations are now impacting the planet to such an extent that they are reducing the ability of ecosystem services to support well-being' (Aoyama et al., 2012, p. 220).

The abilities one favours impact human–human, human–animal, and human–nature relationships. Players involved in the shaping of ecological discourses exhibit ability expectations that influence how they define ecological problems and solutions to the problem, and whom they invite to the table as stakeholders and knowledge producers (Wolbring, 2011b, 2013b, 2014). Naess (1973), for example, described the central objective of the 'shallow ecology movement' as the increase of the ability to enhance the health and affluence of people in developed countries. By contrast, Naess characterized the 'deep ecology movement' to focus on building the ability to promote 'biospherical egalitarianism' (Naess, 1973, p. 95). Ecofeminism is seen to reject the ability expectation of 'dominance, competition, materialism, and technoscientific exploitation inherent in modernist, competition-based social systems' (Besthorn and McMillen, 2002, p. 226) and nourishes the ability expectation of 'caring and compassion and the creation and nurturing of life' (Besthorn and McMillen, 2002, p. 226). It would be interesting for occupational therapy students to investigate where their field stands in relation to human–nature relationships.

ABILITY EXPECTATIONS AND OCCUPATIONAL THERAPY: SOME CHALLENGES

The dynamics around ability expectations pose numerous challenges to the field of occupational therapy.

Language

One challenge is the use of language. Language is an important concern, as the sections engaging with disability studies have already shown. Even if one focuses on abilities, one can use terms, such as *ability defective*, that present the individual as the problem. Terms such as *ability expectation oppressed* or *ability expectation oppression* put a focus on societal framing as the problem. It is up to the occupational therapy field to decide whether to focus on the individual defective or societal framing language. We posit that language that focuses on the societal framing, such as ability expectation oppressed and ability expectation oppression, fits well with concepts such as occupational justice, occupational rights and enablement.

Self-identity Security

Self-identity security means that one has the self-determination of one's identity. Having occupational therapists engage with self-identity security is not only important for people covered within the disability studies discourse but for all kind of social groups that occupational therapy engages with that are defined by others. Engaging with the broad area of self-identity security helps occupational therapists to rectify some of the negative connotations around occupational therapy, specifically that occupational therapy is situated within a biomedical paradigm (Donnelly et al., 2014), and to engage with indicators such as quality of life and the ability to engage in the community.

Power and Privilege

Having certain abilities such as being competitive is a source of power over others and having power allows one to influence which abilities are seen as essential and, in effect, set the tone for how people are treated and who is labelled as ability deficient and of which abilities. Power often allows for privileges. Having certain abilities is the portal to access privileges such as income, political influence and employment (Wolbring, 2014). Hammell (2013) states, '[T]he occupational therapy profession has not engaged in sustained critical reflection about the vulnerability of many clients and the asymmetrical power relations that make meaningful partnerships with professionals inordinately difficult' (p. 145). To reflect on all facets of power related to abilities and ability expectations and the privileges they are linked to will further the ability of occupational therapists to engage with the trends, values and beliefs of their profession, including the advancement of social and occupational justice.

Ability Inequity and Inequality

Inequities and inequalities based on abilities one has access to or exhibits are a global problem (Wolbring, 2010). For both, ability inequity (unjust or unfair distribution) and ability inequality (uneven distribution), two subgroups exist. One group is linked to intrinsic bodily abilities and the other group is linked to external abilities – abilities generated by human interventions that impact humans. These two subgroups of internal and external ability inequities and inequalities are quite distinct in their effects and discourse dynamics, involved stakeholders and goals. Both subgroups pose challenges for the occupational therapy field.

> Definition: 'Ability inequality is a descriptive term denoting any uneven distribution of access to and protection from abilities generated through human interventions, right or wrong'. (Wolbring, 2010, p. 97)
> Definition: 'Ability inequality is a descriptive term denoting any uneven judgment of abilities intrinsic to biological structures such as the human body, right or wrong'. (Wolbring, 2010, p. 97)
> Definition: 'Ability inequity is a normative term denoting an unjust or unfair distribution of access to and protection from abilities generated through human interventions'. (Wolbring, 2010, p. 97)
> Definition: 'Ability inequity is a normative term denoting an unjust or unfair judgment of abilities intrinsic to biological structures such as the human body'. (Wolbring, 2010, p. 97)

If occupational therapists are to advance social and occupational justice, they have to analyse ability-related inequalities and inequities and what role they can play in decreasing such inequities and inequalities. At the same time, occupational therapists have to understand how their actions impact ability inequalities and inequities, and whether their actions might, in fact, increase ability inequalities and inequities.

Ability Security

Ability security (Wolbring, 2010) could be seen as part of the World Health Organization (WHO) framework of human security (Commission on Human Security, 2003) which has seven dimensions: economic security (assured basic income), food security (physical, economic and social access to food), health security (relative freedom from disease and infection), environmental security (access to sanitary water supply, clean air and a nondegraded land system), personal security (security from physical violence and threats), community security (security of cultural integrity), and political security (protection of basic human rights) (United Nations Development Programme, 1994). Ability security means that one can experience all aspects of human security independent of the abilities one has. An occupational therapy field that thinks purely in medical ways and about adding body-linked abilities to the person is ill equipped to ensure ability security. To ensure ability security means in many cases to ensure that the client can experience human security with the abilities they have; adding abilities is often not an option.

ABILITY STUDIES AND OCCUPATIONAL THERAPY

Ability studies allows for the study of multiple subject formations, social relationships and lived experiences based on diverse ability expectations and the actions linked to such expectations. As such, ability studies is useful to investigate many facets of ability expectation factors that impact the beliefs mentioned in Box 23-1, such as the belief that people are social beings. Ability expectations are linked to value, labelling, conflict, choice, identity, motivation, achievement, self-determination, body theories and social constructivism. Ableism is one possible consequence of ability expectations. Ableism is a term developed by the disabled people rights movement and the academic field of disability studies to question the favouritism for species-typical body abilities and the disablement of people labelled as not having these 'essential' abilities (Campbell Kumari, 2001; Carlson, 2001; Overboe, 2007).

This form of ableism adds to the labelling theory discourse which focuses on the linguistic tendency of majorities to negatively label minorities or those seen as deviant from the social norm. We have highlighted the labelling preference in occupational therapy related to people perceived to be impaired. It would be a useful exercise to map the labelling of people with below species-typical abilities within occupational therapy over an extended time frame to observe for any differences. Beyond the impaired labelled group it would be a useful exercise to map out how the field of occupational therapy labels different groups of clients and to outline the biases found.

Although ableism was developed to make visible the active disablement of people with disabilities (Miller et al., 2004), the cultural reality of ability expectations and the disablism experienced by entities not fulfilling ability expectations is a much broader phenomenon. Value theory records what people do value and attempts to understand why they value certain things. Ability expectation is about valuing certain abilities. It would be interesting to map out ability values of occupational therapists and their clients covering the broad scope of occupational therapy involvement outlined in this chapter.

Expectancy-value theory of achievement motivation (the ability desired) is used to analyse dynamics of various discourses. Ability desires are evident within occupational therapy. Cooper states, '[W]e need to show payers, who are increasingly concerned about their own economic viability and who expect return on investment, that occupational therapy services make economic sense' (Cooper, 2012, p. 206). Aoyama et al. (2012) believe:

[W]ith a concern for the ecosystem and sustainable resources, occupational therapists could become advocates for and advisers of the occupations suited to individuals to meet their needs yet to sustain resources and the ecology. The way forward is to be part of the economic and ecological debate, with the occupation for health needs at the forefront of the agenda. It is a different role, but it is the practice of occupational therapy at the global level. (p. 217)

Conflict theory emphasizes possible conflict between social groups. Groups of people with different ability expectations are often in conflict with each other. Indeed, it might be interesting for occupational therapy students to map out ability expectation conflicts evident between different groups involved in the various facets of occupational therapy. Ability expectations influence, and are shaped by, the pillars and carriers of institutions and mechanisms and processes by which institutions persist or change (Scott, 2008). Ability expectations are a factor in many of the components of the discourse-institutionalist framework developed by Genus (2014). It would be interesting to investigate how institutional ability expectations impact occupational therapy to fulfil and support the beliefs listed in Box 23-1. Finally, one chooses between different abilities which can be classified as a 'social choice' problem (Sen, 2013, p. 10). Here, it would be interesting to investigate which social choices impact occupational therapy in which way.

CONCLUSION

According to Hammell and Iwama (2012):

[C]ritical occupational therapy is a committed form of practice that recognizes the impact of inequities such as class, gender, race, ethnicity, economics, age, ability, and sexuality, acknowledges that well-being cannot be achieved by focusing solely on enhancing individuals' abilities, and thus endeavours to facilitate change at both individual and environmental levels. (p. 386)

The field of disability studies investigates ability inequities, inequalities, privileges and disablements, as well as the lack of ability security and self-identity security focusing on body-linked abilities and people labelled as impaired. As such, it has a premise that fits with the beliefs stated in Box 23-1, such as that every person has the right to make choices about life, and every person has the right to self-determination.

Engaging with disability studies allows occupational therapy students and practitioners to engage with the beliefs about the person, occupation and health, and improve the situation of people labelled as impaired.

Ability studies allows the linkage of ability inequities, inequalities, privileges and disablements and the lack of ability security and self-identity security to class, sex, race, ethnicity, economics, age, sexuality, species and nature. Ability studies allows for the investigation of occupational satisfaction, occupational justice, the impact of occupation on behaviour, the impact of ability expectations on occupations, and the impact of ability expectations linked to scientific advancement and technological development on the landscape of occupations. Ability studies also investigates the linkage of humans to nature. As such, it allows the investigation of all aspects of the environment (cultural, institutional, physical and social components) covered in Box 23-1 and the investigation of how the environment influences choice, organization, performance and satisfaction in occupations. Aoyama et al. (2012) state:

A near sacred assumption of both occupational science and occupational therapy has been that occupations support well-being, but we might extend Hammell's (2009) recent critique of this assumption by asking if this is still the case when many contemporary occupations in the industrialized world overexploit ecosystem services and thus weaken the very capability of ecosystems to support our well-being? (p. 220)

Indeed, students and practitioners engaging with the ability expectation framework can ask questions like which occupations are sustainable, and which meanings and frameworks of occupation will still be sustainable?

It is important to seek answers to the question of which occupations still allow one to feel well and have ability security? Will, for example, a system where livelihood is linked to payments for the performance of occupations still be viable? Given the beliefs voiced in Box 23-1, one would expect occupational therapy education to give students the tools to investigate new areas of practice, going beyond the restoration of function. If the trend is indeed holding that occupational therapists should become self-employed and have to find their niche within the field, then the disability

studies and ability studies lens allows for an investigation into the reality of the world that could unearth new fields of engagement. It allows one to also look at the economic viability of one's goal which is seen as increasingly important (Cooper, 2012). Disability studies and ability studies facilitate the ability to act as a change agent, regarded as an important ability of occupational therapists (Hodgetts et al., 2007; Klinger and Bossers, 2009).

REFERENCES

Aoyama, M., Hudson, M.J., Hoover, K.C., 2012. Occupation mediates ecosystem services with human well-being. J. Occup. Sci. 19, 213–225.

Besthorn, F.H., McMillen, D.P., 2002. The oppression of women and nature: ecofeminism as a framework for an expanded ecological social work. Fam. Soc. 83, 221–232.

Buechler, S.M., 1990. Women's Movements in the United States: Woman Suffrage, Equal Rights, and Beyond. Rutgers University Press, New Brunswick, NJ.

Campbell Kumari, F., 2001. Inciting legal fictions: 'disability's' date with ontology and the ableist body of the law. Griffith Law Rev. 10, 42.

Canadian Association of Occupational Therapists (CAOT), 2014a. Current Trends Affecting Occupational Therapy. Canadian Association of Occupational Therapists, Ottawa. Available online at: <http://www.caot.ca/default.asp?pageid=291> (accessed 10.05.16.).

Canadian Association of Occupational Therapists (CAOT), 2014b. Occupational Therapy Values and Beliefs. Canadian Association of Occupational Therapy, Ottawa. Available online at: <https://www.caot.ca/default.asp?pageid=3619> (accessed 10.05.16.).

Canadian Association of Occupational Therapists (CAOT), 2014c. Occupational Therapy – As defined by the Canadian Association of Occupational Therapists. Canadian Association of Occupational Therapists, Ottawa. Available online at: <https://www.caot.ca/default.asp?pageid=3824> (accessed 10.05.16.).

Carlson, L., 2001. Cognitive ableism and disability studies: feminist reflections on the history of mental retardation. Hypatia 16, 124–146.

Chacala, A., McCormack, C., Collins, B., Beagan, B.L., 2014. My view that disability is okay sometimes clashes: experiences of two disabled occupational therapists. Scand. J. Occup. Ther. 21, 107–115.

Commission on Human Security, 2003. Human Security Now. Available online at: <http://reliefweb.int/sites/reliefweb.int/files/resources/91BAEEDBA50C6907C1256D19006A9353-chs-security-may03.pdf> (accessed 10.05.16.).

Cooper, J.E., 2012. Reflections on the professionalization of occupational therapy: time to put down the looking glass. Can. J. Occup. Ther. 79, 199–209.

Daily, S., 2014. Japanese Women Boycott Sex With Any Man Who Votes For Tokyo's 'Menstruating Women Are Irrational' Governor. Daily Star, 7 February.

Donnelly, C.A., Brenchley, C.L., Crawford, C.N., Letts, L.J., 2014. The emerging role of occupational therapy in primary care. Le nouveau rôle de l'ergothérapie dans les soins primaires. Can. J. Occup. Ther. 81, 51–61.

Freeman, A.R., Robinson, I., Cardwell, T., 2014. Proficiency in occupational therapy practice: reflections from the 2013 Occupational Therapy Canada Forum. Occup. Ther. Now 16, 26–28.

Friedland, J., Robinson, I., Cardwell, T., 2000. In the beginning: CAOT from 1926–1939. Occup. Ther. Now 3, 1, 15–19. Available online at: <https://www.caot.ca/pdfs/CAOT1926_39.pdf> (accessed 10.05.16.).

Genus, A., 2014. Governing sustainability: a discourse-institutional approach. Sustainability 6, 283–305.

Green, M.C., Lertvilai, M., Bribbriesco, K., 2001. Prospering through Change CAOT from 1991 to 2001. Available online at: <https://www.caot.ca/pdfs/CAOT1991_2001.pdf> (accessed 10.05.16.).

Hamilton, S., 2013. Book Review: Analyze Anything: A Guide to Critical Reading and Writing. Can. J. Occup. Ther. 80, 120.

Hammell, K.W., 2007. Reflections on … a disability methodology for the client-centred practice of occupational therapy research. Can. J. Occup. Ther. 74, 365–369.

Hammell, K.W., 2009. Sacred texts: a sceptical exploration of the assumptions underpinning theories of occupation. Can. J. Occup. Ther. 76, 6–13.

Hammell, K.R.W., 2013. Client-centred occupational therapy in Canada: refocusing on core values/Recentrer l'ergothérapie au Canada sur les valeurs fondamentales de la pratique centrée sur le client. Can. J. Occup. Ther. 80, 141–149.

Hammell, K.R.W., Iwama, M.K., 2012. Well-being and occupational rights: an imperative for critical occupational therapy. Scand. J. Occup. Ther. 19, 385–394.

Hodgetts, S., Hollis, V., Triska, O., Dennis, S., Madill, H., Taylor, E., 2007. Occupational therapy students' and graduates' satisfaction with professional education and preparedness for practice. Can. J. Occup. Ther. 74, 148–160.

Kielhofner, G., 2005. Rethinking disability and what to do about it: disability studies and its implications for occupational therapy. Am. J. Occup. Ther. 59, 487–496.

Klinger, L., Bossers, A., 2009. Contributing to operations of community agencies through integrated fieldwork experiences. Can. J. Occup. Ther. 76, 171–179.

Miller, P., Parker, S., Gillinson, S., 2004. Disablism: How to Tackle the Last Prejudice. Demos, London.

Naess, A., 1973. The shallow and the deep, long-range ecology movement. A summary. Inquiry 16, 95–100.

Overboe, J., 2007. Vitalism: subjectivity exceeding racism, sexism, and (psychiatric) ableism. Wagadu J. Transnatl. Womens Gender Stud. 4, 23–34.

Panesar, S., Wolbring, G., 2014. Analysis of North American newspaper coverage of bionics using the disability studies framework. Technologies 2, 1–30.

Phelan, S.K., 2011. Constructions of disability: a call for critical reflexivity in occupational therapy. Can. J. Occup. Ther. 78, 164–172.

Scott, W.W.R., 2008. Institutions and Organizations: Ideas, Interests, and Identities. Sage Publications, Thousand Oaks, CA.

Sen, A., 2013. The ends and means of sustainability. J. Human Dev. Capabil. 14, 6–20.

Service Canada, 2013. Occupational Therapists. Government of Canada. Available online at: <http://www.servicecanada.gc.ca/eng/qc/job_futures/statistics/3143.shtml> (accessed 10.05.16.).

Townsend, E., 1993. Occupational therapy's social vision. Can. J. Occup. Ther. 60, 174–184.

Trentham, B., 2001. CAOT during the 1980s. Canadian Association of Occupational Therapists. Available online at: <http://www.caot.ca/otnow/sept01-eng/sept01-history.htm> (accessed 10.05.16.).

United Nations Development Programme, 1994. Human Development Report, 1994. Oxford University Press, New York. Available online at: <http://hdr.undp.org/sites/default/files/reports/255/hdr_1994_en_complete_nostats.pdf> (accessed 10.05.16.).

Van Helmond, M., 1992. Votes for Women: The Events on Merseyside, 1870-1928. National Museums and Galleries on Merseyside, Merseyside, UK.

Wagman, P., 2014. How to contribute occupationally to ecological sustainability: a literature review. Scand. J. Occup. Ther. 21, 161–165.

Wikiquote. Deus Ex: Invisible War. Available online at: <http://en.wikiquote.org/wiki/Deus_Ex:_Invisible_War> (accessed 10.05.16.).

Wolbring, G., 2003. Confined to your legs. In: Lightman, A.S., Chris, Dan Desser (Eds.), Living with the Genie. Island Press, Washington, DC.

Wolbring, G., 2008. Why NBIC? Why human performance enhancement? Innovation (Abingdon) 21, 25–40.

Wolbring, G., 2010. Ableism and favoritism for abilities governance, ethics and studies: new tools for nanoscale and nanoscale enabled science and technology governance. In: Cozzens, S.E., Wetmore, J. (Eds.), The Yearbook of Nanotechnology in Society, vol. II. The Challenges of Equity and Equality. Springer, New York.

Wolbring, G., 2011a. Ableism and energy security and insecurity. Stud. Ethics Law Technol. 5, Article 3.

Wolbring, G., 2011b. Water discourse, Ableism and disabled people: what makes one part of a discourse? Eubios J. Asian Int. Bioeth. 21, 203–207.

Wolbring, G., 2012. Expanding ableism: taking down the ghettoization of impact of disability studies scholars. Societies 2, 75–83.

Wolbring, G., 2013a. Culture of Peace from an ability and disability studies lens. In: Oswald Spring, U., et al. (Eds.), Expanding Peace Ecology: Peace, Security, Sustainability, Equity and Gender; Perspectives of IPRA's Ecology and Peace Commission. Springer, New York.

Wolbring, G., 2013b. Ecohealth through an ability studies and disability studies lens. In: Gislason, M.K. (Ed.), Ecological Health: Society, Ecology and Health. Emerald, London.

Wolbring, G., 2014. Ability privilege: a needed addition to privilege studies. J. Crit. Anim. Stud. 12, 118–141.

24

LIVING AND WORKING AS AN UNDERGROUND OCCUPATIONAL THERAPIST/SCIENTIST IN LOS ANGELES

SUSAN SAYLOR STOUFFER

CHAPTER OUTLINE

Did you start out wanting to be an occupational therapist? Once you heard about occupational therapy, did it resonate with your soul? That is what happened to me. I am a European American woman from Appalachia in the US, with a physical disability, a master's degree in occupational therapy, and a Ph.D. in occupational science. This is the unlikely story of how I became an activist underground occupational therapist, working for occupational justice with a community of children and families in South Los Angeles, California. This work has been shaped in large measure by what I consider my occupational therapy/occupational science habitus[1] (Bourdieu and Wacquant, 1992), an embodied and activated

worldview informed by my years of education, practice and teaching.

BECOMING AN OCCUPATIONAL THERAPIST/OCCUPATIONAL SCIENTIST

I had never heard of occupational therapy until after I graduated from college. Perhaps it was my own encounter with cancer at the age of 11, when I acquired my disability, that created such a powerful attraction to occupational therapy. My husband and I, recently married, applied to the University of North Carolina (UNC) at Chapel Hill. They had an occupational therapy programme for me and a Portuguese programme for my husband. We quit our jobs in Tennessee and moved to North Carolina.

I studied in the occupational therapy programme at UNC Chapel Hill for 2 years and received my

---

[1]Habitus is a concept developed by the sociologist Pierre Bourdieu. It describes a way of being in the world that is an embodiment of dispositions and social structures and that influences and structures thoughts, actions and feelings.

Master's of Science in Occupational Therapy. After graduation, I really wanted to work in the mental health field. With much persistence, some would say stubbornness, I was able to find work in mental health at the UNC Neuropsychiatric Hospital. I enjoyed working there and stayed for 7 years. I worked with excellent, experienced occupational therapists from whom I learned much.

At the same time, occupational therapy practice, and healthcare in general, was changing. I saw the length of stay in all areas of the hospital decline dramatically as insurers took on a larger role in decreasing the cost of care. Healthcare seemed to be becoming less about patient needs and more about reimbursement. I was frustrated and finally decided that, although I had loved my time there, I needed to make a change.

I thought I would like to try teaching occupational therapy. I finally found a good match in an occupational therapy programme at Barry University in Miami, Florida. It was a weekend programme, primarily designed for occupational therapy assistants who wanted to become occupational therapists. I did not always find it easy teaching occupational therapy assistants. They had quite a bit of experience and knowledge, and they were often questioning the professional hierarchy. They were particularly frustrated by new occupational therapists serving as their supervisors, especially when the occupational therapy assistants had more experience. They brought this same edginess to the classroom, and they challenged me in my role as a new occupational therapy professor. I would like to say that I always rose to this challenge; however, that would not be completely true. It was difficult for me at times, and I was sometimes too quick to assume the role given me by virtue of my training and my rank as a university educator. However, I did learn a great deal.

After 2 years of teaching, I decided that, if I wanted to stay in academia, I needed to get my doctorate. I was accepted at the occupational science Ph.D. programme of the University of Southern California (USC). I really liked the idea of studying more deeply the theoretical issues related to occupation. My husband was very supportive, so he and I moved to Los Angeles so that I could begin the Ph.D. programme in occupational science.

Moving to Los Angeles was a much bigger culture shock than moving to Miami had been. We had never even been to California, which is more than 2000 miles away on the other side of the country. Los Angeles, which is the second largest city in the US, is also much larger than Miami, much more crowded and seemed much noisier. Because it was so different and so much further from everything I had known on the East Coast of the US, I was homesick. I cried the first night we spent in USC student family housing and wanted to leave. We stayed!

USC's Ph.D. in occupational science was life-altering. We were given deep and challenging readings in diverse fields ranging from the social sciences to medicine and philosophy. As I was now in my thirties, I found my studies difficult at first. After I settled in, I found that although the programme was indeed challenging, I really appreciated it. During my occupational science studies, I first learned about powerful concepts such as 'whiting out' (Proweller, 1998), performing race (Jackson, 2001), black feminist theory (Lorde, 2007), the 'other' (Mattingly, 2006), and occupational justice (Wilcock and Townsend, 2000). These readings deeply influenced my understanding of the world. I even chose to write a paper about occupational justice as an independent study. Wilcock and Townsend (2000, p. 84) have written that 'whilst social justice addresses the social relations and social conditions of life, occupational justice addresses what people *do* in their relationships and conditions for living'. This idea that everyone should have equitable access to meaningful occupations was very strong and attractive for me. Although occupational justice was a topic of some discussion in our department at the time, it did not seem that all the faculty and students were in agreement about its importance.

CHANGE IN TRAJECTORY: BECOMING AN UNDERGROUND OCCUPATIONAL THERAPIST/OCCUPATIONAL SCIENTIST

I had fully intended to return to academia as an occupational therapy/occupational science professor after I received my Ph.D. However, my trajectory was altered along the way when I became a student intern at the Peace Center of the church I was attending, the United

University Church. United University Church is located on the campus of USC and was founded to serve the campus and community. The church has a long history of social justice work and had started its Peace Center as a programme of the church in the 1980s. The purpose of the Peace Center is to help organize and support attempts to counter war and violence. I had been working as a research assistant in my department, but when I lost that job, I was offered the position of Peace Center Intern. The purpose of this internship was to work with others to organize against the looming war with Iraq[2]. A few years later, before finishing my Ph.D., I became the Peace Center's part-time director. I decided to stay in that role once I finished my Ph.D. Many beloved family and friends were critical of this decision. Why had I spent so much time and money on a master's degree in occupational therapy and a Ph.D. in occupational science if I was not going to use my degrees?

My occupational science curriculum had introduced me to occupational justice and helped me in the process of 'conscientization' (Freire, 1990) to think more critically about issues related to occupational justice. Still, I did not think that I would have the opportunity to work in occupational justice as an occupational science professor/researcher. One of my professors, Gelya Frank, asked why I felt I had to leave occupational therapy/occupational science to work in occupational justice. I believed, based on my experience in my occupational therapy and occupational science programmes, and my work as an occupational therapist, that although a curriculum might be interwoven with occupational justice, there would not be many opportunities for me to help create occupational justice. I felt confident there would have been job opportunities in academia with my Ph.D. from USC, and they would have paid more than I would make as the Peace Center Director. Yet, I still felt the call to work more directly for occupational justice, so I decided to continue working at the Peace Center in order to live more fully in my desire to make a difference.

In my work as Peace Center Director, the new pastor, the Christian Educator and I listened to the requests from the church and the community to provide quality children's programming. Our church and peace centre were located in what was often perceived as a particularly violent part of Los Angeles. There was violence within the community, but there was also systemic economic violence that created many of the difficult conditions with which residents had to live. Our peace centre was working with a broad definition of violence developed by long years of study and practice at a Franciscan nonviolence centre. Violence is 'emotional, verbal, or physical behavior which dominates, diminishes or destroys ourselves or others' (Butigan and Bruno, 1999, p. 13).

In the early years of our peace education programmes, high rates of physical violence in our communities compelled us to address violence as our primary focus. Later, we found ourselves being called to address the issue of poverty as another form of violence. Poverty is violence against the children with whom we are working. It steals many options in the present and undermines their future possibilities. In his powerful poem about racial inequality, Langston Hughes once asked, 'What happens to a dream deferred? Does it dry up like a raisin in the sun? Or fester like a sore?' (Hughes, 1990, p. 268 – Originally published 1951). This question can also be asked in relation to all who live in poverty. We wanted to help these children dream big and to feel that they could actually achieve their dreams, not see them dry up.

We started Peace Camp as a summer educational programme for children that focused on these issues of violence and peace. The first summer, we had 8 to 10 kids, mostly white children from our church, and a few of their friends from the west side of Los Angeles, one of the more affluent regions of Los Angeles. Our Peace Center developed and then offered a week-long programme for the children. I was terrified that the programme would fail and that it would be a great embarrassment for the church and the Peace Center. I had never helped create an original programme before. I worried that I might be fired. Just as I also had a strong dose of persistence, I had a strong fear of failure. The programme did not fail.

In 2016, we began our eleventh year of the programme. We serve around 100 children and youth each year, and even have a waiting list for the now

---

[2]After the September 11, 2001 attacks on the World Trade Center, the US alleged that Iraq was supporting terrorism and harbouring weapons of mass destruction. The US and Great Britain, along with a few others, invaded Iraq in 2003.

4-week summer 'Peace Camp' and the 14-Saturday-per-year 'Peace Kids' and 'Youth Leadership in Peace-making' programmes. The children in these programmes range in age from 5 to 18. The primary focus of these programmes is to help children and youth learn to be peacemakers in an often violent world and community, and to be agents of nonviolent social change. We teach the children/youth peaceful communication and conflict resolution. The children and youth also learn tools for creating change: letter writing, vigils, marches, boycotts, and more. This aspect of experiential learning in our programmes has come in large measure from my occupational therapy training (Nelson and Jepson-Thomas, 2003).

Although participants in the Peace Camp/Peace Kids/Youth Leadership programmes were 90% white when we first started, they have become much more reflective of the neighbourhoods that surround us, as we have intentionally reached out to our neighbours. The response from the neighbourhoods has been positive. Although the programme is offered by the church, it is a nonsectarian programme open to all. It teaches about peace traditions from diverse religious traditions. The children in the programme are now primarily Latinos, with a smaller number of African Americans and a few Asians. Most of the children in our programmes live in poverty, since poverty rates are very high in the neighbourhoods which surround our church. In 2013, the median family income in the closest neighbourhood around our church was US\$22,420 while the California median family income was US\$60,190 (City Data, 2013). In 2011, the Federal Poverty Level for a family of four was US\$22 350 (State of California, Health and Human Services, 2011).

OCCUPATIONAL SCIENCE/ OCCUPATIONAL THERAPY HABITUS

As we have begun to think more deeply about our programme and the challenges the children and families in our programme are facing, my occupational science and occupational therapy training has come to the forefront. In this chapter, I posit that I have been using my occupational science background to function as an occupational scientist as I have studied the issues related to peace and poverty. I am going to use Jackson et al.'s (1998) definition of occupational science as the 'systematic study of the form, function, and meaning of occupation' (p. 327) to support my claim that I have been working as an occupational scientist. I have observed, studied, and researched the issues of peace and poverty in relation to the children and families participating in our Peace Camp/Peace Kids/Youth Leadership programmes. We used the ideas that I bring from my background as an occupational scientist and occupational therapist, supplemented by the assistant director's background as an educator, to create a foundation for understanding the issues with which the children and their families are being challenged.

I further posit that much of my education and practice as an occupational therapist has compelled me to act as an 'underground' occupational therapist in helping to create and implement these programmes. Underground occupational therapy practice is a term that I first encountered in Mattingly and Fleming's (1994) book on clinical reasoning in occupational therapy. In this case, I am using underground occupational therapist to apply to the occupational science/ occupational therapy habitus I mentioned earlier. Since the goal of occupational therapy is 'enhancing participation in roles, habits and routines in home, school, workplace, community and other settings' (American Occupational Therapy Association, 2014, p. S1), and since this has been my training and experience for many years of practice, it is not only compelling that I use this occupational therapy habitus in implementing these programmes, it is also advantageous. I have been well educated in the professional and legal implications of practising as an occupational therapist, so I was not wearing that professional hat for public view, nor charging for occupational therapy services, rather it is my contention that I could not help but wear the occupational therapy hat as I worked on the implementation of these programmes. Thus, I have used the designation of myself as an underground occupational therapist/occupational scientist.

APPLYING OCCUPATIONAL SCIENCE/ OCCUPATIONAL THERAPY TO PEACE AND POVERTY IN CHILDREN AND COMMUNITIES

The Peace Center of United University Church has been very involved in the systemic problems of our neighbourhood and the global community. In many ways, the Peace Center functions as the social justice face of the United University Church. In my work for the Peace Center, I have found that it is one thing to advocate for systemic changes, but another to understand and to address the issues at the level of the individuals and families with which we have been working in our children's programmes. In these programmes, we needed to be working on advocacy to challenge the systemic violence around us and the childhood poverty that is endemic in our neighbourhoods. At the same time, there was a need to be working to address the problems the families were experiencing, arising from the violence and poverty.

Poverty constrains and denies the choices and opportunities of daily activities that are offered to people. It can cause occupational deprivation (Whiteford, 2000). The families living in poverty that we serve are often forced to live in crowded apartments with multiple families. There are often several children sharing a room, so that quiet time to do homework is difficult. The families have increased stress and limited leisure, as the parents work multiple jobs to avoid losing their housing. Schools in these pockets of poverty often have less equipment and less availability of challenging classes than their more affluent counterparts (Oakes et al., 1990). Due to immigration issues, such as lack of documentation and language fluency issues, parents can be forced to take low-paying jobs. The neighbourhoods in these poverty pockets also have fewer parks and green spaces for play than the more affluent neighbourhoods (Wolch et al., 2005). Poverty can also constrain a child's outlook, hopes, and dreams to such an extent that it leads to occupational alienation (Townsend and Wilcock, 2004). When children live in pockets of concentrated poverty, it is difficult for them to imagine possibilities other than poverty. Dreams of becoming high-achieving professionals may be written off as unattainable when economics are experienced as a barrier to good schools and good jobs. The disconnect between young people's dreams and their perception that these dreams are possible may set them up for disconnection from school (Marczuk et al., 2014). Teenage pregnancy and school dropout rates are often high in areas of poverty, creating cycles of poverty (Harding, 2003).

Our programmes began by addressing the most obvious basic issues, such as the immediate physical effects of poverty. The programme began offering a full hot lunch and light breakfast, because most of the neighbourhood children were on the free school breakfast and lunch programme and needed more nutritional support on weekends and in the summer. The programme also added free tutoring on school-year Saturdays, because many of the kids needed help with school but could not afford tutoring.

As we, the staff, built relationships and earned the trust of the children and their families, we discovered some of the sociocultural impact of poverty on their lives. Many of the children had never even been to the beach which is about 20 minutes away, let alone to another state or country. Thus, the programme began to offer programming focused on studying communities all around the world and the issues that impacted them. The staff worked together before each semester of programming to design the curriculum.

The curriculum focuses on the justice issues that confront these global communities such as poverty, violence, environmental challenges, and health challenges in the context of learning through activities. The staff had heard from some of the children in our programmes that they felt uncomfortable when children coming from more affluent backgrounds spoke of their knowledge and adventures in travel around the world. It was our desire as staff that, even if the children never travelled to these other countries, they would be conversant about the issues and the cultures. This would allow them to demonstrate more confidence in social situations.

Over time, the staff also began to recognize that the children in the programmes, although smart and creative, were dealing with other challenges related to living with poverty. The children in the neighbourhoods that surround the campus of USC where the church is located were receiving uneven educational opportunities. Some of the schools in our community were magnet schools that focused on particular programmes such as performing arts, and charter schools which are public schools operated privately and with more freedom in curriculum design. These schools had significant resources from the community to support their focus. Other public schools in our community were struggling to provide similar opportunities. I spoke with a Latina education professor at USC who had been a leader in the movement to provide educational opportunities for local Latino students. She said that many of the children were victims of the *'pobrecitos'* mentality. *Pobrecito* in Spanish literally means 'poor thing' (Pobrecito, 2002, p. 210). Although those who subscribed to this idea might have been well intentioned, the staff of our programmes sometimes heard that 'these children' did not have the background, parental support or English fluency that would allow them to really excel, so teachers and community leaders did not expect too much from them. Unfortunately, these low expectations by teachers and community leaders often turned into self-fulfilling prophecies of low achievement by the students. Thus, the students were subjected to unequal educational opportunities and unequal expectations by the educators.

Working to develop a curriculum to address the issues related to violence and poverty in the lives of the families served by the programme, needed best practices and ideas derived from research. Since I was the only full-time employee of the Peace Center, and because of my doctorate in occupational science, it fell to me to be the researcher. I would research, digest, and disseminate information related to the complex challenges associated with violence and what seemed to be the bigger challenge of the violence of poverty. With this information, our assistant director, our peace teachers, the families with whom we were working, and some of our stalwart supporters in the church could help chart a course and shape the programme. A friend, who had once been a peace teacher in our programme, recommended we read 'How Children Succeed' (Tough, 2012). This book was about the problems that children who were raised in poverty often faced, such as difficulty with delayed gratification and difficulty believing that they could impact their own success or failure. In the KIPP Schools (Knowledge is Power Program) discussed in the book, students were given regular report cards, but also 'Character Report Cards'. These report cards allowed the teachers to talk to the students about such things as 'grit', which involves strong determination, 'self-control', which is about delayed gratification, and 'optimism', which includes a positive expectancy of improvement related to effort. It allowed the teachers to try and help the students with these challenges to

their academic and life success which the teachers saw more frequently with children living in poverty.

Our staff worked together to develop a tool to address issues we saw as challenges such as 'talking about feelings', 'helping others', and 'problem solving'. We worked until we developed 10 such items into a tool for our programme. This tool is based on assets and not deficits. Gorski (2008) talks about the danger of a deficit-based approach. What were the children/youth doing well, and what would they like to and/or need to work on improving? Although most of the children were living in poverty, they were each individuals who brought their own constellation of strengths and challenges. Payne (2008) discussed the need for acquisition of specific skill sets in specific environments to help children living in poverty excel. One example given was that while being very reactive to environmental stimuli might be adaptive in an environment with a lot of challenges, it might also be counterproductive in a school environment where planning and control are valued. This asset-based model, although not always present in occupational therapy, is certainly a thread running through occupational therapy theory (Wilcock, 1998). We believed that helping the children/youth acquire skills in coping would help them be adaptive and resilient agents of change. Indeed, asset-based strategies for increasing resilience in youth can help buffer the effects of community violence (Jain and Cohen, 2013).

As the programme continued to address violence and poverty, the children and staff practised the tools of advocacy in relation to both. The children in the programme were encouraged to write letters about actions needed to address child poverty and violence – to our city councilperson, to the mayor, to our representatives in Congress, to our senators, to our governor and even to the President of the United States. Our programme raised money for causes related to child poverty and violence, and held marches and vigils to raise awareness about these issues. The staff also reached out to other nonprofits, churches, and community leaders to join us in these actions, particularly in the marches and vigils.

PROVIDING PATHWAYS

As the programme continued to develop, it seemed to work well with the younger children. However, it became a challenge to find a role for the older youth as they began to leave the programme at the age of 14 or 15. At these ages, they began to say they were too old for the programme and that they wanted to get a job. They had great difficulty finding jobs due to the economic recession which affected the US starting in 2008 and for several years thereafter. In response, we created a 'youth internship' to give a role to older youth in the programme. It provided them with a small stipend and gave them a way to build their résumé and their professional experience. As some of the first youth interns graduated from high school, the programme was able to hire them to become assistant teachers. In 2014, for the first time, two of the youth, who had worked their way up through the programme, were promoted to lead teachers.

At the time, the staff did not realize that we were creating a pathway for the children. Quiocho and Rios (2000) have discussed the power and potential of having teachers who reflect the communities they serve. The programme had employed Latino and African American teachers, but the real power for the children seemed to come from promoting youth from within their ranks. Now the children have begun to tell the staff that they all expect to become interns and eventually teachers in the programme. Now the programme is potentially facing a great problem to have: too large a pool of potential teachers from within. We, the staff, are now working to help other faith communities start programmes like ours and perhaps our children will one day be the teachers in those programmes.

CONCLUSION: LIVING AS ABOVEGROUND OCCUPATIONAL THERAPISTS/OCCUPATIONAL SCIENTISTS

In conclusion, the pathway that I have taken into this work as an occupational therapist and occupational scientist has been typical in some ways, but uniquely my own in others. What I have learned is the importance of following our own paths, and the importance of using all the tools we acquire to face the challenges we find on our path. I believe it is only in following our particular pathway that we can become fully the occupational beings we aspire to be.

What I have learned for my profession is that, although occupational therapy and occupational science academic training in the US is often interwoven with the thread of occupational justice, academic programmes could better prepare and encourage graduates to actually create occupational justice. I have been out of school for a few years, so I did a quick online search and was rewarded with a few occupational therapy/occupational science programmes in the US that mentioned occupational justice in their programmes. It is my hope that occupational justice will become a core issue in all occupational therapy/occupational science programmes. I believe it is incumbent upon us as occupational therapists and occupational scientists, with our rich history and training, not only to address the particular issues that encumber our clients, but to work hand in hand with them to transform the landscape. Our world needs to cultivate communities that support well and equitably all who live there. In order to create just communities, our discipline needs all occupational therapists and occupational scientists to be able to practise above ground. Occupational scientists and occupational therapists need educational, research, and fieldwork opportunities for occupational therapy and occupational science empowered by occupational justice.

Acknowledgements

The Peace Camp/Peace Kids/Youth Leadership programmes described here were developed originally by the United University Church Pastor Frank Wulf, the church administrator, John Brennan, and me. It was the creative energy of that team and the support and encouragement of the pastor and others at the church, such as Sharon Tool, that were essential in the development and growth of these programmes. After the first 2 years, when our assistant director, Alicia Driscoll, was hired, she became a strong force in the continued development and growth of the programmes. Her background as an elementary school teacher was a great asset in these programmes. I would also like to thank my professor Dr. Gelya Frank, who encouraged me to write this chapter and gave me feedback and support as I worked on it. Of course, without the participation of the hundreds of children, youth and their families from across South Los Angeles, none of this would have been possible. Though these families often struggle under difficult circumstances, they are strong and capable, supportive and gracious in their relationship with our staff and programme. This chapter is dedicated to these families in the hope that one day, none of our children will have to struggle in such difficult circumstances.

REFERENCES

American Occupational Therapy Association, 2014. Occupational therapy framework: domain and process 3rd Edition. Am. J. Occup. Ther. 68 (Suppl. 1), S1–S48.

Bourdieu, P., Wacquant, L.J.D., 1992. An Invitation to Reflexive Sociology. University of Chicago Press, Chicago.

Butigan, K., Bruno, P., 1999. From Violence to Wholeness: A Ten Part Program in the Spirituality and Practice of Active Nonviolence. Pace e Bene, Las Vegas.

City Data, 2013. Onboard Informatics. Advameg, Inc. <http://www.city-data.com/zips/90007.html> (accessed 15.05.16.).

Freire, P., 1990. Pedagogy of the Oppressed. Continuum Publishing Company, New York.

Gorski, P., 2008. The myth of the culture of poverty. Educational Leadership 65 (7), 32–36.

Harding, D., 2003. Counterfactual models of neighborhood effects: the effect of neighborhood poverty on dropping out and teenage pregnancy. Am. J. Sociol. 109, 676–719.

Hughes, L., 1990. Harlem. In: Selected Poems of Langston Hughes. Vintage Books, New York.

Jackson, J.L. Jr., 2001. Harlem World: Doing Race and Class in Contemporary Black America. University of Chicago Press, Chicago.

Jackson, J., Carlson, M., Mandel, D., Zemke, R., Clark, F., 1998. Occupation in lifestyle redesign: the Well Elderly Study Occupational Therapy Program. Am. J. Occup. Ther. 52, 326–336.

Jain, S., Cohen, A.K., 2013. Fostering resilience among urban youth exposed to violence: a promising area for interdisciplinary research and practice. Health Educ. Behav. 40, 651–662.

Lorde, A., 2007. Sister Outsider: Essays and Speeches. Crossing Press, Berkley, CA.

Marczuk, O., Taff, S., Berg, C., 2014. Occupational justice, school connectedness, and high school dropout: the role of occupational therapy in meeting the needs of an underserved population. J. Occup. Ther. Schools Early Interv. 7, 235–245.

Mattingly, C., 2006. Pocahontas goes to the clinic: popular culture as lingua franca in a cultural borderland. Am. Anthropol. 108, 494–501.

Mattingly, C., Fleming, M.H., 1994. Clinical Reasoning: Forms of Inquiry in a Therapeutic Practice. F.A. Davis, Philadelphia.

Nelson, D.L., Jepson-Thomas, J., 2003. Occupational form, occupational performance, and a conceptual framework for therapeutic occupation. In: Perspectives in Human Occupation: Participation in Life. Lippincott Williams & Wilkins, Baltimore.

Oakes, J., et al., 1990. Multiplying Inequalities: The Effects of Race, Social Class, and Tracking on Opportunities to Learn Mathematics and Science, A report of the Rand Corporation. Santa Mónica, CA.

Payne, R., 2008. Nine powerful practices. Educational Leadership 65 (7), 48–52.

Pobrecito, 2002. University of Chicago Spanish Dictionary, fifth ed. University of Chicago Press, Chicago. IL.

Proweller, A., 1998. Constructing Female Identities: Making Meaning in an Upper Middle Class Youth Culture. State University of New York Press, Albany, NY.

Quiocho, A., Rios, F., 2000. The power of their presence: minority group teachers and schooling. Rev. Educ. Res. 70, 485–528.

State of California, Health and Human Services, 2011. New Federal Poverty Levels. <http://www.dhcs.ca.gov/services/medi-cal/eligibility/Documents/c11-16.pdf> (published 11 April 2011, accessed 14.05.16.).

Tough, P., 2012. How Children: Grit, Curiosity, and the Hidden Power of Character. Houghton Mifflin Harcourt, Boston, MA.

Townsend, E., Wilcock, A.A., 2004. Occupational justice and client-centered practice: a dialogue in progress. Can. J. Occup. Ther. 71, 75–87.

Whiteford, G., 2000. Occupational deprivation: global challenge in the new millennium. Br. J. Occup. Ther. 63, 200–204.

Wilcock, A., 1998. An Occupational Perspective of Health. Slack Incorporated, Thorofare, NJ.

Wilcock, A.A., Townsend, E., 2000. Occupational terminology interactive dialogue. J. Occup. Sci. 7, 84–86.

Wolch, J., Wilson, J., Fehrenbach, J., 2005. Parks and park funding in Los Angeles: an equity-mapping analysis. Urban Geogr. 26, 4–35.

25

OCCUPATIONAL SCIENCE INFORMING PRACTICE FOR OCCUPATIONAL JUSTICE

CLARE HOCKING ■ JENNI MACE

Nobel Peace Laureate Desmond Tutu, in his foreword to the second volume of *Occupational Therapies without Borders,* observed that while occupational therapists 'value and work with medical understandings, your main aim seems to go beyond these' to impact 'individual and collective wellbeing' (Tutu, 2011, p. ix). This chapter concerns the contribution occupational science makes to achieving that aim, by challenging occupational therapists to take on a political perspective of the profession's contribution to society, a view deeply entrenched in occupational justice. It is an important concern because, despite decades of literature proposing occupation to be the profession's key concept, the means and ends of practice (McLaughlin Gray, 1998), many therapists struggle to fit their view of what the profession should be into the health contexts in which they work (Wilding, 2010). Crossing the border from practice as it is usually constituted in acute medical, rehabilitation and community health settings to the political practice espoused in this text requires a shift in thinking. Specifically, it

requires broadening occupational therapy's view from the ways health conditions impact everyday life to recognizing and responding to the social, economic and political factors that create healthy lives for some and impose unhealthy patterns of living on others. That shift, we will argue, is supported by ideas proposed and studied by occupational scientists.

OCCUPATIONAL SCIENCE AND A CRITICAL PERSPECTIVE

Proposing that occupational science might help occupational therapy transform itself into a more politicized profession demands an explanation of what the field is about. Stated simply, occupational science is the study of humans as occupational beings. That definition encompasses several interrelated ideas. Firstly, through doing things people experience themselves – their capacities, talents, and temperament. They express their values and beliefs, become what they have the potential to be and, by doing things with and for others, engender a sense of belonging. Over time, human doing creates the physical contexts in which people occupy themselves by modifying the natural world, developing tools and technologies, and building the structures in which they work, live, learn, celebrate, and play. People's collective occupation is an expression of culture, and the means by which culture is transmitted across generations and to newcomers. Further, shared ways of doing generate the kind of society people live in, be that democratic, egalitarian, industrialized, well-educated, secular, conservative, postmodern, collectivist, future-focused, or any number of other ways human societies might be categorized. All of those things together affect the occupations that are available to members of a society, their lifestyle, the manner in which their occupations link together, and their health and well-being (Wilcock and Hocking, 2015).

Occupational science forefronts an occupational perspective, which is 'a way of looking at or thinking about human doing' (Njelesani et al., 2014, p. 226). Applying that perspective to occupational therapy illuminates, in part, the need for more politicized practice. Viewed merely as human activity, occupational therapy practice can be highly repetitive: the same problems are identified and solved over and over again, with each client individually. In some respects, that has advantages. It has enabled occupational therapists to accumulate a wealth of theory, technology, and practical strategies to address a range of daily living problems experienced by people with acute and chronic health conditions. But why keep fixing problems that could have been solved (Hocking, Townsend, et al., 2014)? For example, almost a century after the profession was established, doorways remain too narrow for wheelchairs, workplace accommodations for people with mental illness have not become 'business as usual' and, although many children with disabilities now attend school, they are not routinely included in organized sports.

These problematic aspects of the contexts in which people act could have been rectified. Building codes might have been changed to make standard doorways wider or legislation passed to require employers and sports teams to find ways to include people with special needs. In addition, because clients keep presenting with problems that occupational therapists have the know-how and technology to fix, the profession has tended to focus close-in: on the individual's bathroom at home, but not on the washrooms at the local church or at their friend's house; on an 'accommodating' employer, but not all employers; or on access to the child's classroom, but not to all the venues other children use. Failure to champion systemic change means that social and environmental conditions have not improved for people with disabilities, or not as quickly as they might.

In addition, occupational therapy has remained such a specialized sphere of human activity that knowledge of enabling occupation has not entered people's general knowledge in the way that medical, psychological and dietary information has. Illustrating that point, members of the public are likely to know basic first aid, understand concepts such as intelligence and be aware that they should avoid fatty foods. They are much less likely to appreciate how daily routines can undermine health or the positive impact social and creative occupations can have on well-being. In fact, it might be argued that members of the public now know even less of the relationship between occupation and health than they did in 1917, when occupational therapy was founded. At that time, leading proponents of the Arts and Crafts Movement extolled well-chosen vocation as 'medicine for … body and soul' (Ruskin, cited in Friedland, 2007, p. 295). The lack of transfusion of occupational therapy knowledge into the public domain secures the profession's role and status; by keeping our expertise to ourselves, we close down the possibility of 'self-help' and avoid being snubbed by those who might label our interventions 'applied common sense'. However, it also marks a failure to influence society as a whole. In failing to share what they know, occupational therapists are complicit in perpetuating the disadvantages accrued from being disabled.

Another critique brought to light by an occupational perspective of occupational therapy is that practitioners tend to emphasize the need for their craft – the impairments, risks, and barriers that bring people to therapy – and describe the outcomes in terms of enhancing individuals' functioning. Again, in focusing on the benefits to individuals, occupational therapists have not counted the contribution their efforts make to society; the economic and societal value of prescribing adaptive equipment, modifying homes and workplaces, and enhancing occupational performance. It is telling that the profession is unable to say whether the collective actions of generations of occupational therapists have advanced the right of people with disabilities to attend school, access public buildings and employment, and be supported to participate. There is no account of how much occupational therapy has contributed to making societies more tolerant, inclusive and just for people with different abilities.

OCCUPATIONAL SCIENCE TRANSFORMING PRACTICE

Changing society was not part of the agenda when occupational science was established. Rather, this new field of inquiry was intended to strengthen occupational therapy practice by deepening the profession's knowledge of occupation (Yerxa et al., 1989). Much of the occupational science research achieves exactly that. For instance, Eklund et al. (2012) found that people with mental illness consider their everyday occupations to be a meaningful part of life which generates positive emotions and enhances health. Such findings support a basic premise of occupational therapy: that there is a relationship between the things people do and their health and well-being (Hocking, 2013). Other publications provide insights into the occupational patterns of recipients of occupational therapy (e.g., Connor et al., 2014) and occupations that might be used therapeutically, such as cooking (Hocking et al., 2014), or support concepts that explain how people regain health, such as occupational adaptation (Molineux et al., 2014). Still others lay the foundations for new interventions, such as Erlandsson's (2013) Redesigning Daily Occupations programme for women on long-term sick leave.

Reaching beyond the original goal of generating the knowledge occupational therapists need, two esteemed occupational scientists, Ann Wilcock and Elizabeth Townsend, proposed new explanations of the ways occupation is implicated in ill health. Occupational deprivation (Wilcock, 1998) directs attention to the systemic causes of ill health, while occupational justice (Wilcock and Townsend, 2000) asserts that inequities in participation are a breach of human rights. Their work thus contributes to the politicization of occupational therapy by challenging the profession's benign

view of society and illness causation. To put that knowledge development into context, it is salutary to note that prior to the emergence of occupational science there were perhaps only two occupationally focused concepts to call on to explain how everyday activities might undermine health: occupational imbalance (Townsend and Polatajko, 2013) and deficits in the motor and process skills required to perform tasks (Fisher, 1994). Both of these concepts appear to be 'apolitical', in that anyone's life could get out of balance to such an extent that health was threatened, and anyone could lose skills necessary to do the things they want, need, or are required to do. To correct imbalance, it was assumed that individuals could restore balance by reviewing their lifestyle choices, changing self-defeating values and habits, or learning to manage competing role demands. Equally, therapy proceeded as though it was a simple case of developing new skills, employing compensatory strategies or modifying the environment to support task performance.

Several features of occupational deprivation and occupational justice have been instrumental to their politicizing impact. Firstly, from the outset, both concepts have been framed in relation to marginalized groups of people rather than individuals: prisoners, people who are unemployed, women, immigrants, elderly people, refugees, indigenous people and those living in poverty, people who are homeless, and communities devastated by war and natural disasters. Secondly, the power of these concepts has ignited the imagination of occupational therapists. For instance, in perhaps the first publication to discuss occupational deprivation, Whiteford (1995) vividly described prisoners in a special needs unit within the prison who were subjected to occupational deprivation. They were 'unable to be fully part of the world around them' (Whiteford, 1995, p. 81) and, because humans are innately occupational, were robbed of their humanity. Invoking occupational deprivation is to assert that people literally have little or nothing to do, or are subject to such extreme constraints on valued occupations that a substantive reduction in health is actual or imminent. For a profession dedicated to promoting health, this is a serious accusation.

Thirdly, and perhaps most importantly, occupational deprivation and occupational justice are in themselves political concepts, pointing to systematic disadvantages visited on sectors of the community. Thus, occupational deprivation is defined as being caused by things that individuals cannot control; global events such as economic recessions and environmental degradation, or the entrenched values and beliefs of others – that the people concerned have sub-human capacities, are not welcome or valued, deserve to be punished, are loathsome or cursed, dangerous, dirty, corrupt, foolish, beyond redemption, unpredictable or contagious and, in many cases, that they have brought their misfortunes on themselves (Wilcock and Hocking, 2015). In fact, many people subjected to occupational deprivation are merely female, disabled, impoverished, members of a minority group, or displaced from their homeland. Others fall into occupational deprivation when they lose employment due to economic restructuring, they become homeless or they experience some other misfortune.

Similarly, the concept of occupational justice escalates the idea that occupation can harm people from being a health issue to a matter of human rights. Occupational justice is an aspect of social justice, which is defined as the ethical distribution of opportunities, resources, rights and responsibilities within a society (Commission on Social Justice, 1994). As such, social justice addresses the origins and consequences of injustices, whether people's right to meet their basic requirements is protected and what is done to reduce or eliminate unfair inequities (Commission on Social Justice, 1994). From an occupational justice perspective, that means protecting people from bearing an unfair burden of harmful occupations and questioning whether others have the right to claim a disproportionate share of the benefits. While a basic set of occupational rights has been delineated (Townsend and Wilcock, 2004), more attention has been given to the idea of occupational injustice.

At an individual level, breaches of occupational justice manifest as impaired development, lack of meaning and choice in occupations, exclusion from valued occupations and the privileges they bring, subjection to gruelling or dangerous occupations or enslavement, and the consequent ill health (Stadnyk et al., 2010). At a population level, occupational injustice constitutes an economic burden on the community as a whole, related to failure to develop citizens to

their full capacity and the association between poverty and ill health (United Nations High Commissioner for Human Rights and World Health Organization, 2008), social disintegration and civic disturbance (Stadnyk et al., 2010), and an escalating risk of terrorist activity (Mueller, 2006). Giving credence to the importance of occupational justice for occupational therapists, the World Federation of Occupational Therapists adopted a position statement outlining occupational therapists' skills and responsibility to address it in 2006.

UNCOVERING OCCUPATIONAL INJUSTICE

Occupational deprivation and occupational justice have served as sensitizing concepts that help occupational therapists envisage the possibility of working for society to address health inequities. That remit encompasses populations whose occupations, or limited access to occupation, cause ill health, as well as social issues that are responsive to occupation-focused interventions. Several scholars have supported that vision, offering ways of thinking about and questioning realities that might otherwise be accepted as natural or inevitable. Amongst them, Rudman (2005) revealed how people's assumptions about what is ideal and possible for them to do are subtly shaped by cultural, social, and political discourses. Employing Foucault's concept of governmentality, Rudman analysed content published in 1999 and 2000 in a national Canadian newspaper. Her findings show how the needs, desires, and conduct of older people are channelled towards purchasing leisure and educational opportunities, and remaining in the workforce. As Rudman argues, this positioning privileges some people over others, excluding those with chronic health conditions that preclude active consumer lifestyles or low incomes that necessitate working beyond the age of retirement.

Shifting the focus from the ways people are shaped to how they respond, Angell (2014) asserts that occupation itself is a site where hegemonic societal assumptions about people are reproduced or resisted. Checking how we *look* as we finish getting dressed, for example, is to engage with a cultural discourse about how people like ourselves ought to look. That everyday action signifies the identity and values individuals accept and express, thus perpetuating the gender, ethnic, class, age, and other categories that mask oppression. Another layer of critical thinking about the part occupation plays in preserving the social order was added by Galvaan's (2015) study of the occupational choices of adolescents growing up in an economically deprived community where 'coloured' people had been forced to live during South Africa's apartheid era. She found that historical legacy continues to play out through young people's pattern of poor educational achievement, narrow vocational aspirations, and high rates of unemployment, smoking, and drug and alcohol dependency. The study further demonstrates how people's collective and contextual histories influence the types of occupational choices they make.

In powerfully illustrating that occupation is always a transaction with historic, political, and cultural forces, these authors challenge occupational therapy's assumption that people's potential is realized through engagement in occupation (Asaba and Wicks, 2010). Rather, while some have the freedom to develop to their potential, using creative and constructive means, others are constrained by restrictive contexts and limited resources that thwart the emergence of skills and capacities.

OCCUPATIONAL JUSTICE AS POLITICAL PRACTICE

To illustrate how occupational science can inform political practice, we offer two examples drawn from our own context in Aotearoa New Zealand: one historical and one contemporary. The first is informed by Rudman's (2005, 2012) work, in showing the value of attending to government policy and how it is enacted. It traces the ways the occupational choices of Māori, the indigenous people, have been framed as problems and reveals how broad political goals have detrimentally impacted the occupations they engage in at home. The second is about putting aside occupational therapy's hegemonic assumptions about the context, delivery and outcomes of therapeutic occupation.

As the authors of these accounts, we identify ourselves as occupational therapists with practice experience in mental health services and working with people who have lost their home. These concerns continue to inform our scholarship and research, and influence our selection of the stories to tell in this

context. Perhaps most important, we are *Tauiwi*, non-Māori settlers, which is acknowledged as a limitation in our interpretation of the accounts we have written. To ameliorate the risks inherent in crafting an account that tells both sides of the history of our bicultural nation, we have privileged literature authored by Māori, who have the right to 'hold the pen' in telling their own history. Thus, we issue the following caveat: we are retelling our stories from an occupational rather than an indigenous perspective, with the intent that it is sympathetically and respectfully told.

Colonizing Māori Homes

A home is more than a location. People's homes are their refuge, a place to express themselves and where memories accumulate (Perkins and Thorn, 1999). Homes are historically and culturally situated, with modern homes in Western contexts reflecting values such as privacy, cleanliness, comfort, and fashion (Stanyer, 1994). More than that, homes are the site of an array of occupations: offering hospitality, social gatherings and other forms of entertainment, caring for children and other family members, cooking and domestic work, self-care and sexual activities, gardening, doing homework, car maintenance, and hobbies. Traditional Māori homes, built in tribal villages, were designed for warmth, well-being, and the containment of disease. The *wharepuni* (sleeping quarters), where extended family slept, were low, one-room structures designed for warmth and shelter. They were heated by a fire close to the entrance, with roof ventilation (Wanhalla, 2006). Separate structures and areas existed for garments, tools, food storage, food preparation, and cooking. These designated areas were in keeping with the concepts of *tapu* (restricted or sacred) and *noa* (accessible or ordinary), which maintained hygiene and thus contained the spread of disease (Hall, 2008).

Traditional social and economic life and patterns of healthy living were substantially disrupted through land alienation after Aotearoa New Zealand was colonized by the British (Wanhalla, 2006).

Ever since, Māori have been subjected to moralistic and Eurocentric views about how to live in and look after a home; views closely entwined with being a 'good' citizen. Stimulated by a rapid decline in the Māori population, which had fallen from an estimated 70 000 to 90 000 in 1840 (Pool and Kukutai, 2014) to just 43 000 late in the century, early housing policy was closely linked to health (Dury, 1998). For instance, the Division of Māori Hygiene, which was established under the Health Act (1920), is just one example of policy falsely attributing Māori mortality rates to poor-quality housing rather than the introduction of diseases endemic to European populations (Wanhalla, 2006). Health officials had the power to order occupants to improve their homes on the threat of demolition but were grossly underfunded and unable to erect or improve housing stock (Bierre et al., 2007). In the 1930s, Māori homes were surveyed to assess the need and potential cost of assistance but were measured against European standards for healthy living, including drainage and sewage systems, separate bedrooms to prevent the spread of disease and a stove for indoor cooking (Bierre et al., 2007; Hall, 2008). Housing officers reported not only on the state of housing but also noted what people did in their homes, making special reference to well-kept homes and families who 'lived like Europeans' (Wanhalla, 2006). A recent review of government files clearly shows that families who were considered hard workers or good housekeepers were seen as deserving better housing; those who lived in overcrowded homes who appeared to be doing little to relieve their situation were seen as undeserving (Bierre et al., 2007).

Alienation from traditional ways of living continued with rapid urbanization from the mid-1930s, and particularly after the Second World War, as Māori moved to help with the war effort; access jobs, trade training, higher education, and loans to establish businesses (Nikora et al., 2004); and following family members who had already migrated to towns and cities. In response to the increasingly evident economic disparities between Māori and Pākeha, assimilation policies were enacted (Labrum, 2004). For example, Māori welfare officers, empowered by the Māori Social and Economic Advancement Act (1945) and later supported by the Māori Women's Welfare League, applied European concepts of citizenship, responsibility and home life. This message was reinforced by educational material such as 'Your New Home', published in 1954 by the Māori Affairs Department for Māori households, which gave advice about domestic occupations such as furnishing, decorating, and maintenance.

Opposing these social forces, Māori have reasserted the value of *whakapapa* (genealogy) and the layers of kinship relationships that connect them with tribal land and form a *tūrangawaewae*, a 'place of strength and identity' (Groot et al., 2011). The physical setting and emotional connection to a tribal home provides *wairua* (spiritual attachment) (Davey and Kearns, 1994), with many urban Māori choosing to participate in *tikanga* (shared cultural activities or custom) from their home region. This is referred to as *ahi ka* or keeping the home fires burning (Carter, 2006). Part of this cultural resurgence is a focus on how homes should be designed to accommodate Māori culture and ways of doing. *Ki te Hau Kainga* is a new design guide for Housing New Zealand that incorporates the principles of a *wharenui* (meeting house). It takes into account Māori spatiality (Waghorn, 2009) through concepts of *tapu* and *noa*. For example, toilets are well removed from kitchens, and whilst kitchen and dining areas are open plan, sliding panels can separate the kitchen if the living areas are to be used for *tangi* (funerals). Living areas allow for communal sleeping, as in traditional homes. Areas in front of the home provide spaces in which to welcome people, similar to those of a *marae* (courtyard in front of a *wharenui*) (Hoskins et al., 2002).

Political occupational therapy practice informed by Māori cultural values, the occupations encompassed by Māori homes, and Aotearoa New Zealand's colonial history are positioned in response to this account. A primary consideration is not imposing one's own worldview on others. In particular, it is evident that what is done in a home and how it is done is not just culturally shaped, but imbued with deep cultural significance. Māori concepts of relationship, connection with place and ancestors, spirituality, family, belonging and hygiene are all evident and given power by cultural capital, historical injustices and ongoing resistance to assimilation. The discussion also problematizes culturally embedded assumptions about the features required of a house to support the valued occupations of the people who live there.

Decolonizing Therapy

Health services designed and managed using *kaupapa* Māori (Māori ideology) are becoming more common in Aotearoa New Zealand as evidence mounts that culturally appropriate spaces can positively impact health outcomes for Māori who have lost touch with *iwi* (extended kinship groups) and *tikanga*. For instance, a recent study of patients in a forensic mental health unit showed how engaging in *kapa haka* (performing arts) provided a safe space to express themselves and develop connection to family and ancestors, which in turn built self-identity (Hollands, 2011). One participant articulated the importance of reconnecting to her origins using a metaphor:

> *Life previous to connecting to this part of my being was like being a leaf in autumn. Like the leaf, I was there on the ground, yet I didn't know where I'd come from. Learning waiata in te reo (Māori songs) was like a reclaiming or being welcomed home. It's like being away, not quite knowing who you are, and then finding out this is who I am and this is where I am from … It was like an aspect of who I am finding itself again … It's like the beginning of a journey and yet actually it's a journey of returning.* (Hollands, 2011, p. 47)

Hidden in the background of this account is a decades' long history of Māori resistance to colonizing and hegemonic medical practices. Aligning with Galvaan's (2015) recent work in South Africa, there is awareness that occupational patterns imposed in previous historical periods become self-perpetuating, pushing traditional occupational values and patterns into obscurity, and limiting contemporary occupational choices. There is also resistance, reclaiming and actively using cultural capital to revive traditional ways of doing to improve collective health and well-being. Also hidden are the design of the unit, which creates a suitable space for the performance; the collaboration of Māori and other staff to acknowledge each other's expertise and share resources and time in the programme; and increasing openness to Māori perspectives of health. The transformative power of *kapa haka* aligns with Dewey's ideas of experience and that improvement in living comes from reflection on prior experiences (Frank, 2011). In this example, both patients and staff are called on to reevaluate what has gone before and what is possible now. Most important, through experiencing shared traditional occupations

from a home region, self-identity, belonging, and culture are renewed (Frank, 2011).

CONCLUSION

Occupational justice speaks to the political practice of occupational therapy. It throws a spotlight onto the social forces in play when some people are deprived of or removed from occupations that sustain health and well-being, while others in the same society have privileged access, greater choice and more of the benefits. In this chapter, we have drawn on selected occupational science concepts to illustrate how inequitable access to occupation can be understood, and a pathway forward envisioned. In selecting examples specific to Aotearoa New Zealand, the context in which we are learning and teaching the politics of practice, we have talked of Māori being alienated from occupations that contain, express and pass on cultural values and *wairua*. In this *korero* (talk), we acknowledge our indebtedness to Māori activists and scholars, and especially to the leadership of Māori occupational therapists who are partnering with Pākeha members of the profession as we learn together about the essence of occupation and the impact of the spaces, the time, place, and history in which it exists.

REFERENCES

Angell, A.M., 2014. Occupation-centred analysis of social difference: contributions to a socially responsive occupational science. J. Occup. Sci. 21, 104–116. doi:10.1080/14427591.2012.711230.

Asaba, E., Wicks, A., 2010. Occupational terminology: occupational potential. J. Occup. Sci. 17 (2), 120–124. doi:10.1080/14427591.2010.9686683.

Bierre, S., Howden-Chapman, P., Signal, L., Cunningham, C., 2007. Institutional challenges in addressing healthy low cost housing for all: learning from past policy. Soc. Policy J. New Zealand 30 (3), 42–64.

Carter, L., 2006. Home and location: the problem of place as an ethnic identifier. Int. J. Humanit. 4 (3), 33–44.

Commission on Social Justice, 1994. Social Justice: Strategies for National Renewal. Vintage Books, London.

Connor, L.T., Wolf, T.J., Foster, E.R., Hildebrand, M.W., Baum, C.M., 2014. Participation and engagement in occupation in adults with disabilities. In: Pierce, D. (Ed.), Occupational Science for Occupational Therapy. Slack, Thorofare, NJ, pp. 107–120.

Davey, J., Kearns, R., 1994. Special needs versus the level playing field: recent developments in housing policy for indigenous people in New Zealand. J. Rural Stud. 10 (1), 73–82.

Dury, M., 1998. Whaiora: Maori health development. Oxford University, Oxford.

Eklund, M., Hermansson, A., Håkansson, C., 2012. Meaning in life for people with schizophrenia: does it include occupation? J. Occup. Sci. 19, 93–105. doi:10.1080/14427591.2011.605833.

Erlandsson, L.-K., 2013. The Redesigning Daily Occupations (ReDO) Program: supporting women with stress-related disorders to return to work – knowledge base, structure, and content. Occup. Ther. Ment. Health 29 (1), 85–101.

Fisher, A.G., 1994. Assessment of Motor and Process Skills (Version 8.0), Unpublished test manual. Department of Occupational Therapy, Colorado State University, Fort Collins, CO.

Frank, G., 2011. The transactional relationship between occupation and place: indigenous cultures in the American Southwest. J. Occup. Sci. 18 (1), 3–20. doi:10.1080/14427591.2011.562874.

Friedland, J., 2007. Thomas Bessell Kidner and the development of occupational therapy in the United States: establishing the links. Br. J. Occup. Ther. 70 (7), 292–300.

Galvaan, R., 2015. The contextually situated nature of occupational choice: marginalised young adolescents' experiences in South Africa. J. Occup. Sci. 21 (1), 39–53. doi:10.1080/14427591.2014.9 12124.

Groot, S., Hodgetts, D., Waimarea Nikora, L., Leggat-Cook, C., 2011. A Māori homeless woman. Ethnography. 12 (3), 375–397. doi:10.1177/1466138110393794.

Hall, L., 2008. Māori and Pacific peoples' housing needs in the Auckland region: a literature review. Auckland Regional Council, Auckland, New Zealand.

Health Act, 1920 (**11 GEO V 1920 No 45**) <http://www.nzlii.org/nz/legis/hist_act/ha192011gv1920n45141/> (accessed 14.05.16).

Hocking, C., 2013. Contribution of occupation to health and well-being. In: Boyt Schell, B.A., et al. (Eds.), Willard and Spackman's Occupational Therapy, twelfth ed. Wolters Kluwer/Lippincott Williams & Wilkins, Philadelphia, pp. 72–81.

Hocking, C., Shordike, A., Vittayakorn, S., Bunrayong, W., Rattakorn, P., Wright-St. Clair, V., 2014. Different ways of doing food: cultural influences on food preparation. In: Pierce, D. (Ed.), Occupational Science for Occupational Therapy. Slack, Thorofare, NJ, pp. 133–142.

Hocking, C., Townsend, E., Galheigo, S.M., Erlandsson, L.-K., de Mesquita Chagas, J.N., 2014. Driving Societal Change: Occupational Therapy, Health and Human Rights. Sixteenth International Congress of the World Federation of Occupational Therapists: Sharing Traditions. Creating Futures, Yokohama, Japan.

Hollands, T., 2011. Mental health and consumers' sensory experiences in kappa haka. Unpublished Master's dissertation. Auckland University of Technology, Auckland, New Zealand.

Hoskins, R., Te Nana, R., Rhodes, P., Guy, P., Sage, C., 2002. Ki te Hau Kainga: New Perspectives on Māori Housing Solutions. Housing New Zealand Corporation, Wellington, New Zealand.

Labrum, B., 2004. Developing 'The Essentials of Good Citizenship and Responsibilities' in Māori women: family life, social change, and the state in New Zealand, 1944-70. J. Fam. Hist. 29 (4), 446–465. doi:10.1177/0363199004267322.

Māori Social and Economic Advancement Act, 1945 (9 GEO VI 1945 No 43). <http://www.nzlii.org/nz/legis/hist_act/msaeaa19459gv1945n43381/> (accessed 14.05.16).

McLaughlin Gray, J., 1998. Putting occupation into practice: occupation as ends, occupation as means. Am. J. Occup. Ther. 52, 354–364. doi:10.5014/ajot.52.5.354.

Molineux, M., Strong, J., Rickard, W., 2014. Living with HIV infection: insights into occupational markers of health and occupational adaptation. In: Pierce, D. (Ed.), Occupational Science for Occupational Therapy. Slack, Thorofare, NJ, pp. 121–132.

Mueller, C., 2006. Integrating Turkish communities: a German dilemma. Popul. Res. Policy Rev. 25, 419–441.

Nikora, L.W., Guerin, B., Rua, M., Te Awekotuku, N., 2004. Moving away from home: some social consequences for Tuhoe migrating to the Waikato. New Zealand Popul. Rev. 30 (1–2), 93–109.

Njelesani, J., Tang, A., Jonsson, H., Polatajko, H., 2014. Articulating an occupational perspective. J. Occup. Sci. 21 (2), 226–235. doi :10.1080/14427591.2012.717500.

Perkins, H., Thorn, D., 1999. House and home and their interaction with changes in New Zealand's urban system, households and family structures. Housing Theory Society 16 (3), 124–135. doi:10.1080/14036099950149983.

Pool, I., Kukutai, T., 2014. Taupori Māori: Māori population change – population changes, 1769–1840. Te Ara – the Encyclopedia of New Zealand. Available at: <http://www.TeAra.govt.nz/en/taupori-maori-maori-population-change/page-1> (accessed 11.02.15.).

Rudman, D.L., 2005. Understanding political influences on occupational possibilities. J. Occup. Sci. 12 (3), 149–160. doi:10.1080 /14427591.2005.9686558.

Rudman, D.L., 2012. Governing through occupation: shaping expectations and possibilities. In: Whiteford, G.E., Hocking, C. (Eds.), Occupational Science: Society, Inclusion, Participation. Blackwell, Chichester, UK, pp. 100–116.

Stadnyk, R.L., Townsend, E.A., Wilcock, A.A., 2010. Occupational justice. In: Christiansen, C.H., Townsend, E.A. (Eds.), Introduction to Occupation: The Art and Science of Living, second ed. Pearson Education, Upper Saddle River, NJ, pp. 329–358.

Stanyer, J., 1994. The home: an occupational ideal. J. Occup. Sci. Aust. 1 (4), 31–36. doi:10.1080/14427591.1994.9686390.

Townsend, E.A., Polatajko, H.J., 2013. Enabling Occupation ll: Advancing an Occupational Therapy Vision for Health, Well-Being, & Justice through Occupation, second ed. Canadian Association of Occupational Therapists, Ottawa.

Townsend, E.A., Wilcock, A.A., 2004. Occupational justice. In: Christiansen, C.H., Townsend, E.A. (Eds.), Introduction to Occupation: The Art and Science of Living. Pearson Education, Upper Saddle River, NJ, pp. 243–273.

Tutu, D., 2011. Foreword. In: Kronenberg, F., Pollard, N., Sakellariou, D. (Eds.), Occupational Therapies without Borders, vol. 2. Towards an Ecology of Occupation-Based Practices. Churchill Livingstone Elsevier, Edinburg., p. ix.

United Nations High Commissioner for Human Rights and World Health Organization, 2008. Human Rights, Health and Poverty Reduction Strategies. Author, Geneva. <http://www.who.int/hhr/activities/publications/en/> (accessed 10.04.15.).

Waghorn, K., 2009. Home invasion. Home Cult. 6 (3), 261–296.

Wanhalla, A., 2006. Housing un/healthy bodies: native housing surveys and Māori health in New Zealand 1930-45. Health Hist.

8 (1), 100–120. Available at: <http://www.historycooperative.org/journals/hah/8.1/wanhalla.html>.

Whiteford, G., 1995. A concrete void: occupational deprivation and the special needs inmate. J. Occup. Sci. Aust. 2 (2), 80–81. doi:10.1080/14427591.1995.9686398.

Wilcock, A.A., 1998. An Occupational Perspective of Health. Slack, Thorofare, NJ.

Wilcock, A.A., Hocking, C., 2015. Occupational Perspective of Health, third ed. Slack, Thorofare, NJ.

Wilcock, A., Townsend, E., 2000. Occupational terminology interactive dialogue: occupational justice. J. Occup. Sci. 7 (2), 84–86. doi:10.1080/14427591.2000.9686470.

Wilding, C., 2010. Defining occupational therapy. In: Curtin, M., et al. (Eds.), Occupational Therapy and Physical Dysfunction: Enabling Occupation. Churchill Livingstone Elsevier, Edinburgh, pp. 3–15.

World Federation of Occupational Therapists, 2006. Position Paper: Human Rights. <http://www.wfot.org/ResourceCentre.aspx> (accessed 10.04.15.).

Yerxa, E.J., Clark, F., Jackson, J., Parham, D., Stein, C., Zemke, R., 1989. An introduction to occupational science: a foundation for occupational therapy in the 21st century. Occup. Ther. Health Care 6 (4), 1–17.

26

ENABLING OCCUPATIONAL THERAPY PRACTICE IN MARGINAL SETTINGS

JENNIFER CREEK

CHAPTER OUTLINE

In most countries throughout the world, occupational therapists are employed in healthcare and social care services, where they are often under pressure to work towards outcomes defined by their employers or colleagues. In such circumstances, they sometimes experience erosion of their professional autonomy, leading to frustration and role confusion. However, increasing numbers of occupational therapists are finding a role for themselves in marginal settings, such as war zones (Thibeault, 2005) or areas of poverty (Duncan, 2016). The practice of these therapists suggests alternative interpretations of the purpose of occupational therapy from those dominating mainstream settings. This chapter is based on the findings of a Ph.D. study completed in 2014, which investigated occupational therapy practice on the margins. It discusses the nature of such practice and argues that it has something of value to offer mainstream services.

This chapter begins with a brief account of the emergence of occupational therapy in response to unmet health and social needs at the beginning of the twentieth century and then describes how the profession has developed to maintain its relevance and value to society. The concept of occupational therapy on the margins is introduced, arguing that the margins of society represent important areas of unmet need. A study of occupational therapy on the margins found that certain practitioner characteristics enable effective practice in these settings. Five of these characteristics are described: agency, openness, responsiveness, commitment, and resourcefulness. I propose that, in order to express these enabling characteristics, occupational therapists must be autonomous professionals, with the freedom to carry out their specific role and function.

THE SOCIAL FUNCTION OF OCCUPATIONAL THERAPY

The profession of occupational therapy, which had its formal beginnings in North America and Europe in the early twentieth century, developed 'to fill a specific organizational vacuum – the lack of activity or occupation for long-stay mental patients' (Alaszewski, 1979, p. 437). One of the profession's main goals, as stated in the occupational therapy literature, was to assist patients to reintegrate themselves as far as possible into productive and socially accepted roles in society (Haworth and MacDonald, 1946). In order to meet this goal, occupational therapists engaged people in remedial activities that were appropriate to the patient and to the society of the time. Treatment media were selected as much for their social relevance and value as for their therapeutic potential. For example, in an article about occupational therapy for psychiatric illness, published at a time of full employment in the UK (Philpott, 2012), it was suggested that '[t]he hospital industries are extremely valuable in that they provide a sheltered working environment, one in which the work situation is real and not simulated [and the patient becomes] as capable of a full and efficient day's work as he was before his illness' (Casson and Foulds, 1955, p. 122).

We could say that 'a profession's development is related to the fit between the emerging needs of society and the appropriateness of the profession's response to such needs' (Duncan, 1999, p. 3). After 100 years of development and expansion, the occupational therapy profession is revisiting and restating its goals and purpose in the light of changing patterns of need, current social expectations, and modern healthcare practices. In the twenty-first century, occupational therapists are as likely to advocate for the rights of disabled people as to help them adapt to society's expectations (Whiteford and Townsend, 2011), as likely to be concerned with the needs of communities as with individual dysfunction (Lorenzo and Cloete, 2004), and as likely to focus on health promotion and disease prevention as on remediation or rehabilitation (Wilcock, 2006).

Occupational Therapy on the Margins

In many countries, occupational therapists work outside mainstream healthcare and social care services, with people living their lives on the margins of society.

A margin can be a physical place, a social space or a personal experience on the periphery of the social mainstream or dominant order. For every margin,

there is a centre or core that represents some form or position of authority, power and privilege. Margins exist wherever humans congregate; they affect every form of social grouping, including families, communities, organisations and society, and are constantly changing in response to socio-political, economic, cultural and other forces that marginalise people on the basis of perceived difference. (Duncan and Creek, 2014, p. 460)

The concepts of *margins* and *mainstream* represent a continuum, in that a space or position can be more or less mainstream or marginal. For example, in the UK, unemployed people are marginalized, but not to the same extent as people who are both unemployed and homeless. A particular group of people may be marginalized in some ways, but not in others, such as those who have a mental illness diagnosis but are highly successful in their chosen sphere of work. Furthermore, it is possible for a marginal social position to exist in close physical proximity to a social position of privilege and authority, such as street sleepers in the financial district of a city. Far from being an absolute state, marginality represents a family of conditions that may be experienced by different groups in different ways.

Marginal settings share a number of features, all of which exist in relation to a centre of power, privilege or authority (Duncan and Creek, 2014). These features include social and physical distance from the centre, lack of resources together with inability to access the resources of the centre, and powerlessness relative to the centre. Distance from centres of privilege, lack of resources and relative powerlessness put people in marginal situations at a disadvantage in relation to those in the centre. Professional practice under these conditions makes particular demands on the practitioner, and occupational therapists working on the margins need to display characteristics that will enable them to meet these demands.

As part of my Ph.D. study, I interviewed occupational therapists in nine marginal settings, in the UK and in four countries in southern Africa (since there are low numbers of occupational therapists in some of these countries they are not named to ensure confidentiality). The five settings in the UK were a football league for people with a mental illness diagnosis, film-making with homeless men living in hostels, community-based early intervention for people with a diagnosis of psychosis, horse riding for disabled soldiers and army veterans, and a landscape gardening business employing ex-offenders. The four marginal settings in Africa were community rehabilitation for war disabled people, drama with unemployed youths in an urban area, community mental health outreach in a rural area, and rug making as an income generation project for blind people. Interpretation of the interview transcripts produced a rich description of the nature of occupational therapy practice on the margins and identified that interviewees shared a number of characteristics which enabled them to practise effectively. These enabling characteristics are described in the next section.

FIVE ENABLING PROFESSIONAL CHARACTERISTICS

Occupational therapists practising in marginal settings exhibit five characteristics that make it possible for them to work effectively with disadvantaged groups of people in resource-poor environments. These enabling characteristics are agency, openness, responsiveness, commitment, and resourcefulness. The five terms used to refer to the enabling characteristics, and their definitions, emerged from the study on which this chapter is based. Illustrative examples of each characteristic are taken from the study.

It may be that occupational therapists choose to work in marginal settings because they possess these characteristics and want opportunities to express them in action. On the other hand, practitioners may find that they develop the characteristics while working on the margins. It is likely that the enabling characteristics are further developed through practice even if they are already present, because conditions on the margins require the practitioner to have skills and attitudes that are not necessarily useful in mainstream settings.

Agency

Agency is the capacity to take action towards an end (*Shorter Oxford English Dictionary,* 2002); for example, occupational therapists perceive unmet occupational needs and draw on their knowledge and skills to formulate ways of meeting them, as shown in Box 26-1. All healthcare professionals perceive need through the

---

BOX 26-1
EXPRESSING AGENCY IN ACTION

An occupational therapist volunteered as a prison visitor for several years. Over that time, he observed a pattern in the lives of prisoners: the revolving door syndrome. They would be released after a few months in jail; they would stay out for a while, then reoffend and return to jail. The therapist thought about how he could use his personal and professional skills to break this cycle of imprisonment, release and reoffending. With financial help from friends, he set up a landscape gardening business to employ ex-offenders so that they could learn practical, social and intrapersonal skills that would support fuller participation in society.

---

lens of their own area of expertise; for example, occupational therapists see that physical disability can lead to occupational deprivation, so they formulate the needs of disabled people in terms of overcoming the deprivation rather than the disability. This formulation gives them a role and a focus for intervention.

Agency enables occupational therapists to take action with and on behalf of people whose needs come within their professional domain of concern, which is 'the nature, balance, pattern and context of occupation' in people's lives (Creek, 2003, p. 31). Some people are more agentic than others, that is, they have a greater capacity for action, but agency is never absolute: people might know what they want to do and how to do it but find their actions constrained by the social, cultural, political and economic opportunities available (Sen, 1999). Knowing when to act and when to hold back is an essential aspect of agency.

Agency encompasses the other four enabling characteristics and is demonstrated through them. The occupational therapist working in a marginal setting has to be open to alternative ways of understanding need, responsive to local circumstances, committed to working under challenging conditions, and resourceful in finding the most appropriate ways to act.

Openness

Openness is the ability and willingness to perceive what is there without rigid defences, preconceptions or expectations. It involves looking carefully to see what is there, listening attentively to hear what is being said, questioning received wisdom and being prepared to explore alternative interpretations. The impressions people receive from their surroundings are inevitably influenced by their prior learning and experience, but an open attitude means that this foreknowledge does not act as an undue constraint on their perceptions. For occupational therapists, openness includes taking a broad view of need that goes beyond the individual, carrying out thorough analyses of all aspects of the environment, acknowledging one's own strengths and limitations, and sharing knowledge and power with colleagues and clients.

Being open to new ways of looking and thinking enables occupational therapists to tailor their actions to fit the circumstances. For example, an occupational therapist working in a community mental health team in a rural part of southern Africa recognized that, in order to help individuals with mental health problems, it was necessary to involve their communities, as illustrated by the case example in Box 26-2. This team's ability to conceptualize the wider community as the client depended on their not having an exclusive focus on the needs of the individual but, rather, on thinking more broadly about the context of those needs, recognizing that individuals are shaped by their social contexts and acknowledging that the community is as much a part of the intervention as the individual.

The characteristic of openness enables the practitioner to look at the environment as though from an alien perspective, like an anthropologist on Mars (Sacks, 1995). This is useful for therapists who are working in unfamiliar environments, such as a foreign country, as it allows them to see what is there. Additionally, the employment of an enquiring perspective within a familiar working environment enables occupational therapists to perceive needs that are being missed or ignored by the service.

Responsiveness

When agentic occupational therapists perceive unmet needs, they look for appropriate ways of responding to them. Responsiveness is ability and willingness to take appropriate action as a direct result of some stimulus or influence (*Shorter Oxford English Dictionary*, 2002). In order to make their responses appropriate to the circumstances, occupational therapists have to be flexible, think about what they are seeing, visualize and evaluate alternative responses, let go of habitual ways of thinking and doing things, and be prepared to try out new ideas or new ways of working.

Responsive occupational therapists do not look at the world through the lens of a formal theory or model that directs them towards a particular response or sequence of actions. They take time to make sense of what they are seeing, as described in the case study in Box 26-3, and may choose to accept a degree of risk or uncertainty while postponing action. These therapists avoid simplifying situations, recognizing that multiple factors are intertwined and that by changing any one

---

BOX 26-2
BEING OPEN TO THE CONTEXT

A mental health outreach team, visiting a village in rural southern Africa, saw a young girl with epilepsy. In that area, there was a lot of stigma associated with epilepsy, which was regarded as a mental problem. The child was carried everywhere by her family, she did not go to school and she was not allowed to eat with the rest of the family. Although it seemed initially that the child was the client, the team realized there was a wider issue of social attitudes to epilepsy that could only be addressed by providing education to the family, to neighbours, and to the school. This community intervention was effective and the child was allowed to start school.

BOX 26-3
SEEKING APPROPRIATE WAYS TO RESPOND

An occupational therapist started work at a riding centre for combat veterans and disabled ex-soldiers. Talking to staff and participants, and observing what went on, raised a number of questions that he felt had to be answered before he could decide on his contribution to the project. Participants gained some benefits from attending a 1- or 2-week riding course, but the therapist wanted to know what was going on in other areas of their lives and what happened when they left the centre. He chose to implement a way of measuring the impact that the riding course had on participants – both the immediate effect and how it carried through into other aspects of their lives. This enabled him to identify the areas in which occupational therapy input could be most beneficial: supporting participants through the transition from the riding centre back to their own homes.

factor they might affect any or all of the others in ways that cannot always be predicted.

The characteristic of responsiveness allows occupational therapists to find ways of dealing with unfamiliar situations, solving complex problems, and taking action that is appropriate to the circumstances. Effective practice in marginal settings depends on therapists recognizing and responding to local conditions, customs, and sensitivities. Within mainstream settings, this characteristic raises the possibility of occupational therapists responding to the needs they perceive rather than to the demands of the service or employer.

Commitment

Commitment is the dedication of energy and action, over a period of time, to achieving one's goals. Agentic occupational therapists do not assume that they should follow established routines and processes but take time to collect information, make sense of it and formulate possible responses. Working in this way necessitates commitment of time and energy while acknowledging that the outcomes of intervention are never completely certain.

One of the *Oxford English Dictionary* (2002) definitions of commitment suggests that the action of committing oneself to a course of action can have a moral dimension; for example, it has been claimed that 'occupational therapists have a commitment to everyday justice, specifically social inclusion in the occupations of a society' (Whiteford and Townsend, 2011, p. 68). The moral dimension of occupational therapy incorporates a human rights perspective that focuses on people's rights in relation to occupation: occupational therapists believe that, in a just society, no group is denied access to a range of everyday occupations on the basis of ability or other difference (Townsend and Wilcock, 2004a, 2004b).

In a marginal setting, occupational therapists can face ongoing challenges and barriers to progress and may have to dedicate significant amounts of time and energy to pursuing their goals. A concern with doing the right thing may not be sufficient to maintain this level of dedication over long periods of time, but commitment can bring other rewards, as illustrated in the case story in Box 26-4. These include pride in achievement, pleasure in using one's skills to their full extent,

---

BOX 26-4
THE REWARDS OF COMMITMENT

An occupational therapist volunteered for a project making films with homeless men, most of whom were drug or alcohol dependent. He found it hard to work with people whose behaviour could be chaotic and unpredictable, especially the 14- to 18-year-olds, who were not only very vulnerable but also aggressive and defensive. The therapist observed that the men's repertoire of responses was both very limited and mainly physical: aggression was one of the few ways they had experience of using to indicate that something was wrong and to negotiate a solution. He also perceived that much of their violent behaviour came from feeling insecure about their place in the world and their value to others. The therapist was able to acknowledge that the experience of working with these men presented him with a lot of material for reflecting on his own discriminatory ideas about where the responsibility lies for substance abuse. This recognition of his own deep learning helped the therapist remain committed to working with homeless men, despite the ongoing difficulties.

---

opportunities for new learning and the satisfaction of seeing clients succeed.

Resourcefulness

To be resourceful is to be 'capable, full of practical ingenuity' (*Shorter Oxford English Dictionary*, 2002); resourcefulness means practical ingenuity in using whatever is readily available to solve problems or create opportunities. The resources available to occupational therapists include their own skills, knowledge and experience, together with whatever human and nonhuman conditions are present in the environment. The range of possibilities for action is determined, in large part, by the resources available and the therapist's ingenuity in making use of them.

Margins are, by definition, places or positions that are resource poor in relation to the centre. Occupational therapists working in large hospitals in developed countries can take for granted their access to resources such as equipment, materials, personnel and information. In contrast, many marginal settings lack all of these things and may be situated at a distance from the places where resources can be obtained. This means that occupational therapists have to use their practical ingenuity to locate what is needed or find

BOX 26-5
RESOURCEFULNESS IN PRACTICE

The occupational therapist introduced in Box 26-4 was working on a voluntary basis with homeless men and had no official status within the organization. He therefore had no control over who came into the film group but was expected to accept anyone who wanted to attend. When participants were being especially disruptive and negative, he did not have the status or power within the group to tell them to behave or to leave. At these times, he found himself falling back into a more formal role as a therapist, which he consciously constructed as a way of distancing himself from participants and managing what was going on. Recognizing that this defensive response was unproductive, the occupational therapist began to develop new ways of working with the group and new skills for dealing with these clients. For example, he began to think of the film group as a space in which participants could try out new ways of responding, and negotiated a minimal set of rules with them that would make it a safe space. He found that having the opportunity to make films provided sufficient incentive for participants to accept certain rules.

alternative resources. Sometimes, therapists have to develop their own skills further to meet the demands of the situation, as illustrated in the case story in Box 26-5.

Resources are only useful if they are available to the people who need them, in the right place and at the right time, and if they are effective in meeting one or more needs. Additionally, resources have to be culturally and personally acceptable to participants and used in appropriate ways. Occupational therapists working on the margins have to be imaginative and creative in appreciating the resource potential of their environments and converting that potential into useful resources. For occupational therapists working on the margins, professional resourcefulness is a primary resource.

THE AUTONOMOUS PRACTITIONER

This chapter has described some of the professional characteristics that enable occupational therapists to work effectively within challenging situations. Practitioners in marginal settings, facing complex problems with scarce resources, have to employ all their own skills and resources and work to their maximum potential. This full realization of professional potential is not incidental to practice on the margins; such settings, by their nature, demand that occupational therapists make complete use of their knowledge, skills, attributes, and experience.

In order to express their agency fully, occupational therapists need to work as autonomous professionals. They must be free to plan, in partnership with participants and communities, interventions that are appropriate to the local context. They have to be able to put their plans into action, modifying them as circumstances dictate, without the constraints of targets and protocols imposed by managers, commissioners and funders. When constraints are put on therapists' professional autonomy, this affects both what they can do and the amount of autonomy they can give to their clients.

Healthcare and social care services worldwide are challenged by the volume and complexity of health and social needs arising from conditions such as demographic changes, climate change, human-made disasters, war, and poverty (World Health Organization and World Bank, 2011). In this global context, employing occupational therapists to carry out discharge assessments and short-term interventions is not a cost-effective use of their time and professional expertise. Equally, replacing occupational therapists with unqualified helpers or lower-grade staff is not an effective strategy for dealing with complex needs. Professional occupational therapists working autonomously and innovatively over long periods of time have the capacity to deal effectively with long-term, complex problems, as illustrated by the example in Box 26-6.

Occupational therapists working in marginal settings do not keep their professional skills and knowledge to themselves but try to help the people they work with to develop sufficient understanding and skills to be able to find ways of meeting their own occupational needs. For this to happen, the people who use occupational therapy services need to be involved closely in all aspects of their own treatment, so that they learn both the how and the why in order to be able to do it for themselves. The extent to which the people who use services can be involved is a matter of local and national policy; therefore, occupational therapists

BOX 26-6
CREATING SPACE TO WORK AUTONOMOUSLY

An occupational therapist started a football team for inpatients on the forensic unit where he was working. He then realized that playing football could act as a bridge between the hospital and community, so he set up a minileague, bringing local community teams into the unit to play matches against the inpatients. After one season, his employers decided that the league should be abandoned because he was not being paid to work with community patients. The occupational therapist chose to leave the forensic service and took a job in a community mental health service where, with the agreement of his new employer, one day a week was dedicated to the football league. The project was so successful in engaging people with severe, long-term mental health problems that the service agreed to pay the occupational therapist to work on it full time for 2 years.

need to work with policymakers and managers to ensure that policies do not become barriers to service user involvement.

CONCLUSION

This chapter presented occupational therapy as a profession with a broad remit: to work with people whose occupations are disrupted or curtailed by a health condition, disability, poverty, war, natural disasters, displacement, or social deprivation. Increasing numbers of occupational therapists are choosing to practise in marginal settings where the intersection of all these factors can cause serious occupational deprivation. In my study, I found that practitioners on the margins share certain characteristics that make it possible for them to work effectively in areas of deprivation. These five characteristics enable practitioners to be open to the possibilities and challenges of the social and physical environments in which they operate. Although the characteristics were identified in occupational therapists working in marginal settings, they could also be of value for practitioners employed in mainstream services, as well as those in teaching and learning.

The type of professionalism demonstrated by occupational therapists on the margins can be developed through a dialogue between the theories and skills students learn at university and their experiences during practice placements. Careful thought has to be given to what theories are taught in occupational therapy programmes: procedural and inflexible models may constrain students to think in particular ways, and hence act as barriers to openness and responsiveness. Care should also be taken over how theory is taught, if students are to understand it as part of a dialogue rather than a static reference point. Students need to learn how to think critically about what they are taught, not to believe that theories have universal applicability or that there is a correct approach to use in all circumstances, but to tease out what might be relevant to a particular situation.

While the pedagogy and content of occupational therapy programmes have an influence on what type of practitioners they produce, occupational therapy practice is also shaped by the norms and expectations of service settings, contracts, job descriptions, local and national policies, guidelines, and protocols. Professional autonomy is a necessary condition for the full expression of agency, openness, responsiveness, commitment, and resourcefulness that enable effective practice on the margins.

Acknowledgements

This chapter is based on the findings of a research study carried out at Sheffield University, under the supervision of Professor Jon Nixon and Dr. Sarah Cook, and completed in 2014.

REFERENCES

Alaszewski, A., 1979. Rehabilitation, the remedial therapy professions and social policy. Soc. Sci. Med. 13A, 431–443.

Casson, E., Foulds, E., 1955. Modern trends in occupational therapy as applied to psychiatric illness. Occup. Ther. 18 (3), 113–123.

Creek, J., 2003. Occupational Therapy Defined as a Complex Intervention. College of Occupational Therapists, London.

Duncan, M., 1999. Our bit in the calabash: thoughts on occupational therapy transformation in South Africa. South Afr. J. Occup. Ther. 29 (2), 3–9.

Duncan, M., 2016. Developmental reasoning in occupational therapy community practice. In: Creek, J., Cole, M. (Eds.), Global Perspectives in Professional Reasoning. Slack, Thorofare, NJ.

Duncan, M., Creek, J., 2014. Working on the margins: occupational therapy and social inclusion. In: Bryant, W., Fieldhouse, J., et al. (Eds.), Creek's Occupational Therapy and Mental Health, fifth ed. Churchill Livingstone Elsevier, Edinburgh, pp. 457–473.

Haworth, N.A., MacDonald, E.M., 1946. Theory of Occupational Therapy, third ed. Ballière, Tindall & Cox, London.

Lorenzo, T., Cloete, L., 2004. Promoting occupation in rural communities. In: Watson, R., Swartz, L. (Eds.), Transformation through Occupation. Whurr, London, pp. 268–286.

Philpott, J., 2012. Britain at Work in the Reign of Queen Elizabeth II. Chartered Institute of Personnel and Development, London. Available at: <www.cipd.co.uk> (accessed 06.10.14).

Sacks, O., 1995. An Anthropologist on Mars: Seven Paradoxical Tales. Picador, New York.

Sen, A., 1999. Development as Freedom. Oxford University Press, Oxford.

Shorter Oxford English Dictionary, fifth ed. 2002. Oxford University Press, Oxford.

Thibeault, R., 2005. Connecting health and social justice: a Lebanese experience. In: Kronenberg, F., Algado, S.S., Pollard, N. (Eds.), Occupational Therapy without Borders: Learning from the Spirit of Survivors. Elsevier Churchill Livingstone, Edinburgh, UK, pp. 232–244.

Townsend, E., Wilcock, A., 2004a. Occupational justice. In: Christiansen, C., Townsend, E. (Eds.), Introduction to Occupation: The Art and Science of Living. Prentice Hall, Upper Saddle River, NJ, pp. 243–273.

Townsend, E., Wilcock, A., 2004b. Occupational justice and client-centred practice: a dialogue in progress. Can. J. Occup. Ther. 71 (2), 75–87.

Whiteford, G., Townsend, E., 2011. Participatory Occupational Justice Framework (POJF 2010): enabling occupational participation and inclusion. In: Kronenberg, F., Pollard, N., Sakellariou, D. (Eds.), Occupational Therapies without Borders, vol. 2. Towards an Ecology of Occupation-Based Practices. Churchill Livingstone Elsevier, Edinburgh, UK, pp. 65–84.

Wilcock, A.A., 2006. An Occupational Perspective of Health, second ed. Slack, Thorofare, NJ.

World Health Organization and World Bank, 2011. World Report on Disability. World Health Organization, Geneva.

27

SOCIAL OCCUPATIONAL THERAPY, CITIZENSHIP, RIGHTS, AND POLICIES: CONNECTING THE VOICES OF COLLECTIVES AND INDIVIDUALS

ROSELI ESQUERDO LOPES ■ ANA PAULA SERRATA MALFITANO

CHAPTER OUTLINE

Discussions about the social responsibility of occupational therapists, as well as the resources used to promote the participation and social inclusion of individuals and groups, are becoming increasingly common in occupational therapy. The meaning of social responsibility is not always clear, however. It can sometimes refer to the historical debate about 'social adaptation', founded on uncritical thinking that does not question social structure and its inequalities (Galheigo, 1997) or social injustice contexts (Townsend, 1993). The professional concerns often lie in the integration or reintegration of people into their environment without discussing the reasons for their exclusion and their resistance to reintegration (Galheigo, 1997). The failure of reintegration attempts has been almost always attributed to the types of difficulties the individual is experiencing, the seriousness of their situation, and their family attitudes. The possibility that these social structures may be the causal agents of such failures is being increasingly debated by occupational

therapists. Failure of reintegration can sometimes be the result of a rejection occasioned by the lack of appropriate opportunities that make the best use of people's abilities (Galheigo, 1997).

Therefore, the understanding of macrosocial elements, such as the economic and political factors, has come to be of the utmost importance for occupational therapy interventions, as long as these interventions are planned with the aim of working in the interests of autonomous (in the sense of independence and social interdependence), participative and integrated individuals. Such interventions can create the possibility for people to be subjects who participate in social life in both collective and individual ways. For this reason, familiarity with the issues of citizenship and public policy has become crucial to occupational therapists (European Network of Occupational Therapy in Higher Education, 2013). Occupational therapists need to know about and work with the social rights in their context, which requires services and professionals to be involved in the

245

creation, implementation and evaluation of social policies[1].

The human resources issue is pivotal throughout the whole process of discussing social policy, since it is the professionals in a given area who may have the power to convert political innovation into practice and into real improvements for wider populations (Lopes, 1999). Thus, occupational therapists assume a primary role in mediating access to social commodities when they act as social policy professionals. More specifically, when focusing attention on socially vulnerable groups, the topics of 'citizenship' and 'public policy' are even more central, forming an important theoretical perspective in the development of social occupational therapy in Brazil (Lopes, 2013).

This chapter aims to discuss social occupational therapy in Brazil and to share some experiences developed from this perspective. This subject is important because of the current demands for intervention from many professionals, including occupational therapists. Occupational therapists need to develop skills to improve the social life conditions of many different groups. Occupational therapists have the opportunity to advance outside of the healthcare system (Malfitano, Lopes, Borba and Magalhães, 2014a), dealing with diverse populations, working towards achieving participation for all in society. This chapter explores the relationship among citizenship, social rights and social policies, looking at the possibilities to develop occupational therapy in the social field.

THE CAPITALIST STATE AND SOCIAL POLICIES

One fundamental question that is always current in the analysis of the contemporary State is the understanding of how public policies – and in particular social policies – are generated from existing economic and politico-institutional structures. In the capitalist state, which is based on the private valuation of capital and the selling of labour in the form of a commodity, and in which these structures intrinsically have a class-

related character, what functions can be assigned to those policies?

Democratic capitalist states may be understood as institutional forms of public power based on the structure of classes: people who are owners of the means of production and people who sell their labour force. In capitalist democracies the relations of material production are basically characterized by three functional determinants: the privatization of production, the structural dependence of the accumulation process, and the democratic state. This democratic state is subject to the double determinant of political power: from a materialistic perspective, its content is determined by the development and requirements of the accumulation of capital process. On the other hand, as an institutional form, it is subject to the rules of representative democratic government through the mechanism of periodic elections (Offe and Ronge, 1984).

Therefore, the capitalist state's *public policies* may be defined as a group of strategies through which agreement and compatibility between the structural determinants of the capitalist state are constantly produced and reproduced. However, the state's general strategy of action is aimed at creating the conditions through which each citizen is included in exchange relations (Offe and Ronge, 1984). This definition indicates the strategy that should guide the conception of these policies in order to fulfil the capitalist state's needs. Exchange relations are the source of the wealth and growth on which the state depends, and therefore its policies are conceived towards meeting these needs and ensuring the continuity of its existence (Offe, 1984).

On the other hand, the *social policies* of the capitalist state are defined as a particular case of public policy: They correspond to those relations and strategies organized in a way that creates the conditions for the owners of labour to be included in the exchange relations. To develop social policies, sociopolitical innovations are needed: changes need to be adopted in order to generate, finance and distribute the provision of social services by executive government officers and stakeholders, reconciling the demands made with previously sanctioned needs (Offe and Ronge, 1984). These represent the incorporation of 'human needs' according to the 'interests' of the system. It is important to highlight that conflict is inherent in the capitalist system. A broad acknowledgement of those 'needs'

---

[1]This text is not targeting the service users' dimensions. Our aim is to highlight the professional role, especially that of the occupational therapist, in social policies.

will ensue as a result of the conflicts caused by the balance of power between civil society, political society (Gramsci, 1992), and the system's other social actors (Dagnino, 2007).

The social issue has its origins in the way people organize themselves to produce within a specific social and historical context. This organization is expressed in the social reproduction sphere, which means that the social issue is determined by the specific and peculiar trait of the capital–labour relationship: exploitation. In every struggle against its sociopolitical and human manifestations, the social issue is condemned to face certain symptoms, consequences, and effects without having a major impact on the exploitation mechanisms of the capitalist regime (Netto, 2001).

It is important to analyse the social issue as a political, economic and ideological issue that refers to a specific correlation of power between different classes, integrated into the broader context of the social movement of the struggle for hegemony (Gramsci, 1992)[2]. Some social movements are more favourable to the expression of labour demands and of their admission into society's political scene, demanding their recognition by the capitalist system and the state, resulting in sociopolitical innovations. However, this is constrained by the limits of capitalist society, through citizenship and social rights.

In the following sections we present a theoretical discussion about citizenship, which offers the basis for our notion of a social occupational therapy.

CITIZENSHIP

Concept of Citizenship

The last decade of the twentieth century saw a proliferation of studies on citizenship (Neveu et al., 2011). Thomas Janoski, in *Citizenship and Civil Society*

(1998), highlights three theoretical approaches that deal with phenomena associated with citizenship: Marshall's theory on citizenship rights; the approach by Durkheim[3] on civic culture, already foreseen by Tocqueville[4]; and the Gramscian/Marxist[5] theory on civil society.

The concept of citizenship as the right to have rights, among several other perspectives, is classically referred to in 1949 by Thomas Marshall, who proposed the first sociological theory on the concept by developing the rights and obligations inherent to citizen status. Centred in the British reality of the time, it established a typology of citizenship rights: civic rights, acquired in the eighteenth century; political rights, achieved in the nineteenth century; and social rights, acquired in the twentieth century (Marshall, 1950).

For Durkheim (1972), citizenship is not limited to the form sanctioned by law, and its core characteristic lies in civic virtue. Therefore, enough room is created so that volunteer, private and nonprofit groups in the public sphere make up civil society.

Marxist theories, on the other hand, emphasize the reconstitution of civil society – an idea already put forward by Hegel, reprised by Marx and significantly revisited by Gramsci. The latter created a paradigm shift with his tripartite vision: the State, the market and civil society (Gramsci, 1992). The current reference to civil society carries with it the Gramscian bias of protection against State and market abuses. This

[3]Émile Durkheim (1858–1917), a French philosopher, is considered one of the founders of modern sociology, responsible for the systematization of this new field, outlined in his book *The Rules of Sociological Method* (1895).

[4]Alexis de Tocqueville (1805–1859), was a French social scientist with law knowledge, who held several political and administrative positions. He used the comparative historical method to analyse the historical genesis and sociological and political typology of democratic regimes, both in France and in the United States. His major work was *Democracy in America* (1835).

[5]Karl Marx (1818–1883), a German philosopher, based on the Hegelian dialectic and studies of English economists and French socialism, developed a critique of capitalism. In 1867, he published the first volume of his major work, *Capital*. His *Manifesto of the Communist Party* (1848) had a big impact on European policy. This book, written with Friedrich Engels, is a brief summary of historical materialism and a call to revolution, giving rise to Marxist theory.

[2]Antonio Gramsci, an Italian from Sardinia, was born in 1891 and died in 1937, imprisoned in the jails of Mussolini's fascist regime. He was an original follower of Marxism, which he preferred to call the Philosophy of Praxis. The hegemony notion was created within the Marxist tradition to understand different social settings. For Gramsci, the hegemony concept designates a particular type of domination, the allowed domination, especially of one social class over another. The concepts of the structure and superstructure, and the relationship between them, civil society and ideology, are central in his work (Gramsci, 1992).

could be understood, for some authors (such as Janoski, 1998), as lying halfway between the focus on the State adopted by Marshall and the focus on society-centred civic virtue, mediating between these two different foci.

Civil society theories, concerned with the mediatory institutions between citizen and State, add a wide range of possibilities to the understanding of that relationship. Civil society is mainly formed in the public sphere, where associations and organizations engage in debates, so that most of the struggles for citizenship are conducted within their scope through the interests of social groups. Although civil society might not constitute the locus of citizenship rights, as it is not in the state sphere, it ensures official protection through legal sanctions (Vieira, 2001).

In defining the relationship between civil society and citizenship, political theory and empirical reality need to be discussed. *Liberalism,* which is dominant in Anglo-Saxon countries, with its emphasis on the individual, proposes that most rights involve freedoms inherent to each and every person; despite the individual having obligations (e.g., taxes, military service), civil liberties and property rights are central points. Individual rights are vital. Later, liberalism became the basis for neoliberalism. On the other hand, social rights or group rights represent a break from liberal principles. The relationship between rights and duties is essentially contractual, bearing a heavy load of reciprocity: in general, for each right, there is a corresponding obligation.

Communitarianism prioritizes the community, society and the nation, using solidarity and a sense of common destiny as the cornerstone of social cohesion (Janoski, 1998). Society is based on the actions and support of groups, in contrast to liberal individualism. Its main objective is to build a community based on central values, such as a common identity, solidarity, participation, and integration. This way, obligations become predominant compared with rights. In this perspective of critiquing liberalism, the decline in solidarity between citizens and the absence of a common destiny are important characteristics of modernity. Thus, communitarians assign a character of virtue to citizenship. In the liberal vision, citizenship is an accessory, not a value. In the communitarian vision, individuals are members of units greater than themselves, such as the political community, where social unity and a space for exercising the virtue of participation are created.

Expansive democracy theory (Janoski, 1998) represents a third approach to citizenship, separate from both liberalism and communitarianism. It defends the expansion of individual or collective rights to historically discriminated individuals, especially on account of their class, gender, or ethnicity, claiming an increase in collective participation in decisions and a greater interaction between institutions and the citizen. Despite sharing the criticism of liberalism's privileging of the individual, it emphasizes the right of participation, not accepting the secondary role given to rights, as in the communitarian perspective. It calls for a balance between individual and group rights and obligations, resulting in an identity system built on the concept of the individual as a participant in the community's activities. By 1949, Marshall had already perceived citizenship as a true element of social change in the context of the industrial reality of the time and the associated *welfare state* postwar experience.

The expansion of rights would correspond firstly to the strengthening of previously acquired rights and also to the incorporation of new groups into the State. The territorial basis of citizenship has been transformed though history, moving from the Greek *polis* to the Roman Empire, to the medieval city and, finally, to the modern State. The centralization process that generated the State corresponds to the expansion of the local form to the institutional form of citizenship. From this point of view, the expansion of rights is part of a democratization process, interpreted as an acquisition of rights by the popular classes that were originally created by and for the elites.

Three generations of citizenship rights may therefore be described according to what has been mentioned above, based on Marshall (1950): civil, political, and social. Considering the conflict in the cumulative expansion of rights, Marshall directs his attention to the existing antagonism between civil rights, which grant the individual protection against the State, and social rights, which should ensure the right to a real income through benefits assured by the State. Therefore social citizenship collides with the conditions of capitalism and its practice of generating conflict.

Marshall concluded that social citizenship and capitalism are at war, but argues that citizenship and social class are compatible in a democratic capitalist society, insofar as citizenship has become the source of legitimized social inequality. Such ambiguity would resonate strongly in the debate in the following decades between Marxists and social democrats.

Multiple Citizenships

The present concern is directed towards a search to making the existence of diverse possibilities and grades of citizenship compatible, including life in small communities and the reformulation of citizenship at the nation level or on a global level.

Citizenship under the collective scope can no longer be seen as a group of formal rights, but rather as a way of incorporating individuals and groups into society. With the aim of resolving the conflicting relationship between the multiple traditions of citizenship, based on status, participation, and identity, some authors have sought to formulate a complex system, where access to rights is secured by local, national and transnational institutions (Vieira, 2001).

This chapter highlights two main approaches. The first, from Iris Young (Shafir, 1998), mentions the need for the institutionalization of multiple citizenships as a way to ensure justice and equity. The rights of social groups need to be made real, since under the auspices of universality, exclusion has always existed and will continue to exist: formal equality, paradoxically, creates important inequality. The specific issue concerning several oppressed groups is raised (Afrodescendants, women, Latinos, indigenous peoples, homosexuals, the elderly, the poor, and people with disabilities). The proposal for a differentiated citizenship by Will Kymlicka (1996) advocates that rights should be guaranteed not only to individuals but also to groups. An extension of Marshall's linear scheme is proposed, the guarantee of a fourth generation of rights: the cultural rights of citizenship. Such rights refer to issues related to difference, options, orientations, and cultural aspects of places. If everybody is equal in a society, it is possible that the cultural right of citizenship is the right to a difference.

In the second alternative, by Michael Walzer (1992), the centre for the diversity in citizenship lies precisely in one of the forms of citizenship: politics. The admiration Walzer has for the Greek tradition is evident, where political participation assumes the highest form of humanity as a principle of incorporation and social unity. Walzer (1992) also explores the concept of civil society as a place of challenge: whereas citizenship is the basis of social unity, civil society, by allowing diverse social demands to be articulated, embodies its classical role of generating civility. Respect for diversity and social pluralism should be an integral part of the citizenship discourse.

Citizenship Challenges and the Articulation of Rights

A substantial body of work from the 1990s seems to point in the direction of a unified theory of citizenship. Until now, there has been no one theory, but instead important theoretical contributions have been made regarding the tensions between the diverse elements that constitute the citizenship concept, clarifying the reasons for them being current (Vieira, 2001).

Two interpretations are addressed in this view. In the first, the citizen's role is seen in an individualistic and instrumental way, according to the liberal tradition initiated by Locke[6] (1988). Individuals are considered as private persons, external to the State, and their interests are prepolitical. In the second version, a communitarian conception originating from the political philosophy of Aristotle remains, with the proposition of an active citizenship being central to it. Individuals are integrated into a political community, and their personal identity is a function of traditions and common institutions.

The model derived from Locke's ideas is based on individual rights and equal treatment. The second, based on Aristotelian arguments, defines participation in self-government as an essence of freedom, which is an essential component of citizenship. There would be a passive citizenship, from 'the top', via the state, and an active citizenship, from 'below'. Consequently, there would be a conservative citizenship – passive and private – and another one, a revolutionary one – active and public. It is from that place that we advocate the

---

[6]John Locke (1632–1704) was an English philosopher and physician who is regarded as one of the most influential writers on liberalism theory.

context of citizenship and rights, the broadening of equality and the acknowledgement of differences as the foundations for a social occupational therapy – or, to put it another way, citizenship as an axis, in the words of Sandra Galheigo (1997).

SOCIAL OCCUPATIONAL THERAPY: A COMPLEX FIELD

By the end of the 1990s, we faced a neoliberal avalanche in Brazil. Two main points result in a new configuration of the old social question (Castel, 2003; Donzelot, 1984). First, the growing vulnerability of groups and individuals in the context of a minimalist, privatizing State, and of focused and selective actions in a society that trivializes the word *citizenship*, where democracy seems restricted to the bourgeois precepts of cyclical voting. The second, very fundamental issue, refers to the intense transformations in the world of work that have led to the aggravation of the issue of exploitation of labour and to the degradation of associated protection systems. This transformation process of the social rules has resulted in the emergence of individuals considered as 'conjunctural invalids' (Donzelot, 1977) or 'leftovers' (Castel, 1997), who develop 'deficits of integration' (in work, home, education and culture) and suffer disqualification, social invalidation, dissolution of connections, and even the threat of social exclusion through explicit discriminatory treatment.

In this context, the Metuia project was formed in 1998. This was part of what Denise Barros, Sandra Galheigo and Roseli Lopes describe as the resurgence of the social issue for occupational therapists in Brazil (Barros et al., 2011a). The Metuia group was created by occupational therapy academics, students and practitioners from universities in the São Paulo state. Metuia means 'friend' or 'companion' in the language of the Bororo people, an indigenous community from the centre-west area of the country (Barros et al., 2011b). Metuia members have developed programmes through teaching, research and community engagement based on occupational therapy knowledge. They have been involved with many community populations and have set up several programmes, working with diverse groups (e.g homeless people) and addressing a variety of aims, such as, for example: advocating

against the sexual exploitation of children and young people; and exploring the connections between social policies for the young, culture, and migration.

Barros, Ghirardi and Lopes (2005) identified from a sociological point of view two groups that were targets of a disciplinary discourse, in a Foucauldian way, from both the medical (in the wider sense) and the legal sectors, and that are represented in the population of social occupational therapy:

1. Those who suffer social exclusion processes, where their institutionalization is justified so that they recover, are educated or are repressed. Foucault (2000) critiques the incarceration, surveillance, punishment and other institutional ways of operation. This involves, among others: (a) those who inhabited and continue to inhabit confined and isolated spaces of the community, such as psychiatric hospitals, so-called therapeutic communities, asylums and institutions for people with disabilities, and prisons; (b) poor children and youths; and (c) elderly people in asylums or other residential institutions, who lack civil and social rights.

2. Groups that, due to their social positions, are directly exposed to job precariousness and social vulnerability and, therefore, confined to remaining at the margins, resulting in the rupturing of social networks. For these people, the deficit of integration is associated with the degradation of the labour market and economic consequences on quality of life: difficulty in acquiring a place to live, attaining education and developing sociability and cultural awareness lead to exclusion processes.

Social occupational therapy in Brazil had become noteworthy by the end of the 1990s: the development of occupational therapy was established in healthcare and, therefore, became a necessary mediation between health and disease. The profession had become recognized by other professional groups and was developing services and interventions. The process of promoting social participation created an environment in Brazil that enabled the identification of serious social issues, and a range of social and professional groups, including occupational therapists, were involved in searching for solutions.

Occupational therapy practice reflects what occupational therapy professionals think and produce and the ways they position themselves politically on the social issues that are presented to them. This means that political action is inherent in everyday life and should be strongly related to occupational therapy (Pollard et al., 2008). Occupational therapy methods are tailored for their pertinence to specific problems and their potential solutions. Inequality and poverty are important issues in the context of the global social question. In Brazil, particular social and economic characteristics are developing that require a critical revision of the professional role of the occupational therapists.

Citizenship has been positioned as a principle that has directed the actions of Brazilian occupational therapists since the mid-1980s. Initially, citizenship was the focus of a political struggle through active participation in various social movements, such as health, education, and housing movements. Then, citizenship became a parameter of a new way of acting professionally, transforming itself into the axis which coordinated the actions of the occupational therapist. Individual and collective interventions have, since then, been understood as being rooted in their contextual situation and as part of the historical process of producing meanings and negotiating culture (Barros et al., 2007).

This way, without forgetting that the fight against exclusion entails a combat against the deregulation of labour and in favour of wealth distribution, and without neglecting the fact that actions need to be integrated into a historical and political process, we believe in the knowledge of the participatory and mediative nature of activity. Occupational therapy practice may contribute to the formation of links and action in the social field (Barros et al., 2005).

Barros et al. (2005) defined social occupational therapy in Brazil as the specific knowledge used in occupational therapy to deal with people lacking the social and economic resources to live. Malfitano, Lopes, Magalhães and Townsend (2014b) highlight the context approach:

Social occupational therapy is practiced in the real context where people live and where politics, economic, and cultural aspects of life shape and are shaped by everyday life...The real context can be understood as the locus *for the many sectors of life. In other words, it is the very context within which occupations are realized, subject to the possibilities and limitations imposed by socioeconomic determinants. (p. 2)*

Social occupational therapy emerges from an effort to create links between the social demand from the macrosocial aspects and the accumulated knowledge produced by occupational therapists, regarding the professional function of promoting both social inclusion and autonomy.

Social occupational therapy borrows two fundamental concepts from Paulo Freire: awareness and dialogue (Freire, 1970). Awareness comes from the ability to distance oneself from reality through the experience of having been immersed in it and having moved beyond it in time. It moves beyond awareness by revealing the reasons for the existence of situations, followed by transforming this reality. Freire (1970), as well as Basaglia and Ongaro-Basaglia (1977), does not dissociate technical action from political action.

Since 1999, Brazilian social occupational therapists have been developing various projects of intervention, working together with public governmental and nongovernmental organizations, which act in support of the universalization of citizenship rights and towards strengthening and creating social networks to support populations facing exclusion processes (Castel, 2003). There are distinct demands that imply the need for the building of knowledge and specific methodological procedures, to which current knowledge from the healthcare field provides no real answer.

Social occupational therapy uses the notion of territory and intervention within a specific context, a community space. The territory interventions are oriented to a collective conception of the individual as a community member, rather than towards individual demands. Territorial-based practices are related to the concept of context and environment (Law, 1991) or of community development practices (Leclair, 2010). These ideas originated in Canada and are based on the principle of integrating community spaces of those individuals and groups as a key element of any proposed action. The difference of social occupational therapy is in its conceptualization of space/territory. It not 'only' refers to a consideration of the context and the experiential knowledge (Pollard and Sakellariou, 2014) to measure the action of an individual person, but it also refers to a consideration of the space/territory as the locus of action where the collective dimensions of individual engagements are reached. They are both individual and collective.

Therefore, the social occupational therapist may work in the planning and implementation of policies at the management level, as well as with their articulation in a network, aiming for more effective actions (Malfitano et al., 2014a). The work developed in public schools, in the context of the Brazilian educational policy when working with youth from the periphery, is considered to be an essential action, from a dimension as a collective individual (Lopes et al., 2011b). The work performed with the homeless, having as its central point the political participation of this vulnerable group (Almeida et al., 2012), is another example. The space of cultural policy and its services, used for acting with the most diverse social groups and the access to culture, comprises another area of discussion in Brazilian social occupational therapy, extending its action beyond the services associated with health, education, and social assistance policies (Barros et al., 2013). The discussion about labour and economic and social processes in a society that is suffering important transformations in this regard occupies an important role in the actions of social occupational therapy (Ghiradi, 2012).

On one hand, prioritization is given to the dimension of collective individuals, marked by the concepts of citizenship and rights, and with a focus on action in public policy. This does not mean, on the other hand, that actions with regards to individual people should be less relevant. In contrast, it is through understanding and acting with individuals considered in their collective dimensions that we can improve the work of the occupational therapist in the individual dimension.

With this in mind, the term *individual and territorial follow-up* (Lopes et al., 2011a) was given to an approach linking collective and individual demands, giving priority to the individuals' trajectories and their personal potential for participating in social life. This is a powerful resource for social occupational therapy actions. However, it must be stressed that it distances

itself from a clinical dimension in health. With groups in social vulnerability, such as homelessness, youth living in periphery, and immigrants, the work is developed based on methodologies which emphasize aspects of life, such as narratives, oral history and ethnographic readings, shaping the understanding of reality and of the social occupational therapist's actions. Such methodologies have been used, for example, with youths living in the urban periphery (Bardi and Malfitano, 2014) and with homeless people (Galvani and Barros, 2010), among other practices developed by the Metuia project (Barros et al., 2011a). Through the use of these methodologies, social occupational therapists can explore people's life perspectives and develop interventions/actions to amplify the possibilities for participation in society.

This work aims to collect materials for the building of knowledge based on real aspects of everyday life. Through this, it is possible to develop the potential for occupational therapy practice and also to develop professional education approaches, which address the dimensions of community and territory. These approaches are aimed at developing conviviality (i.e., harmonious living) rather than focusing on the clinical/individual dimension in isolation from the context in which people live. Such radical approaches nonetheless respect individuality because they assume the principles of democracy and rights and duties that arise from citizenship (Lopes et al., 2012).

In present-day Brazil, the realization of enhanced citizenship, in these civil, political and social dimensions, is a process that cannot be avoided, although numerous obstacles still have to be faced. Brazil, despite having enjoyed more than 25 years of democracy, still has not been able to deal with social inequality; in contrast, the forces of conservatism in politics and economic policy threaten to reverse important gains, mainly regarding universality and the comprehensiveness of social rights.

CONCLUSION

In the development of social occupational therapy, the role of professionals and their ethical and political commitment to society is brought into question. If the task of occupational therapy lies in seeking to allow or promote the greater autonomy, participation and social integration of individuals, how should one act professionally without moving away from a core of self-knowledge towards an interdisciplinary, intersectorial and interprofessional field? From our point of view, the answer is by articulating, technically and politically, citizenship, the universality of rights, social policies, the radicalization of democracy, public power, participation in social movements, labour, education, health, justice, housing, art, culture and leisure – in other words, by being in the social field.

REFERENCES

Almeida, M.C., Soares, C.R.S., Barros, D.D., Galvani, D., 2012. Processos e práticas de formalização da Terapia Ocupacional na Assistência Social: alguns marcos e desafios. Cad. Ter. Ocup. UFSCar 20, 33–41. doi:10.4322/cto.2012.004.

Bardi, G., Malfitano, A.P.S., 2014. Pedrinho, religiosity and prostitution: the managements of an ambivalent young man. Saúde e Sociedade 23, 25–35. doi:10.1590/S0104-12902014000100003.

Barros, D.D., Ghirardi, M.I.G., Lopes, R.E., 2005. Social occupational therapy: a socio-historical perspective. In: Kronenberg, F., Algado, S.S., Pollard, N. (Eds.), Occupational Therapy without Borders: Learning from the Spirit of Survivors. Elsevier Science Ltd, Churchill Livingstone, pp. 140–151.

Barros, D.D., Lopes, R.E., Galheigo, S.M., 2007. Terapia ocupacional social: concepções e perspectivas. In: Cavalcante, A., Galvão, C. (Org.), (Eds.), Terapia Ocupacional – Fundamentação & Prática. Guanabara Koogan, Rio de Janeiro, pp. 347–353.

Barros, D.D., Lopes, R.E., Galheigo, S.M., Galvani, D., 2011a. Research, community-based projects and teaching as a sharing construction: The Metuia project in Brazil. In: Kronenberg, F., Pollard, N., Sakellariou, D. (Eds.), Occupational therapy without borders, vol. 2. Towards an ecology of occupation-based practices. Elsevier, Edinburgh, UK, pp. 321–327.

Barros, D.D., Ghirardi, M.I.G., Lopes, R.E., Galheigo, S.M., 2011b. Brazilian experiences in social occupational therapy. In: Kronenberg, F., Pollard, N., Sakellariou, D. (Eds.), Occupational Therapy Without Borders, vol. 2. Towards an Ecology of Occupation-Based Practices. Elsevier, Edinburgh, pp. 209–215.

Barros, D.D., Galvani, D., Almeida, M.C., Soares, C.R.S., 2013. Cultura, economia, política e saber comoespaços de significação na Terapia Ocupacional Social: reflexões sobre a experiência do Ponto de Encontro e Cultura. Cad. Ter. Ocup. UFSCar São Carlos 21, 583–594. doi:10.4322/cto.2013.060.

Basaglia, F., Ongaro-Basaglia, F., 1977. Los Crimines de la Paz: Investigación Sobre los Intelectuales y los Técnicos como Servidores de la Opresión. Siglo XXI, Madrid.

Castel, R., 1997. As armadilhas da exclusão. In: Belfiore-Wanderley, M., Bógus, L., et al. (Org.), (Eds.), Desigualdade e a Questão Social. EDUC, São Paulo, pp. 15–48.

Castel, R., 2003. From Manual Workers to Wage Laborers. Transformation of the Social Question. Transaction Publishers, New Brunswick, NJ.

Dagnino, E., 2007. Citizenship: a perverse confluence. Dev. Pract. 17, 549–556, 2007. doi:10.1080/09614520701469534.

Donzelot, J., 1977. La Police des Familles. Minuit, Paris.

Donzelot, J., 1984. L'Invention du Social: Essai sul le Déclindes Passions Politiques. Fayard, Paris.

Durkheim, E., 1972. Emile Durkheim: Selected Writings. In: Giddens, A. (Ed.), Cambridge Books Online. Cambridge University Press, Cambridge. Available at: <http://dx.doi.org/10.1017/CBO9780511628085>.

European Network of Occupational Therapy in Higher Education (ENOTHE), 2013. Citizenship: exploring the contribution of occupational therapy. Available at: <http://www.enothe.eu/activities/meet/ac13/CITIZENSHIP_STATEMENT_ENGLISH.pdf> (accessed 07.08.15.).

Foucault, M., 2000. Faubion, J.D. (Ed.), Power (Essential Works), vol. 3. The New Press, New York, NY.

Freire, P., 1970. Pedagogy of the Oppressed. Continuum, New York.

Galheigo, S.M., 1997. Da adaptação psicossocial à construção do coletivo: a cidadania enquanto eixo. Revista de Ciências Médicas da PUCCAMP 6, 105–108.

Galvani, D., Barros, D.D., 2010. Pedro e seus circuitos na cidade de São Paulo: religiosidade e situação de rua. Interface Comunicação Saúde Educação 14, 767–779. doi:10.1590/S1414-32832010005000022.

Ghiradi, M.I., 2012. Terapia ocupacional em processos econômico-sociais. Cad. Ter. Ocup. UFSCar 20, 17–20. doi:10.4322/cto.2012.002.

Gramsci, A., 1992. Prison Notebooks, vol. 2. Columbia University Press, New York.

Janoski, T., 1998. Citizenship and Civil Society: A Framework of Rights and Obligations in Liberal, Traditional, and Social Democratic Regime. Cambridge University Press, Cambridge.

Kymlicka, W., 1996. Ciudadania multicultural: una teoria liberal de los derechos de la minoria. Paidós, Barcelona.

Law, M., 1991. The environment: a focus for occupational therapist. Can. J. Occup. Ther. 58, 171–180. doi:10.1177/000841749105800404.

Leclair, L.L., 2010. Re-examining concepts of occupation and occupation based models: occupational therapy and community development. Can. J. Occup. Ther. 77, 15–21. doi:10.2182/cjot.2010.77.1.3.

Locke, J., 1988. Locke: Two Treatises of Government. Laslett, P. (Ed.), In: Cambridge Books Online. Cambridge University Press, Cambridge. Available at: <http://dx.doi.org/10.1017/CBO9780511810268>.

Lopes, R.E., 1999. Cidadania, políticas públicas e terapia ocupacional no contexto das ações de saúde mental e saúde da pessoa portadora de deficiência no município de São Paulo. Doctoral dissertation, Biblioteca Digital da Unicamp. <http://www.bibliotecadigital.unicamp.br/zeus/auth.php?back=http://www.bibliotecadigital.unicamp.br/document/?code=vtls000184393&go=x&code=x&unit=x> (accessed 17.11.14.).

Lopes, R.E., 2013. No pó da estrada. (On the road). Cadernos de Terapia Ocupacional da UFSCar 21, 171–186. doi:10.4322/cto.2013.022.

Lopes, R.E., Borba, P.L.O., Cappellaro, M., 2011a. Acompanhamento Individual e Articulação de Recursos em Terapia Ocupacional Social: Compartilhando uma Experiência. O Mundo da Saúde 35, 233–238.

Lopes, R.E., Borba, P.L.O., Trajber, N.K.A., Silva, C.R., Cuel, B.T., 2011b. Oficinas de Atividades com Jovens da Escola Pública: Tecnologias Sociais entre Educação e Terapia Ocupacional. Interface 15, 277–288. doi:10.1590/S1414-32832011000100021.

Lopes, R.E., Malfitano, A.P.S., Silva, C.R., Borba, P.L.O., Hahn, M.S., 2012. Occupational Therapy Professional Education and Research in the Social Field. WFOT Bulletin 66, 52–57.

Malfitano, A.P.S., Lopes, R.E., Borba, P.L.O., Magalhães, L., 2014a. Lessons from the experience of Brazilian occupational therapists engaged in social policy making and implementation: building a dialogue with Canadian occupational therapists. Occup. Ther. Now 16, 10–12.

Malfitano, A.P.S., Lopes, R.E., Magalhães, L., Townsend, E.A., 2014b. Social occupational therapy: conversations about a Brazilian experience. Can. J. Occup. Ther. 81, 298–307. doi:10.1177/0008417414536712.

Marshall, T.H., 1950. Citizenship and Social Class: And Other Essays. Cambridge University Press, New York.

Netto, J.P., 2001. Cinco notas a propósito da 'questão social'. Temporalis – Revista da Associação Brasileira de Ensino e Pesquisa em Serviço Social (ABEPSS) 3, 41–49.

Neveu, C., Clarke, J., Coll, K., Dagnino, E., 2011. Introduction: questioning citizenships (Questions de Citoyennetés). Citizensh. Stud. 15, 945–964. doi:10.1080/13621025.2011.627759.

Offe, C., 1984. Problemas estruturais do Estado capitalista. Tempo Brasileiro, Rio de Janeiro, Brasil.

Offe, C., Ronge, V., 1984. Teses sobre a fundamentação do conceito de Estado Capitalista e sobre a pesquisa política de orientação materialista. In: Offe, C. (Ed.), Problemas estruturais do Estado capitalista. Tempo Brasileiro, Rio de Janeiro, pp. 121–137.

Pollard, N., Kronenberg, F., Sakellariou, D., 2008. A political practice of occupational therapy. In: Pollard, N., Sakellariou, D., Kronenberg, F. (Eds.), A Political Practice of Occupational Therapy. Elsevier, Edinburgh, UK, pp. 3–19.

Pollard, N., Sakellariou, D., 2014. The occupational therapist as a political being. Cadernos de Terapia Ocupacional da UFSCar 22, 643–652. doi:10.4322/cto.2014.087.

Shafir, G., 1998. The Citizenship Debate: A Reader. University of Minnesota Press, Minneapolis, MN.

Townsend, E., 1993. 1993 Muriel Driver Lecture: occupational therapy's social vision. Can. J. Occup. Ther. 60, 174–184.

Vieira, L., 2001. Os Argonautas da Cidadania. Record, Rio de Janeiro.

Walzer, M., 1992. The civil society argument. In: Mouffe, C. (Ed.), Dimensions of Radical Democracy. Verso, London, pp. 89–107.

28

THE IMPACT OF SOCIAL AND POLITICAL CONTEXTS ON THE DEVELOPMENT OF OCCUPATIONAL THERAPY IN THE REPUBLIC OF CROATIA

SASA RADIC ■ IVANA KLEPO

■ ■

CHAPTER OUTLINE

Occupational therapy in the Republic of Croatia has been developing under specific historical, social, cultural, and political influences. The profession's origins are to be found in the field of psychiatry, though later the profession was introduced to and applied in the rehabilitation of the Croatian First World War veterans. Occupational therapy education started at secondary level but has since progressed to a bachelor's degree course. Significant progress in practice and education has occurred since 1996, collectively accomplished as a result of strategic international networking, exchange of information, and cooperation.

The Republic of Croatia is a country that emerged from a communist sociopolitical system in the early 1990s. Unlike most transitional countries, Croatia's transformation occurred under conditions of war. This has had an effect on the economic and social stratification of Croatian society, which makes it different from other transition experiences (Tomić-Koludrović and Petrić, 2007). An important event in

the Croatian transition was the process of accession to the European Union (EU) and full membership in 2013, which was different and much slower to occur than in other former socialist countries. Croatian society is still experiencing the unfolding socioeconomic and political change as a result of the comprehensive transition process, and this undoubtedly has an effect on the occupational therapy profession as a whole. Pollard et al. (2008) emphasize that in occupational therapy there is a growing awareness of the need to recognize the political context in which practice, education and research occur, and that such political awareness allows occupational therapists a critical understanding of the impact of politics on human occupation and practice. Political and economic status, social norms, the cultural environment and many other contextual factors play an important role in practice, as well as in the development of occupational therapy in the Republic of Croatia. This poses unique challenges but also opportunities for growth.

In this chapter, we will present the multifaceted contextual and significant sociopolitical barriers that collectively have informed and shaped our concentrated efforts and responses in the development of occupational therapy education and practice in Croatia. It is our hope that our lived experience, from the perspective of a small country with a tiny occupational therapy population, can illustrate that the greatest asset in propelling occupational therapy forward, anywhere, is the reliance on human resources, regardless of context.

ROOTS OF OCCUPATIONAL THERAPY EDUCATION AND PRACTICE IN CROATIA

Occupational therapy in Croatia finds its roots in the oldest psychiatric hospital, today known as the University Psychiatric Hospital Vrapče. Brečić et al. (2013) report that occupational therapy in the hospital is as old as the hospital itself, and since its foundation in 1879, patients were involved in agricultural work. Engaging patients in farming activities provided an economic value to the hospital as it served to provide food to all residents. Besides the agricultural engagement, art and crafts were also part of the therapeutic activities later on, and there were established tailor, shoemaker, carpentry, and upholstery workshops. This practice was later introduced in some other psychiatric hospitals.

After the First World War, Božidar Špišić, an orthopaedic surgeon, founded the Disability School that aimed to teach war veterans how to perform familiar and new crafts. According to Špišić (1917), occupational therapy was of special importance in the Disability School because it enabled patients not just to recover but also to develop the necessary skills for daily life.

The consequences of the Second World War, and again a large number of war veterans, prompted the physician Jozo Budak to initiate the establishment of the secondary School of Physical Medicine and Röntgen to educate physiotherapists, occupational therapists and radiographers (Jurinić, 2007). This was the first formal education for occupational therapists with a 4-year curriculum. Forty four occupational therapists successfully graduated from the programme in the 1961/1962 and 1963/1964 academic years. The focus of the occupational therapist was 'to make the

patient interested in one particular job and to distract him from the effects his disease and his limitations and in such a way the therapeutic process is carried out along functional, recreational and sports principle' (Lovrić, 1967, p. 3).

In the 1950s and 1960s, occupational therapy was introduced for the general population in the area of orthopaedics and physical medicine and rehabilitation (Cvitanović-Barišić and Grubić-Jakupčević, 2000; Mandić, 1958; Potrebica, 2000). Describing the importance of occupational therapy in orthopaedics, Ruszkowski (1958) emphasizes the therapeutic use in stretching joint contractures, particularly the fingers and hands, and in the reeducation of motor skills. This type of occupational therapy was called *specific occupational therapy*. On the other hand, 'nonspecific' occupational therapy aimed to distract the patient from illness, and prevent boredom and monotony. Such a reductionist approach to occupational therapy remained prevalent long after that.

Between 1967 and 1986, there was no occupational therapy education programme available in Croatia, so occupational therapists received their education in the neighbouring Yugoslav republics of Slovenia and Serbia. Croatian occupational therapy education at the higher education level was established for the first time in 1986 at the Higher Medical School, a department of the Medical Faculty of Zagreb. A new 2-year curriculum was developed from and embedded in the physiotherapy curriculum[1], leading to a degree in physical therapy with a specialization in occupational therapy. The 2-year programme was structured to include basic science subjects (e.g., anatomy and physiology), physical and rehabilitation medicine subjects, functional occupational therapy, and creativity-based occupational therapy subjects. The joint curriculum created a lot of ambiguity for the profession of occupational therapy in Croatia, not only because of the polysemous degree awarded (Bartolac, 2012), but also because of the dually applicable[2] competencies which have been developed through course content.

---

[1]Students of occupational therapy and physiotherapy had a joint first-year curriculum, with the exception of specific occupational therapy subjects and fieldwork practice.

[2]Competences are applicable across two professions: occupational therapy and physiotherapy.

TIMES OF CHANGE

In the early 1990s, Croatia declared independence and seceded from Yugoslavia, which led to the Croatian War of Independence. Once again, there was a need for the improvement of rehabilitation services, particularly for the implementation of community-based rehabilitation (CBR). International influences ensured the development and improvement of rehabilitation in Croatia. With the initiative of professionals from the Croatian Committee for Physical Medicine and Rehabilitation, appointed by the Croatian Health Minister, Croatian government, and with support from the World Health Organization and the Canadian International Development Agency, a project named Development of Community Based Rehabilitation in the Republic of Croatia was established (Bobinac-Georgievski, 1998b). The main project objectives were the development of new services: CBR team, healthcare professionals educational development, and health policy development (International Centre for the Advancement of Community Based Rehabilitation, 2000).

The project was implemented by Croatian and Canadian experts from Queen's University in the Special Unit for Community Based Rehabilitation, which was part of the General Hospital of the Holy Spirit, Zagreb, in the Department of Physical Medicine and Rheumatology, between 1996 and 1998. Polovina et al. (2007) state that the CBR model of practice, which was implemented, offered various interventions for and with people with disabilities to facilitate their functioning and health within their own environment. This project had a very significant influence on the further development and direction of occupational therapy practice and education in Croatia. With the support of Canadian experts through various activities, new theoretical and philosophical occupational therapy foundations and knowledge in tune with professional legacy and beliefs, were presented and implemented, with a particular focus on the further development of fieldwork practice educators; students were also involved in this process. Some of the outcomes of this project were new occupational therapy solutions for day-to-day practice with people with disabilities. All these developments facilitated the wider consideration of the application of occupational therapy along the rehabilitation continuum.

Analysing the CBR project and its sustainability, Bobinac-Georgievski (1998a) acknowledged that the CBR philosophy can serve as a pillar for a socially responsible and inclusive society, but she also identified prevailing challenges, such as resistance to change, lack of awareness of how to potentially integrate people with disabilities, and a lack of cooperation between the sectors of society involved in healthcare and social care, education, and employment.

Concurrently, in 1997, occupational therapy became an independent course of study (Bartolac, 2012), and in 1998, the School of Health Studies, Department of Occupational Therapy, became a member of the European Network of Occupational Therapy in Higher Education. Through close cooperation with this European organization, and due to a positive climate for change at the School of Health Studies, the study of occupational therapy was structurally changed to a 3-year programme with some minor alteration in the content of the course subjects. During 2002 and 2003, the Department of Occupational Therapy cooperated with Cardiff University and Cardiff and the Vale National Health Service Trust in the UK in an exchange of study visits for students and fieldwork educators, and a workshop focusing on occupational therapy frames of reference, practice models and guiding theories.

These international collaborations raised the need for a more intensive professional development, and they enabled implementation of a model of overcoming barriers in present educational and practice challenges. International cooperation was continued and further developed by a small group of enthusiastic occupational therapists, gathered in the board of the Croatian Occupational Therapy Association, who, since 2006, have implemented a strategy for continuing professional development through organizing educational activities such as lectures, practical workshops, courses and seminars facilitated by a variety of invited speakers. International occupational therapy experts have given a wellspring of innovative occupational therapy knowledge and skills and have collectively served to improve practitioner competencies and the overall standards of service provision to ensure the development of high-quality occupational therapy services.

International cooperation continued through the membership of the Croatian Association of

Occupational Therapists in the Council of Occupational Therapists for the European Countries in 2006, the World Federation of Occupational Therapists in 2010, and the European Network of Occupational Therapy in Higher Education in 2011.

THE LEGAL REGULATION OF OCCUPATIONAL THERAPY PRACTICE

The legal regulation of the occupational therapy profession happened as a result of Croatia's EU entry negotiations and is considered a great milestone for the profession of occupational therapy in Croatia. Close collaboration with international occupational therapy organizations has had a significant impact on that process. Events in the late autumn of 2008 had a snowball effect as they enabled a new path for the profession of occupational therapy in the Republic of Croatia. In late September 2008, while legislating physiotherapy, the Croatian Parliament received a physiotherapy law proposal in which occupational therapy somehow was defined as a part of physiotherapy care. At that moment it was not clear what was the meaning of this and how this could even be possible. The proposed law stipulated that occupational therapists could practise using their own scope of practice, but that they had to do so as part of the physiotherapy profession.

It was immediately evident that upon implementation of that physiotherapy law, the occupational therapy profession in Croatia would completely lose its autonomy, professional integrity and visibility in the eyes of the general public. The physiotherapy law was prepared and sent for emergency discussion and voting procedure due to stipulated reforms in the area of regulated professions as part of Croatia's accession to the EU. For a small group of passionate occupational therapists in the national association, this unfortunate situation was a wake-up call which required them to develop new competences beyond what was expected in the occupational therapy scope of practice. The group realized that they needed to be not just occupational therapist, but leaders, negotiators, politicians, innovators, diplomats, advocates, and catalysts of change if they wanted to change the unfavourable legal working context that the physiotherapy law proposed. Called to action, they mobilized all available resources across a variety of influential bodies, including Croatian occupational

therapy service users, the media, politicians in the government and opposition, members of the European Commission and the European Parliament, all for the purpose of exerting extensive pressure to amending this questionable law. We emphasize the importance of the Council of Occupational Therapists for the European Countries, the European Network of Occupational Therapy in Higher Education, and the World Federation of Occupational Therapists and their then presidents, which contributed to this effort and were mobilized by the Croatian occupational therapy association to strengthen the occupational therapy voice and who jointly helped to influence the Croatian Government and EU Commission. International support was very important, quick and effective, especially given that the implementation of new reforms to achieve EU standards of quality for services users was required, which made members of the international occupational therapy organization crucial opinion makers.

What came out after the law was passed was that it was only applicable to a small number of occupational therapists, all of whom had attained a degree in physical therapy with a specialization in occupational therapy and who were able to practice physical therapy under the proposed law. It was not applicable to any other practising occupational therapists. What was very important was that the parliamentary discussion of the physiotherapy law was turned into a promotion of the occupational therapy profession as a result of intensive lobbying upon members of the parliament by a small group of members of the board of the Croatian Association of Occupational Therapists. During that parliamentary discussion, the Deputy Minister of Health and Social Care made a promise that occupational therapy would become a legally regulated profession in a short period of time. The promise was fulfilled and occupational therapy became a legally regulated profession in July 2009. After that, the Croatian Chamber of Health Professionals was established, which is responsible for registering and licensing occupational therapists and for the regulation of occupational therapy practice.

IS CROATIAN SOCIETY CHANGING?

Maldini (2008) states that trust in the institutions of the democratic system is of vital importance in transitional societies, especially in those who, because of the past, have developed feelings of scepticism and distrust towards institutions. However, research shows that citizens in the Republic of Croatia have little trust in state institutions. A study conducted by the Ivo Pilar Research Institute shows that respondents least trust political parties, government, parliament and the judiciary, while the most trustworthy entities are considered to be the Croatian army and the President of the Republic. Comparing these findings with those of other international research studies, this level of confidence is among the lowest in the European Community (Institute of Social Sciences Ivo Pilar, 2014). Therefore, due to their inefficiency, the agencies that need to implement reforms, enforce and pursue the laws, the ones who need to put the state administration at the service of citizens, and who need to ensure the rule of law and equality, have lost all confidence amongst those they are intended to serve, the Croatian citizens.

After occupational therapy became a legally regulated profession, it was necessary to coordinate bylaws in the health and social sectors, in the labour market as well as in education. Changes to the occupational therapy internship programme (all health care professionals in Croatia are required to undertake a one-year long internship upon graduation in order to be able to sit for the State exam, and get registered and licensed by their regulatory body), the establishment of minimal standards for providing services, and regulation of occupational therapy procedures as part of health insurance reimbursement also needed to be instituted. And, perhaps most importantly, the availability of occupational therapy services at all levels of care, from acute care to CBR, needed to be established.

Since 2010, occupational therapists within the Croatian chamber of health professionals and members of the Croatian Association of Occupational Therapists have been in negotiations, have prepared evidence-based documents, and have held meetings with various key players, but seemingly to no avail. In response, promises by the representatives of various public agencies were made, numerous amendments of the laws and bylaws were asked for, but at the end of the day very little progress was made. Changes are happening quite slowly, and even when they do happen, the results are rather contradictory and confusing. For example, due to a recently implemented regulation applicable to services provided in the social care sector, occupational therapists in Croatia are no longer allowed to utilize an intervention approach that is based on a theory developed by an occupational therapist. It is an intervention approach that is utilized in paediatric occupational therapy practice across the world and requires additional certification. In Croatia, this intervention approach is now legally allowed to be carried out by a profession other than occupational therapy. This is highly frustrating, but to make matters even more confusing, this same intervention approach is legally possible to be carried out by occupational therapists and financed by national healthcare service in the healthcare sector. This incongruence speaks to the high level of misunderstanding and low level of importance of the evidence-based arguments, lifelong learning and quality of provided services[3].

The Croatian experience shows that, as is similar to experiences in other posttransitional former communist countries, changes of political leadership and adoption of new directions at first do not cause significant changes in the deep structures and processes of the social and political system. New institutions tend to adopt the old manner of functioning (Županov, 2011). Of course, this is not a reason to give up; it only gives us more reason to embrace our legacy and values, to be flexible and to step outside our comfort zone.

WHAT WE NEED TO DO – DOING, LEARNING, BECOMING AND BEING CROATIAN OCCUPATIONAL THERAPISTS

As of 2015, there are 357 registered and licensed occupational therapists in Croatia, a ratio of 8.32 occupational therapists per 100 000 inhabitants, which compared with other EU countries is a rather small number (Council of Occupational Therapists for the European Countries, 2015). This also means that occupational therapy services are not available to a large number of

---

[3]During the writing of this chapter, the regulation which defines minimum standards of practice provision of the above mentioned intervention approach was slightly changed so occupational therapists can implement it. But what has happened is that now an intervention approach can be performed by a wide range of professionals from health, social, and educational backgrounds without specialized postgraduate education, which is not in compliance with evidence-based practices.

people who could benefit from them. Croatia's economy has been declining since 2008, the longest period of recession in the EU. According to Eurostat, the unemployment rate is among the highest in the EU (in an EU28 average of 10.2%, the Croatian rate was 16.2%), and of most concern is the very high rate of youth unemployment (41.5%). At the same time, the Croatian employment rate of 54.6% is the lowest in the EU average of 64.9% (European Commission, 2014). According to data from the Croatian Chamber of Health Professionals (2012), the largest representation of occupational therapists is in healthcare (34%), social care (26%), nongovernmental organizations and educational institutions (7%) and, finally, in the private sector (3%). When we talk about health institutions, the largest representation of occupational therapists is in special rehabilitation hospitals (42%), psychiatric hospitals (27%), and university and general hospitals (8%) (SR DRT HKZR, 2012). A very small percentage of occupational therapists is employed at the primary level of healthcare, as well as in the community.

The lack of occupational therapists in the community has been identified by nongovernmental organizations of persons with disabilities who have been trying to ensure the availability of occupational therapists in the natural environment of their clients through various projects (Croatian Association of Occupational Therapists, 2013). As such projects provide occupational therapy services for only a certain number of users, it is essential to systematically address the issue of availability of occupational therapists in the community. There are some occupational therapy services, however, that are innovative for the Croatian context, so nongovernmental organizations and a few public institutions are trying to integrate them into the system through (mostly EU-funded) pilot projects. Such examples are the vocational rehabilitation of persons with disabilities, occupational therapists in schools and kindergartens, and early intervention programmes.

The lack of provision of occupational therapy services was recognized by the new Croatian healthcare strategy 2012 to 2020 (Government of the Republic of Croatia, 2012) and also through the annual report of the Office of the Croatian Disability Ombudsman (Croatian Disability Ombudsman, 2014, 2015). These reports state that in the rehabilitation process occupational therapists provide a link between people and their environment, and with occupational therapy's focus on functionality and participation, there is a qualitative step forward from traditional medical rehabilitation that is focused on disease and injury (Croatian Disability Ombudsman, 2014). One of the reports also mentioned that where there is a need for comprehensive rehabilitation, occupational therapy's unique perspective on humans as occupational beings makes occupational therapists irreplaceable and certainly noninterchangeable with other professionals (Croatian Disability Ombudsman, 2014).

Mihanović (2011) notes that despite positive developments, the biomedical model still prevails in the Republic of Croatia. In such an environment, it is not always easy to point out the importance of biopsychosocial, socioecological or occupational views of human functioning. Croatian occupational therapy practice and educational allegiances to the biomedical model are inextricably linked to and rooted in the educational system, as they are for most Croatian healthcare and social care professions (Havelka et al., 2009). We need to emphasize that there is a rapidly growing community, a 'new wave' of occupational therapists, who think quite differently, who are pushing the boundaries and implementing occupational therapy in accordance with contemporary practices. It is quite clear that occupational therapy is in a way polarized between the 'old' and 'new', and that in Croatia the profession does not yet have a distinctive identity, so some changes should happen if we want to further develop our professional identity. It is therefore important to direct future steps to building knowledge and capacity in the areas of occupational functioning, occupational justice, occupational self-advocacy, client empowerment, and human rights advocacy as key determinants of an inclusive society.

Vertical mobility in education is also one of the challenges for the occupational therapy profession. Occupational therapists are not enabled to go above the bachelor's degree level, but nonetheless they require advanced degrees to become academics and professors. Since there is present lack of occupational therapists in academia, most educators come from other professions, leaving occupational therapy students with a true challenge in terms of developing respect and trust for 'values that are inherent to our profession' (Gilfoyle, 1984, p. 583).

A key challenge that occupational therapy education in the Republic of Croatia is faced with is an overreliance on a teacher-centred learning model versus a student-centred one. This is quite common in the Croatian educational system (Organisation for Economic Cooperation and Development, 2008) and perhaps explains the more dominant presence of a therapist-centred model in practice versus a client-centred one. The authors of this chapter would add to this the recognized issue of 'poor quality of University professors, particularly in terms of teaching and testing methods, not sufficient tuning to the needs of employers and no effective university standards relating to educational processes and learning outcomes' (OECD, 2001). Many of the core philosophies of occupational therapy, such as occupation-based service delivery, and an active and independent involvement in the process of enablement and learning by doing, are provided through continuing professional development activities (provided by professional occupational therapy organizations), and still are not sufficiently developed and implemented in formal occupational therapy education.

Furthermore, the Croatian higher education system is challenged with issues related to *change, innovation* and *accountability* (Lowther, 2004, p. 19). According to the OECD (2001), Croatia espouses a 'rigid, hierarchical and opaque governance and management of its education system' in general, so there is 'very little decentralization, with conflicting authorities, a lack of system-wide focus, and poor management' (Lowther, 2004, p. 19) which has caused several challenges in the further development of occupational therapy education. Croatia has been an active participant in the Bologna process since 2001 and implemented the Bologna structure in occupational therapy education in 2003 (Ministry of Science, Education and Sports of the Republic of Croatia, 2011) which ensured bachelor's level qualification and curriculum enrichment towards European standards. This was still not sufficient, however, to meet the minimum standards set forth by the World Federation of Occupational Therapists, which leaves a constant, perhaps subjective, yet collective doubt[4] among Croatian occupational therapists that they are not sufficiently or are inappropriately qualified to meet the needs of service users.

CONCLUSION

In Croatia, various contextual factors, including social and political factors, have had a specific impact on the development of the occupational therapy profession. While we were trying to enable our profession to flourish, we have developed ourselves. Legal and political competences may not be a crucial part of occupational therapy education. However, our experience shows how important those skills are if there is a need for altering professional identity, integrity and visibility. As occupational therapists, it is necessary to become political in order to influence our professional development and ultimately empower our clients.

The incremental changes that have occurred, and which have been extremely slow to occur, very often create a sense of frustration. On the other side, this enormous frustration gives us so much strength and power to act when the situation demands it from us. While the Croatian context is limiting, international influence tends to be inspiring and has been supportive in the process of shifting boundaries. Getting what is good both for our clients and for our profession requires a very wise approach in all our engagements. It is clear that apart from being occupational therapists, we need to play other crucial roles if we want to be visible on the scene, if we want to influence the context. We need to be politicians and therapists, proactive and flexible, but firm in our position and not at the mercy of the winds, willing to change if the context demands it. Our guide is our belief that through occupation you can enable the person, a group and, ultimately, society. Experience has shown that if occupational therapists want to be competitive and position themselves as opinion makers, they need to be many professions in one: therapists, negotiators, diplomats, change initiators, politicians, researchers, teachers, leaders, analysts, and so much more. Our experience illustrates that if occupational therapists desire a world in which occupational therapy is recognized by everyone, practised in its own right, fully heard and valued by influential decision makers, individual as well as joint efforts need to be present to shape the profession's destiny.

---

[4]This concern about standards is quite common in many parts of the Croatian labour force (Bejaković and Lowther, 2004).

REFERENCES

Bartolac, A., 2012. Using occupational therapy theory in Croatia. In: Boniface, G., Seymour, A. (Eds.), Using Occupational Therapy Theory in Practice. Wiley-Blackwell, Oxford, pp. 128–140.

Bejaković, P., Lowther, J. (Eds.), 2004. Croatian Human Resource Competitiveness Study. Institute of Public Finance, Zagreb, Croatia.

Bobinac-Georgievski, A., 1998a. Community based rehabilitation: a priority model for rehabilitation in Croatia [In Croatian]. Physiotherapy 2 (2), 21–23.

Bobinac-Georgievski, A., 1998b. Community based rehabilitation: development in Croatia [In Croatian]. In: First Croatian-Canadian Conference about Project of Development of Community Based Rehabilitation in Croatia. Book of Abstracts. 20–21 January 1998. Zagreb, Croatia, 1–2.

Brečić, P., Ostojić, D., Stijačić, D., Jukić, V., 2013. From occupational therapy and recreation toward psychosocial methods of treatment of the psychiatric patients in the Hospital Vrapče [In Croatian]. J. Soc. Psychiatry 41, 174–181.

Council of Occupational Therapy for the European Countries, 2015. Summary of occupational therapy profession in Europe 2015. <http://cotceurope.eu/COTEC%20Docs/Summary%20of%20 Profession/Summary%20of%20Prof%202015.pdf>.

Croatian Association of Occupational Therapists, 2013. Croatian OT conference with international participation 'Everyday Rehabilitation in Community'. Book of Abstracts. 15 June 2013. Croatian Association of Occupational Therapists, Zagreb, Croatia.

Croatian Chamber of Health Professionals (SR DRT HKZR), 2012. Strategy for Development of Human Resources in Health-Occupational Therapy. Zagreb, Croatia.

Croatian Disability Ombudsman, 2014. Annual report on the work of the Disability Ombudsman for 2013. <http://www.posi.hr/ index.php?option=com_joomdoc&task=doc_download&gid=20 5&Itemid=98> (accessed 20.06.14.).

Croatian Disability Ombudsman, 2015. Annual report on the work of the Disability Ombudsman for 2014. <http://posi.hr/ index.php?option=com_joomdoc&task=doc_download&gid=29 0&Itemid=98> (accessed 15.03.15.).

Cvitanović-Barišić, V., Grubić-Jakupčević, D., 2000. Special hospital for children with neurodevelopmental and movement disorders [In Croatian]. In: Bobinac Georgievski, A., Domljan, Z., Martinović-Vlahović, R., Ivanišević, G. (Eds.), Physical Medicine and Rehabilitation in Croatia. HLZ, HDFMR, Naklada Fran., Zagreb, Croatia, pp. 504–507.

European Commission, 2014. Eurostatat news release indicators. <http://epp.eurostat.ec.europa.eu/cache/ITY_PUBLIC/3-29082014-AP/EN/3-29082014-AP-EN.PDF> (accessed 15.10.14.).

Gilfoyle, E.M., 1984. Transformation of a profession, Eleanor Clarke Slagle Lecture. Am. J. Occup. Ther. 38, 575–584.

Government of the Republic of Croatia, 2012. National Health Care Strategy 2012-2020. <http://www.zdravlje.hr/content/download/ 10238/74922/file/National%20Health%20Care%20Strategy%20 2012-2020.pdf> (accessed 02.10.14.).

Havelka, M., Despot Lucanin, J., Lucanin, D., 2009. Biopsychosocial model. Coll. Antropol. 33 (1), 303–310.

Institute of Social Sciences Ivo Pilar, 2014. Pilar's barometer of Croatian society 2014. Institute of Social Sciences Ivo Pilar,

Zagreb, Croatia. Available at: <http://barometar.pilar.hr> (accessed 01.10.14.).

International Centre for the Advancement of Community Based Rehabilitation, 2000. Development of Community Based Rehabilitation Project in Croatia. <http://www.queensu.ca/icacbr/ projects/past/cbrcroatia/Full-Project-Details-CBR-Croatia.pdf> (accessed 19.03.15.).

Jurinić, A., 2007. History of physiotherapy in Croatia [In Croatian]. Fizioinfo 8 (2), 7–15.

Lovrić, S., 1967. 20 years of the School of Physical Medicine and Röntgen in Zagrebu. Period: 1947–1967. School of Physical Medicine, Zagreb, Croatia.

Lowther, J., 2004. The quality of Croatia's formal education system. In: Bejaković, P., Lowther, J. (Eds.), Croatian Human Resource Competitiveness Study. Institute of Public Finance, Zagreb, Croatia, pp. 15–27.

Maldini, P., 2008. Political trust and democratic consolidation [In Croatian]. Croatian Polit. Sci. Rev. 45 (1), 179–199.

Mandić, V., 1958. Annual of the hospital department for rheumatoid disease and orthopedic rehabilitation spa Krapinske Toplice 1956–1958. Administration of the spa Krapinske Toplice, Zagreb, Croatia, pp. 59–64.

Mihanović, V., 2011. Disability in the context of a social model [In Croatian]. Croatian Rev. Rehabil. Res. 47 (1), 72–86.

Ministry of Science, Education and Sports of the Republic of Croatia, 2011. Bologna Process and the European Area of Higher Education. <http://public.mzos.hr/Default.aspx?sec=2519> (accessed 12.01.15.).

OECD, 2001. Thematic Review of National Policies for Education: Croatia. OECD, Paris.

OECD, 2008. OECD Reviews of Tertiary Education: Croatia. OECD, Paris.

Pollard, N., Sakellariou, D., Kronenberg, F. (Eds.), 2008. Political Practice in Occupational Therapy. Elsevier Science, Edinburgh.

Polovina, A., Bobinac-Georgievski, A., Jaksić, M., Polovina-Prolosić, T., Grazio, S., 2007. Community based rehabilitation program for people with musculoskeletal conditions. Coll. Antropol. 2, 457–462.

Potrebica, S., 2000. Special hospital for medical rehabilitation Varaždinske Toplice [In Croatian]. In: Bobinac Georgievski, A., Domljan, Z., Martinović-Vlahović, R., Ivanišević, G. (Eds.), Physical Medicine and Rehabilitation in Croatia. HLZ, HDFMR, Naklada Fran., Zagreb, Croatia, pp. 423–428.

Ruszkowski, I., 1958. Meaning and importance of occupational therapy in orthopaedics [In Croatian]. In: Mandić, V. (Ed.), Annual of the Hospital Department for Rheumatoid Disease and Orthopedic Rehabilitation Spa Krapinske Toplice 1956-1958. Administration of the spa Krapinske Toplice, Zagreb, Croatia, pp. 59–64.

Špišić, B., 1917. How we help our disabled. Pictures from orthopedic hospital and disability schools [In Croatian]. Dionička Tiskara, Zagreb, Croatia.

Tomić-Koludrović, I., Petrić, M., 2007. Croatian society – before and during transition [In Croatian]. Društvena Istraživanja 1 (4–5), 867–889.

Županov, J., 2011. Croatian society today- continuity and change [In Croatian]. Croatian Polit. Sci. Rev. 48 (3), 145–163.

29

UTILIZING A SUSTAINABLE COMMUNITY OF PRACTICE MODEL TO BUILD BEST PRACTICE IN WHEELCHAIR PROVISION ON THE ISLAND OF IRELAND

ROSEMARY JOAN GOWRAN ■ JACKIE CASEY ■ JEAN M. DALY

CHAPTER OUTLINE

In this chapter, we introduce the sustainable community of practice (SCOP; Gowran 2012a) model. This conceptual model for sustainable development provides a simplified way of viewing complex systems and their processes through an occupational lens. It adopts a stakeholder-centred approach by using soft systems methodology and the political activities of daily living reasoning tool (Checkland and Scholes, 1999; Kronenberg et al., 2005) connecting service users, providers, and policymakers. The SCOP model creates opportunities for community-led solutions, common meaning, mutual respect, shared identity, knowledge, learning, and cooperation to enable sustainability within a given system. The model provides occupational therapists with a framework to utilize their skills more broadly through stakeholder-centred practice, thus enhancing occupational potential in the longer term for all stakeholders involved. This in turn should lead to better overall services for the wheelchair user, the central tenet of this chapter, to enhance the person's health, participation and occupational well-being, reducing the risk of ill health and inequality of opportunity. If the wheelchair users are left isolated from the process and they receive a wheelchair that is unsuitable, this has devastating effects on their posture and mobility and has major implications upon their independence and daily living. In this chapter, we will illustrate how the SCOP model could be used to build a sustainable community of practice (CoP) in wheelchair provision on the island of Ireland[1], using examples from both the Republic of Ireland (Ireland) and Northern Ireland (NI) (referred to collectively as the island of Ireland). This example is used as both coun-

---

[1]The island of Ireland is made up of two countries: the Republic of Ireland (Ireland) and Northern Ireland (NI), the latter of which is part of the UK and is governed by the UK with some devolved powers. Since the Good Friday Agreement (April 10, 1998) there has been much collaboration between Ireland and NI across various arenas, including health, social, education, and sport and leisure services.

tries have identified the need to develop sustainable wheelchair provision systems. There is also political desire to develop cross-border collaboration to enhance healthcare and social care systems.

SUSTAINABLE COMMUNITY OF PRACTICE CONCEPTS

Sustainable development is most commonly described as development, which facilitates current needs and can serve to meet the future needs of that community and its subsequent generations (United Nations 1987). A sustainable CoP is a community of people who share a common repertoire (e.g., wheelchair provision), understand each other, and recognize that their roles are connected to work together to find ways to meet their combined needs to improve the system in an economically viable, socially acceptable, and environmentally responsible way (Gowran, 2012a; Wenger, 1998).

Traditionally, sustainability concepts are linked with global ecological issues such as climate change and biodiversity impacted by specific local practices relating, for example, to environmental waste or land management. However, according to Gowran et al. (2014), sustainability has no uniform meaning and is dependent upon the context, the dynamics of that community and its ability to create true partnerships to enable a sustainable community (Capra, 2003). The sustainability agenda should encourage diverse and innovative approaches in a nonhierarchical way by facilitating people to work together. Edwards (2005) iterated that it is through having a realization of the full nature and intent of stakeholders, and an honest openness that the CoP is better able to manage complex issues that arise for that community towards sustainable development.

This means that there is a willingness among the wheelchair provision CoP to build alliances, develop community awareness and share an understanding of the key issues (outlined later in the chapter), and actively engage and take responsibility to meet set objectives for sustainable development. Furthermore, stakeholders in any given situation need to work together to challenge the existence of any barriers or borders, both locally and globally, that may deny the meeting of their occupational needs within the CoP (Kronenberg et al., 2005). When using the SCOP

model, the therapist should be able to engage all its stakeholders to identify individual and collective priorities and work together to generate agreement to meet the needs and direction of the CoP. The SCOP model encompasses four dimensions that encapsulate a reflection on processes, and an understanding of key influences and ways of developing a sustainable wheelchair provision CoP. These dimensions are: (a) the valued management of the place, (b) vital meaning for the people, (c) viable maintenance affecting the pace, and (d) visible mindfulness for effective policy (Figure 29-1). These four dimensions are influenced by Seghezzo's (2009) five dimensions of sustainability and are seen as the primary materials for building a sustainable wheelchair provision system. This allows a better understanding among stakeholders when developing a strategy for sustainable wheelchair provision which provides appropriate manual, powered or transit wheelchairs within a system that considers, for example, the wheelchair user's needs, occupational therapy skills set, budget holder constraints, procurement, wheelchair manufacturing, repairs and servicing. The reason for doing this is to meet the needs, for example, of a growing child to have a wheelchair that is the correct size so they can concentrate in school, a young adult following a traumatic injury to push their wheelchair independently and get back to work, or a person whose caregiver needs a lightweight chair to lift in and out of a car so they can go out together to the garden festival.

In the following sections, we will explore what the four dimensions potentially look like for this CoP using examples from both countries.

SUSTAINABLE WHEELCHAIR PROVISION COMMUNITY OF PRACTICE MODEL

In this section, the SCOP model is applied when viewing wheelchair provision on the island of Ireland, integrating the concepts of stakeholder-centred practice, political reasoning, and soft systems.

Firstly, the SCOP model provides a foundation for building a sustainable wheelchair provision platform. Sustainable provision is considered a prerequisite when meeting a wheelchair user's occupational performance needs to allow basic human rights for

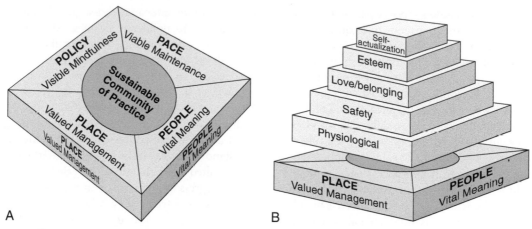

FIGURE 29-1 ■ Model for building a sustainable wheelchair provision community of practice.

personal mobility and occupational potential to be realized. Before applying the model, it is necessary to outline the significance of developing this system, as Gowran et al. (2014) argue that the importance of appropriate wheelchair provision is often misunderstood, because wheelchair use is usually perceived in relation to accessing the built environment such as housing, transport, parking, and public spaces. While this type of accessibility is an essential component for personal mobility, access to the right wheelchair in the first instance is paramount. An appropriate wheelchair is defined by the World Health Organization (2008) as:

[A] wheelchair that meets the user's needs and environmental conditions; provides proper fit and postural support; is safe and durable; is available in the country and can be obtained and maintained and services sustained in the country at the most economical and affordable price. (p. 11)

Gowran (2012b) defines the importance of appropriate wheelchair and seating assistive technology as:

[A]n enabler both extrinsically and intrinsically for people with short-term and permanent posture and mobility impairments of body functions and structures to actively participate across their life span in everyday living. The type and complexity of the wheelchair and seating technology provided will depend on the limitations and restrictions caused to

individuals' posture and mobility to personally participate within their desired environment and context. (p. 2)

The wheelchair is of primary importance to the individual, providing necessary postural support and mobility that will facilitate participation in everyday life tasks (Casey et al., 2013). Providing a wheelchair for children requires continuous monitoring as the child grows, with a constant reexamining of need and meaning to avoid 'learned helplessness' and to promote active participation at every stage of development, through school, at play, and for the teenager who wants to look cool. The wheelchair becomes an extension of the person, so its appearance and ability to fit with the user's personal preferences and lifestyle are essential. Furthermore, for people with a spinal cord injury, for example, who face instantaneous life changes, the wheelchair becomes part of their identity, their ability, and their freedom. The wrong wheelchair overshadows an individual if it does not fit within their physical environment, if adequate backup supports are not provided or if the wheelchair is not repaired on time. This has a major impact when a person is trying to rebuild his or her life and actively participate as a partner, worker, and parent. For example, solid tyres might provide reassurance for a person that they will not get a tyre puncture, antitips bars could provide the user with the support they need to go to the local shop on their own, and flip-away foot plates and arm rests could support a person to transfer safely and without the assistance of another person. The importance of a collaborative approach can mitigate the risk of health implications such as pressure ulcers because of a badly fitting wheelchair, thus reducing the false economy associated with the abandonment of a wheelchair after a short period of usage, and maximize independence, enabling the wheelchair user to be an active citizen in society. Shifting the power dynamic to the middle ground as opposed to a top-down or bottom-up approach allows 'symbiotic relationships' to be established (Capra, 2003, p. 99). Enabling the wheelchair user to be an effective member of the CoP partnership is fundamental to ensuring that the CoP truly recognizes the individualized needs of the wheelchair user and together make the right wheelchair recommendations.

Of note is how the SCOP model, through its advancement of work set out by Rousseau-Harrison et al. (2009), recognizes the significance of wheelchair provision and how the wheelchair is placed as a precursor to survival, as without the wheelchair a person cannot function, remaining in bed and increasing the risk of pressure ulcers, postural deformity, chest infections, and depression. Rousseau-Harrison et al.'s (2009) use of Maslow's (1943) hierarchy of needs theory of motivation emphasizes the importance of meeting an individual's basic physiological and safety needs to enable meaningful occupation with confidence and self-esteem (Bernstein et al., 2003). To this end, a sustainable wheelchair provision CoP is essential to ensuring that this primary need is met, with the wheelchair user's requirements being the central focus of all decision making. Through mutual collaboration and partnership, selection and provision of the optimum wheelchair can be realized across the life course of the user.

Wheelchair provision requires a collaborative approach towards review and development across the island of Ireland. Currently, the country of residence impacts upon how an individual can access a wheelchair and is dependent upon the contextual infrastructure experienced socially (adequate wheelchair service delivery systems, with appropriate education for all), economically (budget allocation, regulating wheelchair procurement costs and cost implications when waiting for the wheelchair), environmentally (adequate

methods of maintenance, reusing, refurbishing, and recycling), and politically (strategy development for all island governance) (Gowran et al., 2011). There is a call on all those involved to work together and to develop acceptable models of service provision (Batavia et al., 2001; Borg, 2011; Eggers et al., 2009; Gowran et al., 2009; Mortenson and Miller, 2008). In addition, the findings of a global survey on government action which addressed the implementation of the Standard Rules on the Equalization of Opportunities (United Nations, 1994) revealed that although some progress has been made in relation to the provision of assistive technology (wheelchairs), good intentions were not backed up by political will (United Nations, 2006). In the following paragraphs, we use the four SCOP dimensions to develop sustainable development solutions.

Valued Management of the Place

This dimension identifies the system and its infrastructures within context. When ensuring appropriate wheelchair provision, the context must be identified and considered and the complexity of the system understood. Specifically, context is defined as:

[T]he dynamic interactive effects between parts of systems; the inherent connectivity that exists between people and events in time space; and the essential unpredictability of human interactions. (Whiteford and Wright-St Clair, 2005, p. 14)

Whiteford and Wright-St Clair (2005) also describe these contextual conditions as part of the complexity of the professional practice landscape within which they are embedded, giving consideration to geographical, political, and temporal developments and how these are connected. Historically, the development of wheelchair provision has evolved for different reasons, as a result of conflicts, natural disasters, congenital impairments, trauma, and disease. Few countries have specifically prioritized wheelchair provision as part of their national government policy and have incorporated policy and services under the assistive technology umbrella (Gowran et al., 2009). When reviewing the island of Ireland, evidence suggests contrasts relating to social, environmental, economic, and political governance between Ireland and NI (Table 29-1). At a

	TABLE 29-1	
	Historical Overview of Wheelchair Provision on Island of Ireland	
Year/Time Period	**Northern Ireland**	**Ireland**
2014	Partnership working with wheelchair users in the design and delivery of NI wheelchair training for occupational therapists Postgraduate degree: Master's in Seating and Pressure care validated at Ulster University	Wheelchair and Seating Provision forum held at the University of Limerick with speakers from NI sharing their experiences of policy and service development Postgraduate certificate: Posture, Seating and Wheelchair Mobility Across the Life Course at the University of Limerick
2013	Regional (NI) Wheelchair Training Coordinator appointed with a recurring training budget National training endorsed by UK professional body, the College of Occupational Therapists	HSE policy on provision of powered mobility equipment for children and adults
2011	Nationally three-tier training model developed (Foundation, Intermediate, Advanced-Master's levels)	Education and training course available through voluntary and corporate sectors; no specific training model at a national level
2009		Medical Devices/Equipment Management Policy (Incorporating the Medical Device Management Standard) published by the HSE (2009) included wheelchair and special support seating
2008	National working group established to implement review recommendations Launch of the proposal for the reform of the NI wheelchair service completed in partnership with service/wheelchair users	General procurement policy published by HSE, to regulate and create sustainable procurement and management of medical devices system
2006	Secretary of State for NI commissioned a review of NI wheelchair service	The Disability Act 2005 set out the entitlement of persons with mobility issues to an assessment and statement of service need for health and education services
1990s	Wheelchair orders from occupational therapists processed via Regional Disablement Services for NI Legislative framework established regional wheelchair criteria for provision and to assist in matching wheelchairs on DHSSPS contract to client needs Wheelchair funding devolved from GPs (community doctors) to occupational therapists	Community occupational therapy service and nongovernment organizations provide assistive technology for those with medical cards and long-term illness cards; Allocation of additional resources through once-off 'Aids and Appliances funding' 1997–1999 (Ireland Department of Health and Children, 2011)
1970s	Chronically Sick and Disabled Persons Act 1970: regional health boards supply medical/technical aids and appliances	The 1970 Health Act introduced eight regional health boards responsible for technical aids and appliances supply to those considered eligible

Abbreviations: DHSSPS, Department of Health, Social Services and Public Safety; GP, general practitioner; HSE, Health Service Executive; NI, Northern Ireland.

glance, evidence intimates that documentation, guidelines, standards, legislation and policy as to the valued management of wheelchair provision in Ireland appears underdeveloped when compared to NI. This is important to understand when considering future developments and collaborations.

Considering this historical context, political drivers of legislation, policy, service design, and location will influence models of practice, and their meaning and impact on the key stakeholders involved. As one example, the Disability Act enacted in Ireland in 2005 legislates for social inclusion as part of the framework for government in relation to equality, employment, and education, yet makes no specific reference to the provision of wheelchair services, entitling a person to an assessment and statement of need despite their ability to pay. However, this does not mean that a wheelchair will be automatically provided if the person does not have a medical card. In contrast, the NI legislative framework entitles an individual to get a wheelchair free of charge where it has been identified that they have a chronic disability impacting upon their mobility. The implementation of legislation such as the Disability Discrimination Act 1995 and Disability Discrimination Order 2006, and the growing numbers of older persons and persons with disabilities have created growing demands on the NI wheelchair service referral system and an increase in the complexity of users needs and technology requirements. This has resulted in the provision of a suitable wheelchair in a timely manner becoming increasingly difficult and variable, leading to a government-led review of regional wheelchair services involving key stakeholders (Department of Health, Social Services and Public Safety, 2008).

Vital Meaning for the People

This dimension identifies the stakeholders, i.e. the people involved in the CoP, and seeks to understand the importance of the wheelchair provision system to them. It provides an opportunity to reflect on and become conscious of the individual and collective aims, needs, interests, and motives in relation to providing an appropriate wheelchair for the person requiring it. For the purpose of explanation, wheelchair provision CoP stakeholders are presented using categories derived from Louise-Bender et al. (2002), Eggers et al. (2009), and Elsaesser and Bauer (2011):

1. People who require the use of a wheelchair as a result of having congenital impairment and/or acquired impairments resulting from traumatic injury, neurological conditions and older age-related conditions. It is important not to generalize wheelchair user stakeholder participation as there can be many independent variables that impact on personal factors or life habits across the life course.

2. Families, caregivers, and personal assistants.
3. Clinical providers including occupational therapists, physiotherapists, and primary care physicians.
4. Rehabilitation engineers and clinical technicians.
5. Product developers/manufacturers/suppliers (vendors).
6. Funding /payers/policymakers.

Effective communication to share perspectives is vital among all stakeholders to establish the connectivity to achieve satisfactory outcomes to address physiological, functional, and lifestyle needs for each individual wheelchair user, and to support personal mobility central to independence, participation, and health. It is paramount to state that wheelchair users are placed as a central voice within the CoP, as every aspect of wheelchair provision has an impact on their life. When utilizing the SCOP model, the occupational therapist acts as a facilitator in this process.

Therefore, in this dimension the therapist embraces the notion of stakeholder-centred practice from an occupational therapy perspective (Gowran, 2012a), working in partnership with the service user (Duncan, 2006; Sumsion 2006; Wilcock 2006). This partnership is usually described as the relationship between the client and the therapist, as therapists traditionally work with individuals whose occupational performance is impacted by illness, disease or impairment, which typically induced a medically focused model of practice. However, drawing from the Canadian Association of Occupational Therapists' definition (2002), a client may refer to either the individual or the organization that weighs upon the occupational roles and performance of a specific population or group. Subsequently, the client here is viewed as the collective CoP that influences the provision process. According to Whiteford (2003), 'this means focussing on developing understandings of what the occupational aspirations of individuals and communities are, and how they can contextually be realised' (p. 44). To this end, stakeholder-centred practice requires occupational therapists to take a new approach to enable stakeholders in identifying their roles and responsibilities within the CoP. Each stakeholder, while sharing a common goal towards wheelchair provision, will have different perspectives and priorities as a wheelchair user, therapist, manufacturer or budget holder, for example.

Therefore, taking into account issues of conflict and collaboration, power, strategic motivation, and social responsibility that exist within systems is essential (Kronenberg et al., 2005).

Consider the following: a teenager requests a wheelchair that blends in with his overall style and personality, is aerodynamic, lightweight, has minimal postural support, is aesthetically pleasing, and easy to manoeuvre. The benefits of the wheelchair to this young person's psychosocial development as an independent adolescent should outweigh the prescription and purchasing costs. The therapist, while wanting to ensure the wheelchair meets the teenager's needs, will also have therapeutic goals: the need to consider growth, long-term postural implications, pressure care, availability of the product, and the costs incurred. The manufacturers may need to develop their current product range or produce a bespoke wheelchair to meet the teenager's request and consider the materials used from an environmental perspective. The budget holder will have certain funding allocation available

and wants to meet the teenager's request. However, these requirements need to be prioritized by the budget holder as to how the budget should be spent to meet needs of the entire wheelchair service user group. By understanding the different perspectives, conflicts can be resolved and compromises made to collaboratively achieve an appropriate wheelchair solution.

As key professionals involved in the assessment, prescription, and management of wheelchair provision, occupational therapists are well placed to manage and facilitate partnerships and collaborations, core elements of occupational therapy practice. The management and facilitation of the process is deemed essential in achieving the successful working of this CoP. Adapting Probst and Borzillo's (2008, p. 344) CoP governance model, eight key elements are identified that contribute to the success of managing communities of practice (see Table 29-2). These encapsulate core occupational therapy skills when working with groups (Finlay 1997), adopting the concept of sustaining organizational change (Buchanan et al., 2005), and

TABLE 29-2
Occupational Therapy Management and Facilitation Skills

Task	Role and Skills
Establish clear aims and objectives	Identification of needs and building of a sustainable CoP
Sponsorship	Occupational therapist identified as having the role and skills enabling planning and coordination of the process
Management	Occupational therapist takes a leadership role engaging stakeholders' participation and collaboration on designated tasks
	Occupational therapist uses good logistical management skills to coordinate interviews in people's homes or work places, to conduct workshops, to ensure accessible venues for all, and to seek personal assistance as required
Facilitation	Occupational therapist uses skills and knowledge of group facilitation, workshop skills, wheelchair assessment and prescription, and therapeutic use of self to empower and support the CoP at every level, while being sensitive to their individual needs
Reflexivity	Opportunity for all to reflect
	Continuous critical self-reflection enables the occupational therapist to be perceived as objective
Crossing boundaries	Occupational therapist provides opportunities for stakeholders from all levels within the system to participate and work together; the occupational therapist ensures the needs of the wheelchair user are upheld within this collaborative process
Building confidence and trust	Occupational therapist provides stakeholders with the opportunity to participate in an environment that feels safe and the opportunity to share their views and debate issues
Strategy development	Occupational therapist utilizes a well-coordinated, systematic framework which should lead to a proposed strategy development to build a sustainable wheelchair provision community of practice

Abbreviations: CoP, community of practice.

considering the key skills for facilitation towards successful and sustainable CoP engagement (Bell, 2005).

These core skills as stakeholder-centred practitioners are essential as they require deliberation to negotiate the diverse complex procedures, interactions, pragmatics of past, present and future conditions that create the narrative of one's occupational performance within wheelchair provision systems (Batavia et al., 2001; Gowran et al., 2010). Taking an occupational perspective, the occupational therapist can act as a catalyst to forge relationships of understanding among the wheelchair provision CoP (Norberg and Boman, 2004). Occupational therapists can apply a political reasoning tool to enable all involved to be individually understood and valued within the system. Kronenberg et al. (2005) note that 'borders' exist between stakeholders in any given context and suggest that these can be renegotiated. Through a political reasoning approach, key political activities of daily living questions can assist in understanding issues of conflict and cooperation between stakeholders as well as the individual narrative (Kronenberg et al., 2005, pp. 69–79).

These questions and concepts are seen as an essential tool when identifying, understanding, and engaging key stakeholders (Gowran et al., 2014). Additionally, community empowerment and the dilemmas faced by the CoP members pursuing collective goals when trying to understand the realities of the wheelchair provision require consideration (Craig and Mayo, 1995). In using the SCOP model, the occupational therapist can focus upon facilitating the processes involved that will lead to an agreed solution.

The therapist provides each stakeholder the opportunity for conscious reflection on what the wheelchair contributes to their being in the world, and what factors enable or inhibit appropriate wheelchair provision. The wheelchair solution will invariably be challenged by social, economic, environmental, and political contexts. However, stakeholders should consider how they can challenge these constraints (Pollard et al., 2009), so that an acceptable and shared solution can be achieved. For the wheelchair user, this could relate to available choices and access to services; for the occupational therapist, this could relate to knowledge, skill, and time available; for the manufacturer, this could relate to sustaining a business while trying

to produce an affordable product; and for the budget holder, it could relate to budgets and to available funding. Incorporating a political reasoning tool and utilizing questions to develop an understanding of all the stakeholders as a part of the SCOP model allows the identification of barriers which inhibit the viable maintenance of the wheelchair provision system. This enables a process that can consensually lead to a proposal for sustainable wheelchair provision within this complex system.

Viable Maintenance Affecting the Pace

This dimension identifies the bottlenecks and barriers affecting the flow of the wheelchair provision system and the impact on all of the stakeholders, with a specific focus on the wheelchair user's occupational performance. Utilizing the World Health Organization guidelines, Table 29-3 presents the wheelchair provision process from referral to follow-up and management, demonstrating similarities between NI and Ireland.

Utilizing the soft systems approach as a chosen methodological framework to apply within the SCOP model, facilitates an understanding of what is happening within the CoP and how stakeholders engage with each other. The soft systems approach acts as a channel for negotiation among stakeholder groups to 'reveal the fundamental purpose' of their partnership (Checkland and Scholes, 1999; Macdonald and Chrisp, 2005, p. 307). Utilization of soft systems thinking creates a logical, structured pathway to review this complex, messy system that is not well defined and needs to accommodate multiple perspectives (Booy, 2005). It is stakeholder-centred and essential when building sustainable systems and communities (see Table 29-4).

The viable maintenance of the current wheelchair provision system affects the overall pace and ultimately temporal quality of the service provision and occupational experiences of all stakeholders involved. Evidence suggests that there are a number of problem indicators which impact on the fundamental freedoms for service users and the working conditions of service providers, particularly those at the grassroots level, with the overall pace of provision affecting everyone's occupational performance (Gowran et al., 2014; Northern Ireland, Department of Health, Social Services and

TABLE 29-3		
Wheelchair Provision: What Happens in Practice		
World Health Organization (2008) Guidelines	**Northern Ireland**	**Republic of Ireland**
Referral and appointment	The user must be recognized as being eligible to register as having a disability that impacts on their ability to walk independently; users are referred to local occupational therapist for assessment	Eligibility is prioritized according to need; availability of services depends on the region of the country a person lives; users are generally referred to local occupational therapist for assessment
Assessment	Individualized assessment of abilities, limitations, and environmental and transport considerations Agree on goal and primary purpose of wheelchair with user	Individualized assessment occurs within the local community care area, in people's homes or in a clinic, depending on where people live and the complexity of need
Prescription (selection)	DHSSPS has a procurement process with a range of wheelchairs on contract; prescription of wheelchair to meet user need is primarily selected from this range, although occupational therapist can go 'off contract' to better meet client needs	HSE has a procurement process; therefore some WSAT are available from the HSE; in complex cases, selection would be accessed directly via suppliers
Funding and ordering	Authorized purchase by occupational therapist's manager (budget holder) Wheelchair ordered via Regional Disablement Services	Budget is categorized in most regions under 'aids and appliances' funding; authorized purchase by occupational therapist's manager (budget holder); wheelchair is ordered via regional stores, direct from manufacturer or suppliers/vendors
Production preparation	Wheelchair configuration and specifications developed to match client, based on therapist and engineer prescription	Wheelchair configuration and specifications developed to match client
Fitting	Appointment to ensure fit of wheelchair and safe usage of wheelchair, at a clinic, school or home depending on client and engineer	Appointment to ensure fit of wheelchair and safe usage of wheelchair, in a clinic or at home depending on needs
User training	Basic level training and written care of wheelchair information are provided at time of handover of wheelchair to user and/or caregiver Skilled wheelchair training available for some depending on clinical condition (e.g. Spinal Cord Injury, SCI) or local availability	Basic training is provided and will vary from region to region
Follow-up and management	Once the wheelchair has been provided there is generally no routine follow-up; however, contact details are provided for the user to self-refer back into the occupational therapy service Contact details for approved repairers are given to the user When the wheelchair is no longer suitable it is returned to regional disabled services for cleaning, refurbishment, and recycling – usually occurs when exchanged for another DHSSPS wheelchair	Once wheelchair has been delivered, the individual will be discharged from the service and is referred as need arises Generally, no routine follow-up Repair, refurbishment and recycling services are contracted via a tender system every 2 years

Abbreviations: DHSSPS, Department of Health, Social Services and Public Safety; HSE, Health Service Executive; WSAT, wheelchair and seating assistive technology.

TABLE 29-4
Adopting the Soft Systems Approach

1. Understand wheelchair provision by identifying and engaging key stakeholders
2. Understand the aims, interests and motive of stakeholders as individuals, through the use of interview
3. As a stakeholder group share experiences and understanding within a workshop to create a visual representation, known as a 'rich picture', identifying the issues that inhibit the flow of the wheelchair provision system
4. Define key issues which require transformation within wheelchair provision system as a CoP, known as 'root definitions' to express the core purpose of the activity (e.g., wheelchair assessment)
5. Create a model of what a sustainable system should look like and compare it to the current system or 'real world' as a CoP known as 'conceptual model'
6. Develop a strategy document for sustainable wheelchair provision as a community of practice

Note: Readers are advised to review the soft systems approach (Checkland and Scholes, 1999) to apply this method fully and also refer to Gowran et al. (2014, 2015) for examples.

Public Safety, 2008). Similar issues are present on the island of Ireland (see Table 29-5).

Within the viable maintenance affecting the pace dimension, efforts are made to ensure the wheelchair is supplied to the user within the timeframe it is required. A number of barriers to the process are outlined in Table 29-5. The importance of mitigating these factors should not be overlooked because of the impact they could have on the wheelchair user's participation. For example, if a person's chair is broken, it is possible they will not be able to get out of bed or move about their home, creating great difficulty in preparing their meals, going to the bathroom or getting to their place of work. In this instance, all stakeholders should be aware of the impact the wheelchair breaking down has on the individual, their family, and their employer, and work towards developing sustainable infrastructures to ensure that adequate emergency repair services and preventative maintenance systems are put in place to prevent any unnecessary impact upon the wheelchair user's health, safety, and ability to participate.

These issues undoubtedly place pressures on the CoP when ensuring a timely and efficient system. In addition, this adds to the overall cost of provision and undoubtedly has the greatest impact on the person

using the wheelchair. Therefore, building a sustainable wheelchair provision system is essential.

Visible Mindfulness for Effective Policy

This fourth dimension generates a collective understanding among the CoP, when working towards the creation of a sustainable strategy for wheelchair provision. The aim is to achieve partnership in the pursuit of a collective understanding of this CoP in the development of indicators for a sustainable wheelchair provision community (Bell, 2005; Morse and McNamara, 2009; Wenger, 1998). Capra (2003, p. 29), along with many other philosophers such as Maturana and Varela (1992, p. 231), talks about 'mind and consciousness' of thought which need to be identified within the individual and communicated to the CoP to generate unified social frameworks to provide 'meaning, purpose and human freedom' (Capra, 2003, p. 72). This is what Gowran (2012a) in this SCOP model names 'visible mindfulness'. Visible mindfulness expands an understanding of human-nature interactions, with personal awareness being essential to promote common responsibility, making visible thoughts, knowledge, and shared understanding to enable the key stakeholders in the community to work together. Wenger (1998, p. 47) states that this includes 'what is said and what is left unsaid; what is represented and what is assumed'. For example, there is an assumption that people understand the wheelchair as being a primary need for survival; however, stakeholder perspectives and understanding in regards to this may differ. Stakeholders reflect on the essentiality of wheelchair provision as a basic human right and its complexity. Stakeholders work together to understand the context and human interaction, which influence the services provided. As a CoP they share individual occupational perspectives, meanings and motivations within the system. There is an opportunity to work together, to be influenced and challenged by, or to accept differences, adopting a universal perspective to position wheelchair provision as 'applicable to everyone and to everyone equally' (Beckinbach, 2009, p. 1112).

By understanding ourselves and others, we as a society could, as Capra (2003, p. 87) suggested, 'create human organisations that mirror life's adaptability, diversity and creativity', to 'bridge the wide gap between

TABLE 29-5
Wheelchair Provision: Problem Indicators and Key Items for Review

Waiting times throughout the flow of the provision process

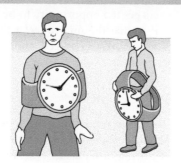

Common language/ communication systems

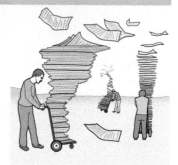

Funding being sanctioned by service provider

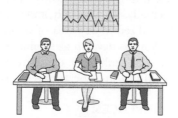

Education for all, at a national and local level

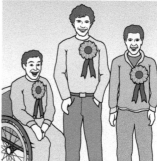

Follow-up and management services

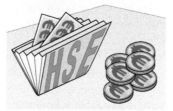

Research and development

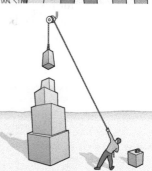

Breakdown/Repair and emergency services

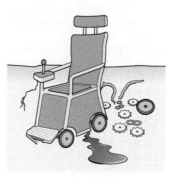

Identifying who takes responsibility for wheelchair provision

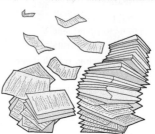

Cleaning, reuse, refurbishment and recycling services

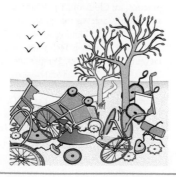

©Rosemary Joan Gowran. Illustrations by Jeroen Timmer.

human design and ecological sustainable systems of nature' (Capra, 2003, p. 86). Stakeholders at all levels of wheelchair provision should unite in partnership and observe wheelchair provision as a 'living system' recognizing 'dissipative structures', being aware of how they flow and change (Capra, 2003, p. 12). This should enable a continuous management of, and adjustment to change 'that determine[s] sustainability ...' (Olsen, 1998, p. 291) in wheelchair provision, allowing the system to operate during stable and austere times (Dervitsiotis, 2005). Table 29-6 identifies a proposed strategy for sustainable wheelchair provision generated from stakeholder-centred practice working in partnership (Gowran, 2012a; Gowran et al., 2014).

While the evidence suggests similarities between NI and Ireland with regards to the proposed strategy development for sustainable wheelchair provision, overall health and social care governance structure in the two jurisdictions differs. Therefore, this proposed strategy is a starting point for negotiation to establish an all-Ireland task force to review and develop an actionable strategy that meets people's primary needs, now and in the future.

It is essential to remember that acquiring a wheelchair is not a luxury item but a tool to enable a person to live their life and be an active citizen in society. It is also important that all wheelchair users and their caregivers get the opportunity to be supported within the CoP so that the final wheelchair provided at the end of this process is agreed upon regardless of where a person lives.

CONCLUSION

There is a need for stakeholder-centred practice in pursuit of real-world action to enhance the health and well-being of all stakeholders involved as individuals and as a CoP. The SCOP model provides four manifold dimensions which are the embedded foundations when building a platform for sustainable wheelchair provision through the community's ownership and action. This type of collective action allows basic freedoms to be achieved, enhancing basic human rights for people who require a wheelchair. This is likely to generate positive payoffs socially, environmentally, economically, and politically. This model can be utilized in any area of occupational therapy when seeking to develop a sustainable CoP which strengthens and enhances the development of sustainable healthcare and social care infrastructures.

TABLE 29-6
Proposed Strategy for Sustainable Wheelchair Provision

Process 1: Access to services (criteria, geographical boundaries)	Process 2: Assessment and delivery
· Referral process · Planning appointments · Keeping appointments	· Assessment process · Delivery and follow-up process · Review process
Process 3: Tracing, tracking and taking care of the wheelchair	**Process 4: Education and research**
· Tracing the wheelchair · Tracking equipment life history · Breakdown service – emergency service · Cleaning and reusing the wheelchair · Refurbishment of the wheelchair · Recycling of the wheelchair	· Education for all stakeholders · Research/technology development/ sustainability indicators

Adapted from Gowran et al. (2014).

REFERENCES

Batavia, M., Batavia, A.I., Friedman, R., 2001. Changing chairs: anticipating problems in prescribing wheelchairs. Disabil. Rehabil. 23 (12), 539–548.

Bell, S., 2005. A Practitioners Guide to 'Imagine' The Systematic and Prospective Sustainability Analysis Blue Plan Papers 3, UK: United Nations Environmental Programme. Available at: <http://planbleu.org/sites/default/files/publications/cahiers3_imagine _uk_0.pdf> (accessed 13.05.16).

Bernstein, D.A., Penner, L.A., Clarke-Stewart, A., Roy, E.J., et al., 2003. Psychology, 6th ed. Houghton Mifflin, USA.

Beckinbach, J., 2009. Disability, culture and the UN convention. Disabil. Rehabil. 31 (14), 111–1124.

Booy, M.J., 2005. Using systems – thinking in health and social care practice. In: Clouston, T.J., Westcott, L. (Eds.), Working in Health and Social Care: An Introduction to Allied Health Professionals. Elsevier Churchill Livingstone, Edinburgh, UK.

Borg, J., 2011. Assistive Technology, Human Rights and Poverty in Developing Countries. Perspectives based on a study in Bangladesh. Unpublished doctoral dissertation, Lund University, Faculty of Medicine, Lund, Sweden. p. 12.

Buchanan, D., Fitzgerald, L., Ketley, D., Gollop, R., Jones, J.L., Saint Lamont, S., 2005. No going back: a review of the literature on sustaining organisational change. Int. J. Manage. Rev. 7 (3), 189–205.

Canadian Association of Occupational Therapists, 2002. Enabling Occupations: An Occupational Therapy Perspective, revised ed. Canadian Association of Occupational Therapists, Toronto.

Capra, F., 2003. The Hidden Connections-A Science for Sustainable Living. Flamingo, London.

Casey, J., Paleg, G., Livingstone, R., 2013. Facilitating child participation through power mobility. Br. J. Occup. Ther. 76 (3), 158–160.

Checkland, P., Scholes, J., 1999, Soft Systems Methodology in Action. Wiley, Chichester, UK.

Craig, G., Mayo, M., 1995. Community Empowerment: A Reader in Participation and Development. Zed Books Ltd, London.

Department of Health, Social Services and Public Safety, 2008. Proposals for the reform of the Northern Ireland wheelchair services. Department of Health, Social Services and Public Safety, Belfast, UK.

Dervitsiotis, K.N., 2005. Creating conditions to nourish sustainable organisation excellence. Total Qual. Manage. 16 (8), 925–943.

Duncan, E., 2006. Foundations for Practice in Occupational Therapy, fourth ed. Elsevier, Edinburgh, UK.

Edwards, A.R., 2005. The Sustainability Revolution. New Society Publishers, Vancouver, Canada.

Eggers, S.L., Myaskovsky, L., Burkitt, K.H., Tolerico, M., Switzer, G.E., Fine, M.J., 2009. A preliminary model of wheelchair service delivery. Arch. Phys. Med. Rehabil. 90 (June), 1030–1038.

Elsaesser, L.-J., Bauer, S.M., 2011. Provision of assistive technology services method (ATSM) according to evidence-based information and knowledge management. Disabil. Rehabil. Assist. Technol. 6 (5), 386–401.

Finlay, L., 1997. Groupwork in occupational therapy. Cengage Learning, Andover, UK.

Gowran, R.J., 2012a. Building a sustainable wheelchair and seating provision community – meeting people's primary needs now and in the future. Unpublished doctoral dissertation. University of Limerick, Limerick, Ireland.

Gowran, R.J., 2012b. Guest editorial. Irish J. Occup. Ther. 39, 2. (special edition wheelchair and seating provision), 2.

Gowran, R.J., McKay, E.A., O'Regan, B., 2009. Creating a forum for planning sustainable services. In: Schmeler, M.R., Trefler, E. (Eds.), Proceeding of 25th International Seating Symposium. Orlando, FL, 12–14 March 2009. Department of Rehabilitation Science and Technology, University of Pittsburgh, Pittsburgh, PA, pp. 71–72.

Gowran, R.J., McKay, E.A., O'Regan, B., 2010. Building sustainable wheelchair service provision communities: phase 1 – 'nothing about us without us'. In: Story, M., Cooper, D. (Eds.), Proceedings of 26th International Seating Symposium. 10–13 March 2010. Sunny Hill Health Centre for Children, Vancouver, pp. 96–99.

Gowran, R.J., McKay, E.A., O'Regan, B., 2014. Sustainable solutions for wheelchair and seating assistive technology provision: presenting a cosmopolitan narrative with rich pictures. Technol. Disabil. 26, 137–152.

Gowran, R.J., Murray, E., Sund, T., Steel, E., McKay, E.A., O'Regan, B., 2011. Sustainable wheelchair provision. In: Gelderblom, G.J.,

Soede, M., Adriaens, L., Miesenberger, K. (Eds.), Assistive Technology Research Series, vol. 29, Everyday Technology for Independence and Care. ISO Press, Amsterdam, pp. 1241–1250.

Gowran, R.J., Kennan, A., Marshall, S., Mulcahy, I., Ni Mhaille, S., Beasley, S., et al., 2015. Adopting a sustainable community of practice model when developing a service to support patients with epidermolysis bullosa (EB): a stakeholder-centered approach. Patient 8 (1), 51–63.

Ireland, Department of Health and Children, (2011) Website [online] <http://www.dohc.ie/> (accessed 24.08.11).

Kronenberg, F., Pollard, N., Sakellariou, D., 2005. Occupational Therapy without Borders – Learning from the Spirit of Survivors. Elsevier Limited, London.

Louise-Bender, P.T., Kim, J., Weiner, B., 2002. The shaping of individual meanings assigned to assistive technology: a review of personal factors. Disabil. Rehabil. 24 (1/2/3), 5–20.

Macdonald, S., Chrisp, T., 2005. Acknowledging the purpose of partnership. J. Bus. Ethics 59, 307–317.

Maslow, A.H., 1943. A theory of human motivation. Psychol. Rev. 50, 370–396.

Maturana, H.R., Varela, F.J., 1992. The Tree of Knowledge – The Biological Roots of Human Understanding, revised ed. Shambhala, Boston.

Morse, S., McNamara, N., 2009. The universal common good: faith-based partnership and sustainable development. Sustain. Dev. 17, 30–48.

Mortenson, W.B., Miller, W.C., 2008. The wheelchair procurement process: perspectives of clients and prescribers. Can. J. Occup. Ther. 75 (3), 167–175.

Norberg, E.B., Boman, K., 2004. User and occupational therapist involvement in development of new assistive devices. Poster presented at Seventh European Congress of Occupational Therapy. September 2004, Athens.

Northern Ireland, Department of Health, Social Services and Public Safety, 2008. Proposals for the reform of the Northern Ireland wheelchair service. <http://www.dhsspsni.gov.uk/proposals_for_the_reform_of_the_northern_ireland_wheelchair_service__pdf_3mb_.pdf> (accessed 30.03.11.).

Olsen, I.T., 1998. Sustainability of health care: a framework for analysis. Health Policy Plan. 13 (3), 287–295.

Pollard, N., Sakellariou, D., Kronenberg, F., 2009. A Political Practice of Occupational Therapy. Elsevier, Edinburgh, UK.

Probst, G., Borzillo, S., 2008. Why communities of practice succeed and why they fail. Eur. Manage. J. 26, 335–347.

Rousseau-Harrison, K., Rochette, A., Routhier, F., Dessureault, D., Thibault, F., Odile, C., 2009. Impact of wheelchair acquisition on social participation. Disabil. Rehabil. 4 (5), 344–352.

Seghezzo, L., 2009. The five dimensions of sustainability. Environ. Polit 18 (4), 539–556.

Sumsion, T., 2006. Client-centred Practice in Occupational Therapy: A Guide to Implementation, second ed. Churchill Livingston Elsevier, Toronto, Canada.

United Nations, 1987. Our Common Future – Brundtland Report. Oxford University Press, Oxford.

United Nations, 1994. The Standard Rules on the Equalisation of Opportunities for Persons with Disabilities. United Nations Publications, New York.

United Nations, 2006. Special Rapporteur on Disabilities. Global Survey on Government Action on the Implementation of Standard Rules on the Equalisation of Opportunities for Persons with Disabilities. South-North Centre for Dialogue and Development, Amman, Jordan, p. 38.

Wenger, E., 1998. Community of Practice, Learning Meaning, and Identity. Cambridge University Press, Cambridge.

Whiteford, G.E., 2003. Enhancing occupational opportunities in communities: politics' third way and the concept of the enabling state. J. Occup. Sci. 10 (1), 40–45.

Whiteford, G.E., Wright-St Clair, V., 2005. Occupation and Practice in Context. Elsevier, Sydney, Australia.

Wilcock, A.A., 2006. An Occupational Perspective of Health, second ed. SLACK Incorporated, Thorofare, NJ.

World Health Organization, 2008. Guidelines on the Provision of Manual Wheelchairs in Less Resources Settings. WHO Press, Geneva.

30

HUMAN-CENTRED DIALOGUE INVOLVING A MAN WITH A SEVERE SPEECH IMPAIRMENT IN OCCUPATIONAL THERAPY EDUCATION

RICK STODDART ■ DAVID TURNBULL ■ DANIEL LOWRIE ■ JESSIE WILSON

CHAPTER OUTLINE

This chapter addresses the problem that arises frequently in healthcare settings, of a person whose entire being is subjected to a process of objectification. We describe a transformative approach, in the context of occupational therapy education, in which dialogue is the means through which the *ontology* of being human is restored. This approach is consistent with the goal of enabling emerging generations of therapists to practise *human-centred* therapy.

SITUATING THE CHAPTER

This chapter is situated broadly in the occupational therapy discourse of *meaningful living* (Hasselkus, 2011; Ikiugu and Pollard, 2015). This discourse brings together traditions of phenomenological and existential humanist thought as it emerged in Europe, and pragmatic instrumentalist thought that emerged most strongly in North America (Kautzer, 2015). Such a connection was made by Rorty (1976), in his comparison of the work of Heidegger and Dewey, and earlier by Schutz (1946, 2013), who linked phenomenology with pragmatism in his sociology of knowledge. A more recent connection between the two traditions has been made in the occupational therapy literature through examining the writings of Viktor Frankl, a Jew who underwent incarceration by the Nazis and who wrote about the existential problem of meaninglessness affecting those prisoners he saw deprived of their familiar routines (Ikiugu and Pollard, 2015).

The uptake of both traditions in occupational therapy is expressed by Wilcock's formulation of occupation as consisting of being and becoming, as well as doing (Whalley Hammell, 2004, 2009; Wilcock, 1999). The notion of *being* connects to the phenomenological idea that human beings have an inner dimension of meaning in their lives that is different to that of mere things. The notion of *becoming* connects to the pragmatic view (from *pragma*, meaning 'deeds done') that the goals of human beings have, to date, only been realized through occupational activity (doing). *Doing* in its more complete sense, involving prospective, and future-directed actions, requires both intention (having a purpose) directed towards a goal and instrumentality (having a project), which provides the means of achieving the goal (Schutz, 2013, p. 278). The pragmatic orientation in occupational therapy emphasizes the instrumentality of occupation as a source of meaning (Ikiugu and Pollard, 2015).

THE ISSUE TO BE ADDRESSED

On the surface, this confluence of traditions within occupational therapy discourse appears unproblematic. However, it is not justifiable to attempt to transfer such thinking into practice when these connections are rendered conventional, as if already given in intelligibility, without any consideration for what the person whose occupational being and doing is in question has to say in response. As Arendt (1998/1958) notes:

> The actor, the doer of deeds, is possible only if he is at the same time the speaker of words. The action he begins is humanly disclosed by the word, and though his deed can be perceived in its brute physical appearance without verbal accompaniment, it becomes relevant only through the spoken word in which he identifies himself as the actor, announcing what he does, has done, and intends to do. (pp. 178–179)

Compounding this universal human need for speech and action is the situation facing people with disability, in particular those whose capacity for saying and doing has been contained within human service delivery systems. Rick is a man with cerebral palsy and a severe speech impairment who knows these systems from firsthand experience. He is an *insider*, one who, as Schutz (1946, p. 476) proposed, 'because he experiences the reported event in a unique or typical context of relevance, knows it better than I would if I observed the same event but was unaware of its intrinsic significance'.

In a variety of situations that Rick, as an insider, has described, there was insufficient time and space given to enabling what constituted meaningful occupations for him (e.g., finding regular work). Rick's sometimes angry response to his lack of occupational opportunities placed him in the situation of being labelled 'difficult' and 'challenging'. Rick's life has been subjected to the restrictions placed on him by the requirements of human service provision and the perceived need to 'fit in'. This creates a form of occupational injustice where Rick's occupational rights are not met, resulting in occupational deprivation and marginalization (Stadnyk, 2007; Townsend and Wilcock, 2004).

At issue is the question of what it takes for people with disability to occupy their place with dignity as equal citizens alongside others. Our concern echoes that raised by Culham and Nind (2003) that efforts towards inclusion (as an overarching goal for people with disability) are hampered by exclusively pragmatic approaches, such as normalization/social role valorization. In such approaches, the achievement of valued social roles is the means by which it is proposed that 'the good things of life' will occur automatically (Wolfensberger, 2011, p. 471). Through the instrumentalities of many people, including some of those who have come into Rick's life for varying periods of time as his service providers, Rick certainly has achieved *some* valued social roles, such as living in his own home in the community and, more recently, making guest appearances as a university lecturer. However, the question remains as to the extent to which such eventualities meet a test of meaningful living and overall life satisfaction that is in accordance with how Rick regards his own situation.

A TRANSFORMATIVE APPROACH

In 2008, Rick and David met and began a dialogue with a hope that it will continue long into the future. We (Rick and David) set out with a transformative project in mind. This is to bring to the attention of medical, therapeutic and other human service personnel, with whom Rick almost exclusively associates, a reminder that there are dimensions of meaningful living that remain beyond the reach of everyday encounters but are intrinsic to our ethical concern.

From 2009 to the time of writing, Rick and David have been delivering guest lectures for occupational therapy students. In the university setting, Rick, to date, is given three opportunities annually. One is a first-year communications lecture that sets the baseline and introduces him as a person with something important to say. A lecture to second-year students covers topics in clinical medicine where Rick discusses his experience of having cerebral palsy and interactions with health professionals. A third lecture is in a course on professional ethics for graduating therapists, where ethical issues arising in advocacy for people with disability are addressed. These three lectures channel the communication with Rick into topics of relevance to occupational therapists.

The goal of including Rick in the occupational therapy teaching programme has been to enable insight into the lived experience of having cerebral palsy and a severe speech impairment. In addition, it is to create opportunities whereby students may encounter firsthand verbal communication taking place without reliance on assistive communication technologies (Antelius, 2009; Hyden and Antelius, 2010; Stoddart and Turnbull, 2015). Beyond these overtly stated goals are unstated, tacit dimensions of the encounter, and it is these we shall begin exploring here.

ASSUMPTIONS AND FRAMEWORKS OF UNDERSTANDING

Rick's appearance in the lecture is tacitly placed within the framework of therapeutic intervention, incorporating the ideal of person-centred practice (Christiansen and Townsend, 2010; Townsend and Polatajko, 2007). This is based upon a phenomenological assumption: that having an insight into what it is like to be a person with a particular lived experience is what matters in understanding the clients with whom therapists work (Wright-St Clair and Smythe, 2013). A further tacit assumption is that through making an empathic connection with these sorts of experiences, students will be familiarized with dealing with the kinds of problems that therapists will engage with throughout their professional careers. This is a pragmatic assumption: that having empathy is a requisite instrument that therapists need in counselling situations that are used to enable clients to reach their occupational goals (Brown et al., 2010; Cole and McLean,

2003; Kayes and McPherson, 2012). The instrumentality of empathy comes to the fore, for example, in the counselling techniques advocated by Carl Rogers (1951, 1961; see also Cameron and McColl, 2015).

These assumptions are an integral part of the conceptual and practice horizon held by occupational therapy staff and students. It is the inadequacy of an exclusive reliance on the phenomenological assumption in combination with the pragmatic assumption that prompts the writing of this chapter. We wish to supplement and also be prepared to critique these assumptions through an emphasis on the dialogical and embodied nature of the encounter with Rick. In dialogue, we are not required to assume an empathic understanding of what it must be like to be Rick. Rick can tell us that for himself, as he sees fit. He is positioned as a person with something important to say on his own terms and with his own voice (Antelius, 2009; Hyden and Antelius, 2010). The recognition of that message requires a *hermeneutical* assumption: that in order to understand or even begin to appreciate the significance of his message a particular process of engagement must be entered into, starting from a recognition of the *embodied standpoint (being here)* he brings to the engagement. For Rick, as for anybody, the question of *who he is* is not an objective fact to be discovered, but rather, an ultimately undefinable mode of being to which he, himself, must attest both in word and in action, in the presence of others (Ricoeur, 1992; Turpin, 2007).

AN ONTOLOGY OF EMBODIED DIALOGUE

What follows is a brief account of the mode of communication David uses with Rick, starting at the level of ontology. The term *ontology* refers to the manner or mode of *being here* in which Rick is as meaningful to himself in relation to others, rather than the manner or mode of being by which Rick appears to others. Rick's appearance to others, *being there* as a wheelchair user and as a person with a speech impairment, is referred to as *ontic*. In *being there,* appearing to others within the other's perspective, may have a different significance for the person whose *being there* it is. This may occur even when the other as a therapist feels *as if* she, as a therapist, having made an empathic connection, understands the feelings of a client. Such an appearance to another may be in considerable tension with the perspective the person holds in relation to their *being here*.

In any embodied dialogical encounter, such perspectives all have a part to play, and no one perspective is final or complete in itself. The supplementary hermeneutical perspective is itself only part of the occupational context in which it occurs.

A BRIEF ACCOUNT OF EMBODIED DIALOGUE

An application of the ontology of embodied dialogue is explained through our account of Rick giving a lecture. At the start of the lecture, David is *here*, about to begin talking with Rick. Rick, the man over *there*, has a severe speech impairment, and the audience is typically unable to understand his words. It is only because David has spent a great deal of time talking with Rick in face-to-face conversation that it is easier for him to understand Rick's speech. In order to dialogue with Rick in this sort of scenario, we have had to devise a way to enable an audience to hear the words that Rick speaks in order to understand his message.

At the beginning of the dialogue, David (from his own perspective, which is different from the audience perspective) is *here* introducing the lecture, and Rick is *there*, remaining silent. The students are also *there* as an audience only, at this stage waiting to be invited into the conversation. David then asks a question and Rick answers, typically embarking on a narrative from his own experience that contains a point that he wishes to make. Throughout the course of the lecture David repeats back to Rick what he thinks Rick said (sentence by sentence), and in doing so the situation is reversed. Rick is now *here* and David is in the position of being *there*. What is now implicitly being asked of David is whether or not he heard the words correctly, and further, whether or not he is able to respond adequately to what Rick has just said.

Communication with Rick is about alternating between *being here* and *being there*, where *here* means a *standpoint* of being in the position of speaking out from a place of one's own thinking and experience, and *there* means in the position of being expected to listen and respond adequately to what one has heard,

doing so as it is regarded from the position of the other. So long as this reciprocal changing of places occurs, there is an opportunity for equality in dialogue.

HOW DOES THIS RECIPROCAL PROCESS OF DIALOGUE ADDRESS THE ISSUE?

The problem in healthcare and other settings is that Rick is often placed under whatever control measures are being expected of him to accept. He is expected to listen since it is assumed his speech is unintelligible, and questions posed to him are typically closed-ended in nature so that Rick only has to indicate in the affirmative or the negative (giving *yes* or *no* responses). Rick experiences himself as positioned, even as a hearer, as being childlike or stupid. Rick's interpretation is based on his being given very simple instructions of the sort given to children and being addressed even as if he is a child. This is evidenced by adult communicators adopting tonalities of voice that are commonly used by parents speaking with very small children.

The aim of the lecture is to model the abolition of such modes of communication and to open up the engagement for further dialogue with the audience. David and Rick do this by demonstrating equality in communication, which they have already established through many hours of interpersonal dialogue. They then demonstrate this mode of dialogue in order to establish a baseline for communication with Rick that is built on a fundamental understanding of ontic and ontological positioning.

The rationale for modelling embodied dialogue is as follows. The issue is not Rick's lived experience as such, or anyone's need to find out about this. 'Lived experience' can be treated as a fact to be discovered, and this be used to reinforce Rick's status as a client. The reciprocal process of dialogue positions Rick not only as a teacher, alongside whoever else is doing the teaching, but as someone whose bodily comportment requires deeper understanding. During the lecture, staff and students are invited into the engagement, and do this by coming forward into Rick's presence to hold a conversation. Students find themselves challenged by their own incomprehension of his speech, and they are invited to explore firsthand the method of communication that has been demonstrated.

REFLECTIONS AND CONCLUSIONS

The challenge for all parties involved in a dialogical encounter such as the one described above is to step out of one's own discourse or worldview and into, or at least towards, that of another. It is easy to pay lip service to this principle, as at face value it seems to resonate harmoniously with much vaunted concepts such as person-centredness, which are recognized as hallmarks of best practice in healthcare (Christiansen and Townsend, 2010; Townsend and Polatajko, 2007). The reality, however, has been that such action is not as easy as it seems. The ability to even partially understand another's worldview requires critical awareness of how a person can remain positioned in the ontic (factual, physical or even phenomenological) dimension of *being there,* as it is this that creates an invisible border (a boundary or barrier) that the other cannot cross. To remove such a barrier, one must engage in a process of honest and, at times, uncomfortable self-reflection in order to evaluate and then overcome the many taken-for-granted assumptions that shape one's own perspective (Phelan, 2011; Stone, 2013).

It would be easy to view Rick as a client. His role as a teacher would be valued in this regard, as someone who might offer insight into the experience and challenges of living with a disability. Rick's involvement in the teaching programme would then represent an attempt to ensure a sense of authenticity on our part as occupational therapy educators by 'enabling' a person with a disability to play a role in shaping the education of those who he (or others 'like' him) may one day encounter as a therapist. It is here that a critical perspective in regards to the ontic comes into play, and that the reflective process begins to become uncomfortable. The risk is that, however well intended, occupational therapists situate themselves in the position of an expert with a preexisting knowledge of the potential learning that Rick has to offer through the act of describing his lived experience (Whalley Hammell, 2015). In a sense, they assume the role of a director with Rick being relegated to the role of an actor, whose contribution to the teaching is bound by

a tightly woven script of having to provide specific answers to specific questions that teaching staff formulate in advance.

Subsequently, therapists' foundational perception of Rick's being there, and by default his potential offering to the students, is forged within (and limited by) this need of theirs to pose questions to which they sense they already have the answers. This subtle regulatory level of role preorchestration is shaped by innumerable factors such as unconsciously held societal depictions of people with disabilities, education, a work history within medically orientated healthcare settings, and a professionally driven desire to 'assist' people such as Rick (Whalley Hammell, 2015). But Rick, like any other individual, is more than this ontic dimension affords him. He is a man with a story of his own that he would like to be heard in his own terms.

The pervasive influence of the ontic world of regulatory mechanisms can only be overcome by stepping into Rick's ontologically meaningful world about which he may wish to speak, and he, in turn, by stepping into that of the therapists', strangers though they may be to each other. To be effective, the process cannot be unidirectional. The same process of reflection and recognition must then be reciprocated in teaching sessions with students in anticipation that they, themselves, will embrace the same sort of iterative, dialogical process in their future roles as health professionals (Fleming-Castaldy, 2015; McCorquodale and Kinsella, 2015; Sakellariou and Pollard, 2013). True, person-focused practice is reliant on this shift in both thinking and process.

While this chapter has explored a dialogical encounter between Rick, David, Daniel and Jessie as education partners, the message it offers is a much broader one. This message is that occupational therapy practice is, at its heart, an encounter between humans. For practice to be meaningful beyond the mere superficiality of an orchestrated production of perceived valued social roles, it must be founded on genuine acceptance of the different standpoints of the persons involved. This cannot occur when one or more participants' voices is restricted. Such restriction of voice occurs due to much more than just difficulties with speech. It is the beliefs and assumptions embedded within the historical perceptions of people with disability that contribute most powerfully in muffling the expression of an individual's being. The risk of this occurring is ever-present in every healthcare encounter. The challenge is thus for professionals to demonstrate the insight and integrity to embrace dialogical processes, such as the one described here, to shape more meaningful and ethical healthcare practice.

REFERENCES

Antelius, E., 2009. Would you like to use one of these or would you rather be able to talk? – Facilitated and/or augmentative communication and the preference for speaking. Scand. J. Disabil. 11 (4), 257–274.

Arendt, H., 1998/1958. The Human Condition. University of Chicago Press, Chicago.

Brown, T., Williams, B., Boyle, M., et al., 2010. Levels of empathy in undergraduate occupational therapy students. Occup. Ther. Int. 17, 135–141.

Cameron, J.J., McColl, M.A., 2015. Learning client-centred practice short report: experience of OT students interacting with 'expert patients'. Scand. J. Occup. Ther. 22 (4), 322–324.

Christiansen, C.H., Townsend, E.A., 2010. An introduction to occupation. In: Christiansen, C.H., Townsend, E.A. (Eds.), Introduction to Occupation: The Art and Science of Living, second ed. Upper Saddle River, NJ, Pearson, pp. 1–34.

Cole, M.B., McLean, V., 2003. Therapeutic relationships re-defined. Occup. Ther. Ment. Health 19 (2), 33–56.

Culham, A., Nind, M., 2003. Deconstructing normalisation: clearing the way for inclusion. J. Intellect. Dev. Disabil. 28 (1), 65–78.

Fleming-Castaldy, R.P., 2015. A macro perspective for client-centred practice in curricula: critique and teaching methods. Scand. J. Occup. Ther. 22 (4), 267–276.

Hasselkus, B.R., 2011. The Meaning of Everyday Occupation, second ed. Slack Incorporated, Thorofare, NJ.

Hyden, L.C., Antelius, E., 2010. Communicative disability and stories: towards an embodied conception of narratives. Health 15 (6), 558–601.

Ikiugu, M.N., Pollard, N., 2015. Meaningful Living across the Lifespan: Occupation-based Intervention Strategies for Occupational Therapists and Scientists. Whiting and Birch, London.

Kautzer, C., 2015. Radical Philosophy: An Introduction. Paradigm Publishers, Boulder, CO.

Kayes, N.M., McPherson, K.M., 2012. Human technologies in rehabilitation: 'who' and 'how' we are with our clients. Disabil. Rehabil. 34 (22), 1907–1911.

McCorquodale, L., Kinsella, A., 2015. Critical reflexivity in client-centred therapeutic relationships. Scand. J. Occup. Ther. 22 (4), 311–317.

Phelan, S., 2011. Constructions of disability: a call for critical reflexivity in occupational therapy. Can. J. Occup. Ther. 78 (3), 164–172.

Ricoeur, P., 1992. Oneself as Another (Blamey, K., Trans.). University of Chicago Press, Chicago.

Rogers, C.R., 1951. Client-centred Therapy. Constable, London.

Rogers, C.R., 1961. A Therapist's View of Psychotherapy on Becoming a Person. Constable & Robinson Ltd, London.

Rorty, R., 1976. Overcoming the tradition: Heidegger and Dewey. Rev. Metaphys. 30 (2), 280–305.

Sakellariou, D., Pollard, N., 2013. A commentary on the social responsibility of occupational therapy education. J. Further High Educ. 37 (3), 416–430.

Schutz, A., 1946. The well-informed citizen: an essay on the social distribution of knowledge. Soc. Res. 13 (4), 463–478.

Schutz, A., 2013. Collected papers VI. In: Barber, M. (Ed.), Literary Reality and Relationships. Springer, London.

Stadnyk, R., 2007. Occupational justice and injustice from the perspective of Robin Stadnyk. In: Townsend, E.A., Polatajko, H.J. (Eds.), Enabling Occupation II: Advancing an Occupational Therapy Vision for Health, Well-being, and Justice through Occupation. CAOT Publications ACE, Ottawa, ON, pp. 80–82.

Stoddart, R., Turnbull, D., 2015. Why bother talking? On having cerebral palsy and speech impairment: preserving and promoting oral communication through occupational community and communities of practice. In: Block, P., et al. (Eds.), Occupying Disability: Critical Approaches to Community, Justice, and Decolonizing Disability. Springer, London.

Stone, S.D., 2013. The situated nature of disability. In: Cutchin, M.P., Dickie, V.A. (Eds.), Transactional Perspectives on Occupation. Springer, London, pp. 95–117.

Townsend, E.A., Polatajko, H.J., 2007. Enabling Occupation II: Advancing an Occupational Therapy Vision for Health, Well-being, and Justice through Occupation. CAOT Publications ACE, Ottawa, ON.

Townsend, E.A., Wilcock, A., 2004. Occupational justice and client centred practice: a dialogue in process. Can. J. Occup. Ther. 71 (2), 75–87.

Turpin, M., 2007. Recovery of our phenomenological knowledge in occupational therapy. Am. J. Occup. Ther. 61 (4), 469–473.

Whalley Hammell, K., 2004. Dimensions of meaning in the occupations of daily life. Can. J. Occup. Ther. 71 (5), 296–305.

Whalley Hammell, K., 2009. Self-care, productivity, and leisure, or dimensions of occupational experience? Rethinking occupational 'categories'. Can. J. Occup. Ther. 76 (2), 107–114.

Whalley Hammell, K., 2015. Client-centred occupational therapy: the importance of critical perspectives. Scand. J. Occup. Ther. 22 (4), 237–243.

Wilcock, A.A., 1999. Reflections on doing, being and becoming. Aust. Occup. Ther. J. 46, 1–11.

Wolfensberger, W., 2011. Social role valorization and, or versus, 'empowerment'. Intellect. Dev. Disabil. 49 (6), 469–476.

Wright-St Clair, V.A., Smythe, E.A., 2013. Being occupied in the everyday. In: Cutchin, M.P., Dickie, V.A. (Eds.), Transactional Perspectives on Occupation. Springer, London, pp. 25–48.

31

OCCUPATION-BASED COMMUNITY DEVELOPMENT: CONFRONTING THE POLITICS OF OCCUPATION

ROSHAN GALVAAN ■ LIESL PETERS

CHAPTER OUTLINE

Critical occupational therapy requires that occupational therapists address the social conditions that limit peoples' participation in human occupation. This involves fully understanding how the inequities that are a result of the preferential treatment of some identities (associated with categories of race, gender, ethnicity, economics, age, ability, and sexuality, among others) impact health, well-being, and participation. Efforts aimed at contributing to changing the status quo of these impacts cannot be focused solely on enhancing individual abilities. Instead, occupational therapy should endeavour to facilitate change at both individual and environmental levels (Hammell and Iwama, 2012). Applied to community occupational therapy, this entails a form of practice where community development (Thibeault, 2002), social inclusion (Galheigo, 2011), human rights and occupational justice are addressed. However, to date, the only occupational therapy practice framework that explicitly focuses on occupational justice and moves beyond individual and occupational performance-oriented approaches is the participatory occupational justice framework (Whiteford and Townsend, 2011).

This chapter will introduce a new framework, the occupation-based community development (OBCD) framework (Galvaan and Peters, 2013), which can act as a guide for occupational therapists working in the domain of community development. This framework has been developed through practice-based evidence and the interpretation of occupational science research.

OCCUPATION-BASED COMMUNITY DEVELOPMENT: AN OVERVIEW

OBCD is 'a value-based form of occupational therapy practice with communities where doing is both the means and ends of actions that are aimed at bringing about changes in human connection and occupational engagement' (Galvaan and Peters, 2013, p. 1). OBCD is underpinned by a deep appreciation of humans, viewing all human beings to be of equal worth, simply because they are human and are deserving of the opportunities (or capability sets) to ensure social inclusion. Social justice thus promotes human dignity through advocating for equitable access to opportunities and freedoms that people require to do and to be in a particular place and time (Nussbaum, 2011). Ecological justice recognizes that human beings are dependent on the sustainability of the environment and that this requires reflection on how human activity affects the environment and climate. Alleviating poverty and social inequality promotes the achievement of environmental sustainability.

In a country like South Africa, where social and economic inequality[1] is prevalent, many people continue to live in poverty. The majority of the South African population, who live in poverty, may be viewed as vulnerable as a result of their exposure to structural oppression and how this has influenced group identities and capabilities to participate. Many people are thus vulnerable since their capabilities to participate in occupations are limited compared to those who are from privileged groups in the same context. Nussbaum (2011) indicates that advancing social justice requires simultaneously addressing individual capabilities, as well as the structural aspects of society (Nussbaum, 2011). For example, although all children have access to basic education, children who attend schools in lower socioeconomic communities are more at risk of dropping out of school and are less likely to be able to access higher education institutions. Also, social protection programmes do not necessarily realize opportunities for occupational engagement and the development of capabilities that contribute to building more meaningful lives. This is because these programmes are not tailored to respond to the way that the politics of human occupation influences participation in daily life for different social groups. Emanating from practice within such a context, the OBCD framework develops interventions that take account of the politics of human occupation in context (we use the term intervention to refer to a collaborative process of change).

OCCUPATION-BASED COMMUNITY DEVELOPMENT: MAIN ELEMENTS

Similar to the participatory occupational justice framework, the OBCD draws on participatory approaches as central to the way the framework is interpreted and actioned. Informed by interpretations of occupational therapy practice in the Global South, OBCD builds upon the participatory occupational justice framework to provide a deeper interpretation of how practice can occur in four key ways.

Firstly, the framework draws on the capability approach, appreciating a human development perspective (Nussbaum, 2011). The capability approach examines the sets of capabilities, also known as substantive freedoms, that each individual requires in order to build lives that they have reason to value (Nussbaum, 2011). It argues that mechanisms should be created in order to realize capability sets for every citizen. Nussbaum (2011) differentiates between internal capabilities that reside within the person and those that reside within the context, with both of these seen as important in their contribution to the human development of individuals and groups. In OBCD, occupational therapists together with communities engage in collaborative processes of naming, examining and cointerpreting the capabilities required to build different lives for themselves. Through these processes, occupation-based approaches are coactioned to support the development of agreed-upon capabilities. The application of the capability approach to guide thinking is beneficial in efforts towards occupational justice (Bailliard, 2014).

---

[1]The Gini coefficient for South Africa, a measure of inequality, shows that economic inequality has increased between 2001 and 2015. Besides different racial distributions in the spread of inequality, class is also shown to influence inequality (van der Berg, S., 2014. South Africa will remain a hugely unequal society for a very long time. The Conversation: Academic Rigour, Journalistic Flair [Online]). Available at: <http://theconversation.com/south-africa -will-remain-a-hugely-unequal-society-for-a-long-time-25949>, (accessed 16 December 2014).

Secondly, the framework draws on development-focused interpretations of action learning (Taylor et al., 1997) as a foundation for the processes of critical reflexivity to be engaged in practice. This demands that occupational therapists reorientate themselves in order to work with communities, coauthoring processes. The notion of the collective identification of needs relative to human occupation in particular contexts is important as different perspectives are explored to uncover multilayered interpretations of the capabilities present or absent in contexts. This collective process means that both the occupational therapist and the community involved engage in ongoing processes of action learning at the core of any intervention. Action learning refers to 'a more conscious form of the natural way that human beings learn from experience, from doing, from living' (Taylor et al., 1997, p. 1). It involves a strategic combination of reflecting on, and learning from, experience and actions so that lessons learnt might be applied to future actions (Taylor et al., 1997). This involves a critical interpretation of how power is produced and reproduced in the daily occupations of communities, and is guided by community development.

Thirdly, intersectionality and an intersectional analysis provide a tool with which to understand the dynamics of oppression (Yuval-Davis, 2006) as evidenced in occupational engagement within contexts. For example, heteronormativity in the discourse of health professions is reflected in the way that gender is approached in occupational therapy, restricting people who have nonconforming gender identities from participating fully. It recognizes that the relationship between each aspect of a person's multiple identities positions them in a particular social space which is mediated through discourses related to their identities, placing people as marginal or privileged (Yuval-Davis, 2006). An intersectional analysis with communities reveals and presents the opportunity to explore how hierarchies of power and privilege are experienced within everyday participation. This intersectional analysis is also applied to the therapist in order to identify their positionality within the OBCD processes and relationships with people. It relies on an understanding of how social divisions associated with identities operate and interact within particular spaces. Through applying an intersectional analysis to the emerging understanding of participation in

occupations in context, the occupations engaged in and the related discourses are revealed.

Lastly, the framework draws on occupational science constructs within its practice processes to explore how human occupation, and its politics, in relation to the nuances in the particular contexts, can be scrutinized. Occupational science constructs are core theoretical concepts developed in the discipline, which allow for the analysis and interpretation of human occupation. Since OBCD focuses explicitly on the location of power in interventions, we are particularly interested in the understanding gained from constructs that speak to the politics of human occupation. Examples of core occupational science constructs include 'occupational choice' (Galvaan, 2015), 'occupational possibilities' (Rudman, 2010), and 'occupational consciousness' (Ramugondo, 2012).

PHASES OF THE OCCUPATION-BASED COMMUNITY DEVELOPMENT FRAMEWORK

The OBCD framework consists of four iterative and parallel phases: initiation, design, implementation, and monitoring, reflection and evaluation (Galvaan and Peters, 2013). The occupational therapist is required to work within and across these phases in an iterative and nonlinear fashion. Although entry into a new community will almost certainly begin with the initiation phase, initiation continues alongside the processes of design, implementation, and monitoring, reflection and evaluation. The design of the intervention is also constantly adjusted and responds to the ongoing action learning process referred to above. Evaluation refines both design and implementation and might push for further and new understandings in initiation.

In the sections that follow, we present an explanation of the phases of the framework and a case example of their application.

THE PHASES OF THE OCCUPATION-BASED COMMUNITY DEVELOPMENT FRAMEWORK IN PRACTICE: THE SCHOOL IMPROVEMENT INITIATIVE

Many school learners in South Africa receive a poor quality of education, reflective of the way that educational opportunities were stratified during apartheid, providing lesser and lower-quality opportunities to those from certain race groups. Although this system of education was abolished with apartheid, its remnants remain in the dual economy of schooling in South Africa (Shalem and Hoadley, 2009). In this dual economy of schooling, enduring economic, structural inequality means that those learners who are capable of paying for better education access this, while those who receive education of a poorer quality have limited access to opportunities after school (Clarke, 2015). The University of Cape Town School Improvement Initiative (SII) responded to this education crisis by building a university–school partnership, working collaboratively with various schools and groupings within and outside of the university (Silbert and Clarke, 2015). This initiative aims to positively influence the quality of schooling for learners in contexts of poverty. Final-year occupational therapy students at the University of Cape Town are placed at an SII primary school (the site selected is negotiated with stakeholders in the community) for their 7-week community development practice learning placement. The example presented here captures the implementation of an intervention in 2014, which was based on the application of the OBCD framework in a school in Khayelitsha township.

Initiation

The aim during the initiation phase of OBCD is to identify challenges to and possibilities for participation. Through applying participatory methods, it unveils new ways of understanding how occupational engagement occurs in context, taking into account the influences of sociopolitical factors on participation. Initiation is viewed as beginning a development process (Taylor, 2003) that is activated through establishing relationships and developing shared understandings of issues related to participation in occupations. This collaborative process is initiated by the occupational therapist but is co-owned by the therapist and participants. What this means, is that the occupational therapist is positioned as the facilitator of a shared process where the occupational engagement in daily life is examined and that, from this, shared meaning develops. The occupational therapist should build a shared understanding through (Taylor, 2003):

- Finding and foregrounding critical questions that are most relevant at the particular time and place.
- Listening and observing deeply.
- Helping others to make sense of their own situations, through storytelling and other creative processes.

Exploring the following three key questions related to the analysis of occupational engagement for a particular group, enables the development of shared understanding. Occupational therapists are tasked with exploring these questions whilst simultaneously facilitating a process where the group of people they are working with have the opportunity to share and critically reflect upon their occupational engagement.

Who Is This Group of People and What Constitutes Daily Occupational Engagement for Them?

Answering this question would involve an analysis of the actual occupations people engage in, in order to identify the dominant and alternate ideologies (including practices and power differentials) informing the participation in occupations. Observing and participating with people in occupations, where possible, assists to deepen the reflective process. In instances where actual participation in occupations is not realistic, alternative methods could be used. For example, photovoice could be applied as a participatory method. This process reveals the common and dominant mindsets about occupations, occupational performance, and what is expected to be done in this community. Critically coanalysing how structural factors (such as cultural, social and economic factors) shape the performance and coselection of occupations, contributes to the understanding of occupations in context. Occupational science constructs are drawn upon in order to inform the analysis inherent in the therapist's reasoning.

What Is Missing From the Range and Types of Occupations Characteristically Engaged In?

Here, attention is given to analysing in detail the factors and reasons which contribute to the gaps in opportunities for people to participate in diverse occupations. The occupational therapist and community or group members should respectfully critique the local values and traditions associated with the preferred ways of participating. Attention is given to exploring the value assigned to certain types and kinds of occupations over others. The reasons why these gaps exist and certain occupations are not participated in are critically considered.

What Is the Potential for Future Occupational Engagement in This Context?

The possibilities for participating differently in a community should be explored by contrasting the actual participation occurring with the gaps in opportunities for participation. This raises questions regarding the potential for future occupational engagement which informs the design of the intervention.

The initiation phase also often highlights other stakeholders who might have a stake in the situation at hand. It is important to examine the perspectives of all these stakeholders. To be able to facilitate the initiation phase successfully, occupational therapists must engage in processes of introspection and critical reflection, focusing on:

- The theories, beliefs, assumptions, and experiences that inform their own conceptualization of the possibilities for change in this context.
- The alternative assumptions regarding occupational engagement for a particular group, who might not have been previously considered in this context both from their own and from the group's viewpoint.
- The influences of their intersectional identity and the intersectional identities of the people with whom they are working.

Working collaboratively with people in analysing their realities assists with building trust, which ensures that real perspectives and reasons would be uncovered towards the design of the intervention. Exploring the political dimensions that influence the way that occupational therapists might work with others and how those people involved in the intervention may respond, is essential in understanding the mechanisms that govern participation (Box 31-1 indicates how the process of initiation is applied in the example of the School's Improvement Initiative).

Design

The design phase draws from mainly occupational science theories to shape an intervention, based on

the emerging needs identified during the initiation phase. The specific occupational science constructs selected depend on the particular need or issue emerging from the analysis during initiation. Different constructs are used as 'lenses' to guide the occupational therapist's reasoning in this process. This allows the occupational therapist to consider the intervention from different theoretical standpoints, shedding light on why occupational engagement might happen in different ways and the reasons influencing this. Following this, one or more constructs are selected to further enhance the understanding gained in the initiation phase and guide the possibilities for intervention.

As in the initiation phase, collaboration to determine the central aim for the intervention is paramount. Certain individuals or groups identified as role players during initiation become partners in designing and implementing the intervention. These partners are engaged actively in the process of design. Once the aim has been codetermined, possibilities for actioning the intervention should be proposed. This is done in consultation with all partners who will be involved. Determining how to access the resources necessary to realize the aim of the intervention takes into account the realities of the context. For example, the occupational therapist and partners involved would first consider what is available to the community and then work to access the resources that are not available but might be central to the achievement of the aim. Mutual advocacy and fundraising are often necessary to access the resources required.

This process involves critical reflection on the following:

- The intervention that would be most effective in bringing about change.
- The way in which the intervention will challenge oppressive power relationships.
- The way in which occupation will be used as both means and end, and how this will embed the intervention in the specific context.
- The mechanisms that should be put in place in order to enhance the longevity of the outcomes.

The analytical reasoning process inherent in the design phase is used to reflect on and evaluate the intervention as it unfolds (Refer to Box 31-2 for an illustration

BOX 31-1
INITIATION IN PRACTICE: UNDERSTANDING THE OCCUPATIONS OF LEARNING AT THE SCHOOL IMPROVEMENT INITIATIVE

The two occupational therapy students placed at the school began by building collaborative relationships with key teachers, the school leadership, school governing body, parents, partner organizations and the learners themselves. They elicited and listened to their perspectives on the learners' needs regarding their participation in the occupations of learning. This included appreciating how social positions operated in context to produce different perspectives regarding how learning happened and what was important to improve upon at the school. The students explored the questions that were part of the initiation process at different points in time with different role players. This exposed a deep analysis of how learning happened in this context and the factors influencing learning. The initial concern raised by the school governing body was that grade 6 literacy and numeracy test results were poor, and the school was worried that these test results reflected learners' poor consolidation of the work in the curriculum and a limited capacity to perform well academically and build a foundation for their futures. This initiated an exploration of the occupations of learning available to learners at the school, what was missing in this repertoire, and how this might correlate with poor performance. The students spent time with teachers in their classes, observing the learners participating, and then engaged in productive conversations (Senge, 2006) with teachers, learners, the school leadership and the school governing body about what they had noticed. These conversations prompted a mutual under-

standing regarding the lack of support for the classroom engagement in learning through complementary occupations, such as homework. The students and teachers asked critical questions regarding why homework was largely absent at the school. This inspired shared understanding that, although homework was given in the past, it was not done. As a result, many teachers had stopped expecting that it should be done. Consequently, valuable time in the classroom was being spent completing homework.

The school culture reflected an assumption that homework could not be completed in this context. Through the process of initiation, role players were able to realize that the reason for this 'gap' in the repertoire of occupations of learning in the school context was also because learners often did not have the necessary support structures, such as a parent to assist them and a place to work, in order to complete their homework. This was the result of the educational legacy that many parents in Khayelitsha faced, due to receiving an inferior education during apartheid. Furthermore, learners had to adjust to being taught in English, rather than their first language (isiXhosa), in the senior grades of primary school. Identifying these factors made the influences of socioeconomic class, culture, and language explicit in terms of how and with whom homework could be completed. Through this process, the various role players did not attribute blame but rather assumed mutual responsibility together with the students to explore viable solutions.

BOX 31-2
DESIGN IN PRACTICE: THE EVOLUTION OF A VERY PARTICULAR KIND OF HOMEWORK PROGRAMME

The occupational therapy students drew on the occupational science construct of occupational choice (Galvaan, 2015) to understand why learners and teachers made particular choices about homework in this school context. In this context, expectations regarding performance in schooling were low and this was accepted as a norm. This enabled the occupational therapy students to realize that, if they were to encourage different occupational choices with regard to homework and participation in school, they would need to influence the learners' sets of dispositions. They would also have to challenge the dominant ways of thinking and doing surrounding homework and participation in school. In thinking about any proposals for interventions that would influence how learners participate in school, consideration of the available resources was critical. Teachers were already stretched with workloads and could not take on additional responsibilities. Taking all of the above into account, the students proposed to the teachers and school leadership that a homework programme was started for grade 6 learners, with one significant difference.

The proposed homework programme was explained as more than simply a space to do homework. It would rely

on the participation of local homework mentors, who would assist the primary school learners to engage in homework. This was important since these mentors would be youth from the same community who were participating in schooling in a way that already challenged the prevailing way occupational choice occurred in this community.

This proposal was well-received and the school leadership dedicated a representative to work with the students to develop the programme further. Together the students and the school representative decided that a local high school nearby the SII primary school had an excellent reputation for academic achievements, with many learners from this school accessing higher education. This school was also an SII-supported school. A process of negotiating with this school regarding their participation in the programme was initiated. The occupation of homework would be used in the programme as both a means and an end in order to promote different occupational engagement in the school. Working closely with the representative that the school assigned and the school leadership also meant that the programme was owned by the school.

BOX 31-3
IMPLEMENTATION IN PRACTICE: THE HOMEWORK PROGRAMME TAKES SHAPE

The occupational therapy students worked with grade 6 teachers and the school leadership to identify two weekly spaces where learners would stay behind after school to complete their homework. Students also negotiated with the closest local high school, inviting grade 11 learners to be involved in this programme. The school agreed that the students' involvement would be incorporated as part of the school's socially responsive activities. Strategically considering how the homework programme could be constituted and to get it off the ground, the students critically explored the occupational engagement of all the key role players. This included the learners, teachers, and parents.

This exposed the relative positions of power that each group held in relation to facilitating learning and the ways in which they wanted to and could be expected to be involved in homework. For example, working with a parent committee, the students facilitated a workshop on a Saturday morning (an accessible time for parents). The workshop was used as a space to consider the usefulness of a homework programme and to explore the parents' possible contributions to the programme. The parents were eager for their children to have the opportunity to participate in a homework programme and were desperate for their children to have the right kinds of opportunities to enhance their education. While they wanted to support the programme, parents felt that the school's expectations of them were unclear. The workshop offered a space where parents could raise their anxieties about their own contribution to their children's homework with teachers and demonstrate their willingness to become involved where they could. Through collectively generating solutions, parents pledged their commitment to encourage their children to attend the homework sessions and to monitor their children's participation in the programme through demonstrating interest.

Ten parents volunteered to become more actively involved in the implementation of the homework programme.

Although the target group of this intervention was the grade 6 learners, the occupational therapy students offered capacity building sessions for the grade 11 homework mentors. The methods selected were based on Kaplan's (2000) strategy for building capacity, which is an approach that focuses on the intangible aspects of capacity alongside those tangible aspects, such as particular skills and physical resources. What this meant was that the occupational therapy students actively developed the grade 11's capacity as leaders and their ideas of themselves as role models with a particular mandate in shifting how the primary school learners thought about and engaged in school. They also worked on developing the mentors' tutoring skills. Action-learning (Taylor, Marais and Kaplan, 1997) was employed here to learn actively from experiences and to apply the concrete learning into ongoing and future capacity development processes. This has evolved into postgraduate teaching students working with homework mentors, focusing on how to teach.

Another consideration in the implementation of the programme was about how to best use the time in the afternoons, since the learners end school at 2:30 PM each day, but the high school learners could only begin the programme at 3:15 PM. The occupational therapy students held the belief that the grade 6 learners needed a balance of opportunities for different forms of occupational engagement, based on the idea of occupational balance (Wilcock, 1998). The kinds of opportunities for participation that learners desired were collaboratively identified and at the time of this writing (2015) include dancing, singing, and games, facilitated by one teacher.

---

of how the design phase would be applied in practice).

Implementation

This phase is entirely dependent on the initiation and design phases. An explanation of the many methods that could be useful in implementation is beyond the scope of this chapter. The selected techniques and methods should promote the execution of the plan and achievement of the identified outcomes developed during the design phase. Organizational learning and development theories and methods can have great utility, given the nature of working with groups of

people as they coconstruct a different reality for themselves (Box 31-3 gives an indication of how implementation could occur in practice).

Monitoring, Reflection and Evaluation

Acknowledging that the outcomes of community-related interventions are difficult to quantify, this phase is reflected in the use of action learning and the iterative nature of the design process. This phase begins early in the process once an aim has been set. It is critical that the occupational therapist negotiates and cooperatively identifies sets of outcomes and indicators of change that can be measured, in

BOX 31-4

MONITORING, REFLECTION AND EVALUATION IN PRACTICE: THE HOMEWORK PROGRAMME BECOMES A PERMANENT FEATURE AT THE SCHOOL AND IS REPLICATED IN OTHER SIMILAR SCHOOL CONTEXTS

The homework programme is in its infancy, and parent and teacher involvement has been growing alongside the involvement of the high school learners. The school librarian, who was identified as the school representative and who is also a community member, was inspired by the programme and worked actively with the students in developing his capacity to establish his role as ongoing homework programme coordinator. He has since grown in this position and is taking full control for the codirection and development of the programme with the SII, ensuring the sustainability of the programme. It is anticipated that the occupational therapy students would continue to support, where required, the ongoing development of this process.

While learners' performance on the year's literacy and numeracy tests and other school examinations will be an important indicator of the contribution of the programme, there have been other small shifts that should be noted through action learning (Taylor, Marais and Kaplan, 1997).

Although the programme has not been evaluated formally, homework is slowly being prioritized for the grade 6 learners and thought about more actively. Learners have been encouraged by the success of their homework mentors and have spoken excitedly about their participation in the programme. This has shifted this occupation of learning to being seen as something that is attractive. Teachers have also begun to have conversations with learners in the classroom regarding their participation in the programme and what they have learnt through this. This is beginning to shift the culture of the school with regard to the way homework is viewed and orchestrated, and has thus made important inroads in challenging the prevailing occupational choices. A particular achievement is thus the ongoing implementation of the homework programme at this school, but also that the programme has been similarly initiated at another similar school in the same community.

order to provide evidence for the validity of gains made (Box 31-4 gives an indication of how Monitoring, Reflection and Evaluation occurred in the example provided).

CONCLUSION

This chapter has provided an explanation of the key theories and components of the OBCD framework. In so doing, it has demonstrated the usefulness of applying such an approach in order to practise critical occupational therapy. The use of occupational science theories that expose and promote a collaborative understanding of the complex nature of the politics of human occupation in the initiation and design phases of the framework, is a key element that directs intervention towards critical avenues for change. Adopting participatory methods complements the value of this analytical lens, advancing opportunities to understand occupational engagement in context. This promotes social inclusion and justice for groups marginalized as a result of their social identities, prioritizing these groups' role in their own processes for change. Importantly, the framework provides a substantial theoretical

lens to guide how occupational therapists may work with communities to confront the politics of occupational engagement and promote occupational justice.

REFERENCES

Bailliard, A., 2014. Justice, difference, and the capability to function. J. Occup. Sci. doi:10.1080/14427591.2014.957886.

Clarke, J., 2015. Access and opportunity: schooling in Khayelitsha, an introduction. In: 'In Schools, in Community': Emerging Lessons from the Schools Improvement Initiative. Khayelitsha, Cape Town, South Africa.

Galheigo, S.M., 2011. What needs to be done? Occupational therapy responsibilities and challenges regarding human rights. Aust. Occup. Ther. J. 58, 60–66.

Galvaan, R., 2015. The contextually situated nature of occupational choice: marginalised young adolescents' experiences in South Africa. J. Occup. Sci. 22 (1), 39–53.

Galvaan, R., Peters, L., 2013. Occupation-based community development framework. <https://vula.uct.ac.za/access/content/group/9c29ba04-b1ee-49b9-8c85-9a468b556ce2/OBCDF/index.html> (accessed 16.12.14.).

Hammell, H., Iwama, M., 2012. Wellbeing and occupational rights: an imperative for critical occupational therapy. Scand. J. Occup. Ther. 19, 385–394.

Nussbaum, M., 2011. Creating Capabilities.The Human Development Approach. Belknap Press of Harvard University, Cambridge, MA.

Ramugondo, E.L., 2012. Intergenerational play within family: the case for occupational consciousness. J. Occup. Sci. 19, 326–340.

Rudman, D., 2010. Occupational possibilities. J. Occup. Sci. 17, 55–59.

Senge, P., 2006. The Fifth Discipline. The Art and Practice of the Learning Organisation. Random House Business Books, London.

Shalem, Y., Hoadley, U., 2009. The dual economy of schooling and teacher morale in South Africa. Int. Stud. Sociol. Educ. 19, 115–130.

Silbert, P., Clarke, J., 2015. 'In schools, In community' – first steps in the enactment of an effective university-school partnership model. S. Afr. J. High. Educ. 29.

Taylor, J., 2003. Organisations and Development: Towards Building a Practice. CDRA, Cape Town, South Africa.

Taylor, J., Marais, D., Kaplan, A., 1997. Action learning for development: use your experience to improve your effectiveness. Juta, Cape Town, South Africa.

Thibeault, R., 2002. Occupation and the rebuilding of civil society: notes from the war zone. J. Occup. Sci. 9 (1), 38–47. Available at: <http://dx.doi.org/10.1080/14427591.2002.9686492>.

Whiteford, G.E., Townsend, E., 2011. Participatory occupational justice framework: enabling occupational participation and inclusion. In: Kronenberg, F., Pollard, N., Sakellariou, D. (Eds.), Occupational Therapy without Borders, vol. II. Towards an Ecology of Occupation-based Practices. Churchill Livingstone Elsevier, Philadelphia.

Wilcock, A.A., 1998. III Occupational risk factors. In: Wilcock, A.A. (Ed.), An Occupational Perspective on Health. Slack, Thorofare, NJ.

Yuval-Davis, N., 2006. Intersectionality and feminist politics. Eur. J. Womens Stud. 13 (3), 193–209.

32

CULTURALLY RESPONSIVE CARE IN OCCUPATIONAL THERAPY: LEARNING FROM OTHER WORLDVIEWS

PAMELA TALERO

Culturally responsive care in occupational therapy refers to equitable, empathetic and contextualized care that is in harmony with the experiences and meanings of diverse peoples, and aims to reduce health inequalities while enabling participation and social inclusion (Gay, 2010; Iwama et al., 2011; Muñoz, 2007; Ring et al., 2008). Caring is 'a value, an ethic, and a moral imperative that moves self-determination into social responsibility and uses knowledge and strategic thinking to decide how to act in the best interests of others' (Gay, 2010, p. 47). Occupational therapy cares about human occupation, for it shapes human existence.

Therapists are working in increasingly different settings, with diverse clients in complex scenarios. It is in these scenarios where therapists may be exposed to diverse cultures. It is also where issues of occupational justice and human rights arise, requiring therapists to understand occupation from other worldviews in order to effectively address people's relevant occupational needs. Such understanding of human occupation depends greatly on the therapist's ability to learn from a worldview different than his or her own. A worldview is defined as 'a set of commonly held values, ideas, and images concerning the nature of reality and the role of humanity within it, that shapes one's emotional, cognitive, and physical (action) responses' (Richardson and MacRae, 2011, p. 343). The way people make sense or perceive the inner and outside world is shaped greatly by culture.

The cultural competence and cultural safety models commonly used in occupational therapy have their origins in other social and health-related professions lacking an occupational perspective, and a critical reflection and awareness of the differences in power and privilege and the inequalities that emerge in social relationships (Talero et al., 2015). Also, some of the major critiques to the current models are related to the limited view of culture as static, treated as a variable that is often conflated with race and ethnicity, and judged from a standard of 'whiteness' or by its vulnerabilities (Kumaş-Tan et al., 2007; Kumagai and Lypson, 2009).

Muñoz (2007) proposed a process-oriented model of 'culturally responsive caring' that results from the interaction of five components: building cultural awareness, generating cultural knowledge, applying cultural skills, engaging culturally diverse others and exploring multiculturalism. Although this model offers a foundation, the areas and components of the model and the learning process need to be further developed.

This chapter describes an entry-level educational model of culturally responsive care in occupational therapy, embedded in service learning. The model aims to guide the development of the required knowledge, skills, behaviours and support systems from a unique occupational perspective. Using this model can help occupational therapists develop critical understanding of the interrelation amongst occupation, justice and enablement, contributing to the development of client centred practices. The model is founded on the participatory occupational justice framework developed by Whiteford and Townsend (2011) and is informed by related and updated published literature, and the professional experiences of the author working in different contexts in the US, Colombia, Guatemala and Cuba.

PRINCIPLES OF CULTURALLY RESPONSIVE CARE IN OCCUPATIONAL THERAPY

Culturally responsive caring is motivated by having a dialogue in which occupational therapists intend to

understand other worldviews of occupation so they can enable participation and foster social inclusion. Thus it is guided by three principles: culture is context specific, cross-cultural encounters are based on recognition of diversity, and the need for a critical examination of occupational therapy's underpinnings.

Culture Is Context Specific

Culture is defined as shared spheres of experience and meaning, as well as the processes involved in creating, ascribing and maintaining meaning to objects and phenomena in the world. Culture is at the core of human occupation, as it is shaped by meaning[1] and thus shapes occupation. One cannot speak about occupation or pretend to understand its complexity without examining culture in a given context (Gray and McPherson, 2005; Iwama et al., 2011; Muñoz, 2007).

Cross-Cultural Encounters Are Based on Recognition of Diversity

Cross-cultural encounters refer to interactions of two or more individuals from different cultural backgrounds (Moran et al., 2011). These encounters are based on the recognition of people's cultural similarities and differences in a horizontal, two-way dynamic, as in a dialogue. All parties involved exchange their worldviews as they interact with each other, both by conveying and receiving a message and by responding to the message in order to recognize each other.

Cultural responsiveness requires that all cultures are critically evaluated by the sociocultural, economic, political and historical power relationships that shape people's worldviews and that constantly influence every cross-cultural encounter. Being conscious of this dynamic allows one to understand different worldviews in context, rather than simply conceptualizing culture as issues of race and ethnicity, or to present 'whiteness' as the standard, excluding it from the concept of cultural diversity (Escobar, 2008; Kumagai and Lypson, 2009; Kumaş-Tan et al., 2007; World Federation of Occupational Therapists, 2009).

---

[1]*Meaning* is defined as the personally or socially constructed sense people make of their living situations; having symbolic or explicit significance (Iwama et al., 2011).

Critical Examination of Occupational Therapy's Underpinnings

A critical examination of occupational therapy's foundational belief system and assumptions is imperative to provide culturally responsive care. Many authors agree that the profession's core values have been historically shaped by mainly Western/Eurocentric, urban middle-class and Anglophone theorists, with limited or no inclusion of other perspectives, which propagates injustice. A critical examination of the profession's underpinnings and their relationship with other worldviews can foster an understanding of self and others (Hammell, 2013; Kantartzis and Molineux, 2012; Pollard et al., 2008; Rudman and Deenhardt, 2008).

These principles guide culturally responsive care in occupational therapy through the profession's lifelong commitment to enabling people's participation and social inclusion in their living contexts. It is necessary to clarify that, just as with the acquisition of new skills, a single cross-cultural service-learning experience will not 'make' one culturally responsive. The process continues throughout one's professional life, rooted in interaction with clients in any setting. Effective culturally responsive care training, however, can provide therapists with the main tools to appropriately think and respond in different cross-cultural encounters.

IT ALL STARTS WITH A CELL: THE DEVELOPMENT OF THE MODEL OF CULTURALLY RESPONSIVE CARE IN OCCUPATIONAL THERAPY, EMBEDDED IN SERVICE LEARNING

The educational model of culturally responsive care in occupational therapy, embedded in service-learning, uses hexagonal shapes to illustrate the relationship between contexts and the delicate balance inside each hexagon. Hexagonal shapes are prevalent in nature and human designs because of their flexibility, efficiency and structural stability (Baltzis, 2011). In a structure made of hexagonal cells, such as a honeycomb, there are no gaps. Each hexagonal cell is unique but interdependent of the borders it shares with other cells.

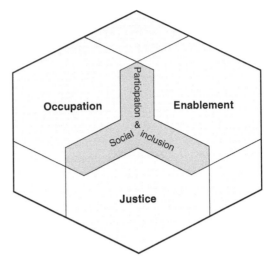

FIGURE 32-1 ■ Using an occupational lens to understand participation and social inclusion in context.

Imagine a world map where coordinates have been traced to locate a place, using a 'hexagon mosaic map' (Carr et al., 1992). This kind of map uses hexagons to form a pattern of tiles that fit perfectly together. Whether zooming in or out, one finds that every particular place is formed by interrelated cells. Each cell represents a context: the habitat of human and nonhuman beings, circumstances, objects or conditions shaped by the experiences of those who form the setting (Moran et al., 2011). Occupation, enablement and justice constitute one's occupational lens: the way therapists picture or read the context, as shown in Figure 32-1. Each context, while different, is interrelated with other contexts through different angles. Caring in a culturally responsive manner in occupational therapy translates into learning through such an occupational lens that one cannot understand oneself without understanding the 'other' (a separate entity from one's own self).

I will exemplify the use of this lens through the use of a hypothetical scenario. Consider a partnership established between an American university and a health clinic located in Bogotá, Colombia. This clinic provides healthcare services, including occupational therapy, to the community of a local authority: Tunjuelito. A service-learning project was established in partnership with the clinic to exchange best practices in occupational therapy. Occupational therapy faculty and students from the US worked with the clinic staff to learn how the profession is practised locally and to help improve the clinic's services[2].

Localize Colombia in the hexagonal mosaic map you have imagined. At first you will see a hexagon as big as the country's territory. If you zoom in you will see that it is made up of multiple cells. Zoom in more and you will find a smaller hexagon: Bogotá. Within that hexagon you will find again multiple cells, one of which is Tunjuelito. This cell will be your main context as it is where the health clinic is located and it represents the community to whom the clinic provides services. How can occupational therapists provide culturally responsive care in this context? First, both faculty and students want to look at how occupations are defined and experienced in Tunjuelito, and to understand what could enable/disable participation in meaningful occupations in this context and how occupational opportunities are negotiated. You will find that in this process, elements of a broader context emerge (e.g., the services provided at the clinic are regulated by the Bogotá district health policies which are articulated with the country's health policy).

This hexagonal occupational lens is always used in collaboration with community partners to address their occupational needs. Following the guiding principles, therapists do not make assumptions about how occupation, enablement and justice are interrelated in a particular context. Instead, therapists allow themselves to explore the interrelation of these areas following a learning process.

AREAS OF THE MODEL AND THE COMPONENTS OF EACH AREA

The areas of occupation, enablement and justice emerge from context. Figure 32-1 illustrates the three interrelated areas of the model. The darker portion

_____

[2]It is important to note that not all encounters may happen in scenarios where occupational therapy is an established profession in the partnering country, region, and/or community. However, it is necessary to investigate if there are academic occupational therapy programmes, licensing boards, professional associations, or local practitioners available, and the conditions under which they are expected to provide services or the possible reasons for the lack of services.

comes into view only through the overlap of the areas. Because care is contextualized (Gay, 2010), one cannot provide culturally responsive care without appreciating these three areas together as they are configured.

Through a lifelong learning process, therapists learn to deconstruct and reconstruct each of the areas and its components in providing culturally responsive care. Each area contains components that characterize its content, as explained below. Notice that although the use of areas and their components provides an organizing structure, the content, per se, will vary upon the uniqueness of the community experience (e.g., Tunjuelito versus another local authority in Bogotá, Bogotá versus another city in the country, or Colombia versus another country in the region or the world).

Occupation

The area of 'occupation' (see Figure 32-1) is conceptualized as meaningful, everyday human activity that happens in a particular time and place, through which humans sustain their livelihoods within a given context (Hammell, 2009; Kantartzis and Molineux, 2012; Pollard and Sakellariou, 2012; Wilcock, 2006) and that can be named in the lexicon of the culture (Clark et al., 1991). Everyday activities are configured differently according to time and place (Escobar, 2008; Pemberton and Cox, 2011; Townsend et al., 2009). For example, eating breakfast is essentially the same as eating lunch: one ingests food. However, the time of the day and the places vary, modifying the experience and what it means to oneself and in comparison to another person.

An understanding of occupation is contingent upon the interplay of its dimensions, namely, doing, being, becoming, belonging and knowing (Escobar, 2008; Pemberton and Cox, 2011; Townsend et al., 2009). Thus occupational therapy education has to aim for developing the practitioners' 'occupational literacy' in the language of cultural diversity. Occupational literacy refers to having an understanding of what one has to do in a particular context (Pollard and Sakellariou, 2012). In order to do so, one has to consider first the multiple meanings that occupation could have.

In reading the experiences of others, one tends to bring one's own ideas of 'what it means' and 'how it is performed'. There is nothing wrong with that, as occupation is indeed multifaceted. However, in culturally diverse contexts, one could easily misunderstand occupation, by ignoring 'what it means': how the language is used and functions in context (Pollard and Sakellariou, 2012). For example, consider the positive connotation that the term *occupation* generally has amongst occupational therapy practitioners. However, occupation may have a tragic connotation in contexts where armed conflict and displacement have been present (e.g., the occupation of a territory by force), or can have a socially 'dark side' or a negative/ill quality or consequences, such as in the case of crime, prostitution, child-soldiering, mining, caregiving, amongst others, respectively (Twinley and Addidle, 2012). This is difficult to learn in a classroom setting; hence the need to learn in a real setting, such as in a service-learning experience.

Occupational literacy should start with a cultural analysis of the dimensions of meanings of occupation. 'Doing' describes the need/opportunity for action; to keep busy; how people structure their living; and habits and routines. 'Being' describes the need/opportunity for a state or quality of people's existence; subjective experience; roles; discovery of oneself; reflection; introspection; meditation; and appreciation of music, arts or literature (Hammell, 2004; Wilcock, 2006). These two dimensions of meaning are typically easier to relate to since the terms *do* and *be* are often used to introduce oneself.

Occupation can also have a meaning of 'becoming' which describes the need/opportunity for changing; transforming; reassessing one's life-priorities; envisioning future selves or possible lives; and exploring new ideas and opportunities (Hammell, 2004; Wilcock, 2006). 'Belonging' describes the need/opportunity to contribute to social interaction; mutual support and friendship; sense of connectedness or being a part of something (Hammell, 2004; Wilcock, 2006). Finally, 'knowing' describes the need/opportunity for perceiving, processing and representing internal and external information; exchanging ideas; acquiring consciousness; and being aware of what and how one knows (Kronenberg et al., 2011). The analysis of the interplay of these dimensions not only allows the therapist to understand occupation from other worldviews; by inquiring about these dimensions through people's

narratives, therapists are also able to monitor the change of those meanings through the therapeutic process, and to contribute to the promotion and improvement of quality-of-life measures widely used in interdisciplinary community development and livelihood projects.

I will return to Tunjuelito to exemplify this area of the model. Eating breakfast in Tunjuelito typically has a different meaning than eating lunch. Breakfast usually consists of *tinto y pan* – black coffee and a piece of bread – where the need for 'doing' is crucial, as it is part of a routine and is described as 'something you need to do to start the day'. Lunch, instead, is the main meal of the day; it has been generally prepared by wives/mothers (an expression of 'being' a wife or a mother in this context, which is in itself a representation of how some occupations are engendered) and usually takes place in a group, with family or coworkers, at school or at the local restaurant. The meaning of lunch is marked by 'becoming' and 'belonging' over the physiological need for ingesting food or 'knowing' how to eat it.

How do people configure their occupations in particular contexts? What component of occupation has more individual and social value and under what circumstances? How is that different between people? Reflecting on questions like these can allow occupational therapists to become culturally responsive.

Enablement

The area of 'enablement' (see Figure 32-1) is conceptualized as providing occupational means or opportunities through participatory practices in a continuum from ineffective to effective, or from disablement to enablement (Whiteford and Townsend, 2011). Enabling occupational opportunities is a complex process. Working with worldviews with which therapists are not familiar challenges them to rethink their ability to respond to a different context, to recognize and empower the voices that often go ignored or oppressed by dominant systems or institutions, and to develop with others alternatives for sustainable participation. Occupational opportunities are determined by power relationships that determine what one can or cannot have access to: the occupational 'right' (Hammell, 2008; Pollard and Sakellariou, 2012; Pollard et al., 2008). Therefore, enablement requires occupational therapy practitioners to play an active role in influencing law and policy.

The participatory practices for culturally responsive care comprise cultural skills, cultural behaviours/attitudes, cultural knowledge/awareness and cultural support systems that differ according to context (Black and Wells, 2007; Kumagai and Lypson, 2009; Muñoz, 2007). Enablement is contingent upon using these practices effectively. When not using these practices effectively, one could inadvertently contribute to disabling occupational opportunities. For example, when pressing for independence in activities of daily living in a context where occupations are shaped by interdependence, one might be isolating people from their community.

Acknowledging that each context determines the possibilities for engagement in occupations, goes hand in hand with recognizing the powers at play and building synergy amongst the participants. This is the result of developing the therapists' cultural skills, behaviours/attitudes, knowledge and support systems through a constant learning process – this is described at the end of this chapter.

The development of 'cultural skills' refers to the acquisition and mastery of techniques, approaches, assessment and intervention strategies, for communicating and interacting with people from different cultures (Black and Wells, 2007; Muñoz, 2007). These strategies include active reading and listening skills, sifting and evaluating evidence (Nussbaum, 1997), culturally responsive interviewing/assessment (Ring et al., 2008) and the therapeutic use of self (Taylor, 2008).

'Cultural knowledge/awareness' refers to seeking information, and analysing and reflecting upon what, who, how, when, where and why one's worldviews (amongst different worldviews) shape human occupations and experiences in a particular context. It includes awareness of sociocultural, political, economic and historical power relationships, ontological and epistemological assumptions that shape worldviews of 'self' and 'other' (Black and Wells, 2007; Muñoz, 2007; Nussbaum, 2010).

'Cultural behaviours/attitudes' refers to personal qualities that enable or disable healthy cultural encounters. Such behaviours include flexibility, open-mindedness, sensitivity, genuineness, empathy, healthy criticism and healthy skepticism (Balcazar et al., 2009; Bazyk et al., 2010).

'Cultural support systems' refers to structural or institutional access or barriers to resources and can include acknowledgement of support/nonsupport from family, community, groups, governmental and nongovernmental agencies, traditional healers and formal healthcare systems (Gray and McPherson, 2005).

Justice

The area of 'justice' (see Figure 32-1) is conceptualized as a vision of society in which all populations have equal access to opportunities, resources, privileges and rights to participate in occupations to their maximum potential in order to satisfy their personal needs and enact full citizenship (Braveman, 2009; Escobar, 2008; Nussbaum, 1997). This justice of difference and social inclusion comprises six nonlinear, interrelated and collaborative enabling processes referred to as 'enablement skills' in the participatory occupational justice framework (Whiteford and Townsend 2011), which for the purpose of the model will be taken as the components of this area as follows:

- *Raise consciousness of occupational justices/injustices* refers to becoming aware of occupational justice as a concern for social inclusion in everyday life.
- *Engage collaboratively with partners* refers to responding to a request, referral, contract offer, or other arrangement, or to initiate a partnership.
- *Mediate agreement on a plan* refers to mediating a plan based on a collaborative partnership.
- *Strategize resource finding* refers to finding human, financial, spatial and other resources for executing a plan based on a collaborative partnership.
- *Support implementation and continuous evaluation of the plan* refers to the consideration of all possible approaches provided by all partners in order to achieve their desired results.
- *Inspire advocacy for appropriate sustainability or closure* refers to fostering leadership among partners, whereby they advocate according to their own needs, to sustain or end the mediated plan, and renegotiate or end the professional relationship.

Negotiating change that is sustainable over time requires working closely with the partnerships one establishes. An authentic service-learning learning experience requires that the benefits to the faculty and the students do not outweigh the benefits for the community partner. A pluralistic view of how occupational rights are achieved is needed to consider other alternatives for development. A successful experience in one context might not be successful in another, considering that power relationships play out differently. Diversity is healthy as it nurtures both thought and action, and should be encouraged rather than hegemonized.

The participatory occupational justice framework (Whiteford and Townsend, 2011) is an excellent tool for exchanging knowledge in the form of meanings of occupation and experiences, through active partnerships. As occupational therapy aims to enable participation in occupation and achieve social inclusion, justice needs to be thought of from an occupational perspective but projected to contribute to a social realm, where occupational therapists collaborate with other stakeholders involved in achieving a greater equity for everyone 'to choose and participate to their potential in their desired occupations' (Whiteford and Townsend, 2011, p. 69).

THE LEARNING PROCESS OF THE MODEL OF CULTURALLY RESPONSIVE CARE IN OCCUPATIONAL THERAPY, EMBEDDED IN SERVICE LEARNING

So how do therapists learn to care in a culturally responsive manner? Experiential learning activities and immersion approaches have shown themselves to be effective methods for culturally responsive care training (Gray and McPherson, 2005). In particular, service learning, an experiential learning approach, has been demonstrated to be more effective than traditional teaching methods, such as lecturing, in developing students' ability to apply what they learned in one setting to another (Billig, 2006).

The learning process of culturally responsive care in occupational therapy, embedded in service learning, follows a revised Bloom's taxonomy: a way to organize thinking skills into hierarchical levels from the most basic to the most complex (Krathwohl, 2002). The six levels of the revised Bloom's taxonomy are organized

in this model into four interrelated but hierarchical phases: narrative imagination, critical reflexivity, critical consciousness and critical action. Each phase studies the interrelation of the areas of occupation, enablement and justice in a particular context at a different thinking level. Furthermore, each phase is related to each of the four main phases of service learning: engagement and design, reflection and plan, reciprocity and implementation, and dissemination and evaluation.

Narrative Imagination

Narrative imagination is 'the ability to think what it might be like to be in the shoes of a person different from oneself, to be an intelligent reader of another person's story, and to understand the emotions and wishes and desires that someone so placed might have' (Nussbaum, 1997, p. 11).

A critical examination of oneself and one's tradition is the starting point for the provision of culturally responsive care. Writing assignments are recommended to cultivate reflection. Keeping a journal in which therapists document critical incidents, their lessons and action steps, can facilitate the process of learning to care in a culturally responsive manner (Bazyk et al., 2010).

Self-reflection about one's worldview and different worldviews can generate fear, anxiety, anger or resentment in the students and/or the faculty. Failure to anticipate different reactions could potentially compromise the success of the training. Thus, therapists must feel safe to engage in an honest dialogue about their own and others' worldviews, articulating the relationship between culture and human occupation, enablement and justice in providing culturally responsive care and critically examining the meaning of dimensions of occupations in time and place and in a particular context. Analysing works of art, literature, music, food or dance, and local news of the context of one studies (Von Wright, 2002) allows one to raise one's own and others' consciousness of occupational justice and injustice by discussing current environmental, sociocultural, historical, political and economic powers that shape human occupation in different context.

Critical Reflexivity

Critical reflexivity is the ability to reflect upon the consistency of one's own and others' discourses and to question the conditions under which knowledge and claims are constructed and accepted (Phelan, 2011; Whiteford and Townsend, 2011). In this phase, therapists demonstrate an understanding of the cultural, social, political, historical and economic considerations that potentially impact the health and wellness needs of diverse populations in a variety of contexts; gain knowledge and appreciation of different worldviews and practices regarding health, illness/disease, participation, and ability/disability and their impact in providing culturally responsive care in occupational therapy; and discuss the implications of historical ontological and epistemological assumptions that have shaped the profession in caring in a culturally responsive manner.

Therapists' reflective journals are used to critically examine commonly held concepts such as occupation, enablement and justice and their different meanings in different contexts. It is crucial to understand that 'knowledge construction is never a neutral process, but rather is influenced by a multitude of social, cultural and political factors' (Rudman and Deenhardt, 2008, p. 153). Using critical disability studies and feminist critical disability studies can help therapists in analysing the cultural views of health, illness/disease and disability that influence participation in occupation in a particular context. Also, in this phase, therapists practise culturally responsive interviewing/assessment by using different mnemonic tools[3] and therapeutic use of self (Taylor, 2008).

Critical Consciousness

Critical consciousness refers to a reflective awareness of power and privilege and their influence in social

relationships (Angell, 2012; Pitner and Sakamoto, 2005) 'and an appraisal of resultant consequences for individual and collective wellbeing' (Kronenberg et al., 2011, p. 2). In this phase, therapists develop and apply cross-cultural knowledge, behaviours/attitudes and skills to mediate agreement on a plan with service-learning community partners, and strategize resource finding with service-learning community partners in a culturally responsive manner.

The fieldwork portion of the service-learning experience should take place at this phase with an active recognition of societal relationships and conflicts and a critical search for appropriate solutions (Angell, 2012). Therapists are exposed to their own prejudices, stereotypes and biases (Pitner and Sakamoto, 2005) through debriefing sessions of at least 30 minutes on a daily basis in which participants discuss critical incidents, strengths and weaknesses and next-step actions of the day. The participation of a community-member representative is useful in the debriefing process as it clarifies possible *descriptive vices* (interpreting what one sees in front of one's eyes only through what looks familiar or by romanticizing it) or *normative vices* (evaluating what one sees in front of one's eyes by judging it, by thinking that one's own culture is best or of the other culture as untouched, or by not formulating an opinion) (Nussbaum, 1997).

A pedagogy of discomfort is exercised when developing critical consciousness as both students/therapists and educators/mentors move outside of their comfort zones, experiencing a cognitive disequilibrium; i.e., encountering unfamiliar or uncomfortable ideas and turning a critical gaze on one's own values and assumptions (Kumagai and Lypson, 2009). Debriefing sessions are crucial to transform the possible discomfort one might feel when being in a different context into critical thinking for engaging with others and with one's own self (Kumagai and Lypson, 2009; Trifonas, 2003).

Critical Action

Finally, critical action is the ability to systematically reflect, pre-, post-, and on action, upon one's work with real people and real issues, improving the appropriateness and justice of: (a) one's own social or educational practices, (b) one's own understanding of these practices, and (c) the situations in which the practices are carried out (Kumagai and Lypson, 2009).

---

[3]Mnemonic tools are helpful in encoding and recalling important information by synthetizing it into a single word or sentence. They are used to explore and understand someone's perspectives and also raise awareness of people's biases. Some of the most commonly used mnemonic tools are: LEARN (Listen, Explain, Acknowledge, Recommend, Negotiate); BATHE (Background/what has happened, Affect/how are you feeling, Trouble/what troubles you the most, Handle/how do you usually handle it, Empathy/provide support); RESPECT (Respect, Explanatory model, Sociocultural context, Power, Empathy, Concerns and fears, Therapeutic alliance/trust); and TRANSLATE, which is used in the presence of an interpreter or other language assistance (Trust, Roles, Advocacy, Nonjudgmental, Setting, Language, Accuracy, Time, Ethical issues).

In this phase, therapists demonstrate professional leadership and creativity in analysing, discussing and addressing occupational issues in cross-cultural scenarios; identifying community participation and social inclusion opportunities and evaluating their potential to enable occupational justice in context; and developing and applying cross-cultural knowledge, behaviours/attitudes and skills to support implementation and continuous evaluation of mediated plan, and to inspire advocacy for sustainability or closure of mediated plan with service-learning community partners in a culturally responsive manner.

This phase should take place during and after the fieldwork portion of the service-learning experience, wherein therapists reflect upon their actions with the service-learning hosting community. Critical action exercises therapists' civic responsibility with other fellow humans in addressing social participation and inclusion in context, creating alternatives to address the occupational needs experienced by the hosting community.

CONCLUSION

Culturally responsive care in occupational therapy is concerned with establishing a dialogue in cross-cultural encounters where knowledge alone is often not sufficient. Behaviours, skills and support systems also shape this dialogue, and the therapist's response can either contribute to enabling or to disabling participation and social inclusion. The main goal of the learning process, facilitated by exposure to different worldviews, is to develop a keen perception for how and why to inquire about others throughout their professional practices as a continuous lifelong pursuit. Since culture is context specific, it is subject to change, as the worldviews of the people who inhabit the context on a daily basis change as well. This requires therapists to welcome and integrate other worldviews in response to the cross-cultural encounters they experience, revisiting elements of each learning phase as needed.

REFERENCES

Angell, A.M., 2012. Occupation-centered analysis of social difference: contributions to a socially responsive occupational science. J. Occup. Sci. 21 (2), 1–13.

Balcazar, F.E., Suarez-Balcazar, Y., Taylor-Ritzler, T., 2009. Cultural competence: development of a conceptual framework. Disabil. Rehabil. 31, 1153–1160.

Baltzis, K.B., 2011. Hexagonal vs. circular cell shape: a comparison analysis and evaluation of the two popular model approximations. In: Melikov, A. (Ed.), Cellular Networks. Positioning, Performance Analysis, Reliability. InTech, pp. 102–122. Available from: <http://www.intechopen.com/books/cellular-networks-positioning-performance-analysis-reliability/hexagonal-vs-circular-cell-shape-a-comparative-analysis-and-evaluation-of-the-two-popular-modeling-a> (accessed 01.09.15.).

Bazyk, S., Glorioso, M., Gordon, R., Haines, J., Percaciante, M., 2010. Service learning: the process of doing and becoming an occupational therapist. Occup. Ther. Health Care 24 (2), 171–187.

Billig, S.H., 2006. Lesson from research on teaching and learning: service-learning as effective instruction. In: Growing to Greatness 2006. National Youth Leadership Council, pp. 25–32. Available from: <http://www.peecworks.org/peec/peec_research/01795BFB-001D0211.1/growing%20to%20greatness%202006.pdf> (accessed 01.09.15.).

Black, R.M., Wells, S.A., 2007. Culture and Occupation. A Model of Empowerment in Occupational Therapy. AOTA Press, Bethesda, MD.

Braveman, B.B.-H.J., 2009. Social justice and health disparities: an evolving discourse in occupational therapy research and intervention. Am. J. Occup. Ther. 63, 7–12.

Carr, D.B., Olsen, A.R., White, D., 1992. Hexagon mosaic maps for display of univariate and bivariate geographical data. CaGIS 19, 228–236.

Clark, F., et al., 1991. Occupational science: academic innovation in the service of occupational therapy's future. Am. J. Occup. Ther. 45, 300–310.

Escobar, A., 2008. Territories of Difference. Place, Movements, Life, Redes. Duke University Press, London.

Gay, G., 2010. Culturally Responsive Teaching. Theory, Research, and Practice, second ed. Teachers College Press, New York.

Gray, M., McPherson, K., 2005. Cultural safety and professional practice in occupational therapy: a New Zealand perspective. Aust. Occup. Ther. J. 52, 34–42.

Hammell, K.W., 2004. Dimensions of meaning in the occupations of daily life. Can. J. Occup. Ther. 71, 296–305.

Hammell, K.W., 2008. Reflections on … well-being and occupational rights. Can. J. Occup. Ther. 75, 61–64.

Hammell, K.W., 2009. Sacred texts: a sceptical exploration of the assumptions underpinning theories of occupation. Can. J. Occup. Ther. 76, 6–13.

Hammell, K.R.W., 2013. Client-centered practice in occupational therapy: critical reflections. Scand. J. Occup. Ther. 20 (3), 174–181.

Iwama, M.K., Thomson, N.A., Macdonald, R.M., 2011. Situated meaning: a matter of cultural safety, inclusion and occupational therapy. In: Kronenberg, F., Pollard, N., Sakellariou, D. (Eds.), Occupational Therapies Without Borders, vol. 2. Towards an Ecology of Occupation-Based Practices. Churchill Livingstone Elsevier, Philadelphia, pp. 85–92.

Kantartzis, S., Molineux, M., 2012. Understanding the discoursive development of occupation: historico-political perspectives. In: Whiteford, G.E., Hocking, C. (Eds.), Occupational Science: Society, Inclusion, Participation. Wiley-Blackwell, West Sussex, UK, pp. 38–53.

Krathwohl, D.R., 2002. A revision of Bloom's taxonomy: an overview. Theory Pract. 41, 212–218.

Kronenberg, F., Pollard, N., Ramugondo, E., 2011. Introduction: courage to dance politics. In: Kronenberg, F., Pollard, N., Sakellariou, D. (Eds.), Occupational Therapies Without Borders. Towards an Ecology of Occupation-Based Practices. Churchill Livingstone Elsevier, Philadelphia, pp. 1–16.

Kumagai, A.K., Lypson, M.L., 2009. Beyond cultural compentence: critical consciousness, social justice, and multicultural education. Acad. Med. 84, 782–787.

Kumaş-Tan, Z., Beagan, B., Loppie, C., MacLeod, A., Frank, B., 2007. Measures of cultural competence: examining hidden assumptions. Acad. Med. 82, 548–557.

Moran, R.T., Harris, P.R., Moran, S.V., 2011. Global leaders and communications. In: Managing Cultural Differences. Leadership Skills and Strategies for Working in a Global World. Elsevier, Burlington, MA, pp. 37–71.

Muñoz, J.P., 2007. Culturally responsive caring in occupational therapy. Occup. Ther. Int. 14, 256–280.

Nussbaum, M.C., 1997. Cultivating Humanity. A Classical Defense of Reform in Liberal Education. Harvard University Press, Cambridge, MA.

Nussbaum, M.C., 2010. Not for Profit. Why Democracy Needs the Humanities. Princeton University Press, Princeton, NJ.

Pemberton, S., Cox, D., 2011. What happened to the time? The relationship of occupational therapy to time. Br. J. Occup. Ther. 74, 78–85.

Phelan, S.K., 2011. Constructions of disability: a call for critical reflexivity in occupational therapy. Can. J. Occup. Ther. 78, 164–172.

Pitner, R.O., Sakamoto, I., 2005. The role of critical consciousness in multicultural practice: examining how its strength becomes its limitation. Am. J. Orthopsychiatry 75, 684–694.

Pollard, N., Sakellariou, D., 2012. Occupational literacy. In: Pollard, N., Sakellariou, D. (Eds.), Politics of Occupation-Centred Practice. Reflection on Occupational Engagement Across Cultures. John Wiley & Sons, West Sussex, UK, pp. 42–50.

Pollard, N., Sakellariou, D., Kronenberg, F., 2008. A political practice of occupational therapy. In: Pollard, N., Sakellariou, D., Kronenberg, F. (Eds.), A Political Practice of Occupational Therapy. Churchill Livingstone Elsevier, Philadelphia, pp. 3–19.

Richardson, P.K., MacRae, A., 2011. An occupational justice research perspective. In: Pollard, N., Sakellariou, D., Kronenberg, F. (Eds.), Occupational Therapies Without Borders, vol. 2. Churchill Livingstone Elsevier, Philadelphia, pp. 339–348.

Ring, J.M., et al., 2008. Curriculum for Culturally Responsive Health Care. The Step-by-Step Guide for Cultural Competence Training. Radcliffe Publishing Ltd, Oxford, UK.

Rudman, D.L., Deenhardt, S., 2008. Shaping knowledge regarding occupation: examining the cultural underpinnings of the evolving concept of occupational identity. Aust. Occup. Ther. J. 55, 153–162.

Talero, P., Kern, S.B., Tupe, D.A., 2015. Culturally responsive care in occupational therapy: an entry level educational model embedded in service-learning. Scand. J. Occup. Ther. 22, 95–102.

Taylor, R.R., 2008. Knowing ourselves as therapists: introducing the therapeutic modes. In: Taylor, R. (Ed.), The Intentional Relationship. Occupational Therapy and Use of Self. F.A. Davis Company, Philadelphia, pp. 67–97.

Townsend, E., et al., 2009. Linking occupation and place in community health. J. Occup. Sci. 16, 50–55.

Trifonas, P.P. (Ed.), 2003. Pedagogies of Difference: Rethinking Education for Social Justice. Routledge Falmer, New York.

Twinley, R., Addidle, G., 2012. Considering violence: the dark side of occupation. Br. J. Occup. Ther. 75, 202–204.

Von Wright, M., 2002. Narrative imagination and taking the perspective of others. Stud. Philos. Educ. 21, 407–416.

Whiteford, G., Townsend, E., 2011. Participatory occupational justice framework (POJF, 2010): enabling occupational participation and inclusion. In: Kronenberg, F., Pollard, N., Sakellariou, D. (Eds.), Occupational Therapies Without Borders, vol. 2. Towards an Ecology of Occupation-Based Practices. Churchill Livingstone Elsevier, Philadelphia, pp. 65–84.

Wilcock, A.A., 2006. An Occupational Perspective of Health, second ed. SLACK Incorporated, Thorofare, NJ.

World Federation of Occupational Therapists, 2009. Diversity Matters: Guiding Principles on Diversity and Culture. WFOT. Available from: <http://www.wfot.org/ResourceCentre.aspx> (accessed 01.09.15.).

33

FACTORS INFLUENCING THE ROLE OF SOUTH AFRICAN OCCUPATIONAL THERAPISTS IN THE OCCUPATIONAL THERAPY INTERVENTION DESIGN PROCESS

PAM GRETSCHEL ■ ELELWANI RAMUGONDO ■
ROSHAN GALVAAN

Designing interventions is an integral aspect of the occupational therapy process. Occupational therapists interact with clients to identify their occupational concerns via various assessment methods and approaches. Interventions are then designed to address these concerns. Occupational therapists are encouraged to pay close attention to how they can contribute to enabling access to meaningful and dignified occupations for marginalized populations (Kronenberg and Pollard, 2006; Pollard et al., 2008). Occupational therapy interventions should be informed by people's diverse and specific occupational engagement and occupational needs. This contributes to the complexity of the intervention design process. To date, the complexity of the occupational therapy intervention design process and specifically the factors that influence the

role of the occupational therapist during the intervention design process have not been explored in South Africa.

The first author aimed to fill this gap through her doctoral research, which explored how a group of occupational therapists designed an intervention for caregivers of HIV-positive children on highly active antiretroviral treatment living in low-income conditions in South Africa. The intervention aimed to improve the self-efficacy of the caregivers to address their children's participation in the childhood occupations of play, learning, and development.

The intersection of social disadvantage and the stigma associated with the HIV diagnosis mean that caregivers and children are a part of a marginalized group in South Africa. The social and living conditions of these caregivers and their children may limit their access to a range of occupations or provide poor opportunities to participate in occupations. This places them at risk of occupational injustice.

Drawing on the intervention design process as a case within a case study design (Stake, 1995, 2008), this chapter will:

- Provide a critique of intervention design within occupational therapy, juxtaposing the occupational therapists designing the new intervention against the caregivers and children for whom the intervention was designed.
- Introduce the concepts of intersectional identity and positionality (Crenshaw, 1995; Yuval-Davis, 2006) and describe how historically located sociocultural factors shape different identities and positionalities across different contexts.
- Encourage a consideration of the social identity and positionality differences between occupational therapists and their clients, as well as how these elements contribute to the complexities of occupational therapy intervention design.
- Put forward questions encouraging occupational therapists' heightened consciousness of, and engagement in, self-reflection to consider the impact of intersectional identity and positionality within the intervention design process.

OCCUPATIONAL THERAPY IN A SOUTH AFRICAN CONTEXT

In South Africa, people are asked to describe themselves in terms of five racial population groups: Black African, White, Coloured, Indian or Asian, and Other/Unspecified (South African National Census, 2011). These five racial population groups stemmed from the apartheid[1] regime's Population Registration Act No. 30 of 1950, which required people to be identified and registered from birth as belonging to a distinct racial group. The Act was typified by humiliating tests, which determined race through perceived linguistic and physical characteristics.

Apartheid, as a system of government in South Africa, attributed inferior value and afforded fewer opportunities to people identified as belonging to the coloured and black race groups. These inequalities persist today despite the abolishment of the apartheid government's policies in 1994. The enduring consequences of social inequalities in post-apartheid South Africa are reflected in the lack of economic and social progress of the majority black South African population. A large proportion of black South Africans live in chronic poverty in disadvantaged townships and informal settlements (South African National Census, 2011). Black South African youth experience the highest unemployment rates in the country, approximately 39.4% compared with the 9.6% unemployed white youth living in South Africa (StatsSA, 2014). The continued social inequalities are also reflected in people's access to higher education. While 36.5% of the white population attain a postgraduate level of education, only 8.3% of black South Africans and 7.4% of coloured people attain a level of education higher than their final year of schooling (South African National Census, 2011). In post-apartheid South Africa, these race categories are also used for Employment Equity[2] purposes and reflect the ongoing experiences of disproportional inequality for black and coloured persons living in the country.

In South Africa, despite shifting demographics, white occupational therapists continue to remain the majority within the profession. The data discussed in this chapter show how the process of occupational therapy intervention design is influenced by differences between the profiles of occupational therapists in South Africa and the identity of the South African population requiring occupational therapy services. With reference to the case group of occupational therapists designing the intervention, it often means discussing the influences on the design process where young, female, white, middle-to-upper income occupational therapists in this study were designing interventions for predominantly black, female, low-income caregivers and their children. This matters to the formulation of occupational therapy practice since a contextually relevant and political practice of occupational therapy should be cognizant of factors of diversity and inequality. South African occupational therapy authors

---

[1]Apartheid was the system of government in South Africa from 1948 to 1994.

[2]Employment Equity refers to policies and programmes aiming to create employment for people disadvantaged by apartheid.

support this view of practice, advocating for the crafting of occupational therapy interventions that attend to the diverse occupational needs of people, which have often been invoked by unique contextual challenges (Galvaan, 2010; Ramugondo, 2009; Watson, 2013).

THINKING ABOUT POWER AND PRIVILEGE AS AN OCCUPATIONAL THERAPIST

The following personal vignette by the first author reflects her personal interest in the role of occupational therapists as intervention designers. This vignette also highlights her conscious consideration of the ways in which sociocultural factors present in her environment shaped her identity and positioning in society and possibly exerted an impact on her interactions with, and interventions designed for her clients.

Prior to becoming an occupational therapy lecturer I, a privileged white female, owned and ran a business in which I acted as a facilitator of caregiver-focused baby developmental groups targeting middle- to high-income mothers and their infants younger than 12 months of age. I gave birth to my first son 3 months prior to purchasing the business and in my interactions with the moms I found that my new entry into motherhood provided a link, which helped me to establish a connection with the moms. I remember thinking often how my facilitation skills would have differed had I not been a mother. I also reflected considerably on the ease with which I interacted with the moms and how this was possibly linked to my 'likeness' to them in terms of race and income status. This was a different experience to my prior interactions with caregivers of children in the public sectors of health and education where I had worked previously. I started to think about how in a diverse context like South Africa, where race and income status often place therapist and client at far distances to each other, different negotiations of interactions forming part of client-centred practice may occur. Furthermore, how would these interactions impact on and inform the interventions that occupational therapists design?

This vignette illustrates the first author's thinking about how power and privilege associated with sociocultural factors may have influenced her therapeutic interactions. Her insights in her own experiences led to her interest in the ways in which differences between occupational therapists and the people that they work with may influence the nature and content of the interventions they design. This interest led to her study of a South African group of occupational therapists' process of designing an intervention for a client population dissimilar to them in terms of race and class positioning.

INTRODUCING THE OCCUPATIONAL THERAPISTS AND THE INTERVENTION

This section will introduce the group of occupational therapists, their client group, and the intervention design process that they engaged in as the case example (Stake, 1995, 2008). South Africa has the largest population of HIV-positive children in the world. An estimated 360 000 South African children under 14 years of age are HIV-positive (UNAIDS, 2013). Despite the rollout of medical treatment in the form of highly active antiretroviral treatment, recent statistics for HIV infection for children are still high, with an estimated 21 000 new infections for children in South Africa in 2012 (UNAIDS, 2013). While prolonging the survival of children, these medical interventions have not eliminated the neurobiological impact of progressive HIV encephalopathy, a common central nervous system disorder in HIV-infected children. Progressive HIV encephalopathy causes a wide array of neurological impairments, placing children at increased risk for developmental and learning difficulties (Blanchette et al., 2002; Ramugondo, 2004; Sherr et al., 2009; Smith et al., 2006).

Adding to the health effects of the virus, HIV has a high prevalence in families living in impoverished circumstances where frequent cases of caregiver illness, depression, and substance abuse are evident (Betancourt et al., 2013; Van Rie et al., 2007). Contextual and family aspects are key contributors to the nature of a child's developmental trajectory. The combined impact of HIV-related encephalopathy and social disadvantage can result in a compromised occupational trajectory for children infected with HIV/AIDS, who often show high rates of school dropout and poor educational outcomes (Blanchette et al., 2002; Cluver et al., 2012; Guo et al., 2012).

In response to these concerns, TOTALCARE[3], a nongovernmental organization, was established in 2001. TOTALCARE aims to provide comprehensive care to children infected with HIV and their caregivers, providing active antiretroviral treatment to more than 1800 children at six sites in Cape Town. Through the implementation of four programmes – Health, Family Preservation (including a Beadwork Income Generating Project), Training, and Early Childhood Development – TOTALCARE aims to address not only the health-related, but also some of the social and economic needs of HIV-positive persons living in South Africa. The four occupational therapists employed by TOTALCARE head the Early Childhood Development programme. In late 2011, these four TOTALCARE occupational therapy employees and two occupational therapists working alongside TOTALCARE were tasked with designing a new occupational therapy intervention directed at caregivers of children infected with HIV. The intervention aimed to build on the caregivers' knowledge and skill in building on the playfulness, learning, and development of their children. Four of the occupational therapists commenced master's studies in occupational therapy, exploring the impact of the intervention on different child and caregiver participation outcomes. The first author's doctoral study explored the occupational therapists' collective processes of designing the intervention.

THE PROCESS OF OBSERVING THE INTERVENTION DESIGN PROCESSES

Over the course of 19 months, the first author joined the group's monthly intervention design meetings, observing and documenting (by means of digital voice recordings and field notes) their process of designing the intervention, paying careful attention to their voiced intent about the structure and content of the intervention, the propositional (theoretical and evidence based) and nonpropositional (personal and professional craft) knowledge (Higgs and Titchen, 2001) they drew on to meet this intent, and factors within the context informing and influencing their decisions regarding the intervention.

Drawing on the participatory methodology of cooperative inquiry (Heron and Reason, 2001), the first author encouraged the participation of the occupational therapists as co-researchers. In this role, the occupational therapists not only pursued the task of designing the intervention but also joined the first author as research partners who reflected on their actions and the outcomes linked to their actions within the intervention design process. The quotes below highlight the group's commitment to their role as co-researchers, through their sharing of emerging insights with the first author about the intervention, as well as their commitment to reflect on the intervention design process (through the means that suited them best, i.e., choosing to meet to discuss the intervention design process, rather than write/only write reflections).

Hi Pam,
I just thought of an important point that would be relevant in your study and our approach to our intervention in the larger sense. [E-mail correspondence sent from Therapist J to first author]

Lindy: Yes, I was also thinking it is all good and well to keep, to document [write reflective notes] on the things but if specially for, thinking for your [principal researcher/first author] research in particular but also for our learning, deeper whatever, we might want a talking space after each [group meeting].

Meredith: The paper doesn't talk back to you. Sometimes you need to take that paper back to another person.

Such a participatory approach was adopted to encourage our (first author included) collective understanding of our practice ontology (ways of bringing ourselves into our practices) and our practice epistemology: what we know, how we know it, and how we create new knowledge.

The first author's emerging insights into the group's intervention design process revealed how the occupational needs of groups of people within a

---

[3]Pseudonym used.

post-apartheid South African context need to be considered through focusing more on the role of the occupational therapist and their consideration of and negotiation of their own identity and positioning. How doing this supports the achievement of more critically considered, contextually relevant and client-centred interventions, will be discussed further within this chapter.

OCCUPATIONAL THERAPISTS' INTERSECTIONAL IDENTITY AND POSITIONALITY: A NEW PERSPECTIVE WITHIN CLIENT-CENTRED PRACTICE

Client-centred practice is a key aspect of best practice in occupational therapy (Law et al., 2001). Client-centred practice is an approach to providing services established through the formation of a partnership with the client. In this partnership, the client and therapist engage together to set therapy goals which address the client's expressed needs (Law et al., 1995). According to Sumsion (2000), 'throughout the process the therapist listens to and respects the client's values, adapts the interventions to meet the client's needs and enables the client to make informed decisions' (p. 308).

To embrace the core aspects of client-centred practice, an occupational therapist must connect with their client and their client's situation to develop an understanding of who they are and how this influences their participation in occupations. Gaining an understanding of the client's social identity and their positioning in society is key to developing this understanding (Galvaan and Peters, 2014). Race, class, gender, sexuality and other points of difference are examples of the social forces interacting to shape our identities (Crenshaw, 1995). An intersectional framework draws attention to the ways in which these multiple social forces intersect to shape how people assume and experience their identities (Crenshaw, 1995; Yuval-Davis, 2006). For example, identity is constructed not only in terms of race, but also gender, class and other characteristics. The identities assumed or prescribed to people differ across contexts and create different positionalities (Crenshaw, 1995). Different positionalities give people access to privilege or oppression. For example, in a South African context, the intersections of race, class, and disability would

position a person of colour with a disability worse than a white person with a disability.

Using the reflection questions below, consider the concepts of intersectional identity and positionality within the contexts in which you work:

> Reflection questions: What social forces [race, gender, class, etc.] operate in your practice contexts? How do these social forces interact to create different social identities of the clients that you work with? How do these identities create different positionalities for your clients?

Client-centred practice is based on the formulation of a partnership. Occupational therapists need to consider and integrate the intersectional identities and positionalities of the clients with whom they work. Occupational therapists, much like the clients with whom they work, cannot be separated from the influence of the historically located sociocultural factors and traditions that exist in their contexts. Thus, in the formation of a client-centred partnership there needs to be a consideration of the intersectional identities and positionalities of the occupational therapists. Their intersectional identity and positionality impacts on who they are, how they enter into a partnership with their clients, and the nature of the interventions they design.

In a South African context, consideration of the influence of the therapists' intersectional identity and positionality has not previously been foregrounded in the process of occupational therapy intervention design. Consideration has also not been given to how the relative intersectional identities and positionalities between the occupational therapists and their clients may affect the partnership formed between them and the interventions designed.

The occupational therapists in TOTALCARE tried to establish a partnership with caregivers, to identify the child-rearing values and goals of the caregivers and include these within the intervention. They sought the support of translators to help them overcome the language barrier between them and the caregivers[4].

---

[4]The caregivers spoke predominantly isiXhosa, one of the official languages of South Africa, while the predominant language of the occupational therapists was English.

Despite this, it was a challenge to connect with the caregivers to identify their concerns about their children's occupational engagement through their traditional means of doing so, that is, conversations, questioning, and standardized assessments.

> **Georgia:** I don't know if, well sometimes the moms finish Matric [the final year of schooling in South Africa, also referred to as grade 12] but don't know if they've been asked or forced to answer those sorts of questions. I mean we've, occupational therapy [as a profession] asks us those questions all the time. So I don't know if education has got a lot to do with it is that they [caregivers] haven't been exposed to that and a lot of those questions do only come out in tertiary education.
>
> **Lindy:** You know, the feedback [from the caregivers] happens more spontaneously. When you ask them questions it is very limited.

The above example illustrates our difficulty in establishing a connection with the caregivers to gain their responses regarding their occupational needs. It also highlights how occupational therapists need to come together to explore different ways of engaging with the clients they work with.

As a result of our struggle to connect with the caregivers to access and gain more insight into their caregiving roles, their concerns about their children and their caregiving needs, we as a group moved towards wanting to share our values and ideals about best practice caregiving practices as shaped by our own personal experiences. It was, however, a challenge to identify how to do this in a way that appreciates the contextual challenges that the caregivers face, as well as how to convey this information in a way that does not seem enforcing or overbearing.

> **Meredith:** So like Georgia was saying their [caregivers'] priorities, [are] food, work, income and almost they [caregivers] are not aware of the values that we hold for child development. Not that we want to impose it, it's something that we want to expose and then hopefully they take on those [values].

The tentative nature of our engagement stems from a difficulty finding resonance with what we observed of the caregiving practices of the caregivers. It was challenging for us to understand the caregivers' lack of direct involvement and engagement with their children though play, their 'wait and see' approach to their children's occupational concerns, and their inconsistent attendance of therapy appointments. These challenges resulted in us struggling to enact our intent to work in a more collaborative manner with the caregivers. We revert back to our familiar and known ways of practice and a child-focused approach becomes central within the intervention we design.

In a South African context, such struggles link to a discomfort in exercising professional power in a context in which power differentials are already so apparent. Here we, as a group of privileged white female occupational therapists, find it difficult to connect with caregiver clients different from us in terms of race and class identities; caregiver clients who continue to be jeopardized by the long-lasting effects of the apartheid regime policies as well as the stigma associated with their and their child/children's HIV diagnosis.

> **Meredith:** Do we *really* [emphasis added] understand what we are asking from them [caregivers]? Do we really understand what [the tasks] we are placing on them [caregivers] financially and personally? With transport costs and missing work? Or having to disclose to their employer that their child/grandchild has HIV in order to get permission to leave work to attend the clinic appointments?

Occupational therapists need to be aware of the several disconnects between them and their clients. They need to consider how these disconnects can influence the resultant decisions that occupational therapists make about the interventions that they provide, as well as issues of congruence and conflict that may arise between them and their clients as a result of these decisions.

The formation of a client-centred partnership requires a consideration of both the clients' intersectional identities and positionalities and of the intersectional identities and positionalities of the occupational therapists. To work towards the formation of this partnership, occupational therapists need to reflect on:

1. How do the therapists' own contexts and the contexts of the people they work with influence occupational engagement? The theoretical lens of cultural-historical activity theory[5] can be drawn on to help identify and explore the impact of these factors on the intervention design process (Gretschel et al., 2015).

2. How do different intersectional identities and positionalities impact on the formation of a partnership between the client and occupational therapist, the structure and content of the intervention designed, and the review of the successes and failures of the intervention?

3. What steps can be taken when differing intersectional identities and positionalities fuel a disconnect?

The above questions are not always considered in the design of an intervention. For occupational therapists working in contexts where there are not many distinct and vast differences in their own intersectional identities and positionalities and those of the people they are working with, posing these questions may not seem so critical. However, given the unique, highly personal nature of occupational engagement, these are essential questions to pose.

CONCLUSION

This chapter has highlighted why a careful consideration of how occupational therapists design interventions needs to take place. The complexities of designing occupational therapy interventions cannot be ignored. It is the seemingly everyday nature of occupational engagement that detracts occupational therapists from the complex diversity of occupational engagement. The case of this particular group of occupational therapists working in South Africa, a homogenous group of white females of economic and social privilege, revealed the challenges they faced in trying to effect a more critically considered, contextually relevant, and client-centred intervention.

The chapter highlights how these challenges need to be interrogated in more depth so that ways to address them can be formulated. As a start, occupational therapists need to recognize and account for the sociocultural factors shaping both their clients' and their own intersectional identities. They need to consider how these identities position them in society, how this positioning determines and influences their occupational engagement, as well as how these relative intersectional identities and positionalities between the occupational therapists and their clients may combine in both positive and negative ways to influence the interventions they design.

The chapter concludes with key reflection questions, which readers are encouraged to apply to their own practice:

- In your engagements as an occupational therapist with the people that you work with, do you explore your intersectional identities and associated positionalities?
- Do you account for the ways in which your practice has been shaped by your intersectional identities and associated positionalities? How much of yourself, your values and your interests do you bring into your practice?
- Do you account for the ways in which your clients' occupational engagement is shaped by their intersectional identities and associated positionalities? How much of your clients' values and interests do you bring into your practice?
- What congruences and conflicts have arisen in this process?
- Have the conflicts been managed? If yes, how?

REFERENCES

Betancourt, T.S., Meyers-Ohki, S.E., Charrow, A., Hansen, N., 2013. Mental health and resilience in HIV/AIDS-affected children: a review of the literature and recommendations for future research. J. Child Psychol. Psychiatry 54 (4), 423–444. doi:10.1111/j.1469-7610.2012.02613.x.

Blanchette, N., Smith, M.L., King, S., Fernandes-Penney, A., Read, S., 2002. Cognitive development in school-age children with vertically transmitted HIV infection. Neurodev. Neuropsychol. 21 (3), 223–241.

Cluver, L., Operario, D., Lane, T., Kgangka, M., 2012. 'I can't go to school and leave her in so much pain': educational shortfalls among adolescent 'young carers' in the South African AIDS epidemic. J. Adolesc. Res. 27, 581–605.

Crenshaw, K.W., 1995. Mapping the margins: intersectionality, identity politics, and violence against women of colour. In: Crenshaw,

---

[5]Cultural-historical activity theory is a cogent conceptual tool guiding thinking about, observations of, and analyses of what people do (Gretschel et al., 2015).

K.W., et al. (Eds.), Critical Race Theory: Key Writings That Formulated the Movement. New Press, New York, pp. 357–383.

Galvaan, R., 2010. A critical ethnography of young adolescents' occupational choices in a community in post apartheid South Africa. Unpublished doctoral dissertation, University of Cape Town, Cape Town, South Africa.

Galvaan, R., Peters, L., 2014. Occupation-based community development framework. Open Educational Resource. <https://vula.uct.ac.za/access/content/group/9c29ba04-b1ee-49b9-8c85-9a468b556ce2/OBCDF/pages/intro.html>.

Gretschel, P., Ramugondo, E.L., Galvaan, R., 2015. An introduction to Cultural Historical Activity Theory as a theoretical lens to understand how occupational therapists design interventions for persons living in low income conditions in South Africa. South Afr. J. Occup. Ther. 45 (1), 51–55.

Guo, Y., Li, X., Sherr, L., 2012. The impact of HIV/AIDS on children's educational outcome: a critical review of global literature. AIDS Care 24, 993–1012. doi:10.1080/09540121.2012.668170.

Heron, J., Reason, P., 2001. The practice of co-operative inquiry: research with rather than on people. In: Reason, P., Bradbury, H. (Eds.), Handbook of Action Research: Participative Inquiry and Practice. Sage Publications, London, pp. 179–188.

Higgs, J., Titchen, A., 2001. Rethinking the practice knowledge interface in an uncertain world: a model for practice development. Br. J. Occup. Ther. 64 (11), 526–533.

Kronenberg, F., Pollard, N., 2006. Political dimensions of occupations and the roles of occupational therapy. Am. J. Occup. Ther. 60 (6), 617–625.

Law, M., Baptiste, S., Mills, J., 1995. Client-centered practice: what does it mean and does it make a difference? Can. J. Occup. Ther. 62 (5), 250–257.

Law, M., King, G., Russel, D., 2001. Guiding therapist decisions about measuring outcomes in occupational therapy. In: Law, M., Baum, C., Dunn, W. (Eds.), Measuring Occupational Performance – Supporting Best Practice in Occupational Therapy. Slack Incorporated, New York, pp. 33–48.

Pollard, N., Sakellariou, D., Kronenberg, F. (Eds.), 2008. A Political Practice of Occupational Therapy. Churchill Livingstone, Oxford.

Ramugondo, E.L., 2004. Play and playfulness: children living with HIV/AIDS. In: Watson, R., Swartz, L. (Eds.), Transformation Through Occupation: Human Occupation in Context. Whurr, London, pp. 171–185.

Ramugondo, E.L., 2009. Intergenerational shifts and continuities in children's play within a rural Venda family (early 20th to early 21st century). Unpublished doctoral dissertation, University of Cape Town, Cape Town, South Africa.

Sherr, L., Mueller, J., Varrall, R., 2009. A systematic review of cognitive development and child human immunodeficiency virus infection. Psychol. Health Med. 14, 387–404.

Smith, R., Malee, K., Leighty, R., Brouwers, P., Mellins, C., Hittelman, J., et al., 2006. Effects of perinatal HIV infection and associated risk factors on cognitive development amoung young children. Pediatrics 117, 851–862.

South African National Census, 2011. Available at: <http://www.statssa.gov.za/publications/p03014/p030142011.pdf> (accessed 30.10.14.).

Stake, R.E., 1995. The Art of Case Study Research. Sage Publications, Thousand Oaks, CA.

Stake, R.E., 2008. Qualitative case studies. In: Denzin, N.K., Lincoln, Y.S. (Eds.), Strategies of Qualitative Inquiry, third ed. Sage Publications, Thousand Oaks, CA, pp. 119–149.

StatsSA, 2014. National and provincial labour market: youth. <http://beta2.statssa.gov.za/publications/P02114.2/P02114.22014.pdf> (accessed 10.09.15).

Sumsion, T., 2000. A revised occupational therapy definition of client-centred practice. Br. J. Occup. Ther. 63 (7), 304–309.

UNAIDS, 2013. Countries and children with HIV. <http://www.unaids.org/en/regionscountries/countries/southafrica> (accessed 30.01.15.).

Van Rie, A., Harrington, P.R., Dow, A., Robertson, K., 2007. Neurologic and neurodevelopmental manifestations of pediatric HIV/AIDS: a global perspective. Eur. J. Paediatr. Neurol. 11 (1), 1–9.

Watson, R., 2013. A population approach to occupational therapy. South Afr. J. Occup. Ther. 43 (1), 34–39.

Yuval-Davis, N., 2006. Intersectionality and feminist politics. Eur. J. Womens Stud. 13, 193–209.

34

THEORETICAL INTERSECTIONS: USING ANTHROPOLOGY, SOCIAL JUSTICE, AND LIFE COURSE PERSPECTIVES FOR ADDRESSING OCCUPATIONAL INJUSTICE

AMY PAUL-WARD

Within occupational therapy, there has always been recognition of the added value of interdisciplinary approaches to understanding human occupation. As the profession has evolved, theories from related disciplines have been used to help occupational therapists define their profession and what services they can provide to help support individuals in their everyday occupations. With the emergence of occupational science, this recognition has taken greater precedence as occupational scientists draw on related knowledge to better understand the cultural, political and economic forces impacting the occupational performance of individuals, communities and society. Florence Clark, one of the early advocates of occupational science, has argued that bringing related knowledge and research to the discipline strengthens the empirical foundations of occupational therapy and can lead to more interdisciplinary research (Clark, 2006).

The goal of this chapter is to illustrate the importance of related knowledge and theoretical intersections in occupational therapy. To best accomplish this goal, I will provide examples throughout the chapter that demonstrate how I use interdisciplinary theories in my research on foster care youth and their transition to adulthood.

BACKGROUND

To give you a brief introduction to my background, I am a cross-trained medical anthropologist with expertise in occupational therapy and disabilities studies. After completing my doctoral studies, I participated in a postdoctoral fellowship in disability studies. As part of this experience, I was given the opportunity to earn a post professional master's degree in occupational therapy, which focused on research and theory. My interest in foster care grew out of my 3-year involvement in a research project that I worked on during my fellowship. The project was looking at how an occupational therapy programme could address the functional deficits that were impacting the abilities of persons with HIV/AIDS in supportive housing as they transitioned to independent living and employment. Several of the participants shared with me that they experienced difficulties in the community as a result of their having been incarcerated. Their stories sparked my interest in conducting research focused on individuals in the criminal justice system and the challenges they faced upon release back into the community. As I explored opportunities for conducting this research from an occupational science/occupational therapy perspective, I realized that many of the individuals in the correctional system had also spent time in foster care as children. This fact led to my interest in foster care. Specifically, I wanted to explore how occupational therapy-based programmes could be designed and implemented to address the independent living and vocational needs of foster care youth in order to decrease their risk of becoming incarcerated in the first place, as well as to improve their long-term quality of life.

So, in my ongoing efforts to understand the needs of this often marginalized group and to develop programmes that have a positive impact, I have found it extremely useful to draw on several interrelated, interdisciplinary theories: social and occupational justice, critical medical anthropology (including structural violence) and the life course perspective. These theoretical areas provide me with a useful framework for studying the issues of marginalized populations with the ultimate goal of affecting positive change. This goal resonates with the values of occupational therapy without borders, especially in light of the fact that we live in a world where aspects of culture, politics and economics at the local level are impacted by global forces, and quickly shifting political and economic conditions impact us all as global citizens. One consequence of these uncertain conditions is the rising number of individuals experiencing psychosocial problems, which in turn is providing more opportunities for occupational therapists to enhance their approach to clinical practice. This instability is also shaping not only how we think about who should receive occupational therapy but also how we can provide services for less traditionally recognized clients, many of whom are significantly at risk for disability and occupational deprivation.

In the next paragraph, I will give a brief overview of several theories underpinning my work. This overview will be followed by a review of the literature on foster care in the US, including my ongoing work on foster care transitions. Lastly, I will provide examples of how these theories help inform this work.

CRITICAL MEDICAL ANTHROPOLOGY

In this section I will discuss medical anthropology generally and critical medical anthropology specifically. Medical anthropology is a subfield of anthropology that seeks to understand human health and disease, healthcare systems and biocultural adaptation. From a medical anthropological perspective, biomedical models are viewed as reductionistic, limiting illness to biological malfunction while ignoring the social factors, which play a crucial role in shaping the illness experience. In order to truly understand health, well-being and health seeking, we need to recognize the importance of the role that society plays in health-seeking processes, as well as in the patient–practitioner relationship.

Critical medical anthropology, an approach within medical anthropology, examines health issues in regard to the political and economic forces that pattern human relationships, shape social behaviour and condition collective experience (Singer, 1986). Singer, an early critical scholar, suggested that central to this approach is the relationship between macrolevels and microlevels of explanation. In order to understand a particular issue, it is necessary to explore microlevel phenomena pertaining to individuals. However, the critical approach views macrolevel structures and processes as the dominant factors in final analyses (Singer, 1986). Further, proponents of critical theory are concerned with the ways in which power differentials shape social processes. Specifically, dominant ideology and practices associated with medical systems are affected by authoritative ideologies outside of medical systems (e.g., religious and political institutions). Therefore, problems within the healthcare system are seen as reflecting the problems of society and the two cannot be separated (Waitzkin, 1981). In short, critical medical anthropology provides us with a way of understanding health and well-being as it relates to the political, economic, social and cultural environment in which health is situated (Paul-Ward, 2009). This perspective is empowering in that it seeks to remediate the oppressive and marginalizing forces that affect the health and well-being of individuals and communities (Castro and Singer, 2004).

Among the available theories within critical medical anthropology is the theory of structural violence. This theory is especially relevant for addressing issues of marginalized or underserved populations in that it seeks to explain constraints on one's potential because of political and economic structures (Winter and Leighton, 2001). From this perspective, people who have unequal access to education, economic security, political participation and adequate healthcare are viewed as victims of structural violence. It is worth noting that structural violence can limit one's life chances and ultimately their life expectancy through its effect, making it a form of 'hidden' violence. Structural violence is problematic because it limits one's ability to fully participate as an equal member of society. It is also important to note that advocates of this perspective have argued that the experience of structural violence places people at increased risk for experiencing physical violence (e.g., Jacobs and O'Brien, 1998; Winter and Leighton, 2001). This theoretical perspective is important to my research because youth in the foster care system are stigmatized on many levels and can easily be labelled as victims of structural violence. Specifically, in my programme of research, I argue that adolescents in foster care are victims of structural violence because they have unequal access to education, economic security and healthcare.

SOCIAL/OCCUPATIONAL JUSTICE

The concept of social justice is not new; historically, the roots of social justice concepts can be traced to early philosophers such as St. Thomas Aquinas, John Locke, David Hume and Jean-Jacques Rousseau. These scholars worked to develop a theoretical understanding of the justice-related issues of their time including individual rights, free society and free will (Braveman and Suarez-Balcazar, 2009). Over time, social justice evolved into a study of the complex relationships among government, society, access and poverty. Not surprisingly, religious scholars have also demonstrated

an interest in justice-related issues. For example, the US National Conference of Catholic Bishops has advocated for a vision of social justice recognizing that people 'have an obligation to be active and productive participants in the life of society and that society has a duty to enable them to participate in this way' (NCCB, Economic Justice for All #71).

In recent years, many disciplines, including anthropology and occupational therapy, have utilized social justice theories to give voice and participation to people regarding the decisions that affect their lives. These theories emphasize the importance of individuals having the ability to control their own life while recognizing that people in positions of power can make it difficult for others to do so (Braveman and Suarez-Balcazar, 2009). The discourse on social justice within occupational therapy encourages practitioners to actively work to overcome the larger societal issues that impact their ability to treat those in need and advocate for and with clients. Although the concept of social justice is embraced across disciplines, occupational therapy has offered its own occupation-based language for discussing justice-related issues, namely, occupational justice. Occupational justice is viewed as the 'rights, responsibilities, and liberties of enablement' (Townsend and Wilcock, 2004, p. 77). This justice-based language has resulted in the development of a framework for categorizing and addressing conditions of occupational injustice. This framework of occupational justice includes four conditions of occupational injustice: occupational imbalance, occupational deprivation, occupational marginalization and occupational alienation (Stadnyk, Townsend and Wilcock, 2010).

THE LIFE COURSE PERSPECTIVE

The life course perspective is a multidisciplinary approach for studying people's lives that takes into account that ageing and development are ongoing continuous processes. As such, a life course perspective provides a context for understanding that we do not develop in a vacuum but are impacted by our relationships, the choices we make, the opportunities presented to us, and the constraints we face from time and place. This notion is further articulated by Danely and Lynch (2013), who posit:

[A] life course approach to aging recognizes that as individuals age, their lives unfold in conjunction with those of people of different ages, and that all of these actors, who occupy different and changing positions and multiple cultural and physical environments over a period of historical time, are shaping and influencing each other in important ways. (p. 3)

The life course perspective more accurately reflects the ever-changing, complex processes that we experience as we grow older. In short, a life course approach provides a broader way of looking at health and well-being over the course of one's life as an integrated whole rather than as disconnected developmental stages that are unrelated to one another. Viewing health and well-being in this way, is useful for thinking about how we establish lifestyles, roles, and habits. If individuals have not established habits in their teen years or even in early adulthood, that support health and well-being, it is less likely that they will establish them in later years. This perspective is very useful in thinking about programme development for adolescents in foster care. In particular, using a life course perspective when working with foster care youth reminds us how important it is to assist them in developing the life skills needed in adulthood. If we do not develop client-centred programmes that incorporate approaches that emphasize the development of these critical skills in adolescence, this population will continue to struggle against societal forces that negatively impact their participation in desired occupations.

The Case of Foster Care

In order to discuss the role that these theoretical perspectives play in my approach to foster care transitions, I must first provide an overview of the context within which my work is situated. In the US, foster care is most commonly defined as '24-hour substitute care for children placed away from their parents or guardians and for whom the State agency has placement and care responsibility', and on any given day there are approximately 400 000 children between infancy and age 18 years in the foster care system (US Department of Health and Human Services, 2015, p. 1). Children and adolescents in the foster care system live in challenging environments (e.g., nonfamilial households, group homes) and as a result often face a great deal of instability. Research has shown that these environments place children and adolescents at risk for numerous negative consequences (e.g., poor academic performance, emotional, behavioural and health-related problems), many of which take on greater meaning when we look at youth who are ageing out of the foster care system into independent adulthood (Bernier et al., 2004; Kools, 1997; Merdinger et al., 2005; Reilly, 2003).

Transitioning Out of Care

In the US, it has been commonly expected that adolescents will finish school, gain independence from their parents and become contributing members of their communities as they transition to adulthood (Arnett, 2000; Hiebert and Thomlison, 1996). However, in recent years, this expectation has changed as ups and downs in the global economy make it increasingly difficult for young adults to be completely self-sufficient after high school (and, in some cases, even after graduating from university). Achieving self-sufficiency is especially more problematic for adolescents transitioning out of foster care. From an occupational therapy perspective, our experience tells us that typically, independent living skills are developed gradually over time, in family environments and through observation, practice and receiving guidance from nurturing adults. However, youth in foster care often do not have the opportunity to acquire these skills developmentally, and the training that is offered is rarely occupation based. It has been reported that only 42 600 foster care youth are receiving independent living services nationwide out of the approximately 170 000 children required to receive them (GAO, 1999; Georgiades, 2005). Eventually, because they lack independent living, vocational and mental health maintenance skills, many former foster care youth wind up receiving services as adults through the criminal justice or the welfare system (Casey Family Programs, 2000; Jonson-Reid and Barth, 2003). This places a huge financial and public health burden on society, and results in negative life consequences for these individuals.

Independent living programmes within foster care agencies are intended to prepare foster children for independence as an adult. These programmes attempt to address a broad spectrum of independent living skills ranging from activities of daily living to education and vocation. While independent living services are legislatively mandated for adolescents preparing to transition out of care, these services are underutilized. They are not designed to be meaningful to teenagers. The number of individuals involved in the conveying of information (e.g., independent living manager, case managers, foster parents, etc.) can be compared to the childhood game of 'telephone',[1] preventing adolescents from staying abreast of all of the programmes available to them at any given time (e.g., information takes too long to reach the intended recipients and is often incomplete). Also, not surprisingly, adolescents are often reluctant to attend because they feel they already have the skills to live independently or do not want to admit not feeling confident (Paul-Ward, 2008, 2009). Having been marginalized and disempowered for much of their lives, many adolescents are tired of having others make decisions for them, and want to leave the foster care system.

Thus recent research has begun to attempt to identify factors contributing to successful transitions out of foster care for these youth (Clark and Davis, 2002; Lemon et al., 2005). In 1986, Congress enacted the Independent Living Initiative to serve as a framework for states to develop services for foster youth to prepare them for transitioning out of care (Reilly, 2003, citing Stoner, 1999). A review by the US Accounting Office, 15 years after implementation, found that the effectiveness of these programmes was unclear. Recent national research reports from the Child Welfare League and Chapin Hall (available at: http://www.chapinhall.org/; http://www.cwla.org) call for new intervention approaches to improve the development of habits and occupational behaviours leading to the mastery of independent living skills among foster care youth. While the obstacles for the

development of independent living skills have been acknowledged, no client-centered, occupation-based interventions have been implemented and evaluated to address this need (Paul-Ward et al., 2014).

The current foster care infrastructure, with variability across state-operated, privatized and community-based systems, is not effectively creating the necessary programmes to provide foster youth with the essential skills for successful transition to self-sufficient adulthood (Krebs and Pitcoff, 2004). Many independent living programmes are one-size-fits-all, didactic and classroom-based programmes emphasizing transition planning and the provision of information on various independent living skills without providing opportunities to actually master skills (Collins, 2001; Paul-Ward, 2009). These programmes are typically housed in office buildings where the physical space does not allow practice of real-world skills, such as learning how to cook in an actual kitchen. Additionally, these programmes are not equipped with the appropriate staff to comprehensively assess each adolescent and provide client-centred services to address individual needs. The result is that the independent living staff frequently do things for the youth rather than assist them in learning how to do things for themselves (e.g., locating and obtaining affordable housing, arranging for assistance when utility bills are not paid). This pattern often results in a cycle of learned helplessness.

My Research Context

South Florida is an excellent natural laboratory for conducting research on issues related to foster care transitions. There are 3500 children in foster care in the system in Miami-Dade and Monroe Counties (Our Kids 2013-2014 Annual Report). From this group, 646 adolescents are eligible to receive independent living/transitional support services as they prepare to 'age out' of the foster care system. From the literature above, it becomes clear that programmes that provide hands-on experiential learning opportunities for independent living and vocational skills are sorely needed to assist foster care youth in transitioning to adulthood.

In response to this need, I have been working with stakeholders in the community to better understand the needs of foster care youth from their perspective, as well as to document the strengths and weaknesses

---

[1]The game of telephone is played with several people sitting or standing in a straight line. One person at the end of the line whispers a word or phrase into the ear of the person next to them. This person will whisper the word or phrase into the ear of the next person and so on until reaching the last person. The last person says the word or phrase out loud and then the first person says the word or phrase. Most of the time the words or phrases are nothing alike.

of existing services. This ongoing programme of research recognizes that the complexities and challenges that adolescents face must be understood from their own perspective, and reflected in the planning of programmes to ensure the successful development of independent living and vocational services. In several phases, foster care youth, foster parents, and staff in foster care case management agencies have been recruited to participate in the research. Their participation has included in-depth interviews, focus groups and participant observations by members of the research team. All of the interviews were conducted by graduate students in the professional master's programme in occupational therapy at Florida International University. Adolescents participating in the study were asked questions about their individual experiences in the foster care system, as well as their knowledge and understanding of programming available to them. They were also asked about their conceptualizations of what it meant to be a successful adult and the types of skills they would need to be a successful adult. Foster parents were asked about their approach to teaching the adolescents in their care life skills, as well as the types of services that were available to them and their foster children through the case management agencies. Lastly, staff in the agencies were asked about the types of independent living and vocational services available, including the strengths and weakness of these services. Data obtained from these interviews have been used to begin developing an occupation-based independent living and vocational skill programme for adolescents transitioning out of care.

Applying These Intersecting Theories to My Work

As described above, adolescents in foster care often have complicated lives and face many challenges. Their foster care 'label' carries an aura of uncertainty as well as the potential for social stigma. The phenomenon of social stigma is typically experienced by individuals who exist on the periphery, limiting their opportunities for social and occupational participation. This concept is especially relevant to foster care in that, by design, these systems tend to devalue and marginalize its members by labelling them as different from other individuals living and developing in the community.

Applying a social/occupational justice perspective has been helpful to me when thinking about how to reframe the everyday experiences of children growing up in the foster care system. By incorporating an occupationally just perspective into how I conceptualize what good foster care should look like for this group, I have become a better advocate for this type of care. This perspective has provided me with a strong argument for why occupational therapists are well suited to work with foster care youth to develop healthy habits and roles, engage in meaningful occupations and participate more successfully as full and equal members within their communities. More broadly, the occupational justice perspective reinforces our individual and collective responsibilities to use the knowledge obtained from population-focused research to effect positive social change for vulnerable children, so they can develop the skills needed across the life course.

The everyday lives of foster care youth have often deteriorated in ways that prevent them from having opportunities to explore and master the skills needed for independent living. Most have come to the foster care system after a traumatic experience that may be characterized by chaotic personal circumstances. From my interviews with youth, it became clear that they are aware that they will eventually be required to move out of foster care, and often hope for that to occur sooner rather than later. However, their confidence for living on their own has been compromised by their experiences of instability and a reactive rather than proactive approach to life.

As a result of their experiences, most foster care youth do not develop strong confidence in their vocational skills, and this affects their vocational interests and motivation. They often lack stable living and employment experiences. While the literature documents that adolescents leaving foster care are not prepared for independence, research exploring the role of motivation and lack of confidence is needed to further understand these experiences.

Most adolescents in foster care have some ongoing functional impairment. They face a variety of physical, psychological and social problems (Courtney et al., 2007; McMillen et al., 2005). Most adolescents lack basic skills required for independent living and forms of employment other than entry-level, minimum-wage jobs. Many have limited education, with only about 31% of these youth having a high school diploma (Reilly, 2003).

We know from the model of human occupation that occupational behaviour is always a result of the interaction of volition, habituation, performance and environment. A single factor in and of itself cannot account for failure or success in the performance and mastery of occupational behaviours (Levin et al., 2007). As a result, in order to understand how any person performs and experiences their life occupations, we must examine the intersection of their volition, habituation and performance abilities with the physical and social environment. Using an example from Levin et al. (2007), if we wanted to understand work as an example of a person's occupation, we would consider how volitional characteristics such as worldview, likes and dislikes, and beliefs about personal capacity, interact with environmental opportunities and barriers to shape the person's choices about the kind of work he or she does, and the level of satisfaction he or she finds in that work. Similarly, a person's performance capacities and learned work habits interact with the demands of doing a particular job in a particular work environment to affect his or her work performance. These explanations of work behaviour and experience present service providers with a holistic understanding of a worker and allow for the development of appropriate vocationally oriented services.

Adolescents transitioning out of foster care are faced with the reality of only temporary support and housing from their foster families. Becoming an independent adult, requires that adolescents develop the skills needed for managing a home. When these youth leave foster care, if they have not yet developed these skills, the process becomes significantly more difficult while they attempt to balance school and work. The development of these skills is challenged by a faltering economy, especially as social services for those who need the most help (e.g., those with disabilities) are often the hardest hit.

Integrally related to this perspective is the inclusion of a social justice lens within the conceptualization of research questions, implementation of the project and building on the research outcomes. As occupational therapy practitioners, it is both an individual and a collective responsibility to use the knowledge obtained from population-focused research efforts to effect positive social change for individuals and groups. For example, in my work, the desired short-term microlevel outcome is the development of client-centred, occupation-based programmes that will assist adolescents transitioning out of foster care in developing the skills they need to be successful independent adults. The desired long-term outcome leading to macrolevel changes is seeing young adults develop into socially conscious adults, who feel empowered to effect positive system changes for themselves and others coming through the foster care system.

CONCLUSION

When we examine the world with an interdisciplinary lens, we are presented with contemporary approaches for understanding real-world barriers that many people face in regards to access, engagement, empowerment and participation. Significantly, this lens allows occupational therapists to more critically examine the role that external forces play in the daily lives of their clients. Recognizing how social, political and economic forces impact individuals and their abilities to meaningfully engage in occupations, challenges occupational therapy practitioners to do more than just serve as advocates; it calls for them to identify strategies that can be used to transform societies. Adolescents in the foster care system are unlikely to access all of the rehabilitative services they need to achieve health, work, and independent living. Utilizing a multidisciplinary theoretical approach, incorporating critical medical anthropology, social and occupational justice and a life course perspective, is providing me with powerful tools for understanding the complex factors that influence the process of transitioning out of foster care. A similar interdisciplinary theoretical approach can be used to better understand the needs of other marginalized populations who could benefit from occupational therapy.

REFERENCES

Arnett, J.J., 2000. Emerging adulthood: a theory of development from the late teens through the twenties. Am. Psychol. 55 (5), 469–480.

Bernier, A., Ackerman, J., Stovall-McClough, K.C., 2004. Predicting the quality of attachment relationships in foster care dyads from infants' initial behaviors upon placement. Infant Behav. Dev. 27, 366–381.

Braveman, B., Suarez-Balcazar, Y., 2009. Social justice and resource utilization in a community-based organization: a case illustration of the role of the occupational therapist. Am. J. Occup. Ther. 63 (1), 13–23.

Casey Family Programs, 2000. Available at: <http://www.casey.org/cnc/fostercare_statistics.html> (accessed 01.10.15.).

Castro, A., Singer, M., 2004. Unhealthy Health Policy: A Critical Anthropological Examination. Altamira Press, Walnut Creek, CA.

Clark, F., 2006. One Person's Thoughts on the Future of Occupational Science. J. Occup. Sci. 13 (2–3), 167–179.

Clark, H.B., Davis, M., 2002. Transition to adulthood: A resource for assisting young people with emotional or behavioral difficulties. Brookes, Baltimore.

Collins, M.E., 2001. Transition to Adulthood for Vulnerable Youths: A Review of Research and Implications for Policy. Soc. Serv. Rev. 75 (2), 271–291.

Courtney, M., Dworsky, A., Cusick, G.R., Havlicek, J., Perez, A., Keller, T., 2007. Midwest evaluation of the adult functioning of former foster youth: Outcomes at age 21. Chapin Hall Center for Children at the University of Chicago, Chicago, IL.

Danely, J., Lynch, C., 2013. Introduction. In: Lynch, C., Danely, J. (Eds.), Transitions and Transformations: Cultural Perspectives on Aging and the Life Course. Berghahn Books, Oxford, pp. 3–20.

General Accounting Office, 1999. Foster Care: Effectiveness of Independent Living Services Unknown. Retrieved from <http://www.gao.gov/new.items/he00013.pdf> (accessed 01.10.15.).

Georgiades, S.D., 2005. Emancipated young adults' perspectives on independent living programs. Fam Soc 86 (4), 503–510.

Hiebert, B., Thomlison, B., 1996. Facilitating transitions to adulthood: Research and policy implications. In: Galaway, B., Hudson, J. (Eds.), Youth in transition: Perspectives on research and policy. Thompson Educational Publishing, Toronto, pp. 54–60.

Jacobs, D., O'Brien, R.M., 1998. The determinants of deadly force: a structural analysis of police violence. Am. J. Sociol. 103, 837–862.

Jonson-Reid, M., Barth, R.P., 2003. Probation foster care as an outcome for children exiting child welfare foster care. Soc. Work 48, 348–361.

Kools, S., 1997. Adolescent identity development in foster care. Fam. Relat. 46, 263–271.

Krebs, B., Pittcoff, P., 2004. Reversing the failure of the foster care system. Harv. Women's Law J. 27, 357–366.

Lemon, K., Hines, A.M., Merdinger, J., 2005. From foster care to young adulthood: the role of independent living programs in supporting successful transitions. Child. Youth Serv. Rev. 27 (3), 251–270.

Levin, M., Kielhofner, G., Braveman, B., Fogg, L., 2007. Narrative slope as a predictor of work and other occupational participation. Scand. J. Occup. Ther. 14 (4), 258–264.

McMillen, J.C., Zima, B.T., Scott, L.D., Jr., Auslander, W.F., Munson, M.R., Ollie, M.T., Spitznagel, E.L., 2005. The prevalence of psychiatric disorders among older youths in the foster care system. J. Am. Acad. Child Adolesc. Psychiatry 44, 88–95.

Merdinger, J.M., Hines, A.M., Osterling, K.M., Wyatt, P., 2005. Pathways to college for former foster youth: understanding factors that contribute to educational success. Child Welfare 84, 867–896.

National Council of Catholic Bishops, 1986. Economic Justice for All: Pastoral Letter on Catholic Social Teaching and the U.S. Economy, #71, 17. Available at: <http://www.usccb.org/upload/economic_justice_for_all.pdf> (accessed 01.10.15.).

Our Kids of Miami-Dade/Monroe, Inc. Annual Report 2013-2104. Available at: <http://www.ourkids.us/SiteCollectionImages/Static%20Data%20Files/OKAR_2013_14.pdf> (last accessed 01.10.15.).

Paul-Ward, A., 2008. Intersecting disciplinary frameworks to improve foster care transitions. Pract. Anthropol. 30 (3), 15–19.

Paul-Ward, A., 2009. Social and occupational justice barriers in the transition from foster care to independent adulthood. Am. J. Occup. Ther. 63, 81–88.

Paul-Ward, A., Lambdin, C., Haskell, A., 2014. Occupational therapy's emerging role with transitioning adolescents in foster care. Occup. Ther. Ment. Health 30 (2), 162–177.

Reilly, T., 2003. Transition from care: status and outcomes of youth who age out of foster care. Child Welfare 82, 727–746.

Singer, M., 1986. Developing a critical perspective in medical anthropology. Med. Anthropol. Q. 17 (5), 128–129.

Stadnyk, R.L., Townsend, E.A., Wilcock, A.A., 2010. Occupational justice. In: Christiansen, C.H., Townsend, E.A. (Eds.), Introduction to Occupation: The Art and Science of Living, second ed. Pearson Health Science, New Jersey.

Townsend, E., Wilcock, A.A., 2004. Occupational justice and client-centered practice: a dialogue in progress. Can. J. Occup. Ther. 71, 75–87.

US Department of Health and Human Services, 2015. Administration for Children and Families, Administration on Children, Youth and Families, Children's Bureau, the AFCARS Report No. 22. <http://www.acf.hhs.gov/programs/cb> (accessed 11.11.15.).

Waitzkin, H., 1981. The social origins of illness: a neglected history. Int. J. Health Serv. 11 (1), 77–103.

Winter, D.D., Leighton, D.C., 2001. Structural violence. In: Christie, D.J., et al. (Eds.), Peace, Conflict, and Violence: Peace Psychology in the 21st Century. Prentice-Hall, New York.

SECTION 4

THE POLITICAL AND FINANCIAL CONTEXT OF OCCUPATION

SECTION OUTLINE

THE DUTY TO AGE WELL: CRITICAL REFLECTIONS ON OCCUPATIONAL POSSIBILITIES SHAPED THROUGH DISCURSIVE AND POLICY RESPONSES TO POPULATION AGEING

DEBBIE LALIBERTE RUDMAN

CHAPTER OUTLINE

The 'ageing population' is a central problematic of contemporary governance within many countries belonging to the Organization for Economic Cooperation and Development (OECD), frequently constructed in various types of texts as a risk to global and national economic and health systems, as well as social cohesion (Mann, 2007). This discursive construction of population ageing as a crisis has been tied to policy responses involving a redistribution of responsibilities, and risks, amongst the state, ageing citizens and business interests (Biggs and Powell, 2001). Such policy responses, while varying within national contexts, have generally been in line with neoliberal rationality, with its emphases on individual responsibility, economic rationality, activation, and austerity (Asquith, 2009). Overall, policy directives in multiple areas, such as

pensions and healthcare, are being employed to remake ageing citizens at risk of state dependency into those who proactively manage their risks (Boudiny, 2013; Cardona, 2008).

Policy directives addressing population ageing have contributed to, and been sustained by, discourses of 'positive' ageing that establish new standards for 'ageing well' and shape new types of 'active' ageing citizens (Asquith, 2009). At first glance, positive ageing discourses seem to open up an array of opportunities for occupation for ageing individuals, and appear to fit well with the key assumption underpinning occupational therapy and science that participation in occupations is a key contributor to health and well-being (Laliberte Rudman, 2006a). However, bringing together a critical gerontological lens and a critical occupational lens, this chapter raises concerns regarding the types of occupational possibilities shaped, and excluded, through positive ageing discourses, as well the occupational injustices and health inequities they may shape and perpetuate. Ultimately, it is argued that the individualization of the 'risks' and solutions of ageing that occurs through such discourses means that while they may open up occupational possibilities for particular types of ageing citizens, they simultaneously shape and perpetuate occupational injustices for those ageing citizens without the capacities and resources to take up the 'duty to age well'.

CONSTRUCTING POPULATION AGEING AS A CRISIS

Demographic statistics convey that population ageing, although unevenly distributed in extent and rate, is occurring on a global scale (Mendes, 2013). The United Nations has estimated that the global population of those 60 years and older will double by the year 2025 (Powell, 2010). To date, much attention has focused on the rapid population ageing occurring in the Global North or 'West' (Polivka and Luo, 2013). For example, in Europe, it is projected that the number of people aged 65 to 79 years will increase by 30% between 2010 and 2030, while those over 90 years will rise by some 57% (Mendes, 2013). However, it is also expected that many nations in the Global South, outside Africa, will experience rapid growth in older segments of their populations over the next 40 years (Neilson, 2003). For example, between 2006 and 2030, while it is projected that the number of older people in Western nations will increase by 51%, this rate is projected to be 140% for countries outside the 'West' (Powell, 2010).

In this chapter, I focus on how population ageing and ageing citizens have come to be discursively constructed, that is, how they are portrayed within various types of texts. How ageing is socially and politically constructed with influential texts shapes how individuals can and do think about their own ageing and that of other people. As well, such constructions provide boundaries within which governments, communities, health professions and other actors structure social institutions, policies and practices (Asquith, 2009; Mendes, 2013). In relation to occupation, such discursive constructions can be seen as ways through which sociopolitical power operates so as to influence

'the ways and types of doing that come to be viewed as ideal and possible within a specific sociohistorical context, and that came to be promoted and made available within that context' (Laliberte Rudman, 2010, p. 55). Through defining the problems of ageing populations in particular ways, texts also promote specific social and individual approaches to managing such problems, while simultaneously excluding or obscuring other possible solutions. For example, such increases could be celebrated as an outcome of social and health initiatives that have promoted longevity and, in turn, could shape policy responses that focus on enabling lives of dignity and meaningful occupational engagement for those in advanced older age (Foster and Walker, 2013; Laliberte Rudman, 2006b).

However, within many types of contemporary texts, such as reports by international organizations, nation-specific policies, and in media, population ageing is often framed as an impending crisis requiring massive transformations in economic, health, and social systems. Terms such as the 'global ageing crisis', 'the baby bust', 'boomageddon', and the 'silver tsunami' circulate within texts aligned with this crisis discourse. Underpinned by an unquestioned assumption that ageing in and of itself as a biological phenomenon means that more money will be required to meet increased needs for health and social services, the problems of population ageing are often framed in relation to economic and intergenerational implications. Simultaneously, very little attention is paid to how various social conditions across the life course, such as access to housing or adequate income, shape health and social needs in later life, that is, to ageing as a sociopolitical phenomenon (Estes and Phillipson, 2002; Koch, 2012; Mendes, 2013).

Within the contemporary context characterized by 'the spread of globalization and the power of global capital' (Estes and Phillipson, 2002, p. 279), the 'crisis construction' of population ageing has gained dominance partly because of the role various international organizations have played in its shaping and circulation (Moulaert and Biggs, 2012). Organizations such as the World Bank (1994) and the OECD (1998, 2009) have taken a lead in this crisis construction, arguing for the need for various states to take a crisis management approach to population ageing in order to reduce the risks posed to economic systems at global to national scales (Estes and Phillipson, 2002; Powell, 2010). Early signs of what would become a common discursive construction of population ageing amongst international organizations appeared in late 1980s. For example, the OECD published a series of reports that articulated a 'burden of ageing discourse' and pointed to the need for various nation states to rein in spending related to healthcare and pensions for ageing citizens (OECD, 1988; Walker, 2009).

Over the 1990s and into the 2000s, international organizations have fed into this 'crisis construction and management' approach. For example, Estes and Phillipson (2002) and Moulaert and Biggs (2012) have pointed to the rise of a global discourse, circulated by the World Bank, the International Monetary Fund, and the OECD, that presents the privatization of pensions schemes and the extension of work lives as essential solutions for ensuring economic and social stability in the face of population ageing. The title of an OECD (2006) synthesis report succinctly articulates this discursive emphasis, 'Ageing and Employment Policies: Live Longer, Work Longer.' At the same time, this discourse largely excludes other alternative solutions, such as an enlarged state role in pension provision to ensure that rates of poverty in later life do not escalate, nor does it critically question the stability of privatized pension schemes or the possibilities available to ageing citizens to continue labour force involvement.

NEOLIBERAL POLICY RESPONSES TO THE 'CRISIS' OF POPULATION AGEING

This 'crisis' discourse of population ageing, in turn, has been actively drawn upon by international organizations to exert pressure on nation states to reconfigure approaches to governing ageing populations and ageing citizens. As will be unpacked within subsequent sections, such reconfigurations have implications for ageing citizens' occupational possibilities.

Aligned with neoliberal ideology, proposed reconfigurations often involve a combination of austerity and activation approaches (Béland and Myles, 2012). As a particular political rationality that has risen to prominence globally since the 1980s, neoliberal rationality is associated with a critique of the welfare state, a prioritization of private market mechanisms, and an emphasis on individual freedom (Brady, 2014; Walker, 2009). Austerity measures encompass state retreat from public expenditures, along with emphases on efficiency, privatization, and individual responsibility (Polivka and Luo, 2013). Activation measures aim to transform citizens viewed as 'at risk' of state dependency into responsible self-reliant citizens who proactively manage personal risks (Rose, 1999). Predicated on the framing of issues, such as ageing, as individual rather than social problems, activation approaches offer up activity-based solutions, tied to self-care, self-improvement, and proactive risk management.

Although it is not argued that neoliberal rationality determines how nation states reconfigure policies and practices, or that this rationality is taken up in homogenous ways (Brady, 2014), it is quite clear that ageing has become a central problematic of contemporary governance and that national responses are increasingly bounded within and reactionary to international, neoliberal pressures (Foster and Walker, 2013; Polivka and Luo, 2013). As an example, with the area of ageing, work, retirement, and pensions, the OECD is producing a series of 'Working Better with Age' briefs that build upon the policy agenda it outlined in the 2006 'Live Longer, Work Longer' document. These briefs will encompass 21 case studies of countries evaluating the impact of work and pension policy reforms and identifying 'good practice' measures that reduce state costs through extending work lives (http://www.oecd.org/els/public-pensions/pensionsataglance.htm). In addition to measures that aim to tackle employer-based barriers and improve older workers' employability, the OECD promotes measures that 'strengthen financial incentives' for continuing working. While such incentives can include offering financial benefits to individuals who delay receipt of public pensions, the OECD (2006) also recommends strategies to minimize state expenditure, such as shutting down or minimizing routes that enable 'early' receipt of public pensions, decreasing the replacement value of public pensions, raising the age of eligibility for public pensions, and creating privatized pension options. By 2013, many countries had reconfigured, or were in the process of reconfiguring, public pensions in ways that align with such recommendations (Foster and Walker, 2013; Polivka and Luo, 2013). In turn, commensurate with the neoliberal tendency to 'individualize the social'

(Laliberte Rudman, 2013), ensuring financial security in later life is increasingly framed as an individual problem and responsibility to be solved through pro-active engagement in the private pension market and lengthier involvement in formal work. In addition, austerity and activation measures have been promoted and implemented in the area of healthcare, in which efforts to control state costs for health and long-term care are accompanied by the development of private healthcare markets and the promotion of individual responsibility for the maintenance of health through responsible lifestyle choices (Estes and Phillipson, 2002; Raymond and Grenier, 2013).

Thus, consistent with neoliberal approaches to governing, 'aging is increasingly understood as a risk for the individual as much as a collective responsibility, with a questioning of the centrality of state provision' (Neilson, 2003, p. 183). This understanding of the problems of ageing has been shaped and sustained by a crisis construction of population ageing, which has provided a justification for the need to reconfigure policies and practices that previously aimed to provide collective solutions to the risks of ageing. In addition, the neoliberal reconfiguration of the governance of ageing, particularly the individualization of problems and solutions associated with ageing, has involved the shaping, circulation and promotion of what have come to be labelled 'positive' or 'active' ageing dis-courses (Boudiny, 2013; Foster and Walker, 2013). The emphasis on 'active aging' at the Second World Assem-bly on Ageing in Madrid in 2002 has been framed as a turning point in policy responses to ageing, and various nation states have incorporated variations of positive ageing discourses into policy agendas (Raymond and Grenier, 2013). For example, within the European Union, reports and guidelines began to prioritize active ageing in policies in the early 1990s and have done so with increasing frequency since the early 2000s (Mendes, 2013).

NEOLIBERAL RATIONALITY AND GOVERNING AGEING AT A DISTANCE: THE DISCURSIVE PROMOTION OF 'POSITIVE' AGEING

Discursive constructions of positive ageing are of par-ticular relevance to occupational therapists and scien-tists given their seeming alignment with the assumption that participation in occupations is essential for health and well-being. Within the remainder of this chapter, I address why it is crucial to adopt a critical stance towards how positive ageing discourses have been taken up within neoliberal approaches to governing in ways that bound occupational possibilities for ageing individuals, individualize the risks of ageing, and shape and perpetuate occupational injustices.

Aligning with Asquith (2009), the term *positive ageing* is used in this chapter to encompass a set of ageing discourses variously labelled, such as active, healthy, and successful ageing, which have increasingly come to prominence. The roots of these discourses are often located in the seminal work of Rowe and Kahn (1997) which defined 'successful ageing' as marked by active engagement with life, low risk for disease and disability, and a high functional level (Dillaway and Byrnes, 2009). Key elements addressed in discourses of positive ageing, which often effectively counter long-standing negative constructions of ageing as a time of decline, disability and inactivity, include good health, social connectedness, and continued activity (Asquith, 2009). Given that active ageing discourses centralize continued activity engagement as essential to health and well-being, at face value, they appear closely aligned with key values in occupational therapy and as potentially providing a means to advocate for policies, programmes and practices aimed at enabling occupa-tional engagement for ageing citizens (Wilcock, 2007). Indeed, some conceptualizations of positive ageing appear to be inclusive of the broad definition of occu-pation taken up in occupational therapy, such as the World Health Organization's (2002) definition of active ageing that encompasses social, economic, cul-tural, spiritual, and civic forms of participation and acknowledges the need for environmental supports to enable ageing individuals with varying capacities and resources to actively age (Walker, 2009; Wilcock, 2007).

However, a more critical engagement is required prior to occupational therapy and science wholeheart-edly aligning with positive ageing discourses, particu-larly as they have been taken up within international and national policies and shaped in contexts in which neoliberal political rationality is dominant. Critical gerontologists, drawing particularly upon a governmen-tality perspective, have conceptualized such discourses as technologies of government which enact neoliberal rationality through enlisting ageing citizens in a duty to age well that permeates everyday life via promoting proactive, responsible, and risk-reducing lifestyle practices (Boudiny, 2013). These critiques highlight how contemporary policies outline a paradigm of positive ageing that is increasingly seen as compulsory, as a 'duty' responsible ageing citizens must take up in order to ensure their own security and well-being, as well as that of society (Carmel et al., 2007; Mendes, 2013). As such, this work raises concerns regarding how positive ageing, predicated on the individualization of the problems of ageing, has been used to govern ageing citizens 'at a distance' in ways that seek to align their actions with broader neoliberal emphases on austerity and activation (Carmel et al., 2007). These authors emphasize that, as taken up with policy, positive ageing discourses highlight the responsibility of ageing individuals to achieve ageing free from disability and to maintain youthfulness, productivity and participation, simultaneously creating space for state retreat from economic, health and social programmes for ageing citizens (Raymond and Grenier, 2013). In the final two subsections of this chapter, I draw on this critical gerontological work and a critical occupational lens to highlight concerns related to how occupational possibilities for ageing citizens are being reshaped through positive ageing discourses and aligned policy initiatives. The critique presented is not an exhaustive consideration of what such discourses and policies may mean for the occupational possibilities of contemporary and future ageing segments of populations. Rather, the primary aim is to illustrate how employing a critical occupational lens can add to existing critiques through considering the implications of the individualization agenda and narrow definition of occupation taken up in positive ageing discourses for occupational possibilities and occupational injustices.

INDIVIDUALIZING THE 'DUTY TO AGE WELL'

Overall, commensurate with the individualization agenda of neoliberalism, positive ageing discourses have been taken up in policies in ways that displace the 'crisis' of population ageing to ageing individuals. In

essence, such discourses convey the message that not only is 'positive ageing' possible for all ageing individuals, but also that it should be continually strived for through making responsible activity, or occupational, choices in relation to various aspects of life, such as work, finances, exercise, and leisure (Dillaway and Byrnes, 2009). What is neglected within such neoliberal reconfigurations is the differential capacity of ageing individuals to engage in the occupations promoted given their differential access to resources over their lifetimes, resulting from social positions and conditions that relate to aspects such as gender, education, and citizenship status (Laliberte Rudman, 2013). Thus, this individualization obscures various ways that occupational possibilities and injustices experienced by ageing citizens are sociopolitically shaped (Carmel et al., 2007; Laliberte Rudman, 2013). As two examples, I consider the differential capacities and resources for women and for people with disabilities to engage in the 'duty to age well'. Through this, while acknowledging that positive ageing discourses open up occupational possibilities for particular types of ageing citizens, I raise concerns regarding how such discourses may 'deprive some groups of older people from the possibilities and experiences of meaningful participation' (Raymond and Grenier, 2013, p. 125).

Individualizing the 'Duty to Age Well': Considering Gender

Within positive ageing discourses, access to physical, socioeconomic, symbolic, and other forms of resources required to participate in the types of occupations promoted as means to work towards and engage in positive ageing, is taken for granted (Raymond and Grenier, 2013). As austerity measures are put in place and states retreat from publicly funded supports and services aimed at ensuring health and financial stability with ageing, individuals are increasingly required to draw on their own financial resources in order to achieve positive ageing (Conway and Crawshaw, 2009). However, women are at greater risk of poverty in later life for several reasons, such as having lower employment rates than men post age 55, being more likely to be engaged in part-time and contingent work, and having greater care responsibilities that lead to periods of either part-time or no engagement in the formal labour force. These factors make it more challenging for women to accrue financial resources over the life course, and policy changes that decrease replacement rates and access to public pensions may perpetuate and further inequalities in income, social security, and quality of life in old age (Foster and Walker, 2013). As well, older women in the Majority World are often deeply affected by the increasing privatization of healthcare and the burden on governments associated with debt repayments to international bodies (Estes and Phillipson, 2002; Powell, 2010).

Thus, the 'duty to age well' may be differentially achievable according to gender, creating inequities in occupational possibilities available due to the differential capacities of men and women to take up the forms of occupation that are promoted as means to age well. In addition, women may experience greater instances of occupational injustices, in which their choices to engage in particular occupations are restricted by sociopolitically produced conditions. For example, given their financial situation and the decreasing availability of public pensions, many ageing women may have less 'choice' to opt out of extended working lives and may be increasingly relegated to low-paying, contingent work as an occupational means to ensure self-reliance in later life (Riach, 2007).

Individualizing the 'Duty to Age Well': Considering Disability

In relation to disability, positive ageing discourses frame impairment and disability with age as 'risks' that can be overcome by individuals through the 'right' lifestyle choices (Mendes, 2013; Raymond and Grenier, 2013). The types of occupations celebrated within such discourses, such as physically active leisure and continued involvement in paid work, often assume that ageing individuals have no physical, cognitive, or other forms of disabilities that would preclude or present challenges to their engagement. Overall, few 'positive' possibilities for occupation are imagined within such discourses for those who are disabled. Such discourses thereby relegate ageing individuals with impairments and disabilities 'to the margins, invisible, or unvoiced' (Raymond and Grenier, 2013, p. 125), and may result in the simultaneous celebration of 'independent elderly people … while the incapacitated elderly are excluded or abandoned in a clear power struggle' (Mendes, 2013, p. 177).

When ageing individuals with disabilities are invisible, or obscured, within and through positive ageing discourses, their occupational needs, and the types of supports and resources required to enable occupational engagement, also become invisible and obscured. Similar to women, persons ageing with disabilities often face challenges to sustainable employment over their lifetimes (Pelkowski and Berger, 2004), affecting their abilities to prepare for retirement, as well as their pension incomes. Consequently, positive ageing discourses may further shape and perpetuate occupational injustices tied to ability status, such that those individuals who age with a disability or acquire a disability as they age have fewer opportunities or supports to engage in meaningful occupations that support their continued participation, health, and well-being (Conway and Crawshaw, 2009; Laliberte Rudman, 2006a, 2006b). As such, rather than fulfilling the promise of combating ageism, 'positive' ageing discourses may reinforce exclusionary and stigmatizing attitudes towards 'oldness', by framing disability and dependency as matters of failed responsibility and, in turn, may support societal retreat from ensuring the occupational rights of all ageing persons.

BOUNDING OCCUPATIONAL POSSIBILITIES: RISK REDUCTION AND PRODUCTIVITY

As noted above, it is acknowledged that some conceptualizations of positive ageing, such as that proposed by the World Health Organization (2002), incorporate a range of occupational possibilities, spanning social, economic, spiritual, and civic forms of participation. However, as taken up within contemporary policy frameworks, these broad conceptualizations have been increasingly narrowed, in particular to a focus on occupations that enable individuals to reduce risks and those that involve productive involvement in the labour market. As such, occupational possibilities, that is, the occupations marked as ideal, possible and responsible for ageing citizens (Laliberte Rudman, 2010), have been increasingly narrowed, bounding the types of occupations that are socially supported and that are promoted as means to age well.

Consistent with the neoliberal emphases on risk management (Rose, 1999), there is a particular emphasis within positive ageing discourses on making proactive occupational choices as a means to reduce one's exposure to the financial, physical, social, and cognitive 'risks' associated with ageing (Conway and Crawshaw, 2009). Thus, in addition to obscuring how collective risks, such as poverty, are often shaped by sociopolitical factors (Mendes, 2013), risk is forefronted as a prime consideration in how ageing citizens should make occupational choices. This focus on the risk-reducing potential of occupation and the forefronting of risk as a primary axis for deciding on occupations creates a narrow frame for occupational choice. This frame neglects the array of meanings and purposes that can be derived from occupation and that, in turn, may contribute to health and well-being (Dennhardt and Laliberte Rudman, 2012). The narrow focus on risk may also create boundaries on the types of health-care services, including occupational therapy, that are funded as means to support the occupational engagement of ageing individuals. Both Wilcock (2007) and Ballinger and Payne (2000) have argued that an emphasis on risk management within occupational therapy, and health services more generally, can inadvertently lead to practice that limits ageing individuals' occupational possibilities in the name of 'protecting' ageing individuals. As well, a focus on risk as something that can and should be managed by individuals through engaging in the 'right' occupations, can facilitate and support victim-blaming when individuals fail to protect themselves from the 'risks' of ageing (Dennhardt and Laliberte Rudman, 2012; Mendes, 2013). When such victim-blaming is drawn upon to justify retreat from health and other services for those who fail to be 'active agers' – that is, those who do experience dependency, disability and poverty – the occupational and health needs of such ageing individuals are increasingly not addressed and situations of occupational injustices may be shaped (Laliberte Rudman, 2006a, 2006b).

Within the broader context of a 'crisis' construction of population ageing, several authors have noted that discourses of positive ageing as taken up in governmental policy have increasingly focused on encouraging productive engagement in the labour market (Foster and Walker, 2013). As summarized by Mendes (2013), 'inclusion increasingly involves having a job and doing paid work, since inclusion through the social security system is less and less desirable' (p. 181).

From a critical occupational lens, this raises concerns about the neglect of other forms of 'productive' and so-called nonproductive occupations, such as caregiving, community leisure activities, and volunteering, through which ageing citizens make contributions to their families and communities. This very narrow definition of valuable occupations, in turn, may mean that such occupations are not socially and politically recognized, valued and supported, further marginalizing the vital caregiving work of seniors and bounding possibilities for volunteer engagement to healthy and well-resourced ageing individuals (Laliberte Rudman, 2006a). As well, the increasing focus on productive occupations, narrowly defined as labour force involvement, works against opening up occupational possibilities for later life, further justifying the retreat from comprehensive ageing strategies that are inclusive of a range of forms of occupational engagement that can promote health and well-being.

Furthermore, Riach (2007) has argued that the primary focus on societal contribution through paid work may mean that ageing individuals not in the labour force are ever more viewed as a 'problematic drain on the economy' (p. 1712). Extended work may be increasingly framed as an obligation of responsible citizenship, particularly for ageing individuals who are unable to be financially self-reliant (Mann, 2007; Mendes, 2013). In turn, promoting extended work as an obligation may further shape and perpetuate occupational injustices experienced by ageing workers in comparison to younger workers and amongst ageing individuals. For example, ageing workers face sociopolitically constructed barriers to continued work and reemployment, such as higher rates of disability, lower rates of receiving workplace accommodations, ageist workplace practices, and ageist workplace relations (MacEwen, 2012; McMullin and Shuey, 2006; Mendes, 2013). These collective barriers tend to be neglected or downplayed in positive ageing policies promoting work, obscuring the need for broader social and political changes to ensure meaningful, health-promoting work options for ageing workers. As well, discourses promoting 'productive' ageing tend to homogenize older workers in ways that align their supposedly shared characteristics, such as being financially secure, with relegation to sectors of the labour market characterized by contingent forms of work that offer little security, benefits, or financial benefit (Riach, 2007). Thus, such discourses may enhance inequities between affluent, highly skilled ageing workers, who can choose to work or not, and disadvantaged older workers who have little choice but to continue to work and whose options may be increasingly narrowed to precarious forms of employment (Ainsworth and Hardy, 2004).

CONCLUSION

Within this chapter, a critical occupational lens was integrated with critical gerontological work to raise concerns regarding the types of occupational possibilities shaped, and excluded, through positive ageing discourses as taken up within the contemporary neoliberal political landscape. In particular, concerns were raised regarding how positive ageing has been taken up with policy agendas in ways that individualize the risks and responsibilities for ageing, shape a duty to age well that is differentially achievable, and create and perpetuate occupational injustices. As well, the types of occupational possibilities promoted as ideal and responsible ways to age 'positively' have increasingly narrowly focused on risk reduction and continued productivity within the formal labour market.

Given the limitations of contemporary approaches to the governing of ageing populations that have been shaped through the intersections of a crisis construction of population ageing and the neoliberal shaping of 'positive' ageing, it is imperative that occupational therapists and scientists critically question what is coming to be increasingly taken for granted about what it means to age 'positively'. Drawing upon a broad conceptualization of occupation and the growing body of knowledge that displays the multiple and complex interconnections among occupation, health and well-being, occupational therapists and scientists have a crucial role to play in advocating for approaches to thinking about and addressing ageing that open up broader occupational possibilities for a diversity of types of ageing citizens. As Walker (Foster and Walker, 2013; Walker, 2009) and Wilcock (2007) have contended, one possible way forward is to return to broader conceptualizations of 'positive' ageing that encompass a range of meaningful pursuits and diverse types of ageing citizens. Another way forward is to work with ageing individuals and collectives to produce

and disseminate critical narratives that raise awareness of the boundaries of contemporary discursive constructions, and bring to light diverse ways ageing individuals engage in occupations and the contributions of such engagement to their lives and communities (Laliberte Rudman, 2013; Raymond and Grenier, 2013).

As a final point, although this chapter has focused on the contemporary governance of ageing, activation-based policies and practices associated with neoliberal rationality are permeating numerous policy areas in international and national spaces (Brady, 2014). Given this, this chapter provides an illustration of how a critical occupational lens can be taken up to consider the implications of such policies and practices, which inherently are about shaping citizens' daily occupational lives, for occupational possibilities and injustices.

REFERENCES

Ainsworth, S., Hardy, C., 2004. Critical discourse analysis and identity: why bother? Crit. Discourse Stud. 1 (2), 225–259.

Asquth, N., 2009. Positive ageing, neoliberalism and Australian sociology. J. Sociol. 45 (3), 255–269.

Ballinger, C., Payne, S., 2000. Falling from grace or into expert hands? Alternative accounts about falling in older people. Br. J. Occup. Ther. 63 (12), 573–579.

Béland, D., Myles, J., 2012. Varieties of federalism, institutional legacies, and social policy: comparing old-age and unemployment insurance reform in Canada. Int. J. Soc. Welf. 21, S75–S87.

Biggs, S., Powell, J.L., 2001. A Foucauldian analysis of old age and the power of social welfare. J. Aging. Soc. Policy 12 (2), 93–112.

Boudiny, K., 2013. 'Active ageing': from empty rhetoric to effective policy tool. Ageing Soc. 33, 1077–1098.

Brady, M., 2014. Ethnographies of neoliberal governmentalities: from the neoliberal apparatus to neoliberalism and governmental assemblages. Foucault Stud. 19, 11–33.

Cardona, B., 2008. 'Healthy ageing' policies and anti-ageing ideologies and practices: on the exercise of responsibility. Med. Health Care Philos. 11, 475–483.

Carmel, E., Hamblin, K., Papadopoulos, T., 2007. Governing the activation of older workers in the European Union. Int. J. Sociol. Soc. Policy 27 (9/10), 387–400.

Conway, S., Crawshaw, P., 2009. 'Healthy senior citizenship' in voluntary and community organizations: a study in governmentality. Health Sociol. Rev. 18 (4), 387–399.

Dennhardt, S., Laliberte Rudman, D., 2012. When occupation goes 'wrong': a critical reflection on risk discourses and their relevance in shaping occupation. In: Whiteford, G.E., Hocking, C. (Eds.), Occupational Science: Society, Inclusion and Participation. Wiley-Blackwell, West Sussex, UK, pp. 117–133.

Dillaway, H.E., Byrnes, M., 2009. Reconsidering successful aging: a call for renewed and expanded academic critiques and conceptualizations. J. Appl. Gerontol. 28 (6), 702–722.

Estes, C.L., Phillipson, C., 2002. The globalization of capital, the welfare state, and old age policy. Int. J. Health Serv. 32 (2), 279–297.

Foster, L., Walker, L., 2013. Gender and active aging in Europe. Eur. J. Aging 10, 3–10.

Koch, T., 2012. Thieves of Virtue: When Bioethics Stole Medicine. MIT Press, Cambridge, MA.

Laliberte Rudman, D., 2006a. Reflections on … positive aging and its implications for occupational possibilities in later life. Can. J. Occup. Ther. 73 (3), 188–192.

Laliberte Rudman, D., 2006b. Shaping the active, autonomous and responsible modern retiree: an analysis of discursive technologies and their links with neo-liberal political rationality. Ageing Soc. 26, 181–201.

Laliberte Rudman, D., 2010. Occupational possibilities. J. Occup. Sci. 17 (1), 55–59.

Laliberte Rudman, D., 2013. Enacting the critical potential of occupational science: problematizing the 'individualizing of occupation'. J. Occup. Sci. 20 (4), 298–313.

MacEwen, A., 2012. Working after age 65. What is at stake? Canadian Centre for Policy Alternatives. <http://www.policyalternatives.ca/sites/default/files/uploads/publications/National%20Office/2012/04/WorkingAfter65.pdf>.

Mann, K., 2007. Activation, retirement planning and restraining the 'third age'. Soc. Policy Society 6, 279–292.

McMullin, J., Shuey, K.M., 2006. Ageing, disability and work-place accommodations. Ageing Soc. 26, 831–847.

Mendes, F.R., 2013. Active ageing: a right or a duty? Health Sociol. Rev. 22 (2), 174–178.

Moulaert, T., Biggs, S., 2012. International and European policy on work and retirement: reinventing critical perspectives on active ageing and mature subjectivity. Human Relat. 66 (1), 23–43. doi:10.1177/0018726711435180.

Neilson, B., 2003. Globalization and the biopolitics of aging. New Centen. Rev. 3 (2), 161–186.

Organization for Economic Co-operation and Development, 1988. Ageing populations. The social policy implications. OECD, Paris.

Organization for Economic Co-operation and Development, 1998. Maintaining prosperity in an ageing society. OECD, Paris.

Organization for Economic Co-operation and Development, 2006. Ageing and employment policies: live longer, work longer. OECD, Paris.

Organization for Economic Co-operation and Development, 2009. Policies for healthy ageing: an overview. OECD Health Working Paper No. 42, OECD Publishing, Paris, pp. 2–32.

Pelkowski, J.M., Berger, M.C., 2004. The impact of health on employment, wages, and hours worked over the life cycle. Q. Rev. Econ. Finance 44 (1), 102–121.

Polivka, L., Luo, B., 2013. The future of retirement security around the globe. Generations 37 (1), 39–45.

Powell, J.L., 2010. The power of global aging. Ageing Int. 35 (1), 1–14.

Raymond, E., Grenier, A., 2013. Participation in social policy discourse: new form of exclusion for seniors with disabilities? Can. J. Aging 32 (2), 117–129.

Riach, K., 2007. 'Othering' older worker identity in recruitment. Human Relat 60 (11), 1701–1726.

Rose, N., 1999. Powers of Freedom: Reframing Political Thought. University of Cambridge Press, Cambridge, UK.

Rowe, J., Kahn, R.L., 1997. Successful aging. Gerontologist 37, 433–440.

Walker, A., 2009. The emergence and application of active aging in Europe. J. Aging Soc. Policy 21 (1), 75–93.

Wilcock, A.A., 2007. Active ageing: dream or reality. N. Z. J. Occup. Ther. 54 (1), 15–20.

World Bank, 1994. Averting the Old Age Crisis. Oxford University Press, New York.

World Health Organization, 2002. Active Ageing: A Policy Framework. World Health Organization, Geneva. Available at: <http://whqlibdoc.who.int/hq/2002/WHO_NMH_NPH_02.8.pdf?ua=1>.

FREEDOMS AND RIGHTS IN AN AGE OF AUSTERITY

HEATHER BULLEN

The recent *age of austerity* was ushered in following the global financial crisis of 2007 to 2008, precipitated by the failure of the deregulated banking sector (Mendoza, 2015). Several governments decided to save the global financial system, through large-scale bailouts to banks, leading to a sovereign debt crisis, whereby trillions of dollars of debt moved from the private sector to appear as deficits on state balance sheets (Blyth, 2013). The cause of the subsequent economic crisis was soon obscured, narrated instead as a problem of overspent states, with voluntary deflation, in the form of austerity measures, presented as the solution (Sen, 2015). These measures included cuts to public and welfare services, higher retirement age and reduced public sector wages. Although higher taxation can also play a role in deficit reduction, in general this was not the chosen option (Blyth, 2013).

Austerity is not a new concept, but this recent age of austerity has provided an opportunity for an exacerbation of the neoliberal ideology that has been increasingly dominant worldwide since the 1990s. During the years since the global financial crisis, austerity has been transformed, in particular within the US and the UK, into an opportunity to further concentrate wealth among the economic elite (Dorling, 2014). Focusing on the experience in the UK, this chapter will consider the impact that an austerity agenda has had on freedoms and rights, considering whose rights are being promoted and whose are undermined. This chapter aims to contribute to a wider debate about the human, societal and occupational cost of austerity and to support a case for alternatives to austerity.

DEFINITIONS OF FREEDOM

Freedom requires deconstructing as there are many assumptions inherent in this term, including Eurocentric perspectives that prioritise individual freedom and autonomy at the expense of more communal perspectives and values (Bauman, 1988, Fineman, 2004). Berlin (2002) conceived freedom as taking two separate forms, positive and negative freedom, and these will be considered next. The former aligns with an individualistic liberal/neoliberal perspective of freedom, while the latter is linked to more communitarian and progressive perspectives (Kelley, 2012).

Negative Freedom

Negative freedom postulates that individuals are free to the extent that no one interferes with their chosen activities (Berlin, 2002). This perspective of freedom is linked to Western liberal philosophy, which emerged at the time of the Enlightenment movement in the seventeenth century and spread globally. Enlightenment thinkers sought to limit the role of the state and postulated the right of the individual to be free in their private domain (Siedentop, 2014). However, although freedom was deemed to be a universal human right, these 'natural rights, in reality, were rights of white European men' (Kallen, 2004, p. 13). Groups such as women and slaves, deemed as lacking rationality, were viewed incapable of achieving freedom: the social order, including chattel slavery and wives as property of their husbands, remained unchallenged (Still, 2012).

Liberal philosophy does not advocate absolute freedom, as one person's chosen activities may impinge on the freedoms of another. Thus, a *social contract* is required, where the individual cedes some freedom to the state in return for protection (Bronner, 2004). The main aim of a liberal government is therefore to support free individuals to be autonomous in their private or family domain, although restrictions may be placed on freedom in the public domain.

Neoliberalism emerged from this philosophy, but focused on a narrower perspective based on the belief that only the capitalist system can deliver prosperity and society therefore needs to be organized around the imperatives of the free market (Gray, 2008). This ideology has been dominant in the UK since the election of Margaret Thatcher as prime minister in 1979. Mombiot (2011) criticises right wing libertarians who use freedom as a cover for exploitation, ignoring the role of bankers, corporations and the wealthy in restricting the freedoms of others. The market requires freedom

juxtaposed with oppression to create 'the symbolic value of difference', meaning that individuals strive to distinguish themselves from others and gain social approval, or risk becoming a 'failed consumer' (Bauman, 1988, p. 70).

Positive Freedom

A contrasting perspective of freedom is *positive freedom*, or the freedom to be one's true self (Berlin, 2002). The concept of positive freedom incorporates ideals such as collective freedom, freedom to earn a living and live a healthy, fulfilled life, and freedom from violence, exploitation and oppression (Kelley, 2012). Here, state interventions can be justified to meet altruistic aims such as freedom from poverty (Sen, 1999). This perspective fits in with the concept of *social citizenship*, whereby the state takes an active role in reducing inequality and protecting citizens against the commodifying effects of the free market. An example of this is the Beveridge Report (1944), where the British government took responsibility for the provision of universal healthcare to the general population and social housing and social security payments to the less well-off (cited in O'Cinneide, 2014). This is not necessarily incompatible with negative freedom, as Beveridge saw this blueprint for a comprehensive welfare state as the fulfilment of the liberal idea of a good society, allowing citizens freedom from anxiety and creating self-confident and autonomous people, able to make free choices (Bauman, 2005).

The risk of a positive perspective of freedom is that the state could impose its definition of how citizens will achieve their true self (Berlin, 2002). However, rather than necessarily requiring state intervention, positive freedom can emerge through a 'collective striving for real democracy' (Kelley, 2012, p. 7). This can happen through, for example, more deliberative forms of democracy, incorporating a wider range of views than the usual aggregate form of democracy that seeks to win an election by maximizing core votes (Young, 2000).

It is important to note that for both types of freedom the state plays a key role, so the debate is ultimately about the goal of state intervention rather than the size of the state (Baker, 2006). Debating these two contrasting views of freedom is important as this concept is central to any discussion of the type of society we wish to live in (Dasgupta, 1986). It also affects prioritization of human rights, as will be discussed next.

FREEDOM AND HUMAN RIGHTS

The Enlightenment, with its liberal notions of human rights, including freedom, became the precursor for formalized declarations such as the Universal Declaration of Human Rights of 1948. This declaration is a statement of principles for protecting fundamental human rights worldwide, setting out the cardinal principles of freedom, equality and diversity as a right for all of humanity (cited in Silvestri and Crowther-Dowey, 2008).

Magdalena Sepulveda, United Nations Special Rapporteur on Extreme Poverty and Human Rights between 2008 and 2014, highlighted how austerity measures taken by states in response to the global financial and economic crises have had devastating impacts on the enjoyment of economic, social and cultural rights worldwide (Sepulveda Carmona, 2014). This makes austerity a critical topic to investigate for occupational therapists, to bring 'an occupational perspective to deep-seated societal issues' (Hocking, 2014, p. 591).

Occupational Rights

Occupational therapy has tended to focus on encouraging people to adapt to existing environments rather than promoting equality of opportunity (Whalley Hammell, 2015), thus ignoring economic, social and cultural rights and freedoms. Although occupational justice has been long-articulated within the profession, it is more concerned with the distribution of resources, rather than addressing the structural causes of injustice or inequality (Whalley Hammell and Iwama, 2012). Occupational rights consider conditions that enable or constrain freedom of action, stating what people have the right to expect, thus providing a clearer mandate for occupational therapy (Whalley Hammell and Iwama, 2012).

AUSTERITY IN THE UK

This section provides an overview of particular forms of *unfreedom* pertaining to economic, social and occupational rights that have been created or exacerbated since the age of austerity.

Freedom of the Market

Since 2008, the private sector in the UK has extended its reach, benefiting from new markets opening in sectors such as education and healthcare (Bell, 2015). Discourses of freedom underpin this privatization; the outsourcing of healthcare services outside the National Health Service, for example, is promoted as giving patients more choice over healthcare, including where to be treated or by whom (National Health Service and Finance Directorate, 2015). However, this has frequently been at the expense of freedom to choose high-quality care: resource cuts have led to tighter eligibility criteria and reduced quality of care (National Health Service Support Federation, 2015). Regional variations and inequalities in access to services could increase cancer mortality rates by nearly 20 000 people per year (National Audit Office, 2015).

Outsourcing public services to private companies has led to behaviours such as 'parking' (or keeping on hold) service users with complex needs and 'creaming off' (taking the best) service users who are cheaper or easier to treat and thus more profitable (Gash et al., 2013). This is a natural effect of increased privatization, without sufficient safeguards or regulation: as private companies are primarily accountable to their shareholders, they have to prioritize making a profit. An ethical dimension within a capitalist framework can only occur through regulation and restricting private companies from maximizing profit at all costs (Brass, 2015).

The privatization of public bodies in the UK has occurred at the expense of reduced public scrutiny and public accountability (Bell, 2015). Private corporations are not democratically accountable to the public: the Freedom of Information Act (2000) only provides public right of access to information for public bodies. Devolving the responsibility for the provision of health and welfare services to the private sector undermines the basic premise of the social contract. In a democracy, the government should be able to step in when things go wrong, to ensure the freedoms of the vulnerable are not undermined (Bell, 2015). Instead, in Austerity UK, the government has given away many of its powers and its responsibility to solve social problems in a time of economic crisis.

Freedom in an Age of Rising Inequality

Freedom only makes sense in contrast to the less free, and thus becomes linked to a differentiation of statuses in society (Bauman, 1988). Over the last 30 years, the UK has become more unequal, with poverty rates doubling despite the economy growing (Oxfam Briefing Paper, 2012). The highest earners have become relatively richer since 2008, with the top 20% of earning households enjoying 37.5% of the income growth (Chakrabortty, 2015).

This is of great concern because income disparity rather than absolute income (above a minimum standard) has been demonstrated to lead to increased health and social problems in more unequal countries. This includes issues as diverse as increased obesity, mental illness, poorer educational performance, homicides and prison rates (Wilkinson and Pickett, 2009). Income disparity affects the occupational rights of both current and future generations. Intergenerational mobility is low in countries with higher income inequality, such as the UK (Corak, 2013).

Rising income inequality can 'stifle upward mobility, making it harder for talented and hardworking people to get the rewards they deserve' (Organisation for Economic Co-operation and Development, 2011, p. 40). Income inequality may impact not only on occupations across the generations, but also on life expectancy. A meta-analysis considering the association between income inequality and health found that mortality over time is greater in less equal countries (Kondo et al., 2009).

With rising inequality, there is an overrepresentation of privileged groups in key jobs 'so stark that it amounts to "social engineering"' (Social Mobility and Child Poverty Commission, 2014a, p. 10). In the first cabinet of the UK coalition government in 2010, 23 of the cabinet ministers were millionaires, and 59% of them attended highly privileged fee-paying schools, compared with 7% of the general population (Jones, 2015). This lack of diversity may lead to less privileged people with equal talent being locked out of access to prestigious employment opportunities (Social Mobility and Child Poverty Commission, 2014a). It can also lead to an illusion of entitlement and an inability to empathize with those in less privileged situations, resulting in repressive policies and attitudes towards those deemed to be from 'inferior' backgrounds (Duffell, 2014). This attitude can be seen in austerity cuts that have focused on the most vulnerable in the UK to the extent of punishing the poor (O'Hara, 2014).

The economic crisis requires not only the restoration of economic growth, but making this growth fairer (Organisation for Economic Co-operation and Development, 2009). This has demonstrably not happened, and occupational rights and engagement, for this generation and subsequent ones, are thereby detrimentally affected. The adverse effects of inequality may also be felt by the more affluent due to spillover effects of psychosocial stress from social comparisons (Kondo et al., 2009). There are risks to social and economic achievement of a society with limited economic security for its citizens (Shiller, 2003). People may choose to remain in a safe but unrewarding role over a more exciting career or limit innovative ventures for a safer existence (Shiller, 2003). Thus, occupational choices become restricted. The following section explores the impact of austerity on people living in poverty.

Freedom in an Age of Food Banks

Freedom of agency of individuals 'is inescapably qualified and constrained by the social, political and economic opportunities that are available to us' (Sen, 1999, p. xii). These opportunities have been detrimentally impacted in the most disadvantaged sectors of society since the global financial crisis (Nolan, 2014). Without resources, an individual is without freedom (Bauman, 1988). Austerity has merely exacerbated a growing trend in neoliberal economy: although the UK is twice as rich as 30 years ago, poverty rates have doubled during this time (Lansley and Mack, 2015). This is a direct consequence of non regulated free market forces.

Austerity cuts can be considered as a form of structural violence, leading to the loss of between 1.3 and 2.5 million years of life annually (Oxfam Briefing Paper, 2012). The cumulative impact of cuts are such that the poorest Britons are detrimentally affected five times more than the general population (Duffy, 2013). Cuts to welfare impact not only the individual recipient, but the entire family. The Welfare Reform Act (2012) that capped benefits at a maximum of £500 a week, regardless of number of children in a family, has been deemed incompatible with the UK's obligations under the United Nations Convention on Rights of a Child to act in the best interests of the child (Social Mobility and Child Poverty Commission, 2014b).

In a neoliberal culture, with a strong emphasis on economic freedom, there are strong pressures to prioritize paid work over voluntary or caring work (Clouston, 2014). The government assumes that paid work equates with empowerment, despite half of the 13 million people in poverty coming from households where at least one person is in work (Mabbett, 2013). Increasingly, families in the UK are living a hand-to-mouth existence, making stark choices between whether to eat or heat their homes (O'Hara, 2014). Food poverty in the UK has been highlighted by 170 medical experts as amounting to a public health emergency, condemning the fact that in one of the world's richest economies the welfare state is increasingly failing to protect citizens from hunger (Ashton et al., 2014). The number of people using food banks run by the Trussell Trust (a charity that coordinates the only nationwide network of foodbanks in the UK, to date) has risen eightfold between 2008 and 2014 (McBain, 2015).

Themes of shame and stigma are central to the experience of living in poverty (Beagan, 2007). Individuals are judged by their choices over what they consume, and can gain or lose cultural capital through this (Bordieu, 1984). Freedom, therefore, becomes a privilege available only to those with adequate monetary resources to create valued identities through 'correct' consumption choices (Bauman, 1988). Leisure choices may also be stigmatized: 65% of those in higher-earning groups see television as a luxury; however, this may be viewed as a necessity by someone lacking resources to access other leisure activities. People may be excluded from activities, such as attending school trips, and may reduce interaction with others through fear of being shamed at not being able to afford to partake in socially valued occupations (Lansley and Mack, 2015). Deprivation thus creates significant inequality in opportunities to participate in occupations that have personal, social or cultural meaning, excluding people from mainstream society (Hocking, 2012).

People choosing to spend social security payments to fit in with the consumer society and media portrayal of essential items, such as the latest brand of trainers, may be condemned for this (McKenzie, 2015). A study on youth subcultures among the white 'underclass', found that on housing estates with limited work opportunities, predatory and excessive occupations, such as drug dealing, may become the only route available that allows youths to purchase status symbols and avoid social shaming (Nayak, 2006). Loan companies are among the beneficiaries of the need to fit into a consumer economy, on top of meeting basic survival needs, with rising numbers of citizens seeking *payday loans*, borrowing in the short-term at excessive interest rates (O'Hara, 2014). This can lead to a downwards spiral of debt and impoverishment (Lansley and Mack, 2015).

Social problems have been increasingly framed in the UK as the responsibility of individuals. This fits with an individualistic, liberal view of poverty as caused through poor lifestyle choices (Lansley and Mack, 2015). There has been a strong sense of moral authoritarianism in the British government that pits neoliberal values of personal responsibility against the 'diminished' values of social security claimants (Bell, 2015). In a neoliberal culture, with a strong emphasis on economic freedom, paid work is prioritized over volunteering or caring work (Clouston, 2014). Those out of work are thus imbued with defects such as 'a culture of worklessness', even though in reality there is no evidence that such a culture exists (Shildrick et al., 2012). This justifies the promotion of freedom through coercive means, imposing cuts to bring about behavioural changes (Bell, 2015).

One study looking at language used within the right-wing media reporting of people with disabilities between 2005 to 2010, found an increase in pejorative terms and in a focus on fraudulent claims (Briant et al., 2013). This representation has impacted on the British public's attitude towards welfare for disadvantaged groups, which has hardened: while 81% of people believed government should ensure a decent standard of living for unemployed people in 1985, only 56% believed so in 2012 (Appleby et al., 2013).

FROM CITIZENS TO DENIZENS

Citizenship has been defined as 'a status bestowed on those who are full members of a community' (Marshall, 1950, p. 149). There is, however, a tension between universal human rights which should apply to all and rights gained in citizenship which are confined to those with a certain status, nationalized rights (Standing, 2014). In the *Origins of Totalitarianism*, considering the stripping away of rights for Jews in Nazi Germany, Arendt (1963, p. 297) considers the importance of the 'right to have rights', arguing the risk that when people are reduced to nothing more than being humans, without political or civil rights, they may no longer be viewed as fellow humans. Increasingly, people in the UK are becoming *denizens*, having a limited range of rights, doing insecure forms of work that are unlikely to help them build a meaningful identity or career (Standing, 2011). *Denizens* was a term that originally applied to foreigners allowed certain rights in their adopted country. The age of austerity is the first time in history where governments are reducing the rights of their own citizens, whilst further weakening the rights of more traditional denizens, such as immigrants (Standing, 2014).

In Austerity UK, civil rights, including social freedom and equality, are under threat for particular groups, including the out-of-work. There has been an increasing penalization of out-of-work individuals through a behaviourist philosophy relying on 'deterrence, surveillance, stigma and graduated sanctions to modify conduct' (Wacquant, 2010, p. 199). A new tier of extremely punitive social security payment sanctions was introduced with the Welfare Reform Act (2012), where payments could be stopped for any period from between 4 weeks (for the first 'offense') to up to 3 years. Over a million people were sanctioned in 2014 for a minimum of 3 weeks, frequently for reasons such as missing an appointment due to bereavement, for failing to look for a job on Christmas Day or for being 5 minutes late (Butler, 2015). The underlying assumption is that such punitive measures can effect behavioural changes, increasing autonomy and 'choice' (Bell, 2015). In situations such as this, where politics works through zones of exclusion, people may be reduced to a hand-to-mouth existence, lacking basic necessities that support life, or give it meaning (Agamben, 1998).

Duffy (2013) condemns the cuts to public expenditure that target disabled people disproportionately: people with the severest disabilities are affected 19 times more than the general population. For example, recent changes to the assessment of individuals unable to work through disability or illness were justified by the UK government as aiming to bring about a 'culture of responsibility' (Wright, 2011). This can cause stress in having to 'prove' a disability to someone who does not understand the full effect of this condition: almost half of people living with multiple sclerosis believed the face-to-face assessments for Employment and Support Allowance caused their condition to deteriorate or relapse (Multiple Sclerosis Society, n.d.). Campaign group Black Triangle (2014) identified over 40 cases directly linking deaths of benefits claimants to the removal or reduction of disability benefits. In a recent case, a 59-year-old man with diabetes, who gave up regular work to look after his mother with dementia, was sanctioned for 4 weeks. He was subsequently found dead. The fridge, where he kept his insulin, was not working as the electricity had been cut off. He had a total of £3.44 in his bank account, and tests showed he had an empty stomach at the time of death (Lansley and Mack, 2015).

Increased labour market flexibility, a requirement of neoliberalism, has led to reduced protection against loss of employment and the rise in zero hours contracts, part-time work and other forms of precarious labour (Standing, 2011). By the end of 2013 in the UK, two thirds of a million public sector jobs had been lost, and wage freezes for the remaining public sector workers were introduced (O'Hara, 2014).

As freedoms are undermined, there is a rising anger at blocked avenues for a meaningful life, despair, chronic anxiety and people feeling alienated from both their work and the democratic process (Standing, 2011). This has the potential to impact on the freedoms and occupations of all, as the varying groups of denizens become a new, dangerous class-in-the-making: floating, rudderless and potentially angry, capable of veering to the extreme right or extreme left politically and backing populist demagoguery that plays on their fears or phobias (Standing, 2011).

CONCLUSION

Freedom can be used to justify many forms of exploitation and inequality, thus supporting the rights of the powerful rather than the vulnerable (Monbiot, 2011). There is a need to move beyond the current narrow perspective of economic freedom (Pedwell, 2010). Instead of an age of austerity and individual freedom, an alternative vision for society needs to be developed: one that promotes political, social and occupational rights and freedoms of all groups, as opposed to promoting agendas of the elite or privileged. For occupational therapists, this must start with the willingness to critically examine and question the validity of collective assumptions and perspectives, both within the profession and outside (Petrenchik, 2006).

In order to play a part in working towards overcoming structural inequalities, educational programmes should be reviewed to train students in 'structural competency', helping them develop the ability to listen to structural stories, as well as individual stories, and consider the 'downstream implications of upstream decisions' made within cultures of oppression and privilege (Hansen et al., 2014, p. 128). Focusing on occupational rights will encourage occupational therapists to promote the rights of all to engage in occupations that contribute to both their own well-being and that of their communities (Whalley Hammell, 2008).

The prevailing ideology of autonomy, self-sufficiency and personal responsibility', promoted through discourses of austerity, allows society to be imagined as made up of self-interested individuals able to manage their own resources (Fineman, 2008, p. 10). Occupational therapists need to play a part in promoting an alternative perspective, where dependency is seen as part of the human condition: We are all born, die, experience infancy or childhood, live with the threat of injury or disease and natural disaster beyond our control (Fineman, 2004). Some of these threats have been exacerbated in an age of austerity, including threats of income or job loss. Therefore we need a society that offers support to those with few resources without stigmatizing them (Fineman, 2004).

Concepts within occupational therapy that focus on independence and autonomy, in line with liberal perspectives of freedom, should be reviewed. Rather than independence, an alternative perspective of humans as inherently vulnerable across the life span (Fineman, 2008) provides a practical model for a radical reorganization of the world and a society that rests on ideals of interdependence (Grear, 2013). Understanding vulnerability as inherent within the human condition and working within a vulnerability model could help promote ideas for a new social contract that supports a less oppressive, more equal society, based on freedom and rights.

REFERENCES

Agamben, G., 1998. Homo Sacer: Sovereign Power and the Bare Life. Stanford University Press, Palo Alto, CA.

Appleby, J., Bryson, C., Clery, E., Curtice, J., Devine, P., Heath, A., et al., 2013. British Social Attitudes: The 30th Report. <http://bsa-30.natcen.ac.uk/contributors.aspx> (accessed 10.10.15.).

Arendt, H., 1963. The Origins of Totalitarianism. Harvest Books, London.

Ashton, J.R., Middleton, J., Lang, T., 2014. Open letter to Prime Minister David Cameron on food poverty in the UK. Lancet 383 (9929), 1631.

Baker, D., 2006. The Conservative Nanny State: How the Wealthy Use Government to Stay Rich and Get Richer. Centre for Policy and Economic Research, Washington, DC.

Bauman, Z., 1988. Freedom. Open University Press, Milton Keynes, UK.

Bauman, Z., 2005. Work, Consumerism and the New Poor, second ed. Open University Press, Maidenhead, UK.

Beagan, B.L., 2007. Experiences of social class: learning from occupational therapy students. Can. J. Occup. Ther. 74 (2), 125–133.

Bell, E., 2015. Soft Power and Freedom Under the Coalition: State-Corporate Power and the Threat to Democracy. Palgrave Macmillan, London.

Berlin, I., 2002. Two concepts of liberty. In: Berlin, I., Hardy, H. (Eds.), Liberty: Incorporating Four Essays on Liberty. Oxford University Press, Oxford.

Black Triangle Campaign, 2014. UK Welfare Reform Deaths: Updated List. October 21st 2014. <http://blacktrianglecampaign.org/2014/10/21/uk-welfare-reform-deaths-updated-list-october-21st-2014/> (accessed 01.11.15.).

Blyth, M., 2013. Austerity: The History of a Dangerous Idea. Oxford University Press, Oxford.

Bordieu, P., 1984. Distinction: A Social Critique of the Judgement of Taste. Routledge, Abingdon, UK.

Brass, T., 2015. Free markets, unfree labour: old questions answered, new answers questioned. J. Contemp. Asia 45 (3), 531–540.

Briant, E., Watson, N., Philo, G., 2013. Reporting disability in the age of austerity: the changing face of media representation of disability and disabled people in the United Kingdom and the creation of new 'folk devils'. Disabil. Soc. 28 (6), 874–889.

Bronner, S.E., 2004. Reclaiming the Enlightenment: Towards a Politics of Radical Engagement. Columbia University Press, New York.

Butler, P., 2015. Benefits sanctions: the 10 trivial breaches and administrative errors. The Guardian. 24 May 2015. <http://www.theguardian.com/society/2015/mar/24/benefit-sanctions-trivial-breaches-and-administrative-errors> (accessed 10.07.15.).

Chakrabortty, A., 2015. Cameron's workers v shirkers scam has at last exposed the Tory law of benefit cuts. The Guardian. 31 March 2015. Available at: <http://www.theguardian.com/commentisfree/2015/mar/31/cameron-workers-shirkers-tory-law-benefit-cuts-deserving-poor> (accessed 20.06.15.).

Clouston, T., 2014. Whose occupational balance is it anyway? The challenge of neoliberal capitalism and work-life imbalance. Br. J. Occup. Ther. 77 (10), 507–515.

Corak, M., 2013. Income inequality, equality of opportunity and intergenerational mobility. J. Econ. Perspect. 27 (3), 79–102.

Dasgupta, P., 1986. Positive freedom, markets and the welfare state. Oxf. Rev. Econ. Policy 2 (2), 25–37.

Dorling, D., 2014. Inequality and the 1%. Verso, London.

Duffell, N., 2014. Wounded Leaders: British Elitism and the Entitlement Illusion: A Psychohistory. Lone Arrow Press, London.

Duffy, S., 2013. A Fair Society? How the Cuts Target Disabled People. Centre for Welfare Reform, Sheffield, UK. Available at: <http://www.centreforwelfarereform.org/library/type/pdfs/a-fair-society1.html> (accessed 20.06.15.).

Fineman, M.A., 2004. The Autonomy Myth: A Theory of Dependency. New Press, New York.

Fineman, M.A., 2008. The vulnerable subject: anchoring inequality in the human condition. Yale J. Law Fem. 20 (1), 1–23. Available at: <http://ssrn.com/abstract=1131407> (accessed 01.11.15.).

Freedom of Information Act, 2000. The Stationary Office. <http://www.legislation.gov.uk/ukpga/2000/36> (accessed 20.10.15.).

Gash, T., Panchamia, N., Sims, S., Hotson, L., 2013. Making Public Service Markets Work: Professionalising Government's Approach to Commissioning and Market Stewardship. Institute for Government, London. Available at: <http://www.instituteforgovernment.org.uk/sites/default/files/publications/Making_public_service_markets_work_final_0.pdf> (accessed 01.11.15.).

Gray, J., 2008. Black Mass: Apocalyptic Religion and the Death of Utopia. Penguin Books, London.

Grear, A., 2013. Vulnerability, advanced global capitalism and co-symptomatic injustice: locating the vulnerable subject. In: Fineman, M.A., Grear, A. (Eds.), Vulnerability: Reflections on a New Ethical Foundation for Law and Politics. Ashgate Publishing Limited, Farnham, UK.

Hansen, H., Borgois, P., Drucker, E., 2014. Pathologising poverty: new forms of diagnosis, disability and structural stigma under welfare reform. Soc. Sci. Med. 103, 76–83.

Hocking, C., 2012. Working for citizenship: the dangers of occupational deprivation. Work 41, 391–395.

Hocking, C., 2014. Editorial: occupational therapists driving societal change. Br. J. Occup. Ther. 77 (12), 591.

Jones, O., 2015. The Establishment and How They Get Away with It. Penguin Books, London.

Kallen, E., 2004. Social Inequality and Social Injustice: A Human Rights Perspective. Palgrave Macmillan, London.

Kelley, R.D.G., 2012. Foreword. In: Davis, A.Y. (Ed.), The Meaning of Freedom: And Other Difficult Dialogues. City Lights Books, San Francisco.

Kondo, N., Sembajwe, G., Kawachi, I., van Dam, R.M., Subramanian, S.V., Yamagata, Z., 2009. Income inequality, mortality and self-rated health: meta-analysis of multilevel studies. Br. Med. J. 339, b4471.

Lansley, S., Mack, J., 2015. Breadline Britain: The Rise of Mass Poverty. Oneworld Publications, London.

Mabbett, D., 2013. The second time as tragedy? Welfare reform under Thatcher and the Coalition. Polit. Q. 84 (1), 43–53.

Marshall, T.H., 1950. Citizenship and social class. In: Manzer, J., Sauder, M. (Eds.), Inequality and Society. Dickinson College, Carlisle, PA, pp. 148–154. Available at: <http://users.dickinson.edu/~mitchelk/readings/marshall-citizenship-and-social-class.pdf> (accessed 20.10.15.).

McBain, S., 2015. The new poor in an age of austerity: why are so many people using food banks? New Statesman. 27 March–9 April 2015. Available at: <http://www.newstatesman.com/politics/2015/03/why-are-so-many-people-using-food-banks> (accessed 20.06.15.).

McKenzie, L., 2015. Estates, Class and Culture in Austerity Britain. Policy Press, Bristol, UK.

Mendoza, K.A., 2015. The Demolition of the Welfare State and the Rise of the Zombie Economy. New Internationalist Publications Ltd, Oxford.

Monbiot, G., 2011. This bastardised libertarianism makes 'freedom' an instrument of oppression. The Guardian. 19 December 2011. Available at: <http://www.theguardian.com/commentisfree/2011/dec/19/bastardised-libertarianism-makes-freedom-oppression> (accessed 01.11.15.).

Multiple Sclerosis Society, n.d. MS: Enough. Make Welfare Make Sense. MS Society UK, London.

National Audit Office, 2015. Progress in Improving Cancer Services and Outcomes in England. Department of Health and NHS England. <https://www.nao.org.uk/wp-content/uploads/2015/01/Progress-improving-cancer-services-and-outcomes-in-England.pdf> (accessed 01.11.15.).

National Health Service and Finance Directorate, 2015. 2015/16 Choice Framework. Department of Health. <https://www.gov.uk/government/uploads/system/uploads/attachment_data/file/417057/Choice_Framework_2015-16.pdf> (accessed 01.11.15.).

National Health Service Support Federation, 2015. NHS for Sale? Proving NHS Privatisation. <http://www.nhsforsale.info/database.html> (accessed 01.11.15.).

Nayak, A., 2006. Displaced masculinities: chavs, youths and class in the post industrial city. Sociology 40 (5), 813–831.

Nolan, A., 2014. Introduction. In: Nolan, A. (Ed.), Economic and Social Rights after the Global Financial Crisis. Cambridge University Press, Cambridge.

O'Cinneide, C., 2014. Austerity and the faded dream of a 'social Europe'. In: Nolan, A. (Ed.), Economic and Social Rights after the Global Financial Crisis. Cambridge University Press, Cambridge.

O'Hara, M., 2014. Austerity Bites: A Journey to the Sharp End of Cuts in the UK. Policy Press, Bristol.

Organisation for Economic Co-operation and Development, 2009. OECD Strategic Response to the Financial and Economic Crisis: Contributions to the Global Effort. Organisation for Economic Co-operation and Development. <http://www.oecd.org/economy/42061463.pdf> (accessed 01.10.15.).

Organisation for Economic Co-operation and Development, 2011. Divided We Stand: Why Inequality Keeps Rising. Organisation for Economic Co-operation and Development. <http://www.oecd.org/els/soc/49170768.pdf> (accessed 01.11.15.).

Oxfam Briefing Paper, 2012. The perfect storm: economic stagnation, the rising cost of living, public spending cuts, and the impact on UK poverty. <http://policy-practice.oxfam.org.uk/publications/the-perfect-storm-economic-stagnation-the-rising-cost-of-living-public-spending-228591> (accessed 01.11.15.).

Pedwell, C., 2010. Feminism, Culture and Embodied Practice. Routledge, Abingdon, UK.

Petrenchik, T., 2006. Homelessness: perspectives, misconceptions and considerations for occupational therapy. Occup. Ther. Health Care 20 (3–4), 9–30.

Sen, A., 1999. Development as Freedom. Oxford University Press, Oxford.

Sen, A., 2015. Amartya Sen: the economic consequences of austerity. New Statesman. 4 June 2015. Available at: <http://www.newstatesman.com/politics/2015/06/amartya-sen-economic-consequences-austerity> (accessed 10.07.15.).

Sepulveda Carmona, M., 2014. Alternatives to austerity: a human rights framework for economic recovery. In: Nolan, A. (Ed.), Economic and Social Rights after the Global Financial Crisis. Cambridge University Press, Cambridge.

Shildrick, T., MacDonald, R., Furlong, A., Roden, J., Crow, R., 2012. Are 'cultures of worklessness' passed down the generations? Joseph Rowntree Foundations. <http://www.jrf.org.uk/publications/cultures-of-worklessness> (accessed 01.07.15.).

Shiller, R.S., 2003. The New Financial Order: Risk in the 21st Century. Princeton University Press, Woodstock, UK.

Siedentop, L., 2014. Inventing the Individual: The Origins of Western Liberalism. Penguin Books, Milton Keynes.

Silvestri, M., Crowther-Dowey, C., 2008. Gender and Crime. SAGE Publications Ltd., London.

Social Mobility and Child Poverty Commission, 2014a. Elitist Britain? <https://www.gov.uk/government/publications/elitist-britain> (accessed 10.07.15.).

Social Mobility and Child Poverty Commission, 2014b. State of the Nation 2014: Social Mobility and Child Poverty in Great Britain. <https://www.gov.uk/government/uploads/system/uploads/attachment_data/file/365765/State_of_Nation_2014_Main_Report.pdf> (accessed 20.10.15.).

Standing, G., 2011. The Precariat: The New, Dangerous Class. Bloomsbury Academic, London.

Standing, G., 2014. A Precariat Charter: From Denizens to Citizens. Bloomsbury Academic, London.

Still, J., 2012. A fictional response to the categorical imperative: women refugees, servants and slaves in Charriere's Trois Femmes. In: Oergel, M. (Ed.), (Re)-writing the Radical: Enlightenment, Revolution and Cultural Transfer in 1790s Germany, Britain and France. Walter de Gruyter, Munich.

Wacquant, L., 2010. Crafting the neoliberal state: workfare, prison fare and social insecurity. Sociol. Forum 25 (2), 197–202.

Welfare Reform Act, 2012. <http://www.legislation.gov.uk/ukpga/2012/5/contents/enacted> (accessed 01.11.15.).

Whalley Hammell, K., 2008. Reflections on … wellbeing and occupational rights. Can. J. Occup. Ther. 75 (1), 61–64.

Whalley Hammell, K., 2015. Quality of life, participation and occupational rights: a capabilities perspective. Aust. Occup. Ther. J. 62, 78–85.

Whalley Hammell, K.R., Iwama, M.K., 2012. Wellbeing and occupational rights: an imperative for critical occupational therapy. Scand. J. Occup. Ther. 19 (5), 385–394.

Wilkinson, R., Pickett, K., 2009. The Spirit Level: Why Equality is Better for Everyone. Penguin Books, London.

Wright, O., 2011. Welfare changes are about changing our culture, says Cameron. The Independent. 23 October 2011. Available at: <http://www.independent.co.uk/news/uk/politics/welfare-changes-are-about-changing-our-culture-says-cameron-2217448.html> (accessed 01.11.15.).

Young, I.M., 2000. Inclusion and Democracy. Oxford University Press, Oxford.

37

STORIES IN TIMES OF CRISIS: REFLECTIONS FROM A PROFESSIONAL DEVELOPMENT AND SUPPORT GROUP IN GREECE

MARIA KOULOUMPI ▪ THEODOROS BOGEAS ▪ EFTYCHIA KALIMANA ▪ IVI KOTSINI ▪ MARTHA KOKKOROU ▪ MARIA ZOUMPOPOULOU ▪ MARIA MARGARI ▪ SOFIA KELEMOURIDOU ▪ MARIA KATSAMAGKOU

We share common philosophies, values of the profession and approaches. We codesign all these and we create a common professional culture.

Eleni, 2014

CHAPTER OUTLINE

I n 2007, some members of the Hellenic Association of Ergotherapists[1] (HEA) actively involved in developing further the profession, initiated discussions regarding the standards of occupational therapy practice in Greece. Inspired by members of the board of the Hellenic Association of Ergotherapists, Sarah Kantartzis and Maria Kouloumpi (coordinators of the continuing professional development programme of the HEA) established a task force group in order to organize actions around the most urgent needs, leading to the development of a continuing professional development programme called 'Learning to Learn 1' (LtL1). Linking theory to everyday practice, LtL1 was focused on the needs of newly qualified occupational therapists. In 2011, 'Learning to Learn 2' (LtL2) followed, attracting professionals from the whole of Greece.

Through a very spontaneous but engaging process, graduates of LtL1 and LtL2 and their tutors developed a discussion group called 'with occupation at the epicentre' (WOE). The initial aim of the group was the exchange of ideas and problem solving in occupational therapy practice. The vision of the group was, and still is, to develop an understanding of occupation in Greece and to promote an understanding of the

---

[1]Ergotherapist is a transliteration of the Greek term εργοθεραπευτής, where *ergo* means 'occupation'.

importance of continuing professional development for occupational therapists.

This chapter aims to share a collection of thoughts and ideas generated through discussions among members of the WOE group regarding their stories and experiences during the early phase of the Eurozone debt crisis in Greece (2008–2014). These reflections form the idea that the WOE group functioned as a counterbalance to members' experiences, within an ongoing crisis situation that had an impact on an emotional, personal, professional, social, occupational, and political level. Being together in the group provided a safe space for all members, helping them deal with feelings of personal disappointment and professional burnout caused by the impact of the financial crisis.

In the paragraphs below, we introduce the WOE group and the context within which it was formed. After that we move on to describe how the participants of the WOE group experience occupational injustice in the form of occupational imbalance, occupational deprivation and occupational alienation (Kronenberg and Pollard, 2005; Townsend and Wilcock, 2004; Whiteford, 2000; Wilcock, 1998), and how adaptation can occur through occupation. In order to highlight the collectivity of the ideas and give life to reflections and experiences as verbalized by the group participants, we will be using direct quotations from group members throughout the chapter (all names used are pseudonyms). Towards the end of the chapter we will describe the importance of the notion of a community of practice as a vision for the future of the group.

CONTEXT: AUSTERITY AND CRISIS IN GREECE

The global economic recession that started in October 2008 triggered the Eurozone debt crisis[2], which resulted in the gradual collapse of the Greek economy. On 23 April 2010, the Greek government announced that Greece had resorted to the help of the International Monetary Fund, the European Commission and the European Central Bank, which formed a joint aid

mechanism for Greece (thereafter referred to as the *troika* or the *establishments*). A series of austerity measures have been declared ever since, including severe cuts in public spending, tax increases, raising the pension age, and the loss of more than 15 000 jobs in the public sector in the first 2 years since the crisis began (Inman, 2012). The annual percentage growth rate of the gross domestic product (GDP) of the country was −0.4% for 2008, −5.4% for 2010, and −8.9% for 2011 (World Bank, 2015). The total household income in Greece was reduced by one-third between 2007 and 2012. The number of people saying they cannot cover their nutritional needs has also doubled (Organisation for Economic Co-operation and Development, 2014). One of the major consequences of the economic crisis is increasing unemployment. The unemployment rate in March 2014, according to Eurostat, was 26.80% while the youth unemployment rate[3] was 57.7% (Eurostat, 2014a, 2014b).

The Organization for Economic Co-Operation and Development (2014) mentioned that, although economic output in Greece was projected to gradually recover, unemployment rates were high while income and the gross domestic product remained far below precrisis levels (Organisation for Economic Co-operation and Development, 2014). Furthermore, job insecurity, income reduction, poverty and an increase in the incidence of mental illness are among the most serious consequences of the crisis. As a result of the increase in the incidence of mental illness, including anxiety and major depression, suicide rates increased by 40% in the first half of 2011, compared with the same period in 2010 (Ifanti et al., 2013). In addition, the incidence of some communicable diseases, such as the human immunodeficiency virus (HIV), has increased significantly. The number of new HIV infections reported between 2007 and 2010 was 10 to 15 every year among injecting drug users. This number increased to 256 in 2011 and to 314 in the first 8 months of 2012 (Quaglio et al., 2013).

Kentikelenis (2014) described several policies which shifted medical costs to patients, such as an increase in

---

copayments for medicines, an additional fee for admission to public hospitals and hidden costs (e.g., increased cost of telephone calls to schedule appointments with doctors). The most crucial point is that social health insurance coverage is linked with employment status. Rapidly increasing unemployment has increased the number of uninsured people, leading to a reduction in healthcare access (Kentikelenis et al., 2014).

A United Nations Children's Emergency Fund (UNICEF) report has revealed the enormous effect of the financial crisis on the living conditions of children in Greece. Of the households of those living below the poverty threshold with children, 74.1% have reported that they cannot cover their basic needs, such as adequate nutrition (Kalmouki, 2014). The crisis has also affected the field of education in a detrimental way. Children of any age experience an inadequate educational environment since there were significant cuts of state funding in primary and higher education, as well as in special needs education (Giavrimis and Papanis, 2011).

HOW THE STORY BEGAN: FROM LEARNING TO LEARN TO THE 'WITH OCCUPATION AT THE EPICENTRE' (WOE) GROUP

The LtL programme was first introduced in 2008, and the need to develop and maintain a lifelong learning culture led to LtL2 2 years later. Both of these programmes ran over 1 year and they combined theory and practice, based on the European competences for occupational therapy (TUNING Occupational Therapy Project Group, 2008). Students in both programmes had to study individually and develop innovative practices (Nikas et al., 2010). Each meeting was divided into lectures (first part) and support/supervision groups (second part) according to each participant's work area (for example, paediatric occupational therapy or psychosocial occupational therapy) (Helena et al., 2009). The second part involved supervision on professional issues referring to the application of theory in daily practice (Helena et al., 2009; Nikas et al., 2010). The topics included generic and occupational therapy competences, learning techniques (mind-mapping or keeping a reflective diary),

processes (clinical reasoning, practice portfolios, project management, ethical practice or evidence-based practice), occupational science, visioning exercises, and more (Helena et al., 2009; Nikas et al., 2010).

At the end of the LtL2 programme, when the first memorandum for national financial help was signed by the then Greek government, the financial crisis had already had a great impact on everyday lives at ethical, personal, professional, social, economic, and political levels. A common need of LtL graduates for communication and peer support led to the creation of the group WOE. In the first few meetings, an open invitation was sent to all participants of both LtL1 and LtL2 programmes and gradually, meeting by meeting, the main group was formed.

The nature of the WOE group, which consisted of ex-tutors and LtL graduates, was, and continues to be, egalitarian; there are no longer students and tutors, and there are no coordinators of the group, as we all participate equally. The format of the group was formulated during these long meetings and facilitated through sharing lunch or dinners that enhanced our bonding. Our discussions have been of a managerial, emotional, practical, political, and economic nature. The group meetings have been taking place anywhere that was available (our homes, national association or public places). From the beginning of the group, we decided to contribute a symbolic amount of money at each meeting to a group fund, which could be used to buy books, to subscribe to occupational therapy associations, to access electronic journals or as seed money for future projects. An exploration of models and frameworks (such as the American Occupational Therapy Framework (American Occupational Therapy Association, 2014)) guided our discussions, helping us explore different concepts and processes while enabling reflections around our practice.

Through the first years of the multifaceted financial crisis, the main function of our group had been to support the practise of our profession and our continuing professional development. This group enacted solidarity to generate opportunities, through knowledge exchange, sharing of experiences and the creation of a safe and trustful atmosphere.

Our monthly meetings provide 'food for thought' to all of us, against the chaotic financial situation (see Table 37-1). Some members of the group live

	TABLE 37-1
	Quotes From the Members of the Group 'With Occupation at the Epicentre'
Pseudonyms	**Quotes**
Eleni	I am seeking my occupational balance among all things. The working hours are for the money, the extra professional hours are for pleasure. It is now clear that our whole life is based on money. Doing – being – becoming has changed to I have – I can – I survive. Difficult situations, like coins, have sometimes two sides: an opportunity and an obstacle.
Elli	My profession is my passion and every day I wholeheartedly dedicate myself to it, doing the best I can. I have been working with children with pervasive developmental disorders and learning disabilities for the past 6 years. I am always next to the children I work with, to help them learn, play, love, feel and come to terms with their difference. My feedback from them is hope, patience, satisfaction, so I become more willing to go on.
Marina	It was not only my personal life that was at stake because of the crisis, or my professional survival through my work. It had also to do with the people I was working with, my clients. I had to digest that feeling of being very small and insufficient to provide them with the services they needed, like I had to be alone and bear the burden of the whole system collapsing around us. My love for working in the mental health sector made me stay longer in a job where the working conditions are deteriorating and the services delivered are compromised.
Mara	I am feeling that the slow and mindful development of this group becomes the counterbalance to the biases and the uncontrolled changes we face in our everyday life.
Elina	My initial desire was to do a master's degree in the UK. Financial constraints changed my plans and made me choose a distance learning course. On the altar of money and survival of the professionals, ethical practice, therapeutic relationship, partnership protocols are forgotten. Roles between professionals are blurred. Caring: this is the core element of everyone in this group. We love to care – ourselves, others, the context we want to live in.
Melina	I live away from Athens and I am a freelance occupational therapist. How am I going to face the everyday challenges of my job with all the demands of continuous professional development when I have to struggle for my economic survival?
Artemis	Since I graduated I had the feeling that I was alone trying to build by myself my way of becoming an occupational therapist. I had to travel 700 km in order to join the continuing professional development programme and be a member in WOE group. I am not satisfied because I have to interact with the others mostly through Skype. Personal contact cannot be replaced.
Eva	As a professional in the paediatric field of occupational therapy in private centres, working with children makes me happier, more playful, childlike innocent and honest. It makes me feel alive and more active in my everyday life. I feel like I gain priceless things from my job. These elements are what I keep in mind when I have an obstacle to overcome in my professional life in this time of economic crisis. Being a member of WOE helps me balance the stress and the concerns raised in my professional practice, and makes me feel a more conscious and responsible therapist. This group helps me to develop not only as a professional but also as a person.
Antigoni	I live in the countryside and try to work with different patients without other occupational therapists in the area. Every day is a new challenge. I have to be creative and make the tools I need for work, because it's difficult to find them at the local market and I cannot buy them online. The WOE helps me to be organized in my job and always in touch with the progress of occupational therapy. The group helps me to grow and mature as a therapist.
Alexia	Above my flat there is a terrace, with an open space between the solar panels. There is a corner wall there where you can stand and see the view around. One summer night I was hot and feeling sad after a long day I had to put up with people that use the crisis in order to exercise power and control. Fed up staying in at home once more, I took a stool and a big glass of iced water and spent some time up there on the terrace. And guess what? The view was great far towards Acropolis and around to Penteli and Ymittos mountains. It felt I was at a luxurious place, for free, having a new perspective of my life. The next time I went up there my neighbours joined me bringing over some music; we felt so rich!! Being rich in times of crisis. This is about occupational enrichment: creating meaning within our identity, creating meaning with others, engaging in collective occupations.

This table contains spoken and written reflections, ideas, experiences, worries and thoughts during the writing process that represent the 'way of being' a member in WOE group, the very personal identity of every participant.

hundreds of kilometres away from Athens, the capital of Greece, and experience professional isolation as the only occupational therapist in their practice. In order to develop an inclusive communication, we use a variety of means including e-mails, video calls, and file sharing. The group meets at weekends, and many times our meetings have some very young listeners – our own children.

NARRATING STORIES THROUGH AN OCCUPATIONAL THERAPY LENS

The Context

This chapter was written in 2014, the sixth continuous year since the financial crisis began. Being an occupational therapist in Greece during those years of crisis provided a variety of perspectives of what austerity means and how it affects everyday life, especially when we are witnessing the human struggle around us, for some more obvious, but for others, covered nicely under dignity and pride.

Many people have seen their salaries being reduced or unexpectedly they have to pay high taxes and *charatsi* (a special tax for land and property), while others have lost their jobs or have no income at all and are surviving with the support of family and friends. Of course, *'having less income not only means that you might not have enough money to buy food, but also that participation in important occupations* [e.g., education, leisure activities] *is restricted'* (Alexia, Melina). Unemployment influences the ability of people to cover their everyday needs and *'provokes negative feelings of insecurity, pessimism, stress, fear, guilt, victimization, and lack of hope'* (Marina, Eleni). It feels that *'we are losing our roles'* (Elli) that go together with a number of routines (e.g., consuming quality food) and habits (e.g., treating friends, eating out) that make life humane and give meaning to everyday life. *'We are losing our identity as we knew it'* (Elli, Elina), and slowly the financial crisis becomes an occupational crisis that drifts the individual into a crisis of identity.

Occupational Challenges

Ideally, an occupationally just society enables access to both opportunities and resources necessary for carrying out occupations (Townsend and Wilcock, 2004). Participation in all aspects of life should be ensured in

a way that all people flourish by doing what is useful and meaningful for them. The financial crisis in Greece has led to restrictions to people's participation through limiting the access to basic resources for survival, meaning, and maintaining or developing identity.

Widening inequality in the distribution of resources, higher rates of unemployment and deteriorating conditions, especially in the big cities (Kentikelenis et al., 2014; Organisation for Economic Co-operation and Development, 2014), create conditions of deprivation. Occupational deprivation is experienced in different ways by different groups of people. The occupational variety of Greek culture and lifestyle is influenced by the crisis both on a financial and on an emotional level. Occupations that require money, such as *'buying books'* (Eleni), *'clothes'* (Antigoni), pursuing *'further education'* (Elina), *'going out to drink or dine'* (Elli, Alexia), *'using transportation, and buying presents'* (Marina, Alexia), were the first to be disrupted or altogether abandoned within our small group, including our families and friends. Some other occupations were affected in subtler ways; for example, before the crisis, going to visit a friend required carrying an expensive present, such as a cake or a bottle of wine. Nowadays, *'we are facing a dilemma of whether to make the visit or not when we realize we cannot afford this anymore'* (Eva, Artemis).

Many questions arise from the current situation: What are the constituents of our everyday life that reflect our values and cultural identities? What does it mean to live in a city in times of a financial, social and occupational crisis? What does it mean to be poor in our times? How could an occupational therapy perspective inform our ideas?

After our group discussions and a search of definitions around poverty, it was striking to realize that poverty in our pluralistic society is not the lack of money, but the lack of a life with choices, feeling of control, opportunities for self-actualization and social participation. Poverty generates an occupational crisis for the individual living in a society governed by a neoliberal value system.

People from vulnerable groups, especially people with disabilities and refugees, are already living in deprivation due to discrimination rooted in disability, ethnicity, poverty and so on, and are often facing occupational deprivation as they are limited in their participation by external factors (Whiteford, 2000). Due to the financial crisis they are facing additional limitations, such as access to basic goods, healthy food, education, health and employment, housing, leisure activities, and transportation (Wilcock, 1998). Vulnerable populations were the first to suffer from occupational deprivation and imbalance, and they are at risk of experiencing occupational marginalization (Kronenberg and Pollard, 2005). The aggravated inability of these people to exercise choice or control over their daily occupations due to the limited resources may be a source of further injustices and poverty (Townsend and Wilcock, 2003). Stories of everyday life in the media are showing persons facing difficult conditions due to lack of electricity, lack of job or feelings of being a burden to family or society.

The impact of occupational deprivation and imbalance is obvious in the *'lack of choices that people are taking for granted and in the lost opportunities for our self-fulfilment'* (Marina). Lack of employment, devaluation of leisure, imposed or unnecessary rest and over-involvement in stressful job-seeking occupations raise the risk of illnesses, burnout or boredom, and challenge our professional belief according to which health is promoted through the balance between work, leisure and rest (Wilcock, 1998). This generates anger and feelings of hostility, especially when the responsibility for resolving the crisis is passed on to citizens through, for example, extra taxation. This is how the financial crisis was followed by a social crisis and already *'gave the chance to extreme right wing political party* [i.e., Golden Dawn] *to enter the Parliament influencing a large part of the population'* (Eleni). As citizens of a European country, *'we have lost our trust in the state, in the government, in politicians as a whole'* (Marina, Eleni). *'Many of our friends have chosen to leave the country to find a better job and a better life abroad, as their skills and talents were devalued and the conditions of work worsened'* (Antigoni, Artemis).

Challenging Occupation

Existing literature (e.g., Humphry and Womack, 2014; Lerner, 2002; Segal, 2014; Watson and Wilson, 2003; Wilson and Landry, 2014) suggests there are life course transitions that are anticipated as normal parts of life: going to school, leaving the parental home, going to university, finding a good job, gaining financial independence, creating a family, and retiring. In Greece, life transitions are similar, but the meaning attached to every stage varies. Studying at university is highly valued for the young person and the family, which has to provide financial support during those years, creating the phenomenon of *prolonged youth* (Kalmouki, 2014; Tsiganou et al., 1999) *'until their children pursue their independence through a good job or the creation of their own family'* (Artemis). For the young Greek, a university degree is an indicator of a socially valued mental determination and a positive prospect of work that fulfils a shared family vision (Kantartzis, 2013). Finding *'a good job makes the person valued among friends, family, and the broader social arena'* (Eva). For example, *'part of the way Greek adults introduce themselves is by naming their job title or their workplace'* (Eleni). A good job gives a person the opportunities to follow a social lifestyle with *'a variety of mostly collective occupations'* (Mara). The above stages *'reflect the identity building of the individual that seems to move towards these constructed social ideals'* (Alexia). The expansion of crisis and the consequent lack of money at every level of society have affected not only the lifestyle but the whole value system attached to these stages towards being a *person*, especially being a young person in pursuit of interests, education and a job.

'There has to be a priority between our financial needs and our social needs to be connected with others as an element of wellbeing, and our cultural value to "have our hands full" when we step in our friends' houses' (Marina, Eleni, Alexia), otherwise, *'we need to develop alternative ways of being with other people'* (Eleni). For example, instead of buying an expensive cake, people often share a homemade one, adding a personal element that shows mindfulness and caring. So rather than not visiting somebody because they cannot afford an expensive present, people will still visit but bake a cake at home, or bring something thoughtful but inexpensive, like a card made by their children. Our need to adapt to a changing environment pushed us to *'discover "alternative actions", exploring what constitutes our inner meanings and prioritizing according to our identity'* (Antigoni, Alexia, Marina). Making these adaptations *'protects us from occupational deprivation and helps us maintain our identity'* (Eleni, Alexia).

The search for meaning and *'occupational enrichment by those members of the group that they persist to *be optimistic is guided by their mindfulness for their loved ones, for their environment and their need to take care of themselves. This generates solidarity and feelings of safety and trust'* (Antigoni). New habits and trends appear, lending elements of well-being and comfort in our everyday occupations. *'Visiting vintage shops and recycling secondhand clothes or other goods is a journey to the familiar habits of our childhood'* (Marina, Elina). We turn to the past of our Greek lifestyle to draw on optimism, to remember the tenderness of our grandmother's cuisine, with loukoumades,[4] halva[5] and vanilla submarine,[6] cheap nostalgic sweets full of smells and familiar memories (Kinti, 2014), to revive intimate experiences and feelings of safety in the unexpected and inconsistent context we are forced to live in. We borrow leisure activities and collective occupations from provincial towns and villages where we used to spend our hot summers: strolling through the squares, spending time with neighbours, planning nights of table games, exchanging plates of the 'dish of the day' with our friends and making handmade presents, expressing our will to take care of the others and our openness to receive care (Kantartzis, 2013), maintaining our values and our identity.

Challenging Crisis

Five years after the crisis began, Greek society in a rather informal way has silently managed to create communities that can offer food for those who do not have money; recycle goods, such as clothes, furniture, toys, shoes, and household goods; and there is always an empty basket at the end of the supermarket aisle that is filled up at the end of the day by the customers who have something to give. Within our microsystem of friends, clients and neighbours we recycle our things to people or groups in need (e.g., refugees or homeless

people). In the streets you may find something left there for the 'unknown user' (for people who are looking in the rubbish to find something useful) while in the metro, tickets are sometimes shared at the end of the journey.

To the eyes of the foreign visitors who walk through the neighbourhoods of the provincial towns, through the narrow streets full of coffee shops and packed restaurants of the big cities, through the beaches of the islands and the buzzing squares of the towns, life seems to be untouched by the lack of money. It is a paradox, as it is often raised by international tabloids. It seems people are still persisting in daily habits and routines, such as going out, sharing time with friends and family, holding long discussions in cafes, in a need for social interaction and networking with different groups of people, because this is the way we perceive ourselves and others. In Greece, our *social self* (Blue, 1999) attributes a special meaning in collective occupations in everyday life. The Greek self – as a social self – historically bases his or her well-being on a small circle of friends and family as a space of protection, generation of knowledge, occupational enrichment, care, and as a way of developing identity (Blue, 1999). It seems that in times of crisis identity expression is challenged by exploring alternatives for a different understanding of the notion of well-being, which may be a strength in order to counterbalance the effects of the crisis. Therefore, occupation needs to be understood not as a concept reflecting Western understandings of a 'healthy' and 'ideal' way of life but contextually, as what people consider an appropriate and healthy way to live (Kantartzis and Molineux, 2011).

'WITH OCCUPATION AT THE EPICENTRE' AS A COMMUNITY OF PRACTICE AND A VISION FOR THE FUTURE

The idea to describe WOE as a community of practice developed after a group member participated in the 12th European Congress of Occupational Therapy in 2012 in Stockholm, Sweden. A community of practice is 'a learning partnership among people who find it useful to learn from and with each other about a particular domain' (Wenger et al., 2011, p. 9). Initially, our

---

[4]Loukoumades: traditional Greek pastry made of deep-fried dough bathed in honey and spiced with cinnamon (Wikipedia, 2015a).

[5]Halva: traditional Greek sweet made from semolina or tahini (Wikipedia, 2015b).

[6]Vanilla submarine: a thick, snow-white and aromatic sweet paste which is made by beating mastic resin with table sugar. When cold, it has the consistency of hard caramel candy: It is meant to be licked like a lollipop as, at body temperature, it gradually becomes softer and more chewable. This is served on a table spoon in a tall glass of ice-cold water (Wikipedia, 2014).

concern was to support ourselves and share our passion for providing quality services to our clients. As time passed, our shared learning became our central link, through collective doing: studying a practice framework and trying to comprehend it, through interpretation and reflection on the Greek context. Writing this chapter has become our most recent project, encouraging us to further develop the group and design future actions. During writing, we had the opportunity to question our practice, reflect on our shared experiences in the group, shape further our vision and express the need to present our outcomes on continuing learning with the rest of our colleagues through workshops. Finally, we spent more time *together* (physically and digitally), which strengthened our sense of membership, recognizing further what we have in common that links us as a group.

As mentioned above, the crisis has economic, social, personal, and political implications, and members of the WOE group found out that through belonging to the group they can stand and bear the difficulties they live through, searching for innovative practices in a desired context of 'an ideal neighbourhood', that of our *community of practice*. Our community finds colleagues who are supportive, who help others overcome barriers, manage burnout and create a sense of belonging. It permits us to imagine how we would like to become, enables us to be less anxious, more organized, and develop professionally to address the professional isolation we felt before joining the group (COmmunities of PracticE = C.O.P.E.). Members feel more confident; they feel valued, often in contrast to what happens in their work settings, where occupational therapy might not enjoy the same recognition as other professions.

Skills-based but culturally inappropriate practice, a strong biomedical focus, and a reductionist approach to intervention that detracts from occupation are some of the reasons why we need to implement a new contextual, culturally sensitive paradigm that is collectively shaped *from* the members *for* the members of the profession who will, consequently, provide appropriate services to users. The type of education we are engaged in is not a formal setup with learning goals, which in Greek is called εκπαίδευση (*ekpedefsi*); our lessons target our moral, spiritual, social and political education, called παιδεία (*paedia*) (Gould and Kolb,

1972). This education counterbalances the lack of choices due to the general crisis and enables us to withstand the lack of control in the current situation.

AS AN EPILOGUE

This chapter aimed to share the perspectives of the WOE group members during the first 6 years of the financial crisis (2008–2014). Through group discussions, the participants communicated their experiences and perspectives of the impact of crisis in the microsystem of their everyday life (close family, friends, colleagues, and service users). Due to the financial crisis there are widespread financial, social and political transitions, as well as identity transitions that have changed occupations in everyday life. The ongoing occupational crisis produces consequences not only in the pluralism of the Greek lifestyle but also in the content of occupations, the meaning attributed to them and the way people prioritize their actions. Poverty is not necessarily the lack of money but the lack of occupations: the lack of meaningful activities that gives people identity, self-fulfilment and a vision for the future.

By the end of the writing of this chapter the crisis had escalated, causing tremendous political dilemmas in Europe and further impacting on life in Greece through capital controls and a climate of distrust and pessimism. This has forced the citizens to pursue alternative resources for managing everyday life (e.g., recycling goods, cultivating gardens or not using cars) and promote volunteering, offering services to vulnerable populations (e.g., free health centres for uninsured citizens, time banks and free meals).

Drawing from the idea of 'where there is a risk – there is an opportunity', this multifaceted crisis can be seen as a chance for people to counterbalance the lack of money by invoking (or triggering) human capital. Observing the ways that the Greek society has been activated in order to survive the crisis may offer an insight to elements of culture that enrich experiences of everyday life and put to question the dominant neoliberal values. The WOE group proposes a lifestyle that supports people to confront issues collectively and exercise values, such as sharing and caring, solidarity and group problem solving that can lead to occupational enrichment. The creation of a new way of *being well* in critical times should be the vision of our profession for the well-being of the people living in occupational crisis.

REFERENCES

American Occupational Therapy Association, 2014. Occupational Therapy Practice Framework: Domain and Process. Am. J. Occup. Ther. 68 (Suppl. 1), S1–S48.

Blue, A., 1999. The Making of Greek Psychiatry (Greek Translation). Exantas, Athens, Greece.

European Commission: Economic and Financial Affairs, 2014. Why did the crisis happen? <http://ec.europa.eu/economy_finance/explained/the_financial_and_economic_crisis/why_did_the_crisis_happen/index_en.htm> (accessed 20.03.15.).

Eurostat, 2014a. EU Labor Force Survey Report, Eurostat. <https://ycharts.com/indicators/sources/eurostat> (accessed 30.07.14.).

Eurostat, 2014b. Harmonized unemployment rate by sex. <http://ec.europa.eu/eurostat/tgm/table.do?tab=table&language=en&pcode=teilm020&tableSelection=1&plugin=1> (accessed 30.07.14.).

Eurostat, Statistics Explained: Glossary. 2014c. <http://ec.europa.eu/eurostat/statistics-explained/index.php/Glossary:Youth_unemployment> (accessed 25.03.15.).

Giavrimis, P., Papanis, E., 2011. Erevna, ekpaideftiki politiki kai praksi stin eidiki agogi. (Research, educational policy and practice in special education.) University of the Aegean, Mytilene, Greece.

Gould, J., Kolb, W., 1972. A Dictionary of the Social Sciences (Greek translation: Panagiotis Lamprias). Hellenic Education, Athens, Greece.

Helena, D., Taha, F., Katsoupa, E., Kouloumpi, M., Koustimpi, M., Kantartzis, S., et al., 2009. Learning to Learn: Programme for support of Continuing Professional Development of newly qualified occupational therapists. In: 5th Panhellenic Congress of Occupational Therapists, Athens, Greece.

Humphry, R., Womack, J., 2014. Transformation of occupations: a life course perspective. In: Schell, B.A., et al. (Eds.), Willard and Spackman's Occupational Therapy, twelfth ed. Lippincott Williams & Wilkins, Philadelphia, pp. 163–172.

Ifanti, A.A., et al., 2013. Financial crisis and austerity measures in Greece: their impact on health promotion policies and public health care. Health Policy (New York) 113 (1–2), 8–12.

Inman, P., 2012. Greek debt crisis: timeline. The Guardian. <http://www.theguardian.com/business/2012/mar/09/greek-debt-crisis-timeline> (accessed 30.07.14.).

Kalmouki, N., 2014. UNICEF, Hundreds of Greek children living in poverty. GreekReporter.com. <http://greece.greekreporter.com/2014/04/03/unicef-hundreds-of-greek-children-living-in-poverty> (accessed 30.07.14.).

Kantartzis, S., 2013. Conceptualizing occupation: an ethnographic study of daily life in a Greek town. Doctoral Thesis. Leeds Metropolitan University, Leeds, UK.

Kantartzis, S., Molineux, M., 2011. The influence of Western society's construction of a healthy daily life on the conceptualisation of occupation. J. Occup. Sci. 18 (1), 62–80.

Kentikelenis, A., Karanikolos, M., Reeves, A., Mckee, M., Stuckler, D., 2014. Greece's health crisis: from austerity to denialism. Lancet 383 (9918), 748–753.

Kinti, S., 2014. Editorial, Foodie 02. Issue. <http://issuu.com/dimitrisalpanezos/docs/foodie2> (accessed 28.03.15.).

Kronenberg, F., Pollard, N., 2005. Overcoming occupational apartheid: a preliminary exploration of the political nature of occupational therapy. In: Kronenberg, F., Simo Algado, S., Pollard, N. (Eds.), Occupational Therapy Without Borders, vol. 1: Learning From The Spirit of Survivors. Churchill Livingstone, Edinburgh, pp. 58–86.

Lapavitsas, C., 2012. Preface. In: Crisis in the Eurozone. Verso, London.

Lerner, R.M., 2002. Concepts and Theories of Human Development, third ed. Lawrence Erlbaum Associates, Mahwah, NJ.

Nikas, N., Lada, M., Makri, K., Kantartzis, S., Kouloumpi, M., Elena, D., et al., 2010. Creating synergy for continuing professional development in a national association: an example of Greece. In: Sharing the World of Occupation from Latin America. Presented at the WFOT Congress, Chile.

Organisation for Economic Co-operation and Development, 2014. Society at a Glance 2014 Highlights: Greece, The Crisis and Its Aftermath. <http://www.oecd.org/greece/OECD-SocietyAtaGlance2014-Highlights-Greece.pdf> (accessed 30.07.14.).

Quaglio, G., Karapiperis, T., van Woensel, L., Arnold, E., McDaid, D., 2013. Austerity and health in Europe. Health Policy (New York) 113 (1), 13–19.

Segal, R., 2014. Dimensions of occupation across the lifespan. In: Hinojosa, J., Blount, M.-L. (Eds.), The Texture of Life: Occupations and Related Activities, fourth ed. AOTA Press, Bethesda, MD, pp. 37–53.

Townsend, E., Wilcock, A., 2003. Occupational justice. In: Christiansen, C., Townsend, E. (Eds.), Introduction to Occupation: The Art and Science of Living. Prentice Hall, Upper Saddle River, NJ, pp. 243–273.

Townsend, E., Wilcock, A., 2004. Occupational justice and client-centred practice: a dialogue in progress. Can. J. Occup. Ther. 71 (2), 75–87.

Tsiganou, J., Daskalaki, K., Frangiskou, A., Georgakarakis, N., Sarris, N., Selekou, O., et al., 1999. Young people at social 'disadvantage'. National Centre for Social Research, Athens, Greece.

TUNING Occupational Therapy Project Group, The, 2008. Reference Points for the Design and Delivery of Degree Programmes in Occupational Therapy. <http://www.unideusto.org/tuningeu/images/stories/Publications/OCCUPATIONAL_THERAPY_FOR_WEBSITE.pdf> (accessed 06.03.15.).

Watson, D.E., Wilson, S.A., 2003. Task Analysis, An Individual and Population Approach, second ed. AOTA Press, Bethesda, MD. American Occupational Therapy Association Inc.

Wenger, E., Trayner, B., de Laat, M., 2011. Promoting and Assessing Value Creation in Communities and Networks: A Conceptual Framework. Ruud de Moor Centrum, Open University of the Netherlands, the Netherlands. Available at: <http://wenger-trayner.com/documents/Wenger_Trayner_DeLaat_Value_creation.pdf> (accessed 30.07.14.).

Whiteford, G., 2000. Occupational deprivation: global challenge in the new millennium. Br. J. Occup. Ther. 63 (5), 200–204.

Wikipedia, 2014. Spoon sweets. Wikipedia, the free encyclopedia. <http://en.wikipedia.org/wiki/Spoon_sweets#Greece> (accessed 22.03.15.).

Wikipedia, 2015a. Halva. Wikipedia, the free encyclopedia. <https://en.wikipedia.org/w/index.php?title=Halva&oldid=655625898> (accessed 22.03.15.).

Wikipedia, 2015b. Lokma. Wikipedia, the free encyclopedia. https://en.wikipedia.org/w/index.php?title=Lokma&oldid=653787795 (accessed 22.03.15.).

Wilcock, A.A., 1998. An Occupational Perspective of Health. SLACK Incorporated, Thorofare, NJ.

Wilson, S.A., Landry, G., 2014. Task Analysis, An Individual, Group and Population Approach, third ed. AOTA Press, American Occupational Therapy Association Inc, Bethesda, MD.

World Bank, The. The World Bank: data, GDP growth (annual %). <http://data.worldbank.org/indicator/NY.GDP.MKTP.KD.ZG?page=1> (accessed 25.03.15.).

38

THE IMPACT OF THE ECONOMIC CRISIS ON THE DAILY LIFE OF PEOPLE IN SPAIN

PABLO A. CANTERO GARLITO ■ DANIEL EMERIC MÉAULLE

From the beginning, occupational therapy has been characterized by presenting a unique approach to analysing and interpreting human behaviour: the occupational perspective. In Spain, the historical development of the profession has led to occupational therapists mainly working in clinical settings rather than in community settings.

Using the financial crisis which started in 2007 (Fontana, 2013) as a context, in this chapter we critically discuss what an occupational perspective might look like. The crisis itself has had a direct impact on the health of citizens, as already reflected in some recent studies (Gili et al., 2013; SESPAS, 2014). Furthermore, the restructuring of health services (through, e.g., staff and service reduction, privatization, changes in eligibility criteria, etc.) have caused changes in the model of universal healthcare for the citizens, as well as difficulties in incorporating and maintaining occupational therapy services in health centres. The aim of this chapter is to present a critical analysis from an occupational perspective of the impact of the crisis on the lives of people in Spain. In this chapter, we also advocate for a greater commitment of occupational therapists to addressing social and occupational injustice.

THE CONTEXT OF THE CRISIS IN SPAIN AND ITS IMPACT ON THE CITIZENS

Spain has experienced a social decline in its historical development since the last century. This regression was promoted by Franco's dictatorship, facilitated by a class-based society, in which powerful groups saw an opportunity to strengthen their hegemony through Franco's government. This class structure continued in the post-Franco era, in institutions such as the monarchy, the church and the business and private banking sectors (Navarro, 2006). Despite efforts to improve the welfare of the population in the 1980s and 1990s, eventually the population began to realize that the development model they had known so far, in which quality of life and opportunities for children tended to be significantly better than those enjoyed by their parents, has been broken. Fear, uncertainty, mistrust of institutions and even despair have become part of the collective subjectivity.

In this sense, Spain has suffered, since about 2007, the consequences of a global crisis that has been lashing the country's economy and social realm with particular virulence. The development of the welfare state, achieved in the years of democracy, and the extension of social rights conquered in the first term of José Luis Rodríguez Zapatero's presidency (2004–2008), have been deeply affected by the crisis. *Anticrisis* or *austerity* measures, proposed by the subsequent socialist (2009–2011) and conservative governments (2012 through to the time of writing (September 2015)), for the management of the *'Gran Recesión'* (Great Recession), not only have questioned the system of economic and social development of the country, but also have had a big impact on the daily life of its citizens.

In May 2010, the socialist government of President Zapatero presented a set of measures involving a series of budget cuts amounting to 15 billion euros, one of the most unpopular and painful economic adjustments in the post-Franco era, signifying the end of an era of prosperity and economic growth. The year 2012 saw the election of a conservative government headed by Mariano Rajoy. This government implemented an austerity plan that has, up to the time of writing, reached 65 billion euros (e.g., cuts in education and health reached 10 billion euros while international development cooperation, culture, justice and research were also affected). The main objective of these measures was deficit reduction and a resulting increase in economic growth. However, this goal is far from complete and has become increasingly distant. In June 2014, Spanish public debt reached and exceeded the historic threshold of 1 trillion euros, accounting for 98.2% of the gross domestic product (in 2010 the debt was 644.692 million euros and accounted for 61.7% of the gross domestic product) (SOMAMFYC, 2014).

The health of communities, as is often the case in situations of economic recession and poverty, has deteriorated as a result of political decisions taken (Segura, 2014). These in turn have increased inequality while benefiting the oligarchies of the country, as we will discuss in the following sections.

Unemployment and Its Effects

Since 2007 unemployment has increased, and at the time of writing (2015) there were more than 6 million unemployed people. The Labour Force Survey puts the percentage of unemployment at 23% for 2015 (Instituto Nacional de Estadística, 2015). The percentage of households with all members unemployed steadily increased by nearly 10% in the first quarter of 2012 (Laparra and Pérez, 2012). Unemployment in young people is particularly significant, reaching 53% for youth under 25 years of age in 2013.

Both the second government of Zapatero and that of Rajoy undertook reforms in labour legislation that deepened the processes of destruction and precariousness of the labour market (Aragón et al., 2012). This, together with wage freezes and declining purchasing power, the increased cost of living, and structural peculiarities of the Spanish labour market (young people without qualifications, adults unprepared for technological change, etc.) (Lima, 2014), set up a social landscape of phenomena that people thought they had left behind in the past, such as evictions and a very high unemployment rate. The profile of people receiving support from the social services has changed, with people who once belonged to the middle classes often requiring assistance. Their difficulties in getting jobs are a factor that must also be now addressed from within a collapsed system.

The worsening of living conditions in general, and in particular those related to access to decent housing, have their greatest expression in evictions. According to the General Council of the Judiciary, over 400 000 mortgage foreclosure proceedings have been initiated since 2008. During this same period, at least 250 000 evictions (Valiño and Simón, 2013) have been conducted. However, due to the complexities of the Spanish legal system, people often remain in debt to the bank and responsible for their mortgage despite the loss of their house.

The weak recommendations of executives on good banking practices did not terminate eviction proceedings, which only stopped after the approval of a 2-year moratorium for groups of 'special vulnerability' (Gobierno de España, 2012a, p. 22493). Paradoxically, these were more restrictive and deeper than the popular legislative initiatives proposed by concerned citizens themselves, following the media coverage of several suicides of desperate citizens who were forced to leave their homes. These properties simply became one more asset for the banks.

THE IMPACT OF THE CRISIS ON CITIZENS' HEALTH

The economic crisis has had a negative impact on the health of the citizens, who are affected by factors such as the extent, nature and duration of the crisis, as well as on the economic and social policies that are in place to mitigate the effects of the recession (Pérez et al., 2014). The effects occur at both individual and population levels, and exert an important influence throughout the population's life cycle. It is important to examine the health effects of the financial crisis, especially regarding the most vulnerable groups (e.g., immigrants, people living in socioeconomic deprivation, women, and youth). The impact on them will be more pronounced as they are more likely to lose their jobs, experience more difficulty finding jobs or depend on precarious work in worse conditions. For example, according to a comprehensive review of the effects and mechanisms of the transmission of poverty that Flores et al. (2014) conducted, it is expected that children who have lived in the crisis period will be affected by it throughout their lives: lower education, lower income, and lower labour opportunities are inextricably linked to lower health indicators (e.g., more chronic conditions including increased risk of cardiovascular disease, cognitive impairment, and dementia).

It is worth noting, given their importance, two aspects related to the living conditions that have important and significant negative health effects: unemployment and housing conditions. The high unemployment rate in Spain is one of the worst effects of the crisis and potentially one of the most dangerous for health. Spain has the second-worst level of unemployment (after Greece) in the EU15[1] (Eurostat, 2015a). Housing problems have a negative impact on mental health: emotional problems, substance abuse, behavioural problems, and lower academic achievement, due to the economic difficulties encountered in meeting other basic needs such as food (Flores et al., 2014).

While there is some disagreement about the effects of the crisis on health, there is a strong consensus that mental health is adversely affected during periods of economic crisis. 'The increased anxiety and depression, and decreased perception and self-esteem, among other factors produced by unemployment, are some of the mechanisms by which the economic crisis could affect health' (Pérez et al., 2014, p. 127). In Spain, the probability of developing mental disorders is three times higher among unemployed men and 1.5 times higher in women (Artacoz et al., 2004; Segura, 2014).

The IMPACT (Gili et al., 2013) study which compared the prevalence of mental disorders in primary care in Spain before and during the economic crisis (2006–2010) shows an increase of mood disorders (19%), anxiety disorders (8%) and alcohol misuse (5%). There has been a significant increase, about 10%, in the consumption of antidepressant drugs between 2009 and 2012.

It might be expected that the minimum guarantees of healthcare and support to people in situations of dependency would have been maintained. However, the essential elements of social cohesion and support from the welfare state (employment, health, education, dependency and pensions) have been the main focus of the austerity measures implemented by the government. Policies to 'ensure the sustainability of the system' (Gobierno de España, 2012b, p. 31290) have served to exclude many citizens from basic healthcare and disability support. Some of these policies include the following:

- The introduction of copayments, whereby service users need to cover, at the point of access, part of

---

[1]The EU15 corresponds to countries that signed their accession to the European Union in 1995 or before: Austria, Belgium, Denmark, Spain, Finland, France, Germany, Greece, Ireland, Italy, Luxembourg, Netherlands, Portugal, United Kingdom, and Sweden.

the cost of healthcare products (e.g., wheelchairs or adaptive equipment) or services (e.g., residential care, occupational therapy services and rehabilitation services). In order to contain public spending, people must make a double contribution to the financing of the system (one through their taxes and another at the time of use), which can clearly have a deterrent effect.

■ The cessation of state contributions to the social protection system fund of carers (Gobierno de la Comunidad de Madrid, 2012) which essentially concerns the protection of women, traditionally responsible for caregiving. This leads to limited access to the labour market, ultimately affecting access to a retirement pension.

■ The end of financial support for some common medicines and some provisions of the national health system (Gobierno de España, 2012b), that are now treated as supplementary or ancillary and thus require copayment. Medicines for chronic illnesses are still covered by public funding, but in recent years the percentage of copayment has changed and now depends on the income and employment of people affected. For example, people must cover 10% of their medication costs if their annual income is less than 18 000 euros, or between 40% and 50% if annual income is between 18 000 and 100 000 euros.

■ Introduction of the pharmaceutical copayment per prescription in some regions of Spain. The so-called Euro prescription is a kind of universal copayment, forcing the user of health services to pay 1 euro for each prescription that the doctor prescribes, regardless of the type of medication, its purpose, its cost or the economic situation of the user. This application has provisionally been stopped by the Constitutional Court.

■ The rupture of the model of universal healthcare, which links the right to healthcare to employment status. Young people over 26 years who have never worked, the unemployed who have exhausted all benefits and subsidies and reside outside of Spain for more than 90 days in a year, and undocumented immigrants, who have been excluded directly from the system, have had their access to healthcare restricted (SOMAMFYC, 2014).

The measures taken by different governments in all areas mentioned above have deepened the inequality gap. Spain has become, after Latvia, the most unequal country in the European Union, where the richest 20% of the population earn 7.5 times more than the poorest 20% (Eurostat, 2015b). The unequal distribution of resources has added to the widespread disaffection for a ruling class that does not take into account the population, motivated, in many cases, by vested interests within the state structures and institutions (political parties, banks and savings banks, municipalities, unions, corporations, the royal house, the courts, etc.). This situation has generated, in everyday life, a renewed interest in politics and the transformation of its institutions as a strategy to position the common good interests of the citizens at the heart of the Spanish political agenda, above the economy.

CITIZEN COUNTERPOWERS AND RESISTANCE EXPERIENCES

A crucial feature in the context of the social and political crisis, which is ongoing at the time of writing (2015), is, according to Errejón (2014), 'the expansion of an inorganic, transversal discontent which is not expressed in the codes of traditional political identities, amid a disorganized civil society in general, a breakdown of community ties and several decades of decline in the values of social cooperation' (p. 1). Spain is faced with a situation in which the majority of the people are becoming poorer while the greater concentration of income and power are in the hands of an economic elite. This is compared with the additional challenge of being the country with a very high youth unemployment, where only one in two young persons works, as well as a society where more than a fifth of the population lives below the poverty line (Instituto Nacional de Estadística, 2015).

In recent years, a process of social change, social activism, has been developing in Spain, working towards the development of new strategies of action and social participation, and reinventing old ones, to propose, to collaborate and to build a fairer society. This is a process of empowerment (Montero, 2003), through which people try to overcome the obstacles that they have experienced in order to find ways to establish community-building processes. In this way, the community members (individuals or groups) become aware of their situation and develop skills and resources together to achieve the transformation of their environment according to their needs and aspirations.

The activities carried out by the *'Plataforma de Afectados por la Hipoteca'* (Platform of People Affected by Mortgages) offer important examples of people trying to resolve the difficult situation a lot of families who have been evicted suffer. Other examples include the green tide mobilizations in defense of public education and against the unstoppable increase of university fees, the crowdfunding driven by '15MpaRato' which served to uncover the bankruptcy of Bankia bank and bring those responsible to justice, or the campaign for voting rights developed by 'Marea Granate'.

The citizens have been able to politicize some of the social problems (e.g., housing and migration), which until then had been treated individually and privately, and to build alternatives from a social, community perspective – from private to public, from public to politics and from politics back into action in everyday life. The politicization of everyday life means leaving behind conceptions of the crisis as an inevitable natural disaster and seeing it rather as a result of specific actions by specific actors (Errejón, 2011). In the same vein, the Commission on Social Determinants of The World Health Organization (CSDH, 2008, p. 34) pointed out that 'the unequal distribution of health-damaging experiences is not in any sense a natural phenomenon but the result of the combination of poor social policies and interventions, unjust economic situations and bad policies'.

Occupational therapists play a role by, for example, participating in the demonstrations in defense of universal public health, developing social entrepreneurship projects for groups at risk of social exclusion, seeking synergy between institutions and creating services for citizens who are expelled from the system. One of the most representative of these practices is Salvador Simó's (2011) projects in Vic, Catalonia.

Occupational therapists are called to reinterpret areas of performance, assumptions about the causes of occupational dysfunction and daily life, from new theoretical and methodological perspectives. They do this together with unemployed citizens at risk of social exclusion, unemployed youth, people who have lost their jobs and have no hope of finding other employment, families who have lost their homes, and immigrants who have been expelled from the healthcare system, among others.

It is important to note that despite the serious difficulties, the social capital of Spanish society has been maintained: social and family relationships have not experienced a deterioration, and even social isolation has been reduced (FOESSA, 2014). As Villasante (2014, p.165) states, 'revolutions of everyday life' are those that ensure longer-term, higher sustainable change. These spaces for participation, creating alternatives and transforming daily life have been spaces in which occupational therapists have offered knowledge, experience and skills for the transformation of everyday life through occupation. Occupational therapists have done this through, for example, the development of dynamic synergies and cooperation with citizens, users and other professionals, which can be the fundamental social laboratories for any sustainable transformation.

15M as an Engine of Sociopolitical Transformation in Spain

On May 15, 2011, just 1 year after the date on which the prime minister presented the main budget cuts that had been made so far in Spain, a decentralized demonstration in different parts of the country was announced online in the same week as local and regional elections were going to be held. Surpassing all predictions, the demonstrations grew exponentially, lending visibility and significance in the 'Occupy Sol Square' movement that occurred in the popular Plaza de Sol in Madrid. That civic space remained occupied until June.

What was this social movement, popularly known as the 'outraged' (*los indignados*), asking for? Some of its basic demands were related to promoting a more participatory democracy far from bipartisanship and the domain of banks and corporations, as well as a genuine separation of powers and other measures intended to improve the daily lives of citizens.

The emergence of 15M Figure 38-1 busted the seams of institutional politics, but it also exploded traditional social movements, as suggested by Sánchez (2013): 'The 15M movement was not born out of

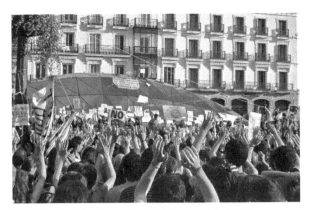

FIGURE 38-1 ■ Puerta del Sol in Madrid during the occupation of the 15M movement.

militancy but out of the crossroads in the journey to politics of a depoliticized generation and a journey to the ordinary of a sad militancy' (p. 24). The 15M movement aroused the sympathy of many people to the extent that it was able to operate within, rather than against, the common sense of the time. Their demands are not ideological, nor supposedly political, but rather are common sense demands because they reside in the daily life experience of a majority of the population (Errejón, 2014), legitimizing a process that, although not yet fully formed, has already achieved remarkable results. An example is the irruption of five seats in the European Parliament obtained by 'Podemos', the political party born within the 15M movement, which has a structure in 'participatory circles'. These working groups of citizens can be territorial (neighbourhoods, towns, cities) or sectoral/thematic (health, education, every job, college, neighbourhood association, cultural, sports, professional or unemployed people, etc.), without the obligation to be part of the membership. These participatory circles may well have to do with the needs of the people served by occupational therapists: they can voice the demands of people with disabilities, including in the political agenda issues related to poverty, quality of life, protection of public health, or take measures to protect the rights of people with disabilities.

The growing of different occupied areas by protesters and citizens, far from clearing out the 15M phenomenon, generated currents of diffusion in other neighbourhoods and in citizen assemblies located in other areas of cities and towns. Even in its latent phase, the 15M movement has been able to break into the media agenda leading to new practices, new discourses and new forms of organization. People's movements such as 'Ahora Madrid' or 'Guanyem Barcelona' function as alternatives to the traditional political parties (oligarchic, opaque, vertical, etc.). These movements have gathered enough supporters to reach positions of power in the municipalities of Madrid and Barcelona.

These transformations in the way of conceiving politics have been pushing the boundaries of what was once possible: what is legal is not necessarily what is legitimate to the extent that what is legal does not always correspond with what is ethical. A good example may be the actions of the 'Plataforma de Afectados por la Hipoteca' (Valiño and Simón, 2013): it may be legal for the bank to repossess your property and have you pay the mortgage on a house you no longer live in, but it is not ethical, and something must be done about it.

Tides of Citizens and Other Forms of Social and Political Participation

One of the best examples of this process of collective construction of actions and knowledge, linking professionals with other citizens, are the *tides* (*mareas*) of citizens. According to Sánchez (2013, p. 12): 'We chose the word "tide" because within the water there are networks, there are channels, there are small organisms changing around them and not staying in it but projecting their examples upstream or downstream.' The tides have achieved goals that were unthinkable not long ago. The White Tide (groups from the public health sector) was able to stop, through legal proceedings, the health privatization in Madrid and the copayment for pharmaceutical products in some regions of Spain.

The 'Plataforma de Afectados por la Hipoteca' has enjoyed a special relevance (Valiño and Simón, 2013). This organization was established in Barcelona in 2009, in order to help those affected. Its main task was to modify mortgage legislation so that ceding one's house cancelled its entire debt. Reaching that goal at that time was especially difficult since other claims were incorporated to prevent the eviction of families and individuals affected, such as getting reasonable alternative relocation and promoting sufficient social rents. Another, especially important, objective was to achieve self-organization by people affected by this problem, creating groups able to defend their rights and fight for their goals.

The last European Parliament elections (2014) in Spain have meant a real electoral earthquake with unpredictable consequences. The collapse of the two hegemonic parties (Partido Popular, Partido Socialista Obrero Español) and the emergence of Podemos, a new party which grew out of the 15M movement and other social movements, signify the development of new political discourses. As Sánchez (2014) stated:

This is the volcano bursting. The results of the European elections were the hole, the crater, so all the magma could flow from the volcano which was about to explode. After some years in which the strength of the underground has collided with every possible wall, occasionally releasing currents through geysers as the Tides, the eruption has been clear and visible from far away. (p. 12)

CONCLUSIONS

The worst tragedy of the crisis is not the impact caused on the economy; the worst tragedy is the unnecessary human suffering. As the last FOESSA report noted (2014, p. 157): 'integration is becoming less full and more precarious, while the social space of exclusion grows both in more moderate and severe levels'. However, in the sociopolitical context in which there has been a sharp rise in inequality, we realize the enormous potential that organized groups may have, trying to change and transform positively the course of history, to cope with the charges of the unfair policies of austerity, and ultimately to improve the daily lives of citizens. Still, we are left to ask ourselves the following questions: What are the challenges that occupational therapists face? What are the lessons that this crisis and the civic resistance are teaching us?

It is now more necessary than ever to reflect on the long-term social impact of political decisions. It is also important to reflect on the role that occupational therapists decide to adopt and how this role can address phenomena such as exclusion or restriction of access to health services, child poverty, evictions, job insecurity, loss of government assistance to people in situations of dependency and their families, unemployment, increased youth emigration, etc.

It is also important that occupational therapists are able to position themselves, to comment on, and create alternatives, in this new context. Occupational therapy discourses have been traditionally constructed from individualistic theoretical standpoints, nested in capitalist systems (Hammell and Iwama, 2012). At this juncture, it is necessary to invest in the construction of critical, social perspectives. As Rivadeneyra et al. (2014, p. 13) note, 'the cuts and privatization policies introduced in different health systems respond to ideological criteria, and not to accumulating evidence. Intelligent pruning must be therefore framed in reforms in order to improve the system in terms of equity, efficiency, quality, accessibility and legitimacy,' with the participation of professionals and different stakeholders.

In conclusion, occupational therapists cannot remain indifferent to the spaces of collective construction in which the interests and needs of users, their families, and other professionals converge. In these spaces, occupational therapists can find the confluence of their own interests as professionals and as citizens affected by the crisis and its management. Occupational therapists need to take risks and develop practices that reflect the transformational power of occupation. Occupational therapy prides itself on its ability to help people construct meaning in their everyday life through their occupations. It seems appropriate, therefore, to reflect on the role of a profession seeking its place in a society which is in crisis and in change.

REFERENCES

Aragón, J., Cruces, J., De la Fuente, L., Martínez, A., Otaegui, A., Llopis, E., 2012. Trabajadores Pobres y Empobrecimiento en España. Fundación 1º de Mayo, Madrid.

Artacoz, L., Benach, L., Borrell, C., 2004. Unemployment and mental health: understanding the interactions among gender, family roles and social class. Am. J. Public Health 94, 82–89.

CSDH, 2008. Closing the gap in a generation: health equity through action on the social determinants of health. Final Report of the Commission on Social Determinants of Health. World Health Organization, Geneva.

Errejón, I., 2011. El 15-M como discurso contrahegemónico. Encrucijadas: Revista Crítica de Ciencias Sociales 2, 120–145.

Errejón, I., 2014. ¿Qué es 'Podemos'? Le Monde Diplomatique, julio, p. 1.

Eurostat, 2015a. Employment up by 0.3% in Euro area and 0.2% in EU28. <http://ec.europa.eu/eurostat/documents/2995521/6993041/2-15092015-BP-EN.pdf/7734df37-e5af-49c9-b165-5e3cff123b93> (accessed 18.09.15.).

Eurostat, 2015b. Inequality of income distribution. <http://ec.europa.eu/eurostat/web/products-datasets/-/tsdsc260> (accessed 18.09.15.).

Flores, M., García–Gómez, P., Zunzunegui, M.V., 2014. Crisis económica, pobreza e infancia: ¿qué podemos esperar en el corto y largo plazo para los niños y las niñas de la crisis? Informe SESPAS 2014. Gac. Sanit. 28 (Suppl. 1), 132–136.

FOESSA, 2014. VII Informe sobre Exclusión y Desarrollo Social en España. Fundación FOESSA, Madrid.

Fontana, J., 2013. El futuro es un país extraño. Una reflexión sobre la crisis social de comienzos del siglo XXI. Ediciones de Pasado y Presente, Barcelona.

Gili, M., Roca, M., Basu, S., 2013. The mental health risks of economic crisis in Spain: evidence from primary care centres, 2006 and 2010. Eur. J. Public Health 23, 103–108.

Gobierno de España, 2012a. Real Decreto-ley 6/2012, de 9 de marzo, de medidas urgentes de protección de deudores hipotecarios sin recursos. Boletín Oficial del Estado, Madrid.

Gobierno de España, 2012b. Real Decreto – Ley 16/2012, de 20 de abril, de medidas urgentes para garantizar la sostenibilidad del Sistema Nacional de Salud y mejorar la calidad y seguridad de sus prestaciones. Boletín Oficial del Estado, Madrid.

Gobierno de la Comunidad de Madrid, 2012. Ley 8/2012, de 28 de diciembre, de medidas fiscales y administrativas por el que se modifica el texto refundido de la Ley de tasas y precios públicos de la Comunidad de Madrid. Gobierno de la Comunidad de Madrid, Madrid.

Hammell, K., Iwama, M., 2012. Well-being and occupational rights: an imperative for critical occupational therapy. Scand. J. Occup. Ther. 19 (5), 385–394.

Instituto Nacional de Estadística, 2015. Encuesta de Población Activa (EPA) Primer trimestre de 2015. INE, Madrid.

Kronenberg, F., Simó, S., Pollard, N., 2007. Terapia Ocupacional sin Fronteras. El Espíritu de los Supervivientes. Editorial Médica Panamericana, Madrid.

Laparra, M., Pérez, B., 2012. Crisis y fractura social en Europa. Causas y efectos en España. Obra Social 'La Caixa', Barcelona.

Lima, A., 2014. I Informe sobre los Servicios Sociales en España. Consejo General del Trabajo Social, Madrid.

Montero, M., 2003. Teoría y Práctica de la Psicología Comunitaria: La Tensión entre Comunidad y Sociedad. Paidós, Buenos Aires.

Navarro, V., 2006. El subdesarrollo social de España: causas y consecuencias. Anagrama, Madrid.

Pérez, G., Rodríguez-Sanz, M., Domínguez-Berjón, F., Cabeza, E., Borrell, C., 2014. Indicadores para monitorizar la evolución de la crisis y sus efectos en la salud y en las desigualdades en salud. Informe SESPAS. Gac. Sanit. 28 (Suppl. 1), 124–131.

Rivadeneyra, A., et al., 2014. Lecciones desde fuera. Otros países en ésta y otras crisis anteriores. Informe SESPAS 2014. Gac. Sanit. 28 (Suppl. 1), 12–17.

Sánchez, J.L., 2013. Las 10 Mareas del Cambio. Claves para Comprender los Nuevos Discursos Sociales. Roca Editorial, Barcelona.

Sánchez, J.L., 2014. Historia de un Volcán: La Izquierda se Revoluciona. Cuadernos ElDiario.es, Núm. 6, pp. 6–12.

Segura, A., 2014. Recortes, austeridad y salud. Informe SESPAS 2014. Gac. Sanit. 28 (Suppl. 1), 7–11.

SESPAS, 2014. Informe SESPAS 2014. Gac. Sanit. 28 (Suppl. 1), 1–146.

Simó, S., 2011. La palabra y la acción: lucha contra la pobreza, salud (ocupacional) y ciudadanía a través de nuevas praxis universitarias. Unpublished doctoral dissertation, Univeristy of Vic, Vic, Spain.

SOMAMFYC, 2014. Informe REDES 2014. Yo Sí Sanidad Universal y Sociedad Madrileña de Medicina de Familia y Comunitaria (SOMAMFYC), Madrid.

Valiño, V., Simón, P., 2013. Emergencia Habitacional en el Estado Español: La Crisis de las Ejecuciones Hipotecarias y los Desalojos Desde una Perspectiva de Derechos Humanos. Observatorio DESC, Barcelona.

Villasante, T., 2014. Redes de Vida Desbordantes. Fundamentos para el Cambio desde la Vida Cotidiana. Los Libros de la Catarata, Madrid.

39

PROMOTING ACTIVE CITIZENSHIP AGAINST POVERTY THROUGH A PARTICIPATORY COMMUNITY INTERVENTION

SALVADOR SIMÓ ALGADO ▪ JORDI DE SAN EUGENIO ▪ XAVIER GINESTA

CHAPTER OUTLINE

Poverty is one of the main challenges faced by society. In this chapter, we discuss the role of occupational therapy in dealing with poverty and promoting active citizenship. To do this, we present a participatory project developed in the town of Manlleu, located in the middle of Catalonia, Spain. The implementation of the project had already started at the time of this writing (October 2015).

The project has three general objectives: to create an inclusive and sustainable community; to design a participatory project in order to deal with poverty; and to create a centre for occupation with the active participation of the users, the citizens, and the third sector. The centre for occupation will develop vocational workshops and will promote personal growing and health through occupations. It will collaborate with local nongovernmental organizations and organizations of the third sector (civil society). Its name, *Molí Mierons* (Mierons Mill), comes from the name of the building, an ancient industrial watermill located near the river Ter.

This project is developing through a strong partnership between the third and the public sectors, with the active participation of local citizens, and it is coordinated by the University of Vic-Central University of Catalonia. The project is multidisciplinary; it is led by the Faculty of Health and Wellbeing of the University of Vic, with the participation of the Faculty of Business and Communication. Two research groups are involved: the Mental Health and Social Innovation Research Group (Faculty of Health and Wellbeing) and the Audiovisual Translation, Communication and Territory Research Group, TRACTE (Faculty of Business and Communication). The project will allow Manlleu's town council to reshape the local place brand. This social project will strengthen different positive tangible and intangible values of the locality in order to promote a more inclusive, tolerant, and respectful city.

POVERTY: A GLOBAL REALITY

More than 2.2 billion people are suffering from poverty worldwide (Green, 2008). More than 15% of the global population is vulnerable to poverty. Almost 80% of the population has no comprehensive social protection

(Green, 2008). Around 12% (842 million) of the global population suffers from chronic hunger, and nearly 50% of the working population (more than 1.5 billion) has precarious employment conditions (United Nations (UN), 2014). Each year, approximately 18 million people die due to the effects of poverty (50 000 people each day), including 34 000 children under the age of 5 years. In Europe, poverty affects 120 million citizens.

This massive and extreme poverty coexists with extraordinary prosperity (Pogge, 2005). For each individual the global economy produces per year approximately $9543 in goods and services, almost 14 times more than the annual $693.5 that defines the extreme poverty experienced by 1 billion human beings. According to the UN, $300 billion is needed globally to escape from extreme poverty. This figure represents a third of the global annual military expenditure (Green, 2008). In 2015, 1% of the world's population will own more wealth than the other 99% put together (Oxfam, 2015). There are the material resources but not the will to eradicate poverty. We refer to this reality as moral poverty, the anaemia of the soul. This refers to the poverty affecting wealthy societies that are indifferent to the suffering, the ones who are merely spectators of human suffering when people's moral responsibility is to be active actors in its resolution.

It is possible to distinguish between three grades of poverty: extreme, moderate, and relative. The condition of extreme poverty means that families cannot fulfil their survival needs. They suffer chronic hunger and they have no access to health or educational services. This grade of poverty is most evident in developing countries. Moderate poverty refers to living conditions where basic needs are covered, but are precarious. Relative poverty refers to people living in rich countries without access to leisure and cultural activities; they have no access to good-quality healthcare or educational services (Sachs, 2005).

Paugan (2007) distinguishes four approaches to measuring poverty: monetary, subjective, living conditions approach, and poverty as the lack of capabilities.

1. The monetary approach is the most common. In Europe, this standard applies to people who live on less than 50% of the national income average.

2. The subjective approach is based on the perception of people experiencing poverty. It focuses on aspects such as personal appearance or being unable to give children a good education.

3. The living conditions approach understands poverty as material deprivation in categories such as food, clothes, electricity, heating, housing conditions, employment conditions, health, education, environment, family leisure activities, and social relationships.

4. Sen (2000) describes poverty as the lack of capabilities. It is the incapacity to control one's own life. Following this approach we can understand how it affects such an important part of the population. For example, how can we have a life project if we do not have a well-paid and secure job? The UN (2014) uses the concept of human vulnerability where people experience the deterioration of their capabilities and options.

Paugan (2007, p. 64) introduced the role of the *assisted* person, somebody who depends on social welfare. From the moment that society takes care of the poor, they receive a concrete social status and start a specific career altering their previous identity. They are stigmatized and defined by a regular and contractual relationship with social services. Stigma and prejudice are very present in this exclusion process. Stigma originally referred to physical attributes that people possessed, associated with certain features, for example, scars shown by slaves (Goffman, 2006). Stigma has cognitive, emotional, and behavioural components.

POVERTY AND CITIZENSHIP

Citizenship is one of the most important, yet most elusive concepts of modern political discourse. It has a long history that starts in Greece. Citizenship is a boundary concept that determines the possession or lack of political, legal, and social rights, as well as the inclusion or exclusion of political communities. The current concept of citizenship comes from the seventeenth and eighteenth centuries, from the French, English, and American revolutions and civil wars. Within these traditions there are two main components of citizenship:

1. Political citizenship involves a relationship between an individual and a community, under

which the individual is a full member of that community and owes loyalty. The idea of citizenship as a form of participation originated from Athenian democracy: the citizen is one who deals with public issues and recognizes discussion, rather than violence, as the means to solving disputes. The tradition of citizenship as a legal status comes from Rome: the citizen acts within the law and in return expects the protection of the State (Cortina, 2005).

2. Social citizenship implies that the citizen is a person who enjoys social rights (such as work, education, housing, health and social benefits in times of vulnerability). These social rights would be guaranteed by the welfare state.

Poverty is related to citizenship. The solution to poverty requires transferring real power and capacities to the people (Sen, 2000). The experience of poverty includes a feeling of helplessness and exclusion from decision-making processes. People need power over their own destiny and over the factors that influence them, like political powers. Active citizenship refers to a combination of rights and obligations that links individuals to the State; these can include the payment of taxes, obeying the laws, and access to social, civil, and political rights. Active citizens use these rights to improve the quality of political or civic life, through their engagement in the decisions related to economy or politics, or through collective action (Green, 2008). Active citizenship involves political activism.

OCCUPATIONAL THERAPY AND POVERTY

Occupational therapists need to contribute to the Millennium Goals and the Post 2015 Development Agenda (UN, 2015). These are global goals, whose object was to have reduced poverty by 50% by 2015 and to have eradicated it by 2025.

Occupational therapists understand human beings as occupational beings (Wilcock, 2006) and work to address situations of occupational dysfunction. Occupational dysfunction may be caused by physical, psychological, social or environmental factors, and one of these factors is poverty, which can have a direct impact on activities of daily living. Poverty is closely related to

unemployment or to insecure types of work, and it determines people's self-maintenance and leisure occupations.

Sen (2000) describes poverty as the lack of capabilities. From this definition it is easy to understand the vital role that occupational therapy has in addressing poverty. The profession is based on the science of capacitation (Townsend and Polajatko, 2007), from an empowerment model. If people cannot control their own lives, they cannot develop a meaningful life. Frankl (1964) suggests that the consequences of this lack of meaning are depression and suicide, aggression or addiction, which are some of the biggest challenges of contemporary society. Occupational therapists can help individuals and communities develop meaningful life projects, which can be done through helping people to access meaningful occupations. The first author defines meaningful occupations as the occupational intersection between the needs, the potential, and the spirit of the person (Simó Algado, 2010). Spirit is people's true essence and is expressed through occupations (Egan and Delat, 1994). Spirituality is related to the dimensions of meaning and connection with oneself and the others (Simó Algado and Burgman, 2004).

The UN (2014) affirms the need to distribute capabilities to enable people to live a decent and worthwhile life. To achieve this, it is necessary to reduce persistent vulnerabilities and instead promote resilience, the human capability to confront adversity. Occupational therapists need to advocate for fair access to basic services, such as health and education, more solid social protection, and full employment. Occupational therapists can especially focus on promoting well-being and job inclusion, a basic dimension of human productivity.

Occupational therapists are called to be social activists promoting inclusive and sustainable communities, and empowering their users as active citizens through user-centred models. Considering the constant violation of human rights at a global scale, and its impact on human well-being, it is necessary to incorporate the human rights approach into occupational therapy (Guajardo and Simó Algado, 2010).

It must be understood that the emergence of poverty and of unemployment are directly related to economic and political structures. Occupational therapists cannot talk about occupational justice, understood as the promotion of a social and economic change to ensure access to meaningful occupations (Simó Algado and Townsend, 2015), without considering the origins of injustice. The contemporary context is framed by globalization. Unfortunately, we cannot talk about a globalization of human rights. The dominant form of globalization has concerned the financial markets, promoting and imposing neoliberal values at a global scale. The economic context is marked by a neoliberal capitalism.

Neoliberal economy refers to the resurgence of nineteenth-century ideas associated with laissez-faire economic liberalism. Beginning in the 1970s and 1980s, its advocates supported extensive economic liberalization policies such as privatization, fiscal austerity, deregulation, free trade, and reductions in government spending in order to enhance the role of the private sector in the economy (Duménil and Lévy, 2004). Neoliberal economy promotes consumerism, competition, individualization, hedonism, and the advance of severe economic inequalities.

Neoliberal economy is often presented as the only possibility since the collapse of communism. This is the central idea of the theory of the end of history (Fukuyama, 1993). This theory is unacceptable. It is the theory of winners who intend to extend forever their domination. To look for alternatives is not only possible, it is necessary. Pikkety (2014) affirms that the existing neoliberal system causes the concentration of wealth and this unequal distribution of wealth causes social and economic instability. Piketty proposes a global system of progressive wealth taxes to help reduce inequality and avoid the vast majority of wealth coming under the control of a tiny minority.

Neoliberal economy condemns to exclusion and unemployment ever larger sections of the population. The result of neoliberal economy is the consolidation of wealth among elites, who become unable to perceive the need to organize or to distribute wealth in order for their economic system to be sustainable from a social and ecological point of view. This system condemns a vast part of the population to poverty and exclusion. Some authors refer to globalization as 'feudalization' or as a 'social fascism' (Sousa Santos, 2005, p. 235). Ecologically, it is endangering the capability of human beings to survive. People need to develop an intergenerational and intragenerational solidarity, taking care of present and future needs for survival.

For Bauman (2005), the concept of unemployment is changing its meaning from a temporary to a permanent situation. Unemployment is accompanied by the constant worsening of the job market. Beck (2000) explains how the European job market is promoting bad working conditions. Workers are losing their rights and social protection. Almost 20% of Europeans are working poor, due to the low salaries they receive.

As occupational therapists are aware that the economic system is causing occupational injustice, they must start thinking about new paths for human development. Occupational therapists need to promote an economic system based on people, not on the accumulation of capital. Latouche (2009) proposes a *serene degrowth (decline), la décroissance sereine,* based on the commitment to reduce, reevaluate, reconceptualize, relocate, and reuse. Social entrepreneurship promotes enterprises whose main goal is to create meaningful jobs for people solving social and ecological problems through innovation. In both cases, human occupation linked to productivity is the key factor.

OCCUPATIONAL THERAPY AND PLACE BRANDING

Place branding is the creation of a strategic brand identity based on a place's main active value (identity), with the aim of subsequently placing it on the market by optimizing the main passive value (image) (Govers and Go, 2009). The practice of place branding should be based on three fundamental instances: place identity, place image, and the consumer experience in the place. Anholt (2010) contends that the direct objective of place or city branding is not defined by economic gains, but rather the brand aims to achieve a positive reputation for the place, which in turn will generate economic and social benefits. The most significant differences between a place brand and a commercial brand generally arise from the economic dynamics linked to the implementation of place brands. Furthermore, the social implications of a place brand in comparison to the market interests of a commercial brand are another of the conceptual divergences between the two types of branding.

The Molí Mierons project is helping the town of Manlleu to reshape its image. For this reason, the contribution of the research group on Communication and Territory is important to give the participants in this project a framework, in order to understand how their actions to fight poverty can be useful in a place or city branding campaign (de San Eugenio, 2012).

Occupational therapy can help in the development of the human and social dimensions of place branding, helping to construct inclusive and sustainable places (communities). It is in that sense that, as the following section details, we, the authors, understand this project as a clear social place branding strategy (Nolan and Varey, 2014). The creation of a centre for occupation can contribute to the creation of an inclusive and sustainable community allowing citizens to design together a participatory policy to confront poverty in their city. In addition to these general objectives, other specific objectives to be implemented with this project include: empowering citizens to confront poverty, improving employability in the city, enabling people to develop a meaningful life project, creating a system of compensation for people who receive social assistance, reducing social stigma and prejudice against poor people, and, finally, promoting occupational justice, health, and social inclusion. The fulfilment of these objectives can contribute to reshaping the image of the city; Manlleu's local brand could be strengthened with the creation of an occupational centre. The centre will improve the brand not only for its citizens, who will perceive a more fair and cohesive city, but also among external stakeholders.

THE PROJECT

The project[1] has been inspired by the participatory occupational justice framework (Whiteford and Townsend, 2011). At the time of writing (October 2015), the first phase of the project has finished. The main goal of this stage has been to develop a participatory assessment process to identify the main problems of the city at a social level, and to design the centre for occupation. Some of the issues that are considered at this stage include: what activities will be developed,

who will lead them, when will they happen, how will they be developed, and what resources are needed. The occupational therapist (first author) has written several proposals to secure funding for the project. A communication policy is being created. At present, the renovation of the building has started, with the active participation of users and citizens.

The Molí Miarons project is located in the town of Manlleu. It is a town of 20 435 inhabitants located in the region of Osona. According to the Catalan Database Organization (Idescat, 2014), 29.27% of the town population are immigrants, while poverty and unemployment rates are close to 30%. Although 15% of the population has no access to secondary education (16–18 years), the town has two public libraries and several cultural associations. The economy of the region had been closely connected to the textile industry since 1980s, but was in crisis at the time of this writing (2015) and the industrial activities moved to other economic sectors, such as the metallurgic, food, and chemical industries.

The town's symbol is the river Ter, so it is meaningful that the project is located near the river, in an old industrial watermill. The renovation of the Molí Miarons is the first stage, as it will be the headquarters of the project. The University of Vic-Central University of Catalonia is a participant in the project through a transfer of knowledge contract signed with Manlleu town council. The communication strategy of this project has been designed by the Faculty of Business and Communication, where students attend workshops on the practice of journalism. In these courses, students manage the corporate media of the faculty, a radio station, a blog, a digital magazine, and the faculty's social media (a Twitter account).

The first author's responsibility in the project has been to coordinate it and to design the future Centre for Occupation (Box 39-1), based on a participatory process, with the third sector, the city council (social, welfare and occupational services), a group of citizens, and representatives of the users. A Delphi method has been used, developing participatory action research beginning with the definition of the problems and deciding the design of the centre. Another responsibility has been to empower the professionals of the city council, the citizens, and the clients. This has been done through capacitation courses. Poverty is

---

[1]See www.salvadorsimo.org (Section: projects).

BOX 39-1
THE CENTRE FOR OCCUPATION

During the participatory process, the citizens have decided what they want to happen in the centre. The building has three floors, an annex building, and a 3000-m^2 vegetable garden. The associations of the third sector will have their own space in the centre, and they will lead the projects. Professionals in the organization will contribute some of their working time to managing the project.

The basement floor will be a space intended for recycling furniture and small appliances. On the ground floor, there will be a bar to serve organic food at affordable prices. It will be connected to the vegetable garden and offer training in the culinary sector, which is very important in Spain. The space will hold different workshops:

- World cuisine: people from diverse cultures will share their culinary knowledge.
- Cookery for adolescents: cookery courses for teenagers who want to be independent.
- Tasty and healthy: a course on how to develop healthy and tasty menus on a limited budget.

On the first floor, there will be a health space and the 'Agora' space. The health space will be an assessment area for well-being (with links to primary healthcare), offering advice on issues such as pregnancy. The Agora will be a meeting point, a place for debate, where all the associations and citizens will be able to congregate. The second floor will host two bedrooms. It will be used in case of exchanges, meetings, etc., when people need to stay over. Finally, the third floor will be customized as 'the art of living', a space for different activities such as:

- Music (percussion, music of the world, etc.).
- Art and expressive media (painting, sculpture, comics, graffiti, etc.).
- Body expression (yoga, tai chi, relaxation, Pilates, emotional intelligence, etc.).
- Theatre (related to the theatre of the oppressed[2]).

The centre will have some annex buildings and spaces:

- Vegetable garden.
- Solidarity wardrobe: a local nongovernmental organization will collect and distribute clothes for poor citizens; they will organize courses about clothes making and patchwork.
- Bike world: a space to repair bikes and provide training in mechanics.
- Capacitation space: future users have asked for a variety of professional courses, such as sports refereeing, sports coaching, gardening and landscaping, languages, computing, painting, introduction to economy or ecological horticulture.
- Ready to work: this space will offer guidance and support to those who want to find a job, psychological support during unemployment, communication and assertiveness skills, etc.

It is important to note that the building and its surroundings will be based on the principles of universal design[3]. The cleaning and maintenance of the mill will be done by the users of the project.

[2]Inspired by Augusto Boal, this theatre deals with the social problems through dramatic collective techniques.
[3]Refers to a broad-spectrum ideas meant to produce buildings, products, and environments that are inherently accessible to everybody.

---

understood as the lack of capabilities (Sen, 2000). One of the main topics with the professionals has been 'how to develop a client centred approach', moving from a deficit model towards an empowering model.

REFLECTIONS

One of the key points for community interventions is the development of a partnership policy. We are developing partnerships between the public, private, and third sector. The private sector contributes with its dynamism and funding. The public sector contributes legitimacy and sustainability to the project. The city council has donated the building and is contributing partially to the funding for the renovation. The third

sector, civil society, is composed of the associations that do not belong to the state or to the market. It offers volunteers and gives a sense of belonging, creativity, and commitment. The following third sector organizations are involved in this project: FCMPPO (mental health foundation); Caritas, a religious charity organization; ADFO (Physically Disabled People's Association of Osona); Sant Tomas, an association for people with learning disabilities; Women for Solidarity; and ADFMMO, an association of people with mental health problems and their families. The project is also in contact with other organizations, such as leisure centres, civic centres, and local libraries.

This participatory methodology has involved a great deal of time dedicated to meetings with all the community actors. Occupational therapists need to adapt to the different rhythms of the partners without delaying the project, as poverty is an urgent problem whose confrontation cannot be postponed. Finding a common goal is necessary.

When developing community interventions, therapists must take into account different competences that will add value to the final outcomes: project design, community diagnosis, transcultural interventions, social entrepreneurship, job-creation initiatives, coordination, writing funding proposals, dealing with mass media (television, radio, and the digital newsstand, etc.) and social networks, negotiation skills, etc.

An important challenge for the occupational centre is not to become a ghetto for people experiencing social exclusion. It is important to design and implement an attractive occupational programme with the active participation of all the citizens, both in the community and in the centre. For this reason, we are involving the third sector in the management of the centre.

One of the strengths of the project so far has been the leadership developed by the town council's social services. However, although the project is an initiative of the Manlleu town council, it is not a priority on the political agenda. This has translated into a lack of initial funding and slow progress. Within the town council some departments are very supportive, such as Social Services, but not all the departments have the same attitude. This causes delays in project development, affecting the motivation of the community leaders involved in the project.

CONCLUSIONS

Bauman (2006) argues that civilization was born through the compassion and care of others. Sometimes people need to be reminded of their common interdependence. They need each other as human beings, and they need the ecosphere. We need to develop a *personalist* revolution, following the ideas of Mounier (1968), a transformation of human values and their expression through socioeconomic structures. Mounier called for the recovery of human values, such as solidarity, cooperation and justice, that extreme capitalism is destroying, transmuting them into values of competition, exclusion, and injustice.

This revolution of values must come together with a transformation of the unfair political and economical structures. We need to build an economic system centred on human beings and their well-being, in a sustainable way.

To deal with poverty, occupational therapists need to understand this complex reality and its connections to the economic neoliberal context. It is necessary to move away from paternalistic approaches and towards empowerment models. Occupational therapists need to promote active citizenship from a human rights approach and help people control their own life through guaranteeing access to meaningful occupations.

Occupational therapists in partnership with other professionals, in this case economists and communication experts from the TRACTE research group at the University of Vic-Central University of Catalonia, can develop strong alliances with the public, private, and third sector to confront poverty. The citizens are the main protagonists of this process from an empowerment approach based on participation. Our goal is to construct healthy, inclusive, and sustainable communities where everybody can contribute to the community using their potential, despite any occupational dysfunction due to the presence of any kind of physical, psychosocial or ecological issues. Human occupation is central in this process.

REFERENCES

Anholt, S., 2010. Places: Identity, Image and Reputation. Palgrave Macmillan, Basingstoke, UK.

Bauman, Z., 2005. Vidas Desperdiciadas. La Modernidad y sus Parias. Paidós, Barcelona.

Bauman, Z., 2006. Confianza y Temor en la Ciudad. Convivir con Extranjeros. Arcadia, Barcelona.

Beck, U., 2000. Un Nuevo Mundo Feliz. La Precariedad del Trabajo en la Era de la Globalización. Paidós, Barcelona.

Cortina, A., 2005. Ciudadanos del mundo. Paidós, Barcelona.

de San Eugenio, J., 2012. Teoría y Métodos para Marcas de Territorio. Open University of Catalonia, Barcelona.

Duménil, G., Lévy, D., 2004. Capital Resurgent: Roots of the Neoliberal Revolution. Harvard University Press, Cambridge, MA.

Egan, M., DeLaat, D., 1994. Considering spirituality in occupational therapy practice. Can. J. Occup. Ther. 61 (2), 95–101.

Frankl, V., 1964. El Hombre en Busca de Sentido. Herder, Barcelona.

Fukuyama, F., 1993. The End of History and the Last Man. Penguin, London.

Goffman, E., 2006. Estigma. Amorrortu, Bilbao.

Govers, R., Go, F.M., 2009. Place Branding: Glocal, Virtual and Physical Identities, Constructed, Imagined and Experienced. Palgrave Macmillan, Basingstoke, UK.

Green, D., 2008. De la Pobreza al Poder. Ediciones Octaedro, Barcelona.

Guajardo, A., Simó Algado, S., 2010. Hacia una terapia ocupaiconal basada en los derechos humanos. Revista Tog 7 (12), 25. Available at: <http://www.revistatog.com/num12/pdfs/maestros.pdf>.

Idescat, 2014. Manlleu city's statistics. <http://www.idescat.cat/emex/?id=081120&lang=es> (accessed 10.05.14.).

Latouche, S., 2009. Petit Tractat Sobre el Decreixement Serè. Tres i Quatre, Valencia.

Mounier, E., 1968. La Petita por del Segle XX. Edicions 62, Barcelona.

Nolan, T., Varey, R.J., 2014. Re-cognising the interactive space: marketing for social transformation. Mark. Theory 14 (4), 431–450.

Oxfam, 2015. Richest 1% will own more than all the rest by 2016. <http://www.oxfam.org.uk/blogs/2015/01/richest-1-per-cent-will-own-more-than-all-the-rest-by-2016> (accessed 10.02.16.).

Paugan, S., 2007. Las Formas Elementales de la Pobreza. Alianza editorial, Madrid.

Pikkety, T., 2014. The Capital for the XXI Century. Harvard University Press, Cambridge, MA.

Pogge, T., 2005. La Pobreza en el Mundo de los Derechos Humanos. Paidós Ibérica, Barcelona.

Sachs, J., 2005. El fin de la Pobreza. de Bolsillo, Barcelona.

Sen, A., 2000. Desarrollo y libertad. Planeta, Barcelona.

Simó Algado, S., 2010. Universities and the global change. In: Kronenberg, F. et al. (Eds.), Occupational Therapy without Borders. Elsevier, Oxford, pp. 357–367.

Simó Algado, S., Burgman, I., 2004. Children survivors of war. In: Kronenberg, F., et al. (Eds.), Occupational Therapy without Borders: Learning from the Spirit of Survivors. Elsevier, Oxford, pp. 246–261.

Simó Algado, S., Towsend, E., 2015. Eco-social occupational therapy. Br. J. Occup. Ther. 78 (3), 182–186.

Sousa Santos, B., 2005. El Milenio Huérfano. Ensayos para una Nueva Cultura Política. Editorial Trotta, Madrid.

Townsend, E., Polajatko, H., 2007. Enabling Occupation II: Advancing an Occupational Therapy Vision for Health, Well-being and Justice through Occupation. CAOT Publications, Toronto.

United Nations, 2014. Human development report. <http://hdr.undp.org/sites/defahttp://hdr.undp.org/sites/default/files/hdr14-report-en-1.pdfult/files/hdr14-report-en-1.pdf> (accessed 10 November 2014.).

United Nations, 2015. Objetivos de Desarrollo del Milenio. <http://www.un.org/en/ecosoc/about/mdg.shtml> (accessed 02.10.15.).

Whiteford, G., Townsend, E., 2011. Participatory Occupational Justice Framework (POJF 2010). In: Kronenberg, F., et al. (Eds.), Occupational Therapy Without Borders, v.2. Elsevier/Churchill Livingstone, Edinburgh.

Wilcock, A., 2006. An Occupational Perspective of Health, second ed. Slack Incorporated, Thorofare, NJ.

40

INEQUALITY AND SOCIOECONOMIC DISCRIMINATION OF INDIGENOUS PEOPLE: THE CASE OF RAPA NUI (EASTER ISLAND)

ELENA S. ROTAROU

CHAPTER OUTLINE

Historically, dominant groups and cultures have discriminated against indigenous peoples, a fact that has often led to their economic, social and political exclusion (United Nations, 2009). This chapter deals with issues of socioeconomic inequalities faced by indigenous people, and in particular it presents the case of the Rapanui, the indigenous people of Easter Island, Chile. Since the island's colonization in the late eighteenth to early nineteenth centuries, the Rapanui identity has been under threat; more recently, the occupation of their lands and the dramatic growth of the tourism industry have led to a series of economic, social and political problems, and have endangered the Rapanui traditions, occupations and beliefs.

The aim of this chapter is to present the challenges faced by indigenous people and how the discrimination they experience leads to higher levels of poverty, identity loss and poor performance regarding socio-economic indicators such as health, education, employment, and political and civic participation. It is argued that government policies regarding indigenous people need to be adjusted in order to better protect indigenous people's property, culture and occupations, as well as to improve their standard of living.

Globally, indigenous people number more than 370 million and represent approximately 5000 distinct peoples in more than 90 countries. While they account for about 5% of the world population, they represent nearly 15% of the world's poor, and about one-third of the world's 900 million extremely poor rural people (International Fund for Agricultural Development, 2007). There is no official or universal definition of what 'indigenous' means, mainly due to the fact that indigenous people reject any definitions proposed by external agencies because of the long history of political repression and assimilation policies by states

(Gigler, 2009). The term *indigenous* refers to 'distinct peoples who have been pursuing their own concept and way of human development in a given geographical, socioeconomic, political and historical context' (International Labour Organisation (ILO), 2007, p. 3). It has come to include people who:

■ 'identify themselves and are recognised and accepted by their community as indigenous
■ demonstrate historical continuity with precolonial and/or presettler societies;
■ have strong links to territories and surrounding natural resources;
■ have distinct social, economic or political systems;
■ maintain distinct languages, cultures and beliefs;
■ form nondominant groups of society; and
■ resolve to maintain and reproduce their ancestral environments and systems as distinctive peoples and communities' (World Health Organization, 2007, no page).

Indigenous people can be found in all regions of the world; however, roughly 70% of them live in Asia. About 45 to 48 million indigenous people live in Latin America, representing approximately 10% of the region's population (Montenegro and Stephens, 2006). The ethnic composition of Latin America is very diverse and includes, besides the indigenous population, people of European ancestry, European-Amerindians or mestizos, Amerindians, blacks and mulattos (Latinobarómetro, 2011).

An interesting point to make is that while the official statistics often show a specific percentage of the population as being indigenous, various surveys indicate a different picture: due to the different methods used to identify indigenous people, estimates vary greatly (Patrinos et al., 2007). Also, depending on the country, people tend to identify themselves as indigenous in a lower percentage if compared with official data. Figure 40-1 proves this point. In a 2011 survey in Latin America, for example, only 27.3% of the Bolivians interviewed saw themselves as indigenous compared with the official number of 55%, and only 6.9% of Peruvians interviewed identified themselves as indigenous compared with the official number of 45%; the majority saw themselves as mestizos (in this

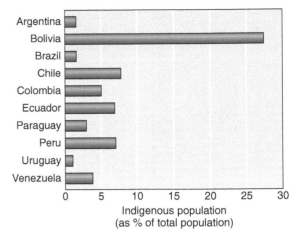

FIGURE 40-1 ■ Percentage of people identifying themselves as indigenous in Latin America (2011).

case, 57.3% of Bolivians and 76% of Peruvians) (Latinobarómetro, 2011)[1].

One of the reasons behind this discrepancy – besides the various methodologies employed – is the widespread discrimination that has led many indigenous people to seek to assimilate with the dominant population. This assimilation process started in many Latin American countries in the twentieth century, when governments initiated programmes for the promotion of the Spanish language among indigenous communities and the inclusion of these communities in the mainstream (Madrid, 2012). As a result, many indigenous people opt to identify themselves as mestizos rather than indigenous (or in some cases, both), since they perceive that they would have more economic opportunities in life, instead of being associated with poverty, illiteracy and primitivism (Albó, 2008; de la Cadena, 2000; García, 2005; Madrid, 2012).

[1]The existence of *mestizaje* between various racial and ethnic groups has led to ambiguous ethnic identities in the region. Surveys have shown that which ethnic group people identify themselves with depends on the choices available, thus leading to large variations among different surveys. In the majority of Latin American countries, people will pick *mestizo*, when the choice is given (Madrid, 2012; Reyles, 2008). In most cases, invisibility of indigenous groups in official statistics and systems indicates the inferior situation in which these groups often live (Ñopo, 2012).

INEQUALITY AND INDIGENOUS PEOPLE

Inequality is multidimensional and refers to 'fundamental disparities that permit one individual certain ... choices, while denying another individual those very same choices' (McKay, 2002, p. 1). These dimensions of inequality may include education, health, security, gender, political power, social inclusion, income or consumption, and assets. Large inequalities in a society can lead to deterioration in social relations (increase in social conflict, violence, imprisonment, lack of trust), health (decrease in life expectancy, and increase in drug abuse, infant mortality, mental illness, obesity) and human capital (decrease in child well-being, perseverance of unequal educational opportunities, low social mobility, teenage births) (McLaren, 2007; Pickett et al., 2005; Subramanian and Kawachi, 2004; Wilkinson and Pickett, 2009). Overall, high inequality is considered a serious threat to human development, since it harms growth, poverty reduction efforts, and the quality of social and political engagement (United Nations Development Programme, 2014).

Historically, one of the groups most affected by inequality has been indigenous people. This discrimination and socioeconomic exclusion are manifested in violation of their basic rights to their ancestral lands, language, culture and self-governance, as well as limited or nonexistent access to basic social services (such as education, health and housing), and the fundamental material conditions for a satisfying quality of life (Gigler, 2009; Partridge et al., 1996; Tauli-Corpuz, 2005). Extensive research into indigenous populations has shown that indigenous people are among the poorest in terms of income with regards to national averages, and that they are severely disadvantaged according to a series of socioeconomic indicators (Alesina and LaFerrara, 2005; Borland and Hunter, 2000; Gundersen, 2008; Hall and Patrinos, 2010; Maani, 2004; United Nations, 2009).

Governments, decision-makers and development agencies – in their effort to promote poverty reduction, food security, sustainable development and the national economy – often consider indigenous people's traditional occupations as outdated and unproductive, while at the same time they disregard indigenous people's lifestyle, values and customs (ILO, 2007). As a result, indigenous people experience inequality within the economic, social, cultural, civil and political areas. According to the International Work Group for Indigenous Affairs (IWGIA, 2012), indigenous people often face:

1. *Socioeconomic inequality:* Indigenous people have generally little access to formal employment and decent living, and many of them work as unskilled labourers, without social protection and with lower wages than the legal minimum. Indigenous women and children are particularly vulnerable to exploitation and abuse; in the worst cases, this abuse may extend to sexual exploitation, trafficking, and child labour.

2. *Civil and political inequality:* Indigenous populations often have fewer civil and political rights than dominant ethnic groups and may even be denied citizenship or hold no identification documents. They are often excluded due to poverty, low education, inability to speak the dominant language, geographic isolation, and different lifestyles and traditions. As a result, they have more difficulty in accessing justice, participating in political decisions, standing for election, voting or getting elected.

3. *Lack of recognition of indigenous people's collective land rights:* Indigenous people face serious violations of their rights to their land, territories and natural resources, which form an important part of their subsistence as well as their spiritual and cultural well-being. This comes as a result of land appropriations by states and private companies, and the exploitation of natural resources by extractive industries, such as mining.

4. *Unequal access to public services:* Indigenous people suffer from discrimination with regards to health access[2] and public services, including

[2]Various studies indicate that indigenous people do not have adequate access to health services and health prevention programmes, and that services are often culturally inappropriate (Athais, 2004; Sanchez, 2004). Some of the most important obstacles to healthcare access are structural and economic factors (distance and location of healthcare facilities, geographical isolation of indigenous communities) and cultural insensitivity of healthcare systems and providers (disrespect for traditional healing practices, language and religious barriers, and impersonal environment of hospitals) (Montenegro and Stephens, 2006).

clean water supply, sanitation, schools, and clinics. Consequently, they generally have lower literacy rates, have higher dropout rates, suffer from poorer health, experience disability and are more likely to die at a younger age. The reasons behind this discrimination include geographic marginalization, nomadic lifestyle, cultural barriers, as well as social and political marginalization.

5. *Contempt for indigenous people's culture:* Indigenous cultures have often been regarded as inferior and primitive, compared with mainstream and dominant cultures. Despite a growing recognition of indigenous cultures in humanity's heritage, many indigenous cultures are on the verge of extinction, while others are threatened by modernization, urbanization, and tourism.

6. *Gender-based inequality:* Indigenous women face discrimination both within mainstream society – due to the fact that they are indigenous and often poor – and from their own societies, especially those that are very conservative and patriarchal; for example, they may have less access to education and training, may have little control over their bodies and may be forced to obey male rules regarding marriage, reproduction and harmful customary practices. They may also be excluded from land ownership and inheritance, as well as from decision-making processes in their community.

However, what are the reasons behind the socioeconomic exclusion and discrimination of indigenous people? According to Hall and Patrinos (2010), a review of the main literature has revealed six main theories on the causes of the inequality and discrimination faced by indigenous people (Table 40-1).

Indigenous people themselves have cited five reasons behind their current status, those being the 500-year-old colonial encounter, the establishment of postindependence states, modernization, economic globalization, and the current crisis of biodiversity loss and climate change (United Nations, 2009). Many communities have been indeed marginalized due to land grabbing, illegal poaching, population transfer, large-scale projects and establishment of protected areas. As a result, they have lost control over their own

TABLE 40-1	
Main Theories of Discrimination of Indigenous People	
Theory	**Explanation**
Spatial disadvantage	Geographic characteristics, including climate, vegetation and remoteness, explain poverty disparities
Human Capital Theory	Lack of education opportunities and poor health, which result in limited labour productivity, lead to low income
Asset-based explanations and poverty traps	Lack of human capital assets and of a minimum asset threshold, together with vulnerability, reduces the possibility of exiting poverty
Social exclusion and discrimination	Lack of social capital and access to key 'networks' leads to social exclusion of the poor, while discrimination limits their access to services and credit
Cultural and behavioural characteristics	The poor are influenced by their own behaviours, including 'culture of poverty', stigma, group-level influences and peer effects
Institutional path dependence	Inequality is reproduced through the social and political status quo and exploitation from the elites

development, while their economy is undermined on account of external control and management of their land and resources (ILO, 2007).

The following section presents the current situation of the Rapanui, the indigenous population of Rapa Nui (Easter Island), as a case of historical discrimination against a particular group of indigenous people by a state/government (in this case, Chile). It provides a useful insight into the modern history of the island that is helpful in order to understand the existing problems and conflicts between Rapa Nui and the Chilean state.

RAPA NUI AND ITS INDIGENOUS PEOPLE: PAST AND PRESENT

The Rapanui are officially recognized as one of the nine indigenous groups of Chile. The country's indigenous people amount to 1 565 915 individuals, that is, 9.1% of the total population (Ministry of Social Development, 2015a). As it is often the case with indigenous populations worldwide, the poverty rates of indigenous population in Chile are higher than the rates of the nonindigenous population. They are, however, falling and converging: while in 2006 the poverty rate of indigenous people was 44% and that of nonindigenous people was 28%, both rates experienced an impressive decrease, and by 2013 the poverty rate of the indigenous population was 23.4% and that of nonindigenous population was 13.5% (Ministry of Social Development, 2015a).

With about 5000 individuals – the majority of whom live on Easter Island, 3512 km away from continental Chile – the Rapanui account for a mere 0.3% of the country's entire indigenous population (Ministry of Social Development, 2015a). Despite their small number, the Rapanui are known worldwide due to their impressive megalithic statues – the Moai – that attract tens of thousands of tourists every year, who are fascinated by the island's archaeological heritage and natural beauty.

During the last few decades, tourism has become the island's main economic motor, with the number of tourists increasing rapidly every year: thus while there were only 27 305 tourist arrivals in 2002, in 2014 this number had reached 65 064 people (CONAF, 2015). Rapa Nui's popularity and the subsequent arrival of an increasing number of tourists have led to a higher income for the local population; it is estimated that in 2012 the annual per capita income may have been in the range of US $8064 to US $15 572 (Figueroa et al., 2013).

Research on the island shows that local people acknowledge the central role that tourism plays in improving their living standards and that they support the further development of the tourism sector, since they have seen visible improvements in their life (Ecopolis, 2010; Figueroa et al., 2013). This positive change has taken place, on the one hand, due to local people's increasing purchasing power – on account of the massive growth of tourism – that has allowed them to invest more in housing, education or family businesses. On the other hand, another reason has been the heavy investment in infrastructure from the Chilean government, not only because

Rapa Nui lagged behind other regions in the mainland but also due to its significant touristic importance that reflects the country's image, especially to foreign visitors.

Despite the central role that tourism plays for Easter Island's economy, tourism has been accused of causing overpopulation, destroying cultural heritage, adding extra pressure on scarce natural resources, and increasing pollution. The growth of the tourism industry is also largely held responsible for an increase in individualism, the weakening of family ties, the introduction of consumer mentality, and an increase in crime and drugs.

Brief History

The history of the Rapanui people has been one of marginalization, discrimination and socioeconomic exclusion that goes back to the eighteenth century and the island's 'discovery' by Western explorers[3]. This discovery was followed by centuries of exploitation and plundering of Rapa Nui's lands and resources. The existing conflict between the Rapanui and the Chilean government cannot be understood outside its historical context, since much of the current dissatisfaction of the Rapanui with the Chilean rule stems from a long history of oppression of the indigenous population.

This history officially began in 1888, when Chile obtained sovereignty over the island through the signature of a treaty with the Rapanui authorities. This agreement remains a thorny issue in the Rapa Nui–Chilean relationship, since many Rapanui reject it completely and claim that it should be declared invalid since the Rapanui community never agreed to handing over their territory and there were differences between the text in Spanish and the one in Rapanui (Fischer, 2005). After 1888, the Rapanui were submitted to conditions of semislavery, abuses, forced exclusion in a small area of the island and mistreatment until the 1960s.

One of the most serious violations of the rights of the Rapanui was the usurpation of their territory, which took place in 1933 when the entire island was registered in the name of Chile, since it 'had no other

---

[3]This chapter does not intend to provide a detailed history of Rapa Nui. For more information on its history, see Diamond (2005), Fischer (2005), Foot (2005) and IWGIA (2012).

owner' (Aylwin, 2005, p. 6). Later on, the Chilean government embarked on a process of assimilation or 'Chilenisation' of the Rapanui, and refused to recognize the separate identity of their culture and language[4]. Nevertheless, during the 1960s, the government increased its efforts to erase the island's former 'colonial' status and to improve the living conditions of the population. According to Porteous (1981), 'infrastructural improvements were motivated on the one hand by the need to provide basic standards for a nascent tourist industry, and on the other by feelings of guilt regarding Chile's neglect of the island during the previous eighty years' (p. 176).

The Rapanui's civil and political rights were acknowledged in 1966 with the introduction of the Easter Island Law (Ley Pasqua), with which the Rapanui gained Chilean citizenship and other benefits, such as tax exemptions, certain land rights and prohibition of land sales to non-Rapanui (Aylwin, 2005). Their rights were further reinforced through the 1993 Indigenous Act that recognized the Rapanui's rights as an indigenous ethnic group and the responsibility of the State to safeguard those rights. In 2007 a constitutional reform was approved, according to which Easter Island is declared 'Special Territory' for the purpose of its government and administration. Finally, in 2009, Chile ratified Convention No. 169 of the International Labour Organisation on Indigenous Peoples, which states that no plans or programmes that affect the life of the Rapanui can be undertaken without first consulting the Rapanui themselves.

Although the socioeconomic condition of the Rapanui people has improved and they have a much more active role in decision-making processes, they still have a long way to go to achieve their goal of self-determination, as better analysed in the section below.

Current Situation on Rapa Nui: Land Restitution and Other Demands

Historically, on account of the island's geographic isolation, the survival of the Rapanui has been based on the self-supply of goods. Their traditional occupations, which are deeply embedded in their culture, include fishing, agriculture and – more recently – livestock. However, with the vast increase in population and tourist numbers, local produce is no longer enough to cater for the demand. This demographic change has led to the vast majority of products being imported from mainland Chile and the Rapanui turning away from their traditional occupations in order to engage in the much more profitable tourist sector[5].

The general socioeconomic data for Rapa Nui reveals that the island has a stable economy, with unemployment very low or nonexistent (Delaune, 2012; Figueroa et al., 2013). Several sources underline that tourism is the main economic base and that most of the community is employed in this sector (Azócar and O'Ryan, 2011; Ecopolis, 2010; Pérez and Rodriguez, 2011).

With regards to poverty rates, in 2013 poverty in Easter Island was 14.1%, a figure which is lower than the regional average (15.6%) and the national average (14.4%), as well as much lower than other regions of Chile, such as in La Araucanía (27.9%), Los Ríos (23.1%) and Maule (22.3%) (Ministry of Social Development, 2015b). Information regarding housing, education, and health also indicate that the living conditions of the Rapanui have improved significantly in the last two decades; while there is still much room for progress, especially with regards to health services (mostly sewer and wastewater treatment) and the provision of specialist doctors to cater to the island's health needs or emergencies[6], most indicators show a positive image, compared with regional or national averages (Ministry of Health, 2013; Ministry of Social Development, 2014).

Nevertheless, in spite of this recent progress and the relative better position they enjoy with regards to other indigenous groups in Chile, the Rapanui still feel

---

[4]The 'Chilenisation' campaign continued during the 1970s and 1980s, with a large increase in Spanish-language television and radio, government offices and education (Porteous, 1981).

[5]A traditional activity that tourism has revitalized is Rapanui dancing, due to the increase in the number of restaurants and the revival of traditional festivals.

[6]It is expected that the construction of the Hanga Roa Hospital, which was inaugurated in October 2012, will greatly improve healthcare, on account of its modern infrastructure and equipment.

marginalized and lacking political power. An issue of great concern to the Rapanui is the uncontrolled immigration by mainland Chileans and foreigners, who decide to live permanently on the island. Since the island is a closed, fragile and small ecosystem, the Rapanui fear the change in the demographics that could result in the slow death of Rapa Nui culture, lifestyle and customs, as well as in irreversible environmental damage. As a result, after consultation with the Rapanui people, an Immigration Control bill was introduced to Congress in 2009, the application of which would regulate the flow of tourists to the island, as well as limit the stay or residence of persons outside the community (Azócar and O'Ryan, 2011). This bill is still pending.

However, the Rapanui's main demand from the Chilean state and the greatest cause of conflict is the restitution of their lands. For the Rapanui, land is of a particular significance due to their socioeconomic and cultural attachments to it. It is not simply a utilitarian relationship; the success of their lifestyle and their own happiness depends on the 'harmonious relationship with the land which bound humans, nature, religion and economics into an indivisible unit' (Jensen, 1993, p. 13). Being pushed by dominant groups into marginal lands of little economic value prevents indigenous people from staying true to their identity, continuing with their traditional occupations, as well as renewing themselves (Frank, 2011). Their disadvantaged position leads to significant disempowerment and lack of self-determination.

In the Rapanui's case, all the lands are claimed as ancestral territory held collectively by the different clans of the island (IWGIA, 2012). Currently, more than 70% of lands remain in the hands of the Chilean state, including the Rapa Nui National Park. The Rapanui's demand includes the right for self-administration of their lands, including the National Park; currently, the income generated by the park is not employed for various development projects on the island, but instead is forwarded to mainland Chile. The occupation of the majority of their lands has not only disrupted their traditional lifestyle but also has forced them to become increasingly dependent on the newly introduced economic structures, that is, tourism, which has had a negative impact on their social organization, worldviews and traditions through the adoption of imported ideas, work practices and even destructive behaviours, such as drinking and drug abuse[7].

As a result of the perceived lack of dialogue with the Chilean government concerning their lands, the Rapanui have initiated a collective demand of restitution of their territory. In order to make their voice heard, various clans proceeded to the occupation of public and private buildings on the island between August 2009 and February 2011. Their demands were suppressed by the Chilean state through the mobilization of emergency police force, violent evictions and the criminalization of the protests (IWGIA, 2012)[8]. This created further discontentment from the Rapanui and increased their distrust in the government, with voices being heard of autonomy and even independence from Chile and the establishment of a Polynesian nation[9].

CONCLUSIONS AND FINAL REMARKS

Indigenous people represent a rich diversity of cultures, traditions, lifestyles, religions, languages, and histories. Nevertheless, they often experience discrimination and serious socioeconomic inequalities; underlying social, economic, historical and environmental factors and structural barriers are the main drivers behind the indigenous people's higher poverty rates, informal employment status, forced displacement,

---

[7]Many mental health problems, including depression and suicide, have been connected either to historical colonization or neocolonization practices and the dispossession of the indigenous people, which in turn has led to the disintegration of indigenous economic, social, political and cultural institutions (United Nations Permanent Forum on Indigenous Issues, 2015).

[8]The demonstrations for land restitution and greater administrative power continued in 2015 when the Rapanui blocked the entrance to the island's main archaeological sites. The demonstrations were peaceful and concluded with a preliminary agreement regarding the administration of the Rapa Nui National Park by the Rapanui themselves.

[9]Gatter Espinosa (2011) concludes that the independence movement is highly unlikely to succeed due to the economic integration between Rapa Nui and the mainland, the lack of official external support for the independence movement, and the extensive migration of mainland Chileans to the island. Interviews on the island further confirmed this conclusion; the vast majority of Rapanui are against independence from Chile but in favour of greater autonomy (Figueroa et al., 2013).

poorer health, fewer education and training opportunities, and limited voice in decision-making processes. They often face racism and lack of cultural sensitivity not only by official governments but also by society in general, that may view their customs, lifestyles and beliefs as primitive. The issues of the usurpation of indigenous lands by governments and private corporations or illegal poaching and habitat destruction are one of the central concerns for many indigenous groups. Land conflicts are often coupled with plundering of resources, cultural and legal discrimination, and a lack of official recognition of their own institutions.

In recent years, there has been progress in the protection of the rights of indigenous people, as well as increased attention from the part of governments to the impediments faced by indigenous populations worldwide. As a result, in many cases, such as, for example, the Rapanui, indigenous people have acquired more rights concerning self-administration, together with better access to education and health, especially since their protests have become much more visible than in the past, due to fast media coverage.

In the case of the Rapanui people, the recent measures that have been adopted by the Chilean state to promote their rights have been generally considered as uncoordinated and unhelpful to resolve the problems brought along by massive migration and tourism, and the individual land claims (IWGIA, 2012). There has been no real effort to address the historical disputes and conflicts with the Chilean state over land, and the constant demands of the Rapanui for self-determination and more political participation. Consequently, the relationship between Rapa Nui and the Chilean state can be characterized as strained and lacking cooperation and trust.

What is needed in the Rapanui's case – but also in the case of most indigenous people – is consultation between communities and government or dominant groups, not imposition of norms and practices of mainstream society. States can and should intervene to reduce inequality and discrimination through a number of policy interventions, including the introduction of accountable institutions of governance, civic engagement and collective mobilization, affirmative action, formal incentives and preventative laws (United Nations Development Programme, 2014).

Community-based projects could also be introduced, which could rely on community control and decision making, cultural appropriateness of work, skill acquisition and economic improvement; thus these programmes can help indigenous people develop skills, improve administration infrastructure in the community, expand social services, improve housing, reduce violence and crime, improve health of communities and create a stronger bond with their culture and traditions (Jensen, 1993).

Overall, in order to address the inequality and socioeconomic discrimination of indigenous people, it is important that research, interventions and policies are better integrated and more pluralistic than at present. It is indispensable to address historically rooted attitudes against indigenous peoples through campaigns, laws and educational measures that will build tolerance, promote inclusion and equity, and therefore support social cohesion and mobility. Governments, policymakers, professionals and researchers need to include in their decisions the world vision, culture and traditions of indigenous populations, and to provide them with the opportunity to represent their own perspectives on all matters that affect their community, such as health, education or employment. There is an increasing need for systems to be appropriate within the indigenous context with the establishment of mechanisms of cooperation among government officials, communities, and policymakers. Addressing socioeconomic inequalities of indigenous people needs to be part of a wider development agenda that takes into account and respects the particularities of indigenous communities and their traditional structures and practitioners.

The introduction of ILO's Convention No. 169 by many governments was a first step towards increasing the self-determination of indigenous people and reducing the neocolonialist practices of governments or dominant groups. However, depending on each case, it needs a much better implementation in order to give a louder voice to the indigenous people and a real opportunity to shape their own policy priorities, and in the end, their future.

REFERENCES

Albó, X., 2008. The 'long memory' of ethnicity in Bolivia and some temporary oscillations. In: Crabtree, J., Whitehead, L. (Eds.),

Unresolved Tensions: Bolivia Past and Present. University of Pittsburgh Press, Pittsburgh, PA, pp. 13–34.

Alesina, A., LaFerrara, E., 2005. Ethnic diversity and economic performance. J. Econ. Lit. 63, 762–800.

Athais, R., 2004. Indigenous traditional medicine among the Hupd'ah-Maku of Tiquie River (Brazil). In: Indigenous Peoples' Rights to Health: Did the International Decade of Indigenous People Make a Difference? London, 9–10 December 2004. London School of Hygiene and Tropical Medicine, London.

Aylwin, J., 2005. Pueblos Indígenas de Chile: Antecedentes Históricos y Situación Actual. Instituto de Estudios Indígenas, Universidad de la Frontera, Temuco, Chile. Available at: <http://www.archivochile.com/Pueblos_originarios/hist_doc_gen/POdocgen0004.pdf> (accessed 08.08.14.).

Azócar, C.C., O'Ryan, P., 2011. Desafíos y Oportunidades de Desarrollo Sostenible de Isla de Pascua Basadas en el Turismo. RedSur Consultores and NGO POLOC, Santiago.

Borland, J., Hunter, B., 2000. Does crime affect employment status? The case of indigenous Australians. Economica 67 (265), 123–144.

CONAF, 2015. Estadísticas de Visitantes Años 2004-2014. CONAF, SNASPE, Santiago. Available at: <http://www.conaf.cl/parques-nacionales/visitanos/estadisticas-de-visitacion/> (accessed 24.06.14.).

de la Cadena, M., 2000. Indigenous Mestizos: The Politics of Race and Culture in Cuzco, Peru, 1919-1991. Duke University Press, Durham, NC.

Delaune, G., 2012. Rapa Nui on the verge: Easter Island's struggles with integration and globalization in the information age. Berkeley Plan. J. 25 (1), 126–139.

Diamond, J., 2005. Collapse: How Societies Choose to Fail or Succeed. Viking, New York.

Ecopolis, 2010. Hacia una Rapa Nui Integrada y Sustentable. Ecopolis, Hanga Roa, Easter Island.

Figueroa, E., Rotarou, E., Aguilar, M., Salazar, A., Gutiérrez, P., Mellafe, R., 2013. Impacto Económico del Establecimiento de un área de Protección Marina en la Provincia de Isla de Pascua-Chile: Informe de Avance. PEW Foundation (PEG-Chile), CESUCC and CENRE, University of Chile, Santiago.

Fischer, S.R., 2005. Island at the End of the World: The Turbulent History of Easter Island. Reaktion Books, London.

Foot, D.K., 2005. Easter Island: a case study in non-sustainability. Greener Manage. Int 48, 11–20.

Frank, G., 2011. The transactional relationship between occupation and place: indigenous cultures in the American Southwest. J. Occup. Sci. 18 (1), 3–20.

García, M.E., 2005. Making Indigenous Citizens: Identities, Education, and Multicultural Development in Peru. Stanford University Press, Palo Alto, CA.

Gatter Espinosa, K.M., 2011. Isla de Pascua or Rapa Nui? Easter Island and the Prospects of Independence. Center for Latin American and Latino Studies, American University, Washington, DC.

Gigler, B.S., 2009. Poverty, inequality and human development of indigenous peoples in Bolivia. Working paper series no. 17. Georgetown University, Center for Latin American Studies,

Washington, DC. Available at: <http://pdba.georgetown.edu/CLAS%20RESEARCH/Working%20Papers/WP17.pdf> (accessed 12.02.15.).

Gundersen, C., 2008. Measuring the extent, depth, and severity of food insecurity: an application to American Indians in the USA. J. Popul. Econ. 21 (1), 191–215.

Hall, G., Patrinos, H.A., 2010. Ch.9 Conclusion: Towards a better future for the world's indigenous. In: Hall, G., Patrinos, H.A. (Eds.), Indigenous People, Poverty and Development. Draft manuscript. World Bank, Washington, DC, pp. 310–339.

International Fund for Agricultural Development, 2007. Statistics and Key Facts about Indigenous Peoples. IFAD, Rome.

International Labour Organisation, 2007. Eliminating discrimination against indigenous and tribal peoples in employment and occupation: a guide to ILO Convention No. 111. ILO, Geneva.

International Work Group for Indigenous Affairs (IWGIA), 2012. The human rights of the Rapa Nui people on Easter Island. IWGIA Report 15, Report of the International Observers' Mission to Rapa Nui 2011. IWGIA, Santiago, Chile. Available at: <http://www.iwgia.org/iwgia_files_publications_files/0597_Informe_RAPA_NUI_IGIA-Observatorio_English_FINAL.pdf> (accessed 20.06.14.).

Jensen, H., 1993. What it means to get off sit-down money: community development employment projects (CDEP). J. Occup. Sci. 1 (2), 12–18.

Latinobarómetro, 2011. Analysis online: Valores – Raza y discriminación: Raza a la que pertenece. Latinobarómetro, Santiago, Chile. Available at: <http://www.latinobarometro.org/latOnline.jsp> (accessed 21.07.14.).

Maani, S.A., 2004. Why have Maori relative income levels deteriorated over time? Econ. Rec. 80, 101–124.

Madrid, R., 2012. The Rise of Ethnic Politics in Latin America. Cambridge University Press, New York.

McKay, A., 2002. Defining and measuring inequality. Briefing Paper No 1. Overseas Development Institute and University of Nottingham. <http://www.odi.org/sites/odi.org.uk/files/odi-assets/publications-opinion-files/3804.pdf> (accessed 18.08.14.).

McLaren, L., 2007. Socioeconomic status and obesity. Epidemiol. Rev. 29, 29–48.

Ministry of Health, 2013. Estadísticas de Salud: Estadísticas por Tema. Department of Statistics and Health Information, Ministry of Health, Santiago, Chile. Available at: <http://www.deis.cl/> (accessed 02.09.14.).

Ministry of Social Development, 2014. Reporte Comunal: Isla de Pascua, Región de Valparaíso. Serie Informes Comunales No 1. Ministry of Social Development, Santiago, Chile.

Ministry of Social Development, 2015a. CASEN 2013: Pueblos Indígenas, Síntesis de Resultados. Government of Chile, Santiago, Chile. <http://observatorio.ministeriodesarrollosocial.gob.cl/layout/doc/casen/publicaciones/2011/pobreza_casen_2011.pdf> (accessed 17.03.15.).

Ministry of Social Development, 2015b. CASEN 2013: Situación de la Pobreza en Chile. Government of Chile, Santiago. <http://observatorio.ministeriodesarrollosocial.gob.cl/documentos/Casen2013_Situacion_Pobreza_Chile.pdf> (accessed 17.03.15.).

Montenegro, R.A., Stephens, C., 2006. Indigenous health in Latin America and the Caribbean. Lancet 367, 1859–1869.

Ñopo, H., 2012. New Century, Old Disparities: Gender and Ethnic Earnings Gaps in Latin America and the Caribbean. Inter-American Development Bank and World Bank, Washington, DC.

Partridge, W.L., Uquillas, J.E., Johns, K., 1996. Including the Excluded: Ethnodevelopment in Latin America. World Bank, Washington DC.

Patrinos, H.A., Skoufias, E., Lunde, T., 2007. Indigenous peoples in Latin America: Economic opportunities and social networks. World Bank Policy Research Working Paper 4227. World Bank, Washington, DC.

Pérez, M., Rodriguez, C., 2011. Impactos ambientales generados por el desarrollo turístico en la Isla de Pascua. RIAT 7 (1), 42–48.

Pickett, K.E., Mookherjee, J., Wilkinson, R.G., 2005. Adolescent birth rates, total homicides, and income inequality in rich countries. Am. J. Public Health 95 (7), 1181–1183.

Porteous, J.D., 1981. The Modernisation of Easter Island. University of Victoria, Victoria, BC.

Reyles, Z.D., 2008. Oversimplifying identities: the debate on what is *indigena* and what is *mestizo*. In: Crabtree, J., Whitehead, L. (Eds.), Unresolved Tensions: Bolivia Past and Present. University of Pittsburgh Press, Pittsburgh, PA, pp. 51–61.

Sanchez, G., 2004. I render services for science don't I? … and I am an indigenous descendant. In: Indigenous Peoples' Rights to Health: Did the International Decade of Indigenous People Make a Difference? London, 9–10 December 2004. London School of Hygiene and Tropical Medicine, London.

Subramanian, S.V., Kawachi, I., 2004. Income inequality and health: what have we learned so far? Epidemiol. Rev. 26, 78–91.

Tauli-Corpuz, V., 2005. Indigenous people and the Millennium Development Goals. In: 4th Session of the UN Permanent Forum on Indigenous Issues. New York, 16–27 May 2005. United Nations, New York.

United Nations, 2009. State of the world's indigenous peoples. Department of Economic and Social Affairs. United Nations, New York.

United Nations Development Programme, 2014. Human development report 2014 – sustaining human progress: reducing vulnerabilities and building resilience. UNDP, New York.

United Nations Permanent Forum on Indigenous Issues, 2015. Thematic Issues: Health. United Nations, New York. <http://undesadspd.org/IndigenousPeoples/ThematicIssues/Health.aspx> (accessed 03.03.15.).

Wilkinson, R., Pickett, K., 2009. The Spirit Level: Why More Equal Societies Almost Always Do Better. Allen Lane/Penguin, London.

World Health Organization, 2007. Health of indigenous people. Fact sheet no. 326, October 2007. World Health Organization, Geneva. <http://www.who.int/mediacentre/factsheets/fs326/en/> (accessed 05.03.15.).

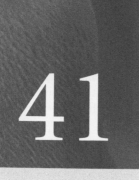

41

FACES OF CAREGIVING IN A SOUTH AFRICAN CONTEXT

THAVANESI GURAYAH ■ PRAGASHNIE GOVENDER ■ DESHINI NAIDOO ■ DEBORAH LEIGH FEWSTER ■ THANALUTCHMY LINGAH

In this chapter, we discuss the lived experiences of caregivers within a South African context. A caregiver is defined as 'an unpaid person who helps an adult or child with physical care or coping with disease' (Hunt, 2003, p. 28) and is a key role player in enabling the care recipient to live in the community (Nalder et al., 2012).

Caregiving can be understood as a purposeful and meaningful occupation. The role of caregiving can be as a result of an occupational choice, or imposed as a moral duty or obligation, and can shape occupational behaviour both positively and negatively. Addressing the needs of caregivers is an emerging field of practice for occupational therapists due to the recognition of the caregiver as an invisible client. Caregivers are at risk for illness themselves, and the stressors they face in fulfilling their role are often not given adequate attention.

In this chapter we use five phenomenological studies (Barr, 2013; Fewster, 2014; Gurayah, 2015; Ive et al., 2013; Kharva et al., 2013) to paint a picture of the caregiving experience in South Africa. The people who participated in these studies were spouses, children, siblings, extended family members and neighbours who provided care predominantly to people with chronic illness. Our aim in this chapter is to illustrate the nuances of caregiving and contribute to the development of occupational therapy intervention for caregivers.

In exploring caregiving as an occupation, we used Molineux's (2010) proposal of recognizing the key characteristics of occupation, which include active engagement in occupation, occupation as purposeful and meaningful, occupation as contextualized and that engagement in occupation is a key characteristic of being human. The studies explored the lived experiences of caregivers, and in particular caregivers of children with autism spectrum disorders (Fewster, 2014), cancer (Kharva et al., 2013) and Down syndrome (Barr, 2013). Further studies of caregiving of individuals with dementia (Gurayah, 2015) and other mental illnesses (Ive et al., 2013) were included to understand the experiences in caregiving from a child's perspective, where the child takes on the role of caregiver.

CAREGIVERS: THE INVISIBLE CLIENTS

Increasingly, caregivers are being recognized as the 'hidden patient' or 'invisible client' in the healthcare system, as they often have neglected health needs (Moghimi, 2007, p. 227). Caregiving activities are labour intensive, with caregivers providing frequent physical handling of the adult or child in their care, despite little training. Caregivers are often faced with the challenges of finding a balance between work and family responsibilities, managing their emotional and physical stress, as well as negotiating access to healthcare for the care recipient (Moghimi, 2007). Systematic reviews by Hunt (2003) and Rigby et al. (2009) reported that caregivers tend to neglect their own health needs, due to a lack of awareness of the effects of caregiving on their mental and physical health.

Caregivers could experience fatigue, changes in their roles and relationships, emotional changes and fluctuations in engagement with daily occupations due to the exigencies of providing care (Nalder et al., 2012). Many caregivers voice uncertainty about the future, a lack of belief in their own skills, as well as feelings of doubt, guilt, sadness and anxiety (Hasselkus and Murray, 2007). The adoption of the caregiver role is time consuming and can result in the neglect of other roles, often causing a lifestyle imbalance. Caregiving can sometimes lead to strained relationships between spouses or other family members (Morgan et al., 2002).

The challenge for occupational therapists is to recognize caregiver needs and to develop methods for intervention that incorporate caregivers. There is also a need to initiate more research focusing on caregivers, to understand the culture-specific impact of caregiving (Pattanayak et al., 2010).

One of the cornerstones of occupational therapy intervention is holistic management. In a client-centred approach, it is essential to consider the characteristics of the individual receiving intervention, as well as the support systems and the environment in which they reside, among other considerations. Liaison with the caregiver is often included in occupational

therapy programmes. However, we propose that this be considered in the foreground of the intervention process. For this to occur, occupational therapists need to understand the occupation of being a caregiver and how intervention for caregivers fits into the process of occupational therapy. We consider it the health professional's responsibility to explore the challenges that caregivers face.

THE ROLE OF CAREGIVING: IMPOSED OR A CHOICE?

Caregivers can be motivated by feelings of affection or obligation. This motivation may be influenced by strong identification with culture, values and beliefs. Moghimi (2007) highlighted that caregivers can be motivated by an altruistic need to reduce other people's distress and improve their welfare. Caregivers can also be motivated by an ego-driven need to help others to gain a feeling of power, receive a reward or improve their social contacts or standing in the community (Moghimi, 2007). The role of caregiving may be an imposed occupation when there is no one else to take on the responsibility. This can lead to feelings of resentment in the caregiver, which is an underreported aspect of caregiving.

Parents are caregivers by virtue of the relationship with their children. Disability or illness places an additional burden to the caregiving relationship. The impact of caregiving responsibilities is illustrated in this example of a mother of an adolescent son with autism (Fewster, 2014, p. 56):

> [It's] an incredible impact on your life, I mean you have this career and you have your life laid out before you and suddenly you are winded. This just comes and lands in your lap, you know…and it changes your life direction, because your focus then becomes that child and getting the support and help for that child… (Shiela)

The following example of Nadia's experience further illustrates: 'You know our kids are not able to help themselves, they need assistance for everything…so for me that is my biggest worry, my biggest fear…' (Fewster, 2014, p. 74).

This attests to the human, innate need to take on the occupation of caregiving. Although the caregiving role in the case of a child with a special need may initially be an imposition on the parent and family as a whole, often the caregiving role becomes a choice. The choice to actively take on the occupation of caregiving resulted in positive experiences and joy for the study participants.

Research in different contexts around the world explores caregiver stress and the effect that the stress has on one's health. Depression, anxiety, social isolation and financial stress are often reported as the main issues (Sherwood et al., 2005). Caregiver burden is the resultant negative consequence of caregiving on the caregiver's personal, social and occupational roles (Given et al., 2001). Similarly, Braithwaite (1996) defined caregiver burden as the conflict that arises from caregivers trying to meet the demands of the caregiving role, to the detriment of meeting their own or their family's basic needs.

We realized from interacting with participants in our studies that the entire family is affected by the consequences of caregiving, both positively and negatively. The following quotes give voice to three parents' reflections on their children's reaction to having a sibling with a disability. These examples from Barr (2013, p. 80) and Fewster (2014, p. 78) highlight family tensions.

> My 13 year old said to me...he has never gone by car when going to school but this child goes with a car... (Thando)

> They also love her but there is that jealousy when my other son asks why I always buy (gifts) for her and I have to explain that it is because she is always in hospital and I tell him I will also buy (gifts) for him when I get the chance. (Fanele)

> She feels neglected...she says we love Andrew and we don't love her. She has started to vocalize that now. She has become very needy. (Andrea)

Conversely, some parents reported that siblings presented with resilience and were impacted positively by the challenges they faced. In Fewster (2014, p. 76), a mother of a child with autism voiced: 'I must say they have become very responsible and very socially aware with people' (Shiela).

Sometimes, spouses found the occupation of caregiving a strain on their relationship, often resulting in separation or divorce. However, some spouses found that facing the challenge of caregiving seemed to forge a new bond that strengthened their love and commitment to each other (Fewster, 2014). The following example from Fewster (2014, p. 79) illustrates the effect of caregiving on the parents' relationship:

> We are fortunate that we've been able to stay together for so long, in many cases the marriage does not last, we are just lucky that we have been able to work through the issues together. It has been a huge challenge...let me tell you right now. (Pieter)

Research has highlighted that caregiving may have positive spin-offs for some caregivers, who report a renewed meaning and purpose in life. Povee et al. (2010) and Mhlanga (2013) found that despite the challenges experienced when caring for a child or adult, caregivers reported finding meaning and joy in their role as a caregiver. Social support, internal locus of control, and optimism were some of the critical factors that contributed to positive coping outcomes in caregiving (Cappe et al., 2011). Narratives about caregiver well-being often allude to finding new meaning in caregiving, the satisfaction or confidence linked to feelings of competence about caregiving and a change in worldview. Positive concepts in caregiving have been linked to caregiver esteem relating to task satisfaction. The occupation of caregiving enhanced the caregiver's experience of their own spirituality and enriched their worldview (Hunt, 2003). Similarly, Moghimi (2007) found that the caregiver role can lead to the development of meaning, spiritual satisfaction, companionship and fulfilment. The following example from Fewster (2014, p. 52) illustrates these deeper concepts further:

> It's also given me a different perception of disabilities, [of] people out there. I think if we didn't have children with special needs, we would not have appreciated others with special needs...Learning to accept people that are different [is] very rewarding. (Nadia)

*I guess having a child with autism you start
knowing the meaning of life. I think appreciating
even the smallest things…'hey mommy see it's
a bird'…and I can spend a few minutes looking
at that bird where once I wouldn't have done it,
so we start to appreciate, I see a lot of life
through his eyes…and life is not a bad thing…*
(Shereen)

THE OCCUPATION OF CAREGIVING

Engagement in occupation is central to developing a
person's sense of identity and competence. Most caregivers had occupations that were fulfilling before
becoming caregivers. Caregiving is described as:

> [T]he provision of extraordinary care, exceeding the
> bounds of what is normative or usual in family
> relationships. Caregiving typically involves a
> significant expenditure of time, energy, and money
> over potentially long periods of time; it involves
> tasks that may be unpleasant and uncomfortable
> and are psychologically stressful and physically
> exhausting. (Prince et al., 2012, p. 671)

Caregiving Contextualized

Caregiving practices may vary across contexts and cultures. The cultural dynamics that are present in the
multicultural context of South Africa embody the filial
responsibility that exists within the Asian and African
cultures. *Ubuntu* is an African concept which values
the rights of the collective over the rights of the individual (Chaplin, n.d.). People are defined by their
interconnectedness with others. The interests of the
individual are seen as subordinate to the interests of
the group, and hence the group constitutes the focus
of individual activities (Du Preez, 2010).

Caregivers are a heterogeneous group of people,
constituting spouses, children, siblings, extended family
relatives, neighbours and volunteers who provide care,
a role which is often seen as a social and moral duty
(Pattanayak et al., 2010). This form of caregiving is
informal and unskilled, as many of these individuals
do not have the necessary training and education to
provide care for the adult or child in their charge
(Buckwalter and Davis, 2011).

Caregiving as a Purposeful and Meaningful Occupation

Caregiving is viewed as purposeful as there is a goal
that the caregiver intends to achieve in the process of
caring. These goals can include daily care of the individual, fostering relationships, aiding recovery, attaining appropriate milestones, and facilitating therapy
and medical interventions. The purpose in caregiving
is driven by an acceptance of the situation which was
identified in an example from Fewster (2014, p. 104):

> *Don't procrastinate. Your child is just a child but
> autism is just that, and a child is still a child, his
> personality, his character all that makes him…Just
> (to) embrace your child and it's just a journey.
> (Nadia)*

Caregiving is meaningful. The meaning people
attribute to caregiving is dynamic and in flux, which
is in keeping with the nature of occupations. Meaning
is also subjective and is constructed through engaging
in caregiving (Pierce, 2001). Meaning-making is closely
linked to choice and control, and meaning motivates
occupational performance (Townsend, 2002).

The notion that choice and control can be linked
to meaning-making and occupational performance,
as posited by Townsend (2002), is illustrated in the
lives of parents who opted to cease working or made
a change in their career focus. This active engagement
in caregiving is concretized by the daily roles, tasks
and routines caregivers assume. Despite the child's
disability or illness, the parental roles of nurturing
and protecting, for example, are clearly seen in the
studies referred to in this chapter. The following
example from Barr (2013, p. 77) speaks to the protective parenting role of a mother of a child with Down
syndrome:

> *Myself, I choose where Sonto must go…Sonto you
> can't go to that person, to that house…especially
> that house because I don't know what was going to
> happen when I'm not there…and I can't just leave
> her with anyone; I have to leave her with a
> person…the one that I rely on her…that she is
> going to look after her the way I look after her.
> (Busi)*

The caregiving role extends beyond just being a parent or caregiver, at times encompassing advocacy (Fewster and Gurayah, 2015). An emerging role of advocacy in caregiving was evident in our studies. Through assuming an advocacy role, the caregivers moved from being passive recipients of society's negative views on illness and disability, to evoking change to these negative perceptions. This was described by a mother of a child with Down syndrome (Barr, 2013, p. 89):

You must love your child so much that the other people next to you will love your child…and you must accept the child so that the others can do the same…and you must be strong, because if you are strong, if there's anybody talking something, telling silly stories you will not listen to them… (Nozipho)

This advocacy role was reiterated by a mother of two children with autism (Fewster, 2014, p. 104):

Don't hide your child away.…Go out there and carve that spot in society. They deserve it, you deserve it and you need to empower yourself with everything you need to know to reach that stage… you can invest in them. Knowledge is power. (Nadia)

Caregiving Shapes Occupational Behaviour

Clarke et al. (2005) reported that caregiving is often full-time work that can consume caregivers' lives to the extent that it leaves little time for other activities. The occupation of caring for another person can be a physically and psychologically demanding task, and can lend itself to occupational risk factors (Schulz and Martire, 2004). Caregivers are especially prone to occupational imbalance and deprivation. According to Whiteford (1997), occupational deprivation may be defined as a state of prolonged preclusion from engagement in occupations of necessity or meaning, due to factors such as geographic isolation, incarceration or disability, which may be outside the control of an individual.

Often caregivers experience role strain from having to balance their caregiver role with their other roles, for example, being a mother or girlfriend (Hunt, 2003). This may result in occupational imbalance,

which manifests when individuals feel that their health and quality of life are compromised due to time constraints from the numerous roles they have to fulfil (Backman, 2010). In a study with children of parents with mental illness (Ive et al., 2013), caregiving was seen as being part of their daily lives. They oscillated between being cared for when the parent was stable and taking care of the parent when he or she relapsed. The eldest sibling was expected to move between child and adult occupations when the parent was unable to care for themselves. The following example is from Jabu, a child of a mother with a mental illness in Ive et al.'s study (2013):

The thing is she [the parent] is very passive, whereas my other siblings, whom are older than me…are more authoritative and stuff…yeah and they disciplined us more. (p. 47)

This occupational disruption was primarily noted in play, leisure and socialization of the children, whose time was taken up by caregiving. In this context, going to school took on an added meaning as a source of comfort and focus, as success at school implied normality. The following quote by Tom (Ive et al., 2013) is indicative:

I was a good student because whatever I didn't have at home, I tried to come and like, you know, get that out of school. I made the most out of my schooling career. (p. 55)

Despite the occupational disruption, a sense of occupational adaptation (Schkade and Schultz, 1992) in these children was noted. The merging of adult and childhood roles was seen as an opportunity to become more independent in making decisions for their own care. The elder sibling would often check homework, provide meals and ensure safety and security (Ive et al., 2013). The first example below is of a mother who was caring for her child with cancer in the hospital, thus demonstrating the shift in roles at home (Kharva et al., 2013, p. 44). The role shift may also encompass a sibling assuming a disciplinarian role, which is illustrated by the second example (Fewster, 2014, p. 78), a father in relation to his daughter's response to her older brother who has Asperger syndrome:

My eldest child, but their father also helps out especially when it comes to cooking. I am very troubled since most of the work has to be done by my eldest child who is only 14 years of age. (Andiswa)

She [sibling Katie] is 12 years old, got to the point where she has to be prescriptive with Andrew… e.g. she would say, 'No, don't do that…' (Darren)

Occupation of Caregiving as a Cultural Construct

The cultural context forms the lens through which people assign meaning to their occupations and influences how they interpret the occupation (Whiteford, 2010). The studies mentioned in this chapter highlight the occupation of caregiving as a cultural construct. The caregivers' behaviour, their feelings of acceptance and the decision to share information about health status was influenced by the community's belief systems. Below, we describe a few of the cultural influences that appeared to shape the occupation of caregiving.

Traditional African beliefs about illness impact community and caregiver perceptions and behaviours. Often, the condition or disease is considered to be a 'curse' by the ancestors for ill-doing on the part of the parents. Ancestor worship is common in Zulu culture (von Kapff, 1997). Ancestors are relatives of the family who have passed away and are relegated to the spirit world, and are seen as links between the living and the dead. They must be remembered at all times, and if forgotten may bring misfortune on the family, which may be in the form of an illness (von Kapff, 1997). The following quotations are indicative of the beliefs of some of the caregivers about Down syndrome (Barr, 2013, p. 70) and (Kharva et al., 2013, p. 36):

I did feel guilty because like I think there was something wrong I did to God, why God must give me a child like this? Because I was thinking everything I am doing, I am doing okay, but I was like maybe there is this thing I did wrong, that's why I got a child like this…or maybe my ancestors are punishing me for something that I did not know. (Thandi)

[T]hey have the belief that it is not only hereditary, some believe it is a traditional illness [ancestors]… [but] we tried traditional healers and still there was no result. (Philile)

There was also the belief that traditional beliefs may have negatively influenced a child's condition. The following quotations from participants (Kharva et al., 2013, pp. 37–38) demonstrate tensions that may exist between different belief systems, and the potential impact arising out of these tensions.

The community does not even believe it is cancer because the child loses weight, they assume it is HIV/AIDS…. (Nosipho)

Sometimes I blame myself for my child's condition since when I was pregnant the doctor had given me pills to take but I kept throwing them away…. (Thabi)

The caregivers often felt rejected by families and communities due to the traditional beliefs held (Barr, 2013, pp. 83–84):

You find that the child will come back from the neighbour crying or the other kids will chase the child away…they are not accepted in the community…the community is not educated about children with Down's. (Thembi)

Even the community can't accept, can't accept. Even the neighbours and the small kids hit the babies. It's hard, it's hard, it's hard. (Lungi)

Yet, they remained hopeful for acceptance from family members and the community. The following quotation from a parent of a child with Down syndrome highlights this need for acceptance (Barr, 2013, p. 78):

So you need to pray and hope for the family to accept the child because you can accept…because it is your child but the family can be very un-accepting. (Bongi)

Silence in the community about certain health or disease states was another interesting observation from our studies. When there was nondisclosure of the illness, we noticed that the communities were not in a position to practise discrimination. Many caregivers reported not feeling comfortable in sharing the condition or diagnosis with their community members. Some expressed fear at not knowing how the community would react, and restricted disclosure to family and close friends only. As such, the sense of the collective, of *ubuntu* appeared lost. Following are some voices of caregivers of children with cancer (Kharva et al., 2013, pp. 36–37):

I am the only one in the community with the child with cancer. (Neliswe)

I was really hurt when my child was diagnosed since I had not ever heard in my community that there is a child with cancer, I was going to be the first one. (Phume)

The community does not accept it very easily that a young child has cancer, especially when no one in the family has ever had cancer. (Eunice)

IMPLICATIONS FOR OCCUPATIONAL THERAPY PRACTICE

Assessment

A comprehensive and culturally sensitive assessment of the caregiver is needed before intervention. Some of the areas that need to be considered include the following:

- Physical and mental health conditions that may affect the caregivers' ability to perform the required tasks.
- The scope and nature of the caregiving duties.
- The potential occupational risk factors.
- The social and physical support available from the extended family and community.

Intervention

Caregivers need to be both a part of the multidisciplinary team and recipients of care.

Being Part of the Team

To be an effective member of the multidisciplinary team, caregivers need training to improve their mastery

of daily activities required by the role and to decrease the perceived sense of caregiver burden. This burden of care is further compounded by the stigma related to illness and disability. Caregivers might benefit from training in how to identify and deal with issues relating to stigma. This training should include advocacy, awareness and education of caregivers, who will use these skills and knowledge to empower both the family and their communities.

Being a Recipient of Care

In order to be effective in their role, caregivers need to manage their physical and emotional health, as well as understand and address occupational risk factors. Intervention strategies that occupational therapists could employ include setting up peer support and mentoring programmes for the caregivers to deal with issues such as the management of guilt, self-blame, vicarious pain and acceptance.

Furthermore, occupational therapists need to improve their awareness of the risk factors to assist individuals to maintain good levels of health, well-being and participation in their occupational choices, with an emphasis on occupational balance being crucial to good health.

These intervention strategies would assist occupational therapists in working more effectively with caregivers to allow them to balance their caregiver responsibilities and to tailor their own personal occupations in such a way that they achieve occupational balance.

CONCLUSION

Caregiving is a complex phenomenon with negative and positive consequences. Caregivers are a heterogeneous group of people including spouses, children, siblings, extended family, neighbours and volunteers, and practices may vary across cultures and contexts. While caregiving can be a purposeful and meaningful occupation for some, for others it may cause occupational disruption. Caregiving may be an imposed occupation for some, but others show resilience by choosing this as a way to add meaning to their lives. Occupational therapists need to be mindful of the unique problems that caregivers face to effectively address them.

REFERENCES

Backman, C.L., 2010. Occupational balance and well-being. In: Christensen, C., Townsend, E. (Eds.), Introduction to Occupation: Art and Science of Living. Prentice Hall, Upper Saddle River, NJ.

Barr, M.D., 2013. The experience of raising a child with Down's syndrome: perceptions of caregivers in KwaZulu-Natal. Master's thesis. University of KwaZulu-Natal, Durban, South Africa. <http://hdl.handle.net/10413/11132>.

Braithwaite, V., 1996. Understanding stress in informal caregiving: is burden a problem of the individual or of society? Res. Aging 18 (2), 139–174.

Buckwalter, K.C., Davis, L.L., 2011. Elder caregiving in rural communities. In: Talley, R.C., et al. (Eds.), Rural Caregiving in the United States: Research, Practice, Policy. Springer Publishing Company, New York, pp. 33–46.

Cappe, E., Wolff, M., Bobet, R., Adrien, J.L., 2011. Quality of life: a key variable to consider in the evaluation of adjustment in parents of children with autism spectrum disorders and in the development of relevant support and assistance programs. Qual. Life Res. 20 (8), 1279–1291.

Chaplin, K., n.d.. The Ubuntu spirit in African communities. <http://www.coe.int/t/dg4/cultureheritage/culture/Cities/Publication/BookCoE20-Chaplin.pdf> (accessed 10.04.15.).

Clarke, J.N., Fletcher, P.C., Schneider, M.A., 2005. Mothers' home health care work when their children have cancer. J. Paediatr. Oncol. Nurs. 22 (6), 365–373.

Du Preez, R., 2010. An ethnographic study of caregiving at a day care centre for developmentally challenged children. Master's thesis. University of South Africa. Available at: <http://uir.unisa.ac.za/bitstream/handle/10500/4685/dissertation_depreez_r.pdf?sequence=1> (accessed 10.04.15.).

Fewster, D.L., 2014. A Qualitative Study to Understand the Experiences and Coping Processes of Primary Caregivers of Children with Autism Spectrum Disorder. <http://researchspace.ukzn.ac.za/xmlui/handle/10413/10979> (accessed 05.13.16.).

Fewster, D.L., Gurayah, T., 2015. First port of call: facing the parents of autism spectrum disorder. S. Afr. Fam. Pract. 57 (1), 31–34. doi: 10.1080/20786190.2014.995917.

Given, B.A., Kozachik, S., Collins, C.E., DeVoss, D.N., Given, C.W., 2001. Caregiver role strain. In: Maas, M.L., et al. (Eds.), Nursing Care of Older Adults: Diagnosis, Outcomes and Interventions. Mosby, St. Louis, MO, pp. 679–695.

Gurayah, T., 2015. Caregiving for people with dementia in a rural context in South Africa. S. Afr. Fam. Pract. 57 (3), 194–197. doi: 10.1080/20786190.2014.976946.

Hasselkus, B.J., Murray, B.J., 2007. Everyday occupation, well-being, and identity: the experience of caregivers in families with dementia. Am. J. Occup. Ther. 61 (1), 9–20.

Hunt, C.K., 2003. Concepts in caregiver research. J. Nurs. Scholarsh. 35 (1), 27–32.

Ive, C., Abbott, K., Williams, L., Feng, P., Lubbee, C., Paruk, H., 2013. The study of adult offspring's lived experiences, with a mentally ill parent, where the parent is receiving intervention at King Dinizulu Hospital. Bachelor's thesis. University of KwaZulu-Natal, Westville.

Kharva, N., Mamane, T., Mtolo, S., Stott, T., Trend, S.J., 2013. The psychological effect of having a child with cancer: life through the eyes of mothers at CHOC Durban. Bachelor's thesis. University of KwaZulu-Natal, Westville.

Mhlanga, S., 2013. Positive experiences of mothers of a child with Down syndrome in the Western Cape. Unpublished Masters dissertation, North-West University, Potchefstroom. Available at: <http://dspace.nwu.ac.za/bitstream/handle/10394/9593/Mhlanga_S.pdf?sequence=1> (accessed 10.04.15.).

Moghimi, C., 2007. Issues in caregiving: the role of occupational therapy in Caregiver Training. Top. Geriatr. Rehabil. 23 (3), 269–279.

Molineux, M., 2010. The nature of occupation. In: Curtin, M., et al. (Eds.), Occupational Therapy and Physical Dysfunction: Enabling Occupation. Churchill Livingstone-Elsevier Ltd., New York.

Morgan, J., Robinson, D., Aldridge, J., 2002. Parenting stress and externalizing child behaviour. Child Fam. Soc. Work 7 (3), 219–225. doi: 10.1046/j.1365-2206.2002.00242.x.

Nalder, E., Flemming, J., Cornwell, P., Foster, M., 2012. Linked lives: the experiences of family caregivers during the transition from hospital to home following Traumatic Brain Injury. Brain Impair. 13 (1), 108–122.

Pattanayak, R.D., Jena, R., Tripathi, M., Khandelwal, S.K., 2010. Assessment of burden in caregivers of Alzheimer's disease from India. Asian J. Psychiatr. 3 (3), 112–116.

Pierce, L., 2001. Untangling occupation and activity. Am. J. Occup. Ther. 55 (2), 138–146.

Povee, K., Roberts, L., Bourke, J., Leonard, H., 2010. Family functioning in families with a child with Down syndrome: a mixed methods approach. J. Intellect. Disabil. Res. 56 (10), 961–973.

Prince, M., Brodaty, H., Uwakwe, R., Acosta, D., Ferri, C., Guerra, M., 2012. Strain and its correlates among carers of people with dementia in low-income and middle-income countries: a 10/66 Dementia Research Group population-based survey. Int. J. Geriatr. Psychiatry 27 (7), 670–682.

Rigby, H., Gubitz, G., Phillips, S., 2009. A systematic review of caregiver burden following stroke. Int. J. Stroke 4 (4), 285–292.

Schkade, J.K., Schultz, S., 1992. Occupational adaptation: toward a holistic approach in contemporary practice, Part I. Am. J. Occup. Ther. 46, 829–837.

Schulz, R., Martire, L.M., 2004. Family caregiving of persons with dementia: prevalence, health effects, and support strategies. Am. J. Geriatr. Psychiatry 12 (3), 240–249.

Sherwood, P.R., Given, C.W., Given, B.A., von Eye, A., 2005. Caregiver burden and depressive symptoms. J. Aging Health 17 (2), 125–147.

Townsend, E., 2002. Enabling Occupation. An Occupational Therapy Perspective. C.A.O.T. Publications ACE, Ottawa.

von Kapff, U., 1997. Zulu 'People of Heaven'. South Africa Holiday Africa Publications, South Africa.

Whiteford, G., 1997. Occupational deprivation and incarceration. J. Occup. Sci. 4 (3), 126–130.

Whiteford, G., 2010. Occupation in context. In: Curtin, M., et al. (Eds.), Occupational Therapy and Physical Dysfunction: Enabling Occupation. Churchill Livingstone-Elsevier Ltd., New York.

42

OCCUPATIONAL DEPRIVATION FOR ASYLUM SEEKERS

ANNE-LE MORVILLE ■ LENA-KARIN ERLANDSSON

A man without occupations is a dead man.
—Citation from a 26-year-old Afghan farmer and asylum seeker

CHAPTER OUTLINE

On a global level, the number of people forcibly displaced by war, civil unrest or danger of persecution is rising. The United Nations Refugee Agency (United Nations High Commissioner for Refugees, 2015) estimated that in 2014, 59.5 million people were forcibly displaced due to conflict and persecution, 13.9 million people were newly displaced, and another 38.2 million people were internally displaced, and the numbers keep rising. In 2014 alone, 1.7 million people were seeking asylum (United Nations High Commissioner for Refugees, 2015). The increased number of armed conflicts and wars seen since 2001, and especially since 2010 and until the time of this writing (2015), has made the presence of asylum seekers and refugees increasingly common in clinical settings all over the world (United Nations High Commissioner for Refugees, 2015). Forced migrants, and among them asylum seekers, experience a major change in their daily life by fleeing their homeland. They often leave following traumatic incidences of persecution, war, armed conflict, and human rights violations. This disruption and often deprivation of daily occupations and routines and the consequences for asylum seekers is the focus of this chapter. We describe the deprivation that asylum seekers and refugees living in detention can experience and how it affects their everyday lives, in combination with factors such as trauma, health, exposure to war-related crimes, and legal status. The term *asylum seeker* in this chapter denotes a person who has fled his or her own country in order to seek asylum in another country, but has yet to receive a residence permit.

Occupational therapists and other healthcare workers primarily meet asylum seekers in ordinary practice, which seldom leaves room for the specialized treatment that may be needed. Due to the lack of knowledge and maybe even avoidance of including such matters as consequences of war-related crimes, human rights violations, and trauma into occupational therapy research and practice, there is a risk of delivering inadequate or no treatment. In addition, cultural and language barriers may obstruct rehabilitation. This group of clients often experience different aspects of occupational imbalance due to the process of fleeing and relocating in a new environment. We find it imperative that occupational therapy practice and research is aware of this group, no matter where one's clinical practice is located. The two cases presented here are fictional but are based on real-life stories about daily life of asylum seekers in Denmark (Case 42-1 and 42-2).

THE OCCUPATIONAL CONDITIONS OF BEING AN ASYLUM SEEKER

People seeking asylum can be disadvantaged and vulnerable, due to their exposure to traumatic incidents, and their legal and social situation. They are an economically and medically disadvantaged group as they often do not have the same access, if any, to work, healthcare and rehabilitation as the resident population in the host country. There are large national differences in the legal, economic, and housing possibilities for asylum seekers. In Denmark, asylum seekers live in shared rooms or small apartments with at the most four occupants. If they are a family, they have the right to have two rooms and are free to come and go as they wish (Danish Immigration Service, 2013). In other countries, refugees and asylum seekers are in detention centres and are not allowed to leave

CASE 42-1

Alaia's Story

Alaia was a medical doctor and mother of four who had fled her country with her youngest son, Ramir, 14, but leaving her three grown sons and their families behind, including two beloved granddaughters. She had been abducted and flogged for working as a paediatrician at a hospital run by a foreign charity. With the aid of family and friends they were smuggled across the border and then left for Denmark. Ramir started school at the centre 2 weeks after arrival and Alaia started a group for families with small children. She explained that it was needed, because all these young women and men did not have their families around to support them. She also assisted as interpreter and medical advisor for the nurses at the centre's medical clinic. Alaia soon had 'office hours' outside what the medical clinic could offer, and felt that what she did now was maybe even more meaningful than what she had done before. She kept a strict daily routine for herself and her son, including taking part in language classes, and after a few months both could have a basic conversation in Danish. After they received their residence permit, Alaia has been busy working on getting a Danish authorization as a doctor, taking courses and doing clinical practice. Ramir is in a Danish primary school, has a growing circle of friends and is a hero of the local football team.

CASE 42-2

Ali's Story

Ali was a young teacher who had to flee his homeland, family, friends and girlfriend due to political persecution. Before he managed to flee he was both arrested and tortured. In Denmark, he ended up in an asylum centre where there was a hair salon, though without a hairdresser. The room contained the necessities for shaving and giving haircuts, and Ali took on the responsibility for taking care of the room and applying for new materials, when needed. He also started to cut the hair of other residents at the asylum centre, and soon called himself 'chief hairdresser'. Ali was then moved to another centre, but took the bus every morning to 'go to work', though he was never paid for what he did. He also helped with interpreting for the other asylum seekers. After a few months in the centre Ali had stopped working and just sat in his room or went for walks. He did not participate in the available activities at the centre and did not feel that there was meaning in what he did. He said that he had only taken on the role as hairdresser in order 'not to go crazy' and keep busy. He wanted to teach again but did not want to work for free; he did not, however, have the qualifications or permission to work in the centre's school. Ali has been unemployed since he gained his residence permit 2 years ago and has given up on learning Danish and being a teacher. He spends most of his time alone in his apartment.

these facilities, where they have to share small rooms with 15 to 20 or more other asylum seekers. In Denmark, a mother like Alaia and her son Ramir (Case 42-1) would have two rooms, a private bath and a kitchenette, a key to lock their door and the ability to maintain their privacy, whereas, for example, in Austria, they would have to stay in a room with six others, with unlocked doors, no personal keys and no access to privacy (Danish Immigration Service, 2013; Steindl et al., 2008). Access to work and education also differ between countries, but all asylum seekers experience a major upheaval and change in their daily lives (Bennett et al., 2012; Bhugra and Becker, 2005; McElroy et al., 2012; Morville and Erlandsson, 2013).

What most asylum seekers have in common is that they are forced to leave behind their occupational repertoire, that is, the opportunity to belong and participate in work, family relations and network, and the occupations connected to these (Bennett et al., 2012; McElroy et al., 2012; Morville and Erlandsson, 2013; Townsend and Polatajko, 2007). Ali (Case study 42-2) lost his roles as worker, son, boyfriend, brother, uncle, and friend, depriving him of the familiar occupations which he valued and that gave meaning in his life. Alaia, on the other hand, kept her role as a mother and as a doctor, which made her loss of roles and occupations less severe.

Asylum seekers often spend months, if not years, in asylum centres with limited opportunities to pursue former occupations or develop new ones. They describe their lives as interrupted, on hold, or blown off course (Bhugra and Becker, 2005; Burchett and Matheson, 2010; McElroy et al., 2012). The structural elements that underlie occupations, such as legal, institutional, social, cultural, and geographic factors, block opportunities for engagement in meaningful and valued occupations. These losses might trigger marginalization and a string of negative events for both the individual and the group, and even on a societal level (Townsend and Polatajko, 2007). By losing the opportunity to maintain and pursue familiar and valued occupations over a longer period of time, asylum seekers are in danger of experiencing a state of occupational deprivation. This is due to the move from a known environment and legal restrictions. However, some may adapt to or even change their new environment, as can be seen with Alaia and

Ramir, who both managed to adapt to their new environment, as well as gain new occupations.

Asylum Seekers and Occupational Disruption

Occupational disruption is described as the act of delaying or interrupting continuity in everyday life, or in other words something which creates disorder (Whiteford, 2000). The serious and demanding disruptions that asylum seekers experience influence their opportunities for making choices regarding occupations (Bennett et al., 2012; McElroy et al., 2012). Ali lost his familiar networks, not to mention the loss of roles and routines, and the occupations connected to those roles. The feeling of being a capable and valuable person through occupations is lost, and many experience a major change in occupational identity due to this loss, as did Ali, as his opportunity to keep busy and have something valuable and meaningful to wake up to were missing (Hammell, 2004; Morville and Erlandsson, 2013; Townsend and Polatajko, 2007). The lack of meaningful and valued occupations can result in a major shift not only in daily occupations, but in roles, social relationships and status, giving way to a change in occupational identity (Morville and Erlandsson, 2013). This occupational alienation leaves the asylum seekers in a void of not belonging in the cultural and social environment in their host country and the experience of a life out of control, even though the cases here illustrate that people try to stay in control (Morville and Erlandsson, 2013). While Alaia manages to keep control, Ali loses control after a period of time. People seeking asylum find themselves in a new country, often without the means or opportunities to continue their previous daily life with valued occupations. This is on a basic level such as having the opportunity to perform a familiar task, like cooking a meal. This activity may be unavailable because one is obliged to eat in a canteen or because the environment does not support the habitual way of cooking (Martins and Reid, 2007; Steindl et al., 2008). Some centres in Denmark use the obligation to eat in a canteen as a deliberate punishment, denying the opportunity to perform such basic occupations as making a meal, in order to make the stay in Denmark less attractive. Also, expressing oneself in one's own language, the amount of clothes to put on when in different climates (Whiteford, 2004) and different ways of structuring daily life are influenced by this change in environment (McElroy et al., 2012; Morville and Erlandsson, 2013). However, occupational disruption can be a temporary state and one that, given supportive conditions, can resolve itself (Whiteford, 2000).

Some may gain control and adapt to the new environment if it supports the opportunity to regain old occupations or develop new ones, such as in Alaia's case, where she was able to find something meaningful to do. However, most asylum seekers in Denmark are in an environment that does not support the opportunity to engage and participate in new or former valued occupations. This reduces their choice and range of occupations available, and they may subsequently develop a state of occupational deprivation, and this in turn has consequences for their psychological and physical health and well-being, and their life quality (Morville et al., 2015a; Whiteford, 2005).

Asylum Seekers and Occupational Deprivation

Occupational deprivation is a state of preclusion from engagement in occupations due to factors that stand outside the immediate control of the individual (Whiteford, 2000). When discussing occupational deprivation in relation to asylum seekers, it is important to note that this pattern of deprivation may have begun as persecution or marginalization in their homeland and during the flight, and is not just a state they experience exclusively in an asylum centre. Ramir (see Case 42-1) revealed that he did not play with other kids in his homeland, as he was afraid that someone might slander and persecute his family; Alaia was persecuted and punished for working as a doctor, due to the occupational marginalization of female doctors in her homeland. Whether people experience occupational alienation and deprivation may differ between the different locations where they seek asylum, as in each there are different structural factors, such as rules and legislations regarding the rights and obligations of being an asylum seeker.

Studies have shown that these profound changes in environment, life roles, and daily occupations influence the meaning and purpose of familiar occupations to such an extent that it influences people's identity (Huot and Rudman, 2010; McElroy et al., 2012; Morville and Erlandsson, 2013). People build their identity through occupations; a lack of positive experiences and opportunities to seek meaning and purposeful occupations can distort this formation and continuing development of a positive identity. Ali's case shows that the loss of his identity as a teacher and the adoption of his new identity of being a hairdresser influenced his identity and occupational status negatively. The challenges and knowledge needed for being a hairdresser in the camp were not comparable with the profession he had as a teacher. Accepting jobs below their formal education, competences and experience is a situation that a majority of refugees find themselves in after they have gained refugee status in their host country, due to language barriers, for example.

A part of occupational deprivation is taking part in occupations that do not serve any purpose or give meaning. Kronenberg and Pollard have described this as occupational absurdity (Kronenberg et al., 2005), which can reinforce the deterioration of an occupational identity. A study by Morville and colleagues (2015b) indicated that asylum seekers in centres who spend a large proportion of their time doing nothing, or merely filling time with activities that have a minimal potential for being engaging or meaningful, reported a very low level of satisfaction with daily occupations. It is likely that the reported dissatisfaction reflects occupational deprivation and alienation, as opportunities for feeling engaged, challenged, and competent through occupations are missing or low.

In relation to asylum seekers' experience of occupational deprivation, one should be aware that the quantity of activities is not in itself an indication of whether a person perceives general satisfaction with daily occupations, self-rated health, and well-being. Even so, having more to do is positively related to health and well-being, but it seems to depend on the area of activity, for example, work/study, leisure, home chores and self-care, which all influence the satisfaction in different ways (Eklund and Leufstadius, 2007; Morville et al., 2015b). Time spent in paid work has been shown to be an especially important aspect of the actual activities that are of importance to self-rated health and well-being and the healing process (Mollica, 2006; Rosenthal et al., 2012).

The lack of opportunities to spend time on work and studies might play a large role in the asylum seekers' experience of occupational deprivation. A study by Morville et al. (2015b) showed a positive relation between quantities of activities, satisfaction with occupations and well-being in a group of asylum seekers, even though the asylum seekers in general rated their satisfaction with daily occupations as low. The passivity, boredom, lack of purpose and meaning often go hand in hand with the contextual factors, and can draw asylum seekers into discomfort and undermine their health and satisfaction with occupations (Morville and Erlandsson, 2013; Morville et al., 2015b). Thus, it seems to be better to have something to do than having nothing to do. Even though Alaia did not receive pay for her work at the centre, she had work-like occupations, which might have been a factor that helped her to adapt to a new life in a new country. Ali, on the other hand, was not able to have a meaningful sustainable worker role, which might be a factor in the occupational dysfunction that developed in his situation, since she now had a role which did not reflect his education and status in his home context.

Morville et al. (2015b) reported that those people who had higher education reported having more activities than those without. People with a higher level of education seem to cope better with the time in detention and lack of occupations (Morville et al., 2015b; Quiroga, 2005).

Asylum Seekers and Occupational Dysfunction

A string of negative incidents and occupational deprivation leads to occupational dysfunction and can have an impact on occupational performance (Whiteford, 2000). The capacity to perform occupations is based on whether the person possesses the skills to act (Fisher and Jones, 2011; Kielhofner, 2007). Even if the person possesses those skills, occupational deprivation over a longer period of time may reduce both the person's skills and their experience of health and well-being, that is, they might develop a state of occupational dysfunction (Whiteford, 2000). Several studies (Morville et al., 2014, 2015a, 2015b) have shown that some asylum seekers already had a decreased activities of daily living (ADL) ability on entrance to the host country. The experience of deprivation over a

longer period of time not only reduced their opportunity to maintain occupations and satisfaction with their doing on a daily basis, but for some people also severely decreased their ability to perform daily tasks and maintain routines (Morville et al., 2014). One of the problems regarding ADL ability that asylum seekers encounter, seems to be primarily in process skills, which are needed in order to plan and execute an occupation (Morville et al., 2014, 2015a). This change threatens the asylum seeker's ability to adapt to the new environment, in order to maintain some daily routines. Furthermore, this development is worrisome as the asylum seekers' decreased ability to plan and execute a daily activity may influence their ability to adapt to a new environment and transition into society when they gain asylum, as was seen in Ali's case.

An occupational therapy-guided intervention enabling opportunities to include some of the lost daily and meaningful tasks that he missed in his daily repertoire, might lessen Ali's dysfunction. He had, however, been deprived for so long that his dysfunction had become a more or less chronic state. Subsequently, he had difficulties getting a job and lost his ability to engage in occupations, experiencing a further decrease in ADL ability. A case such as Ali's shows that the consequences of the time spent in a centre and the experience of occupational deprivation and loss of hope might negatively influence the possibility of a transition back to a balanced and satisfying daily life, once the asylum seeker is granted his or her residence permit.

This string of events that has such a negative impact on the lives of people seeking asylum is mirrored in the problems with maintaining a daily life and getting employment once asylum in the host country has been gained. The negative influence on not just the individual but also the group and society is severe, as both social and economic problems surface due to the deterioration in skills and competences of those having gained asylum.

ASYLUM SEEKERS WITH TRAUMA

One fact, seldom discussed in occupational therapy, is that war-related crimes and the subsequent traumas are an important factor in the health and occupational problems that some asylum seekers display (Black, 2011). Occupational therapists often meet traumatized survivors of war-related crimes in their clinical practice, but lack the instruments and knowledge to provide appropriate services.

Asylum seekers have often been exposed to armed conflicts or war-related traumatic incidents, which influence their health and well-being. Many studies have shown that asylum seekers may experience depression, anxiety, post-traumatic stress and pain, and that their health can deteriorate further while being in an asylum centre without opportunities to pursue valued occupations (Hallas et al., 2007; Masmas et al., 2008; Williams et al., 2010). Those who have been subjected to war-related crimes, such as torture, have a larger prevalence of both psychological and physical symptoms (Masmas et al., 2008). Torture is one of the most serious violations of human dignity. It is not directed only against individuals, but also their societies, with the goal of destroying the community (Quiroga, 2005). It makes examples of individuals and their families and it terrorizes the entire community into submission. For example, its influence on a child like Ramir, who did not dare to talk to his friends, shows how the whole community could be exposed to occupational deprivation as a result. Both the survivors and the witnesses to such crimes could be at higher risk of being afflicted by ill health and occupational deprivation and eventually develop occupational dysfunction, such as the reduced ability to perform daily tasks, for example, cleaning or cooking a meal, in a safe and independent manner.

Morville and colleagues (2014) found no difference in occupational performance of daily tasks or satisfaction with the opportunities for occupations available at the centres between tortured and nontortured asylum seekers, when they were newly arrived at the asylum centre. However, when assessed for occupational performance after 10 months, they found not only a severe decline in occupational performance, but also that the number of torture methods the asylum seeker had been exposed to was associated with a decline in ADL motor skills (Morville et al., 2015a). It is important to note that war-related traumas may manifest themselves in many ways. Asylum seekers may integrate into the host society, for example, working, taking care of family, pursuing leisure

interests, etc., and after a number of years experience post-traumatic stress, depression, and physical symptoms, due to the incidents they experienced before or during their flight and the time spent in the asylum centres.

This leaves a group of people requiring appropriate rehabilitation, since traumatized victims of war and human rights violations often experience long-term health-related consequences (Carlsson et al., 2006; Coffey et al., 2010; Egloff et al., 2013; Morville et al., 2015a, 2015b; Williams et al., 2010).

Several countries have ratified the United Nations Convention against Torture (2012) and by doing so are committed to providing rehabilitation to survivors of war-related traumas. However, the convention is not generally followed. One of the consequences of restrictions on access to healthcare and rehabilitation is that asylum seekers living in centres, over time could develop a persistence of both the physical and the psychological symptoms that are seen after traumatic incidences. These in turn contribute to, among other factors, the decrease of ADL ability and loss of those occupations which provide meaning in daily life (Morville and Erlandsson, 2013; Morville et al., 2015a).

Need for Occupational Therapy Intervention

The need for occupational therapy might be even greater in the asylum-seeker population who have survived war-related crimes than among other asylum seekers. Unfortunately, specialized centres for rehabilitation of traumatized asylum seekers often lack occupational therapists, even though the skills and knowledge that occupational therapists possess are well suited to fit this group's need for rehabilitation. It is even rarer to have occupational therapists in asylum centres who recognize the specific occupation-related needs of asylum seekers. The lack of medical and especially rehabilitation professionals in asylum centres is foremost a structural and political issue. In general, the centres are for people who are waiting either for permission to stay or to be deported from the country. In this phase, rehabilitation is not prioritized. At the same time, maybe due to occupational therapists' avoidance of the tales of torture or other human rights violations, this is so far an unchartered area within occupational therapy. However, some organizations, such as Occupational Opportunities For Refugees and Asylum

Seekers (http://www.oofras.com/), have helped bring attention to the problems that asylum seekers and refugees experience.

It is urgent for occupational therapists to address the health issues experienced by asylum seekers and refugees and to start using their skills and knowledge about occupation, designing specific occupational therapy interventions for and with asylum seekers who experience ill health and limitations due to war-related traumas. Identifying and targeting those at risk or in need of rehabilitation at arrival and applying adequate intervention before the transition into the host country, would enhance quality of life for the asylum seeker, and possibly make the transition easier. Preventing development of further occupational inability would have a positive influence not only on the individual, but at the group and society level as well.

Another problem that is often encountered within healthcare is that asylum seekers and refugees are excluded from research due to problems with participation and communication. Many develop a distrust of authorities, as they might have experienced violation of human rights through, for example, doctors taking part in executing torture. A recent literature review indicates that a general problem within healthcare research and practice is that ethnic minorities seldom participate in research, both due to lack of invitation to participate and language/interpretation issues (Morville and Erlandsson, 2016). This leaves asylum seekers and refugees at risk, due to a lack of appropriate healthcare and intervention methods, as the interventions have not been developed with the target group (Pooremamali, 2012; Pooremamali et al., 2012). To conclude, there is a lack of research and documentation of group-specific assessment instruments and interventions, which has an impact on the availability of appropriate actions within rehabilitation in general and for occupational therapists specifically.

What to Do?

Guided by the aim of enabling occupations, the appropriate occupational therapy intervention might not be very different from the services provided to other clients. Furthermore, asylum seekers can face several issues in common with other individuals experiencing occupational deprivation, for example, individuals on long-term unemployment or those in prison (Farnworth et al., 2004; Fazel and Baillargeon, 2011; Rosenthal et al., 2012). Many of the clients that occupational therapists often work with, such as war veterans, can also have traumatic pasts and suffer from many of the same symptoms as traumatized asylum seekers. The most specific condition related to asylum seekers can often be that they are newcomers to the host country. Therefore, the challenge for healthcare professionals is to adapt assessments and interventions to fit the clients' needs and context, while acknowledging the fact that many asylum seekers have additional war traumas and have been subjected to violations of human rights.

Exposure to war-related crimes and the subsequent traumas is a sensitive issue, both for the therapists and the survivors. The fear of triggering flashbacks or other strong reactions, and an avoidance of dealing with such an unpleasant issue as torture may lead to the therapist neglecting the fact that the person might have been subjected to human rights violations. Much has been written about cultural differences: truly client-centred occupational therapy is culturally sensitive. This demands, however, that occupational therapists are well aware of their own cultural expectations and ethnocentric perspectives, in order to attain cultural safety. Cultural patterns are reflected in one's daily occupations. What is perceived as a valued and appropriate occupation is related to, for example, the community, country, gender, past experiences, social relations, and roles in daily life. There are often invisible norms and expectations about, for example, who should participate in which occupations, how, when and where. The right and ability to express one's culture in the pattern of daily occupations seems crucial to one's identity but also well-being. Culture and the structure in which we live our lives are important factors in what makes daily occupations meaningful and valued. By honouring the different occupational needs, abilities, interests, and social situations, the occupational therapist shows respect and can subsequently be an agent of change in order to enable reorganization of daily occupations and routines for the individual, and to reach integration and participation in a new context without a loss of valued occupations.

CONCLUSION

Asylum seekers are exposed to severe occupational deprivation and some subsequently develop the need for occupational therapy intervention during the asylum seeking period. There is a great need for more knowledge about the occupational problems that people seeking asylum experience and also for development of occupational therapy interventions for this group. Support in finding meaning and purpose through occupations, structuring daily life, and maintaining ADL ability is needed and is often sought by asylum seekers, some of whom are survivors of war-related crimes.

It is important to remember that even though human occupation is universal, both interventions and research should be adapted to suit the group in question. Asylum seekers should not be treated as a uniform category. They embody a variety of genders, ages, nationalities, educational levels, cultures, and life experiences, and the content and daily structure with valued occupations vary between groups and individuals. The importance of a daily repertoire of valued occupations is essential for all humans in order to gain and maintain a sense of coherence and meaning in life. By providing the tools for enabling occupations, occupational therapy interventions can help asylum seekers build resilience and have an easier transition to daily life in new surroundings.

Acknowledgements

The authors wish to thank Professor Mona Eklund, Lund University, Sweden, for her profound support and participation in the main part of the thesis work on which this chapter is based.

REFERENCES

Bennett, K.M., Scornaiencki, J., Brzozowski, J., Denis, S., Magalhaes, L., 2012. Immigration and its impact on daily occupations: a scoping review. Occup. Ther. Int. 19, 185–203.

Bhugra, D., Becker, M.A., 2005. Migration, cultural bereavement and cultural identity. World Psychiatry 4, 18–24.

Black, M., 2011. From kites to kitchens. Collaborative community-based occupational therapy with refugee survivorsof torture. In: Kronenberg, F., Pollard, N., et al. (Eds.), Occupational Therapies Without Borders. Churchill Livingstone, London.

Burchett, N., Matheson, R., 2010. The need for belonging: the impact of restrictions on working on the well-being of an asylum seeker. J. Occup. Sci. 17, 85–91.

Carlsson, J.M., Olsen, D., Mortensen, E., Kastrup, M., 2006. Mental health and health-related quality of life: a 10-year follow-up of tortured refugees. J. Nerv. Ment. Dis. 194, 725–731.

Coffey, G.J., Kaplan, I., Sampson, R.C., Tucci, M.M., 2010. The meaning and mental health consequences of long-term immigration detention for people seeking asylum. Soc. Sci. Med. 70, 2070–2079.

Danish Immigration Service, 2013. Conditions for Asylum Seekers. Danish Immigration Service, Denmark. Available at: <http://www.nyidanmark.dk/en-us/coming_to_dk/asylum/conditions_for_asylum_applicants/conditions_for_asylum_applicants.htm> (accessed 29.04.13).

Egloff, N., Hirschi, A., von Kanel, R., 2013. Traumatization and chronic pain: a further model of interaction. J. Pain Res. 6, 765–770.

Eklund, M., Leufstadius, C., 2007. Relationships between occupational factors and health and well-being in individuals with persistent mental illness living in the community. Can. J. Occup. Ther. 74, 303–313.

Farnworth, L., Nikitin, L., Fossey, E., 2004. Being in a secure forensic psychiatric unit: every day is the same, killing time or making the most of it. Br. J. Occup. Ther. 67, 430–438.

Fazel, S., Baillargeon, J., 2011. The health of prisoners. Lancet 377, 956–965.

Fisher, A.G., Jones, K.B., 2011. Assessment of Motor and Process Skills, vol. 1: Development. Standardization, and Administration Manual. Three Star Press, Fort Collins, CO.

Hallas, P., Hansen, P., Staehr, M., Munk-Andersen, E., Jorgensen, H., 2007. Length of stay in asylum centres and mental health in asylum seekers: a retrospective study from Denmark. BMC Public Health 7.

Hammell, K.W., 2004. Dimensions of meaning in the occupations of daily life. Can. J. Occup. Ther. 71, 296–305.

Huot, S., Rudman, D.L., 2010. The performances and places of identity: conceptualizing intersections of occupation, identity and place in the process of migration. J. Occup. Sci. 17, 68–77.

Kielhofner, G., 2007. Model of Human Occupation: Theory and Application, fourth ed. Lippincott Williams & Wilkins, Baltimore, MD.

Kronenberg, F., Simo Algado, S., Pollard, N., 2005. Occupational Therapy without Borders: Learning from the Spirit of Survivors. Elsevier, Churchill Livingstone, London.

Martins, V., Reid, D., 2007. New-immigrant women in urban Canada: insights into occupation and sociocultural context. Occup. Ther. Int. 14, 203–220.

Masmas, T.N., Moller, E., Buhmannr, C., Bunch, V., Jensen, J., Hansen, T., et al., 2008. Asylum seekers in Denmark—a study of health status and grade of traumatization of newly arrived asylum seekers. Torture 18, 77–86.

McElroy, T., Muyinda, H., Atim, S., Spittal, P., Backman, C., 2012. War, displacement and productive occupations in Northern Uganda. J. Occup. Sci. 19, 198–212.

Mollica, R., 2006. Healing Invisible Wounds: Paths to Hope and Recovery in a Violent World. Harcourt Books, Orlando, FL.

Morville, A.-L., Erlandsson, L.-K., 2013. The experience of occupational deprivation in an asylum centre: the narratives of three men. J. Occup. Sci. 20, 212–223.

Morville, A.L., Erlandsson, L.-K., 2016. Methodological issues when doing research with ethnic minorities – a scoping review. Unpublished manuscript.

Morville, A.L., Erlandsson, L.K., Eklund, M., Danneskiold-Samsøe, B., Christensen, R., Amris, K., 2014. Activity of daily living performance amongst Danish asylum seekers: a cross-sectional study. Torture 24, 49–64.

Morville, A.L., Amris, K., Danneskiold-Samsøe, B., Eklund, M., Erlandsson, L.K., 2015a. A longitudinal study of changes in asylum seekers ability regarding activities of daily living during their stay in the asylum center. J. Immigr. Minor. Health 17 (3), 852–859.

Morville, A.L., Erlandsson, L., Danneskiold,-Samsoe, B., Amris, K., Eklund, M., 2015b. Satisfaction with daily occupations amongst asylum seekers in Denmark. Scand. J. Occup. Ther. 22 (3), 207–215.

Pooremamali, P., 2012. Culture, occupation and occupational therapy in a mental health care context. The challenge of meeting the needs of Middle Eastern immigrants. Unpublished thesis, Malmø University, Malmø, Sweden.

Pooremamali, P., Eklund, M., Ostman, M., Persson, D., 2012. Muslim Middle Eastern clients' reflections on their relationship with their occupational therapists in mental health care. Scand. J. Occup. Ther. 19, 328–340.

Quiroga, J.J., 2005. Politically-motivated torture and its survivors: a desk study review of the literature. Torture 16, 3–101.

Rosenthal, L., Carroll-Scott, A., Earnshaw, V., Santilli, A., Ickovics, J., 2012. The importance of full-time work for urban adults' mental and physical health. Soc. Sci. Med. 75, 1692–1696.

Steindl, C., Winding, K., Runge, U., 2008. Occupation and participation in everyday life: women's experiences of an Austrian refugee camp. J. Occup. Sci. 15, 36–42.

Townsend, E.A., Polatajko, H., 2007. Enabling occupation II: advancing an occupational therapy vision for health, well-being and justice through occupation. Canadian Association of Occupational Therapists, Ottawa.

United Nations Convention against Torture. 2012. General comment no. 3. <http://tbinternet.ohchr.org/_layouts/treatybodyexternal/Download.aspx?key=92g0+9FnI5fX/ePqHxWObJmyT0S1LMuCPjfHU49c1zxSWySlkYHXFFxu6hcdyx33&Lang=en> (accessed 30.09.13).

United Nations High Commissioner for Refugees, 2015. Global Trends 2015. UN Refugee Agency. <http://www.unhcr.org/556725e69.html> (accessed 10.30.15.).

Whiteford, G., 2000. Occupational deprivation: global challenge in the new millennium. Br. J. Occup. Ther. 63, 200–204.

Whiteford, G., 2004. Occupational issues of refugees. In: Molineux, M. (Ed.), Occupation for Occupational Therapists. Wiley-Blackwell, Oxford.

Whiteford, G., 2005. Understanding the occupational deprivation of refugees: a case study from Kosovo. Can. J. Occup. Ther. 72, 78–88.

Williams, A.C., Peña, C., Rice, A., 2010. Persistent pain in survivors of torture: a cohort study. J. Pain Symptom Manage. 40, 715–722.

43

EMPOWERING SOCIAL INCLUSION IN CHALLENGING TIMES

THEODOROS BOGEAS ▪ SARAH KANTARTZIS ▪
MARION AMMERAAL ▪ LILIYA ASENOVA TODOROVA ▪
SALVADOR SIMÓ ALGADO ▪ MARIJKE C. BURGER ▪
VARVARA APOSTOLOGLOU ▪ DIMITRIOS KARAMITSOS ▪
MARIA KARAMPETSOU ▪ STEFANOS LAZOPOULOS ▪
KATRIEN MEERMANS ▪ VASILIKI TSONOU

I feel free, but I cannot fly. My wings are gone.

—*ELSiTO member*

CHAPTER OUTLINE

This chapter presents the reflections of some of the members of the Empowering Learning for Social Inclusion Through Occupation (ELSiTO) network, upon the notion of social inclusion during the European economic crisis, which began in 2008 and is still ongoing at the time of writing in 2015 (Thomson et al., 2014). In this chapter, we will reflect on the changes we have experienced in relation to our understanding and lived experiences of social inclusion.

Following a brief introduction to the ELSiTO network, the experiences of members from Belgium, Bulgaria, Greece, the Netherlands and Spain will be explored. The discussion will be framed against background information regarding the crisis and will incorporate quotes from the authors (presented anonymously). The chapter will conclude with proposals for practical approaches towards social inclusion, developed from our own experiences. Throughout the chapter when referring to 'we', we are referring to the writing group.

THE PAST AND THE PRESENT

ELSiTO was initially established as a European collaboration in 2009[1] to explore, in partnership with persons from vulnerable social groups (particularly persons experiencing mental health problems), the nature and processes of social inclusion. Specific

---

[1]Partners of the programme were the Hellenic Association of Occupational Therapists (HAOT) (Greece), Actenz/GGZinGeest (the Netherlands) and the Hogeschool-Universiteit Brussel (Belgium). Collaborative partners were the University of Ruse (Bulgaria), Universitat de Vic (Spain), University of Teeside (UK) and the European Network of Occupational Therapy in Higher Education (ENOTHE). Local partners were, in Greece, the Municipality of Iraklion Attikis-Centre of Ergotherapy Services and the Panhellenic Union for Psychosocial Rehabilitation and Work Integration (PEPSAEE), and in Belgium, the café Polparol-Leuven.

objectives included to empower all members to develop competences relevant to social inclusion, to identify collaborative learning strategies, and to disseminate our lived experiences to the wider community (Ammeraal et al., 2011). ELSiTO was funded as a Grundtvig Learning Partnership under the European Union's Lifelong Learning Programme for 2 years (2009–2011), during which time four international visits were realized, a booklet was produced[2] and a website was created (www.elsito.net). Several presentations were made to international congresses, and two 1-day public seminars were organized. Three articles were published, collaboratively developed by ELSiTO members (Ammeraal et al., 2013; Kantartzis et al., 2012; Nikaki and Bogeas, 2010).

ELSiTO thrived under the important notion of our equality as ELSiTO members-learners, regardless of our professional and personal roles, age, sex and abilities. This standpoint stemmed from the important question posed at the beginning of the partnership: 'Who are the experts on mental illness?'

We came to understand social inclusion to have three components (see Figure 43-1). Objective conditions include laws, financial resources and accessibility. Subjective conditions refer to personal feelings of safety, trust, opportunities to grow and to 'be yourself'. The third component is the daily, ordinary activities that people do together, are meaningful for them, promote well-being and help people feel connected. These three elements are interrelated and all three are essential components of social inclusion (Ammeraal et al., 2011).

After the funding period ended, the ELSiTO partnership continued formally in Greece under the hospices of the Hellenic Association of Occupational Therapists, informally in the Netherlands and in Belgium, and internationally across Europe. The Greek group, meeting monthly, keeps its mixed shape of service users, family members and professionals, working equally as 'ELSiTO members'. In the Netherlands, members meet informally and work in pairs on an irregular basis, for example, holding lectures and discussions with students, or working towards

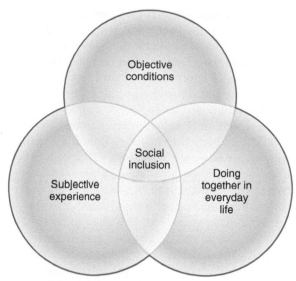

FIGURE 43-1 ■ The three components of social inclusion. *(Figure adapted from Ammeraal, M., Kantartzis, S., Vercruysse, L. (Eds.), 2011. Doing Social Inclusion. ELSiTO. Uitgeverij Tobi Vroegh, Amsterdam, p. 8.)*

community projects. The Healthy Bite projects[3] continue in a number of neighbourhoods, involving both service users and community members. In Belgium, service users, professionals and occupational therapy educators, students and people living in the neighbourhood continue to meet once a week in the Polparol community café (www.polparol.iseral.be), where there is a place for everybody and everyone is equal. In Spain, the gardeners of the Miquel Martí I Pol project[4] continue working with occupational therapy students, maintaining a garden and developing activities in the natural environment, with one gardener describing how 'I am happy in the garden project because I can contribute with something beautiful to the community'. This cooperation is formally included in the curriculum of the occupational therapy programme of the University of Vic. In Bulgaria, students from the

---

[2]Available at: http://elsito.net/wp-content/uploads/2011/05/elsito-booklet-totaal-+-cover.pdf

[3]For further information on the Healthy Bite, Polparol Café and other projects working towards social inclusion, see the ELSiTO website (www.elsito.net). There are, of course, many other projects working towards social inclusion.

[4]http://www.salvadorsimo.org/CA/proyectos/miquel-marti-i-pol

University of Ruse organize group work, doing things together with the service users at the mental health centre once a week during the spring period. Internationally the network exists informally and irregularly, for example, to inform each other of personal events, when we meet at conferences or as we were working together on this chapter.

The invitation to write this chapter was sent to all ELSiTO members. Fifteen writers from five countries completed a one-page reflection on their experiences of social inclusion. An outline with several questions derived from these narratives was sent to all authors. The answers, emanating from group discussions or individual reflections, were published in words and pictures on an interactive web page, enabling everyone involved to read, add and comment on all contributions. In this way, we were able to work with single and group stories from multiple perspectives. All writers commented on the final draft chapter. For writers wishing to write in their own language, other members helped with translation to English. Several key themes were identified from the written narratives, and reflections that we saw could be discussed within the three-part structure of social inclusion that we had developed during the original project. These themes are presented in the following sections.

EXPERIENCES OF INCLUSION

Objective Conditions

The year 2008 is generally regarded to be the year in which the economic crisis started (Thomson et al., 2014). While at the time of this writing (2015) there is a suggestion that economic recovery is beginning (Eurostat, 2015a), many would argue that the effects continue to be far-reaching (Ötker-Robe and Podpiera, 2013). Although the crisis is affecting many countries throughout the world, the discussion here will be limited to the impact on Europe. The conditions that are particularly relevant to this discussion are employment, mental health services and community services (such as municipal services that offer opportunities for leisure activities).

Employment

Between 2008 and 2014, unemployment throughout Europe rose, from 6.8% early in 2008 to 9.9% by December 2014 (EU28), with youth unemployment rising from 15.8% to 23.4% (Eurostat, 2014). While this is alarming for the European Union (EU) as a whole, the figures for the countries of many of the authors are even more revealing. Between 2008 and 2013 unemployment rose in Greece from 7.7% to 27.3% (youth unemployment to 57.3%) and in Spain from 11.3% to 26.1% (youth unemployment to 54.9%). Even those countries considered less affected saw rises: in Belgium from 7.0% to 8.4% (youth unemployment to 23.9%) and in the Netherlands from 3.1% to 6.7% (youth unemployment to 11.4%). In Bulgaria, outside the Eurozone, unemployment rose from 5.6% to 13.0% (youth unemployment to 28.1%) (Eurostat, 2015b). At the same time, income inequality is increasing (although to varying degrees) throughout Europe (Organization for Economic Cooperation and Development, 2014). Vulnerable groups such as mental health service users face additional challenges, such as finding a job in a country with 25% unemployment. Unemployment for mental health survivors in Spain is around 90% (Sánchez, 2013).

Employment conditions have also changed, although with considerable variation between countries. In Greece, the minimum wage was reduced by about 20% between 2012 and 2014, whereas in Bulgaria it increased by 25% and in Spain for the same period has slightly increased by 0.5% (Eurostat, 2015c). Part-time employment increased by 30% between 2011 and 2013 in Greece and by 4% in the Netherlands (Eurostat, 2015d). However, these figures can be misleading, as in Bulgaria, where the rate of the cost of living is rising faster than the minimum wages.

Employment was one of the main themes of the discussion for both professionals and service users. The focus was to find, to have and to keep a paid job. Rising unemployment created a general sense of unease and insecurity. Some members discussed how their salaries had been reduced over the past years, while some were required to work longer hours. Members also experienced irregular payment, often without knowing when they would be paid over a period of weeks or even months. For example, Greek members working in the tertiary mental health sector remained unpaid for about a year between 2012 and 2013, and one ELSiTO member worked for 6 months in a European-funded programme in 2014 without being paid. At the same time, taxes have increased in Greece, the Netherlands and Spain (Eurostat, 2014).

Several training and employment vouchers (coupons provided by local governments and the European Social Fund, to provide short-term employment directly to the private sector) have been created (Hellenic Ministry of Labour, Social Security and Welfare, 2014). The insurance and financial benefits are not always to the advantage of the employee, with one member noting:

> I applied for a training voucher for 500 hours. After that, the company will hire me for only 3 months. I worked out that this means for me: unemployment, no social bursaries, 3 months' salary and 60 days of social security. I believe that a good opportunity for me to start work again would be a 1-year contract, both for financial and security reasons, such as the availability of my health insurance.

Mental Health Services

Health services in general have been affected by the economic crisis, with many countries reducing health budgets, but also with health insurance schemes suffering reduced income from falling payroll contributions, as in Greece (Thomson et al., 2014). Both Greece and Spain have reduced both the number of healthcare staff and the salaries of those staff (Thomson et al., 2014).

Evidence from earlier recessions, suggests there is a link between recession and reduced health, influenced by a combination of increased household vulnerability (usually due to unemployment) and reduced government services. In Greece, state funding for mental health decreased by 20% between 2010 and 2011, and by a further 55% between 2011 and 2012, constraining the ability of mental health services to cope with the 120% increase in the use of services between 2011 and 2014 (Kentikelenis et al., 2014). There has been an estimated 2.5% increase in the prevalence of major depression between 2008 and 2011, with economic hardship as a major risk factor (Simou and Koutsogeorgou, 2014).

In the Netherlands and Belgium, mental health reform continues. This has two aspects: one is the vision of reduced hospitalization with a focus on the benefits of living and participating in the community,

and the other is using this transition for budget reduction. In the Netherlands, funding to prevent the exacerbation of chronic illness decreased from €14 million in 2011 to €6 million in 2014, while simultaneously funding for community-based services increased (within the same €6 million reduced budget), leading to changes in the services available for those with mental illness. In the Flemish part of Belgium, the number of local health networks responsible for the promotion of mental health was reduced in 2010 from 26 to 15 (European Commission, 2013). In Bulgaria in 2012, only 2% of the health budget went to mental health, with no budget to enhance community services or preventive programmes (European Commission, 2013). Moreover, although some countries did not face severe economic difficulties, funding to the healthcare sector was reduced due to fear that the financial crisis might affect them, too, despite the evidence that the crisis increases the number of people affected by mental health problems (Greek Presidency of Europe, 2014).

The economic crisis has affected both those using and those working in mental health services. Professionals had fewer opportunities for work and the quality of work changed either positively or negatively according to the particular circumstances of the service. One of the professionals, speaking for many of us, commented:

> How can you deal with the need and the demands for sustainability (i.e., the funding and availability of mental health and community projects) with ongoing changes at levels you have no influence on (such as governmental decisions)?

For service users, due to a reduction in personnel and in some cases the closure of services, they had to terminate their therapy or have reduced access to services, as one commented: 'We take less care of our health because of difficulties in accessibility in the health system. Unemployment, fear, insecurity, an image of neglect.'

Community Services

Besides the availability of mental health services there is also a need for community services, available to all citizens, including persons with mental health problems. Many of us support the view that 'the services should follow people and provide support in their own community, not take them out of the community'.

There is considerable variation between our countries regarding whether closing services are being replaced by community services. In the Netherlands, several laws support the transition from healthcare to community participation, with local authorities getting increased responsibilities for creating opportunities (Vereniging van Nederlandse Gemeenten and G32, 2011). In Bulgaria, it is noted that there is a lack of true community-based services:

> Objective conditions are not really supporting the inclusion process. The first problem is defining the community. Though the services are community-based they are located on the territory of the mental health centre.

The availability of community services was particularly expressed in the notion of 'safe places': the importance of having small, local places where the person could experience a sense of belonging and safety. There was also concern for the availability of housing.

> I mostly worry about clients finding a place to live and trying to participate in life … It's so hard to find a place because everything is so expensive or because of the social stigma.

Subjective Conditions

The changing objective conditions, fuelled by the economic crisis, have led to a range of subjective experiences, both positive and negative. Negative feelings were discussed many times in the group, particularly anger, feelings of insecurity and powerlessness, and lack of trust. Stress for the future has increased, feelings of uncertainty as to whether we will be able to offer what we feel we need to, according to our roles and ambitions: 'I'm afraid that I won't be able to support my children in the future, when they will need it'.

The ongoing economic instability, leading to annual increases in taxation, reductions in salaries and cuts in services, perpetuated this stress. Some members expressed a loss of faith not only in the political system,

but also with particular political parties and politicians in whom they previously had confidence and had supported. Their faith that politics can turn the situation around has weakened. In addition, some feel that due to the crisis they had lost opportunities for employment, rehabilitation and development. Changes in taxation and the provision of health services were, in some cases, seen to be discriminatory:

> The introduction in 2012 of a personal contribution in mental healthcare services, but not in other parts of healthcare, caused a reduction in referrals. And although the measure stopped due to protest, people felt discriminated and stigmatized. So did I.

However, positive outcomes were also mentioned, such as experiencing closer relationships with others, a feeling of increasingly working together. The change required to respond may lead to positive results (although these may be really difficult to recognize at times). At a personal level, some have advanced their skills according to the opportunities offered:

> So the crisis influenced me positively as I understood that I was not alone in this and I was motivated to participate in a citizens' local group whose philosophy is to try to change some things that are going wrong in the community.

Others felt creative as they developed competences that could be used in innovative projects. Psychological resilience is present as living conditions are adverse. Some found the opportunity to take courage and adopt new social roles through participation in social groups (formal and informal) promoting solidarity. A member from a gardening project writes: 'I feel I am part of a community'. The following section discusses participation in the doing of everyday life, the third element of social inclusion.

The Doing of Everyday Life

Members discussed in particular their experiences around their employment, the nature and availability of mental health services and the impact on their everyday life, their relationships with others, and the need to find 'small worlds' where they can have positive experiences. Current circumstances imposed changes in daily lifestyle, having the possibility to purchase only poorer-quality or free products and services; one member described how 'I've changed supermarket and I'm very careful of what I buy. I changed brands due to price'.

Employment

With reductions in funding to the mental health sector, some members experienced deteriorating working conditions, such as a reduction in cleaning services and money for external activities and increasing pressure to address needs with reduced resources:

> As manager of the home [for young people] my worries are not anymore about the quality of life and the services provided to the residents but how to find the necessary money for heating during the winter.

There was increased pressure for the individual to work harder and more effectively as there was a sense that one was replaceable. Consequently, tension developed between colleagues with a gradual loss of trust. Outside work there are also tensions, as one ELSiTO member describes: 'I feel I do not have the right to talk about my negative experiences at work, with so many unemployed'. Uncertainty in the future restrained new professional beginnings, such as applying for other jobs, despite professional burnout and a desire for professional development.

Relationships With Others

Several authors felt that their relationships have changed. For example, some described how they hide things they have done for themselves which might be perceived as luxurious by others: 'I went to the dentist and I'm afraid if my colleagues see that I have repaired my teeth …'. Different social classes are recreated: the employed versus the unemployed, those whose businesses are closing and those that are in prosperity, and finally those who pay many taxes and those who do not (creating a sense of tax inequality).

The crisis influenced our relationships due to living under different conditions or due to political arguments. Some members have moved for employment to other European countries or experienced family members and friends emigrating within the same or another country. While offering opportunities, this forced migration causes a rift in existing relationships and history. While the mobility of the workforce is regarded as an advantage of the EU, it is also less of a possibility for people experiencing mental illness, creating further inequality and disadvantage.

Finding Small Worlds

> Reading, companionships, strolls, cinema, are small daily things that give value to my life. I will add the fellowship of ELSiTO … a small parallel pathway through time. It is a pleasant interactive circumstance that foretells continuity.

A significant part of our discussion was related to the importance of having small worlds or special places where we feel we belong. For some of us this seemed to have become more significant due to the increasing sense of powerlessness and insecurity regarding macro-level social, political and economic structures. The importance of family, friends and colleagues was mentioned, but also the ELSiTO group, the Polparol café, the Healthy Bite and the Miquel Martí I Pol garden. These were places where we feel we belong, have relationships that are equitable, where communication is honest and clear. These places seem to be those most effective in tackling issues of stigma, which is about relationships with others, but also with the self: 'Social inclusion is about feeling [as] normal as the rest of the people'.

There was some discussion as to whether such safe places are increasingly under threat due to reduced funding:

> The evaporation of mental healthcare in our countries is becoming a very inconvenient truth and very bad for our emancipation. Mental health requires very subtle connections and a very open eye to soft signals. It's really important to create small and very honest spaces.

EMPOWERING INCLUSION IN CHALLENGING TIMES

Our reflections on our experiences of the changing world in which we are living lead us again to see the relevance of the three elements of social inclusion discussed in the earlier work of the group. The economic crisis that began in 2008 influenced in various ways and to various degrees the objective conditions within our countries, influencing in turn both subjective conditions and the doing of everyday activities. This reflects discussions on the social determinants of health (Commission on Social Determinants of Health, 2008), but also discussions of capabilities as depending on both external and internal conditions, enabling people to have the freedom 'to choose between different ways of living that they can have reason to value' (Sen, 1990, p. 114).

There are a number of further points to discuss. First, we discuss the changes taking place in mental health services. These seem to be both an effect of the economic crisis as well as part of ongoing changes to health services towards the community and to an increased focus on self-management. The change towards the community is positive under the condition that these services are accessible for all who need them. The question is: 'What is good community care and is self-management possible?' Healthcare has been delegated to families and service users, and this will continue in the future. In that way, the state is relieved from its legal and financial obligations for healthcare for their citizens, without necessarily offering the required means for this shift. From the statistics mentioned earlier (Eurostat, 2014; Eurostat, 2015b, 2015c, 2015d; Organization for Economic Cooperation and Development, 2014; Sánchez, 2013), it may be seen that the resources available to enable each person to have the same possibility to choose and to act (Nussbaum, 2011) differ greatly from country to country. Limited resources or no access to choices enabling 'what a person can do or be' hinders functioning in what a person can actually manage to do (Sen, 1990, p. 114).

One other point, is the frequently discussed importance of 'safe havens'; small, personal spaces or places for persons who are seen as 'different' in society's ordinary environments (Kal et al., 2012; Pinfold, 2000). The creation of spaces that are emotionally supportive can enable meaningful activities and nurture people's self-worth. This is looking at social participation, not from a macro perspective (which might be challenging), but at the local level in the relationships between people, in a restoration of reciprocity, where people can participate according to their needs and capacities (van Eijken et al., 2012). Many small projects organized by different stakeholders, such as client organizations, local government, social entrepreneurs and educational institutions of various kinds, have been developed. Such projects can create local places, constructed and enacted through occupation, which become part of the stories and discussions of the members. They may be their only places where people feel included or safe.

Even when I sit passively in the group, I feel that I'm included and by that way I communicate. I feel satisfied even on days that I'm not well.

It has given me a sense of freedom, leisure, and my mental health has improved a lot thanks to the garden. It has allowed me to participate in society and meet people from the city and break my isolation, this is important, because solitude is very bad.

Being able to participate in occupations is very important, for example when I'm in the garden I have no paranoid thoughts, my mind relaxes and I feel great. Being in the garden brings me well-being, to be in a beautiful place, when I am in touch with life I feel alive!

A third discussion point is the possible change in power relations between service users and professionals that the crisis may be bringing. Some of the available services described are under pressure due to lack of resources. In our discussions it seemed that the professionals were often more concerned with the loss of these services than the service users. We questioned whether this is because of the time and effort needed to develop these places, the time and effort to build relationships, or personal pride or fear of losing a job? Are professionals finding greater problems than service users in these changing situations in which they feel powerless, living in a world we cannot control due to evaporating resources? Perhaps this sense of losing control, of powerlessness, is a feeling that service users have had for a long time and perhaps these shared experiences can open new ways of working together, as one member commented: 'I have more in common with other people, now we feel the same crisis. I was more confused before the crisis'.

Experiences of loss of control link to discussions of mental health and poverty, an inability to control one's life without access to materials and resources (Sen, 1990) and stigma. Poverty and mental illness are both stigmatized, being framed as a certain identity from an outside force. Both societal and internalized stigma were mentioned in our discussions. Members told each other how society speaks more openly about mental illness, but that lack of knowledge or rejection remains obstinate as 'people understand more, yet there is no acceptance.' Internalized stigma can limit opportunities for developing one's true potential. Providing opportunities for places of meaningful occupations, where persons are seen with their capabilities and where internalized opinions may change, is important.

We suggest that being connected has an influence on fighting stigma, by sharing hope, respect, recognition and a feeling of justice beyond the crisis. The need to feel connected as the central part of social inclusion is highlighted in the literature and also in our discussion of the three elements of social inclusion. Since Aristotle, 'man' has been recognized to be a social animal, while Baumeister and Leary (1995) discussed people's fundamental need to belong. Connection includes feeling valued and having respect for each other, having a variety of supporting relationships, acknowledging expertise, and collaborating. It is not only an important emotional experience but leads to standing up for oneself and for one's group and engaging with the social world.

Finally, regarding paid work, the possibility for us all to work, to be part of environments with the potential for growth and development, remains urgent and necessary. We recognize and acknowledge this importance, yet state that despite the fact that we live in times of crisis, the focus of social inclusion should not be only on work, but also on other life domains, such as community ties and our social and political way of life. It is essential to be and to feel accepted, to feel that we belong somewhere and are recognized, creating an environment or a space that we can share and live together. This can also combat the feelings of powerlessness and loss of control that poverty and mental illness can bring.

As part of our critical discussions, there emerged the conclusion that there are several small things that can be done to strengthen social inclusion (see Box 43-1). Our proposals are presented in four sections: 'Empowering social inclusion' requires acknowledging that even small incidents may occasionally influence the world, while 'empowering others' recognizes that all people should feel connected, and it is achievable through small steps.

Together, we made suggestions on how to 'empower the occupational therapy profession' and the 'future mental health service users'. For the first it is necessary to develop a clear viewpoint that will promote inclusive and sustainable communities, guided by human rights' objectives. For the latter, service users are encouraged to take initiatives, learn their rights and exploit all the opportunities that they have at all levels.

CONCLUSION

In this chapter we have shared some reflections on social inclusion in challenging times, based on the experiences of members of the ELSiTO network across five European countries. The discussion supports an understanding of the complex and dynamic nature of inclusion, with the change and its impact taking place across all levels, from the structural to the immediately personal.

When social inclusion is seen as the interrelationship of objective conditions, subjective experiences and everyday doing, it may be seen how significant changes in one area (such as the objective conditions of the financial crisis) may be counterbalanced by changes in the other conditions. At the micro level, subjective experiences supported through shared doing and within safe places seem to be powerful enough to enhance social inclusion that is threatened due to crisis. This is of course not to say that objective conditions such as unemployment, the provision of adequate health services, and community projects creating safe places do not need to be addressed.

In the healthcare sector, services and projects are fighting for their sustainability. On the one hand, the move to community services is valuable and potentially offers enormous potential towards more inclusive communities. However, there is vast inequality

BOX 43-1
SMALL THOUGHTS AND ACTIONS TOWARDS SOCIAL INCLUSION

EMPOWERING SOCIAL INCLUSION

- Offer your help when needed, instead of waiting to be asked.
- Try new things and places more than once. It is also helpful to do the things that we are good at and we enjoy.
- Walk and learn the city and the spaces we live in.
- Organize the environment, our commitments and our time.
- Give feedback, express how much you enjoy each others' company, share your small steps and endeavour to feel intimacy and trust.
- Be aware of the impact of the outside world on what you can do and how you feel.
- Find the balance between the material and nonmaterial world and empower your choices linked to your roles, regardless of the crisis.

EMPOWERING OTHERS

- Accept that current social challenges are not individual problems but are a broader phenomenon. Work with others and this may give you hope.
- Offer help and learn to accept help when it is necessary: 'Everybody needs somebody!'
- Belong to one or more groups, where you feel connected and a sense of belonging.
- Engage with other people, such as neighbours, that we have never spoken to, or employees in the supermarket we go to, just by greeting them. They will then acknowledge our existence and so we will by sharing the same world. Later on, we may ask them how they are doing.
- Prepare the appropriate words that help to get closer to other people, who perhaps we see as different and with whom we would not usually interact. Try many times and do not be afraid of failure. Perhaps these people may be vulnerable, too, and hide behind a mask.

EMPOWERING THE OCCUPATIONAL THERAPY PROFESSION

- Reorientate practice away from functional skills towards well-being, social and human rights' objectives.

- Work to change societal attitudes and provide health-promotion programmes to combat stigma in the community.
- Gain political influence at a macro level.
- Follow politics in the community (or at a higher level) and be political, for example, in collaborating with agents that you never thought that you would.
- Recover professional values such as solidarity and respect for diversity. Strengthen other values, unifying them in one notion of 'living together well'.
- Be open to collaborations and teamwork.
- Offer love to the profession and consequently offer love to the service users.
- Listen and learn how to learn from the service users as they show trust and therefore you should offer opportunities to be critiqued. Step out of your role and work together without neglecting to pay attention to each member of the group. Learn from each other.
- Go on, no matter how hopeless it seems, and make all positive results widely known to society.

EMPOWERING FUTURE MENTAL HEALTH SERVICE USERS

- You became ill; that does not mean that it is the end of life.
- Social inclusion is therapeutic, so give it a try just by sharing e-mail addresses with members of a group you attend and making appointments to do things together.
- Be aware that there is discrimination related to mental illness and you must battle for diminishing it.
- Ask for help and make the next steps.
- Learn about your rights and find the benefits you have the right to have. Discover the offered services and make good use of them.
- In ELSiTO we have the courage to say our opinion, new ideas spring up and every idea becomes important. These new ideas help us develop. You must be open-minded.
- Go out, be in the world, try new places. Realize that most people are vulnerable and hide behind a mask; it takes time to connect.

---

between countries regarding the budget available for these, the existing differences in services, together with considerable differences in the income and living conditions of individuals within and between each country. This inequality indicates the need for an equitable approach to ensure that all have the

opportunities 'to do and to be' their capabilities (Nussbaum, 2011, p. 20).

ELSiTO has been experienced until now as a project, as a pilot study and as a unique way of living together. It is one of those inclusive spaces that many members recognize as important for our sense of belonging. We have come to believe that in order to sustain social inclusion we must take action. We must work every day, take small actions, be strategic and join other small islets of inclusion. We have to be social activists and fight for our rights, through engaging in shared occupations. Fighting for our rights may refer to a variety of activities, from daily communication and interactions with our neighbours and colleagues, to participation in collective occupations such as demonstrations, public meetings and rallies. Central in this process is sharing together, acting together, with an honest and inclusive communication. This raises issues around roles, power sharing and equity of opportunities, particularly between professionals and service users, who may become equal partners. Social inclusion, the creation of healthy, inclusive and sustainable communities, is greatly influenced by the challenging times Europe faces today. Therefore, it is more necessary than ever to recognize each other as citizens, sharing a common world.

POSTSCRIPT

This chapter was written between the summers of 2014 and 2015. During the final writing stage of this chapter, Europe agreed to a new memorandum for the financial aid of Greece (July 2015), affecting intensely the relationships among EU members. We cannot yet know the sequel to these events and their impact on the structure of the EU. The consequences for social inclusion are similarly unknown, yet it is our firm belief that the impact and the processes that have been discussed in this chapter will be relevant in the future.

REFERENCES

Ammeraal, M., Kantartzis, S., Vercruysse, L. (Eds.), 2011. Doing Social Inclusion. ELSiTO. Uitgeverij Tobi Vroegh, Amsterdam.

Ammeraal, M., Kantartzis, S., Burger, M., Bogeas, T., van der Molen, C., Vercruysse, L., 2013. ELSiTO. A collaborative European initiative to foster social inclusion with persons experiencing mental illness. Occup. Ther. Int. 20, 68–77.

Baumeister, R.F., Leary, M.R., 1995. The need to belong: desire for interpersonal attachments as a fundamental human motivation. Psychol. Bull. 117 (3), 497–529.

Commission on Social Determinants of Health, 2008. Closing the gap in a generation: health equity through action on the social determinants of health. Final Report of the Commission on Social Determinants of Health. World Health Organization, Geneva.

European Commission, 2013. European profile of prevention and promotion of mental health (EuroPoPP-MH). <http://ec.europa.eu/health/mental_health/docs/europopp_full_en.pdf> (accessed 24.02.15.).

Eurostat, 2014. Taxation Trends in European Union. Taxation and Customs Union, European Commission. <http://ec.europa.eu/taxation_customs/resources/documents/taxation/gen_info/economic_analysis/tax_structures/2014/report.pdf> (accessed 25.02.15.).

Eurostat, 2015a. EU28 current account surplus 33.4 bn. 20 February 2015. <http://ec.europa.eu/eurostat/documents/2995521/6643067/2-20022015-AP-EN.pdf/25f0eb29-3bd2-4926-8ba5-ba8e05cbead5> (accessed 23.02.15.).

Eurostat, 2015b. Unemployment statistics. <http://ec.europa.eu/eurostat/statistics-explained/index.php/Unemployment_statistics> (accessed 30.01.15.).

Eurostat, 2015c. Minimum Wages. <http://ec.europa.eu/eurostat/tgm/table.do?tab=table&plugin=0&language=en&pcode=tps00155> (accessed 24.02.15.).

Eurostat, 2015d. Labour Force Survey Main Tables. <http://ec.europa.eu/eurostat/tgm/table.do?tab=table&init=1&language=en&pcode=tps00159&plugin=1> (accessed 24.02.15.).

Greek Presidency of Europe, 2014. Informal meeting of health ministers. Economic crisis and healthcare. Discussion paper. 28–29 April 2014. <http://gr2014.eu/sites/default/files/Athens%20Informal%2028-29.4%20-%20Session%20II%20-%20Economic%20crisis%20and%20healthcare.pdf> (accessed 27.10.14.).

Hellenic Ministry of Labour, Social Security and Welfare (Υπουργείο ασφάλισης, κοινωνικής εργασίας και πρόνοιας), 2014. επιτάγή επαγγελματικήσ κατάρτισησ (Training Vouchers). <http://voucher.gov.gr> (accessed 28.10.14.).

Kal, D., Post, R., Scholtens, R., et al., 2012. Meedoen gaat niet vanzelf. Kwartiermaken in theorie en praktijk (Participation is not easy. Creating space for otherness in theory and practice.). Tobi Vroegh, Amsterdam.

Kantartzis, S., Ammeraal, M., Breedveld, S., Mattijs, L., Geert, L., et al., 2012. 'Doing' social inclusion with ELSiTO: empowering learning for social inclusion through occupation. Work 41, 447–454.

Kentikelenis, A., Karanikolos, M., Reeves, A., McJee, M., Stuckler, D., 2014. Greece's health crisis: from austerity to denialism. Lancet 383, 748–753.

Nikaki, I., Bogeas, T., 2010. A learning partnership through occupation: ELSITO. Ergotherapeia 43, 89–94, (in Greek).

Nussbaum, M.C., 2011. Creating Capabilities. The Human Development Approach. Harvard University Press, Cambridge, MA.

Organization for Economic Cooperation and Development, 2014. Income inequality update. Rising inequality: youth and poor fall further behind. <http://www.oecd.org/social/OECD2014-Income-Inequality-Update.pdf> (accessed 10.05.15.).

Ötker-Robe, I., Podpiera, A.M., 2013. The social impact of financial crises. Evidence from the global financial crisis. World Bank. <http://www-wds.worldbank.org/external/default/WDSContentServer/IW3P/IB/2013/11/14/000158349_20131114113429/Rendered/PDF/WPS6703.pdf> (accessed 23.02.15.).

Pinfold, V., 2000. 'Building up safe havens … all around the world': users' experiences of living in the community with mental health problems. Health Place 6, 201–212.

Sánchez, O., 2013. Espacios para el desarrollo profesional. (Spaces for professional development). Asociación canaria de rehabilitación psicosocial, Las Palmas, Spain.

Sen, A., 1990. Justice: Means versus Freedom. Philos. Public Aff. 19 (2), 111–121.

Simou, E., Koutsogeorgou, E., 2014. Effects of the economic crisis on health and healthcare in Greece in the literature from 2009 to 2013: a systematic review. Health Policy (New York) 115, 111–119.

Thomson, S., Figueras, J., Evetovits, T, Jowett, M., Mladovsky, P., Maresso, A., et al., 2014. Economic crisis, health systems and health in Europe: impact and implications for policy. WHO Regional Office for Europe/European Observatory on Health Systems and Policies (Policy Summary 12), Copenhagen. <http://www.euro.who.int/__data/assets/pdf_file/0008/257579/12-Summary-Economic-crisis,-health-systems-and-health-in-Europe.pdf?ua=1> (accessed 15.01.15.).

van Eijken, J., van Ewijk, H., Staatsen, H., van Doorn, L., Fruytier, B., Grundemann, R., et al., 2012. Samenleven is geen privé zaak (A good society is more than just a private affair). Boom Lemma, Den Haag, the Netherlands. Available at:: <http://www.kwartiermaken.nl/english> (accessed 05.09.15.).

Vereniging van Nederlandse Gemeenten and G32, 2011. Van Zorg Naar Participatie. (Association of Dutch municipalities. From care to participation). <https://vng.nl/files/vng/publicatie_bijlagen/2012/20110714_visie_van_zorg_naar_participatie.pdf> (accessed 25.04.15.).

SECTION 5

PRACTICES OF TRANSFORMATION

44

JUST HOW DO YOU WORK WITH 'THE COMMUNITY'?

MARTIN O'NEILL

Public policy is increasingly based on the belief that there is a need to involve communities in healthcare and social care initiatives. This belief is based on the understanding that if such initiatives are going to be effective, then the people who are their focus need to be engaged with, and take some form of 'ownership' of, the delivery of these initiatives. However, what is often less clear within such policy directives is how such involvement is to be achieved, what it might mean, and how it might impact on the various partners concerned. Meaningful community engagement requires that new ways of working and interacting be developed by all stakeholders involved.

This chapter is based on over a decade's experience of working in a number of poor, disadvantaged, postindustrial communities in the South Wales area of the UK. It will explore the intricacies and issues involved in developing effective and meaningful engagement. This will be illustrated using concrete examples of initiatives where community members,

healthcare professionals, and other stakeholders have co-productively developed effective initiatives and interventions aimed at addressing issues faced by those in the community.

CONNECTING WITH THE COMMUNITY

The importance of 'working with the community' is often and increasingly invoked as a desirable requisite of various aspects of healthcare and social care delivery (Andersson et al., 2006; Syme, 2004). The word *community* is a term often used in various combinations, such as community action, community care, community initiatives, community development, community projects, community centres, community groups, and probably the most enigmatic of all, 'community engagement'; however, what this term means exactly and how it is put into practice is often far from clear. In order to more fully understand what is meant by this concept, it is necessary to interrogate what is meant by these essentially abstract notions of 'community' and 'engagement', and how the two can be brought together in a practical and sustainable way.

This belief in the importance of involving communities in policy delivery has emerged against a backdrop of the increasing political dominance, particularly in the UK, of neoliberal approaches in the wider political environment (Campbell and Pedersen, 2001). Whether it be the Blair's Labour Government's 'Third Way' or Cameron's Conservative 'Big Society', this approach is categorized by market deregulation, state decentralization, and reduced political intervention. Therefore, within this more contemporary political environment, it appears the community now has more of a role to play by stepping in and providing those functions that were previously fulfilled by local and national government. However, it is worth considering that any community consists of a collection of individuals who, while sharing certain characteristics, will also have marked differences to others in the community.

THEORIZING THE NATURE OF MODERN COMMUNITIES

From such early theorists as Tönnies (1887) and Roper (1935), some have argued that modernity would see the death of traditional notions of community. This is an argument perpetuated by more recent theorists, who appear to believe that traditional notions of neighbourhood are being replaced by new imagined communities in a 'postindustrial' environment, which individuals can choose to belong to or not.

Lash and Urry (1994), for example, argue that modernity is characterized by a globalization of economic and social life, and that this contemporary global order is now best categorized as a 'structure of flows' a 'decentred set of economies of signs and space' (1994, p. 4). These flows are increasingly subject to 'time-space distanciation' (Giddens, 1990, p. 21), where time and space empty out. Capital, labour, commodities, information, and images are all increasingly disembedded from concrete space and time, as their mobility steadily expands. Lash and Urry (1994) argue that 'post-Fordist' restructuring of manufacturing and service industries is illustrative of this feature of modernity. They feel this has led to a flattening out of economic, social, and political life and hypothesize

that with the privatization of social life, old neighbourhoods and communities are being replaced by new communities. Lash and Urry (1994) state:

To a greater or lesser extent we are not so much thrown into communities, but decide which communities to throw ourselves into ... the invention of communities is a sort of conduct which we more frequently enter into, new communities are being ever more frequently invented so that such innovation becomes almost chronic. (p. 316)

Although they do not completely discount physical proximity, they believe that information technology and greater mobility have, for the most part, made this factor redundant. It may be true, to an extent, that we are witnessing the construction of new types of invented communities, examples of which may be seen in the emergence of 'neighbourhood watch' schemes, for example, or in a more virtual dimension, the growth in the importance of social media, such as Twitter and Facebook, in peoples' lives. However, as to the nature of modern communities, the question that needs to be asked of this analysis is whether this choice is equally available to all, and do people replace their old communities with these new forms or just use them to augment traditional communities?

As long ago as the mid-1980s, Cohen (1985) had already highlighted the importance of the symbolic in the nature and construction of community. In his analysis of change in modern society and how it impacted on contemporary communities, he argues that communities around the world are becoming increasingly influenced by factors outside their boundaries, such as industrialization, urbanization, mass production, centralization of markets, spread of the mass media and of centrally disseminated information, and general increased mobility of both people and markets. He believes that all of these combine into a process that undermines social encapsulation where people only socially interact within the physical boundaries of their neighbourhood or locality that was a feature of more traditional forms of community. He sees this process as flattening any difference in cultural forms, such as language, family structure, political and educational institutions, economic processes, and religious and recreational practice. He does not believe, however, that these apparent similarities mean that old community boundaries have become redundant and anachronistic. His main argument is that the more outside pressure there is on communities to conform and blur their boundaries, the more they reassert their boundaries symbolically. As Cohen (1985) states:

> The structural bases of boundary become blurred, so the symbolic bases are strengthened through flourishes and decorations, aesthetic frills and so forth. (p. 44)

Cohen (1985) further goes on to suggest that this model of the outside world enveloping neighbourhoods or bounded communities is too simplistic. A neighbourhood does not simply consume the influences of larger society, but rather through a system of communal bricolage transforms the alien structural forms that originate from outside, in a process of importation, reconstitution, and negotiation with indigenous meaning.

Although new imagined forms of community may be emerging in certain areas of society, the experience of working with a number of communities does not appear to support the theory that they are universally replacing more traditional forms of community. New and emerging trends of devolution, regionalism, and nationalism would tend to reinforce this analysis (Swendan, 2006), and as Cohen has rightly pointed out, community is what we all belong to more immediately than the abstract concept we call society. Although in modern-day society nations can be conceptualized as imagined communities in the Benedict Anderson (2006) sense of the term, the importance of immediate neighbours appears to be no less diminished (O'Neill, 2003). The neighbourhood sense of community is something that most people experience on a daily basis.

The purpose of this proceeding discussion is to highlight some of the complex nuances incorporated into the notion of community. As time passes there may be fundamental changes in the nature and make up of society but the notion of community remains central to the way people behave and live their lives. Any community is a highly complex and nuanced social entity, and this complexity needs to be understood if effective engagement is to be achieved.

UNDERSTANDING A MODERN COMMUNITY

Probably the most common understanding of what community means is the classic geographic community of a group of people living in one district or area, a neighbourhood. However, it takes very little consideration of this description to realize that it is somewhat inadequate. The notion that a location possesses some sort of sense of community implies that there is more to this than individuals simply realizing that they live in the same place. Therefore, together with this sense of place there is a sharing of other factors, such as interests, problems, or a sense of belonging. A classic academic definition of what 'community' means is 'an area of social living marked by some degree of social coherence. The bases of community are locality and community sentiment' (MacIver and Page, 1961, p. 8).

However, this definition is again problematic as it assumes consensus within the community. If agencies, professionals or individuals talk of 'working with the community' or of 'the needs of the community', who in the community do they mean? By definition, as the previous discussion highlighted, any such community consists of a number of individuals whose wants and desires need not necessarily coincide. If we go back to the notion of a community being centred on a particular locality, within any such locality there is most probably going to be a number of divisions. For example, gender, age, lifestyle, religion, and ethnicity divisions are all likely in any community, and these divisions and classifications can often be defined locally.

Often, the reality of initial stages of working with the community means in practical terms working with already established community groups as they are relatively easy to engage. However, by definition those involved in such community groups are the activists of the community. Additionally, often such groups have their origins in other social networks centred around other community concerns such as neighbourhood watch schemes, mother and toddler, bingo, old age or faith groups, so often people who are involved in such groups have other priorities, which may not be shared by all of those in the community or even the majority. For example, a community group dominated by middle-aged and elderly men will probably have different priorities and views as to what is important to a group that consists predominantly of young to middle-aged women. Both groups could well have very different ideas of what they want to see in their community, even though they inhabit the same space and live very close to each other.

Another consideration in relation to what constitutes a community is its boundaries: how they are defined and how they are negotiated. Getting these boundaries wrong or misunderstanding them can have disastrous consequences for the process of community engagement. Where does one community end and another one begin? Where do the boundaries of community lie? Are these boundaries physical, or are they more readily understood as conceptualizations inside the minds of community members? The way that communities might be defined by outside agencies may be very different from the way they are understood by those who are part of the community. It takes very little time interacting and talking to members of any community to get a sense of the understanding that people have of their own communities: where are the good places, where are the not-so-good places, where are the safe places, and where are the not-so-safe places.

Any notion of community as some sort of homogenous and easily defined entity is problematic. Within any locality, neighbourhood or community there are dynamics of cooperation and conflict and alliances and antagonisms; that is just the nature of community and needs to be understood in formulating any approach to working with the community. Also, defining the boundaries of a community, particularly for the outsider, is highly problematic. The boundaries to such communities do not exist in the lines on paper drawn up by bureaucrats through wards or constituencies, but in the heads of the individuals who belong to them. This is where the notions of inclusivity and exclusivity reside: who are us and who are them?

'Mapping' the Community

To return to some of the considerations posed in the introduction to this chapter, within the notion of 'working with the community' there are a number of questions that need to be asked. Some of these questions are: Who in the community? How is the community defined? Whose definition of community?

However, although any straightforward notion of community is problematic, the notion of community, and indeed working with the community, is a very useful and powerful approach when executed effectively. Additionally, there are other more macro dimensions to any community that need to be considered, which can and will most probably extend outside any geographic location, can also have significant implications for engaging with any community, and can be connected to larger social networks. For example, the 'Asian' community could refer to those from a particular locality or country and could also be defined quite differently by those either inside or outside of that community, but what is important is that these definitions are explored and made explicit, so that people can accept or reject them. These social networks will often have community, regional, national, and global dimensions and will, in turn, have implications for the nature and influence on local communities. Therefore, community is a multifaceted entity that has both micro and macro dynamics, all of which have implications as to its nuances, nature, and significance. A comprehensive understanding of these internal and external dimensions and networks is fundamental in formulating a sustainable and effective approach to community engagement.

Communities are often defined by criteria imposed by outsiders. For example, in the UK these may be electoral wards or even postal districts. However, the way local people define their own particular area can have very different borders and boundaries than those defined by official classifications. Additionally, those classifications will not be shared by all members of the community. Understanding the importance of these mind maps held by members of the community is important to any successful approach to engaging the community.

Writers such as Bourdieu (1977) and De Certeau (1984), have addressed some of these tensions between outsider definitions of a community and how it may contrast with insiders' understanding of the same community. To illustrate this point, Bourdieu uses the analogy of the use of street maps. People who know the geography of an area within which they live, do not need or use street maps to organize their routes from place to place. It is only the outside observer who feels a need to construct such a map. He argues that in the study of community, it is important to realize and understand that local people do not regulate the way that they navigate the community in reference to any abstract map constructed by outsiders in their attempt to navigate the community.

What this analysis highlights is that there is a tension between the spontaneous, subjective, and instinctive cartographic sense of the locals and the abstract, objective, and rational knowledge of the detached observers. Both Bourdieu and De Certeau realize that it is more complex than simply replacing an objectivist perspective with a subjective one. It is not only local people who have access to the maps which direct their actions. This approach advocates that people do make strategic choices and plans of routes but within the context of 'objective' maps and guidelines, which have been generated and developed within their own localities. So, the external observer can perceive the totality of the actions of local community members in a way which may not be accessible to the members themselves. However, the external observer needs to reflect on and assess the extent to which observations derive from their own particular position. There is then a chance that the account of what is happening and why, developed by the 'outsider', might coincide with and reflect a reality recognized by the community member. The strength of this approach to analysis is that it highlights that any explanation devised by the researcher to explain how a community is organized and works, has no existence for those who live and work in any such community. Such external analyses do not, therefore, regulate behaviour, but may make explicit the implicit parameters within which those in the community make the choices on how to navigate their way through everyday life.

PRACTICAL APPROACHES TO REALIZING MIND MAPS

A useful approach to engaging with and understanding these mind maps of how local people understand and navigate their community is community mapping. The concept behind this approach is to move away from top-down maps, often adopted by local or national government. A community map is very much what it sounds like – it is a map created by members of a community. The map should show areas of interest or concern. The map created should reflect the local knowledge of those who were involved in creating it, as they are the experts in this particular area.

Community maps can be created in a number of ways, by starting with a traditional two-dimensional representation of the geographic area and asking community members to mark or put stickers on those areas where, for instance, they might go to socialize, or to access healthcare services, or where they might feel safe/unsafe. Another approach that can be utilized is to ask community members to draw their community from scratch. The strength of this approach is that community members are able to define their own boundaries of the community and indicate where a community starts and where it ends. Whichever technique is adopted, a good approach is to use a large-size map, at least A1 (594 × 84 mm), but preferably larger. The process should be characterized by all participants crowding around a table and contributing to the construction of the map through discussion and negotiation and an exploration of why people categorize areas as they do. It is important that the finished map is recorded somehow, either photographically or by retaining the map itself. Additionally, it is important to keep a record of the discussions that emerge around the production of the map as within those there is a wealth of information to understand how the community works, how it ticks. This might be done by recording the conversations and discussions or by a note-taker recording the relevant points. Community maps create a comprehensive picture of an area, of a community, through the eyes and minds of those who inhabit the space and who are part of the community, and they can be an incredibly useful resource for gaining insight, understanding, and engagement with a community.

Participatory mapping as a form of research and fostering community engagement is an approach that has gained in popularity over the past 30 years (Chambers, 2006, pp. 2–3) and had its roots in the developing world and development studies (Chambers, 2008, p. 299). The strength of this approach for community members is that it is 'visual and tangible and usually performed by small groups', and the maps created can be 'social or census, showing people and their characteristics, resource ... and mobility maps showing where people travel for services' (Chambers, 2008, p. 298). The approach should also be a participatory exercise in itself, where the facilitator (or professional) works as an equal coproducer of the community map who values the perspective and analysis of local people as much as their own (Chambers, 2008, pp. 298–299).

Community Engagement: A Case Study

In recent years, this approach to community mapping has been utilized together with community development principles to ensure that it can effectively bring about social change. Professionals from fields such as healthcare, social care, and academic research can work with communities to not only carry out community mapping but also to instigate interventions and projects aimed at addressing the issues identified. A project in North Merthyr Tydfil in South Wales in the UK used this approach to address issues of confidence as a barrier to accessing employment in a stigmatized area categorized as disadvantaged and hard to reach under official indicators (Welsh Index of Multiple Deprivation, 2015).

Merthyr Tydfil is a community facing many of the same problems and challenges that confront other postindustrial areas throughout the UK, whose economies were dependent on traditional heavy industries, such as iron and steel production, and mining. As a result of the long decline throughout the twentieth century and the eventual demise of these heavy industries in the 1970s and 1980s, the area, like many others in South Wales (Bennett et al., 2000), is now characterized by long-term unemployment, low incomes, poor housing, and all the problems typically associated with social exclusion. Geographically, the town is located in the upper reaches of the Taff valley on the northern boundary of the former South Wales coalfield. The area consists of a number of distinct neighbourhoods, such as old Gurnos, new Gurnos, Galon Uchaf, Penydarren, and Dowlais. Although each neighbourhood has its own distinct identity, they are all categorized as deprived under official indicators (Welsh Index of Multiple Deprivation, 2015).

As an example of the issues such areas face, the housing in the Gurnos area was initially constructed during the late 1950s and early 1960s to rehouse the population displaced by the clearance of the industrial slum areas, in Penydarren and Dowlais, that had grown up around the former iron works during the industrial revolution. At this time, the estate was seen as a symbol of renewal and regeneration, with modern housing offering hot and cold running water and indoor bathrooms and toilets. The neighbourhood continued to expand until the late 1970s, but the loss of industrial production and rising levels of unemployment in the area were followed by corresponding increases in social problems, such as crime, educational underachievement, and substance dependence.

At the time of this writing (September 2015), the Gurnos Estate comprises more than 2500 councilbuilt properties, managed by a housing association. Property ownership in the area remains relatively low, with only 27.5% of local residents exercising their right to buy. The areas of Gurnos and Penydarren, which constitute most of the area of North Merthyr Tydfil, are both within the top 10% of the most deprived communities in Wales, as categorized by the Welsh Index of Multiple Deprivation. In addition to the formal statistical evidence; the social reality of the area is also informed by a certain reputation and notoriety well beyond the immediate locality. In recent years, there have been a number of sensational news and media stories about the area, such as a number of episodes of Channel 4's *Skint*[1] screened in April 2015, which portrayed the area in less than favourable terms. Such representations compound the sense of inequality and injustice among local residents which is made all the more understandable by the fact that the area is only 24 miles from economically buoyant Cardiff.

The important point to take from this discussion is that the residents of the neighbourhoods that make up the communities of northern Merthyr Tydfil are themselves only too conscious of the area's reputation and deprivation. They know how it is regarded, and they also know that this can contribute to the already harsh

---

[1] *Skint* is a UK 'reality' television programme which claims to represent the reality of people living in the nation's poorest communities. One example of public reaction to the programme can be found at: http://www.walesonline.co.uk/whats-on/whats-onnews/channel-4s-skint-reaction-please-9038002.

difficulties many of them face. It also means that often there is a high degree of suspicion and cynicism regarding the attentions of outsiders, and this makes it difficult to develop of any sort of research-based development initiatives led by people classed as outsiders to the area.

Insider participatory research was an approach developed in the area under the Triangle Project, an initiative funded under the Welsh Assembly Government's Sustainable Health Action Research Programme. Via this project, which ran from 2000 to 2005, the School of Social Sciences at Cardiff University developed an approach that sought to work with local groups to identify, employ, and train local people in the role of community-based action researchers. The Triangle Project was specifically aimed at tackling health inequalities and was particularly successful in developing a number of sustainable initiatives that effectively engaged with local community members in developing joint initiatives for addressing problems that local people faced (O'Neill and Williams, 2004). As the effectiveness of this approach had been demonstrated through the experiences of the Triangle Project, the same approach was used to identify and tackle the barriers to employment faced by the local population, to understand the factors contributing to the social exclusion of many, and to continue the participatory research process. As argued elsewhere (O'Neill, 2001), in all social research there is a reciprocal nature to the relationship between the observer and the observed. For the researchers to gain the acceptance needed to collect data, there is a necessity to enter into social relationships with those that they research. This is particularly the case within the epistemological model of participatory research, which accepts that the researchers are not a value-neutral entity and need to immerse themselves in a process of 'subjective soaking' (Clammer, 1984). Therefore, it is important to understand where the researcher is socially located in relation to that which is the focus of the research.

Through community mapping and developing reciprocal and participatory relationships with the community, it was possible to identify that one of the major barriers to accessing employment and also making employment sustainable, concerned the psychological dimension of the confidence of people who often had not been in employment for a considerable period of time. The participatory research approach identified, in consultation with the group, what interventions could be developed to address this lack of confidence. Many of the group reported that their lack of confidence related to their basic reading and writing skills and interpersonal skills of being in a group, as many had been confined to the house for a number of years because of child-rearing responsibilities. Again, through talking to the group it became clear that they did not want formal literacy training, as many had bad memories of their time in formal education. What they asked for was a softer peer-to-peer support approach, supported by a mentor to assist in developing their overall confidence and their literacy skills.

Over time, the above approach proved to be very successful. The vast majority of participants remained involved in the group for a number of years, although during this time a number faced significant challenges in their personal lives due to a number of reasons. It was particularly at these times of individual personal challenge that the group very much coalesced into an informal but powerful support network that individuals valued highly. As time progressed, some were successful at accessing and retaining employment, while others successfully completed access to further and then higher education courses, and eventually completed degrees. This enabled them to access employment that would otherwise have been inaccessible to them. This case study illustrates the effectiveness of community engagement and a participatory approach to working with communities, and highlights its sustainability.

CONCLUSION

Communities are complex, difficult, and continually evolving and changing. Successful community engagement has the potential to deliver innovative, effective, and sustainable models of change. As the work of Cohen (1985) highlights, the concept of community is something we all understand more immediately and more concretely than those more imagined ethereal notions, such as society or nation. We know and interact on a daily basis with those who belong to our community or neighbourhood, while society or nation remain abstract, imagined notions. As Crow and

Allen (1994) state in relation to neighbourhood and community:

> *People are embedded in local relationships to different degrees and in different ways … equally the manner in which people were incorporated was shaped by their own circumstances and social identities. Within the communities fine gradations separated those whom outsiders looking in at the community might tend to lump together (p. 186)*

Cohen (1985) argues that although community is largely a mental construct, its character is sufficiently malleable that it can accommodate all of its members' selves without feeling their individuality to be overly compromised; attachment is a great help in this respect. He argues that communities are best approached as 'communities of meaning'. In other words, 'community' plays a crucial symbolic role in generating people's sense of identity and belonging (Crow and Allan, 1994). For Cohen (1985), 'people construct community symbolically, making it a resource and repository of meaning, and a referent of their identity' (p. 118). This, and the discussion in the earlier part of the chapter, pose three questions to those who want to foster community engagement and participatory coproductive approaches to achieving change:

- How is a community defined by both outsiders and insiders?
- What internal and external social networks are working within the community?
- How does community membership impact on personal behaviour?

Initial community engagement and working with the community usually involves working with the activists of the community who are sometimes called the 'usual suspects', as they are as much part of the community as anyone else, and they can provide the initial connection to the community. The aim should be to move beyond the usual suspects and work with as wide a cross section of the community as possible. Strategies, such as community mapping, can be useful in doing that by identifying those who are not already engaged and where it might be possible to engage with them and what activities they might be involved in.

Working with and engaging with communities can be messy, difficult, and time consuming, but it is by far the most effective way of making meaningful and sustainable change. As this chapter has highlighted, by working with the 'experts', that is, community members, and utilizing their expertise by developing a co-productive approach, meaningful and sustainable community engagement and meaningful and sustainable change can be achieved.

REFERENCES

Anderson, B., 2006. Imagined Communities Reflections on the Origin and Spread of Nationalism. Verso, London.

Andersson, E., Tritter, J., Wilson, R., (Eds.), 2006. Healthy Democracy: The Future of Involvement in Health and Social Care: 2006. National Health Service, London.

Bennett, K., Beynon, H., Hudson, R., 2000. Coalfields Regeneration: Dealing with the Consequences of Industrial Decline. Policy Press, Bristol, UK.

Bourdieu, P., 1977. Outline of a Theory of Practice. Cambridge University Press, Cambridge.

Campbell, J., Pedersen, O., 2001. The Rise of Neoliberalism and Institutional Analysis. Princeton University Press, Princeton, NJ.

Chambers, R., 2006. Participatory mapping and geographic information systems: Whose map? Who is empowered and who disempowered? Who gains and who loses? EJISDC 25 (2), 1–11.

Chambers, R., 2008. PRA, PLA and pluralism: practice and theory. In: Reason, P., Bradbury, H. (Eds.), The SAGE Handbook of Action Research: Participative Inquiry and Practice, second ed. Sage, London.

Clammer, J., 1984. Approaches to ethnographic research. In: Ellen, R. (Ed.), Ethnographic Research. Academic Press, London, pp. 63–85.

Cohen, A., 1985. The Symbolic Construction of Community. Tavistock, London.

Crow, G., Allen, G., 1994. Community Life: An Introduction to Local Social Relations. Harvester, Weatsheaf, London.

De Certeau, M., 1984. The Practice of Everyday Life. University of California Press, Berkeley.

Giddens, A., 1990. The Consequences of Modernity. Polity Press, Cambridge, UK.

Lash, S., Urry, J., 1994. Economies of Signs and Space. Sage Publications, London.

MacIver, R., Page, C., 1961. Society. Macmillan, London.

O'Neill, M., 2001. Participation or observation? Some practical and ethical dilemmas. In: Gellner, D., Hirsch, E. (Eds.), Inside Organizations: Anthropologists at Work. Berg, Oxford.

O'Neill, M., 2003. Family and social change in an urban street community. In: Davies, C., Jones, S. (Eds.), Welsh Communities: New Ethnographic Perspectives. University of Wales Press, Cardiff.

O'Neill, M., Williams, G., 2004. Developing community and agency engagement in an action research study in South Wales. Crit. Public Health 14 (1), 37–47.

Roper, M.W., 1935. The City and the Primary Group. University of Chicago Press, Chicago.

Swendan, W., 2006. Federalism and Regionalism in Western Europe: A Comparative and Thematic Analysis. Palgrave Macmillan, New York.

Syme, S.L., 2004. Social determinants of health: the community as an empowered partner. Prev. Chronic Dis. Available from: <http://www.cdc.gov/pcd/issues/2004/jan/03_0001.htm>.

Tönnies, F., 2001 (Originally published 1887). In: Harris, J. (Ed.), Community and Civil Society: Texts in the History of Political Thought. Cambridge University Press, Cambridge. <http://www.cambridge.org/gb/academic/subjects/politics-international-relations/texts-political-thought/tonnies-community-and-civil-society>.

Welsh Index of Multiple Deprivation, 2015. <http://gov.wales/docs/statistics/2015/150812-wimd-2014-revised-en.pdf> (accessed 20.10.15.).

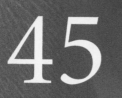

45

MIND THE GAP; ADDRESSING INEQUALITIES IN HEALTH THROUGH OCCUPATION-BASED PRACTICES

HANNEKE E. VAN BRUGGEN

CHAPTER OUTLINE

'Mind the gap' is a refrain that any passenger on undergrounds and trains will have had drilled into their brains. In development and human rights, one of the most controversial issues is how to deal with the dangerous governance gap between the powerful globalizing forces in our economies, often led by large companies, and the often weak capacity of societies to cope with the problems and damage these forces can cause for health and participation in different areas of life and society. Economic inequality is a catastrophic waste of talent. By denying the poor the opportunity to fulfil their potential, inequality not only reduces well-being, but also strangles the supply of human capital needed to drive a resilient and innovative economy (Shaheen, 2014).

The report 'Closing the Gap in a Generation' (World Health Organization (WHO), 2008) concludes that health inequities are determined by the conditions in which people are born, grow, live, work, and age and the inequities in power, money, and resources that give rise to these conditions. Relative deprivation impacts on a person's ability to participate in or have access to employment, occupation, education, recreation, family and social activities, and relationships, which are commonly experienced by most people.

If occupational therapists seriously study the global context, figures, and facts on disability, then they can question if what they do is effective and whether there are alternative strategies to achieve better results in participation and social inclusion of occupationally deprived people.

There are globally more than a billion people with disabilities, about 15% of the world's population, and rates of disability are increasing due to population ageing and increases in chronic health conditions (WHO, 2015). However, The World Federation of Occupational Therapists (2014) has stated that there are only 417 235 occupational therapists. Furthermore, 80% of those with disabilities live in developing countries, while more than 80% of the occupational therapists work in developed countries. This demonstrates that there is a lack of occupational therapy services for many persons with disabilities, and that the distribution of therapists is unequal, even in the developed world. For example, while in Sweden there are 9400 practising occupational therapists for 9.503 million inhabitants (99 in 100 000), in Bulgaria there are 15 practising occupational therapists for 7.265 million inhabitants (0.2 in 100 000) (World Federation of Occupational Therapists, 2014). Between 2010 and 2012, the risk of poverty rate rose by 0.4 percentage points on average in the European Union (EU), with considerable differences between member countries. The largest increases in inequality were registered in the Baltic countries, followed by other Central and Eastern European countries. This trend of increasing inequality is attributed to a number of factors such as a skill-biased technological change, the deregulation of the financial sector, and the globalization of financial operations (European Commission, 2014). Between 2005 and 2015, the gap in health between rich and poor has widened, according to an international study of nearly half a million adolescents from 34 countries across Europe and North America (Elgar et al., 2015).

These figures demonstrate that if occupational therapists want to address socioeconomic and health inequalities, they must have a commitment to occupational justice and operate in a socially accountable way at community and population levels (Watson and Swartz, 2004). These issues cannot be resolved only by individual solutions and traditional clinical reasoning, but require professional strategic reasoning in a socioeconomic and political context of health and the use of occupation-based collective approaches in which *all* individuals find their place.

In this chapter, I discuss certain international and European contexts and policies which are relevant for occupational therapy and which give guidance to a socially accountable and community oriented way of working. This is an essential step towards combating poverty, inequality, and occupational deprivation and developing the concepts and practices necessary for an inclusive, occupationally just community (van Bruggen, 2010).

CONTEXT MATTERS

Context matters for community development outcomes, yet there is little understanding of how exactly 'context' affects outcomes and which contextual factors matter most. The critical task, of course, is how to identify which are the critical contextual factors (Joshi, 2013).

A two-pronged approach to the study of context in community development seems to be emerging. On the macro side, there is an approach that examines patterns of enabling and constraining contextual factors in broad domains (O'Meally, 2013). On the other hand, there is an approach that attempts to unpack particular causal chains and the microcontextual conditions that seem to make them work.

On the macro side, accountability processes need to take into account larger histories of citizen-state engagement and related political processes. At the micro level, local factors can clearly drive the way certain social accountability interventions unfold and the extent to which they are successful, even within otherwise broadly similar contexts (Joshi, 2013). It is important that practitioners use longer time horizons, take account of global influences on accountability, build on existing processes, and make issues of inequality, inclusion, and exclusion more central to accountability processes, defending these choices to their employers or political administrators. The essence of accountability is answerability (Brinkerhoff, 2004): being accountable means having the obligation to answer questions regarding decisions and actions (Schedler, 1999). Social accountability has, at least in theory, the potential to empower people who have traditionally been excluded or marginalized to claim entitlements and rights more effectively (United Nations (UN) Children's Emergency Fund, 2014).

Growing Inequality and Its Impacts

One of the most influential contextual factors on a global, European, national, or local scale is inequality.

This is inequality not only in terms of money and possessions, but also in education, health, occupation, housing, and other factors (WHO, 2010). Income inequality leads to uneven access to health and education, and therefore to unequal social opportunities, creating poverty traps, wasting human potential, and resulting in less dynamic, less creative societies (UN Department of Economic and Social Affairs, 2013).

Inequality is also an issue of social justice. It impacts on educational access and achievement, individual employment opportunities and labour market behaviour, household joblessness, living standards and deprivation, family and household formation/breakdown, housing and intergenerational social mobility, individual health and life expectancy, and social cohesion versus polarization (Growing Inequalities Impacts, 2012).

Inequality and Disadvantaged Groups

Despite the tremendous improvements in overall health and life expectancy during the past century, there are presently indefensible gaps in health for many vulnerable groups, including racial and ethnic minorities and the poor (Marmot, 2016). These gaps in health prosper in a climate of economic and social inequities. These inequities create the conditions that adversely affect the health of individuals and communities by denying individuals and groups the equal opportunity to meet their basic human needs (Levy and Sidel, 2006). There is a particularly large body of evidence linking greater inequality to worse population health (Pickett, 2013).

It is important to address group inequalities that are socially embedded and defined in terms of social characteristics such as ethnic background, culture, language, disability status and so on. Such inequalities constitute a large component of overall inequalities within countries (United Nations Research Institute for Social Development, 2010) and tend to be more persistent over time than economic inequalities between individuals. Factors that matter most are intergenerational transmission of poverty, educational attainment of the parents, growing up in a workless household, and place of residence (Serafino and Tonkin, 2014). Furthermore, unequal access to resources can affect the well-being of the individuals belonging to disadvantaged groups. In addition, many individuals belong to more than one disadvantaged group, and inequalities across dimensions often reinforce each other.

Both young people and older people across the globe experience a broad range of disadvantages that are associated with their age. Unemployment is a particularly severe problem for youth. The most recent rate of global youth unemployment stood at 13% in 2015, amounting to 74 million young people unemployed, and it is set to rise (International Labour Office, 2015). Inequities in older people's health and well-being relate to a considerable extent to differences in conditions experienced earlier in their lives. Older persons are disproportionately at risk of inadequate and insecure income, insufficient access to quality healthcare and other services, such as accessible transportation and housing. They are also at risk of discrimination on the basis of their age (United Nations Department of Economic and Social Affairs, 2013).

Recent systematic reviews suggest that many European migrant groups have poorer self-reported health than the majority population (Nielsen and Krasnik, 2010). Migrants also face manifold disadvantages, including discrimination. Disadvantages are greater among women than among men within these groups. Indigenous peoples generally fare worse than the non-indigenous in every socioeconomic dimension (United Nations Department of Economic and Social Affairs, 2013).

There are also significant social inequalities between persons with disabilities and the general population in educational and health outcomes and in access to full and productive employment and decent work opportunities. The World Bank estimates that 20% of the world's poorest people have some kind of disability and tend to be regarded in their own communities as the most disadvantaged (WHO, 2011). According to the European Disability Forum, 75% of people with severe disabilities lack the opportunity to fully participate in the European labour market. Persons with disabilities have less access to education, have the highest unemployment rates, and generally live on significantly lower incomes. They often cannot move around freely, go to work, go to a restaurant, shop, meet friends, or take part in any other daily activity, due to inaccessible public transport, pavements, or buildings and attitudinal barriers. More than 200 000 disabled persons in Europe are forced to live in closed institutions deprived of the most fundamental human rights. Among disabled persons, one out of two persons has never participated in leisure, cultural, or sporting activities, and has never had access to theatres, to cinemas, to concerts, or to libraries (European Disability Forum, 2015).

Inequality may result in, and at the same time be caused by, lack of political power. Addressing inequalities in the social determinants of health faced by disadvantaged and marginalized social groups is not only an imperative, but also a practical entry point to combating inequality in society (Marmot, 2016; United Nations Department of Economic and Social Affairs, 2013).

Health Inequality, Social Injustice, and Social Exclusion

Framing health as a social phenomenon emphasizes health as a topic of social justice more broadly. Consequently, health equity described by the absence of unfair and avoidable or remediable differences in health among social groups (WHO, 2010) becomes a guiding criterion of health.

The system of social injustice has contributed to disparities not only in health but also in other sectors, such as transportation, work, and housing. Social injustice underlies many public health problems throughout the world. It is manifested in many ways, ranging from various forms of overt discrimination to wide gaps between the 'haves' and 'have-nots' within a country, and between rich and poor countries. It leads to higher rates of disease, injury, disability, and premature death. Health professionals need a clear understanding of social injustice in order to address these problems (Levy and Sidel, 2006). Improving global health requires a new generation of professionals who understand the many complex dimensions of health, healthcare, global institutions, and processes and can reason ethically about the many difficult moral dilemmas they present.

Inequality is inherent to social exclusion and is closely related to extreme poverty. Social exclusion has been defined by the Department of International Development (2005) of the UK as 'a process by which

certain groups are systematically disadvantaged because they are discriminated against on the basis of their ethnicity, race, religion, sexual orientation, caste, descent, gender, age, disability, HIV status, migrant status or where they live' (p. 3). Discrimination occurs in public institutions, such as education and health services, as well as social institutions. Relative powerlessness is a common experience of all excluded groups. According to the Social Exclusion Knowledge Network (2008):

> [E]xclusion consists of dynamic, multidimensional processes driven by unequal power relationships interacting across four main dimensions – economic, political, social and cultural – and at different levels including individual, household, group, community, country and global levels. It results in a continuum of inclusion and exclusion characterised by unequal access to resources, capabilities and rights which leads to health inequalities. (p. 2)

The above-mentioned contextual information demonstrates the influence of inequality on health and social development. At the same time, these issues are a matter of human rights, health ethics, and equity-oriented policies. It is imperative that health services should meet the needs of individuals and populations in an equitable and efficient manner.

What Can Be Done to Reduce Inequality?

Inequities in health cannot be reduced without addressing inequities in the causes of ill health. These causes include the conditions of daily life and the distribution of power, money, and resources (WHO, 2012). Human rights approaches support giving priority to improving health and reducing inequities. This requires definitive action on the social determinants of health; the costs of health inequities to health services are such that no society can afford inaction (WHO, 2014a; WHO, 2008). Health in All Policies (HiAP) is a whole government-system approach on what is needed to tackle health inequities (WHO, 2012).

According to the WHO (2014b):

> HiAP is an approach to public policies across sectors that systematically takes into account the health implications of decisions, seeks synergies, and avoids

harmful health impacts in order to improve population health and health equity. As a concept, it reflects the principles of: legitimacy, accountability, transparency and access to information, participation, sustainability, and collaboration across sectors and levels of government. (p. 1)

HiAP addresses the effects on health across all policies such as agriculture, education, the environment, fiscal policies, housing, and transport. It seeks to improve health and at the same time contribute to the well-being and the wealth of countries and communities through structures, mechanisms, and actions planned and managed mainly by sectors other than health (Ståhl et al., 2006). Health needs to be embedded in the mindset and the general policy developments that feed into overarching social goals (Leppo et al., 2013). The HiAP approach is not only for governments but can also be applied at neighbourhood or project level. And yet, hardly any (local) government is ready to address structural issues of redistribution of resources.

Advancing HiAP as occupational therapists in the community will depend greatly on the ability to actively seek opportunities to collaborate with and influence other sectors. 'The ability to communicate effectively across and within sectors with politicians, civil servants, key civil society organizations, and the private sector is crucial' (WHO, 2014b, p. 12). This requires knowledge of global, European, and national development policies.

Global Policies: The Millennium Goals

The Millennium Development Goals (MDGs) served as a milestone in global development since their inception in 2000. The MDGs were specifically designed to address the needs of the world's poorest citizens and the most marginalized populations. Yet, there is a striking gap in the MDGs: persons with disabilities are not mentioned in any of the eight goals and inequality has deepened (United Nations, 2011). Persons with disabilities have not benefited from much of the progress brought about by the MDGs, and their living standards may actually have declined in relative terms (Wapling, 2012). Only by making specific reference to disability and including disability as a cross-cutting target with measurable indicators can the post-2015

framework redress the effects of discrimination and exclusion. In 2013, for the first time, persons with disabilities were invited to participate in the development of the new Sustainable Development Goals (SDGs), which were determined in September 2015.

The post-2015 era demands a new vision and a responsive framework, which embraces the integrated essential elements of dignity, people, prosperity, planet, justice, and partnership.

- *Dignity* to end poverty and fight inequalities.
- *People* to ensure healthy lives, knowledge, and the inclusion of targeted groups such as women, children, and persons with disabilities.
- *Prosperity* to grow a strong, inclusive, and transformative economy.
- *Planet* to protect our ecosystems for all societies and our children.
- *Justice* to promote safe and peaceful societies, and strong institutions.
- *Partnership* to catalyse global solidarity for sustainable development (United Nations, 2014, p. 16).

The agenda itself mirrors the broader international human rights framework, including elements of economic, social, cultural, civil, and political rights, as well as the right to development (UN, 2014).

Compared with the MDGs (2000–2015), the following topics have been added in the new SDGs: promotion of equality of opportunity, inclusive and sustainable growth, access to decent employment and social protection, universal healthcare coverage, addressing environmental challenges, and contribution and participation of all people in national and local governance (UN, 2015).

The SDGs include seven targets, which explicitly refer to persons with disabilities, and several others refer to persons in vulnerable situations, including persons with disabilities. For example, target 4.5 aims to 'by 2030, eliminate gender disparities in education and ensure equal access to all levels of education and vocational training for the vulnerable, including persons with disabilities, indigenous peoples, and children in vulnerable situations' (UN, 2015, p. 19).

The most important message of the MDGs beyond 2015 is: 'Leave No One Behind' (UN, 2013). The impact of this new vision will depend on how the elements are translated into specific priorities and actions. The history of development policy, however, is a history of the replacement of slogans without any noteworthy consequences for development practices. Whether it was called modernization or social change, trade instead of aid, support focused on basic needs, sustainability or good governance or human rights, the reference frame always remained the growth-oriented, resource and energy-intensive economic and social model of the Northern Hemisphere (Mabanza, 2015). A reorientation is necessary and will only be reached by constructive cooperation. What is needed are real changes, corresponding to the various local and national necessities. These have to come from the people themselves and through new kinds of solidarity between the North and the South (Mabanza, 2015).

European Policies 2010 to 2020

The key targets of the EU Strategy 2020 comply with the world vision on sustainable and inclusive development. This vision promotes social inclusion, in particular through the reduction of poverty and social exclusion. Concretely, the EU aimed for five ambitious objectives to be reached by 2020:

1. *Employment*
   ■ 75% of the 20- to 64-year-olds to be employed.
2. *Research and Development (R&D)/innovation*
   ■ 3% of the EU's gross domestic product (public and private combined) to be invested in R&D/innovation.
3. *Climate change/energy*
   ■ Greenhouse gas emissions 20% lower than 1990.
   ■ 20% of energy from renewables.
   ■ 20% increase in energy efficiency.
4. *Education*
   ■ Reducing school dropout rates to below 10%.
   ■ At least 40% of 30- to 34-year-olds completing higher education.
5. *Poverty/social exclusion*
   ■ At least 20 million fewer people in or at risk of poverty and social exclusion (European Commission, 2015).

These targets are interrelated and mutually reinforcing and need to be translated into national targets. The first years of the Europe 2020 strategy coincided with a severe financial and economic crisis which had a significant impact on progress towards the goals of the strategy. At the time of writing (September 2015), the credibility of the EU and the fight against poverty are facing a serious crisis: the EU and its member states are not delivering on the poverty target of the Europe 2020 Strategy (lifting at least 20 million people out of the risk of poverty). On the contrary, over 8 million more people find themselves at risk of poverty with the biggest increase in material deprivation (Eurostat, n.d.). Youth unemployment figures (23% average, 55% in Greece, Eurostat, n.d.) are unacceptable, and the reduction in funding is having a detrimental effect on the quality and impact of essential public, social, and healthcare services. Promoting good health is an integral part of Europe 2020, whereby the following linked strategic objectives are explicitly mentioned:

■ Improving health for all and reducing health inequalities.
■ Improving leadership and participatory governance for health (WHO, 2013).

The WHO EU review advises governments and healthcare workers to do something, do more, and do better, in order to decrease the social causes of inequalities (WHO, 2014a).

If taken seriously, the SDGs and the EU agenda will require profound changes in policies as well as governance. In particular, the implementation requires fundamental changes in fiscal policy. Occupational therapists can try to work through organizations such as the World Federation of Occupational Therapists (WFOT) and the Council of Occupational Therapists for the European Countries to influence these policies. They can also make use of the development goals and keep governments accountable.

The World Bank as well as the EU Commission and national governments ensure some money for all these goals, although this is often not enough. If occupational therapists can demonstrate that they can contribute concretely to the goals, they may receive funding.

For instance, in 2010 four Polish universities in partnership with the ministries of health and education and disability organizations received 2 million euros from the EU Commission for the establishment of occupational therapy. Within 2 years of the award of the funding this should guarantee higher education for 200 young people and employment in occupational therapy, and improve quality of life and employment for persons with disabilities.

The global and European context offers chances for occupational therapists to engage in the implementation of policies for development and social change, in partnership with relevant stakeholders. In doing so, occupational therapists need to ask for social accountability from their educational and practice services towards all stakeholders.

Social Accountability

The concept of accountability is at the heart of both democratic, rights-based governance and of equitable human development. Social accountability refers to a form of civic engagement that builds liability through the collective efforts of citizens and civil society organizations to hold public officials, service providers, and governments responsible for their obligations (Houtzager and Joshi, 2008). It describes the principle of a vibrant, dynamic, and accountable relationship between states and citizens underpinning efforts to ensure equitable development (United Nations Development Programme, 2013). It is important to emphasize that social accountability is the operationalization of a number of key principles, which are at the heart of both democratic governance and a human rights-based approach to development.

Elements of social accountability are:

■ *Voice,* which refers to a variety of mechanisms, formal and informal, through which people express their preferences, opinions, and views and demand accountability from power-holders/service delivery.

■ *Civic engagement,* which is a concept encompassing a number of different mechanisms through which citizens or their representatives engage with and seek to influence public processes in order to achieve civic objectives and goals (United Nations Development Programme, 2010).

The WHO (1995) defines social accountability of health professionals' training as:

[T]he obligation to direct their education, research and service activities towards addressing the priority health concerns of the community, region and/or nation that they have a mandate to serve. The priority health concerns are to be identified jointly by governments, healthcare organizations, health professional and the public.

The education of health professionals must go beyond care for the individual to instil the importance of community advocacy and the ethic of practising in areas of the greatest need (Wen et al., 2011). Five steps are proposed by Wen et al. (2011) for every health professional training programme to help align their programme with societal needs:

■ An explicit social mission needs to be established.

■ Community learning and service should be integrated into the curriculum.

■ The importance of primary care deserves particular emphasis.

■ There needs to be a service option in exchange for free health education.

■ Health professionals need to be engaged in social accountability throughout their education.

Using an accountability lens: (a) helps to generate a system-wide perspective on health sector reform, and (b) identifies connections among individual interventions. These results support synergistic outcomes, enhance system performance, and contribute to sustainability. A systemic view of accountability highlights the interdependencies among health actors (Brinkerhoff, 2003).

Occupational therapists should strive to be socially accountable agents of change in order to contribute to closing the health inequalities gap. This has implications for the use and choice of theory, the reasoning and methods which are used in practice, as well as for research. Also, professional organizations should partner with disability organizations in order to achieve social reform.

CONTRIBUTING TO CLOSING THE GAP

Today's extremes of inequality are bad for everyone. The problems of health inequity and poverty reduction cannot be solved simply by individual treatment plans or by traditional clinical reasoning. If occupational therapists want to play a role in the constantly changing healthcare and social care world and make a contribution to reducing health inequities and poverty in order to prevent disability, they need to have a commitment to occupational justice. As Whalley, Hammel and Iwama (2012) state, 'the ability and opportunity to engage in occupations is an issue that concerns rights' (p. 385).

The profession, therefore, needs an underpinning by a critical occupational science, which enhances awareness of occupational inequities and injustices, impacts on social transformation, and understands occupation as a human right (Rudman, 2013). Furthermore, different ways of reasoning and occupational therapy practice are needed, for example, strategic reasoning and a social developmental framework for occupation-based community/population practice.

Critical Occupational Science

Occupational science is the science of everyday living. As a discipline, it is able to make a cogent contribution to global phenomena which are essentially occupational, such as reducing inequality and enhancing social inclusion. For Whiteford and Hocking (2012), 'Occupational Science, in particular constructions of occupational justice, which foreground difference and diversity in capabilities, has a substantive contribution to make across arenas of disability, health and welfare' (p. 7).

Occupational therapists need to commit to occupational justice to mobilize resources with the aim of creating occupationally inclusive communities and societies, based on people and their need and right to *do*. For Townsend (1999), 'occupational justice is concerned with economic, political and social forces that create equitable opportunity and the means to choose, organise and perform occupations that people find useful or meaningful in their environment' (p. 154).

If occupational therapists are concerned with social reform and reducing health inequalities, they need to develop a transformative discipline, in which occupation is contributing to social changes. The necessity of such disciplinary development has involved scholars advocating an 'emancipatory agenda' (Whiteford and Hocking, 2012, p. 3) of social reform in which the power of occupation is emphasized. As summarized

by Laliberte Rudman (2014), 'there is a growing number of voices-from diverse geographical locations-pointing occupational science in transformative directions' (pp. 375–376). An agenda for social reform through occupation needs underpinning from occupational science as well as strategic reasoning to achieve inclusive development goals.

Strategic Reasoning for Inclusive Development

There is agreement among researchers (see, e.g., Bonn, 2005; Liedtka, 1998; Pisapia, 2009; Senge, 1990) that systems thinking, creativity, and vision are key elements of strategic thinking (see Figure 45-1). Systems thinking enables the identification and clarification of patterns and supports effective change, thereby increasing creativity. Vision helps to provide meaning and gives a sense of direction in the decision-making process. Strategic thinking is at the intersection of these three elements (Bonn, 2005); it is not just an individual activity but is influenced by the individual's environment and social interactions.

A systems perspective also demands that the strategic thinker has knowledge of the external context as well as the internal environment of the community or population (van Bruggen, 2016). How can an

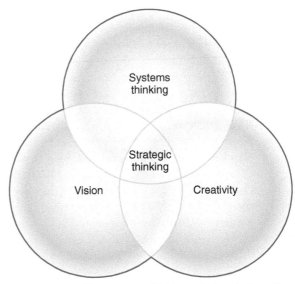

FIGURE 45-1 ■ Strategic thinking. *[Adapted from Bonn (2005).]*

occupational therapist reason strategically, for example, in the case of a single poor mother, who is attending a rehabilitation centre with her child with learning disabilities in a country where there is little or no social protection? Should the child be treated individually and then sent with the mother back to the same situation from which they came? What different perspectives can be explored? How can the mother and her child be understood in their situation? If our vision is social inclusion and poverty reduction through occupational participation for all, how can improvement be made in this situation? It is important to think in different systems and at different levels, for example, health, education, employment, and legal systems. Using creativity in finding participatory strategies and solutions can result in:

- A social network where mothers take turns to take responsibility for the care of the children and others can work.
- An advocacy parent group lobbying for inclusive education.
- Stakeholders' participation in developing an inclusive school as a pilot project.
- An occupational therapist appointed as policymaker for inclusive education in the Ministry of Education.
- A renewed curriculum for primary teachers with one obligatory year on inclusive education (with occupational therapy input).

These results can follow directly from the occupational therapist looking beyond the immediate problem, considering the broader picture and thinking strategically. Strategic reasoning is not enough to achieve social inclusion or to reduce health inequalities; strategic planning and implementation and community-based approaches are needed as well.

Community-Based Approaches

There is growing evidence from developed and developing countries that community-based approaches are effective in improving the health of individuals and populations, especially when the social determinants of health are considered in their design (Kelly et al., 2007). That means working in partnership at local level to improve the social conditions in which we are born, live, grow, work, and age. Empowering individuals and communities and giving people a voice is integral to addressing health inequalities.

Case studies have shown that synergy between all elements (including antipoverty strategies, non-government organization–government collaboration, empowerment and fostering EU wide standards, certification of e-health development, and active health programmes) is probably the most effective way to improve health and development outcomes (WHO, 2006). When implementing community-based programmes, there are several strategies that occupational therapists may use. These are discussed in the following paragraphs.

Establishing Partnership

Establishing partnerships is important in order to enable different groups of people and agencies to collaborate, cooperate, and coordinate to solve problems and share resources. Partnerships take place at different levels (local, regional, national, or international). A partnership is a cross-sector collaboration in which organizations work together in a transparent, equitable, and mutually beneficial way towards a sustainable development goal and where those defined as partners agree to commit resources and share the risks as well as the benefits associated with the partnership (Tennyson, 2011). Cross-sector (business, not-for-profit organizations, government, academia, media) partnering is an important mechanism for addressing critical and sustainable development issues such as health, employment, social inclusion, and development.

A systematic partnership or stakeholder analysis helps to define whom, and how, to involve in the design of a multistakeholder process and find out whose occupational needs must be considered. Various tools can be used to identify stakeholders, such as brainstorming, interviews with key informants, or focus groups.

Building Capability for Development Through Engagement in Occupation

Another strategy identified within community development is capacity building, based on the theory of the economist and philosopher Amartya Sen, who has outlined an alternative approach to appraising the success of development interventions. Sen (1999) argues for the necessity of going beyond the conventional development targets and measures of success to take into account improvements in human potential. Development, from this perspective, is fundamentally about fostering the capabilities of people by increasing the options available to them. This can be done, in part, by focusing on the freedoms generated by conventional outcomes rather than just on the outcomes themselves. These freedoms come in the form of capabilities that people can exercise to choose a way of life they value. The emphasis here is on what individuals are able to do (i.e., *capable* of). Sen's (1999) definition of poverty is individual: it is deprivation of basic capabilities, always defined as individual capabilities. Sen's capability approaches are individualistic in methodology, derived from microeconomics and generalized by adding problems of access to non-market-related entitlements. However, concepts of development are required that recognize and emphasize the collective rights of marginalized communities to find alternative routes to 'development as freedom' (O'Hearn, 2009).

The development scientists Baser and Morgan (2008) defined capacity as the emergent combination of individual competencies *and* collective capabilities that enable a human system to create developmental value. Capacity can be conceptualized as being built on five core collective capabilities, which can be found in all organizations, communities or systems. These are the capability to commit, engage, and act; generate development results; relate; adapt and self-renew; and, finally, balance diversity and achieve coherence. All five capabilities are necessary to ensure the optimum overall capacity of a community (Baser and Morgan, 2008).

Changes observed in these five dimensions at relevant levels in the system – individual, organization, network, or the system as a whole – feed into broader capacity and performance changes. Figure 45-2 illustrates the various capabilities and how they relate to capacity (Baser and Morgan, 2008).

Crucial to the process of capacity development is the energy, commitment and ownership of all partners to engage in a process of change. Ownership is everything! (Box 45-1)

Over the past 15 years, the European Network of Occupational Therapy in Higher Education in

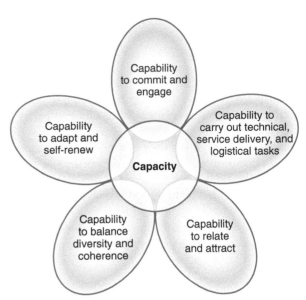

FIGURE 45-2 ■ Elements of capacity.

BOX 45-1

Now try to apply the above-mentioned theory and strategies in the following situation: you are asked as an occupational therapist to contribute to improving quality of life in a disadvantaged neighbourhood. Some of the problems are: children drop out of school before 16 years, and there is high criminality and high youth employment. Demonstrate how you can engage with them, with whom you want to partner and how you can build neighbourhood capacity.

---

collaboration with national and local governments, universities, practitioners, disability, and other marginalized groups with the support of funding of the EU has systematically facilitated capability development with the following results (van Bruggen, 2011):

■ Development of eight new occupational therapy schools in different Eastern European countries: Bulgaria, Georgia, Armenia, Romania, and Poland.

■ Development of six new occupational therapy associations in the Czech Republic, Bulgaria, Georgia, Armenia, Romania, and Poland.

■ Strengthening and establishment of associations of marginalized groups.

■ Changing laws towards more rights for persons with disabilities in employment and education.

CONCLUSION

The role of occupational therapists needs to go beyond the traditional role of working with individuals with occupational needs in the healthcare sector, to working with communities on capability development through engagement in occupation and facilitating inclusive communities. A systematic approach of implementing community development theories in occupational therapy in the transition countries in Europe has demonstrated the changes in the rights of persons with disabilities and their families (van Bruggen, 2011).

Working with communities implies that the individual is considered as a citizen within the community, with rights as well as responsibilities and obligations. This vision and way of working has consequences for the content of the curriculum and for the educational strategies used in the education of occupational therapists, as well as for research.

In order to prepare its members to work with communities rather than only with individuals, the profession of occupational therapy needs to engage with questions, such as: Are occupational therapists able to work on inequalities in complex communities? Is occupational science underpinning occupation-based practice for development and social reform? Are students, teachers, and researchers seeing the bigger picture? Are they thinking globally and acting locally?

REFERENCES

Baser, H., Morgan, P., 2008. Capacity, Change and Performance Study Report. ECDPM Discussion Paper 59B. European Centre for Development Policy Management, Maastricht, the Netherlands.

Bonn, I., 2005. Improving strategic thinking: a multilevel approach. Leadership & Organization Development Journal 26 (5), 336–354.

Brinkerhoff, D.W., 2003. Accountability and Health Systems: Overview, Framework, and Strategies. The Partners for Health Reformplus Project, Abt Associates Inc, Bethesda, MD.

Brinkerhoff, D.W., 2004. Accountability and health systems: toward conceptual clarity and policy relevance. Health Policy Plan. 19 (6), 371–379.

Department for International Development, 2005. Reducing Poverty by Tackling Social Exclusion: A DFID Policy Paper. Department for International Development, Glasgow.

Elgar, E., Pförtner, T., Moor, I., De Clercq, B., Stevens, G., Currie, C., 2015. Socioeconomic inequalities in adolescent health 2002–2010: a time-series analysis of 34 countries participating in the Health Behaviour in School-aged Children study. Lancet 385 (9982), 2088–2095.

European Commission, 2014. Memo Poverty and Inequalities: Frequently asked Questions. <http://europa.eu/rapid/press-release _MEMO-14-572_en.htm> (accessed June 2016.).

European Commission, 2015. Europe 2020, Targets. <http://ec.europa.eu/europe2020/targets/eu-targets/index_en.htm> (accessed June 2016.).

European Disability Forum. <http://www.edf-feph.org/> (accessed June 2016.).

Eurostat, n.d. <http://ec.europa.eu/eurostat/statistics-explained/index.php/Main_Page> (accessed June 2016.).

Growing Inequalities Impacts, 2012. Flyer. <http://www.gini-research.org/system/uploads/400/original/GINI_at_a_glance_November_2012.pdf?1353928051> (accessed June 2016.).

Houtzager, P., Joshi, A., 2008. Introduction: contours of a research project and early findings. IDS Bull. 38 (6), 1–9.

International Labour Office, 2015. World Employment Social Outlook. International Labour Office, Geneva. Available from: <http://www.ilo.org/global/research/global-reports/weso/2015/WCMS_337069/lang–en/index.htm> (accessed June 2016.).

Joshi, A., 2013. Context Matters: A Causal Chain Approach to Unpacking Social Accountability Interventions. IDS Bulletin Volume 45 Number 5 September 2014. Wiley, Oxford.

Kelly, M.P., Morgan, A., Bonnefoy, J., Butt, J., Bergman, V., 2007. The social determinants of health: developing an evidence base for political action, final report to WHO CSDH. NHS, London. <http://www.who.int/social_determinants/resources/mekn_final_report_102007.pdf> (accessed June 2016.).

Laliberte Rudman, D., 2014. The 2013 Ruth Zemke Lecture in Occupational Science: embracing and enacting an 'occupational imagination': occupational science as transformative. J. Occup. Sci. 21, 373–388.

Leppo, K., Ollila, E., Peña, S., Wismar, M., Cook, S., 2013. Health in All Policies Seizing opportunities, implementing policies. Ministry of Social Affairs and Health, Finland.

Levy, B.S., Sidel, V.W., 2006. Social Injustice and Public Health. Oxford University Press, Oxford.

Liedtka, J., 1998. Strategic thinking; can it be taught? Long Range Planning, 31(1). Elsevier, London, pp. 120–129.

Mabanza, B., 2015. From MDGs to SDGs: An African Civil Society Perspective on the Gap between Claim and Reality, Issue 728, AfricAvenir <http://www.pambazuka.org/governance/mdgs-sdgs-african-civil-society-perspective-gap-between-claim-and-reality> (accessed June 2016.).

Marmot, 2016. The Health Gap, The challenge of an Unequal World. Bloomsbury, London.

Nielsen, S., Krasnik, A., 2010. Poorer self-perceived health among migrants and ethnic minorities versus the majority population in Europe: a systematic review. Int. J. Public Health 55 (5), 357–371.

O'Hearn, D., 2009. Ámartya Sen's development as freedom: ten years later. Policy Pract. 8 (Spring), 9–15.

O'Meally, S.C., 2013. Mapping Context for Social Accountability: A Resource Paper. Social Development Department. World Bank, Washington, DC.

Pickett, K., 2013. Reducing inequality: an essential step for development and wellbeing. J. Progress. Econ.

Pisapia, J., 2009. The strategic leader. Information Age Publishers, Charlotte, NC.

Rudman, D.L., 2013. Enacting the critical potential of occupational science: problematizing the 'individualizing of occupation'. J. Occup. Sci. 20 (4), 298–313.

Schedler, A., 1999. Conceptualizing accountability. In: Schedler, A., Diamond, L., Plattner, M.F. (Eds.), The Self-Restraining State: Power and Accountability in New Democracies. Lynne Rienner Publishers, Boulder, CO, pp. 13–29.

Sen, A., 1999. Development as Freedom. Oxford. Oxford University Press, Oxford.

Senge, P., 1990. The Fifth Discipline. Doubleday, New York, NY.

Serafino, P., Tonkin, R., 2014. Intergenerational transmission of disadvantage in the UK & EU. The National Archives, Kew, London. Office for National Statistics. <http://www.ons.gov.uk/ons/dcp171766_378097.pdf> (accessed June 2016.).

Shaheen, F., 2014. Mind the gap: why UN development goals must tackle economic inequality. The Guardian, UK. <www.theguardian.com/global-development/poverty-matters/2014/jul/01/mind-gap-un-development-goals-economic-inequality> (accessed June 2016.).

Social Exclusion Knowledge Network, 2008. Understanding and Tackling Social Exclusion. <http://www.who.int/social_determinants/knowledge_networks/final_reports/sekn_final%20report_042008.pdf?ua=1> (accessed June 2016.).

Ståhl, T., Wismar, M., Ollila, E., Lahtinen, E., Leppo, K., 2006. Health in All Policies, Prospects and Potentials. Ministry of Social Affairs and Health, Finland.

Tennyson, R., 2011. Partnering Toolbook. International Business Leaders Forum, London.

Townsend, E., 1999. Enabling occupation in the 21st century: making good intentions a reality. Aust. Occup. Ther. J. 46 (4), 147–159.

United Nations, 2011. Disability and the Millennium Development Goals; A Review of the MDG Process and Strategies for Inclusion of Disability Issues in Millennium Development Goal Efforts. UN, New York.

United Nations, 2013. A New Global Partnership: Eradicate Poverty and Transform Economies through Sustainable Development. UN, New York.

United Nations Department of Economic and Social Affairs, 2013. Inequality Matters, Report of the World Social Situation 2013. UN, New York.

United Nations Development Programme, 2010. Fostering social accountability: from principle to practice, guidance note. <http://www.undp.org/content/dam/undp/library/Democratic%20Governance/OGC/dg-ogc-Fostering%20Social%20Accountability-Guidance%20Note.pdf> (accessed June 2016.).

United Nations Development Programme, 2013. Reflections on Social Accountability. UNDP, New York. <http://www.undp.org/content/dam/undp/documents/partners/civil_society/publications/2013_UNDP_Reflections-on-Social-Accountability_EN.pdf> (accessed June 2016.).

United Nations, 2014. General Assembly Sixty-ninth Session, The Road to Dignity by 2030: Ending Poverty, Transforming All Lives and Protecting the Planet-A 69/700. Synthesis report of the Secretary-General on the Post-2015 Sustainable Development Agenda. UN, New York.

United Nations, 2015. Transforming Our World. The 2030 Agenda for Sustainable Development. UN, New York.

United Nations Research Institute for Social Development, 2010. Combatting Poverty and Inequality: Structural Change, Social Policy and Politics. UNRISD, Geneva.

van Bruggen, H., 2010. Working towards inclusive communities. In: Curtin, M., Molineux, M., Supyk-Melsson, J. (Eds.), Occupational Therapy and Physical Dysfunction, Enabling Occupation. Churchill Livingstone/Elsevier, London.

van Bruggen, H., 2011. Eastern European transition countries: capacity development for social reform. In: Kronenberg, F., Pollard, N., Sakellariou, D. (Eds.), Occupational Therapy without Borders, vol. 2. Churchill Livingstone Elsevier, London.

van Bruggen, H., 2016. Strategic thinking and reasoning in occupational therapy. In: Cole, M.B., Creek, J. (Eds.), Global Perspectives in Professional Reasoning. Slack, Thorofare, NJ.

Wapling, L., 2012. Disability in the post 2015-framework; addressing inequalities the heart of the post 2015 development agenda and the future we want for all, global thematic consultation. <http://www.beyond2015.org/sites/default/files/Disability%20in%20the%20post%202015%20framework.pdf> (accessed June 2016.).

Watson, R., Swartz, L., 2004. Transformation through Occupation. Whurr Publishers. London, UK.

Wen, L.S., Greysen, S.R., Keszthelyi, D., Bracero, J., de Roos, P.D., 2011. Social accountability in health professionals' training. Lancet 378 (9807), e12–e13.

Whalley Hammell, K.R., Iwama, M.K., 2012. Well-being and occupational rights: an imperative for critical occupational therapy. Scand. J. Occup. Ther. 19 (5), 385–394.

Whiteford, G.E., Hocking, C., 2012. Occupational Science: Society, Inclusion, Participation. Blackwell, Oxford.

World Federation of Occupational Therapists, 2014. Human Resources Project. <http://www.wfot.org/ResourceCentre.aspx> (accessed June 2016.).

World Health Organization, Boelen, C., Heck, J.E., 1995. Defining and Measuring the Social Accountability of Medical Schools. WHO, Geneva.

World Health Organization, 2006. Regional Office for Europe's Health Evidence Network (HEN) 2006. What is the evidence on effectiveness of empowerment to improve health? WHO, Copenhagen, Denmark.

World Health Organization, 2008. Closing the gap in a generation: health equity through action on the social determinants of health: final report of the Commission on Social Determinants of Health. WHO, Geneva.

World Health Organization, 2010. A Conceptual Framework for Action on the Social Determinants of Health. WHO, Geneva.

World Health Organization and World Bank, 2011. Disability Report. WHO, Geneva.

World Health Organization, 2012. Health 2020: a European policy framework supporting action across government and society for health and well-being. WHO Regional Office for Europe, Copenhagen, Denmark.

World Health Organization, 2013. Health 2020, a European Policy Framework and Strategy for the 21st Century. WHO Regional Office for Europe, Copenhagen, Denmark.

World Health Organization, 2014a. Review of social determinants and the health divide in the WHO European Region: final report. Copenhagen, DK. <http://www.euro.who.int/__data/assets/pdf_file/0004/251878/Review-of-social-determinants-and-the-health-divide-in-the-WHO-European-Region-FINAL-REPORT.pdf> (accessed June 2016.).

World Health Organization, 2014b. Health in All Policies (HiAP); Framework for Country Action. WHO, Geneva.

World Health Organization, 2015. Factsheet no.352 Disability and Health <http://www.who.int/mediacentre/factsheets/fs352/en/> (accessed June 2016.).

46

WORKING ON A HUMAN SCALE TO REVITALIZE THE COMMUNITY WE LIVE IN

LAURA PARRAQUINI ■ FEDERICO BARROSO LELOUCHE

This chapter describes the authors' experience: we are a young professional couple motivated by a strong social commitment, who decided to settle in a small town in Argentina to address sanitary and socio-cultural issues by starting the San Francisco de Bellocq Community Project. This project aims to strengthen the fabric of society through learning activities in a number of distinct interrelated areas: permaculture, art, communication, and occupational therapy.

Living in the community, we became acquainted with the way it worked and detected its needs. Nourished by all those who are actively involved in the proposal, we can help improve the quality of life of the place we work in, which is also the place we live in, a not-so-common trait in community occupational therapy, which we will share below.

AN INTRODUCTORY WALK AROUND TOWN

San Francisco de Bellocq is a town located in the south of the province of Buenos Aires, Argentina. It is only eight by four blocks, surrounded by agricultural fields and crossed by dirt streets. Its 567 inhabitants live in low houses with big gardens, and they all know their neighbours.

Kids go to school on foot or by bike. If a kid is engaged in any mischief that might harm others, some passing neighbour calls him by his name and invites him to behave and work for the common good. An old man suffering with Alzheimer's takes a daily walk and gets lost every day, but everybody knows who he is and how to guide him home. In the afternoons, boys play soccer in the local club; some girls train with them, but they are not allowed to compete on the weekends as the championship is a 'men's thing'.

From the opposite side of the street, the unsuspecting visitor might confuse the town library with a bike shop; in front of its vibrant façade, several bicycles without locks line up in the sidewalk. The colour and movement are an invitation to go in and discover what is going on inside. It is the meeting point of kids and teenagers, the place where they borrow books, do their homework, use the computers, participate in art workshops, and get English lessons to complement the ones that they have at school.

When they are at home, children spend most of their time alone with their mothers as men are generally expected to work and enjoy social gatherings. One does rarely come across them in the streets during the day: most men work in the fields with animals, cultivating the ground, installing fences, or transporting the harvest. Others are municipal workers: they are in charge of maintenance work in the town, they are clerks or they work in the Urban Solid Waste Management Plant. Yet others work in the local electric cooperative, doing administrative work or grid maintenance. And some are self-employed and work as blacksmiths, tyre dealers or car mechanics.

One can catch a glimpse of women in the streets only when they go shopping at the grocery store, to pick their children up from the kindergarten, or to attend a school meeting. They then spend the rest of the day at home without having consciously chosen to be housewives. Few women have had the chance to study, to empower themselves, or to acquire skills. Those who have, provide services in the fields of teaching or healthcare, or they are employed in some store; those who did not have the opportunity to study and decide to work, are maids in neighbouring towns. Without men noticing, many women have, slowly and painstakingly, done their best to acquire skills, to meet, and learn to debate. They occupy decision-making positions in local institutions and different civil society organizations, and return home pleased at having met others, acted on their desires, and decided their own path.

HISTORICAL AND POLITICAL CONTEXT

The town of San Francisco de Bellocq was born and developed around the train station, inaugurated in 1929. The town is the commercial hub for the agricultural products grown and harvested by criollos[1] and immigrants (Italians, Basques, Dutch, and Danish) who settled in this part of the Pampa Region (Gil de Jiménez, 2002).

Both the population and social assistance programmes increased continuously from the arrival of the railways until 1963, the year the train stopped running and the network was dismantled, responding to international economic interests. The people who worked for, or in some way depended on, this important means of transportation, moved gradually to urban centres. The exodus left many dwellings empty and their proprietors with little hope of ever being able to sell or rent them, since nobody would look for a house in a place from which opportunities for employment, consumption, health, and cultural experiences had vanished.

In spite of the situation, the residents who had any connection to rural work or who provided services to the agricultural or rural sector remained in San Francisco de Bellocq and witnessed the consolidation of an economic model that markedly worsened their living conditions. The industrialization of agriculture made it a barely profitable business for those who did not have a significant expanse of land. As a result, farmworkers were left unemployed, cooperatives were closed down, and small- and medium-scale producers either sold their fields to big companies or rented them under unfavourable conditions (Pousa and Pinella, 2004).

For the next few years, the town continued to deteriorate considerably. It suffered the constant flight of its inhabitants until the onset of the worst crisis in Argentina's neoliberal economy, which reached its peak in December 2001 with the outbreak of violent riots in the country's biggest cities and the president's abdication. The town residents followed these events on television, waiting for the ripple effects that would eventually arrive at their doors.

Out of this crisis arose an autonomous organizing process that the country had rarely seen before, led by several integrated social sectors. Argentina began to revive. The people in San Francisco de Bellocq had not had the chance to promote change, since most of the

---

[1] Men of European descent born in the former Spanish colonies in the Americas.

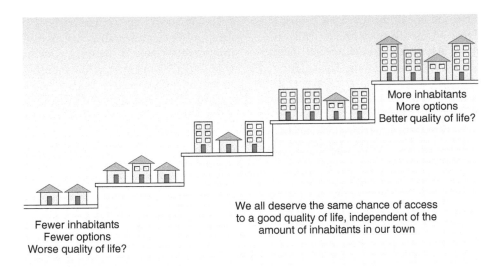

Fewer inhabitants
Fewer options
Worse quality of life?

More inhabitants
More options
Better quality of life?

We all deserve the same chance of access
to a good quality of life, independent of the
amount of inhabitants in our town

FIGURE 46-1 ■ Occupational injustice ladder.

inhabitants with skills in management and with a degree of social engagement had emigrated. Once again, the town received the ripple effects, but this time they brought new opportunities in the form of work and access to social benefits.

Since then, a lot of work has been done and still a lot more is left to be done in terms of healthcare, education, occupational justice, gender equality, defense of the rights to land and seeds (food sovereignty), and a decentralized, sustainable production. But something has undeniably become clear after all this economic and sociopolitical turmoil: San Francisco de Bellocq will not disappear, it will not turn into a ghost town; it can be brought back to life if the fabric of society is mended.

SOCIO-OCCUPATIONAL SITUATION OF THE POPULATION

In Argentina, most occupational opportunities (in education, entertainment, art, sports, social activities, work, etc.) are usually found in the big cities. For the inhabitants of San Francisco de Bellocq, these opportunities are 40 kilometers away, in the city of Tres Arroyos, which is not accessible by rail or by any other means of public transport.

This inequality in opportunities will continue to prompt the exodus towards the cities, backed by the fact that the government interventions which are intended to improve the quality of life seem to be aimed at the areas where the population is concentrated, generating the false idea that the more inhabitants there are, the better the lifestyle. Thus, a kind of *occupational injustice* (Townsend and Wilcock, 2004) ladder appears: the towns that are less densely populated occupy the lowest step, and the city with the highest population occupies the top step (Figure 46-1).

Everybody looks upwards, and see how the step directly above them enjoys more options in terms of education, healthcare, work, consumption, etc. Few manage to look inwards, to promote a Local Endogenous Development[2] (Capalbo, 2011, p. 170) that would change the established order and improve the living conditions, encouraging equality of opportunities thanks to the joint work of town and government.

Throughout the years, some governments have forgotten San Francisco de Bellocq; others have taken care

[2]This model seeks to foster the community's inner capacities to strengthen society from the inside out. Lucio Capalbo's proposal, in his book *Decrecer con equidad*, is to promote cooperative processes in the civil society, its institutions, and local governments in small- or medium-sized towns. He also points out that for the development process to be truly endogenous, neighbours must be able to trust in their peers and in their abilities for real participation.

of the people living here through welfare policies. In neither of these two scenarios has civil society allowed itself to decide its own destiny; maybe because it did not know how, maybe because it did not have enough self-esteem, or maybe because it had climbed onto the *occupational injustice* (Townsend and Wilcock, 2004) ladder and had accepted the situation that as long as the population did not grow, change would not come.

The outcome of this is a society which is poor in opportunities and lacking social rights (Pacto Internacional de Derechos Económicos, Sociales y Culturales, 1976), trapped in a paternalistic model through which the town does not participate in the decision-making process. Many people do not know what occupation they find meaningful, they are unable to express their needs or wishes, and they are inclined to accept what others decide for them. This situation cannot be addressed if the people do not have the opportunity to get to know themselves and to express their expectations. The situation will not improve unless the government decides to find out what is best for the population.

In this small town, occupational injustice (Townsend and Wilcock, 2004) is an issue many have become accustomed to living with. Making it visible and naming it, enabled us to start putting into practice specific interventions that can help promote change.

Following the Brazilian occupational therapist Galheigo (2006), we, the authors, set out to develop a community project with a view to empowering the people of the town, groups, and institutions, awakening participatory action, and promoting self-management. Having interviewed prominent representatives of the community and having listened to their needs, we designed proposals for the people according to their own context, proposals that could favour the development of their identity, reinforcing the perception of their own skills, giving them opportunities to express their feelings, recovering and preserving their cultural roots, trying to find new ways of building a fairer society.

THE COMMUNITY PROJECT OF SAN FRANCISCO DE BELLOCQ

To put into practice what we had planned, to be actively involved in the community, we decided to settle in San Francisco de Bellocq. When you are part of the town, it is possible to work on the sanitary and sociocultural issues with a comprehensive and holistic perspective. Given the demographic characteristics of the town, its history, and its inhabitants' lifestyle, it is possible to make interventions on a *human scale* (Max-Neef et al., 2010) (Box 46-1), a factor that fosters face-to-face contact among neighbours, and thus develops each person and the group's potential for a supportive communal life.

In 2013, we went to live in the town and started the Community Project of San Francisco de Bellocq, in a wooded plot of land covering 2.5 acres. With the goal of improving the quality of life of everybody involved and of strengthening the fabric of society, each intervention is transdisciplinary, drawing on occupational therapy, art, communication, and permaculture principles (Box 46-2).

BOX 46-1

DEVELOPMENT ON A HUMAN SCALE

Meeting human needs, providing for autonomy and an organic coordination among people, nature and technology are the fundamental goals of the development on a human scale model. To achieve them, people are required to be the real protagonists favouring the diversity and independence of each area of participation. Transforming the person-object into a person-subject is a question of scale given the difficulty of participating in a huge system hierarchically organized from top to bottom (Max-Neef et al., 2010).

BOX 46-2

PERMACULTURE

This is a design system that seeks to develop self-sufficient perennial human settlements over time. The design is carried out applying a series of principles so that inhabitants meet their basic needs in their own environment without contaminating or depleting it; thus, future generations will be able to live there and a permanent culture will be achieved. It is based on the observation of how natural ecosystems work; it draws on the wisdom of traditional cultures as well as on current scientific knowledge and technology. It is applied to agricultural systems, architecture, economic structures, education, and to the recovery of already established communities.

In this work environment, academic titles become blurred; they are intertwined to be able to meet each task with a perspective that also integrates the multiple components of *popular knowledge*[3]. By discovering that all people are holistic beings, we try to see others in the same way: moving away from specificity and close to multiplicity.

Using and valuing diversity (Holmgren, 2012) is not just a principle the community project employs during its interventions; it is rather a motto that permeates and nourishes it. Applying this perspective to the economic side, this project finds financial aid in various sources: most of the activities are subsidized by the municipal and national governments (which in turn are represented by different political parties). The rest of the activities are financed with funds coming from civil society organizations (such as the local development centre, public library, etc.), with product exchanges and with the work of volunteers. Moreover, most of the interventions encourage long- or medium-term self-sufficiency in order to free ourselves from the ups and downs extraneous to the project. The saying 'don't put all your eggs in one basket' expresses the fact that diversity provides security against the unexpected in nature, governments, markets, and everyday life.

Aimed at different groups and people, the principles of the cooperative workshop (Box 46-3) guide many diverse activities, including: pregnancy and upbringing meetings, workshops to promote respect and equality, a kite day, cinema classes, a mural workshop, or a writing workshop. The interventions to be conducted are based on specific needs that can be observed both because we live in the same community in which we work and because of the feedback we receive as a result of our proposals, which encourage the community's active participation in the demands for change.

Aiming at autonomy as a seed for empowering people, the Community Project of San Francisco de Bellocq fosters their interventions, effectively communicating through collective activities with a view to improving listening and promoting nonviolence[4]. For

---

BOX 46-3
COOPERATIVE WORKSHOPS

According to Janine Vigy (1980), in her book *Organisation Coopérative de la Classe*, the methodology of the Cooperative Workshop aims not at coordinators giving a class, but rather at their making suggestions, and providing means and tools necessary to fulfil the goal of each encounter, making sure everybody participates and is able to listen and find common interests through different channels of communication. This pedagogic method gives the opportunity to learn to organize oneself, to be committed and to become aware of one's own and the group's possibilities and limitations. It is a kind of work that, in the long run, fosters solidarity and confidence, encouraging people to share their ideas, fears, and proposals with their peers and the community.

---

example, every Thursday we hold an Agro-ecological Garden Workshop for sixth-grade children from the local elementary school. They arrive with their school teacher, eagerly awaiting the outdoor activities, so different from the ones they are used to doing in the classroom. We start by greeting one another with a kiss and a hug, we make a circle, and we sing the welcome song. The group thus tunes in, which encourages close contact, caring relations, and a good attitude towards the teamwork we are about to embark on. Once everybody understands the task at hand, each one chooses the activity they like the most: collecting earth, transplanting, harvesting, preparing organic fertilizer, or watering. Each and every person in the group guides the learning process. At the end, we make the circle again to listen to individual experiences. In this closing circle, it becomes immediately apparent how this way of working lets us share the necessary knowledge to produce healthy food, and renewable resources, to develop new knowledges, and, last but not least, foster good human relations.

Using sustainable practices that do not harm the environment, every proposal brought forward by the

---

[3]Popular knowledge is a form of social knowledge one shares as a member of a group or community. It is grounded in observation without the need to check contents. It is acquired through social interaction and is passed down from generation to generation.

[4]Nonviolence (in Sanskrit *ahiṃsā*, nonviolence, 'lack of desire to harm or kill') is the personal practice of being harmless to self and others under every condition. It comes from the belief that hurting people, animals, or the environment is unnecessary to achieve an outcome and refers to a general philosophy of abstention from violence based on moral or spiritual principles.

San Francisco de Bellocq Community Project favours the development of undertakings that generate new income sources for local inhabitants by creating the appropriate environments for gathering. The Clothing Recycling Workshop further illustrates this fact. We needed a sewing machine, and we had the money to buy it as the National Ministry of Education finances the purchase of materials and tools. However, the young girls who took part in this activity decided to manufacture backpacks with recycled fabric, sell them and use the money raised to buy the sewing machine. Together they pulled it off, they learned to organize themselves, and to kick-start a business venture which grew and started functioning independently from the Community Project.

HANDS IN THE MUD

Illustrating a Life-Changing Experience

Every year, when summer arrives, the occupational possibilities move to the beach. A 15-minute drive separates the town from a coastal city where houses overlooking the sea are rented at high prices. Tourists from big cities settle there; they enjoy street shows, cinema projections, theatre plays, games, and sporting events. For a couple of months, the beach town will climb many steps up the occupational justice ladder (see Figure 46-1). Few inhabitants of San Francisco de Bellocq can, or allow themselves to, take advantage of these opportunities in spite of their proximity to the city; some barely manage to go, even on a sunny day, to have a swim in the sea.

It is a scorching hot Wednesday afternoon in San Francisco de Bellocq. In some gardens and backyards, canvas swimming pools help people to cool off for a while and entertain the kids. Many people are taking a nap, waiting for the sunset to bring down the temperature so they can go out on the streets. At 5 PM, in the wooded piece of land where the community project takes place, some laughs and joyful shrieks are heard as people start to arrive. We make a circle of greetings and hugs, and we welcome everybody to the natural building workshop.

Guided by permaculture ethics of earth care and people care (Holmgren, 2012), the initial circle seeks to make sure everyone is at the same distance from the centre; together we build what takes place inside that

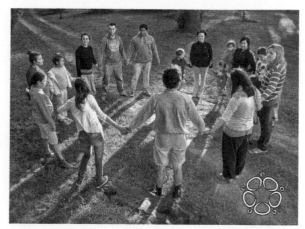

FIGURE 46-2 ■ The circle.

circle (Figure 46-2). The circle lets us build the collective wisdom sharing our knowledge horizontally. From a bird's-eye view, we represent the icon of the design principle No. 8 of Permaculture: 'Integrate rather than segregate' (Holmgren, 2012, p. 293). We are a group of people holding hands; the space in the centre could represent the whole being greater than the sum of the parts that will enable us to obtain big material and spiritual benefits thanks to the different synergic relationships that will develop when coming together in this integrated system.

Leaving aside age and social differences, we are all invited; we take care of each other and we encourage everyone to find their role in the work that gathers us in this circle. The game rules are reprised. Having fun, feeling comfortable, listening and being listened to, focusing on the positive rather than on the negative is allowed. Actions and behaviours which discourage participation are not allowed, for example, lying, aggression, segregating activities according to gender differences, undermining proposals or opinions, or laughing at the person next to us without this person participating in the laughter.

The work starts. In the natural building workshop we are building a sculpture with adobe (an ancient material prepared mixing earth, water, and horse manure). To make it, we find inspiration in the totems from native peoples from all over the world, and in the animals indigenous to our bioregion. We learn to model and build using an eco-friendly technique, the same used by men and women who trod this land many years ago.

We made the design for the totem by drawing on the observation of our environment. Through games and group dynamics, we took our time to experience nature from different perspectives, to interact with it, and to discover the other beings we live with. Learning to observe and then interact fosters a creative, autonomous thinking that enables us to apply suitable solutions to our specific situation. Trusting in our skills of observation and in the sensory interaction will help us to find the best path in our quest for innovative ideas to the everyday problems of the town.

A group of people knead the mud with their bare feet while others bring tools and carry the adobe from the *pisadero*[5] to the monument. Some are already starting to soak more straw in the adobe and to add it into the structure. Little by little, the silhouettes of the animals drawn start to appear and are welcomed with joy. We are discovering that everyone has artistic skills and that you just have to help them wake up with an interesting activity that involves us all emotionally (Figure 46-3).

The totem is erected on the sidewalk of our land. Neighbours who do not participate in the natural building workshop pass by on bikes or cars and try to discover what has drawn the attention of other neighbours who have already gone by and commented in the grocery store that something was happening in this corner of town. We receive many visits during which approval and surprise abound. Those verbal expressions come accompanied with a positive energy that is received and multiplied, nurturing the trust and the self-esteem, encouraging us to work better.

The proposal recovers a regional home-building technique which is very common and accessible to all, but which has been ousted and spurned by the laws of the market. In applying it, we use and value local and renewable resources, making the best use of the abundance of the nature to reduce our dependence on non-renewable resources (Holmgren, 2012). See Box 46-4 for comments by one of the participants.

The work continues at a good pace. Chats and laughter overlap, the mate[6] goes from hand to hand among the participants. Concentrating, a boy sings while he moulds the beak of a hornero[7]. Suddenly, he stops. He seems to have discovered something important. He looks up and suggests: 'What if we build a house?' We all look at him to listen attentively; he then elaborates: 'If we can do a two-meter sculpture all together, we can also build our own houses.' We are overwhelmed by emotion.

With his 12 years and this transformative experience, Juan Cruz managed to be empowered. His hypothesis makes us think how very pertinent it is to combine occupational therapy and permaculture in an artistic activity. Moreover, it represents a true challenge for the next cooperative workshops of the Community Project of San Francisco de Bellocq.

CONCLUSION

Trusting in the potential transformative power inherent to circular spaces of meaningful occupations, the Community Project of San Francisco de Bellocq continues to foster encounters of this kind. Gradually, the community starts to sense that it is not necessary to emigrate to more populated cities to improve their quality of life, because in this small community where the work on a human scale (Max-Neef, et al., 2010) is real, they can generate proposals to meet each person's needs.

Day after day, we walk the streets of our town and we greet every person we see. We are part of these people, of their fabric of society; the community project belongs to the community. As coordinators, the meaningful occupation that keeps us healthy is generating spaces where the circle is formed, where we hold hands and the circle starts to turn around. Whoever comes into the circle must act with

---

[5]Site where you mix sand, clay, water, and some kind of fibrous or organic material (straw or manure) by treading it in with your feet. The result is also used for natural building of houses or for making mudbricks.

[6]Characteristic Argentine infusion, made with the leaves of *yerba mate* (*Ilex paraguariensis*). It is served in a small gourd or wood container and it is drunk hot using a straw called a *bombilla*.

[7]A big inspiration for bio-architects and natural builders, the hornero, or *Furnarius rufus,* is an indigenous bird that builds its nest with a round shape (similar to that of a clay oven), using a very efficient technique and local materials, such as mud and straw.

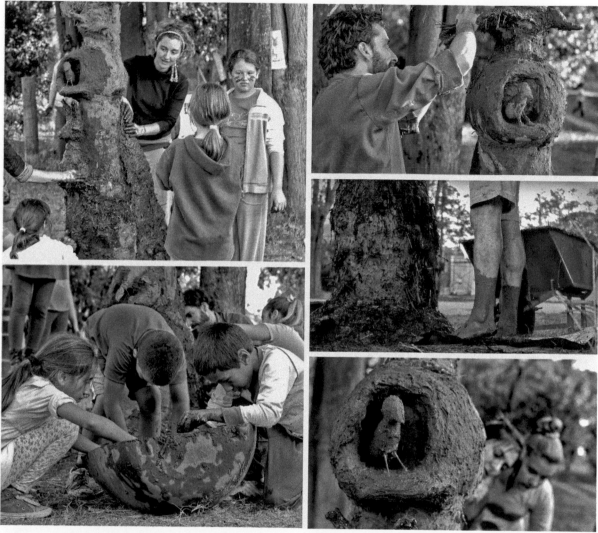

FIGURE 46-3 ■ Building a sculpture with adobe.

BOX 46-4

'We learned the whole process: how to dig a hole to get the earth, how to shake it, mix it with water...a whole lot of things, of live teaching, with living materials, that is different to a class at school. It's satisfying to learn and, in turn, to see how others learn, their faces when they say: "Oh, look at that!" That's when you realize they have learnt it. That's the moment.'

—MARÍA ANGÉLICA, 42 YEARS OLD

commitment, participating actively, looking people in the eye, and establishing healthy social relationships. In each workshop they choose to attend, people enjoy a sense of belonging, their interests and motivations are respected, they find an occupational opportunity that they like and that is in harmony with the environment. Boys and girls, free from prejudices and avid for new experiences, show the highest commitment; they also become the main spokespeople of this new conscience of moving towards change.

In every activity held by the community project, people have become used to hugging and being hugged.

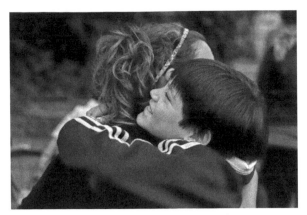

FIGURE 46-4 ■ A hug builds, comforts, and unites.

Bodies have gradually adapted to neighbouring arms. We are surprised and happy to see that this energy transcends a specific intervention and flows into the streets, into the families, into the school, and into the library. Physical contact is not only pleasant; it is necessary for our psychological, emotional, and physical well-being, and it improves the individual and society's health. Hugging is a very special way of coming close that makes you accept yourself better and feel accepted by the rest (Keating, 2000). We do not need

fancy tools to revitalize a community; if we work on a human scale, the length of our arms is enough because the hug builds, comforts, and unites (Figure 46-4).

REFERENCES

Capalbo, L., 2011. Decrecer con equidad: nuevo paradigma civilizatorio. Ciccus, Buenos Aires.

Galheigo, S.M., 2006. Terapia ocupacional en el ámbito social. Aclarando conceptos e ideas. In: Kronenberg, F., Simó Algado, S., Pollard, N. (Eds.), Terapia Ocupacional sin Fronteras: Aprendiendo del Espíritu de Supervivientes. Médica Panamericana, Buenos Aires.

Gil de Jiménez, S.M. (Ed.), 2002. Recuperar la memoria. Tres Arroyos, Argentina.

Holmgren, D., 2012. Permacultura: Principios y Senderos Más Allá de la Sustentabilidad. Kaicron, Buenos Aires.

Keating, K., 2000. Abrázame. El Abrazo es Amor y Alegría. Javier Vergara, Buenos Aires.

Max-Neef, M., Elizalde, A., Hopenhayn, M., 2010. Desarrollo a escala humana. Opciones para el Futuro. Biblioteca CF+S, Madrid.

Pacto Internacional de Derechos Económicos, Sociales y Culturales. 1976. <http://www.ohchr.org/SP/ProfessionalInterest/Pages/CESCR.aspx> (accessed 11.10.14.).

Pousa, J., Pinella, R. (Eds.), 2004. Abandonos. Teina, Tres Arroyos.

Townsend, E., Wilcock, A., 2004. Occupational justice and client-centred practice: a dialogue in progress. Can. J. Occup. Ther. 71 (2), 75–87.

Vigy, J.L., 1980. Organización cooperativa de la clase. Talleres permanentes con niños de 2 a 7 años. Cincel-Kapelusz, Madrid.

47

OCCUPATIONAL JUSTICE AND ADVOCACY: WORKING WITH FORMER REFUGEES AND ASYLUM SEEKERS AT PERSONAL AND COMMUNITY LEVELS

YDA SMITH

■ ■ ■ ■ ■ ■ ■ ■ ■ ■ ■ ■ ■ ■ ■ ■ ■ ■ ■

'Without attention to cultural and systemic barriers, occupational therapists are operating without the tools to provide an environment conducive to healing and personal success' (Smith and Munro, 2008, p. 23).

CHAPTER OUTLINE

This chapter describes an occupation-based fieldwork programme in Salt Lake City, Utah, in the US working with former refugees and asylum seekers. This programme is shaped by concepts in alignment with the participatory occupational justice framework (POJF) developed by Whiteford and Townsend (2011). Issues at an individual level are addressed, but this community-based programme goes beyond the constraints of a person-based, or even family-based, approach. Using the POJF supports the expansion of occupational therapy principles into work that facili-

tates goal achievement of groups of people and communities as well as providing a supportive framework for addressing issues of occupational justice and advocacy for individual human rights (for more information about POJF, refer to Whiteford et al., 2016). The various settings occupational therapy students are assigned to during fieldwork will be described, with examples of how occupational therapy is engaged with individuals, families, groups, and communities. In addition, examples of how occupational therapy has been involved in manoeuvres against unjust treatment as well as in advocacy for policy change will be described.

FORCED MIGRATION AND RESETTLEMENT OF REFUGEES AND ASYLUM SEEKERS

The number of refugees worldwide, according to the United Nations High Commissioner for Refugees (UNHCR), was 16.7 million in 2013 with an additional 1.2 million asylum seekers (UNHCR, 2014). A refugee is defined by the UNHCR (2005) as a person who:

> [O]wing to well-founded fear of being persecuted for reasons of race, religion, nationality or political opinion, is outside the country of his [or her] nationality and is unable or, owing to such fear or for reasons other than personal convenience, is unwilling to avail him [or her]self of the protection of that country. (UNHCR, 2005, p. 5)

Millions of people around the world have been forced to flee their homes due to political unrest and persecution, but only those who have crossed an international border into a second country qualify for UNCHR refugee services. Fewer than 1% are settled in a third country. Of these, more than half come to the US where they are supported by government and community services (Ott, 2011). Asylum seekers also arrive in the US, but in much smaller numbers. These are people who arrived in a foreign country without refugee status. They have been through many of the same experiences as refugees but must find ways to survive without the support of government programmes that provide former refugees with financial and case management support. Refugees and asylum seekers placed in the state of Utah come from a wide range of countries including Somalia, Burma, Bhutan, Afghanistan, and Iraq. Approximately 1000 refugees arrive in Utah each year (United States Office of Refugee Resettlement, 2013).

According to the US Office of Refugee Resettlement (2013), 58 238 refugees were settled in the US in 2012. They have often witnessed the death of loved ones, may have been subjected to torture, and most have endured the confinement and harsh conditions of refugee camps for years, sometimes decades. While confined to these camps, they experience occupational deprivation, a form of occupational injustice (Townsend and Wilcock, 2004). Occupational depri-

vation is 'the result of individuals being denied the opportunity and resources to participate in occupations' (Wolf et al., 2010, p. 15).

When powers outside of the individual limit a person's ability to participate in activities and occupations that are important and meaningful, the person is forced into a condition of occupational deprivation. Refugee camps are a dramatic example of a context in which this occurs. Refugees are cut off from their former livelihoods. Family and community networks are disrupted. Roles are altered, and new routines have to be established. Education and healthcare are limited, and employment is most often not available or not even permitted. When individuals are given an opportunity to work to support their most basic needs, they may still suffer from a state of occupational deprivation (Townsend and Wilcock, 2004).

COMMON PROBLEMS FACED DURING RESETTLEMENT

The transition to life in a host country is challenging at best and often overwhelming. People from refugee backgrounds, in particular women and the elderly, may become isolated in their homes, unable to navigate their community and unable to participate in familiar and meaningful occupations. Language barriers restrict their abilities to interact with others and often deny access to education and employment (Haines, 2010; Mitchell, 2009; Mitschke et al., 2011). In some cases, people arriving with refugee status are highly educated, having had professional careers in their home countries, and are frustrated with their inability to practise in these professions because their diplomas and credentials are not validated in the US (Rabben, 2013). Occupational restrictions and occupational deprivation are commonplace even among former professionals who were employed in urban environments (McAllister et al., 2010; Whiteford, 2000). Adaptation to a new culture and environment can be extraordinarily stressful, often resulting in further traumatization (Haines, 2010; Mitchell, 2009).

A reduction in stressors during this transition can be facilitated through work from an occupational perspective in very practical ways. Life skills training can assist with the adjustment process through targeted person-centred, occupation-based life skills training with individuals and groups (Suleman and Whiteford, 2013).

THE PARTICIPATORY OCCUPATIONAL JUSTICE FRAMEWORK WITHIN A REFUGEE RESETTLEMENT CONTEXT

The participatory occupational justice framework (POJF) has a focus on occupational justice and concerns for positive or negative engagement in everyday life, or everyday occupations, of individuals, families, groups, communities, organizations, and populations (Whiteford and Townsend, 2011). Use of the framework has been helpful in programming as it generates an expansive view of how to address health-promoting participation in occupations moving within and beyond the historical and usual parameters of occupational therapy services. For example, Article III, one of the six key features of POJF, states, 'Occupational therapy objectives ideally address the means and ends of social inclusion for the people whom they work with who are, or may be at risk of becoming, marginalized, disadvantaged or oppressed' (Whiteford et al., 2016; see Chapter 18, p. 167).

The remainder of this chapter will describe the University of Utah Division of Occupational Therapy Immigration and Refugee Resettlement Fieldwork Program, the community sites where programming takes place, and some of the projects facilitated by students in these settings, in alignment with, and further inspired by, the principles of POJF.

THE FIELDWORK SETTING

The Immigration and Refugee Resettlement Fieldwork Program was established in 2004. It began with the idea that the fundamental skills of the occupational therapy profession would be beneficial for those entering the US with refugee or asylum seeker status. There are abundant barriers for this population that impact participation in everyday life simply due to unfamiliarity with US home and community environments, institutional systems, and cultural expectations. The programme is designed to address the multiple barriers former refugees and asylum seekers face on a daily basis and to recognize their strengths and capacity for rebuilding their lives (Smith et al., 2013). The value of occupational therapy has been demonstrated within several community settings, and agency personnel at fieldwork sites have developed a strong appreciation for occupational therapy after seeing how their clients benefit from occupational therapy services.

University of Utah students, as well as students from schools in other parts of the US, participate in this programme, with supervision provided by an occupational therapist employed by the University of Utah. Programming is developed and implemented in collaboration with culturally diverse populations living in the local community and community organizations, including University Neighborhood Partners-Hartland Partnership (UNP-Hartland), the International Rescue Committee, and Utah Health and Human Rights Project (UHHR).

University Neighborhood Partners-Hartland Partnership

Located on the west side of Salt Lake City, UNP-Hartland provides a home base for the occupational therapy fieldwork programme. The mission of UNP-Hartland is 'bringing together University and west side resources in reciprocal learning, action, and benefit' (University Neighborhood Partners, n.d.).

In 2004, the University of Utah Division of Occupational Therapy began to offer student fieldwork opportunities in collaboration with UNP-Hartland within the grounds of the Hartland Apartments. This large apartment complex has long been home to people with refugee backgrounds, who have been trying to build a new life. They often struggle with everyday life skills within and outside their homes and face tremendous obstacles in access to higher education and employment opportunities. With the location of the centre within their apartment complex, transportation to necessary services was easy and referrals to additional community resources could be provided. The centre also created a sense of community where residents come together and share their stories and advice. UNP-Hartland is a collaborative setting where students from social work, occupational therapy, nursing, and other disciplines work together with residents and local nonprofit organizations to provide programming and opportunities identified as needed by the residents. Occupational therapy life skills programming fits well with the UNP-Hartland mission as it was designed to be collaborative with those partici-pating in services involved in all aspects of goal-setting and prioritizing of activities. Occupational therapy students began to offer classes and individual sessions with content focused on everyday activities such as money management, home maintenance, use of public transportation, and computer skills. The first class offered was predriving, a class designed to help people learn the rules of the road and prepare for successful completion of the written Utah state driver's license examination.

In 2007, events occurred at the Hartland Apart-ments and the Hartland Partnership Center that provide an example of how occupational therapists can work with communities to contest social and occupational injustices. Staff employed by a new apart-ment management company informed a great many families that they would not be able to renew their annual apartment leases. Home maintenance and cleanliness were the most common reasons cited when explaining to residents they would have to leave. This event was a tremendous problem for a large number of families who did not have the resources to move to another apartment. Families had no sense of how to defend themselves against what appeared to be dis-criminatory practices and became desperate for ideas on how to avoid becoming homeless.

With UNP-Hartland located within the apartment complex, the opportunity arose for staff at the centre to begin conversations with management regarding how to appropriately deal with this situation. If the claim against a family involved issues of cleanliness, management was asked to allow the occupational therapy students time to train families in home main-tenance. Management staff were put to the task of defending their claims against particular families. Accusations were often made that seemed to have more to do with cultural norms than anything else. On more than one occasion there were accusations of home cleanliness deficits when, in fact, the 'problem' was the scent of cooking spices that were unfamiliar to Western noses (Smith and Munro, 2008).

Occupational therapy students contributed to this project by helping residents learn how to clean their apartments to meet the standards of apartment complex management. Working on home mainte-nance also opened up opportunities to provide educa-tion on apartment leases, resident rights, and how to communicate with the apartment manager when home repairs were needed.

Due to the involvement of Hartland Center person-nel and occupational therapy students, management often felt obligated to give residents extra time to learn home cleaning techniques with a follow-up inspection a month later. This allowed several families the oppor-tunity to stay in their apartments for a longer period of time. In some cases management claimed that damage had been done to the apartment. Occupa-tional therapists were in a position to check on this damage and if none existed, they guided families through the process of reporting this back to manage-ment. A greater level of cleanliness was required in some homes to avoid cockroach infestation, but in many cases the accusations of damage could not be substantiated.

Negotiations and open communication required management to become accountable for their claims and to reconsider lease renewals. In the end, the major-ity of families were forced to move, but at the very least, the process delayed eviction, providing sufficient time for families to relocate. Not one of these families became homeless because of this incident. After resi-dents relocated, occupational therapy students were available to provide training in public transportation so they could return to access the centre as well as access other community resources. They also helped residents learn to create résumés and fill out job appli-cations in order to increase incomes to a level that would cover additional rental fees.

The Hartland Partnership provided a space for families to turn to when they were desperate for help and gave them a voice in the public sphere. Rosemarie Hunter, Director of University Neighborhood Part-ners, reflected back on this incident:

[W]e always thought it was a great thing that occupational therapy was doing [public transportation training] but we didn't understand the power of it in terms of self-empowerment of people until [the evictions] happened and we saw them take the power in their own hands to get on the bus because they knew how to do that and come back to the classes here. (Smet, 2014, p. 65)

During the housing crisis, occupational therapy training was focused on the basic life skill of home maintenance, but this was taking place within a context of power dynamics. As mediators between cultural systems and advocates for members of marginalized groups of people, occupational therapists can do more than just teach people how to clean their homes. They can support them emotionally, sharing in their frustrations. They can speak with management with the resident present, providing a model of self-advocacy, defending their rights as tenants. Often, just having a white, middle-class, English-speaking adult advocating for a particular resident puts management on alert that someone who knows the system is aware of what they are doing. Renters are frequently taken advantage of by landlords who are well aware of the fact that tenants with refugee backgrounds are, most often, not able to read the lengthy rental contracts and do not have experience with renting an apartment. They become easy targets for abuse including unwarranted evictions, unreasonable fines, and loss of housing deposits when they move. Teaching residents about their rights as tenants and demonstrating for them how to advocate for themselves can help those new to the country learn to take action to protect themselves from these abuses and 'raise consciousness in others of occupational injustice' (Whiteford et al., 2016; see Chapter 18, p. 168).

As illustrated above, there was great benefit to embedding occupational therapy services within the context of a particular community event where tenants were being treated unfairly and without compassion by an apartment management system that was primarily interested in its own financial profits. Involvement of the Hartland Partnership, including occupational therapy, resulted in more favourable outcomes and created learning opportunities for residents to understand their rights and to recognize that they are not entirely powerless against such institutions.

Situations like this demonstrate the need for broader responsibility in the field of occupational therapy and highlight how limited the usual scope of occupational therapy is. Tremendous opportunities exist for occupational therapists to address the societal barriers that limit occupational performance. It is necessary for the profession to train students to recognize societal forces that create and perpetuate systemic inequalities.

Certainly, within the US, medical systems employing occupational therapists do not view this as a reimbursable role. Much is lost in fostering independence and full participation by not addressing these barriers. By pushing the occupational therapy profession in this direction, healthier communities can be fostered with improved quality of life for those who have been traditionally marginalized by dominant social groups.

Work at the Individual and Family Levels With International Rescue Committee and Utah Health and Human Rights Project

The Immigration and Resettlement Fieldwork Program works with two agencies that focus on individual and family case management for those who arrived in the area with refugee status or are asylum seekers. These agencies are the International Rescue Committee and UHHR.

The International Rescue Committee is a federally funded refugee resettlement agency that provides services for newly arrived refugees during their first 2 years in Salt Lake City. Other than a weekly predriving class, occupational therapy students work in the community with individuals. Occupational therapy sessions begin with an informal interview, asking questions about the person's daily life and priorities in what they would like to learn and access. Individual sessions are structured to address these expressed interests and needs. Often people wish to have more mobility within the community and would like to learn about public transportation. They also want to know how to grocery shop, pay their bills, and take care of their homes. Frequently, occupational therapy students are asked to help with medication management and other concerns related to health issues such as diabetes, cognitive impairments due to head injuries, or physical disabilities. As Whiteford and Townsend (2011) have stated, 'Concerns about occupational injustice start with a focus on everyday life' (p. 67) as individuals strive to gain personal skills and to engage with family, friends, and members of their communities. Occupational therapy, in this setting, addresses occupational justice at the individual level by enabling individuals to function effectively and safely within new environmental contexts.

UHHR has provided occupational therapy students with additional learning opportunities. UHHR offers mental health services and case management for refugees and asylum seekers who are survivors of torture. The most common diagnoses include post-traumatic stress disorder, major depressive disorder, and generalized anxiety disorder. The same training mentioned above may be provided, but therapy may also focus on mental health specifically. This generally involves facilitating engagement in meaningful occupations within the home or community that are enjoyable, decrease stress, improve sleep, and are designed to decrease pervasive, disturbing thoughts and memories. Staff at UHHR also request cognitive assessments, in particular memory assessments, due to the high incidence of mild-to-moderate brain trauma caused by injuries sustained during imprisonment or torture experiences in home countries. Therapists at UHHR report that these assessments are helpful in their treatment planning and are used to support requests for disability funding and citizenship examination waivers.

In addition to working with individuals, occupational therapists work with families. In one case students worked on relationship building with a mother and her children. This mother was suffering from severe posttraumatic stress disorder and depression. She rarely interacted with her young children and they seemed to pay little attention to her. Games were brought into the home and with the mother sitting on the couch, rather than lying in bed. They worked on integrating her into playtime with her children with the husband present so he could observe ways he could encourage these interactions without the occupational therapy students present.

The sections above provided examples of work with individuals, families, and a residential community. The following sections provide examples of enabling with both groups and organizations.

THE KAREN WEAVERS

The first principle outlined by the World Federation of Occupational Therapists in its position statement on human rights is that 'people have the right to participate in a range of occupations that enable them to flourish, fulfil their potential and experience satisfaction in a way consistent with their culture and beliefs' (World Federation of Occupational Therapists, 2010 p. 1). With this general concept in mind, a weaving programme was initiated in 2008 to support the desire

of Karen women in Salt Lake City to continue their traditional practice of backstrap weaving. The Karen are an ethnic group in Burma whose people have been brutally attacked by the Burmese military government for decades. Thousands have been forced to flee their homes to seek refuge in Thailand. Many have been relocated from there to other countries including the US (UNHCR, 2010).

Several Karen women were living in the Hartland Apartments in 2008 and were asked if they were weavers. They responded that they did weave but were unable to access the necessary tools and supplies. Over the course of the next year, with support from UNP-Hartland Partnership, occupational therapy students researched and located appropriate materials and the Karen weaving group began. As the group developed, it became apparent that backstrap weaving is a fundamental aspect of identity construction for many Karen women and can impact mental health status. They take pride in their skill and see their work as representative of their Karen culture. Karen women have expressed the importance of wearing Karen clothing and the need to pass this skill on to the next generation. As one woman said, 'If you are Karen, people sometimes they will come talk to you. "You are Karen people? Do you have a culture? Show me about your culture." We need to show that because we are Karen people' (Stephenson et al., 2013, p. 228).

In working with the Karen women it has been apparent that there is a role for occupational therapy in assisting groups to achieve goals that support the group's mission as well as its individual members. From the very beginning, the Karen weavers made it clear they wanted to work in a communal style rather than developing as individual entrepreneurs. Education has been provided on how to market their products, purchase needed supplies, maintain a website, and on financial management. It has been of vital importance to support the women in their preferred management style 'rather than attempting to set goals that standardize and universalize what everyone does in life or in a service context' (Whiteford and Townsend, 2011, pp. 71–72). By not pushing the women towards conforming to American cultural standards and supporting their control of the decision-making process, opportunities for Americans to learn about alternative organizational systems have been created.

SYSTEM CHANGE AFFECTING COMMUNITIES

Many Karen maintained gardens while living in refugee camps or foraged for vegetables in areas near the camps. At the Hartland Center, a group of Karen were shown photographs of plants that had been growing in a large garden at the Mae La Refugee Camp in Thailand. At that time, they spoke little English so the photographs were critical in helping to understand what plants they wanted to grow. They showed a great deal of enthusiasm for some plants and no interest in others. A plant they were particularly interested in was *Ipomoea aquatica*, also known as *phak bung* in Thai and water spinach in English. *I. aquatica* is considered an invasive species in the US and can cause significant issues in areas of the US where temperatures remain relatively warm in the winter. There are a few states where permits have been issued for legal planting and harvesting, but Utah was not one of them. *I. aquatica* is a very popular Asian leafy vegetable and is a great source of vitamins A and C. Being able to grow and purchase this familiar food could help the Karen feel more comfortable in their new environment as well as provide them with a nutritious key ingredient for many of their meals.

Evidence was located on the nature of *I. aquatica* and the impact of the local environment on its ability to proliferate. The state agency in charge of regulation of plants grown in Utah was contacted and provided with documents showing that it would be safe to grow *I. aquatica* as long as the seeds did not leave the state. By making the correct contacts and supplying evidence in support of the request to allow seeds into the state, permission was eventually granted. It is now legal to grow *I. aquatica* in Utah, if grown in a greenhouse and managed appropriately. In the meantime, occupational therapy supported the Karen community in gaining access to a community garden space and worked with members of the community in getting the gardens started. Several Karen families are now able to grow fresh food and are now gardening annually without occupational therapy support. Efforts are still under way to access a greenhouse in order to grow *I. aquatica* locally. Addressing state laws that limit occupational engagement in this way fits with Article VI of POJF which states, 'Occupational therapists

strive to work with others in pursuit of the ideal of occupational justice irrespective of attendant political and economic challenges and current environmental limitations. Hope, and a vision of possibility, underpins their efforts' (Whiteford et al., 2016; see Chapter 18, p. 167). Working with the Karen community in this way, advocating for issues that are important to them, demonstrates that occupational therapy can make significant contributions to policy changes that impact occupations and quality of life.

SYSTEM CHANGE WITHIN THE OCCUPATIONAL THERAPY PROFESSION

The fundamental principles of occupational therapy have tremendous potential for enhancing services in a wide range of settings where occupational therapists are not employed at this time. Occupational therapists can play a role in advocating for change within systems to include occupational therapy services in new practice arenas. Advocacy for expansion of occupational therapy to environments outside of healthcare facilities often requires volunteer work and a long-term commitment to personal involvement with staff and administrators in a particular setting. The University of Utah Immigration and Resettlement Fieldwork Program has been an effective tool for change within the local refugee resettlement community. Staff at local agencies have seen how their clients have benefitted from occupational therapy services and how valuable an occupational therapy perspective can be in their work setting. It has taken many years of involvement, but the agencies the programme has been involved with increase their referrals every year and some are looking for ways to fund occupational therapy services. It is hoped that continued advocacy for occupational therapy services with refugee populations will lead to a positive change in the standard of service provision for this population.

CONCLUSIONS

Working with newly arrived residents with refugee backgrounds has provided ample opportunity to see how a shift towards work with advocacy and justice in mind can benefit and empower the people occupational therapists interact with in their professional settings. In addition, experiences doing this work have demonstrated the powerful role occupational therapy can play engaging with groups and communities.

Townsend and Marval (2013) ask if occupational justice can be enabled by occupational therapists. This chapter provides several examples of how occupational therapists can address everyday injustices people living in our communities face. Occupational therapy practitioners need to understand how institutional barriers and power relationships play out in the lives of the people they work with and how these barriers can negatively impact health and participation in home and community life. This knowledge supports therapists in their efforts to help the people they work with push against the constraints created by societal power dynamics, leading towards greater opportunities for successful community integration.

REFERENCES

Haines, D.W., 2010. Safe haven: a history of refugees in America. Kumarian, Sterling, VA.

McAllister, L., Penn, C., Smith, Y., Van Dort, S., Wilson, L., 2010. Fieldwork education in non-traditional settings or with non-traditional caseloads. In: McAllister, L., Paterson, M., Higgs, J., Bithell, C. (Eds.), Innovations in Allied Health Fieldwork Education: A Critical Appraisal. Sense, Rotterdam, the Netherlands, pp. 39–47.

Mitchell, A., 2009. Reflections on working with South Sudanese refugees in settlement and capacity building in regional Australia. In: Pollard, N., Sakellariou, D., Kronenberg, F. (Eds.), A Political Practice of Occupational Therapy. Elsevier, London, pp. 197–205.

Mitschke, D.B., Mitschke, A.E., Slater, H.M., Teboh, C., 2011. Uncovering health and wellness needs of recently resettled Karen refugees from Burma. J. Human Behav. Soc. Environment 21, 490–501.

Ott, E., 2011. Get up and go: refugee resettlement and secondary migration in the USA. United Nations High Commissioner for Refugees, Geneva. Available from: <http://www.unhcr.org/cgi-bin/texis/vtx/home/opendocPDFViewer.html?docid=4e5f9a079&query=refugeeadmissions> (accessed 27.05.15.).

Rabben, L., 2013. Credential recognition in the United States for foreign born professionals. Migration Policy Institute, Washington, DC.

Smet, N., 2014. Advocating the role of occupational therapists with immigrants and refugees. University of Toledo, OTD. Toledo, OH.

Smith, Y., Munro, S., 2008. Anthropology and occupational therapy in community-based practice. Pract. Anthropol. 30 (3), 20–23.

Smith, Y.J., Cornella, E., Williams, N., 2013. Working with populations from a refugee background: an opportunity to enhance the occupational therapy educational experience. Aust. Occup. Ther. J. 61 (1), 20–27.

Stephenson, S.M., Smith, Y.J., Gibson, M., Watson, V., 2013. Traditional weaving as an occupation of Karen refugee women. J. Occup. Sci. 20 (3), 224–235.

Suleman, A., Whiteford, G., 2013. Understanding occupational transitions in forced migration: the importance of life skills in early refugee resettlement. J. Occup. Sci. 20 (2), 201–210.

Townsend, E., Marval, R., 2013. Can professionals actually enable occupational justice? Cadernos de Terapia Ocupacional da Ufscar 21 (2), 215–228.

Townsend, E., Wilcock, A.A., 2004. Occupational justice and client-centered practice: a dialogue in progress. Can. J. Occup. Ther. 71 (2), 75–87.

United Nations High Commissioner for Refugees, 2005. Self-study module 2: refugee status determination. Identifying who is a refugee. UNHCR, Geneva. Available from: <http://www.unhcr.org/cgibin/texis/vtx/home/opendocPDFViewer.html?docid=43144dc52&query=refugee%20definition> (accessed 10.11.14.).

United Nations High Commissioner for Refugees, 2010. UNHCR helps thousands of Karens fleeing fighting in Myanmar. UNHCR, Geneva. Available from: <http://www.unhcr.org/4cd94a076.html> (accessed 11.11.14.).

United Nations High Commissioner for Refugees, 2014. War's human cost: UNHCR 2013 global trends. UNHCR, Geneva. Available from: <http://reliefweb.int/report/world/unhcr-global-trends-2013-wars-human-cost> (accessed 10.11.14.).

United States Office of Refugee Resettlement, 2013. Fiscal year 2012 refugee arrivals. UNHCR, Geneva. Available from: <http://www.acf.hhs.gov/programs/orr/resource/fiscal-year-2012-refugee-arrivals> (accessed 10.11.14.).

University Neighborhood Partners, n.d. <http://partners.utah.edu/home/> (accessed 12.11.14.).

Whiteford, G., 2000. Occupational deprivation: global challenge in the new millennium. Br. J. Occup. Ther. 63, 200–204.

Whiteford, G., Townsend, E., 2011. Participatory occupational justice framework (POJF 2010): enabling occupational participation and inclusion. In: Kronenberg, F., Pollard, N., Sakellariou, D. (Eds.), Occupational Therapies without Borders, vol. 2. Towards an Ecology of Occupation-Based Practices. Elsevier, New York, pp. 65–92.

Whiteford, G., Townsend, E., Bryanton, O., Wicks, A., Pereira, R., 2016. The participatory occupational justice framework: salience across contexts. In: Sakellariou, D., Pollard, N. (Eds.), Occupational Therapies without Borders: Integrating Justice with Practice, second ed. Elsevier, London.

Wolf, L., Ripat, J., Davis, E., Becker, P., MacSwiggan, J., 2010. Applying an occupational justice framework. Occup. Ther. Now, 15–18.

World Federation of Occupational Therapists, 2010. Human rights position paper. <http://www.wfot.org/wfot2010/docs/WI_04_Elizabeth%20Townsend.pdf> (accessed 10.11.14.).

48

OCCUPATIONAL THERAPY IN CHILE: AN EXPERIENCE AGAINST OCCUPATIONAL INJUSTICE OF MOTHERS WITH INTELLECTUAL DISABILITIES

CONSTANZA DEHAYS PINOCHET ■
MELISSA HICHINS ARISMENDI ■ VANESSA VIDAL CASTILLO ■
CRISTIAN ARANDA FARÍAS ■ WILSON VERDUGO HUENUMÁN ■
ANDREA YUPANQUI CONCHA

CHAPTER OUTLINE

Love, tolerance, brotherhood, and respect are values that have mobilized occupational therapy since its beginning. Promoting social change, working to overcome inequalities and poverty, as well as overcoming differences between social classes are social responsibilities to society that occupational therapy has had from its beginning. Occupation, that is, participation in society, is considered to be a human right, and there are specific roles and responsibilities for occupational therapists in situations where the right to occupation is threatened (World Federation of Occupational Therapists, 2006).

In the south of Latin America, occupational therapy has strongly assumed the defence of human rights,

under the influence of the social and political history that has marked our countries (Galheigo, 2011; Salazar, 2010), exemplified through situations of extreme violence and rights violations (dictatorships, bad distribution of resources, social segregation). In this context, occupational therapy has had its part in the political and social reconstruction of our countries leading to more just, inclusive, and supportive societies. Occupational therapists are still working with the persistent aftermath of the heritage of historic rights violations, related to discrimination, racism, and social inequality. These violations become evident through unequal access to education, health, housing, and commodities in much of the population, particularly for social minorities. In Chile, these important attitudinal and physical barriers that threaten the safety, survival, and health of people have negatively affected many people by limiting their participation in meaningful occupations, leading to occupational injustice. This concept is defined as injustice that occurs when 'participation in occupations is barred, confined, restricted, segregated, prohibited, undeveloped, disrupted, alienated, marginalized, exploited, excluded or otherwise restricted' (Townsend and Wilcock, 2004, p. 77).

Historically, Chile has recognized people with disabilities as receivers of charity and assistance. This has been driven strongly for the last 40 years through television campaigns, focused on collecting money to support rehabilitation centres in the country. This has helped to develop a general vision amongst Chileans of people with disabilities as 'other dependent beings, not as subjects of rights' (United Nations (UN), 2012, p. 6). Against this context, occupational therapy has worked hard to encourage the transition from a negative perception of people with disabilities as victims to an approach of dignity and empowerment, focusing on human rights.

The aim of this chapter is to highlight the experiences of women with intellectual disabilities[1] as they try to defend their fundamental rights in this society on a daily basis. In this chapter, we discuss how a team of occupational therapists support these women in their need to fulfil their role as mothers, despite the many barriers that society daily imposes on them.

MAKING IT VISIBLE: WOMEN WITH DISABILITIES AND THEIR EXPERIENCES OF HUMAN RIGHTS VIOLATIONS

Disability is a multidimensional phenomenon, reflecting the negative aspects of the interaction between people with a health problem and the characteristics of the society in which they live, such as lack of social support (Worth Health Organization, 2001). Therein lies the common obstacle to all people with disabilities worldwide, which particularly affects women with disabilities: discrimination and exclusion from society, which in turn increases their vulnerability to violence, abuse, and exploitation (Worth Health Organization/World Bank, 2011). Their greatest risk of violence is directly related to 'factors that increase their dependence on others, these make them vulnerable and deprived them of their rights', as stated by UN Women (2012, p. 6).

Gender and disability are often combined with violence. The sexual and reproductive rights of disabled women have been historically violated worldwide, forcing them to mass sterilization (Peláez et al., 2009; UN, 2012; Women with Disabilities Australia, 2011), forced abortions, and the involuntary surrender of their children for adoption (Llewellyn, 2010).

Women with intellectual disabilities, particularly mothers, are exposed to situations of daily violence linked to the perception society has towards them, considering them as people without skills, unintelligent, submissive, and timid. Consequently, these women are not regarded as credible when they report abuses (UN Women, 2012). There is a prevalence of myths and stereotypes about these mothers and their sexual and reproductive rights, suggesting that their desire to be mothers is unacceptable and unrealistic and that their behaviours are harmful to their children (Sheerin et al., 2013).

Sexual expression is a basic right of every individual irrespective of medical condition and is an inherent part of the human experience (Sakellariou and Simó Algado, 2006). In Chile, recognition and guarantees for women with disabilities are still in the process of development; evidence of this is the lack of national statistics on the relationship between gender, disability, and violence. The country also has no statistics on mothers with intellectual disabilities, which also hinders their social visibility and ability to generate national intervention strategies. At the moment (October 2015) it is not part of local collective knowledge that sexual rights are fundamental human rights (see Box 48-1), which disproportionately affects this most vulnerable population. However,

[1]Intellectual disability is a diagnosis characterized by impairments of general mental abilities that impact adaptive functioning in conceptual, social, and practical areas. The symptoms begin during the developmental period and are diagnosed based on the severity of deficits in adaptive functioning (American Psychiatric Association, 2013). The term *intellectual disabilities* is equivalent to what is commonly called *learning disabilities* in the UK or *learning difficulties* in the US.

BOX 48-1

What are sexual and reproductive rights? Sexual rights embrace human rights that are already recognized in national laws, international human rights documents and other consensus statements. They include the right of all persons, free of coercion, discrimination, and violence, to:

1. Have access to the highest attainable standard of sexual health treatments including access to sexual and reproductive healthcare services;
2. Seek, receive and impart information related to sexuality;
3. Sexuality education;
4. Respect for bodily integrity;
5. Choose their partner;
6. Choose to be sexually active or not;
7. Consensual sexual relations;
8. Consensual marriage;
9. Decide whether or not, and when, to have children; and
10. Pursue a satisfying, safe and pleasurable sexual life.

Source: *Reprinted with permission from World Health Organization, 2006. Defining sexual health. Report of a technical consultation on sexual health. WHO, Geneva, p. 5.*

various movements and groups have been commissioned to denounce the violence and discrimination that seriously affect women and girls with disabilities, a violation of human rights that remains invisible in Chilean society (Benavides, 2014).

INFRINGEMENT OF SEXUAL AND REPRODUCTIVE RIGHTS OF MOTHERS WITH INTELLECTUAL DISABILITIES

The concept of intellectual disabilities focuses on the individual characteristics of each person and their close relationship with the demands of the environment, along with the support they need to perform their activities optimally (Verdugo and Schalock, 2010). The violence that affects mothers with intellectual disabilities has to do with the limited social participation that the environment affords them, which undermines the exercise of their basic human

rights and generates situations of occupational injustice.

From the inception of the occupational therapy department at the University of Magallanes in 2003, disabilities and respect for basic human rights of people in the region have been the main motivation and focus of its activities. In 2011, a groundbreaking study at regional and national levels on gender, disability, and violence was carried out there[2]. The recognition given to this study by local and national institutions focused the attention of Chilean parliamentarians on this social problem and gave it visibility for the first time in Chile.

This work demonstrated the existence of acts of repeated and systematic violation of human rights of women with intellectual disabilities (Dehays et al., 2012, p. 17). It showed that the local situation is similar to the international findings (Blacher and Baker, 2002; Llewellyn, 2010; Peláez et al., 2009; Sheerin et al., 2013; UN, 2012; Women with Disabilities Australia, 2011), and mothers with intellectual disabilities experience a social invisibility and discrimination because of their disability and motherhood. As a consequence, they are victims of triple discrimination and occupational injustice.

After identifying the issues affecting women with intellectual disabilities in the region, a research team was established in the occupational therapy programme at the University of Magallanes to look for research-based solutions. The team was composed mainly of occupational therapists with the support of other professionals, with the participation of occupational therapy students. Based on evidence from

---

[2]This first regional work has been rewarded and recognized by various bodies, such as:

- First place in the national contest 'Count Your Thesis in Human Rights', the Human Rights Institute of Chile.
- Third place in the national contest 'Abstracts: Gender Dissertation', the National Women's Service of the Government of Chile.
- First Regional Congress in Scientific Initiation for Professionals and Students from the University of Magallanes.
- Regional Distinction of the Chamber of Deputies of the Chilean Government.
- Regional Recognition of the Inclusive Higher Education Network of Magallanes.

numerous studies (e.g., Blacher and Baker, 2002; Díaz, 2013; Llewellyn, 2013; Peláez et al., 2009; Verdugo et al., 2002), this team started a programme based on sexual and reproductive rights education for women with intellectual disabilities. The programme offered support in access to services, information, and intervention tailored to the national, geographic, cultural, and contextual characteristics and needs of these women.

THE PROGRAMME

The first stage of the programme focused on securing funding. Financial support was granted by the Regional Government of Magallanes in partnership with the University of Magallanes. Connections were also developed with regional and national networks working in this area in order to educate and raise awareness of human rights neglects in this population of women. The programme had two main areas, which are described below.

Area 1: Education on Sexual and Reproductive Rights for Young Women With Intellectual Disabilities and Their Families

The programme focused on the prevention of violence and promotion of sexual and reproductive health. The programme was offered in three local institutions serving young people with disabilities. In order to empower young people and their families, the programme generated educational examples that emphasized basic knowledge in social and emotional skills, self-care, sexual and reproductive health education, and the prevention of violence and sexual abuse. At the same time, an annual community educational activity was created, called the 'Women, Disability and Violence' seminar, which aimed to develop education and community awareness and offer training for future professionals and regional organizations working in this area. These activities take place in the University of Magallanes.

Area 2: Support for Mothers With Intellectual Disabilities

The activities aimed at supporting motherhood (both before and after birth) in women with intellectual disabilities were implemented in two stages. During the prenatal stage, the main objective was to strengthen the mothers' role in order to validate their rights and also to encourage family support. In this regard, we worked on the following areas:

1. Structuring routines and habits related to self-care activities, such as respecting meal times; promotion of healthy eating; maintaining hygiene and personal care; care and vigilance during leisure; and observing sleep times.
2. Organization of weekly routines in activities of daily life, regarding health checks (ultrasound and other prenatal care procedures); the acquisition and administration of drugs and new responsibilities; strategies for requesting external support; support networks to accompany them in health checks as well as coordination with teams of professionals and referral to various community networks.
3. Education on sexual and reproductive rights by providing educational and adapted information; strengthening the aspects of self-concept and self-image, together with the recognition and acceptance of body changes as a natural process of pregnancy.
4. Adaptation of the physical environment to decrease the risk factors of accidents at home.
5. Education and childbirth, recognizing the stages of labour (the time between contractions as an indication of different stages), and the types of labour and birth; guided visits to the hospital to familiarize themselves with the physical location of the process and to ask about the process.
6. Tailored education on prenatal care through various techniques, for example, through the use of a weekly diary on prenatal exercises, or the use of music and aromatic oils, to establish communication with and attachment to the unborn baby. In addition, education about the importance of a healthy lifestyle during pregnancy, recognizing the baby's movements in the womb in the ultrasound images.

In the postnatal period, activities focused on strengthening the skills related to the role of mother in order to validate the women's basic human rights, foster family support, and promote the optimal psychomotor development of the baby. The activities at this stage focused on:

1. Structuring routines and habits linked to motherhood, including techniques for breast-feeding; food preparation and proper management; and diapering; dressing and bathing the baby.
2. Adaptation activities and physical spaces at home through the use of educational materials with images for better understanding by the mother; development and adaptation by creating sequential notebooks showing daily tasks pertaining to motherhood, such as diapering, through images that mothers could follow to familiarize themselves with the appropriate steps for each task and any necessary materials.
3. Education on healthy habits (including eating habits) and promoting respect for the sleep of mother and baby.
4. Education to decrease risk factors for accidents in the home, such as preventing falls; education regarding the importance of the baby having its own space and sleeping in its crib rather than in the same bed with its mother; or positioning the bathtub securely, for example, on a table instead of in the shower.
5. Education for comprehensive early psychomotor development of the baby through specific weekly exercises, building support through use of an activities guide; this guide contained psychomotor stimulation activities through the use of playing techniques, primarily with toys or readily available household objects.
6. Promoting the membership of mothers and children at health centres so that they can qualify for all the available benefits which are often unknown to these women and their families; to observe required health checks, and also to have access to the managed network of support for women in cases of necessity or emergency.
7. Education on sexual and reproductive rights, providing information in an accessible format, especially on the importance of postnatal maternal care, control of fertility and the identification of situations of violence against women.

Programme Results

Area 1: Education on Sexual and Reproductive Rights for Young People With Intellectual Disabilities and Their Families

Before the beginning of the programme, the participating women were characterized by their experiences of a disregard of their human rights and, in particular, sexual and reproductive rights. Within families, and particularly in the case of young people, there had not been a previous instance of human rights education. The intervention programme addressed this issue, facilitating, for the first time in the region, an educational process on sexual and reproductive rights. Young people acquired basic knowledge of sexuality, human emotions, and violence prevention. One notable result was the initial recognition of their rights, understanding for the first time the existence of these rights in all human beings and regarding their sexuality from a rights perspective. Families also learned to recognize the value of human rights education and the importance of violence prevention and prevention of discrimination against women. Finally, an important result is that most of the regional institutions concerned with the formal educational needs of young people with disability included the issue of sexual and reproductive rights in the training of their students. To sustain the results of this programme, it is vital to instigate a process of cultural change and maintain sexual rights as a permanent item in the agenda of healthcare and social care organizations.

Area 2: Support for Mothers With Intellectual Disabilities

The triad of interacting factors of being a woman, experiencing disability, and violence, is linked with situations of poverty, illiteracy, and difficulties accessing health information, education, and work, combined with a lack of support from public services. All these elements precipitate a situation of occupational injustice that affects these women, and it becomes a vicious circle which is almost impossible to break. Society demands the separation of these women from their role as mothers. Social prejudice is a major barrier that limits their possibility of exercising motherhood. This multiple discrimination is present in all the daily occupations of these women and their families.

This intervention has succeeded in demonstrating that intellectual disability is not an obstacle to developing the maternal role in women. They are able to develop a clear and strong mother–child relationship and support the protective and secure attachment, through which the comprehensive development of a human being is achieved. One noted example is a mother who had to face a series of legal disputes over the recognition of legal guardianship about her daughter and several attempts to force her to give her baby up for adoption. The University of Magallanes, together with the regional government, managed to successfully defend the right to maternity of this particular woman through more than a year of intervention.

Probably one of the most important results of this intervention is its contribution in making the triad of womanhood, disability, and violence visible, conceptualizing it as a macro issue of human rights, both locally and nationally. Furthermore, the this programme highlighted a lack of regional support networks for parents and families, few opportunities for education about human rights at either a local or a national level, and a lack of forums and community education awareness for the rest of the population.

At the institutional level, the study found that the information provided by various services was not adapted or accessible to women with intellectual disabilities. They regularly receive inadequate answers from professionals, questioning their skills and decisions, which suppresses them and violates their rights. They feel afraid of losing their children. Professional practices are predominantly characterized by the negative prejudices of public institutions, repeatedly demonstrating their ignorance about disability, their lack of attention to human rights–based approaches, and the presence of myths and negative stereotypes (coinciding with the point made by Sheerin et al., 2013). All this influences professional decisions, which explains why the rights of these women in diverse health and social care services are repeatedly violated. The factors mentioned above are the main agents responsible for the occupational injustice affecting these women, persistently denying women with intellectual disabilities the possibility of motherhood.

At the governmental level, there are no public policies that protect this population. Consequently, another positive result has been the support of the Honorable Senator of the region of Magallanes, Ms. Carolina Goić, in requesting that the Health Committee of the Senate of the Republic of Chile addresses and makes the situation of women and mothers with intellectual disabilities and their families visible, so as to realize their constitutionally guaranteed rights.

Following on from the results of this experience, there has been new research on knowledge of sexual abuse prevention in young people with intellectual disabilities in the region. Preliminary results indicate that young people between 13 and 24 years old have less knowledge in the areas 'Taking care of one's own body' and 'Safety and emergency maintenance' (American Occupational Therapy Association, 2014, p. 631), which may prevent them from identifying abusive behaviour and exposure to violence[3].

In addition, the Department of Occupational Therapy at the University of Magallanes has also reported positive results from this experience. It has brought great benefits to both students and users who have participated in the intervention. The students expressed high appreciation and satisfaction with the experience, which was recognized as very significant and enriching, and as an important means of achieving a comprehensive professional development that allows the acquisition of specific skills training.

CONCLUSIONS AND RECOMMENDATIONS

The exposure of the violation of the human rights of persons with disabilities is an unavoidable necessity for occupational therapists around the world, whose professional duty includes working with others to combat all forms of rights violations and injustices. Services cannot pretend to be inclusive of people with disabilities if they cannot stop them from experiencing daily violations of their fundamental rights. It is necessary

---

[3]A study (publication forthcoming) by Joselyn Guichapani, Jazmín Muñoz, and Catherine Orellana, occupational therapy students at the University of Magallanes, focuses on the knowledge of three specific areas related to the activities of daily living: changes of the own body, taking care of one's own body, and safety and emergency maintenance.

to ask whether services, or indeed society as a whole, are doing enough to combat these violations, and whether what is being done is consistent with the ideals of the occupational therapy profession. A truly inclusive society involves the articulation of policy in the common interest of the people, primarily social policies but also economic policies. However, most policies are focused on the economic and commercial components of our societies, whereas the social aspects, and therefore matters such as rights, become matters of secondary importance.

The programme presented in this chapter has shown an effective response to the violation of human rights and gender violence suffered by these women; even though this is an initial battle, there is no end date for this matter. In this chapter, we also provided information on the specific types of violence to which these women are exposed, such as denial of adapted information through public services, and the denial of support to access and participate in a significant occupation (if not the most significant for many of them), as is the exercise of motherhood. In Chile as well as many other countries, there is an obligation to deliver according to international regulatory framework governing this matter[4].

In conclusion, these issues require urgent attention:

- The promotion of education, through accessible and understandable language for parents with intellectual disabilities and their families, regarding all aspects relating to pregnancy, childbirth, and upbringing of their children.
- The education of society at all levels on human rights, through a thorough review of educational curricula at all educational levels: kindergarten, primary, secondary, and higher education level.
- The explicit incorporation of human rights education in occupational therapy educational curricula, with a focus on all people, including those whose needs often remain invisible.

- Training on gender issues, disability, and violence directed at healthcare and social care professionals.
- The promotion of public policies on gender, disability, and violence. This will contribute to a real understanding of sexual and reproductive rights as fundamental human rights by society as a whole.
- The development of person-centred supports to women with intellectual disabilities in Chile (similar to those reported by Sheerin et al., 2013, p. 194) guided by a human rights perspective, to respond to their needs.
- It is important that the laws of the Chilean state and its institutions recognize the fundamental rights of these women, for example, to health and education. This statutory recognition will be the only way for the financing of these programmes which cannot rely solely on the third sector or the ad hoc financing of projects, but rather on services offered by the state
- The promotion of research in occupational therapy with emphasis on issues of justice, human rights, and the politics of occupation (Laliberte Rudman, 2014; Ramugondo and Kronenberg, 2013; Stadnyk et al., 2010). The duty of occupational therapists is to continue to expose existing social inequalities and propose solutions based on research evidence. The 'concern for social justice, inclusion and participation can never truly be separated from the study of occupation' (Cutchin and Dickie, 2012, p. 34).

The task of this team in Magallanes continues to develop, in order to continue generating social change in favour of inclusion and non-discrimination of these women. The greatest outcome and success of this project is empowering women with intellectual disabilities to defend their rights, and to feel strong and happy loving and taking care of their children.

The essential is invisible to the eyes.
—Antoine De Saint-Exupery

Acknowledgements

Writing for this book has been a real honour, a great gift, and an opportunity to work from the end of the

---

[4]'Article 4 (a) of the Convention on the Rights of Persons with Disabilities requires States parties to take all appropriate legislative, administrative and other measures to prevent and punish violence against women and/or domestic violence, including violence against women and girls with disabilities' (United Nations, 2012, p. 15).

world (or maybe the beginning) in the development of our beloved profession. We gratefully acknowledge the support of the University of Magallanes, the Regional Government of Magallanes, occupational therapy students at University of Magallanes, and Daniela Mandiola Godoy, faculty member of the Department of Occupational Therapy at the University of Magallanes.

REFERENCES

American Occupational Therapy Association, 2014. Occupational therapy practice framework: Domain and process (3rd ed.). Am. J. Occup. Ther. 68 (Suppl. 1), S1–S48.

American Psychiatric Association, 2013. Diagnostic and Statistical Manual of Mental Disorders: DSM-5. American Psychiatric Publishing, Arlington, VA.

Benavides, M., 2014. Introducción a género, discapacidad y violencia (Introduction to gender, disability and violence). Seminario Género, discapacidad y violencia. Segundo Seminario Mujer, Discapacidad y Violencia, Universidad de Magallanes, Punta Arenas, Chile, 1 Diciembre 2014 (in Spanish).

Blacher, J., Baker, B.L., 2002. The Best of AAMR: Families and Mental Retardation: A Collection of Notable AAMR Journal Articles Across the 20th Century. American Association on Mental Retardation, Washington, DC.

Cutchin, M.P., Dickie, V.A., 2012. Transactionalism: occupational science and the pragmatic attitude. In: Whiteford, G.E., Hocking, C. (Eds.), Occupational Science: Society, Inclusion, Participation. Blackwell, West Sussex, UK, pp. 23–37.

Dehays, P.M., Hichins, A.M., Vidal, C.V., 2012. Análisis del significado de las ocupaciones atribuidas a ser mujer y madre para mujeres con discapacidad intelectual en la ciudad de Punta Arenas (Meaning analysis of occupations attributed to be a woman and mother for women with intellectual disability in the city of Punta Arenas). Revista Chilena de Terapia Ocupacional 12 (2), 1–18. doi:10.5354/0717-5346.2012.25301 (in Spanish).

Díaz, E., 2013. El reflejo de la mujer en el espejo de la discapacidad (The reflex of the woman in the mirror of disability). Grupo Editorial Cinca, S. A., Madrid (in Spanish).

Galheigo, M.S., 2011. What needs to be done? Occupational therapy responsibilities and challenges regarding human rights. Aust. Occup. Ther. J. 58, 60–66.

Laliberte Rudman, D., 2014. Embracing and enacting an 'Occupational Imagination': occupational science as transformative. J. Occup. Sci. 21 (4), 373–388. doi:10.1080/14427591.2014.888970.

Llewellyn, G., 2010. Parents with intellectual disabilities: past, present and futures. John Wiley, Chichester, UK.

Llewellyn, G., 2013. Parents with intellectual disability and their children: advances in policy and practice. J. Policy Pract. Intellect. Disabil. 10 (2), 82–85. doi:10.1111/jppi.12033.

Peláez, A., Martínez, B., Leonhardt, M., 2009. Maternidad y discapacidad (Maternity and disability). Grupo Editorial Cinca S.A., Madrid (in Spanish).

Ramugondo, E.L., Kronenberg, F., 2013. Explaining collective occupations from a human relations perspective: bridging the individual-collective dichotomy. J. Occup. Sci. 22 (1), 3–16. doi:10.1080/14427591.2013.781920.

Sakellariou, D., Simó Algado, S., 2006. Sexuality and disability: a case of occupational injustice. Br. J. Occup. Ther. 69 (2), 69–76.

Salazar, G., 2010. Bicentenario: 200 años de daño transgeneracional (Bicentenary: 200 years of transgenerational damage). Reflexión 38, 11–15, (in Spanish).

Sheerin, F.K., Keenan, P.M., Lawler, D., 2013. Mothers with intellectual disabilities: interactions with children and family services in Ireland. Br. J. Learn. Disabil. 41, 189–196. doi:10.1111/bld.12034.

Stadnyk, R., Townsend, E.A., Wilcock, A., 2010. Occupational justice. In: Christiansen, C., Townsend, E.A. (Eds.), Introduction to Occupation: The Art and Science of Living, second ed. Prentice Hall, Thorofare, NJ, pp. 329–358.

Townsend, A., Wilcock, A.A., 2004. Occupational justice and client-centred practice: a dialogue in progress. Can. J. Occup. Ther. 71 (2), 75–87. doi:10.1177/000841740407100203.

United Nations, 2012. Thematic study on the issue of violence against women and girls and disability. Report of the Office of the United Nations High Commissioner for Human Rights. March 2012, General Assembly UN, New York. Available at: <http://www.ohchr.org/Documents/Issues/Disability/ThematicStudyViolenceAgainstWomenGirls.pdf>.

United Nations Women, 2012. Forgotten sisters: violence against women and girls with disability, speech of Opening of Lakshmi Puri. General Subsecretary and Executive Attached Director of UN Women in the Panel of Debate on Prevention and Eradication of the Violence against the Women with Disability, New York, October 23, 2012. Available at: <http://www.unwomen.org/es/news/stories/2012/10/forgotten-sisters-violence-against-women-and-girls-with-disabilities#sthash.YyNbFZkZ.dpuf>.

Verdugo, M.A., Schalock, R., 2010. Últimos avances en el enfoque y concepción de las personas con discapacidad intelectual (Changes in the understanding and approach to persons with intellectual disability). Revista Siglo Cero 41 (4), 7–21, (in Spanish).

Verdugo, M.A., Alcedo, M.A., Bermejo, B., Aguado, A., 2002. El abuso sexual en personas con discapacidad intelectual (Sexual abuse of people with mental retardation). Revista Psicothema 14, 124–129, (in Spanish).

Women with Disabilities Australia, 2011. Sterilization of women and girls with disabilities: an update on the issue in Australia. March 2011, WWDA, Tasmania. Available from: <http://www2.ohchr.org/english/bodies/cedaw/docs/cedaw_crc_contributions/WomenwithDisabilitiesAustralia.pdf>.

World Federation of Occupational Therapists, 2006. Position Statement on Human Rights. 2006. WFOT, Western Australia. Available from: <http://www.wfot.org/ResourceCentre.aspx>.

World Health Organization, 2001. International Classification of Functioning, Disability and Health. WHO, Geneva.

World Health Organization, 2006. Defining sexual health. Report of a technical consultation on sexual health. January 2002. WHO, Geneva. Available from: <http://www.who.int/reproductivehealth/publications/sexual_health/defining_sexual_health.pdf>.

World Health Organization/World Bank, 2011. World Report on Disability. WHO/World Bank, Geneva.

49

OCCUPATIONAL THERAPY FOCUSING ON SOCIAL CHANGE: AN EXPERIENCE IN DISABILITY-INCLUSIVE DEVELOPMENT IN TUNISIA

HETTY FRANSEN-JAÏBI

Health, occupation, and participation are influenced by many determinants, largely by factors outside the medical, technical, or public health domain, such as social, economic, and political conditions (World Health Organization (WHO), 1978). These social phenomena are of major interest in understanding the health, occupation, and participation of people in society and determining how improvements may be developed.

Occupational therapists working with communities are inspired and informed by theories and models from different fields and disciplines. Many issues will lead occupational therapists in the choice of a social approach, such as: What kind of social change is possible to improve daily health, occupation, and participation? What environmental factors will influence changes? What competences are needed to support social change in a specific situation? How can occupational therapists engage with the issues and enact changes?

This chapter discusses occupational therapy focusing on social change in the specific context of disability-inclusive development. It is in part a follow-up of a previously published work (Fransen, 2005). My aim in this chapter is to address strategies to tackle inequities and injustice through community changes and to translate these strategies into concrete, workable actions. A transformative approach to inclusion and participatory citizenship is adopted and explained. In the second part of the chapter, the focus is on participatory approaches in practice using the example of a project addressing accessibility of public transport in the rural south of Tunisia. Rather than draw generalizable conclusions, the aim of the chapter is to enhance the readers' and practitioners' own creative and critical thinking in order to encourage and empower them to find appropriate solutions to the particular challenges they face (Hurrell et al., 2006).

A VISION OF HEALTH, OCCUPATION, AND PARTICIPATION FROM A SOCIETY PERSPECTIVE

Understanding Social Influences

Recently there has been increased attention on persistent differences in health between different social classes and groups, for example, through inequalities in material resources (poverty), working conditions, or access to health and education. These inequalities are the biggest cause of widespread ill health and exclusion of people (Commission on Social Determinants of Health, 2008; Irwin and Scali, 2010). At the macro level, the gap between countries and within national borders in income levels, opportunities, health status, life expectancy, and accessibility of care is widening (Blas and Kurup, 2010).

In 2005, the WHO set up the Commission on Social Determinants of Health. They performed many activities and published several useful documents. The rainbow model of Dahlgren and Whitehead (1991) has become well-known and is commonly used to identify in a simple way the key determinants of health. Changes in these determinants can promote health, enable occupation, and prevent disability. These changes can be achieved by legislation and changes in policy, capacity building, and technical developments, and through improved access to healthcare, rehabilitation, education, support services, and employment. Occupational therapy and occupational science value social justice

and recognize the importance of addressing health inequities and occupational justice. However, the question remains how to do this in practice and make steps forward and contribute to a more just society.

Strategies to Tackle Inequities in Health and Participation

The Convention on the Rights of Persons with Disabilities, adopted in 2006, has as its aim 'to promote, protect and ensure the full and equal enjoyment of all human rights and fundamental free property by all persons with disabilities, and to promote respect for their inherent dignity' (United Nations, 2006, http://www.un.org/esa/socdev/enable/rights/convtexte.htm). Equality in health is seen as a human rights issue and is defined as the absence of unfair and avoidable differences in health between social groups (Blas and Kurup, 2010).

Political awareness and the willingness to do something are necessary conditions to progress. The paradigm of human rights has a transformative approach: critical of society and emancipatory in nature. In other words, disability is a human rights issue because many people with disabilities experience structural inequality (in health, education, work, etc.) and participate less in society. Therefore, people with disabilities are often victims of violations of their human dignity and do not enjoy full citizenship rights (Fransen et al., 2015). This human rights perspective needs to guide policies and measures to foster a greater equality in health.

The Commission on Social Determinants of Health developed a framework to tackle the existing gaps and persisting inequities (Solar and Irwin, 2010). This is a big step forward, while it aims to translate knowledge into concrete, operational strategies and measures. An innovative aspect is that the healthcare system is also seen as a social determinant, influencing health and being a possible cause of health inequity and exclusion. Three broad approaches are defined in public health by the Commission on Social Determinants of Health to combat socioeconomic health differences (Solar and Irwin, 2010). These approaches are:

1. Specific programmes for disadvantaged or vulnerable populations (e.g., people with mental illness, refugees, single elderly, homeless, low-skilled, people with multiple disabilities).

2. Fighting the gaps in health between 'worse' and 'better' or more fortunate people (e.g., differences in life expectancy depending on income, education or geographic location)

3. Focus on the social determinants of health for the entire population (e.g., loneliness and social cohesion, alcohol abuse and addictions, obesity and heart disease).

These approaches are complementary, that is, they may coexist and have a synergic effect on each other. Within these broad approaches, specific strategies have their place, such as preventive measures or improvement of accessibility measures through attention to diversity and activities aimed at health promotion. The results of the approach depend on the quality of intrasectoral collaboration (different sectors working together to achieve common goals), working towards increased social participation of civil society and empowerment of disadvantaged groups. Policies and actions take place at a micro level (individual interaction), meso level (community, organizations, workplaces), and/or macro level (society and overall laws and politics).

Including Disability in Development

Inclusive development encourages participation for all marginalized groups. Disability-inclusive development respects the diversity that disability brings and appreciates that it is an everyday part of the human experience. Disability-inclusive development sets out to achieve equality of human rights for people with a disability as well as full participation in, and access to, all aspects of society (CBM, 2012).

Awareness raising, participation, comprehensive accessibility, and the twin-track approach are the core guiding principles (WHO, 2010). A twin-track approach is a core element in disability and development policy and includes specific actions for people with a disability in conjunction with mainstream inclusion. It promotes concurrent action across two broad sets of initiatives. One set is through disability-specific activities that are targeted directly for people with a disability; the other is through the mainstreaming of disability into broader activities. Interventions on either track alone will not provide the breadth of involvement, integration, and support needed for

people with a disability to fully participate. Genuine inclusion and empowerment can only occur when both tracks are employed together (CBM, 2012; Fransen, 2005; WHO, 2010)

INCLUSIVE COMMUNITIES: STRIVING FOR PARTICIPATORY CITIZENSHIP

A Rights-Based Participatory Approach Based in Community-Based Rehabilitation

Occupational therapists working with communities use diverse strategies in striving for an inclusive society, for example, in community-based rehabilitation (CBR) or community development. Disability needs to be included in the mainstream of all policies (WHO and World Bank, 2011). Poverty reduction is explicitly emphasized in the latest guidelines on CBR (WHO, 2010).

Great emphasis is put on the multisectoral strategy, referring to the need for participation of all relevant stakeholders. Stakeholders are people with disabilities, their families, their communities, administrators (local, provincial, national), nongovernmental organizations, organizations of persons with disabilities, social workers from the health, education and social services, and the private sector.

Nowadays, CBR, operating within community development, has integrated a rights-based participatory approach to disability inclusion through rehabilitation, poverty reduction, social inclusion, and equity of opportunity. CBR aims to remove disabling barriers, address the causes of disability, and bring people with and without disabilities together with an overarching contribution to poverty reduction and improved quality of life for all.

From Working *in* to Working *with* the Community

Over the last decades, in several countries, there has been a change from institutional care to more community-located care. There are several causes for these changes, including the following: an increasing emphasis on cost-saving, and social changes with regards to people with disabilities and their perceived needs. A multitude of types of care are located in the community: home care, home treatment, day care, health education, and mental health programmes.

These can often be guided by conventional healthcare traditions. It is therefore understandable that confusion exists between 'care located in the community' and 'community development' (Fransen and Kronenberg, 2012). The shift in the vision of CBR no longer aims to deliver 'service in the community' but envisions 'development and management *by* the community' (Fransen et al., 2011; Scaffa and Brownson, 2005).

Transformation and Participatory Citizenship

An inclusive society is 'a society for all', that is, a society where everyone has rights, responsibilities, and an active role to play. A critical perspective enables examination of the processes of inclusion and exclusion, and facilitates a better understanding of what transformations are necessary to achieve equality of human rights as well as full participation for people with disabilities. In other words, this means being able to realize access to all aspects of society and 'to act as a citizen'. Participatory citizenship implies the active involvement of citizens, including all people, in the life, in the activities, in decisions regarding their communities, being interconnected and shaping the world together. Health and inclusion can be understood as collective issues, transcending an individual rights-based approach (Fransen et al., 2013, 2015).

PROJECT METHODOLOGY IN PRACTICE: A CASE STUDY ON 'ACCESSIBILITY OF PUBLIC TRANSPORT'

This section presents a case study from Tunisia, in which the emphasis is on the participatory process and the methodology of doing a project. The structure follows the phases of the project management cycle: Phase 1: Situation analysis; Phase 2: Planning and design; Phase 3: Implementation and monitoring; and Phase 4: Evaluation and lessons learned (Blackman, 2003; The World Bank, 2005).

A Student Project in the South of Tunisia

The starting point for the project was the observation that in Tunisian society people with reduced mobility were neglected in the design of public spaces and services. The lack of accessibility in the environment forms a barrier for simple activities of daily life, whether in travel, housing, working, education, leisure, or community activities. The general objective of the project was to facilitate access to public transport for people with disabilities and improve their life conditions. Two occupational therapy students carried out the project for their final study assignment for their Bachelor's of Occupational Therapy at the Tunisian School for Health Sciences and Techniques of Tunis in 2014, during a period of 12 weeks in the rural south of Tunisia. Both students originated from that region. They were inspired by the project 'A town for all: improved accessibility for people with disabilities to public and private transport' carried out by the Tunisian Association of Occupational Therapy and Handicap International in two towns in the north of Tunisia (Association Tunisienne d'Ergothérapie, 2014). Knowledge and expertise supporting people with disabilities was structurally lacking in both towns.

Phase 1: Situation Analysis

The students started their fieldwork in a centre for physically disabled children. A group of teenagers, four girls and three boys, between 14 and 16 years of age, were interested in the project and willing to participate. They lived in the surrounding rural area at a distance of 12 km or more and used wheelchairs. Most of them were fairly independent in carrying out daily life activities, despite their physical impairment. The teenagers were in a disabling situation with regard to their mobility and the use of public transport.

The Assessment of Life Habits (International Network on the Disability Creation Process, 2005) revealed that without the help of an accompanying person they found themselves incapable of realizing their life habits, such as participation in education, leisure, and cultural activities and community life, or spending time with friends. Nothing was accessible: neither the public parks, the youth's houses, the sidewalks, nor above all, the means of transportation. A lot of teenagers with disabilities in the area lack access to the wider world because of their low autonomy, non-accessible public buildings, and parental overprotection. Hence the boys spent significantly more time at cafés than in other leisure activities. Furthermore, adapted public toilets were lacking, as were leisure activities for girls with disabilities and recreational spaces adapted for persons with a visual impairment.

Problem tree

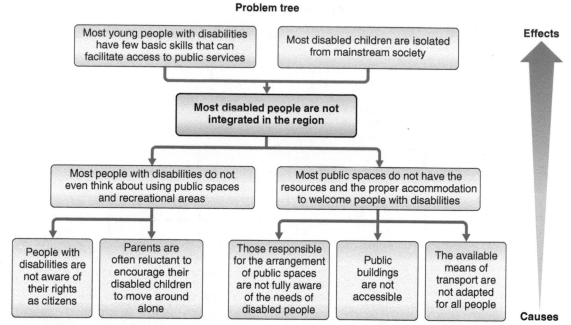

FIGURE 49-1 ■ The problem tree. *Adapted from Ben Moussa, N., Rais, O., 2014. Le rôle de l'ergothérapie dans l'aménagement des espaces de transports pour personnes à mobilité réduite. Unpublished Bachelor's in Occupational Therapy dissertation. Higher School for Health Sciences and Technics of Tunis, Tunisia.*

Facts collected about people with disabilities reveal that there are 4007 people with disabilities registered in the area, distributed over four types of disability: motor disability (39%), learning difficulties (28.92%), visual disability (13.85%), and hearing disability (12.62 %) (Ministry of Social Affairs, 2002). Information was also gathered about the legislative and institutional framework. Tunisia ratified the Convention on the Rights of Persons with Disabilities, which acknowledges participation in cultural life, recreation, leisure, and sports as a fundamental right for disabled persons (United Nations, 2006) through its Article 30. Tunisia has initiated a number of significant legal and institutional reforms to promote the academic and economic integration of disabled persons (United Nations, 2011). However, these measures are not always applied. Effective controlling mechanisms are missing and the means to implement them are scarce, leading to a disconnection between these policies and the reality experienced by Tunisians with disabilities.

Meetings with stakeholders were held, involving the teenagers, their families, the director of the centre, the regional delegates, and the management and employ-ees of the bus station. The project and the occupational therapy profession were represented. Viewpoints and experiences were gathered and exchanged. Collaboration started.

A problem analysis was undertaken: the main problems, their root causes and effects or consequences were identified with the stakeholders. Building a shared understanding and purpose was important. A 'problem tree' (see Figure 49-1) was used as a tool to visualize the situation with its specific set of problems (Blackman, 2003; WHO, 2010; World Bank, 2005).

An objectives analysis was undertaken, involving the reformulation of the identified problems into objectives. The problem analysis presented the negative aspects of the existing situation, while the analysis of the objectives dealt with positive aspects of a desired future. An 'objectives tree' was used to identify options for the project (see Figure 49-2).

Resources were analysed: the project had no external financial resources. The students boosted their competences and confidence by connecting with, participating and learning in the 'A town for all' project. Every 2 weeks a face-to-face meeting took place at the

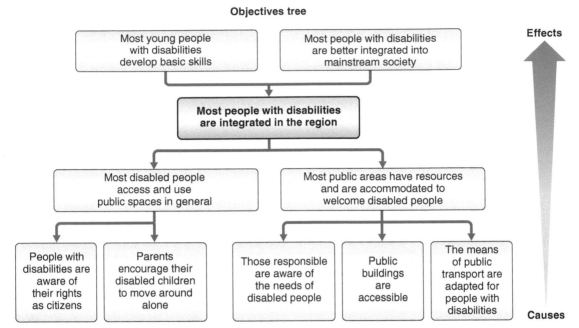

Objectives tree

FIGURE 49-2 ▪ The objectives tree. *Adapted from Ben Moussa, N., Rais, O., 2014. Le rôle de l'ergothérapie dans l'aménagement des espaces de transports pour personnes à mobilité réduite. Unpublished Bachelor's in Occupational Therapy dissertation. Higher School for Health Sciences and Technics of Tunis, Tunisia.*

university with student peer groups and supervision to give students the necessary support.

Guiding Frameworks for Practice

Guiding frameworks for practice were decided upon along the way. The principles of disability inclusion and inclusive community development framed the overall approach, based in a paradigm of social justice and human rights, and enacted through its core principles of awareness, participation, comprehensive accessibility, and a twin-track approach.

The disability creation process model (Fougeyrollas et al., 1998) was used to build a shared understanding of disability and handicap as a dynamic process. This human development model has little technical or specialist terms, which may exclude people. Together with people with disabilities, the students identified facilitators and obstacles for the realization of daily life activities, like access to transportation, and the consequences of these issues for their social participation.

This social enterprise and its implementation and management were supported by the project management cycle (CBM, 2012; WHO, 2010). The methodo-

logical approach is used to frame the important elements to take into account and to make the indicators for good practice explicit. In this case, it guides the inclusive approach through all the phases and helps to manage the project as a whole (Spreckly, 2006). The important elements in this project were related to awareness raising, participation, comprehensive accessibility, and the twin-track approach in practice. The indicators for good practice help in evaluating the progress made towards the formulated goals.

Phase 2: Strategic Choices: Planning and Design

Awareness raising and information sharing about the situation of people with disabilities in the area and about the stakeholders' perspectives was needed in order to plan and design the specific objectives, activities, and results to be achieved and to set strategic choices. To enable this, the centre organized a thematic day, 'together for better accessibility for people with specific needs', to which stakeholders were invited. Invitations were personally delivered to those responsible for public transport, the president of the regional association for solidarity and development, all people related to the association, the parents of the children and adolescents of the association, and the representatives of a connected disability centre in Libya. During the day, information was provided about the convention of rights for people with disabilities, about accessibility and handicap, about occupational therapy, about the reality of inaccessible public spaces in the area and of potential solutions which had been realized in other parts of Tunisia. Photos and a video (with written permission and informed consent) made with the adolescents showed their access difficulties at the bus station.

The presented findings were reviewed and discussed over the second part of the day, and options and priorities were determined together. Another analysis tree, the 'strategic tree', helped stakeholders to focus on what was possible and most needed in the short term, within the available resources and time, and also where the potential for relevant and appropriate change may exist (see Figure 49-3).

The strategic choices made were the following:

1. A global objective: for people with reduced mobility to be able move around independently in the area.
2. A specific objective: that most of the public spaces are adapted to accommodate and welcome people with reduced mobility.

The expected outcomes were that:

1. People responsible for transport are aware of the rights of people with disabilities to use public transportation.
2. All public services are accessible for people with reduced mobility.
3. The regional bus station is accessible for persons in a situation of disability.

For the planning of the project, activities a logical framework 'logframe' (Blackman, 2003; WHO, 2010; World Bank, 2005) was developed to describe goals, purposes, outcomes, and activities.

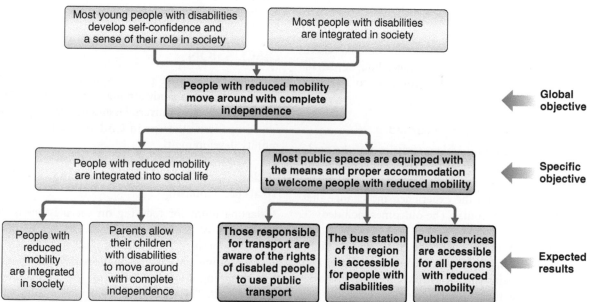

FIGURE 49-3 ■ The strategic tree. *Adapted from Ben Moussa, N., Rais, O., 2014. Le rôle de l'ergothérapie dans l'aménagement des espaces de transports pour personnes à mobilité réduite. Unpublished Bachelor's in Occupational Therapy dissertation. Higher School for Health Sciences and Technics of Tunis, Tunisia.*

Phase 3: Implementation and Monitoring

Detailed work plans were developed. Informed consent was obtained from all the stakeholders and permission sought to make a detailed analysis at the site of the bus station.

The planned activities were carried out. These included:

- Revisiting the site of the bus station and taking photographs of obstacles.
- Obtaining the existing technical drawings of the site.
- Verifying if the drawings corresponded to the actual site and collecting complementary data.
- Taking measurements on-site and inputting the data in a computer programme.
- Developing a video explaining the various barriers that the teenagers in wheelchairs faced in taking the bus to go shopping.
- Synthesizing the difficulties and barriers and proposing solutions.
- Realizing an appropriate and detailed plan.
- Presenting and discussing the proposal with the stakeholders and advocating for its implementation.
- Disseminating the findings.

A budget was needed for the realization of all this, but the project came to an end before this could be raised. The students intend to make a detailed budget plan of the adapted propositions and continue to strive to raise interest and funding.

Evaluation and Lessons Learned

An evaluation was undertaken at the end of the field-work period by the students themselves. Their focus was on the results obtained (outcomes), and on the lessons learned from the experience and change that has taken place (outputs). The outcomes included:

- Increased awareness of the disabling situations people with disabilities encounter in the area to realize their daily activities and participate in social life; their problems were made visible and there was a common understanding about the existing barriers, especially regarding the inaccessibility of public spaces.

- Increased awareness and knowledge about the rights of people with disabilities and the importance of this knowledge for policy formation.
- Increased motivation in the community to improve quality of life and do something about the exclusion of people with disabilities.
- Increased knowledge about occupational therapy, its technical expertise, and its focus on occupation, health, and participation in being a partner for inclusion.
- Realization of a detailed proposal of an accessible bus station, elaborated with rigour and precision, and disseminated to all the stakeholders.

However, given the short period and the lack of budget, the proposed adaptations were not realized. The site was recently restored and a new budget will only be allocated 4 years from the time of this writing (October 2015). The managers have expressed their intention to discuss the proposal in the municipal council. In response, the students worked out possible adaptations to realize in the short term, such as a ramp at the entrance, an office window to buy tickets no more than 1.20 metres high, small mobile wooden ramps, and the fixation of handrails. These temporary solutions are low budget and can improve accessibility pending the final implementation.

DISCUSSION

Although the example presented above presents only one particular case study among many others, it identifies and highlights universal issues that are important for occupational therapy in CBR and inclusive community development.

Sociopolitical Reasoning, Partnering, and Strategic Thinking

A starting point for focusing on social issues is the recognition of their sociopolitical nature. Working with a framework for inclusive development begins with actioning the desired changes through valuing and attending to the quality of the participatory process itself. The more the core principles of awareness raising, participation, comprehensive accessibility, and a twin-track approach are effectively realized, the more sustainable the empowerment and inclusion will be. Although the results of this project evaluation are small and modest, change has started and future developments are envisioned.

Working with marginalized or excluded groups of people requires respect and recognition of them as fellow citizens and taking full account of how they perceive their world and live their lives. It is necessary to be explicit about motives and interests and to be able to communicate these actively, in order to develop a working relationship based on trust and open communication.

Both students showed positive partnering behaviour and communication. They were engaged and committed, genuinely interested in other peoples' views, experiences, and priorities. They were prepared to take their share of responsibility for establishing an effective working relationship and were willing to be held accountable. And they were open to new ideas and to new ways of approaching tasks, while maintaining commitment to consensus and consultation (McManus and Tennyson, 2008).

Strategic thinking is required. This means looking far ahead (policy level), connecting through accessible language, scaling down to a concrete idea, and becoming an attractive partner (by being a solution). The methodological approach in this case study was based on the project management cycle. The tools are widely used by international agencies, for example, the World Bank and the European Commission. They are helpful in making projects transparent and participatory. Often they are a prerequisite for the funding which is necessary for effective implementation, such as the realization of adaptations or upscaling. To be effective agents in these developmental projects, occupational therapists need to demonstrate management skills and master the logic, the terminology, and the tools. However, caution is always needed with the use of tools. They may be taken as recipes, a means of focusing on the details without systematic thinking, which encourages a reductionist approach (Blackman, 2003).

Cultural Compatibility and Cultural Grounding of Frameworks and Models

All activities must be rooted in a thorough understanding of the local culture, especially when the objectives include awareness raising and changing attitudes. Firstly, all developmental activities take place within a cultural context. Secondly, in communities where people with disabilities are not seen as a priority for development nor included in mainstream programmes, an awareness of cultural issues surrounding disability is a key point for integrating disability into the general developmental process (Coleridge, 2000).

In this case, both students originated from the region and were part of the larger community. The guiding frameworks are in line with the basic commitment to human rights and justice and with the core belief of occupational therapy that human beings as active subjects are able to shape their daily lives. The framework of the disability creation process has rich potential for building shared understanding of disability, occupation, and social participation.

Most occupational therapy frameworks or models originate from Western countries, although new horizons have arisen with alternative and complementary approaches, for example, the Kawa model using the metaphor of life as a river (Iwama, 2006). Developing and disseminating culturally grounded models in a real-life context is necessary and important, given that most of the disabled people in the world live in developing and non-Western countries. Their daily realities also require very practical and concrete actions which respond to their basic needs of survival, dignity, and quality of life. In this case study, the metaphor is a strong olive tree, especially relevant in the rural areas of Tunisia. The olive tree is a symbol for life, peace, prosperity, and the sacred.

The Process Is as Important as the Product

The specific project objectives were to raise awareness about the rights of people with disabilities, to show the role of the occupational therapist in accessibility, and to provide a detailed proposal for the modification of a bus station to make it accessible for people with disabilities. In conclusion, looking at the evaluation and lessons learned, the outputs of the project are much broader. The problems of the daily life situations of people with disabilities in the area were made visible and given a voice. A shared understanding and purpose were built with community stakeholders, and motivation increased to tackle the existing barriers to social participation. Possible solutions for realizing them were identified.

The students defined increased knowledge of occupational therapy as an explicit goal, but there should be some critical distance about how important it is for project beneficiaries to have knowledge of occupational therapy and whether this self-promotion is ethical. However, within partnering processes, the partners have to know each other to engage and see the utility to make the alliance. The key focus here was on social reform rather than occupational therapy.

Capacity Building and the Social Responsibility of the University

After finishing the project, the students intended to continue their activities of awareness raising and of motivating people and the community to improve the accessibility of the bus station. They felt more experienced in occupational therapy, universal design, and project implementation, and they wished to link this experience with their future practice.

Occupational therapy education in Tunisia aims to confront students with different situations and practice paradigms. The profession in Tunisia operates in multiple contexts, from university hospitals, private clinics and social care, to poorly resourced infrastructures in regions where people live in poverty. Graduates need to be prepared for their future role in society and be proactive towards emerging practice opportunities for the benefit of the wider community, as well as for the benefit of all people with significant occupational needs (Fransen-Jaïbi, 2012). Some students explore emerging domains of practice and engage in a community-university-partnership, like the students in this case study.

Collaboration with communities has frequently been identified as an approach that can facilitate occupational therapists to address the social, political, and cultural aspects of occupational participation for all citizens. However, the complexities of community–university collaboration should not be underestimated, and the need to ensure that balance is achieved between the needs of students and communities has been noted (McGrath et al., 2013).

CONCLUSIONS

This chapter focuses on social change, addressing inequalities in health, occupation and participation.

These issues can feel as if 'everything is connected to everything else', resulting in a confusion of intertwined concepts, paradigms, and practices whereby relevance to a strategic connection can be lost. To avoid this, in this chapter a real-life example was used. Although the experience presented is very specific and context related, it provides knowledge, insight, and information. This may be significant in the situations occupational therapists face and a source for encouragement to engage with issues of social responsibility, creative thinking, professional development, and the building of skills. We close the cycle and come back to where we started with the words of the students:

Improving accessibility for people with disabilities is to act on the means necessary to achieve, without exclusion or discrimination, for every citizen, the freedom of movement and access to a place, a space or a service independently. Furthermore, it enhances for all the inhabitants...the quality of services and activities.

Acknowledgements

With gratitude and genuine recognition to Nesrine Ben Moussa, Ons Rais, Hajer Kanoun, Moez Boulila, Tared Ben Zaied, and all the partners of the project for their engagement.

REFERENCES

Association Tunisienne d'Ergothérapie, 2014. Guide de référence à l'intention des organismes du transport public/privé et aux usagers [Reference Guide for Organisations of public/private transport and for users]. ATE, Tunis.

Ben Moussa, N., Rais, O., 2014. Le rôle de l'ergothérapie dans l'aménagement des espaces de transports pour personnes à mobilité réduite [The role of occupational therapy in the adaptation of spaces for transport for persons with reduced mobility]. Unpublished Bachelor's in Occupational Therapy dissertation. Higher School for Health Sciences and Technics of Tunis, Tunisia.

Blackman, R., 2003. Project cycle management. Tearfund, Teddington, UK. Available from: <http://tilz.tearfund.org/Publications/ROOTS/Project+cycle+management.htm> (accessed 05.05.10.).

Blas, E., Kurup, A.S., 2010. Equity, social determinants and public health programmes. World Health Organization, Geneva. Available from: <http://whqlibdoc.who.int/publications/2010/9789241563970_eng.pdf>.

CBM, 2012. Inclusion Made Easy: A Quick Program Guide to Disability in Development. CBM Australia, Melbourne. Available from: <http://www.cbm.org/article/downloads/78851/CBM_Inclusion_Made_Easy_-_complete_guide.pdf>.

Coleridge, P., 2000. Disability and culture. Selected readings in CBR. Series 1. Asia Pacific Disabil. Rehabil. J. 21–38 .

Commission on Social Determinants of Health, 2008. Closing the gap in a generation: health equity through action on the social determinants of health. Final Report of the Commission on Social Determinants of Health. World Health Organization, Geneva. Available from: <http://whqlibdoc.who.int/publications/2008/9789241563703_eng.pdf>.

Dahlgren, G., Whitehead, M., 1991. Policies and Strategies to Promote Social Equity in Health. Institute of Futures Studies, Stockholm.

Fougeyrollas, P., Cloutier, P., Bergeron, H., Côté, J., St Michel, G., 1998. The Quebec Classification Disability Creation Process. International Network on Disability Creation Process (INDCP)/CSICIDH, Québec.

Fransen, H., 2005. Challenges for occupational therapy in community-based rehabilitation: occupation in a community approach to handicap in development. In: Kronenberg, F., Simo Algado, S., Pollard, N. (Eds.), Occupational Therapy without Borders: Learning from the spirit of survivors. Elsevier-Chuchill Livingstone, Edinburgh.

Fransen, H., Kronenberg, F., 2012. Ergotherapie gericht op sociaalmaatschappelijke veranderingen [Occupational therapy focusing on social and societal change]. In: le Granse, M., van Hartingveldt, M., Kinébanian, A. (Eds.), Grondslagen van de Ergothérapie. Elsevier, Amsterdam.

Fransen, H., Hartingveldt, M., Kinebanian, A., Logister-Proost, I., 2011. Ergotherapie gericht op maatschappelijke veranderingen? Naming and framing [Occupational Therapy focusing on society changes? Naming and framing]. Wetenschappelijk Tijdschift voor Ergotherapie (4), 46–49.

Fransen, H., Kantartzis, S., Pollard, N., Viana Moldes, I., 2013. Citizenship: exploring the contribution of occupational therapy. Position statement. <http://www.enothe.eu/activities/meet/ac13/CITIZENSHIP_STATEMENT_ENGLISH.pdf> (accessed 10.06.16.).

Fransen, H., Pollard, N., Kantartzis, S., Viana-Moldes, V., 2015. Participatory citizenship: critical perspectives on client-centred occupational therapy. Scand. J. Occup. Ther. 22 (4), 260–266. doi:10.3109/11038128.2015.1020338.

Fransen-Jaïbi, H., 2012. Evolution de l' ergothérapie en Tunisie: histoire d'une profession [Evolution of occupational therapy in Tunisia: history of a profession]. Ergothérapies 46, 65–72.

Hurrell, S., Hussain-Knaliq, S., Tennyson, R., 2006. The case study toolbook. Partnership case studies as tools for change. <http://thepartneringinitiative.prg/w/resources/toolbook-series/the-cas-study-toolbook/> (accessed 10.06.16.).

International Network on the Disability Creation Process, 2005. Assessment of Life Habits (LIFE H 3.0). <http://thepartneringinitiative.org/publications/toolbook-series/the-case-study-toolbook/> (accessed 10.06.16.).

Irwin, A., Scali, E., 2010. Action on the social determinants of health: learning from previous experiences. Social Determinants of Health Discussion Paper 1 (Debates). World Health Organization, Geneva. Available from: <http://whqlibdoc.who.int/publications/2010/9789241500876_eng.pdf>.

Iwama, M., 2006. The Kawa model: culturally relevant occupational therapy. Churchill Livingstone/Elsevier, Oxford.

McGrath, M., Viana Moldes, I., Fransen, H., Hofstede-Wessels, S., Lillenberg, K., 2013. Community-University Partnerships in occupational therapy education: a preliminary exploration of practice in a European context. Disabil. Rehabil. 36 (4), 344–352. doi:10.3109/09638288.2013.788220.

McManus, S., Tennyson, R., 2008. Talking the Walk: A Communication Manual for Partnership Practitioners. IBF, The partnering Initiative, Oxford, UK. Available from: <https://business.un.org/documents/resources/talking_the_walk.pdf> (accessed 10.06.16.).

Ministry of Social Affairs, 2002. Statistics of Persons with Disabilities in Tunisia. Ministry of Social Affairs, Tunisia. Available from: <www.cnipe.nat.tn> (accessed 10.06.16.).

Scaffa, M.E., Brownson, C., 2005. Occupational therapy interventions: community health approaches. In: Christiansen, C.H., Baum, C.M., Bass-Hagen, J.D. (Eds.), Occupational Therapy: Performance, Participation and Well-being, third ed. Slack Incorporated, Thorofare, NJ, pp. 476–493.

Solar, O., Irwin, A., 2010. A conceptual framework for action on the social determinants of health. Social Determinants of Health Discussion Paper 2 (Policy and Practice). World Health Organization, Geneva.

Spreckly, F., 2006. A project cycle management and logical framework toolkit: a practical guide for equal development partnerships. EQUAL. Local livelihoods Ltd, Birmingham, UK. Available from: <http://portals.wi.wur.nl/files/docs/ppme/gpg_pcm_toolkit%5B1%5D.pdf>.

United Nations, 2006. Convention on the Rights of Persons with Disabilities. New York, United Nations.

United Nations, 2011. Concluding Observations of the Committee on the Rights of Persons with Disabilities: Tunisia. Available from: <http://www2.ohchr.org/SPdocs/CRPD/5thsession/CRPD-C-TUN-CO-1_en.doc> (accessed 10.06.16.).

World Bank, The, 2005. The logframe handbook: a logical framework approach to project cycle management. World Bank, Washington. Available from: <http://www-wds.worldbank.org/servlet/WDSContentServer/WDSP/IB/2005/06/07/000160016_20050607122225/Rendered/PDF/31240OLFhandbook.pdf> (accessed 02.03.07.).

World Health Organization, 1978. The declaration of Alma Ata. Available from: <http://www.who.int/hpr/NPH/docs/declaration_almaata.pdf>.

World Health Organization, 2010. CBR-guidelines: towards community-based inclusive development. WHO, Geneva. <http://www.who.int/disabilities/cbr/guidelines/en/> (accessed 10.06.16.).

World Health Organization and World Bank, 2011. World Report on Disability. World Health Organization, Geneva.

50

OCCUPATIONAL JUSTICE FOR ASYLUM SEEKER AND REFUGEE CHILDREN: ISSUES, EFFECTS, AND ACTION

CONCETTINA TRIMBOLI

In an ideal world, people would have access to conditions and resources that enable them to not only survive, but flourish. If we consider children, these conditions are likely to include being in a safe environment, being surrounded by family and friends, playing, and going to school. However, the reality in today's volatile world is quite different. The second decade of the century has been witness to a time of political instability, contributing to unprecedented numbers of refugees and asylum seekers. Children are particularly vulnerable to forced displacement and to the resulting occupational injustices that prevent them from living a meaningful life that promotes health and well-being.

The purpose of this chapter is to bring to light issues of occupational injustice that are experienced by refugee and asylum seeker children, and to identify the detri-mental, and potentially long-lasting, effects of forced migration on children. Practising Occupational therapists and occupational therapy students are encouraged to consider the tools that they have at their disposal to address the mental health and developmental issues that these children may experience, being aware of the importance of cultural and ethnic sensitivity. Both a participatory occupational justice framework and the Person-Environment-Occupation (PEO) model are used to provide some structure on how to identify and provide input for these children at a micro, meso, and macro level. Lastly, relevant World Federation Occupational Therapists position papers and statements are identified to demonstrate that occupational therapists have a professional responsibility to ensure that human rights are upheld during human displacement. All names and personal details discussed in this chapter have been changed to protect anonymity.

THE JOURNEY

A journey of a thousand miles must begin with one step.

— Lao Tzu

Refugees and asylum seekers are often in fear for their own lives and for the lives of their loved ones. Escaping from a country which may be in turmoil or war is often not a matter of choice for them. The experiences for each individual, whether it be an adult or child, may differ in their details, but there are many similarities: upheaval and disruption to people's daily lives and routines, deprivation, uncertainty, and constant fear (Gupta and Sullivan, 2013; Lustig, 2010).

Under the Geneva Convention Relating to the Status of Refugees, in order to be classified as an asylum seeker, people must show that they have a well-founded fear of persecution due to their race, religion, nationality, political opinion, or membership of a particular social group, and are unable or unwilling to seek protection from the authorities in their own country (United Nations High Commissioner for Refugees (UNHCR), 1954). Children make up a significant percentage of people forced to flee their country. Of the estimated 14.2 million refugees worldwide, 41% are believed to be children under the age of 18 years, and of the 24.5 million people internally displaced because of conflict, 36% are children (United Nations Children's Emergency Fund, 2007). More recently, by the end of 2013, refugee information disaggregated by age was available for 7.5 million refugees, 64% of the total population. The available evidence indicated that refugee children constituted 50% of the global refugee population (UNHCR, 2014).

The journey of an asylum seeker is not an easy one. These people are faced with continuous challenges and dangers as they cross country borders with few or no official papers, often hiding from authorities and threatening situations. Once arrived in a country of safety, the challenges are not over. They will be placed in refugee camps or immigration detention centres until their refugee claims are processed, which may vary from months to years (Lustig, 2010). Only once a positive decision on their asylum claim is reached will their status change to 'refugee', and they can begin their next journey of resettlement and acculturation.

OCCUPATIONAL JUSTICE

Occupational therapy's theoretical underpinnings stress that engagement in meaningful occupations promotes health and well-being (Law et al., 1998). Occupational justice is a concept developed by Townsend and Whiteford (2005) which emphasizes the rights that enable individuals to experience health and well-being through engagement in a wide variety of occupations that satisfy personal, health, and social needs. In developing this concept, the authors envisioned an occupationally just world where people would be supported by health services and social initiatives regardless of age, ability, gender, or social class (Townsend and Wilcock, 2004).

The unfortunate reality is that we do not yet live in an occupationally just world. Occupational injustices occur in many forms, including deprivation (being denied opportunities and resources to participate in occupations), alienation (being required to participate in occupations individuals find meaningless), marginalization (individuals lacking the power to exercise occupational choice), and imbalance (having too few or too many occupations) (Townsend and Wilcock, 2004). Refugees are a group highlighted as being particularly at risk of occupational deprivation (Whiteford, 2000).

To illustrate an example of occupational injustice, a fictional, though based on personal experience, scenario will be presented. Ahmed was 6 years old when he and his family fled Syria. They arrived in Australia speaking no English and were put into a remote detention facility by authorities, while their application for residency was being processed. Ahmed was not permitted to leave the facility to attend school and he had limited opportunities to play in appropriate areas or with age-appropriate toys. Ahmed spent a lot of time sleeping, had nightmares, and started wetting his bed in the detention centre. Ahmed did not see any health professionals in the detention centre.

We can identify that in the detention centre, Ahmed had limited opportunities to engage in age-appropriate occupations. He experienced occupational deprivation in the form of being confined to the detention facility and inability to engage in developmental and culturally appropriate occupations such as attending school or a mosque. His confinement meant that he could not access appropriate health services or have access to play areas. He was unable to make age-appropriate choices, for example, where to play or what to play with, constituting occupational marginalization. In addition to psychological distress, Ahmed's excessive sleeping may have been attributed to not having sufficient activities to participate in, thus resulting in occupational imbalance. We will later take a look at how an occupational justice framework can be used to provide occupational therapy intervention for Ahmed on various levels.

THE IMPACT OF FORCED MIGRATION ON CHILDREN

'Migration is considered one of the major life events which often involves profound changes ... It challenges the adaptive capacity of the families collectively and each of their members individually' (Roebers and Schneider, 1999, p. 125). These words reflect the challenges of free-choice migration; however, for those forced to escape from their country due to physical danger or possible death, the impact can be even more profound and long-lasting (McIntyre et al., 2011).

Children are in a very vulnerable position when forced to migrate, for a number of reasons. They may lack travel paperwork, restricting their access to services, and they may not have access to basic necessities such as food, appropriate shelter, sanitation, and safe water (Davidson and Farrow, 2007). Children generally have fewer and less well-refined coping mechanisms than adults, and in addition to dealing with the multiple stresses related to displacement, they also have to cope with many developmental changes (Adjukovic and Adjukovic, 1993). They may have also been abused, tortured, forced into military recruitment or witnessed violence (Simó-Algado et al., 2002). Unaccompanied young women and children with disabilities are particularly vulnerable to sexual and gender-based violence and discrimination. Young women are often subject to sexual exploitation and are marginalized in terms of decision making. Children with disabilities are reported to be at a greater risk of violence, abuse, exploitation, and neglect. The lack of privacy in some situations, such as a lack of access to latrines and bathing areas, increases the risk of abuse (UNHCR, 2011).

Various studies have been conducted investigating the effects of forced migration on children during the different phases of their migration process; however, few of these have been conducted in the field of occupational therapy (Copley et al., 2011; Driver and Beltran, 2010). Potential reasons for this may include that this is an emerging area of practice for occupational therapy with relatively few occupational therapists working in this area, as well as methodological and ethical issues concerned with conducting research into this population (Whiteford, 2005).

Using immigration detention centres as an example, research clearly shows that these restrictive environments can affect children's development, as well as their physical and psychological health and school performance (Cleveland et al., 2012; Mares and Jureidini, 2004; Robjant et al., 2009; Sultan and O'Sullivan, 2001). These effects included anxiety, disruptive conduct, nocturnal enuresis, sleep disturbances, and impaired cognitive development (Sultan and O'Sullivan, 2001). In Mares and Jureidini's study (2004), developmental delays were noted in children aged less than 6 years. Among the children in the older age range, mental health difficulties included posttraumatic stress disorder, depression, suicidal ideation, and self-harm behaviours. It is likely that children's parents also experience psychological difficulties as a result of their forced migration and may not be able to cope with providing appropriate care for their children. This can sometimes result in children prematurely taking on a role of increased responsibility disproportionate to their age, adding further stress to an already stressful situation (Robjant et al., 2009).

Although the physical environment might improve upon release into the community, children may continue to experience various difficulties including interacting with others, establishing friendships, and settling into a new way of life. Settlement issues include children needing to become orientated to a new environment, a new language, different values, attitudes, and cultural norms. Driver and Beltran (2010) identified that students' occupational performance may also be affected. In their study, children commonly demonstrated aggressive behaviour attributed to their difficulty with the host country's language. They also had difficulties in performance component areas such as concentration, attention, and fine-motor coordination, affecting activities such as handwriting, using scissors, art activities, and reading.

An example of these difficulties upon release in the community can be seen in the case study of Shala. Shala is an 8-year-old girl from Iran, and was in an immigration detention centre with her family on Christmas Island before being released into the Australian community. She has been out of detention for over a year but continues to experience many negative effects of her detention, such as inability to sleep, delayed motor development, and constant anxiety. Shala's mother explains that her daughter will not go to the bathroom and will hold on until she is in pain or wets herself. When Shala goes to the bathroom, she needs her mother to be there, as she does not like to be by herself and she never shuts the door as she is scared of feeling closed in. While in the detention centre, Shala had limited opportunities to play and witnessed people attempting to harm themselves.

Whilst the negatives of forced migration abound, there is some promising research investigating resilience in maltreated children and children exposed to war (Fernando and Ferrari, 2013). These findings suggest that children are highly resilient and can often find ways to cope. By drawing strength from their families and communities, and by learning, playing, and having space to explore their talents and skills, children can become active members of the community (UNHCR, 2012).

ACTION FOR OCCUPATIONAL THERAPISTS

Do what you can, with what you have, where you are.

— Theodore Roosevelt

The United Nations Convention on the Rights of the Child (Office of the High Commissioner for Human Rights, 1989) states that children have the right to the highest attainable standards of health and education and the right to be free from discrimination, exploitation, and abuse. Occupational therapists considering working with refugee and asylum seeker children may find the prospect of doing so daunting, given that there has been very little occupational therapy involvement and literature published in this field to date. In this chapter, I propose that working with asylum seekers and refugees should be seen as an emerging area of occupational therapy practice with many exciting possibilities and rewarding opportunities. Smith (2005) acknowledges the anxieties occupational therapists may feel when working with refugees, due to feeling ill prepared. In order to help alleviate this anxiety, she proposed that the solution lies in transferring existing skills to this area and taking a proactive stance. In addition to this, occupational therapists have a versatile tool kit at their disposal in the form of frameworks, models, skills, and knowledge to help them work with refugee and asylum seeker children.

Within an occupational justice framework, occupational therapists may consider what opportunities exist to influence issues at a micro (individual), meso (practice environment), and macro (structure and organization) level (Townsend and Wilcock, 2004). When possible reasons for the occupational injustices that Ahmed experienced are considered, it becomes clear that Australia's policy of mandatory, indefinite detention for all people, regardless of age, is a significant political barrier to him experiencing occupational justice (macro level). In addition, the detention centre staff were not adequately trained to deal with the trauma associated with forced detention in children, nor in cultural diversity issues (meso and macro level). Ahmed did not have access to specialist healthcare services (meso and macro level). By applying a participatory occupational justice framework, we can help address some of these examples of occupational injustice.

At a *micro* level, occupational therapists might want to consider volunteering or, if the opportunity exists, working in a detention centre within the occupational therapist's own country to provide Ahmed and other children in similar situations with opportunities for occupational engagement. Here, they can address any developmental delays or psychological issues they might observe by drawing on their knowledge of occupation, meaningful activities, art or play therapy given the age and the psychological needs these children may have. Activity and creativity can bridge cultural gaps and reduce dependence on language (Shackman and Reynolds, 1993). Countries will have their own protocols for visiting immigration detention facilities and will most likely involve completing a visitor application form. As in some countries detention centres are run by private companies, access may be difficult. Working through a nongovernmental organization may offer support and facilitate access.

At a *meso* level, occupational therapists could consider the appropriateness of liasing with and providing education to the detention centre staff, alerting them to issues associated with child forced migration, and providing strategies on ways that they can interact empathetically with these children, highlighting the need for suitable occupational participation and cultural sensitivity. Occupational therapists could also suggest that health professionals associated with the detention environment become involved and educate them on the potential of occupational therapy in the detention centre if no occupational therapy input currently exists. Again, being able to engage staff in these situations may be difficult as there is no prevailing enabling culture. As occupational therapists might observe or be informed of abusive practices, their efforts may be undermined or sabotaged in some situations, particularly if they are working unsupported. Occupational therapists should be aware of the need to negotiate changes with various stakeholders, from political decision-makers, to detention centre staff, and the refugees themselves.

At a *macro* level, occupational therapists could become advocates, liaise with appropriate community organizations, or become politically active and lobby/educate politicians and the public about the impact of forced migration on children and what can be done. While few studies have been conducted by occupational therapists in this area, research from other professions has identified that children in detention receive limited age-appropriate stimulation and exhibit developmental delays and mental health issues including posttraumatic stress disorder, depression, and anxiety (Cleveland et al., 2012; Mares and Jureidini, 2004). Occupational therapists could also consider conducting research investigating the occupational impact of forced migration on children, and consider publication and dissemination of their findings. By simultaneously working towards occupational justice at an individual and societal level, occupational therapists can take a proactive stance and bring the issues of occupational injustice to light.

USING THE PERSON-ENVIRONMENT-OCCUPATION MODEL

Now, let us imagine Ahmed is released into the community with his family and begins attending school. Ahmed is referred to occupational therapy services as his teacher has concerns about his progress. The referral reports that Ahmed is experiencing developmental delays in the areas of cutting, writing, and bilateral activities. His teacher notes that he rarely plays with other children in the playground during break times. Using an occupational lens, what are some of the things occupational therapists might need to consider?

Occupational therapists are aware that being client-centred often involves liaising not just with the client, but also everyone who comes into contact with them. In the case of child forced migration, this will most likely involve their parents, teachers, other children, and possibly support workers. The occupational therapist makes an appointment to visit Ahmed at school and to meet with his parents to talk about the things he docs at home, his level of independence, and what their expectations are. She arranges for an interpreter, if necessary.

In order to gain Ahmed's trust and develop rapport, the occupational therapist attends the school on two occasions. The first time is to just observe Ahmed in class and in the playground, and the second visit is to do some one-on-one intervention. She uses the PEO model (Law et al., 1996) to guide her assessment and intervention.

Although it may feel reassuring to go in and assess Ahmed using standardized occupational therapy tools, the reality is that it is more important to use everyday skills: listening, demonstrating respect, and seeing Ahmed as an individual with a unique identity (Whiteford, 2005). These children and their families will initially be searching for empathy more than an answer to their complex problems and needs (Keyes and Kane, 2004).

As a *person*, Ahmed is viewed holistically from a mind, body, and spiritual perspective. He is observed in class and during break times, and the occupational therapist acknowledges the impact that his background may have on his performance. For example, she notices that he has difficulty writing left to right.

She also observes that some of the children make fun of him because of his clothing and the lunches he brings to school. When observing Ahmed, the occupational therapist assesses him from a range of perspectives including motor, sensory, social, and cognitive. She keeps in mind the cultural limitations of the assessments she has; for example, that they have not been validated with children from non-Western backgrounds, and thus the results may not be reliable, and the fact that Ahmed's first language is not English. The occupational therapist opts to use observational tasks and reports from his teachers and parents, rather than standardized assessments. Ahmed does indeed demonstrate developmental delays in the areas noted by his teacher, in addition to a lack of confidence when faced with unfamiliar tasks. Socially, he seems to have only one friend who he sometimes plays with during break time and he can be seen smiling when they play together.

The occupational therapist has a meeting with Ahmed's teacher, which enables her to ascertain the teacher's level of empathy, her understanding of Ahmed's cultural background, and the impact of his deficits on his occupational performance. The occupational therapist also highlights Ahmed's strengths. In addition to this, the occupational therapist engages in self-reflective practice to identify any potential biases or prejudices that may impact on her interactions with Ahmed and his parents.

The occupational therapist considers Ahmed's *environment* from many perspectives: cultural, socioeconomic, institutional, physical, and social. She identifies that he attends the mosque weekly with his family and enjoys this, including socializing with the other children there, but is not yet friends with anyone in his neighbourhood. Ahmed's mother expresses concern that Ahmed might be made fun of either at school or in the neighbourhood, because of his ethnic and cultural background. She also reports that she feels helpless in their new host country as she does not yet speak the language. Ahmed's father states that he would like to be able to drive to take Ahmed to school and extracurricular activities. In addition to speaking with Ahmed's family, the occupational therapist considers the teacher's and fellow students' sensitivity towards Ahmed and their cultural awareness. Occupational therapists should also be aware that conflict may not only exist between refugees and asylum seekers and the host culture, but may also come from other ethnic groups.

The PEO model identifies the areas of *occupation* as self-care, productivity, and leisure (Law et al., 1996). Wilcock (1993) argues that a varied and full occupational lifestyle will maintain and improve health and well-being if it enables people to be creative and engage physically, mentally, and socially. The occupational therapist identifies that Ahmed used to enjoy playing football but now plays no sport. During her observations, she also notes that he enjoys art and this is a time when he seems to take pride in his achievements.

Following the occupational therapist's observations and liaison with Ahmed, his teacher, and his parents, they all identify some goals that everyone wants to work towards. These include:

- Supporting Ahmed to improve his performance in the areas of cutting, writing, and bilateral activities through a programme developed by the occupational therapist.
- Ahmed to join a school football team and a neighbourhood art course.
- The occupational therapist to liaise with Ahmed's school to consider the appropriateness of a school day that celebrates ethnic diversity; this could involve music, food, traditional clothing, and games.
- Ahmed's mother to attend an English course for migrants; the occupational therapist to support her with public transport training and investigating childcare options.
- Ahmed's father to look into getting his driver's licence.

As previously mentioned, the occupational therapist considered Ahmed from, among other things, a cultural and ethnic perspective. This is very important as occupational therapists need to recognize any underlying values, beliefs, or prejudices they have, which may affect their interactions and expectations of people from differing backgrounds, such as refugees and asylum seekers. There is no single solution to identifying and addressing the needs of clients from different ethnic and cultural backgrounds; however, occupational therapists can actively listen, reflect, and seek appropriate and timely support to ensure that their interactions are relevant and meaningful.

Many practitioners are very concerned that they may make a cultural faux pas when working with clients from different cultures to their own. While it is wise to be well informed and sensitive to cultural issues, one should not allow being oversensitive to stop oneself from trying to help. Where anxieties about cultural differences may exist, knowledge about the individual and his or her country of origin can be developed; however, remember that within ethnic groups, culture may differ dramatically. Refugees can often be seen as a homogeneous group and yet they are an extremely diverse population with diverse needs, so occupational therapists should avoid generalizations. Occupational therapists should not be afraid to ask questions and admit to gaps in their understanding.

THE RIGHT TO ENGAGE IN OCCUPATION

The international occupational therapy community has expressed its concern about the issues of marginalized and at-risk populations by releasing a position statement on human rights (World Federation of Occupational Therapists, 2006) and more recently a revised position paper on human displacement (World Federation of Occupational Therapists, 2014). Whilst these documents do not use the terms *occupational justice*, they closely align with people's right to engage in a range of occupations, including educational, social, creative, and spiritual activities to enable them to maintain health, to flourish, and create. In order for occupational therapists to fulfil their mandate to promote human rights and respond to the occupational needs of displaced people, they need to make occupational injustice visible, and increase awareness of underlying conditions, attitudes, and policies that give rise to and sustain occupational injustices.

RESOURCES

There is considerable support and resources available for occupational therapists considering working in this area. Occupational Opportunities for Refugees & Asylum Seekers Inc. is a network of occupational therapists whose focus is to enable people with refugee experiences to participate in daily occupations, life roles, and in their community. They have also produced the *IdiOT's Guide to Working with Refugees* (Occupational Opportunities for Refugees & Asylum Seekers Inc., 2006) which is an orientation to the field of working with refugees. Their Web page has an extensive list of references available (www.oofras.com). In addition, UNHCR and United Nations Children's Emergency Fund are two of the leading authorities taking a proactive stance to improve public awareness and conditions for refugees and asylum seekers. Lastly, OT frontiers (http://www.otfrontiers.co.uk) provides some useful resources.

CONCLUSION

Do not be put off from working with refugee and asylum seeker children by all that you think you do not know. Occupational therapists do have a role to play in bringing occupational injustice issues of refugee and asylum seeker children to light, and they have a transferable skill set that enables them to view not just the individual, but the big picture, and all the factors that prevent occupational justice from being achieved. By using existing models and frameworks, skills, and knowledge, they are in a unique position to enable children who have experienced the traumas of forced migration to not only survive, but thrive.

Acknowledgements

I would like to thank Ms Tara Watts, whose passion for refugee and asylum seeker children, and our fruitful discussions, inspired this writing. I would also like to thank the editors and reviewers for their helpful feedback, and last but not least, Ms Kate Zakaria and Mr Volker Paelke for being great sounding boards.

REFERENCES

Adjukovic, M., Adjukovic, D., 1993. Psychological well-being of refugee children. Child Abuse Neglect 17, 843–854.

Cleveland, J., Rousseau, C., Kronick, R., 2012. Bill C-4: the impact of detention and temporary status on asylum seekers' mental health. <http://oppenheimer.mcgill.ca/IMG/pdf/Impact_of_Bill_C4_on_asylum_seeker_mental_health_full-2.pdf> (accessed 21.06.15.).

Copley, J., Turpin, M., Gordon, S., McLaren, C., 2011. Development and evaluation of an occupational therapy program for refugee high school students. Aust. Occup. Ther. J. 58, 310–316.

Davidson, J., Farrow, C., 2007. Child migration and the construct of vulnerability. <http://www.childtrafficking.com/Docs/savechild_07_cmcv_0108.pdf> (accessed 18.03.15.).

Driver, C., Beltran, R.O., 2010. Impact of refugee trauma on children's role as school students. Aust. Occup. Ther. J. 45, 23–38.

Fernando, C., Ferrari, M., 2013. Handbook of Resilience in Children of War. Springer, New York.

Gupta, J., Sullivan, C., 2013. The central role of occupation in the doing, being and belonging of immigrant women. J. Occup. Sci. 20, 23–35.

Keyes, E.F., Kane, C.F., 2004. Belonging and adapting: mental health of Bosnian refugees living in the United States. Issues Ment. Health Nurs. 25, 809–831. doi:10.1080/01612840490506392.

Law, M., Cooper, B., Rigby, P., Letts, L., 1996. The person-environment-occupational model: a transactive approach to occupational performance. Can. J. Occup. Ther. 63, 9–23.

Law, M., Steinwender, S., Leclair, L., 1998. Occupation, health and well-being. Can. J. Occup. Ther. 65, 81–91.

Lustig, S.L., 2010. An ecological framework for the refugee experience: what is the impact of child development? In: Evans, G.W., Wachs, T.D. (Eds.), Chaos and Its Influence on Children's Development: An Ecological Perspective. American Psychological Association, Washington, DC, pp. 239–252.

McIntyre, T., Barowsky, E.I., Tong, V., 2011. The psychological, behavioral, and educational impact of immigration: helping recent immigration students to succeed in North American schools. <http://aasep.org/fileadmin/user_upload/Protected_Directory/JAASEP/Fall_2011/Psychological_Behavioral_Educational_Impact_of_Immigration.pdf> (accessed 21.01.15.).

Mares, J., Jureidini, J., 2004. Psychiatric assessment of children and families in immigration detention – clinical, administrative and ethical issues. Aust. N. Z. J. Public Health 28, 520–526.

Occupational Opportunities for Refugees & Asylum Seekers Inc., 2006. The idiOT's Guide to Working with Refugees. <http://oofras.files.wordpress.com/2011/03/idiots-guide.pdf> (accessed 27.03.14.).

Office of the High Commissioner for Human Rights, 1989. Convention on the Rights of the Child. <http://www.ohchr.org/en/professionalinterest/pages/crc.aspx> (accessed 27.01.15.).

Robjant, K., Hassan, R., Katona, C., 2009. Mental health implications of detaining asylum seekers: systematic review. Br. J. Psychiatry 194, 306–312. doi:10.1192/bjp.bp.108.053223.

Roebers, C.M., Schneider, W., 1999. Self-concept and anxiety in immigrant children. Int. J. Behav. Dev. 23, 125–147.

Shackman, J., Reynolds, J., 1993. Refugees and mental health: issues for training. <http://www.freedomfromtorture.org/sites/default/files/documents/Shackman-Refugees%26MentalHealth.pdf> (accessed 27.03.15.).

Simó-Algado, S., Mehta, N., Kronenberg, F., Cockburn, L., Kirsh, B., 2002. Occupational therapy intervention with children survivors of war. Can. J. Occup. Ther. 69, 205–217.

Smith, H.C., 2005. Feel the fear and do it anyway: meeting the occupational needs of refugees and people seeking asylum. Br. J. Occup. Ther. 68, 474–476. 2005.

Sultan, A., O'Sullivan, K., 2001. Psychological disturbances in asylum seekers held in long term detention: a participant–observer account. Med. J. Aust. 175, 593–596.

Townsend, E., Wilcock, A.A., 2004. Occupational justice and client-centred practice: a dialogue in progress. Can. J. Occup. Ther. 71, 75–87.

Townsend, E., Whiteford, G., 2005. A participatory occupational justice framework: population-based processes of practice. In: Kronenberg, F., Simo-Algado, S., Pollard, N. (Eds.), Occupational Therapy without Borders: Learning from the Spirit of Survivors. Elsevier Churchill Livingston, Toronto, pp. 110–126.

United Nations Children's Emergency Fund, 2007. Progress for children: a world fit for children statistical review. <http://www.unicef.org/progressforchildren/2007n6/files/Progress_for_Children_-_No._6.pdf> (accessed 07.12.14.).

United Nations High Commissioner for Refugees, 1954. The United Nations conference of plenipotentiaries on the status of refugees and stateless persons: convention relating to the status of refugees. <http://www.ohchr.org/EN/ProfessionalInterest/Pages/StatusOfRefugees.aspx> (accessed 27.01.15.).

United Nations High Commissioner for Refugees, 2011. Working with persons with disabilities in forced displacement. <http://www.unhcr.org/4ec3c81c9.html> (accessed 27.02.15.).

United Nations High Commissioner for Refugees, 2012. A framework for the protection of children. <http://www.unhcr.org/50f6cf0b9.pdf> (accessed 27.02.15.).

United Nations High Commissioner for Refugees, 2014. Demographic and Location Data. <http://www.unhcr.org/54cf9a8f9.html> (accessed 09.06.15.).

Whiteford, G., 2000. Occupational deprivation: global challenge in the new millennium. Br. J. Occup. Ther. 63, 200–204.

Whiteford, G., 2005. Understanding the occupational deprivation of refugees: a case study from Kosovo. Can. J. Occup. Ther. 72, 78–88.

Wilcock, A., 1993. A theory on the human need for occupation. J. Occup. Sci. 1, 17–24.

World Federation of Occupational Therapists, 2006. World Federation of Occupational Therapists (WFOT): Position statement: human rights. <http://www.wfot.org/ResourceCentre.aspx> (accessed 03.08.14.).

World Federation of Occupational Therapists, 2014. World Federation of Occupational Therapists (WFOT): Position paper: human displacement revised. <http://www.wfot.org/ResourceCentre.aspx> (accessed 03.08.14.).

51

COMMUNITY CRAFTS: A SUSTAINABLE RESOURCE CONTRIBUTING TO HEALTH, WELL-BEING, AND COMMUNITY COHESION

JANE DIAMOND ■ IMOGEN GORDON

CHAPTER OUTLINE

This chapter explores the potential benefits and influence of craft and craft groups, in a community setting. It refocuses on the sometimes forgotten power of traditional occupations and their cultural influence, recognized more frequently in the majority world rather than within Western culture. The research discussed in this chapter (Diamond, 2014) highlights the need for ongoing community development where occupational therapy has the potential for a vital role.

Occupational therapy recognizes that individuals live and act within their environments, be it the immediate physical and social, or the wider political, cultural, and economic environments (Kielhofner, 2008). It is these environmental factors that impact upon occupations, defining the form, function, and meaning of them for the individual at any given time (Hocking, 2009; Wilcock and Hocking, 2015). These environ-

ments are often represented by the communities in which people actively and passively engage. Labonte (2012) considers the definition of community as a combination of physical place (geography), our roles and habits (identity), life challenges, and social relationships (institutional relations). These reflect the environments described in occupational therapy theory and can be the greatest cause of occupational deprivation (Whiteford, 2011).

Arts on prescription, a commissioned time-limited arts-based therapy, is recognized for its benefit to people's health and well-being (Crone et al., 2012; Stickley and Hui, 2012). The arts are also being increasingly identified as tools with which communities can organize themselves to support their health and well-being. McDonald and coworkers (2012) propose that community organization, the shared process of identifying community issues and goals and the resources needed to address them, comes from within the culture of a given community. Built upon past actions and future hopes, and expressed through various art forms, community organization is critical to forming identity and creating awareness. Using examples of arts-based projects being utilized by communities to explore their issues and strengths in an effort to increase participation, organize, and effect change, McDonald and colleagues (2012) describe community organization as including the collective resources of a community. In doing so, they describe the notion of social capital in which individual skills and social relationships present within a community are combined to create assets that can be used to achieve a common goal (Ennis and West, 2010; Vyncke et al., 2013). Asset-based community development (Ennis and West, 2010) builds on social capital and similarly relies upon social networks – those vital social connections, relationships, and resources found both within and outside of any given community and which are necessary for building social capital (Ennis and West, 2010; Vyncke et al., 2013). Asset-based community development is goal orientated, assesses strengths, considers environmental factors, and seeks to provide meaningful choices and autonomy. Aspects of social capital and asset-based community development are the implicit influences affecting our community craft groups and were instrumental in the analysis of Jane's research, which will be described below.

RESEARCHING COMMUNITY CRAFT GROUPS

Building on previous research (Diamond, 2013), the study presented in this chapter (see also Diamond, 2014) explored benefits to the well-being of members of two community craft groups (see Case 51-1), based within a suburban, inner-city housing estate. The study focused on the reasons for attendance, perceived benefits to individuals, interactions between the groups and the community, and their sustainability. In addition, the relationship between the groups' functioning and their contribution to the community was explored. All members, irrespective of the presence or not of a medical diagnosis, were invited to participate, in recognition that social determinants can equally affect well-being (World Health Organization, 2011). Jane undertook this research as part of

her occupational therapy Masters degree, and was supported by Imogen as her research supervisor.

In the UK, at the time of the research, there was growing recognition of the importance of well-being for health (HM Government, 2010a), becoming evident within health and social policy (Department of Health, 2014). This policy targeted health promotion and ill-health prevention at a community level (HM Government, 2010b). In addition, there has been a long-standing drive to move occupational therapy to the promotion of health (College of Occupational Therapists, 2013). In this study, carried out 4 focus groups, with a total of 19 participants from two craft groups. In addition, as a worker within the community, Jane was able to draw on interactions from the preceding 12-month period with the participants outside of the focus groups. Sampling was purposeful and homogenous, seeking participants from two specific community craft groups. The only inclusion criterion was to be a member of one of the craft groups. It was not the intention to sample only those with diagnosed health conditions. The community as a whole experienced a higher number of lifestyle diseases and lower life expectancy than the UK national average. Interpretive interactionism (Denzin, 2001) was used to analyse and interpret the data, which were considered within the socioeconomic context of the community in which the groups were located. We considered not only the immediate human relationships between the group members and their immediate geographic community, but also the social, cultural, economic, and political backdrop to that community.

The Community Setting: The Local Context

The community in which the research project was conducted is based in a multicultural English city. This community is a largely white, blue-collar population, despite the multicultural nature of the wider city. The land was originally a private estate gifted to the city with the remit of providing affordable, good-quality housing, and it still retains a large park area at its centre. Whilst the parkland is an asset, it also divides the community because of its geographic location, with people having to cross the park to get to services on the other side. The area was declared as economically deprived in 2000 and was provided with substantial funding under the then UK Government's New

CASE 51-1

The 'Needlecrafters' and the 'Knitters'

The Knitters and Needlecrafters (pseudonyms reflecting the activities of the groups) are community craft groups. At the time of writing (October 2015), the Needlecrafters had been established for over 5 years, originally to develop needlecraft and textile skills, such as sewing and knitting, with and for women from the community. A weekly membership fee was charged, which paid for the room hire at a local community centre and for refreshments. They were a constituted group[1], enabling them to apply for external funding, which paid for specialist equipment and supplies. This meant that a member could engage in any available craft for the weekly membership of £2, only paying extra for optional trips to craft exhibitions and events. The group also held and attended craft fairs to raise awareness and additional funds through the display and sale of their own made products.

The Needlecrafters began with two founder members, but quickly increased to four and grew rapidly thereafter. With time, the group became better known locally and was invited to take part in community and city projects, using their combined skills to explore their community identity (McDonald et al., 2012). Greater awareness of the group attracted individuals from the wider community and they began to accept men into the group. At the time of the research they had one male crafter and one noncrafting male participant. This group had recently secured funding for new equipment and supplies that would allow them to expand into paper crafts, such as card-making and quilling, thereby broadening their skill base and appeal.

The Knitters had been running for approximately 2 years, meeting on a weekly basis at a community café established and run by two local women interested in promoting cross-generational activity within their community. The founders supported a number of local groups by providing space and facilities, including a home-education school group, set up and run by local families for their children, and a social group for older adults, set up by a local foundation and supported by its volunteers. There was no charge to attend the Knitters, with current members providing wool and needles for new members from personal donation and some fundraising. However, it was expected that individuals would buy their own wool and needles after an initial period of attendance. Despite being held in a community café, people were allowed to bring their own food and refreshments, but most bought something from the café, recognizing the need to support this local initiative.

The founders had hoped to build textile-based skills within the local community and bring people together. Running the community café, the two founders had a venue for the group but not the skills. Hoping to learn as much themselves, they had co-opted a local woman who had the skill set to offer free and informal teaching of some textile crafts. From this initial starting point the group had become focused on knitting and crocheting through the choices of its members. The group attracted women of all ages, daughters bringing mums along, mums bringing young children with them, and so their target of cross-generational activity was met. By holding the group within the café, not in a separate room, nonmembers were introduced to the group and joined in on the day, or joined up and came more often. In addition, working together with the home education group widened the scope of activity and facilitated interactions between the different groups' members. Each group taught the other new skills, thereby increasing and developing social capital.

---

[1]In the UK, if a community group wishes to apply for funding, it generally requires a bank account. In order to hold a bank account, the group needs to be constituted. A constitution is the written process by which the group commits to abide, setting out the group's aims and intentions. The group will consist of a minimum of three officers – a treasurer, a secretary, and a chairperson – but can include other roles as defined and required by the group, such as vice/deputy roles. The Needlecrafters are a constituted group and consequently have successfully applied for funding available from the local foundation, as well as other sources. This has allowed them to invest in specialist equipment and pay for transportation to events and activities.

Deal for Communities Scheme (NDC), part of the European Social Fund. The NDC considered deprivation at a smaller community level rather than looking at the wider local authority average, which could hide the extent of deprivation in these smaller areas (Fordham, 2010). The scheme provided 39 of the most deprived communities in the UK with funds to be spent within a 10-year period (Fordham, 2010). A community-based group, now a foundation, was established to oversee the spending and investment. This group worked in partnership with the community, engaging them in the decision-making process to identify what would be required in terms of facilities and services to promote urban regeneration. The NDC sought to address three place-based issues – housing and the physical environment, community, and crime – and three person-based issues – worklessness, education, and health (Batty et al., 2010). These were also identified as key areas of need by people within this specific community.

Being several years beyond the funding period, the foundation in the community now consists of a business arm and a charitable arm. The business arm of the foundation has a focus on income generation to support ongoing community development in the area. As a result of the initial and ongoing investment there have been some notable successes. There has been a marked reinvestment and improvement of available housing in both private and social sectors, educational qualifications of children have improved, and there has been a reduction in the rates of crime and antisocial behaviour. As expected in a relatively short time frame, whilst improved, unemployment and lifestyle-related health conditions remain higher than the national average, there is a lower life expectancy (Fordham, 2010), and there is still a significant gap in gross disposable household income levels compared with the national average (Office for National Statistics, 2013). Despite being located in a developed country, this community experiences the results of poverty. This may be exacerbated by the global economic crisis and national political response resulting in a series of austerity measures and changes to the social benefit system. The Joseph Rowntree Foundation (Hastings et al., 2015) has stated that those with the greatest need are being most affected by the cuts, and that the efforts by staff and services at a local level to counter those

effects will be unsustainable in the longer term. The Joseph Rowntree Foundation further identifies that it is preventative and developmental services which are most at risk, and the impact of the loss of these services will likely be more costly in meeting resultant needs in the future. The community perceived the application of austerity measures by the UK Government as having had a negative impact on their lives, particularly for those on a low working wage. One such example, was the introduction in 2013 of under-occupancy rules, known as 'the bedroom tax' (Wilcox, 2014), which applied to social housing tenants in receipt of housing benefit. This meant those living in houses with more bedrooms than the government identified as necessary began to be charged for any additional rooms, or had to move to smaller accommodation. Due to the predominant type of available houses in the area, this could take them away from their immediate social networks, developed over decades, and from family which they may have relied upon or who provided support for child and/or adult care. The breakdown of such social networks may result in a reduction in intergenerational integration, asset sharing, and community cohesion (Ennis and West, 2010).

The Community Setting: National Context

As the NDC funding period came to a close, this community was also experiencing a changing political backdrop. In 2010, the UK Government published the 'Building the Big Society' policy document (Cabinet Office, 2010), setting out policy drivers that would include giving communities greater power and encouraging individuals to be active within their own communities, in a sense reframing previous social policy around this topic. However, being accompanied by austerity measures, this new policy was seen by some as a cloak for financial cuts (Williams, 2012), putting those with greatest need at risk of greatest deprivation (Hastings et al., 2015). A number of health and social policy documents (Department of Health, 2010a; HM Government, 2010a, 2010b) followed, demonstrating the potential for strategic cohesion with 'The Big Society', but with considerable criticism levelled at a lack of substance and practical application (Williams, 2012).

The Big Society notion of building communities as an asset for their own growth, is not a new concept.

Social capital as a conceptual theory dates back to the 1960s and can be defined as the existing or potential capital within a community, which can by that community to address common issues and encourage development (Vyncke et al., 2013). Long-standing exponents across history have highlighted the need for a cohesive and equitable society informed by education, arts, political justice, and fairness in industry (Condorcet, 1796). The aim of such a society would be to ensure happiness through engagement in meaningful occupations and social activity.

FINDINGS FROM THE RESEARCH

The following key themes emerged from the research: the purpose of the groups, the motivations of individuals to join, benefits of engaging in craft-making, and attending the craft groups.

Both groups had begun with a community focus, aiming to provide access to textile-based crafts at an affordable level. Acting for the benefit of themselves and others from within their community, provision was made for all abilities and capabilities. There were multiple reasons for people joining their craft group. Many had joined the Needlecrafters through personal recommendation and one had heard of the group through a supermarket campaign supporting local initiatives. With the Knitters, word of mouth and accessing the venue for other activities were common ways of finding out about the group, and three participants were keen to point out that their enrolment on a locally provided volunteering course had given them the confidence to join in other community activities and groups. Mostly, people joined to learn new skills, refresh unused skills, or develop and improve existing ones. Being part of a group gave them access to practical advice and support, and this was reported as being more useful than reading about a technique in a book.

Most participants were keen to meet new people and increase their social activity. Phrases such as 'getting out' and 'meeting people' were common reasons given for joining the group. This was particularly common among the people with reported health conditions or social factors that would otherwise isolate them in their homes. However, for some, a real appreciation of the social aspect only came once they had joined and developed friendships. One woman mentioned how she would stop and talk to one mum and son in the street, having met them through attending the same group. She felt that she would not have otherwise had the opportunity to meet them and felt less isolated because she could greet someone in the street. She also felt more confident about attending the café alone at other times, more certain of meeting people she now knew. Others used social media to exchange tips outside the group and developed friendships from there, especially if they had other things in common, such as caring for young children or starting their own businesses.

The research built on previous research findings on crafting (Diamond, 2013). Similar to previous findings from Mee, Sumsion and Craik (2004), participants reported the same sense of achievement when completing a project and gaining recognition. In addition, in line with the findings of Reynolds (2004), increased confidence came from learning new skills and perfecting existing ones, and parallel working maximized opportunities for choice, providing a sense of autonomy. References were also made to physical health benefits, as also found by Haltwinger and coworkers (2011), and an increased overall sense of well-being when crafting, as identified by Dickie (2011). This supports the use of a range of crafts as therapeutic media for intervention. In addition, emphasis was placed on the passing on of skills and traditions, of making links to the past, and using those skills to create lasting objects for the future, also found by Haltwinger et al. (2011) and Pöllänen (2013). Art and craft traditions are often recognized for their contributions to physical, emotional, spiritual, and social well-being. Examples include the traditional weaving, lace-making, and painting of Cretan women (Tzanidaki and Reynolds, 2011) or the attempt by Inuit tribes to balance traditional stone carving, hunting, and gathering skills alongside computer technology (Thibeault, 2002). By contrast, traditional occupations in modern Western culture appear less valued (Chard, 2007), and yet the preservation of these traditional craft skills was important for many of the participants. Even those who spoke of 'modern methods', felt it was important to pass on this knowledge to the next generation. The traditional skills became adapted to the needs of the next generation and were made sustainable.

Other benefits arose from attending the craft group more than from crafting alone. The social aspect, more than the acquisition of skills, was most valued once people had joined their group. Similar to the findings of Perruzza and Kinsella (2010), coming to the group was a driver to getting out and engaging with like-minded adults, especially for those with young children at home or for those who were retired. Several participants felt their group provided emotional as well as practical support, particularly when facing a challenging personal circumstance or having a difficult day. The group was somewhere participants could come and 'leave stuff at the door'; it was a break from the daily routine, a safe place to come and 'de-stress'. These additional benefits are also reported by Crone et al. (2012) and Stickley and Hui (2012) in their arts-based therapy groups, and demonstrate how a community-based group can give the same social benefits as a prescribed arts programme.

Through the mutual identification of purpose and need, the groups sought to bring people within the community together and to teach or share skills in an organized way. The founders of both groups sought to alleviate economic circumstance as a barrier to participation. This consideration of one barrier to occupational participation was a significant act in terms of enabling members of the community to access a desired occupation, and it produced a significant result in terms of confidence, self-esteem, and well-being. The findings supported the notion of groups providing a means of being heard, as 'having a safe space to meet, providing mutual support and gaining the knowledge, confidence and skills to engage more widely' (Blake et al., 2008, p. 2). Participants were provided with access to skill acquisition and a place for social participation; the groups built social capital through asset sharing within the community, thereby enhancing cohesion and development (Ennis and West, 2010). Through their interactions with each other, with other groups and the wider community, each craft group developed wider social networks at a group level and for its individual members.

DISCUSSION

Much has been written about the benefits of using craft and creative activities for therapeutic purposes in both formal and informal settings (Crone et al., 2012; Dickie, 2011; Haltwinger et al., 2011; Mee et al., 2004; Perruzza and Kinsella, 2010; Reynolds, 2004). However, whilst engaging in craft-making was described as a valuable and meaningful occupation for individuals, during the study the importance of group membership was afforded greater importance and benefit by the participants. Additional benefits to members' sense of well-being arose from crafting with a group, rather than alone. These benefits included social interaction within and beyond the groups and an increased confidence in the ability to socialize. The groups provided practical support towards finishing a challenging project and achieving a goal, resulting in increased self-efficacy. Group members were able to actively share their skills, and their assets, thereby building social capital within their groups and the wider community. Unexpected skills arose from group membership; the process of setting up a group, organizing, and running a weekly group, and having an awareness of the possible needs of potential members relating to accessibility and ability, were factors both groups faced. The Needlecrafters had a formal structure requiring additional member responsibilities such as the keeping of accounts, organizing group activities, and managing the venue. However, some of these members had commented on how they felt obliged to maintain these roles in the absence of other members being willing to take on the additional responsibilities. Even those without a formal role could identify a role for themselves within each group. In the Needlecrafters, the husband of one member joined in the social aspect of the group and had built a practical role for himself by managing refreshments, moving supplies, and making friendships. Whilst at the Knitters, people were able to support and enable new members to become more skilled. Subsequently, these members provided a welcome to the wider community, acting as ambassadors for the community in their more public, open venue.

Membership of craft groups offered some a means to challenge their health conditions in a positive and productive way. Participants in this study formed close friendships within their groups. Social consciousness was increased as members became more aware of each other's health and well-being needs, more able to offer emotional as well as practical support which was afforded great value. Hammell (2009) considered how occupations that encourage social connections and allow participants to contribute to others and foster a sense of belonging are key factors in creating well-being. Members spoke about needing to encourage more people to come, to make the group bigger, wanting to reach more people who were socially isolated.

Participants felt part of a community of crafters, but were also part of other overlapping, intertwining communities that provided them with a sense of identity and gave them additional roles. Social networks were developed between individuals and groups, something which is vital for building social capital and community cohesion. By building relationships both within and out of the community, individuals had greater awareness of their community and began to take ownership of it. For example, the Needlecrafters set up a petition to save their building which was under threat to be closed. The founders of the Knitters opened their doors to other groups. These acts of community responsibility and ownership helped to increase community cohesion through asset sharing and tackle the issues identified by the NDC and the community itself, further demonstrating social capital. This study reinforced how important social interaction is for community group members. The occupation needs to be meaningful to participants in order to attract them to the group initially, but the feeling of ease with other members and of belonging are the factors that maintain people's attendance.

CONCLUSIONS

UK health policy is recognizing the importance of well-being to promote good health, reduce the need for acute services, and thereby provide a more sustainable health and social care service for the future. Service provision is being targeted at a community level in order to address the specific issues that lead to ill health within communities. Community groups that are supported by an occupational therapist can provide local, low-cost interventions which address social and well-being issues, thus reducing the need for medical intervention. The role of an occupational therapist is in helping set up the structure of the group,

supporting members to identify their capacity, skills and assets, but ultimately giving control of the group to its members, empowering them to become a sustainable resource that other community members can have access to (see, e.g., Ripat et al., 2010).

The combination of an informal community group with an occupation-specific focus and the support of an occupational therapist would be more effective in meeting long-term needs, tackling the social determinants of health at a preventative stage. However, the occupational therapist would need to let go of the control, empowering the community members to own their group, and develop it as they see fit to match their needs as individuals and members within the local context of their community. Social occupational therapy emerged from social inequality in Brazil in the late twentieth century. It addressed the impact of changes to traditional families, social networks and unemployment (Barros, Ghirardi, Lopes, et al., 2011). Occupational therapy would benefit by learning from this to address health, disability, and disadvantage. This re-emphasizes the opportunity for occupational therapy to move beyond community development into wider healthcare, to grasp health promotion at a community level, and to learn from and with local communities.

REFERENCES

Barros, D., et al., 2011. Brazillian experiences in social occupational therapy. In: Kronenberg, F., Pollard, N., Sakellariou, D. (Eds.), Occupational Therapy Without Borders, vol. 2. Elsevier Churchill Livingstone, Oxford, pp. 210–215.

Batty, E., Beatty, C., Foden, M., Lawless, P., Pearson, S., Wilson, I., 2010. The New Deal for Communities Programme: A Final Assessment. The New Deal for Communities National Evaluation: Final report, vol. 7. Department for Communities and Local Government, London.

Blake, G., Diamond, J., Foot, J., Gidley, B., Mayo, M., Shukra, K., et al., 2008. Community Engagement and Community Cohesion. Joseph Rowntree Foundation, York.

Cabinet Office, 2010. The Big Society. <https://www.gov.uk/government/uploads/system/uploads/attachment_data/file/78979/building-big-society_0.pdf> (accessed 12.01.14.).

Chard, J., 2007. Computer games and karate: the arts and crafts of today. Br. J. Occup. Ther. 70 (8), 329.

College of Occupational Therapists, 2013. Written evidence from the British Association and College of Occupational Therapists (LTC 46). <http://www.publications.parliament.uk/pa/cm201415/cmselect/cmhealth/401/401vw43.thm> (accessed 28.04.15.).

Condorcet, N.M.J.A., 1796. Outlines of an historical view of the progress of the human mind. <http://oll.libertyfund.org> (accessed 01.05.15.).

Crone, D.M., O'Connell, E.E., Tyson, P.J., Clark-Stone, F., Opher, S., James, D.V.B., 2012. 'Art lift' intervention to improve mental wellbeing: an observational study from UK General Practice. Int. J. Ment. Health Nurs. 22, 279–286.

Denzin, N., 2001. Interpretive Interactionism, second ed. Sage Publications Ltd., London.

Department of Health, 2010a. Equity and Excellence: Liberating the NHS. The Stationery Office Limited, London.

Department of Health, 2014. Wellbeing: why it matters to health policy. <https://www.gov.uk/government/uploads/system/uploads/attachment_data/file/277566/Narrative__January_2014_.pdf> (accessed 12.06.14.).

Diamond, J., 2013. What are the perceived benefits of engaging in craftwork / handicrafts to the health and wellbeing of adults with chronic or life-threatening health conditions? Unpublished BSc dissertation. Coventry University, Coventry.

Diamond, J., 2014. How does the attendance of a community owned craft group benefit the wellbeing of group members? Unpublished MSc dissertation. Coventry University, Coventry.

Dickie, V.A., 2011. Experiencing therapy through doing: making quilts. OTJR Occup. Participation Health 31 (4), 209–215.

Ennis, G., West, D., 2010. Exploring the potential of social network analysis in asset-based community development practice and research. Aust. Soc. Netw. 63 (4), 404–417.

Fordham, G., 2010. The New Deal for Communities Programme: Achieving a Neighbourhood Focus for Regeneration. The New Deal for Communities National Evaluation: Final report, vol. 1. Communities and Local Government, London.

Haltwinger, E., Rojo, R., Funk, K., 2011. Living with cancer: impact of expressive arts. Occup. Ther. Ment. Health 27, 65.

Hammell, K.W., 2009. Self-care, productivity and leisure, or dimensions of occupational experience? Rethinking occupational 'categories'. Can. J. Occup. Ther. 76 (2), 107–114.

Hastings, A., Bailey, N., Bramley, G., Gannon, M., Watkins, D., 2015. The cost of the cuts: the impact on local government and poorer communities. Joseph Rowntree Foundation, York.

HM Government, 2010a. Confident Communities, Brighter Futures. Department of Health, London.

HM Government, 2010b. Healthy Lives, Healthy People: Our Strategy for Public Health in England. The Stationery Office Limited, London.

Hocking, C., 2009. The challenge of occupation: describing the things people do. J. Occup. Sci. 16 (3), 140–150.

Kielhofner, G., 2008. The environment and human occupation. In: Kielhofner, G. (Ed.), Model of Human Occupation, fourth ed. Lippincott Williams & Wilkins, Baltimore, pp. 85–100.

Labonte, R., 2012. Community, community development, and the forming of authentic partnerships. In: Minkler, M. (Ed.), Community Organizing and Community Building for Health and Wellbeing, third ed. Rutgers University Press, London, pp. 95–109.

McDonald, M., Catalani, C., Minkler, M., 2012. Using the arts and new media in community organizing and community building: an overview and case study from post-Katrina New Orleans. In: Minkler, M. (Ed.), Community Organizing and Community Building for Health and Wellbeing, third ed. Rutgers University Press, London, pp. 288–304.

Mee, J., Sumsion, T., Craik, C., 2004. Mental health clients confirm the value of occupation in building competence and self-identity. Br. J. Occup. Ther. 67 (5), 225–233.

Office for National Statistics, 2013. Regional Profile of East Midland – Economy, June 2013. <http://www.ons.gov.uk/ons/dcp171780_314403.pdf> (accessed 24.05.14.).

Perruzza, N., Kinsella, E., 2010. Creative arts occupations in therapeutic practice: a review of the literature. Br. J. Occup. Ther. 73 (6), 261–268.

Pöllänen, S., 2013. The meaning of craft: craft makers' descriptions of craft as an occupation. Scand. J. Occup. Ther. 20 (3), 217–227.

Reynolds, F., 2004. Textile art promoting wellbeing in long-term illness: some general and specific influences. J. Occup. Sci. 11 (2), 58–67.

Ripat, J.D., Redmond, J.D., Grabowecky, B.R., 2010. The Winter Walkability Project: occupational therapists' role in promoting citizen engagement. Can. J. Occup. Ther. 77 (1), 7–14.

Stickley, T., Hui, A., 2012. Social prescribing through arts on prescription in a UK city: participants' perspectives (part 1). Public Health 126, 574–579.

Thibeault, R., 2002. Fostering healing through occupation: the case of the Canadian Inuit. J. Occup. Sci. 9 (3), 153–158.

Tzanidaki, D., Reynolds, F., 2011. Exploring the meanings of making traditional arts and crafts among older women in Crete, using interpretative phenomenological analysis. Br. J. Occup. Ther. 74 (8), 375–382.

Vyncke, V., De Clerq, B., Stevens, V., Costongs, C., Barbareschi, G., Jónsson, S.H., et al., 2013. Does neighbourhood social capital aid in levelling the social gradient in the health and well-being of children and adolescents? A literature review. BMC Public Health 13 (1), 1–18.

Whiteford, G., 2011. Occupational deprivation: understanding limited participation. In: Christiansen, C.H., Townsend, E.A. (Eds.), Introduction to Occupation: The Art and Science of Living, second ed. Pearson Education Ltd., London, pp. 303–328.

Wilcock, A.A., Hocking, C., 2015. An Occupational Perspective of Health, third ed. Slack Incorporated, Thorofare, NJ.

Wilcox, S., 2014. Housing Benefit Size Criteria: Impacts for Social Sector Tenants and Options For Reform. Joseph Rowntree Foundation, York.

Williams, B., 2012. The big society: post-bureaucratic social policy in the twenty-first century? Polit. Q. 82 (Suppl. 1), 120–132.

World Health Organization, 2011. Rio Political Declaration on Social Determinants of Health. <http://www.who.int/sdhconference/declaration/Rio_political_declaration.pdf?ua=1> (accessed 04.05.15.).

52

COMMUNITY HEALTH PROMOTION IN A RESOURCE-CONSTRAINED SETTING: LESSONS FROM MALAWI

HIDENORI MATSUO

CHAPTER OUTLINE

In recent years, the role of occupational therapy has been expanded to include disease prevention and health promotion. Many studies have discussed occupational therapy's role in and its contribution to health promotion (e.g., Finlayson and Edwards, 1995; Jaffe, 1986; Moll et al., 2013; Scaffa et al., 2010; Scriven and Atwal, 2004). Health promotion and occupational therapy often share the same goals, and the synergy between them can improve the health and well-being of individuals, communities, and larger populations (Tucker et al., 2014). However, little has been reported on the potential contribution of occupational therapists to community health promotion in resource-constrained settings, such as in sub-Saharan African countries.

As an occupational therapist with 3.5 years of clinical experience, I had the opportunity to expand my horizons when I decided to work on a community health project in Malawi as a volunteer. My duties included conducting a health needs survey, improving health education and promotion, and most importantly, contributing to capacity development of Malawian health workers and other stakeholders at the community level. While facing several difficulties throughout the process, this experience stimulated my interest in the ways occupational therapy and health promotion are interlinked and how occupational therapists can contribute to community health promotion in developing countries.

The aim of this chapter is to explore how occupational therapists might be able to work in community health promotion in resource-limited settings, utilizing their unique knowledge and perspective. After setting the background, I introduce my experience in Malawi. Lastly, I discuss the role of occupational therapy in community health promotion and make recommendations for further developing that role.

PROMOTING HEALTH AND WELL-BEING IN THE COMMUNITY

Paradigm Shift Towards Health Promotion

The concepts of disease prevention and health promotion have changed drastically over the course of time and they continue to evolve. The epidemiological transition (Omran, 1971) is characterized by a radical shift in human mortality and morbidity from infectious diseases to chronic diseases as the leading cause of death. Medical advances played an important role in the epidemiological transition but these cannot always address human behaviour and lifestyle changes. Changes in human behaviour are complex and associated with historic development. As the field of medicine struggled to develop strategies to effect behavioural change, there was a renewed interest in socioenvironmental factors. The socioenvironmental approach focuses on communities and environments, and its main strategies are 'encouraging community organization, action and empowerment, political action and advocacy' (Baum, 2008, p. 445).

Community Approaches in Health Promotion

The World Health Organization (1986, no page number) defines health promotion as 'the process of enabling people to increase control over, and to improve, their health'. The Ottawa Charter for health promotion emphasized the importance of social determinants of health, beyond risk factors for diseases. The Ottawa Charter also outlined the central role of health promotion and described some appropriate strategies to achieve this, including creating supportive environments, strengthening community actions, and developing personal skills (World Health Organization, 1986). With the emphasis shifting towards the social and environmental determinants of health, several concepts, such as community participation, equity, and empowerment, emerged in the new health promotion movement in the 1980s, which changed the discourse of health promotion theory and practice (Robertson and Minkler, 1994). However, these bottom-up strategies require different skills from health promoters (Naidoo and Wills, 2009). In addition, due to the nature of health promotion, such practices are far more complex than the more traditional top-down medical approach and are difficult to accomplish. The complexity of factors influencing community participation reveals the difficulties in identifying the direct link between health outcomes and such approaches (Rifkin, 2014). It can be argued that community involvement approaches should be understood as a process supporting concrete interventions to improve health outcomes, rather than as an intervention-driven perspective or predecided, imported intervention protocols (Rifkin, 2014; South, 2014; Trickett et al., 2011). However, much remains to be understood about the nature of successful community approaches in health promotion and the influencing factors (South, 2014).

THE SYNERGY OF HEALTH PROMOTION AND OCCUPATIONAL THERAPY

The principles of health promotion overlap with the goal of occupational therapy. Occupational therapists traditionally focus on understanding health-related needs of people, focusing on occupation and environment, and respecting people's self-determination. Occupational therapy is one of the health professions to have at its heart a consideration of both bodily function and physical and sociocultural environments, and how these interact. These important concepts of occupational therapy are clearly shown in the definition of occupational therapy by the World Federation of Occupational Therapists (2012, no page number):

> Occupational therapy is a client-centred health profession concerned with promoting health and well-being through occupation. The primary goal of occupational therapy is to enable people to participate in the activities of everyday life. Occupational therapists achieve this outcome by working with people and communities to enhance their ability to engage in the occupations they want to, need to, or are expected to do, or by modifying the occupation or the environment to better support their occupational engagement.

Tucker et al. (2014) highlighted the similarities between health promotion and occupational therapy for enabling people to improve the control they have over their own health. Finlayson and Edwards (1995) state that 'health promotion is helping people help themselves – within health promotion, people identify their health needs, and utilize available tools/information to elicit change in their own lives' (p. 72). They also emphasized the importance of grassroots ownership in health promotion and the influences between the individual and the environment. These basic principles of health promotion fit naturally with occupational therapy's approach. The clients of occupational therapy may be communities, organizations, or populations (Canadian Association of Occupational Therapists, 2008). Occupational therapists can be in a better position as facilitators of the health of individuals and populations with a focus on community participation, empowerment, and the importance of purposeful, productive, and meaningful occupation (Scaffa et al., 2010; Tucker et al., 2014).

A CASE STUDY IN MALAWI

Personal History

Why did I get involved in the public health project in Malawi as a volunteer? Since my college days, I have been interested in personal and environmental factors in human life. After graduation, I began working in a hospital in Japan as an occupational therapist. I mainly supported rehabilitation for people dealing with the effects of stroke or hypertension. I recognized that many people were suffering from lifestyle-related diseases and chronic illnesses as a result of rapidly changing lifestyle patterns; these are usually due to a complex mix of economic, social, and cultural change (leading to increased consumption of fatty and sugary foods, a sedentary culture of passive entertainment, more smoking and drinking, more intense working practices etc.), which in turn are often the result of the development and the adoption of a Western-style consumer culture. This experience made me understand the importance of disease prevention and health promotion in a broader perspective. Moreover, I was interested in working in developing countries with my expertise of occupational therapy as a profession concerning human life, in order to broaden my horizons. Consequently, I applied for an opportunity to volunteer in community health in Malawi. Throughout my stay in Malawi, I faced several challenges, including changing the way of thinking about the traditional

therapist–patient relationship and applying the knowledge of occupational therapy in the public health field.

Health Situation in Malawi

Malawi, located in Southeastern Africa, is considered to be one of the world's poorest countries (World Bank, 2015). The country is facing numerous challenges, such as a high burden of infectious disease, including HIV/AIDS and malaria, a high incidence of maternal and child health problems, and a growing prevalence of noncommunicable diseases (World Health Organization, 2009). In 2004, the Malawi government initiated a health sector-wide approach in collaboration with donors, which led to the reprioritization of the Essential Health Package, which focuses on 11 major health conditions (vaccine-preventable diseases; acute respiratory infections; malaria; tuberculosis; sexually transmitted infections including HIV/AIDS; diarrhoeal diseases; schistosomiasis; malnutrition; ear, nose, and skin infections; perinatal conditions; and common injuries) throughout the country (Ministry of Health Malawi, 2011a; World Health Organization, 2009). The Malawi government and various donors are working together to tackle these burdens. The national health strategic plan for 2011 to 2016 was launched in 2011 to address the burden of disease by encouraging health promotion and community participation (Ministry of Health Malawi, 2011a). Furthermore, the health promotion policy was established in 2013 to deal with the social determinants of health, including empowerment for social behaviour change and other wider socioeconomic and environmental factors, in order to tackle the current burden of diseases (Ministry of Health Malawi, 2013). This health promotion policy was led by the African Regional Health Promotion policy adopted by the World Health Organization Regional Committee for Africa (Ministry of Health Malawi, 2013; World Health Organization Regional Office for Africa, 2013).

The Japan International Cooperation Agency (JICA) is one of the donors who support the health sector in Malawi. More than 1500 JICA volunteers, mainly working at the community level, have been dispatched to Malawi in different technical fields, including health, nutrition, HIV/AIDS, and community development (JICA, 2012). I worked as a JICA volunteer at a rural health facility in the district of Mzimba.

Project Overview

Located in the north of Malawi, Mzimba is the largest district in the country. Mzimba South Health District includes 31 health facilities serving a population of 524 000 (Ministry of Health Malawi, 2011b). The Mzimba district hospital oversees the training of community health workers with the purpose of improving health services at the community level. The community health workers, who are called health surveillance assistants (HSAs), play a central role in the Essential Health Package as grassroots healthcare providers (Ministry of Health Malawi, 2009). HSAs are responsible for promoting healthy lifestyles and healthy environments at the community level while working with other community-based workers across different sectors (Ministry of Health Malawi, 2011a). However, it was difficult to provide high-quality services since the HSAs would only train for 10 to 12 weeks in total. Therefore, the government requested several volunteers to help support several health centres located in the Mzimba South Health District in order to improve the health workers' skills. Volunteers were expected to support and collaborate with HSAs at the local level, but also to exchange information with other volunteers at the district hospital level. During this time period, volunteers worked under the coordination of the JICA's local field coordinator.

As one of the JICA volunteers, I was assigned to a health centre located in the Mzimba South Health District from June 2011 to December 2012. The health centre is located in a town near the border with Zambia, in the southern part of Mzimba district, with 15 000 people living in this area. Ten HSAs cover this area. The health centre accepts outpatients and provides basic healthcare and obstetrical services. The health centre has six health posts, which are the focal points for providing basic health services at the community level. These health posts are located 6 to 14 km away from the health centre. The community health workers, called health surveillance assistants (HSAs), are responsible for providing the following community-based healthcare tasks:

- Conducting under-5 clinics (immunization, growth monitoring, and vitamin A distribution for children under 5 years old and their mothers).

- Promoting antenatal/postnatal care and family planning.
- Conducting health education.
- Organizing and managing village health committees.
- Monitoring safe water supply.
- Conducting surveys of seasonal infectious diseases.
- Implementing various campaigns about cholera and other diseases.

In addition, the HSAs and other community-based health workers are expected to raise awareness about health promotion interventions at household and community levels (Ministry of Health Malawi, 2013).

The project activities mainly focus on community-level approaches, including enhancing the under-5 clinics, encouraging relevant health education, and promoting capacity building among health workers and communities. At the time of my involvement (2011–2012), the HSAs were facing tremendous difficulties in their workload which was directly related to the health situation in remote areas. Therefore, the project priority was focusing on the HSAs' day-to-day work in order to improve the quality of health services and health-promotion interventions at the community level.

Within the project framework, I encouraged a process of 'thinking and acting on our own' (Japan Overseas Cooperative Association, 2012) for sustainable interventions, with the collaboration of HSAs and communities. Figure 52-1 shows the conceptual model of this approach.

The main concepts of the approach include:

- Identifying the health-related needs in the community and clarifying the problems which can be solved within the available resources by HSAs and community members.
- Conducting effective health education and interventions with community members according to their needs.
- Strengthening the cooperation between health workers and community members.

Project Results

At the end of the dispatch period in December 2012, several positive changes were observed. The main

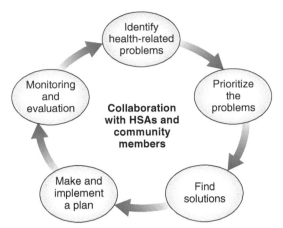

FIGURE 52-1 ■ Community-led intervention model. The model emphasizes a continuous process for effective health education and community participation.

positive results included an increase in vaccinated children, an increase in the number of participants in the nutrition programme, and an improvement in hygiene conditions in some villages in the catchment area. HSAs and community members dealt with health-related needs, using the locally available resources, and they implemented these processes independently of JICA volunteers. For example, HSAs, village health committees, and under-5 clinic volunteers organized village inspections and health education sessions in each village. Afterwards, there was an increase in the numbers of pit latrines, refuse pits, and hand-washing facilities. HSAs visited some households individually and conducted health talks whenever they saw any health-related problems. Although these changes were small, HSAs and community members collaborated together and they were able to deal with health-related problems at the village level.

DISCUSSION

This case study raises two questions when examining occupational therapy's role in community health promotion: (a) how the specificity of the context affects health promotion practices in the community, and (b) how an occupational therapy perspective can be applied in such practices. Although the project was not structured based on a conventional occupational therapy framework, it is important to discuss these questions and current challenges in order to expand the contribution of occupational therapists in community health promotion.

It is important to consider the importance of community empowerment. High dependency on donors in Malawi raises concerns regarding the uses of external funding. Asking communities to implement programmes that are planned and evaluated in someone else's terms may lead to commitments that are maintained only for 'as long as the money lasts' (Green and Kreuter, 2004, p. 268). In addition, the long history of external support might have caused a dependency mind-set in the community, which would be resistant to the efforts of the government and the donors to improve health-related conditions in Malawi. Moreover, there are difficulties in achieving sustainable changes within the donor's framework, which require the necessity of showing the impact of projects over a relatively short-term period. As a result, the aid from donors has mainly focused on medical or disease-specific aspects. For these reasons, health promotion practitioners are required to work as facilitators, beyond the traditional expert-led relationship, to improve the community's ownership and to focus on other social and environmental determinants of health and well-being. The client-centred principle of occupational therapy can contribute to enabling all people to improve the control over their health and well-being.

Occupational therapy values can shed light on the issues which have been overlooked by the current aid flows in Malawi. The outcomes of the project only focused on some specific aspects of health in the community, such as immunization, nutrition, and sanitation, among others. Although these aspects have a major impact on health, other important dimensions of health and well-being (e.g., participation in society) can be more emphasized to improve the quality of life. In addition, the project might have missed opportunities to include more vulnerable populations in the community, such as people with disabilities. This raises concerns that community members from a particular population may have been excluded from the benefits of the project. The occupational perspective should be emphasized as an essential element for health promotion (Scaffa et al., 2010) to increase the awareness of the benefits and risk factors associated with occupational engagement across the lifespan (Moll et al., 2013). For these purposes, occupational therapy's values should be enhanced to consider the influence of meaningful and purposeful occupation and the environment. Although there is little awareness in the public health field regarding the role of occupational engagement (Moll et al., 2013), the inclusion of an occupational perspective might help address the complexities of health and well-being in the community. The existing challenges in community health promotion relating to the need for evidence-based practices, offer an opportunity for occupational therapy to contribute by evaluating health and well-being, considering the meaning and purpose to life, beyond the traditional health indicators which are commonly used.

There are a number of challenges when adopting occupational therapy's knowledge in such practices. Occupational therapy values are not widely recognized from other health professionals in the international development assistance field. Moll et al. (2013) discussed the challenges to promoting occupation related to the language used to communicate occupational therapy ideas and the multidimensional nature of occupational outcomes. This suggests that occupational therapists should develop a system to show occupational therapy's values to other health professionals in a clear way. Furthermore, more role models are necessary to demonstrate how occupational therapists can work from a health promotion approach in practice (Holmberg and Ringsberg, 2014; Leclair, 2010). Additional training and educational opportunities are needed to complement therapists' occupation-based knowledge in health promotion on the societal level (Holmberg and Ringsberg, 2014; Tucker et al., 2014). Finally, a new framework is required to describe occupational therapy's added value in community health promotion, considering the analysis of occupation at the community level. To achieve this, occupational therapists need to examine the most effective way to capture the health-promoting value of occupation for all clients, from the individual to the community level (Leclair, 2010; Moll et al., 2013). Traditional categories of occupation, such as self-care, productivity, and leisure, should be reconsidered so that occupational therapists may identify

closer correlations between occupational engagement and well-being (Hammell, 2009).

Overall, there are important reasons why it would be useful to increase occupational therapy's role in community health promotion in resource-constrained settings. By considering the current challenges, occupational therapists might contribute to the improvement of health and well-being with their unique knowledge and perspectives.

CONCLUSION

In this chapter, I presented my experience working in a health promotion programme in Malawi and explored potential contributions of occupational therapists in community health promotion in resource-constrained settings. Although the role of occupational therapy in the international development field is underdeveloped, I believe that occupational therapists can help improve community health and well-being through an occupational perspective. Developing a clearer system to describe the value of occupation will allow occupational therapists to work more effectively in community health promotion.

Acknowledgements

I would like to thank Professors William Sherlaw and Eric Breton for their helpful advice and critical suggestions on earlier drafts of this chapter. I also wish to thank Gavin Foster McDonough, Aleksandra Dysko, and Fabienne Azzedine for reviewing an earlier version of this chapter.

REFERENCES

Baum, F., 2008. The New Public Health, third ed. Oxford University Press, Oxford.

Canadian Association of Occupational Therapists, 2008. CAOT Position Statement: Occupations and Health. <https://www.caot.ca/pdfs/positionstate/occhealth.pdf> (accessed 26.04.15.).

Finlayson, M., Edwards, J., 1995. Integrating the concepts of health promotion and community into occupational therapy practice. Can. J. Occup. Ther. 62 (2), 70–75.

Green, L., Kreuter, M., 2004. Health Program Planning: An Educational and Ecological Approach, fourth ed. McGraw-Hill, New York.

Hammell, K.W., 2009. Self-care, productivity, and leisure, or dimensions of occupational experience? Rethinking occupational 'categories'. Can. J. Occup. Ther. 76 (2), 107–114.

Holmberg, V., Ringsberg, K.C., 2014. Occupational therapists as contributors to health promotion. Scand. J. Occup. Ther. 21, 108–115.

Jaffe, E., 1986. The role of occupational therapy in disease prevention and health promotion. Am. J. Occup. Ther. 40 (11), 749–752.

Japan International Cooperation Agency, 2012. Annual Report 2011. <http://www.jica.go.jp/malawi/english/office/others/c8h0vm000001k4nx-att/report2011.pdf> (accessed 11.03.15.).

Japan Overseas Cooperative Association, 2012. JOCA Malawi Project for Farmers' Self-Reliance towards Community Empowerment in Mzimba 2005-2012. <http://www.joca.or.jp/upload/item/1227/File/malawi_brochure._en.pdf> (accessed 11.03.15.).

Leclair, L.L., 2010. Re-examining concepts of occupation and occupation-based models: occupational therapy and community development. Can. J. Occup. Ther. 77 (1), 15–21.

Ministry of Health Malawi, 2009. Health Surveillance Assistant Training Manual Facilitator's Guide. <https://www.advancingpartners.org/sites/default/files/malawi_health_surveillance_assistant_training_manual_facilitators_guide.pdf> (accessed 11.03.15.).

Ministry of Health Malawi, 2011a. Malawi Health Sector Strategic Plan 2011–2016. <http://www.medcol.mw/commhealth/publications/3Malawi HSSP Final Document (3).pdf> (accessed 11.03.15.).

Ministry of Health Malawi, 2011b. Mzimba District Implementation Plan. Unpublished report, Malawi.

Ministry of Health Malawi, 2013. Health Promotion Policy. <http://healthpromotion.gov.mw/index.php/2013-08-12-12-52-31/2013-08-12-12-52-32/policies-strategies?download=5:malawi-health-promotion-policy> (accessed 25.04.15.).

Moll, S.E., Gewurtz, R.E., Krupa, T.M., Law, M.C., et al., 2013. Promoting an occupational perspective in public health. Can. J. Occup. Ther. 80, 111–119.

Naidoo, J., Wills, J., 2009. Foundations for Health Promotion, third ed. Elsevier, London.

Omran, A.R., 1971. The epidemiologic transition. A theory of the epidemiology of population change. Milbank Mem. Fund. Q. 49 (4), 509–538. <http://www.ncbi.nlm.nih.gov/pubmed/5155251> (accessed 06.09.15.).

Rifkin, S.B., 2014. Examining the links between community participation and health outcomes: a review of the literature. Health Policy Plan. 29, ii98–ii106.

Robertson, A., Minkler, M., 1994. New health promotion movement: a critical examination. Health Educ. Q. 21 (3), 295–312.

Scaffa, M.E., Van Slyke, N., Brownson, C.A., 2010. Occupational therapy services in the promotion of health and the prevention of disease and disability. Am. J. Occup. Ther. 62 (6), 694–703.

Scriven, A., Atwal, A., 2004. Occupational therapists as primary health promoters: opportunities and barriers. Br. J. Occup. Ther. 67 (10), 424–429.

South, J., 2014. Health promotion by communities and in communities: current issues for research and practice. Scand. J. Public Health 42 (15 Suppl.), 82–87.

Trickett, E.J., Beehler, S., Deutsch, C., Green, L.W., Hawe, P., McLeroy, K., et al., 2011. Advancing the science of community-level interventions. Am. J. Public Health 101 (8), 1410–1419.

Tucker, P., Vanderloo, L.M., Irwin, J.D., Mandich, A.D., Bossers, A.M., 2014. Exploring the nexus between health promotion and occupational therapy: synergies and similarities. [Explorer le lien entre la promotion de la sante et l'ergotherapie: Synergies et similarites.]. Can. J. Occup. Ther. 81, 183–193.

World Bank, The, 2015. GDP per capita (current US$). <http://data.worldbank.org/indicator/NY.GDP.PCAP.CD?order=wbapi_data_value_2013+wbapi_data_value&sort=asc> (accessed 05.09.15.).

World Federation of Occupational Therapists, 2012. Definition of occupational therapy. <http://www.wfot.org/aboutus/about occupationaltherapy/definitionofoccupationaltherapy.aspx> (accessed 20.04.15.).

World Health Organization, 1986. The Ottawa Charter for Health Promotion. <http://www.who.int/healthpromotion/conferences/previous/ottawa/en/> (accessed 21.04.15.).

World Health Organization, 2009. WHO Country Cooperation Strategy 2008–2013 Malawi. <http://www.who.int/countryfocus/cooperation_strategy/ccs_mwi_en.pdf> (accessed 11.03.15.).

World Health Organization Regional Office for Africa, 2013. Health Promotion: A Strategy for the African Region. <http://www.afro.who.int/index.php?option=com_docman&task=doc_download&gid=7972&Itemid=2593> (accessed 25.04.15.).

53

INCLUSIVE EDUCATION IN THE FRAMEWORK OF AN INTERNATIONAL COOPERATION PROJECT: A COMMUNITY APPROACH FOR THE INCLUSION AND PARTICIPATION OF CHILDREN

ESTHER DOMINGUEZ VEGA

■ ■ ■ ■ ■ ■ ■ ■ ■ ■ ■ ■ ■ ■ ■ ■ ■ ■ ■ ■

CHAPTER OUTLINE

This chapter summarizes the experience of an occupational therapist who contributed in an inclusive education project in a rural area in the south of Senegal for 2 years. The account presented here comes from my reflections on my involvement in the project. The aim of this chapter is to highlight the development of a community-based approach to intervention, based on the needs and resources available within the community. More specifically, in this chapter I will present a project which aimed to increase access to schooling for disabled children in a rural area of Senegal.

Approximately one third of the 72 million children who are deprived of access to education in the world experience some kind of disability (Handicap International, 2012; Organisation des Nations Unies pour l'Education, la Science et la Culture, 2007). However, this percentage may vary considerably from one country to another. In countries of middle to low income, such as Senegal, the schooling of disabled children takes place mainly in specialized centres, generally found in the major cities. This educational system inevitably excludes poor families, in particular those coming from rural areas, and accentuates the vicious cycle of poverty and disability. Inclusive education projects are intended to address this problem by reducing exclusion and finding effective solutions to the individual needs of the students (Handicap International, 2012, United Nations Children's Emergency Fund, 2013, 2014).

In Senegal, there is a general idea that school is no place for disabled children. The absence of technical and human resources that can address the social causes of disability contributes to the fact that people are often not aware of the causes or the origin of the disability, and do not know which interventions are available to improve the development of disabled children. Disability is perceived as an unchangeable status and families can do little or nothing about it. Hence, the general thought is that disabled children do not have the necessary abilities to learn at school to improve their situation. The origin of the disability is usually attributed to the violation of certain social standards by the family, which creates a stigma within the community. Consequently, many families accept the situation with shame and guilt, which leads them to manage it exclusively within their household.

Furthermore, the lack of economic resources drives the families to sacrifice the enrolment of disabled children in school in favour of the rest of the children under their care, seeing that they cannot meet schooling expenses for all of them. Similarly, the girls' enrollment in school is undermined by the social priority of boys in the family unit.

The lack of resources within schools is another aspect that hinders access to education by disabled children. Teachers face the inclusive education policies with uncertainty and scepticism, due to the high ratio of students per class and the lack of technical and material resources they have in hand to address the inclusion of disabled children.

THE RELEVANCE OF AN INCLUSIVE EDUCATION PROJECT

In order to address the situation, a cooperative development project was implemented in a rural area in the south of Senegal. This project was managed by an international organization. The objectives of the project were to facilitate the access of disabled children to the regular education system and to transform schools into inclusive facilities with technical and material capacity adapted to the needs of the students.

During the 4 years of implementation, 100 schools were involved in the project.

My involvement in the project began 2 years after it had started. In those 2 years, the organization had already made significant progress in raising awareness, within both the educational community and the social and family environments. The project team had detected a great number of children who were excluded from the educational system. These workers developed awareness-raising within the families and teachers in order to facilitate the access of the children to school and their inclusion in school. The organization covered schooling expenses, thus addressing a main obstacle to participation. Once a student had enrolled at a school, the project team would develop an individualized health and rehabilitation action plan.

However, there was still an important obstacle to overcome. The children who presented high levels of physical impairment limiting their mobility were finding it hard to get involved in school activities. My task in this project was to foster the children's participation in the school and family environments through ergonomic adaptations, support products, and the removal of architectural boundaries.

OCCUPATIONAL THERAPY CONTRIBUTION TO AN INCLUSIVE EDUCATION PROJECT

When we visited his school, Idrissa (all names used in this chapter are pseudonyms) was 8 years old. He presented with spastic tetraparesis and dysarthria. What the teacher told us clearly showed how his inclusion in the school was managed:

Idrissa is a pleasant boy, we all love him in the school. At first, he came every day and sat there, in the first row. He is very active and is constantly drawing the attention of the other students while they are working. That's the reason why I decided to sit him in the last row. He can barely sit still on his chair, and he cannot write yet, he cannot even grab the pencil because of his disability. He has trouble speaking and I cannot always understand him; it is very difficult to work with him.

Thanks to the work of the project team, the boy had surpassed the cultural, social, and economic boundaries that prevented him from accessing the school. However, the lack of adapted material and the architectural boundaries did not allow him to be involved in its activities. Due to inactivity, caused by the lack of resources allowing the child to participate, he answered by drawing attention from his classmates and making it difficult for them to carry out their work. The teacher decided that Idrissa should sit alone at the back. This decision made it even harder for him to participate.

Such situations contribute to the representation of disabled children as those 'who cannot integrate in the educational system'. Hence the disabled children's inclusion process is given an exclusively charitable and caregiving nature. Failed attempts at inclusion can generate frustration in children, who might perceive the school environment as hostile. This brings out their 'incompetence' when it comes to achieving the requirements imposed by their environment to enjoy full participation.

Idrissa's case is an example of the limited opportunities for participation that can be available to children with physical impairments. Projects which aim to increase inclusion need to develop strategies aimed to overcome both sociocultural boundaries, but also material solutions to transform the schools into accessible spaces.

Cooperation projects have a specific duration. Once the project is over, the children continue school if families assume the costs of schooling. Teachers no longer receive support. In view of this situation, it was important to develop an inclusive and sustainable project in which parents, teachers, and children perceived a change in their welfare and development. To ensure the sustainability of the project outcomes (i.e., children remaining in school after the completion of the project), it was important to network with the local community. This was necessary, because families and teachers assume the effort to keep children with disabilities at school if there are positive results in its development and prosperity. The community had to see that school is a resource for everyone to develop to the fullest.

CONTEXT ANALYSIS

My visits to the community made it clear that it was necessary to obtain more detailed information about the context in order to analyse the socioeconomic situation of the families and the health and educational services available to them. Beyond the material factors, there was also the social and cultural environment that largely determined the daily activities of people and marked the regulations for the basic activities of life. The sociocultural environment plays a decisive role in how activities such as eating, clothing, personal hygiene, writing, and praying are performed. Understanding these factors was essential in order to facilitate the occupational performance of the children and their participation within their community.

Close collaboration with the project workers was a key factor to get to know the context. Although they did not have healthcare experience, local workers had a defined social profile and a profound knowledge of the environment. Furthermore, they had established a privileged trust relationship with the families. Working together with the local team, made it easier to access the families and obtain valuable information. I paid special attention to the availability of support devices, to the characteristics of education facilities and functional rehabilitation services, and to the natural, social, and cultural environment.

The Natural Environment and Changes Derived From Human Activity

The south of Senegal is a tropical region, rich in natural resources, that suffers from the effects of an armed conflict that has been going on since 1982. The intermittent clashes between the rebels and the military, the presence of mines, displaced population, and physical and psychological consequences are part of this context.

The absence of basic infrastructure in many areas and the apparently makeshift growth of towns and cities can have a big impact on the possibilities for mobility, even within urban areas. The heavy downpours during rainy season and the sandy nature of the ground, for example, can present a big obstacle for people with reduced mobility.

The Social and Cultural Environment

The place of residence and the income source of each family are decisive factors to access the locally available services. In many cases, the family unit acts as the

Binta

Binta is the eldest daughter of a large family. Apart from going to school every day, she takes care of her brothers when her mother goes to work in the market. As a result of the poliomyelitis she suffered when she was small, she uses two tall crutches to move around. Under the project's offer, Binta's family accepted for her to go to the hospital. There, the medical team determined that the best option was to perform surgery in order to be able to use an orthotic device to enhance movement. The fear of surgery and the fact that she would be far away from home during the months of rehabilitation, made the family decide against the offer, although all costs would be covered by the project. However, the possibility of using a wheelchair was well-received. It did not mean away time for the child, it allowed moving more easily to school, and it made it possible for her to help her mother move goods to the market.

decisive factor in the choice of intervention. The example provided in Case 53-1 is a case in point.

This example comes to illustrate how interventions exclusively based on biomedical protocols are not always appropriate. Mistrust towards healthcare service quality, the lack of guarantees that it would make them reach functional movement within an environment where long journeys over irregular surfaces were required, the long-term costs that the family had to face for maintaining and renewing the orthosis once the project was over, and the family's desire that the girl should follow a particular occupational pattern, all had an influence on the choice of intervention. The use of a locally made wheelchair should facilitate maintenance and repair within the community, without high costs involved for the family once the project was over. It did not mean an invasive intervention from healthcare services with scarce human and material resources. This intervention also enabled Binta to fulfil the socially recognized role of being able to help in household tasks and in taking care of others. Furthermore, it made it possible for her to move independently and safely.

Awa

Awa suffers from right-side hemiparesis. Although she can walk by herself, travelling the long distance from her home to school involves a great deal of effort. She is part of a community in which following the rules of usage of right and left hand for different activities is essential. In her school, there is a free canteen service for all students. This service was implemented to improve child nutritional status and avoid the lack of assistance during those hours in which the children who lived faraway had to go home to eat. As she cannot use her right hand to eat, Awa is deprived of participating in a collective activity with her fellow students and instead needs to go back home to eat, missing the afternoon classes.

The parameters that decide the appropriate ways of carrying out daily life activities are other aspects to consider. The food and tools used to eat, the clothes, the extent of personal hygiene, the importance of participating in religious events, leisure, gender-assigned roles, and each person's personal tasks are defined by culture, which determines not only the type of activity that is expected of each person, but also the way in which such activities should be performed.

Depending on the cultural context, the meaning of being able to carry out an occupation or not can vary. Generally speaking, the act of eating is carried out in Western societies with both hands and it requires the use of several utensils depending on the type of food eaten and at least one plate per person. In Senegal, this activity is a collective act of special significance in which all family members sit around the bowl to eat. They all use their right hand to eat, sometimes using a spoon. The right hand is also used for other important tasks, such as writing or greeting. In contrast, the use of the left hand is associated with personal hygiene after urination or defecation. The importance of this is illustrated by Case 53-2.

The analysis of everyday activities, considering social and cultural aspects, is fundamental to explore the impact that physical impairment can have. The participation difficulties Awa faced came from the interactions between hemiparesis and sociocultural expectations associated with eating. Awa rejected the option of eating with her left hand in public, so she had to go back home to eat. In this context, this deficiency, which has little impact on participation within other societies, generates a disabling situation. Without a comprehensive occupational analysis, this situation could have gone undetected. The simple act of adapting a locally made piece of cutlery to allow Awa to use her right hand not only improved her social participation within the school, but it also improved her nutritional condition and facilitated her attendance at school in the afternoon.

Schools and Functional Rehabilitation Services

The lack of adapted school furniture and material, the absence of school transport, and the presence of architectural boundaries often generated a high dependency for children with physical impairments. Activities such as moving around the school, going from home to school, accessing the playground, or even going to the toilet depended on the availability of their classmates. The toilets on school grounds were built inside 50-centimetre aboveground pavilions. These latrines did not have any type of adaptation for reduced-mobility people. Many families were reluctant to expose their children to be aided by their classmates in the absence of specialized caregivers within the school. Some of the children did not drink or eat during the whole school day just to avoid using the toilet.

Accessibility issues were not limited to the school environment. Rehabilitation services in the area were located in two regional hospitals. The distance and the cost of these services are two important barriers for a population. On the other hand, the healthcare teams from local health infrastructures (healthcare clinics and posts) often lack the specialized skills and expertise necessary to address the needs of disabled people; disability and its effects are often seen as 'untreatable' and people with disability as being beyond help. The combined effect of these factors might explain why many children have never accessed specialized services, leading to the absence of a medical diagnosis.

The limitations of access to public rehabilitation services increase the state of uncertainty with which the family confronts its unawareness of the aetiology,

evolution and the possibilities for improvement of the physical and functional conditions of their children. They also favour the search for other therapeutic alternatives, whether through traditional medicine or religious practice. They looked for solutions by relying on the resources available in their communities.

Support Devices and Available Technologies

In the south of Senegal, there is no formal distribution or industrial manufacturing of supportive devices, although there is artisanal production. Disused imported devices could often be found in hospitals and even in some homes. The export of wheelchairs, crutches, or custom-made orthoses from countries in the North to countries in the South is an extended common practice. This practice is the result of a charitable understanding of the concept of aid and is often quite ineffective. These devices, which can hardly be adapted to the personal features of the new users, often end up unused. When they are used, they often have short durability due to the fact that the environment is not the same as the one they were designed for, and there is a shortage of spare parts.

The export of support products to southern countries as a strategy to solve the functional limitations of the inhabitants reveals how such measures oriented towards impairment, overlooking the broader environment, often fail. These strategies seem to consider the deficiencies as the sole origin and cause of the disability. They ignore the complex nature of the situation created by the interaction between individual characteristics and needs and the physical, cultural, and social environment in which people live.

PLANNING THE INTERVENTION

Participation Assessment and Analysis of Needs

The fact that I did not speak the local languages required me to communicate via the project workers, who acted as interpreters. The project workers often directed interactions according to the information needed and they promoted interaction with the families who could communicate in their own language with a person they knew and with whom they shared cultural references. Project workers not only acted as interpreters but also as cultural brokers.

The project workers often provided me with guidance as to how to address certain intimate or taboo subjects. The direct questions to the families on disability onset, its connection with potential problems during childbirth, domestic accidents, or genetic inheritance could be interpreted as seeking responsibilities over the child's situation. Disability can also be seen as a form of transgression, as a punishment of the family, and therefore it is sometimes a source of shame and remains hidden (Agbovi, 2009). However, this information was of vital importance to determine the progressive or nonprogressive nature of the disability, since there was no diagnosis to guide intervention. Hence, it was important to create an environment of trust and consider the cultural factors. Some women, for instance, refused to talk about subjects related to maternity in front of men.

Another important aspect that came up during the need identification process was to avoid creating false expectations. We had to highlight the fact that our intervention was not aimed to cure or improve motor alterations. Our job was to facilitate the performance of those activities that they deemed important by using certain support devices.

The process took place within both the child's family and school environments, following semi-structured interviews and direct observation. The main question at first was focused on the activities carried out in a general manner by the children with whom they shared the same range of age. My purpose was to get to know the expected occupational pattern in that specific context and to identify activities with limitations. The next step was to know in what way that limitation was important in performing these activities. Subsequently, I analysed the environmental and personal factors, including deficiencies in infrastructures and organic functions that influenced the performance of the activities. The list of questions followed an established order. Starting with participation and ending with deficiency, the environment was regarded as the core of the intervention, and deficiencies were one among many factors to be considered.

Next, I studied the solutions that the community had provided up to that moment, and those that they thought to be the ideal solutions. Pictures of the devices that could help improve the occupational performance of the child were shown to the family, emphasizing the associated requirements of the manufacturing process and their later use. The idea was to assess any possible stigmatization or rejection that could come with the use and/or the changes in the way of carrying out the activity (wheelchair, adapted cutlery, writing with the mouth, etc.). This process ended with negotiation and consensus between both parties.

Design and Manufacture of Devices

The various devices were produced in close collaboration with local craftsmen (blacksmiths, carpenters, upholsters, tanners, etc.). The use of low-cost technology and materials available locally, as well as the high level of freedom in the design, ensured the devices addressed the unique needs of each child in their specific context.

All devices were easy to repair and reproduce within the community and did not require a long process of training in their use. The craftsmen were fully aware of the intended use of each device through instructions such as these:

Aliun cannot stand up or squat. He needs a special seat that adjusts to his latrine. The seat has to have the same height of the wheelchair to allow him to move from the chair to the seat. It is important that it be well-polished and that all bindings are well-protected to avoid abrasion during movement. The chair will have one armrest on the right side. This way, he will set the chair on the left side to move comfortably. By setting the armrest on the right side, he can hold himself up with his right hand while using his left hand for personal hygiene.

Adjustments, Delivery, and Follow-Up

To avoid situations such as the one detailed in Case 53-3, the project workers were trained to carry out follow-up visits. The fact they lived in the same area as the beneficiaries offered the chance of carrying out a continuous follow-up. The project workers learned to identify the nondesired effects of inappropriate use of the devices and the need for readapting them, plus the care and maintenance they required. The continuity in the use of adaptations and support products depended

Moussa

Moussa fell from a tree when he was playing with his friends. Due to the lack of economic resources and the distance to the hospital, the family decided to visit a traditional healer to treat his injured leg. However, the child's health began to deteriorate. The family asked family and friends for help and they took him to the hospital where he had his leg amputated. A nongovernmental organization paid the costs of a prosthesis and he was able to go home after he was able to walk again. We visited Moussa 2 years later. His prosthesis had barely been used; nobody had explained to him how to put it on, or let him or the family know that the device required modifications as a part of the follow-up.

on the transmission of this information to families and teachers.

CONCLUSION

When I was offered the possibility to work in an inclusive education project in Senegal, I committed myself to it with the intention of designing strategies that would continue once the project was over. My objective was to promote the effective inclusion of disabled children within schools and to facilitate a change of perception within the community about the needs and abilities of disabled children.

The nature of the intervention, based on environmental adaptation, combined with the lack of a health-care and rehabilitation network, led me to rule out those interventions focused on improving performance skills using a medical-rehabilitation approach on body structures and functions. Guided by the holistic nature of occupational therapy, I focused on both the physical and cultural environment and the personal and social context. For the first time in my professional career, I designed an intervention plan focused not on an individual, but on a community.

The analysis of the environment, revealed the factors responsible for the participation issues the children with disabilities often encountered. Furthermore, it highlighted the resources and opportunities the context offered to enable participation. I considered the sociocultural differences and the limited resources that were available, as a chance to develop other intervention methods. This experience allowed me to develop an in-depth understanding of the impact of the material, cultural, and social factors in the participation of the people within their community.

REFERENCES

Agbovi, K.K., 2009. Handicap International. Représentation et perception du handicap par les cadres de l'administration publique et les autorités locales. Projet DECISIPH – Bénin, Burkina Faso, Mali, Niger, Sénégal, Sierra Leone, Togo.

Handicap International, 2012. L'éducation Inclusive. Document Cadre, Lyon, France.

Organisation des Nations Unies pour L'éducation, la Science et la Culture (Unesco), 2007. L'Education pour Tous en 2015. Un Objectif Accessible? UN agencies, Paris.

United Nations Children's Emergency Fund (UNICEF), 2013. Estado mundial de la infancia 2013. Niños y niñas con discapacidad, New York, USA.

United Nations Children's Emergency Fund (UNICEF), 2014. Tous les enfants à l'école d'ici 2015. Initiative mondiale en faveur des enfants non scolarisés. Rapport Régional. Afrique de L'Ouest et du Centre, Paris.

54

PEOPLE WITH DISABILITIES IN EAST TIMOR: SOME CONSIDERATIONS FOR OCCUPATIONAL THERAPY PRACTICE IN DEVELOPING COUNTRIES

JANE SHAMROCK

CHAPTER OUTLINE

Globalization and ease of travel inspire an increasing number of occupational therapists (Humbert et al., 2011) and occupational therapy students (Humbert et al., 2012) to work or volunteer in other countries, including developing countries. Occupational therapists are learning that activities of daily living may vary from culture to culture and even from household to household, depending on levels of poverty, resources available, and in the instance of disability, the capabilities of individuals and their families. However, occupational therapists almost exclusively absorb their professional knowledge from models which arose within Western societies (Iwama, 2007; Whiteford and Wilcock, 2000). Theories of disability and occupation are generally developed in Western or 'minority world' settings (Barnes and Sheldon, 2010; Grech, 2009), while the remaining 83% of the world's population, that is,

the 'majority world', live in environments where beliefs and constructs, and connection with occupation and the practice of daily life may be significantly different (Hammell, 2011).

In this chapter, I describe some of my experiences as an Australian occupational therapist working and researching in East Timor. I worked in East Timor intermittently as an occupational therapist between 2000 and 2008, and since that time I have been undertaking doctoral research on the lived experience of physical disability in East Timor. In this chapter, I describe some of the challenges of cross-cultural practice, using the voices of East Timorese people with disabilities to illustrate some of the points.

My aim in this chapter is to discuss:

- The importance of a community-centred approach.

- The role of occupational therapists in community-based rehabilitation (CBR).
- The importance of taking time to begin to understand the host culture.
- Some considerations regarding translation and language.
- Some considerations regarding personal safety.

BACKGROUND

East Timor is a small and recently independent Asian country accessible from Australia by plane on an 1-hour flight from Australia's main northern city, Darwin. In East Timor, the dilemmas of cross-cultural practice are experienced by the occasional occupational therapist and by aid workers on a daily basis.

East Timor was a colony of Portugal for approximately 400 years. However, in 1975, the colonial period ended with a few months of independence, followed by annexation and a 26-year occupation by Indonesia. During that time, reports filtered through of the suppression of local resistance organizations (Molnar, 2010), including the deaths of five Australian journalists attempting to report on these and other human rights violations (O'Shaughnessy, 2000).

In August 1999, a referendum was held by the Indonesian administration in East Timor, in which 78% of the population chose independence from Indonesia. In the lead up to the vote and within hours after the announcement of the results, paramilitary forces began attacking civilians in and around the capital city, Dili. United Nations (UN) observers fled and many Timorese families escaped to the mountains. A systematic destruction of property and infrastructure was carried out until the arrival of UN forces in September 1999. The militia activity reduced over the next few months under the administration of the International Force for East Timor (INTERFET). However, by the time peace returned, most of the country's infrastructure and many public and private buildings were destroyed.

I first visited the country as a young traveller in 1972. At that time, it was still a colony of Portugal and I stayed with a Timorese family who had a child with multiple disabilities. My interest in East Timor remained during the Indonesian occupation, and I returned as an occupational therapist and humanitar-

ian volunteer in early 2000. Since 2000, I have been involved in several projects, staying up to 4 months at a time and working with people with disabilities.

EAST TIMOR SINCE 2000

There is a hint of the complexity of the small country of East Timor in the following speech by Xanana Gusmão, Prime Minister of East Timor from 2002 to 2007.

> *Both the catholic faith and the Portuguese language took up roots in our existence, assuming more visible presence during the period of the Indonesian occupation and becoming an important instrument for the Timorese resistance. It was from this meeting of cultures and civilisations that our small half-island, with an enclave inside the other half, within an archipelago composed of over 14 thousand small and large islands of Indonesia that our Country, Timor-Leste, affirmed itself as a People. (Gusmão, 2014, p. 3)*

I wanted to know what happened to the family who had hosted me in earlier years. I returned to Dili in 2000 to find a town unlit at night, with the burnt-out shells of shops and businesses and the streets full of rubble. As an occupational therapist and humanitarian volunteer, I felt almost out of my depth in the small medical clinic where I was volunteering. With the help of interpreters I listened for hours to family members describing how they lived their lives and managed at home with whatever barriers they were experiencing, while trying to regain a normal life. Alita's (pseudonyms are used throughout the chapter) story is an example from that time (Case 54-1).

Disability in East Timor

Forty-one percent of people in East Timor live below the poverty line and there is a 'hungry season' each year as a result of traditional cropping practices worsened by erratic rainfall (Barnett et al., 2007). Services for people with disabilities have gradually developed in recent years but are mostly limited to the capital city. Families generally love and care for a disabled family member, but that is the limit of everyone's expectations. During 2012 and 2013, a research project

CASE 54-1

The story of Alita

Alita was a young woman determined to go to her newly restored school despite her diagnosis of tuberculosis. Her difficulties arose firstly from fatigue and secondly from lack of furniture in the classroom. All the girls in Alita's class carried a stool from home each day as the school chairs had all disappeared and any new chairs brought into the classroom also disappeared overnight. Alita was not strong enough to carry a stool to and from the school. My occupational therapy intervention with Alita and her mother was simply to explore strategies to manage fatigue together with options for getting a stool to and from the school; I was surprised that this simple discussion seemed to be helpful. I concluded that the recent trauma made lateral thinking and problem solving difficult for Alita and her mother.

---

entitled 'the lived experience of physical disability in East Timor' aimed to investigate the barriers faced by people with disabilities. For example, there is a common assumption in East Timor that the disabled person will never get married, work or contribute to society, and thus normal occupations are out of reach. Sylviana was ambitious but frequently experienced a lack of support in her quest for an education:

> The people said to me, you have no life, you are disabled, why do you go to school, why do you want that, when you finish school what can you become? (Sylviana, September 2013)

For those who managed to get an education there were problems with employment:

> After school graduated I just tried to seek opportunity to work…I tried many times but I could not pass…I tried to apply to technical school but they have the criteria that they will not allow people with physical disability to apply. (Mauricio, September 2013)

Disability is a strong predictor for the presence of physical or sexual abuse throughout the world, both in resource-poor and in resource-rich settings. At times during my work in East Timor, I sought advice from a local nongovernment organization (NGO) which specialized in trauma and abuse. If I suspected abuse, the NGO staff was helpful, promising to visit the family and attempt to understand if the person about whom I had concerns was at risk.

CROSS-CULTURAL CONSIDERATIONS FOR OCCUPATIONAL THERAPY PRACTICE

Occupational therapists have at times insisted that patients and clients adapt to Western cultural norms, rather than seeking to understand how their clients and patients live and experience their own worlds (Iwama, 2007). The 'cultural safety' approach to cross-cultural work has been developed to help occupational therapists understand how power relationships may affect client and patient outcomes (Nelson, 2007; Thomas et al., 2011). When planning a new occupational therapy service in the United Arab Emirates, Awaad identified a range of influences on cross-cultural practice, for example, that culture is dynamic and may be different in different family contexts, and that the practitioner needs to consider details such as modes of address and conversational etiquette, body language, personal space, the amount of information that individuals are willing to divulge, and the effects of using family members as interpreters (Awaad, 2003). For those planning to practise occupational therapy in communities with a colonial past, a questioning of power relating to Western ethnocentric assumptions is needed (Smith, 1999). Together with these considerations, occupational therapists need to consider their own beliefs stemming from their own ethnic background, religion, class, gender, relative or perceived wealth, and age (McGoldrick and Hardy, 2008; Mullings, 1999).

In isolated communities, the arrival of a foreigner can be an interesting and public spectacle. When visiting remote communities, I often met with people with disabilities together with family and neighbours present, making privacy impossible and putting pressure on those being interviewed. East Timor has a hierarchical society and people with disabilities are placed towards the lower end of the ladder. When I met people with disabilities together with their family, especially in a remote setting, the discussion at times appeared difficult and uncomfortable. I assumed that perhaps people were wary in front of an outsider like myself.

LANGUAGE

Over 20 languages are used in East Timor, including many local languages. Tetum (an indigenous language) and Portuguese are the national languages, while English and Indonesian are classed in the constitution as working languages. Most people in and around Dili and in most of the districts of Timor can speak Tetum and around Dili Tetum is sprinkled with Portuguese words. English is used in foreign aid workplaces in Dili but is little understood away from the capital.

Translation and understanding in cross-cultural practice is also much more than simply word-for-word transmission of language (Temple and Young, 2004). Although Tetum is the most commonly used language, words from English, Indonesian, and Portuguese are often used to manage communication about contemporary matters such as computers, the processes in planning health projects or in trade and business. Skilled interpreters need time to gain familiarity with specific professional terminology. When using interpreters, I found that the concerns of the occupational therapist such as the details of daily life appeared so insignificant that at times the interpreters felt that they could save time and answer such basic questions for the person being interviewed. I had to explain that as a foreigner I did not know these details. For example, I needed to know how the person gets to the bathroom, is it near the house, and is it necessary to crawl in the dirt, and I really wanted to hear directly from people how they managed at home.

Temple and Young (2004) extend their concerns regarding power in cross-cultural communication to those who do not speak the dominant language in a country. Interpreting is also much more than transmission of information through an interpreter. The interpreter has agency, may feel aligned with either the therapist or the interviewee, is embedded in a particular culture, and can be a member of a more or less dominant social group (Angelelli, 2004).

When working with interpreters, I made use of some or all of the following strategies:

- I consulted with a cultural mentor before visiting a remote district to check if I could safely ask my planned questions.
- At times, I engaged my interpreter in a role-play to ensure that he or she understood my questions and to get any other relevant feedback.
- As I seldom had a female interpreter, I first asked advice of a female cultural mentor about how I could approach women with a male interpreter.
- I found that laughter, at times related to cultural differences, was a way to develop relationships and keep a fresh focus on the work at hand.

THE COMMUNITY-BASED REHABILITATION TRAINING IN EAST TIMOR

I was involved in planning the first CBR training programme funded by Australian foreign aid in East Timor (2006–2007), together with two Australian physiotherapists. There were no locally trained allied health professionals in East Timor at the time, and we felt that Timorese trained in CBR would be able to start to provide basic services in local communities with a CBR grassroots approach. Twenty-five people started the training and most were either school-leavers or local health workers wanting to add to their skill base.

> *Community-based rehabilitation (CBR) focuses on enhancing the quality of life for people with disabilities and their families; meeting basic needs; and ensuring inclusion and participation. It is a multi-sectoral strategy that empowers persons with disabilities to access and benefit from education, employment, health and social services. CBR is implemented through the combined efforts of people with disabilities, their families and communities, and relevant government and non-government health, education, vocational, social and other services. (World Health Organization, n.d.)*

CBR is a term covering a range of programmes based on principles of health promotion which include enablement, social justice, importance of a meaningful lifestyle, and respect for cultural difference (Fransen, 2005). In East Timor, we used the Community Approaches to Handicap in Development (toolkit) described in 'Disability in Development' (2006) as the basis for the training programme. We made changes to ensure that the training was culturally specific to East Timor, for example, by describing typical Timorese life and families when discussing a case study. The toolkit provided outlines of teaching modules such as basic anatomy, basic communication skills and safe feeding techniques for people with severe disabilities, and interviewing skills and assessment skills, among many other topics. The training programme was designed to run for one year based on one week of classroom activity per month, followed by a period of supervised practical work. The story of Fatima, illustrates some of the difficulties in the life of a person with disabilities, as well as some of the dilemmas of cross-cultural practice (Case 54-2).

An evaluation of the training programme carried out in 2008, revealed positive results together with some difficulties. While the CBR workers were contributing to the general welfare and occupational engagement of their clients, the role of the CBR worker was not easy. For example, many felt isolated after the training ended due to the departure of the expatriate trainers (Shamrock, 2009).

Personal Safety

Specialized training programmes conducted by NGOs are available in Australia for people going to work in dangerous environments. Participants can learn strategies for managing personal safety such as making preparations for emergency departure, strategies for survival as a hostage or when threatened physically. An occupational therapist planning to work in a dangerous developing country may be offered training in personal security. Even when specific training is not necessary, an awareness of personal security is advisable for those working in a new culture. For example, both men and women may find that dress considered suitable by the locals will help reduce cultural gaps and promote a collegiate relationship. Details of what constitutes suitable dress can be discussed with a cultural mentor.

Towards the middle of 2006, during the first 3 months of the CBR training, tension began to develop

> ### CASE 54-2
> #### *Story of Fatima*
>
> Amando was a trainee CBR worker and I was Amando's supervisor. Amando was expected to undertake home visits and carry out simple interventions as a part of his fieldwork between modules of the CBR training programme.
>
> We visited Fatima and her mother about 2 weeks after they were discharged from the residential facility outside of Dili. Fatima was a very small 8-year-old child with a large head and stick-thin arms and legs who had previously arrived in the residential facility with her mother. She demonstrated developmental delay, general weakness, contractures, and malnutrition. They both lived in a hut at the edge of her community as her mother was ostracized by the community for having a disabled child. Fatima was so malnourished that her mother could easily carry her inside the home, although she was too heavy to carry to the distant garden where her mother worked growing a few vegetables to eat or to sell; for much of her day Fatima was at home, alone and immobile. They stayed together at the rehabilitation centre for 3 weeks and during that time Fatima's smile broadened every day as she and her mother ate plenty of nutritious food and for the first time Fatima played with toys. She listened to music and had others around her to communicate with.
>
> Fatima and her mother eventually returned to their hut at the edge of the village. At the time of our home visit, Fatima's mother reported that initially she could no longer carry Fatima around because of her weight gain; however, Fatima had since lost that weight. Both were further ostracized by the community for having received help and extra food. They returned to the rehabilitation centre for further problem solving within the CBR programme, this time by finding ways for Fatima's mother to better connect to her community and by starting a process of increasing community understanding of disability and community advocacy. The importance of community engagement could clearly be seen in this instance.

in Dili as a faction of the army, representing mostly personnel from the west of the country, complained of discriminatory practices relating to salaries. Many of this group deserted the army, taking with them a quantity of weapons, and gathered in a remote rural centre. On their return to Dili, there were armed clashes which resulted in at least five deaths. Unemployed youth joined the fighting around the centre of the town and markets, and at times houses of those suspected of hiding the opposition or opposition sympathizers were set on fire. By the end of May, homes were frequently burnt and shooting in the main marketplaces became commonplace. Trainees and trainers were fearful and preoccupied and the CBR training temporarily closed. By early June, many Timorese had fled and many were housed in internally displaced persons camps, while most expatriates were evacuated.

For a few weeks, fighting was commonplace in and around Dili and near to the rehabilitation facility where I lived together with two other foreigners and some of the CBR trainees. Timorese who had been traumatized in the past during the Indonesian occupation were quickly fearful again. As foreigners, we were unsure whether we would be targets in the general atmosphere of fear and distrust, or would we simply be ignored in an internal conflict. Timorese either stayed indoors or fled into the neighbouring hills.

The rehabilitation facility had an intermittent phone service. This was the only phone in the local district, and people came into the facility hoping to be able to make phone calls to trace missing family members. The phone was located in a central community room and some people remained in the room gathering comfort from the presence of others. I saw the fear and general distress of the people who came to the community room and found a large jigsaw puzzle to spread on the dining table. The puzzle provided a simple distracting leisure activity and invited communication between people without requiring concentration or complex problem solving. I also observed the power of play for the children who lived in the facility. Frightened by the gunfire, a small group of children were gathered together by one of the volunteers. She and the children found that fear was easier to manage with activity which reflected the source of their fear. While the guns sounded in the distance, the

children marched around the compound with imaginary guns, shouting words of songs or nonsense words, or counting out loud, anything to make a noise and to be active.

OCCUPATIONAL THERAPY AND DISABLED PEOPLE'S ORGANIZATIONS

Disabled peoples organizations (DPO) are those where 51% of the board members are people with disabilities. DPOs are involved in activities such as self-help and self-advocacy groups and provide advice at local and national levels (Hurst, 2003). One of the DPOs in East Timor has been involved in practical projects such as water, health, and sanitation projects (see Inclusivewash, 2011), and I found that my relationship with DPO members enriched my understanding of disability in East Timor. DPO members were usually people with disabilities who could describe the experiences of stigma, exclusion, and problems with mobility common to most disabled East Timorese. They also considered themselves as role models for people with disabilities in rural areas, where negative attitudes and stigma were more common.

In East Timor, the movement had a very modest beginning in 2006 with a sole representative sitting in committee meetings when the CBR training was being discussed. By 2013, the DPO had representatives in all the districts of East Timor and consisted of approximately 14 staff, most of whom had disabilities themselves. It was a difficult transition for some members who experienced stigma in the past to actively advocate for others and themselves:

> ...so at the start I'm very shy, I'm a little ashamed...working with this organisation, when I look at myself it seems like shame. I am disabled and it feels like that I am going to talk about myself. (Jacinto, October 2013)

Some of the DPO members were trained in group facilitation techniques to train staff in government and NGOs about disability rights and barriers, in line with the National Disability Policy. Augustina's story illustrates some of the common experiences of members of the DPO in East Timor including interrupted education, stigma, and exclusion which she

Story of Augustina

Augustina is a small, attractive woman who walks confidently supporting her shortened leg with one hand while holding a stick in the other. She is unusual as she was always encouraged and supported by her family. She is now a powerful member of the DPO in Timor and uses a three-wheeled motorbike to move around Dili:

> Sometime they say that the people with the disability can't do anything. And they can just stay at and home and they can just... eat and sleep. I just say it's true, but you can see my condition and you can make an example from me...I can teach you and I can drive the motorbike. You can look at me. (Augustina, September 2013)

Augustina completed her high school education, although she missed a lot of school time during the Indonesian occupation of Timor when schools were closed or barely functioning, and she now works with a disability organization. She is attending university part-time, and she plans to get married eventually and have children. She is a trainer and leader in disability rights and a change agent within her community, yet people at times still question her right to these universal roles and occupations. Augustina has made a powerful difference in her work as an advocate for people with disabilities; she has conducted training sessions with staff from government ministries, giving them blindfolds and canes or crutches to get firsthand experience with mobility problems.

However, Augustina is relatively inexperienced. She left school 1 year before getting her job with the disability NGO, so she had to rapidly learn the concepts and processes which are embedded in foreign NGO projects such as needs assessments, consultation with beneficiaries and stakeholders, monitoring and evaluation, and report writing. Augustina is still learning all of this on the job. In her consultations with foreign NGOs she needs to explain her culture while having these concepts at her fingertips. Augustina is courageous and confident; however, women with her level of confidence are uncommon in the conservative society of East Timor. When I worked beside Augustina I had unique insights from the viewpoint of a woman, a person with disabilities, and a Timorese.

---

manages in her work while rapidly learning new ideas (Case 54-3).

The occupational therapist can provide professional knowledge to community health workers on issues, such as childhood milestones, and facilitate development of specific skills, such as how to do a home assessment. When learning is linked to the local context by a person with a disability, the message is much more potent. Augustina manages many barriers and she can explain to others, such as visiting occupational therapists, what these barriers are and how they affect her life.

CONCLUSION

In this chapter, I described some of the challenges in cross-cultural practice in East Timor and some of the strategies used to address these challenges. Occupational therapists can often be well positioned to work with these challenges. Therapists need to be aware of the need to:

- Adopt a community-centred approach.
- Take time to understand the new culture and in particular the origins of barriers to participation.
- Establish a relationship with one or more people as cultural mentors.
- Allow time to develop a good working relationship with translators.
- Be thoughtful regarding personal safety and personal presentation.

Working in a context one is not familiar with is a complex process. Occupational therapists must take time to meet people, listen to stories, ask naïve questions, study the local language, understand the role of humour, and consider the acceptable speed of change, in order to make positive contributions.

Acknowledgements

I would like to thank Natalie Smith and the Leprosy Mission of East Timor (TLMTL) for their whole-hearted and generous support of my recent work and research in East Timor.

REFERENCES

Angelelli, C.V., 2004. Medical Interpreting and Cross-Cultural Communication. Cambridge University Press, Cambridge.

Awaad, T., 2003. Culture, cultural competency and occupational therapy: a review of the literature. Br. J. Occup. Ther. 66, 356–362.

Barnes, C., Sheldon, A., 2010. Disability, politics and poverty in a majority world context. Disabil. Soc. 25, 771–782.

Barnett, J., Dessai, S., Jones, R.N., 2007. Vulnerability to climate variability and change in East Timor. Ambio 36 (5), 372–378.

Disability in Development, 2006. <http://www.cbm.org/article/downloads/54741/CAHD_-__Disability_in_Development_-_Experiences_in_Inclusive_Practices__-_full_document.pdf> (accessed 26.02.15.).

Fransen, H., 2005. In: Kronenberg, F., Simo Algado, S., Pollard, N., Eds.), Occupational Therapy without Borders: Learning from the Spirit of Survivors. Elsevier/Churchill Livingstone, Edinburgh.

Grech, S., 2009. Disability, poverty and development: critical reflections on the majority world debate. Disabil. Soc. 24, 771–784.

Gusmao, X.K., 2014. Speech by H. E. the Prime Minister, Kay Rala Xanana Gusmão. 16 July 2014. <http://timor-leste.gov.tl/wp-content/uploads/2014/07/Timor-Lestes-Policy-during-its-leadership-of-the-CPLP_-UNTL-Conference-16.7.2014.pdf> (accessed 03.01.15.).

Hammell, K.W., 2011. Resisting theoretical imperialism in the disciplines of occupational science and occupational therapy. Br. J. Occup. Ther. 74, 27–33.

Humbert, T.K., Burket, A., Deveney, R., Kennedy, K., 2011. Occupational therapy practitioners' perspectives regarding international cross-cultural work. Aust. Occup. Ther. J. 58, 300–309.

Humbert, T.K., Burket, A., Deveney, R., Kennedy, K., 2012. Occupational therapy students' perspectives regarding international cross-cultural experiences. Aust. Occup. Ther. J. 59, 225–234.

Hurst, R., 2003. The International Disability Rights Movement and the ICF. Disabil. Rehabil. 25, 572–576.

Inclusivewash, 2011. <http://www.inclusivewash.org.au/Literature/Case%20Study%2007_Building%20skills%20in%20disability%20inclusive%20WASH.pdf> (accessed 30.04.15.).

Iwama, M., 2007. Culture and occupational therapy: meeting the challenge of relevance in a global world. Occup. Ther. Int. 14, 183–187.

McGoldrick, M., Hardy, K.V., 2008. Re-visioning family therapy: race, culture, and gender in clinical practice. Guilford Press, London.

Molnar, A.K., 2010. Timor Leste. Routledge, London.

Mullings, B., 1999. Insider or outsider, both or neither: some dilemmas of interviewing in a cross-cultural setting. Geoforum 30, 337–350.

Nelson, A., 2007. Seeing white: a critical exploration of occupational therapy with Indigenous Australian people. Occup. Ther. Int. 14, 237–255.

O'Shaughnessy, H., 2000. Reporting East Timor: Western media coverage of the conflict. The East Timor Question: The Struggle for Independence from Indonesia. I.B.Tauris, London, pp. 31–40.

Shamrock, J., 2009. Evaluation of a pilot community based rehabilitation training programme in East Timor. Asia Pac. Disabil. Rehabil. J. 20, 17–31.

Smith, L.T., 1999. Decolonizing Methodologies: Research and Indigenous Peoples. Zed Books, New York.

Temple, B., Young, A., 2004. Q'ualitative research and translation dilemmas. Qual. Res. 4, 161–178.

Thomas, Y., Gray, M., McGinty, S., 2011. Occupational therapy at the 'cultural interface': lessons from research with Aboriginal and Torres Strait Islander Australians. Aust. Occup. Ther. J. 58, 11–16.

Whiteford, G.E., Wilcock, A.A., 2000. Cultural relativism: occupation and independence reconsidered. Can. J. Occup. Ther. 67, 324–336.

World Health Organization (WHO), n.d. Community-based rehabilitation (CBR) disabilities and rehabilitation section. <http://www.who.int/disabilities/cbr/en/> (accessed 26.02.15.).

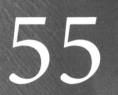

55

CROSSING THE PRACTICE BORDER FOR CHILDREN WITH DISABILITIES: PARTICIPATION-ENABLING SKILLS IN COMMUNITIES

MARGARET JONES ■ CLARE HOCKING

P articipation is essential to people's health and development, and the concept itself points to a societal perspective of functioning (World Health Organization, 2001). However, children with disabilities, who are one of the more vulnerable groups in society, face significant participation challenges, with consequent long-term health issues as they move through to adulthood (Mesterman et al., 2010). Research reveals that these children participate less often, in a smaller range of occupations and contexts, and with fewer people than their peers (Bedell et al., 2013; Michelsen et al., 2014). One of the most prominent concerns raised by children and their parents, is the barrier posed by negative attitudes from others in the children's social environment (Anaby et al., 2013). This chapter presents new insights into the ways people can work to assist one another to take part in occupations. The

discussion is underpinned by an understanding that disability is fundamentally a transactional process that occurs 'when one group of people create barriers by designing a world only for their way of living, taking no account of the impairments other people have' (Minister for Disability Issues, 2001). We argue that the ideas we present, derived from a study undertaken in Aotearoa (New Zealand), provide a foundation from which occupational therapists may develop interventions to drive changes at a community level for improving participation.

Barriers to children's participation have an effect beyond individual lives, arguably disadvantaging society as a whole. Social capital theory directs attention to the benefits that accrue to communities when people collaborate and network through engagement in occupation. This body of knowledge holds that the social connections that people form with one another are an asset to communities and have an inherent, collective value in terms of cooperation, trust, reciprocity, resources, and opportunities (Putnam, 2000).

In particular, social capital that links people from different social groupings enables them to access knowledge and resources that lie outside their immediate social circle (Putnam, 2000). However, skill is required to form bonds with people from other walks of life (Field, 2008). The ability to engage with changing and diverse social groupings provides a source of support for addressing challenges faced throughout adulthood (Pahl and Spencer, 1997). When negative attitudes prevent the participation of children with disabilities, not only are those children deprived of social connections which are the building blocks for their future health, but others in the community miss valuable opportunities to develop skills and resources for embracing a range of human perspectives and capabilities, and for overcoming future barriers.

To date, however, rehabilitation for children with disabilities has largely ignored these wider concerns, focusing at an individual level, on remediating impaired structures and functions or adapting the physical environment. Although emergent research suggests that addressing participation issues at the level of the individual may not necessarily solve the problems they face (Wright et al., 2008), limited information has been generated about how communities can effectively involve children with disabilities in occupations. Accordingly, occupational therapists have lacked the groundwork from which to make change in the social environment and support children with disabilities to participate more fully (Rosenbaum, 2010).

OUR OCCUPATIONAL THERAPY PRACTICE CONTEXT

Margaret's years of occupational therapy practice with children who have sustained traumatic brain injuries sensitized her to the extent to which their participation is suddenly and unexpectedly disrupted as the result of an accident. The changes that take place for these children and their families are momentous, but in her day-to-day practice, she also got hints that the changes extend through to those in the children's communities with whom they participate. She noticed that the things that people usually do when they engage in

occupations with a child are no longer effective and that it takes community members a long time to come to grips with ways to participate with someone who often seems like a different person.

However, Margaret also observed that interventions designed to improve the children's performance of particular occupations result in some tensions. They do not directly address families' fears about their children beginning to participate again in school and community life, and time spent in rehabilitation seems to be time spent away from participation with peers and other families in the community. As a means of tackling these concerns, we undertook a study to find out about the aspects of participation that were important for children after traumatic brain injury, and to learn about the facilitators and barriers to their participation.

THEORETICAL UNDERSTANDINGS INFORMING THE STUDY

The notion of participation draws attention to the interrelationships of people and their occupations in context. John Dewey's pragmatist philosophy has raised occupational therapists' awareness of the concept of transaction as a means of understanding these relationships (Cutchin and Dickie, 2013). Transaction is embedded in an understanding of continuity of people with their environments through time. As people act in connection with the environment, changes take place in those who act, but so too are aspects of the environment changed. In this way, it can be seen that when a child sustains a traumatic brain injury, there will not only be an effect on the child, but the accident event and the changes in the child will also have an effect on others in their community.

STUDY METHODOLOGY

Given this understanding, an approach was sought to guide the study that provided a view of the person and their participation as continuous with the environment. Case study methodology was adopted because of its ability to generate in-depth information about complex phenomena as they occur in social life, and to take account of changes that occur. The interpretive case study approach developed by Robert Stake (1995,

2006) stresses the meaning of events and experiences situated in real-life settings and time. Drawing on Stake's approach, we obtained range and depth of understandings about phenomena such as the influences on people's actions and the impact of those actions over time.

STUDY DESIGN

Six case studies were undertaken, each centring on a child aged 9 to 12 years who had sustained a traumatic brain injury. For every case, parents and teaching staff were interviewed. Those children who were able to, took photographs of objects that represented important occupations in which they had taken part, and were interviewed in the process of developing their photographs into a poster. Children were also observed participating in a range of meaningful occupations, and documents were reviewed to provide information about the aspects of participation prioritized by rehabilitation providers. Data from each case were first analysed using a mapping process (Northcott, 1996), then, when individual case reports had been written, a cross-case analysis was undertaken.

STUDY FINDINGS

By adopting a research design that attended to key people and occupations involved in the children's participation, information was generated from a variety of perspectives about relationships and processes that took place. The excerpts presented here illustrate those perspectives. They are drawn from the case study of Anton, an 11-year-old boy who sustained a severe traumatic brain injury when he was 6 years old (all names are pseudonyms). Anton lived with his parents and brother in a semirural setting on the outskirts of a city and attended a special education classroom attached to a mainstream school. Although Anton was independently mobile, as a result of his injury he had frequent seizures, minimal speech, jerky limb movements, and impulsive behaviour. He required a high level of support with personal care activities.

Shared Occupation

The concept of 'shared occupation' was of central importance to participation. Shared occupation

referred to people taking part alongside others in an activity that had meaning for them.

Here is free play, happy chaos. The noise levels are high, kids all different ages, all chattering, catching up, standing around in small groups. Anton and his friend chase each other. 'Stop, stop'. The boy drops to all fours, Anton stops without falling over him. Anton runs with arms and legs all out of synch, but with force and perseverance, his mouth open in a big grin. His friend is laughing as well. Soon a smaller younger boy joins in.

A lady and her daughter come in and sit down beside me. They are pleased to see Anton, and explain they are still getting to know him, but seem welcoming of him being part of the group.

The boy stops suddenly and turns around and hugs Anton who promptly falls over. He helps pick Anton up. Then the boy falls over. Anton stops in time and looks at him. More running, then both boys fall and roll. Anton grabs another boy who drops to the floor. This seems to be a loosely coordinated game of tag. (Observation, Scouts)

Although activities were meaningful when they reflected a child's choice, at times, children were also required to take part in activities that adults identified as meaningful for their future health and development. Shared occupation was seen as an essential component of the children's well-being, both in the present and looking forward into the future.

It's him being part of the landscape, being part of the group of children who go, and not being cosseted or separated off. (Mother interview)

It's good for him to do things with other people… You could say he's living in his own world, and of course we want to shake him out of that, and you know, let him experience that he can have fun when you do things you know, games with other people. (Father interview)

Children reflected a strong drive to share occupations with others, and occupation was seldom carried out in isolation. Occupations were shared with adult family members, siblings, teachers, rehabilitation providers, peers, and sometimes with other adults in the community. Where others were not available to share occupations, children actively sought to share their occupations with pets, TV or movie characters, insects or toys. When left to his own devices, Anton spent time absorbed with the characters in his two favourite videos, or murmuring to the doll in his small toy car.

Occupation was shared both directly and indirectly. Directly shared occupation occurred in parallel with others, such as when children all carried out a similar individual activity at the same time. On other occasions, the occupation was shared collectively, where people directly collaborated in an occupation, or where a person directly carried out a task which contributed to the function and well-being of a wider group. However, occupations were also shared indirectly with others, or vicariously. In these situations, children provided information as they were able about their participation experiences using words, written language or with symbols such as drawings, photographs, and artefacts such as awards or keepsakes.

Participation-Enabling Skills

The study found that children and adults all demonstrated varying levels of skill for helping one another to take part in occupations. 'Participation-enabling skills' were defined as the ability of people, both adults and children, to act to enable members of a community to be involved in and carry out a shared occupation. People's participation-enabling skills reflected their understandings about others, and about the value of others' involvement in a shared occupation. In this way, stronger participation-enabling skills meant that more diverse perspectives, experiences, roles, and skills could be contributed to the shared occupation. It was important that actions used by group members treated people in the same way, so that individuals were not singled out. To support participation, participation-enabling skills needed to be used by the whole group towards one another, rather than being directed solely towards a child with a disability. Illustrating that, Anton's mother described the way families of children with disabilities helped children who were new to a soccer game to take part.

There's parents involved, and they mix into the team. Everybody's rustling around and kicking the ball and it comes to Anton…'Stop. Anton's turn.' Anton kicks the ball to someone, they make sure he kicks, then they all keep going at the normal speed, and then it's back to Anton and 'Stop'. So he's very much in the early stage, but they're very welcoming and they're helping him to be established. (Interview)

Sometimes, an adult, such as a teaching assistant or caregiver, remained close to a child with traumatic brain injury and took full responsibility for involving them in shared occupation. At these times, the child's peers held back, seeing that it was the role of the adult to support the child to participate and not their own. In these situations, the participation-enabling skills of peers were not put to optimal use. At other times, adults deliberately held back, to facilitate children to use their own participation-enabling skills.

During the relays, Anton looks over to Joe, his caregiver, who is across the room. At this point, Sally, one of the other children, takes Anton onto the floor and shows him how to roll, helping him. This is hard for Anton, but he copies Sally as best he can, crawling up to the front, then standing up. Sally seems to enjoy helping Anton. Her assistance is entirely voluntary. (Observation, Scouts)

Skills for enabling participation were not unique to those without disabilities and there were instances where those children with disabilities demonstrated higher levels of skill than their peers or than the adults involved.

At the soccer game, Kathleen, Anton's mother encourages him to sit beside another boy with a disability. The other boy greets Anton; they are in the same class at school and Kathleen is friendly with his mother. Anton looks at the boy's face, then relaxes beside him. The boy rubs Anton's back gently seeming to sense how tired he is today. The boy is aware of Anton's presence, and has learned how to interact with him in a way that fits for Anton. (Observation, Soccer)

Variation in participation-enabling skills was also observed across different communities, reflecting cultural attitudes and practices towards participation, and the value placed on participation in particular occupations by that community (e.g., rugby, water sports, kapa haka[1]). The specific participation-enabling skills observed and reported were driving, leading, including, and performing shared occupations.

The Participation-Enabling Skill of Driving

'Driving' refers to people's ability to envision, source opportunities, seek out information about, weigh up, plan and prepare for, and press someone to share in an occupation. Although the role of driving was often taken on by adults, children were also observed to 'drive' some of their shared occupations themselves.

Communication was an important aspect of 'driving a shared occupation', and was reflected in the way people networked to identify opportunities and resources, exchanged information, and established strategies and processes that assisted children to express their preferences, or to 'have a say' in what they wanted to do. Thus, driving was a skill that enabled children to try out and experience a range of occupations, often referred to by participants as 'having a go'. Anton's mother described the way she and a caregiver, Joe, were 'driving' an opportunity for him to participate in the occupation of kayaking.

Joe has been involved in Sea Scouts for years and he thought Anton would enjoy it. He thought that because Anton's got a strong upper body he would be good at kayaking. My husband said 'what happens if he has a seizure in the canoe?' Joe said if he does, which is unlikely, we've got his medication, we'll give him that and let him rest, and then we'll keep going. My husband's saying 'what if, what if' and Joe's saying 'why don't we start thinking about what he can do, not what he can't do. Let's just start to think about the positives, what can be achieved and what we're aiming for'. I tend to feel a bit that way. I'm not quite as concerned about negative eventualities because I think we will get past them. (Interview)

Driving needed to be delivered judiciously, and, as seen above, people who were drivers of shared occupation opportunities carefully considered the pros and cons before proceeding. For children with traumatic brain injury, opportunities were needed that attended to their safety needs, and which held the possibility of fitting with their abilities.

Not all attempts at shared occupation were enjoyed or successful. Some of the children with a traumatic brain injury were not confident, and many were reluctant to drive new shared occupations, preferring the familiar and the safe. For these children, adults played an important role in 'driving their shared occupation', and familiarization, practice, and trial runs were an essential part of the driving process. For others, even though not all attempts at shared occupation were enjoyed or successful, they were simply satisfied with the opportunity to try a particular occupation out and the chance to learn that it was not something they enjoyed.

The Participation-Enabling Skill of Leading

People in a position of responsibility within a shared occupation, showed different levels of skill for directing, guiding, teaching, modelling, and coaching others in ways to facilitate group members' involvement. People with skills in 'leading' also took responsibility for structuring, regulating, and adjusting shared occupations to promote involvement. In this way, leading involved not only teaching others, but also creativity and problem solving in relation to occupations and their context.

People with 'leading' skills might model ways to deliver physical or verbal assistance, ensure people were given the opportunity to express their views or have a turn, establish rules or boundaries for behaviour towards others, reinforce positive actions towards others, or might create special roles within a shared occupation. They were seen to adjust the physical parameters, objects used within or the timing of the occupation. Joe used his leading skills during a scout meeting to facilitate Anton's involvement.

Joe goes over to Rob, one of the scouts, and encourages him to help Anton when he goes off track. He demonstrates how to hold Anton, and explains what to do if Anton is

---

[1]Kapa haka is a New Zealand Maori cultural performing group (Moorfield, n.d.).

wandering out of line, or running when he's not meant to.

Later during a group discussion, Rob brings the thick, bundled up rope from the tug-of-war over to Anton and places it on his lap. Anton happily begins sorting the knotted rope out. Joe explains to me that Anton really likes undoing and "dismantling" things, so he ensures that others give him this job. (Observation, Scouts)

Both adults and children demonstrated skills for leading, although children sometimes needed prompting by adults to assume a leading role. When there was a lack of people with leading skills, participation in shared occupation was hampered and was dominated by some group members, with other group members ignored.

The Participation-Enabling Skill of Including

Findings from the study indicated that inclusion was not simply a concept or being physically placed in a setting with other people, but that it involved people's actions towards one another. Moreover, people showed different levels of ability to act in ways that 'included' other people.

'Including' refers to the actions used by adults and children to involve each other into a shared occupation. A number of specific including actions were identified, such as noticing another's need for assistance or to be involved, greeting, introducing, inviting, touching, listening, asking, explaining, offering and sharing resources, turn-taking, providing and receiving help, reciprocating, encouraging, and praising.

When Anton's mother took him to the playground, other children used their 'including skills' to involve him in their game.

He likes football. I've seen him going up to one or two children on the field – they're ones who know him because there's a group around his age. They'd say 'Anton, do you want to kick the ball?' Or throwing hoops with the basketball, he would go over and want to observe, or try and get the ball and have a turn. So there was a bit of interaction. (Interview)

When including actions were used, children became observably more integrated into a shared occupation. On the other hand, when including actions were not used, children were observed to be on the outer of a group and were excluded from contributing.

The Participation-Enabling Skill of Performing

The ability to 'perform' an occupation was also an important participation-enabling skill. 'Performing' refers to people's capacity to carry out and achieve a shared occupation. This was an aspect of participation typically emphasized in rehabilitation documents. A range of 'performance skills' was observed in classrooms and in community activities. The children in the study who had traumatic brain injury experienced some reductions in their performance skills, but had retained the ability to follow others' actions, and often used this ability to support their own 'performance'. Peers with strong performance skills, therefore, performed an important role in supporting shared occupation by modelling ways to carry out the occupation. For instance, during the tug-of-war, Anton imitated the actions of other children and this helped him to take part successfully.

Now the two teams are changing ends. Anton knows to swap over, and moves with the others to the new position. They are trying to get the knot centred over the line again. Anton backs up with the others in his team and his friend, perhaps a little confused, but following suit. 'Right, PULL!!!' Anton is not really pulling, still not getting it, but keeps his hands on the rope, and watches his friend in front of him. (Observation, Scouts)

Learning Participation-Enabling Skills

As children and adults shared occupation with one another, it could be seen that there was an exchange of information. 'Learning' gradually took place about one another's experiences, and about one another's needs and abilities in relation to that occupation. Learning was optimal where a group incorporated some people with strong participation-enabling skills in the areas of driving, leading, including, and performing. Learning occurred in these situations through observation, trial and error, coaching, and modelling. It could be seen that learning participation-enabling skills was cyclical. Where people shared occupation together, learning brought about an increase in their participation-enabling skills and further shared occupation was facilitated. Anton's teacher described the way children from the mainstream classes learned how to participate when they visited Anton's class for children with special needs.

I have buddies coming in here as well – they read and play games together. Buddies are great, they love our kids. At first, if you've got kids who haven't worked with your kids, they get nervous. And they'll keep their distance until they warm up. It's just because our kids are so new for them, a lot of mainstream kids have never been in a special needs classroom. But when they get used to it, they just come in and they get to know the kids as people. (Interview)

Conversely, where people had seldom participated together, learning did not take place, and when needing to share an occupation, they were at a loss as to how to go about supporting one another's involvement. This was often seen in situations of sudden change, such as a transition to a new school or a move to a new home in another area.

PARTICIPATION-ENABLING SKILLS: A FOOTHOLD TO CHANGE PRACTICE

The presence of participation-enabling skills among those who share occupation is lent credence by themes present in earlier occupational therapy and occupational science literature. In 1973, Anne Cronin Mosey proposed that individuals develop group interaction skills for cooperating and interacting with others when performing tasks. Ruth Humphry (2005) has also noted the way communities create occupational opportunities, and that individuals within those communities use a range of strategies to bridge gaps in others' performance. By attending to the things that people do to support one another to participate in shared occupation, our understandings about people's attitudes can be reframed; the notion of participation-enabling skills, instead, suggests that the ways people

think and act towards those who are different can be changed through learning. What is more, learning occurs experientially in the context of shared occupation. In this study, attitudes were not fixed, and shared occupation prompted the evolution of other's understandings about the involvement of diverse team members and the development of new ways of going about occupations together.

Consistent with the tenets of social capital theory (Field, 2008), it was apparent in the study that children and adults who shared in occupations with the children with traumatic brain injury gained knowledge and skills that equipped them for engaging in situations where others brought different abilities and perspectives, and where development of creative solutions to problems was demanded. In recognizing, naming, and describing the range of participation-enabling skills, important leverage is gained for shifting the focus of occupational therapy practice from the individual to communities who take part in occupation. To promote participation, our occupational therapy intervention needs to move outside the border that has traditionally encompassed children and their families, and bring about change in the wider environments with which they are connected.

The possibility is opened up for evaluating the skills that different people in a community might contribute to support children to participate, and for considering people's participation-enabling skill levels when making decisions about placement or whether a shared occupation is a reasonable participation option for a child. Practitioners might identify those in the environment who have stronger participation-enabling skills, and draw on those skills in the context of shared occupation to extend the knowledge to others and support children's participation in a sustainable way. Because specific strategies were identified within the participation-enabling skill areas, intervention could target particular actions that can be learned to support participation. The findings indicate there is value in occupational therapists working directly with groups of children who are sharing in an occupation. In this way, practice allows for modelling of strategies that people can use to support one another to participate, whilst ensuring opportunities for others to use their skills at driving, leading, including, and performing.

CONCLUSION

Making change to ways of doing things is never straightforward. Extending practice with children outside traditional boundaries to bring about change in the wider social environment, will require occupational therapists to chart new territory. The chapter, has provided an initial outline of a map to guide the way beyond that boundary. As others begin to travel that way, the map can be adjusted and refined. To support the future health of children with disabilities, therapists must now open out that map and face the challenge of taking that first step on the journey.

REFERENCES

Anaby, D., Hand, C., Bradley, L., Direzze, B., Forhan, M., Digiacomo, A., et al., 2013. The effect of the environment on participation of children and youth with disabilities: a scoping review. Disabil. Rehabil. 35, 1589–1598.

Bedell, G., Coster, W., Law, M., Liljenquist, K., Kao, Y.C., Teplicky, R., et al., 2013. Community participation, supports, and barriers of school-age children with and without disabilities. Arch. Phys. Med. Rehabil. 94, 315–323.

Cutchin, M.P., Dickie, V.A. (Eds.), 2013. Transactional Perspectives on Occupation. Springer, New York.

Field, J., 2008. Social Capital. Routledge, New York.

Humphry, R., 2005. Model of processes transforming occupations: exploring societal and social influences. J. Occup. Sci. 12, 36–44.

Mesterman, R., Leitner, Y., Yifat, R., Gilutz, G., Levi-Hakeini, O., Bitchonsky, O., et al., 2010. Cerebral palsy: long-term medical, functional, educational, and psychosocial outcomes. J. Child Neurol. 25, 36–42.

Michelsen, S.I., Flachs, E.M., Damsgaard, M.T., Parkes, J., Parkinson, K., Rapp, M., et al., 2014. European study of frequency of participation of adolescents with and without cerebral palsy. Eur. J. Paediatr. Neurol. 18, 282–294.

Minister for Disability Issues, 2001. New Zealand Disability Strategy. Ministry of Health, Wellington.

Moorfield, J.C., n.d. Te Aka Māori-English, English-Māori dictionary and index. Available from: <http://www.maoridictionary.co.nz/> (accessed 09.06.16.).

Mosey, A.C., 1973. Activities Therapy. Raven Press, New York.

Northcott, N., 1996. Cognitive mapping: an approach to qualitative data analysis. J. Res. Nurs. 1, 456–464.

Pahl, R., Spencer, L., 1997. The politics of friendship. Renewal 5, 100–107.

Putnam, R.D., 2000. Bowling Alone: The Collapse and Revival of American Community. Simon & Schuster, New York.

Rosenbaum, P., 2010. Improving attitudes towards children with disabilities in a school context. Dev. Med. Child Neurol. 52, 889–890.

Stake, R.E., 1995. The Art of Case Study Research. Sage, Thousand Oaks, CA.

Stake, R.E., 2006. Multiple Case Study Analysis. Guilford Press, New York.

World Health Organization, 2001. International Classification of Functioning, Disability and Health (ICF). WHO, Geneva.

Wright, F.V., Rosenbaum, P.L., Goldsmith, C.H., Law, M., Fehlings, D.L., 2008. How do changes in body functions and structures, activity, and participation relate in children with cerebral palsy? Dev. Med. Child Neurol. 50, 283–289.

56

DISASTER SUPPORT ACTIVITIES AFTER THE GREAT EAST JAPAN EARTHQUAKE IN FUKUSHIMA

YOSHITAKA SHIINO ■ KEIICHI HASEGAWA

On 11 March 2011, the Pacific side of East Japan, including Iwate, Miyagi, and Fukushima prefectures, suffered a heavy impact by the Great East Japan Earthquake. The earthquake and the tsunami that followed devoured a lot of buildings, household effects, and human lives in an instant. Furthermore, in Fukushima, many people were forced to leave their hometowns and communities as a result of the earthquake and the ensuing accident at the Fukushima I (Daiichi) Nuclear Power Plant. At the time of this writing (March 2015), most of those affected are still forced to live as evacuees. It is difficult to know when and how they can rebuild their lives. Unlike the other prefectures, Fukushima has taken a different path and developed support activities as a response to the nuclear accident and its consequences. Living and working in Fukushima, we observed that in the aftermath of the disaster occupational participation became restricted for many people. Therefore, occupational therapy had an important role to play.

The first section of the chapter gives an overview of the Great East Japan Earthquake and the disaster support activities developed by occupational therapists in Fukushima. The aim of the chapter is to reflect on our support activities, discuss new possibilities for occupational therapists, and increase awareness of the potential for occupational therapy after disasters. It is important to make use of the lessons learnt in order to be prepared for future large-scale disasters.

OVERVIEW OF THE EARTHQUAKE AND DAMAGE IN JAPAN

At 14:46 on 11 March 2011, an earthquake occurred about 130 kilometres east southeast of the Oshika

Peninsula of Miyagi prefecture. The magnitude indicating the scale of the earthquake was 9.0. It was the most powerful earthquake ever recorded to have hit Japan. The epicentre was immense. It was approximately 500 kilometres from north to south, and approximately 200 kilometres east to west. The Japanese government named the disaster 'the Great East Japan Earthquake' on 1 April 2011 (Ministry of Land, Infrastructure and Transport Meteorological Agency, 2011a, 2011b).

The earthquake triggered a powerful tsunami with a wave height of more than 10 metres (Japan Weather Association, n.d.). Devastating damage occurred on the Pacific coast of Japan. In addition to the huge tsunami, there were aftershocks, solid liquefaction, subsidence, breaches in dams, and major disruption on various infrastructures such as electricity, water, gas, road, and rail. Moreover, about 1 hour after the earthquake, the Fukushima I Nuclear Power Plant lost its power supply due to the tsunami and the active cooling systems stopped, resulting in a meltdown of Units 1, 2, and 3 of the plant's six nuclear reactors. Parts of the roof were blown by hydrogen-air explosions. Massive amounts of radioactive materials leaked out, causing the largest nuclear incident in Japan.

The evacuation period for residents from the area around the plants has been extended due to the nuclear disaster. At the peak period immediately after the disaster, the number of evacuees was more than 340 000, and more than 220 000 people were still unable to return to their hometown in March 2015 (Reconstruction Agency, April 8, 2015). In August 2014, the number of dead and missing due to the earthquake and tsunami was estimated to be about 20 000, with about 400 000 buildings totally and partially collapsed (Ministry of Internal Affairs and Communications Fire and Disaster Management Agency, 9 March 2015).

CHARACTERISTICS OF THE GREAT EAST JAPAN EARTHQUAKE FROM AN OCCUPATIONAL PERSPECTIVE

The life of an evacuee is presented through the Person-Environment-Occupation model (Yoshikawa, 2011). The performance occurs in the circuit of the three circles representing 'person', 'environment', and 'occupation'. In the case of this earthquake, the circle of

environment was restricted because residents were forced to move from their hometown due to the nuclear accident. As a result, participation became difficult or impossible. The evacuees' physical activities have been reduced, and both physical and mental functions diminished due to disuse over time. Therefore, the circle which describes the quality of being a person is also restricted, because evacuees may have lost many of the facilities through which they engage in daily experiences that reinforce the sense of doing, being, and belonging.

As a consequence of the sudden environmental change, people lost their jobs in industries such as fishing, forestry, or agriculture in which they had been engaged before the earthquake. In addition, most of the occupations associated with cooking, washing, cleaning, and shopping were not necessary in the evacuation shelters and children could not go to school. The evacuees could not do leisure activities such as gardening, repair or maintenance of their houses. In other words, their roles, purpose of life, pleasures, and many valuable occupations were lost. Furthermore, the community collapsed because the local residents of each city, town, and village unit in Fukushima were dispersed throughout Japan.

In the evacuation shelters, many people who were utter strangers now lived in shared spaces and slept under the same roof. They lost communication with neighbours and close friends, and lost the opportunities to go shopping to familiar shops. Consequently, they went out less frequently. They had nothing to do in their daily lives and became depressed. These issues were not only physical and mental problems, but major social and vocational problems. Even though they have moved from the shelters to temporary housing or houses rebuilt or rented by local government, these problems have continued for some evacuees.

SUPPORT ACTIVITIES BY THE FUKUSHIMA ASSOCIATION OF OCCUPATIONAL THERAPISTS

Initial Response

Our first response was to confirm the safety of our families, relatives, acquaintances, and occupational therapy colleagues. In the period immediately after the earthquake it was difficult to make connections through telephones and e-mail and most people took refuge some distance away.

On Starting the Support Activities

The Fukushima prefecture was in a condition of fear and anxiety due to the nuclear accident, while the supplies of gasoline and food were short too. While they still worked, most occupational therapists were troubled every day with anxious and confused feelings about their own lives: 'Is it okay to stay here or should we evacuate now?' During the first month after the disaster, the Fukushima Association of Occupational Therapists had as its primary concern to establish the well-being of its members, and therefore it could not support or coordinate other professional activities.

Support Activities in the Primary Evacuation Shelters

By April 2011, supplies such as gasoline were almost restored. Support activities started from the inland area; because of its distance from the epicentre there was relatively less damage. Using some holidays in April, we visited the gymnasium which was being used as a primary evacuation shelter and asked evacuees about the difficulties they had experienced: 'Isn't there anything you have had trouble with?' Many answers were unexpected, for example, 'We do not have any problem in particular.' Also, there were several who answered, 'We do gymnastic activities along with a radio broadcast in the morning and evening', 'Dance and yoga instructors come and teach us some exercises'. Indeed, taking the lesson from other past disasters, many public workers, such as health visitors (public health nurses), and volunteers from other organizations were aware of disuse syndrome and deep vein thrombosis and acted appropriately to prevent these issues. Thus, for some time we were doing nothing for the evacuees but just saying 'please contact us if you have any trouble'. However, we understood later that this was a big mistake.

Over the course of time, an eagerness to do something real to make the lives of evacuees more pleasant gained momentum; thus, we changed our approach and decided that we should develop activities for people in evacuation shelters. As a result, we prepared materials for beanbags and origami, colouring books,

etc., and revisited the evacuation shelters during the May holidays.

Although the participants were few at first, as the ice was broken by having fun, they started speaking about their problems: 'Actually, my hand is clumsy due to a stroke 5 years ago. Here at the shelter, it gets worse because there are no household chores to do', 'Here I wear slippers [slippers are worn indoors in Japan, not shoes], it is difficult to walk, and I stumble often. The other day, too. I slipped and fell down in the restroom', 'I decided not to drink water, so that I don't need to go to the restroom because it's scary to walk', 'I was sleeping in a bed at home, and it is difficult to get up from the floor mat here', and so forth. They spoke out about their problems all at once. We hurriedly did simple checks on balancing ability and other physical functions and were surprised to find some problems in almost everyone, particularly the elderly and disabled people who were showing signs of disuse syndrome. Those who kept saying 'it's okay', actually experienced severe conditions, about which they began to speak due to the relaxation achieved through occupational therapy activities. We would not have known the truth by just coming to a shelter. We reflected on and radically revised our plans and started support activities from that moment.

The objectives of support activities were: (a) to prevent the progression of disuse syndrome by using the knowledge and implementation of occupational therapy interventions, and (b) to make opportunities for enjoyment and health available to people forced to live at evacuation shelters.

The contents of the support activity were: (a) to recommend physical exercises (Figure 56-1), to advise evacuees on some ideas to support reengagement in daily life occupations, and to provide aids and adaptations to those people who may be frail, vulnerable or at risk of falls; (b) to offer places where they could do creative activities; and (c) to maintain communication with the people (especially with the elderly) who declined physical activity interventions. We visited the evacuees every day, collaborated with physiotherapists and prosthetists, and brought welfare equipment, such as shoes and canes. For people whose cane, for example, did not fit, we cut and adjusted the height of the cane or provided a new one. For people who had difficulty walking in slippers, we evaluated the functioning of

4. 新聞紙でストレッチ！〜リング体操〜

身近な道具を使って車椅子や椅子に座ったまま行え、簡単に身体のストレッチができます。

1. 用具
新聞紙…2枚、ビニールテープ…1つ
作り方…新聞紙を二枚重ねて丸め、両端をテープで貼れば完成！！

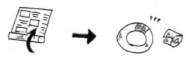

2. 方法
①椅子に座った状態でリングを両手で掴みながら
万歳するように真上にあげて深呼吸をします。
深呼吸はリラックス効果があります。

②真上にあげた状態で左右に身体を倒し身体の筋
肉を伸ばします。脇腹が伸びるように意識して
ください。

③リングを掴んだまま胸の前に持っていき、車の
ハンドルを回すように両腕をねじります。主に
肩と腕の筋肉が伸ばされ鍛える事が出来ます。

FIGURE 56-1 ■ Physical exercises using a newspaper.

their lower limbs and provided proper shoes. We advised individually about their life rhythm and activities of daily living based on the information from public health nurses. For creative activities, we made beanbags, cloth sandals, basket, origami and some traditional crafts products, and played Japanese traditional games.

As mentioned above, we talked to several people at first and worked with a small number of people at the primary evacuation shelters. Once participants were inspired and the activity space was energized, a large number of people gradually gathered and had begun to participate in those activities voluntarily. Men were unfamiliar with and were negative about crafts like origami, but actively participated in the work-like activities, such as making cloth sandals and baskets.

Some even willingly helped and taught others who were unused to making them. A woman who had had a stroke improved her finger movement. The evacuees showed improvements in their health and occupational engagement, even after working with occupational therapy for only a short while. Some people made craft items as presents to their families and their families appreciated their work very much. We worked on supporting, always cooperating and sharing information with other professionals, such as public health nurses, physiotherapists, care managers, and social workers in each evacuation shelter.

Support Activities in the Secondary Evacuation Shelters

The evacuees gradually moved from the gyms which were primary evacuation shelters to the hotels and inns which were used as secondary evacuation shelters. Although these were improvements in their living environment, there were new problems of tripping on unfamiliar steps and also that evacuees shut themselves away in their private rooms. We continually visited each room with colleagues from social services to provide support. We performed evaluations and gave daily living advice, offering welfare equipment according to the needs of each evacuee.

Support Activities in the Temporary Housing

Temporary housing was completed around August/September in 2011 and many people moved from evacuation shelters to temporary housing. We shifted our focus and started support activity for people in their temporary housing at around the same time. At first, we began with the advice on structural issues regarding the temporary housing, including repair of handrails and eliminating steps. There were many problems such as the big front step, impractical handrails, and a deep, small bathtub. We advised on these issues, in cooperation with physiotherapists, to administrative officers, such as public health nurses and care managers.

Then, we focused on wellness and prevention of social withdrawal at the support centre. We provided exercises and activities focusing on fitness, recreation, and fun. In addition, we coached the staff of the support centre in understanding the point of the activities so that they were able to facilitate them even after the occupational therapist team had left. As our support activities became known to the evacuees, the number of participants increased and they voluntarily attended as they enjoyed participating. Due to the limited number of available occupational therapists, the support activities were done in only a few temporary housing sites and were greatly appreciated by evacuees, administrative officers, and volunteers.

Other Support Activities

Making a Brochure ('Winter Living') and Instruction Lectures (Figure 56-2)

Fukushima prefecture is the third largest prefecture in Japan and the climate is different between inland and coastal regions. While the inland part experiences heavy snowfalls, the coastal region on the Pacific side is warm. During the heavy winter snow, it is necessary to be able to walk on the snow-covered roads and to clear the snow. Evacuees from the warmer coastal regions were challenged by living inland in such an unfamiliar environment.

Moreover, the risk of falls was high, especially for the elderly and disabled people. They needed to be very careful. Therefore the occupational therapists who were used to living in the heavy snowfall area made a brochure titled 'Winter Living', cooperating with physiotherapists, and distributed it to all of the evacuees' homes. In addition, we organised an instruction lecture using the brochure before the snowfall season came. These actions led to the development of interventions with a specific focus on winter life (Figure 56-3 illustrates some strategies for safe walking on ice and snow).

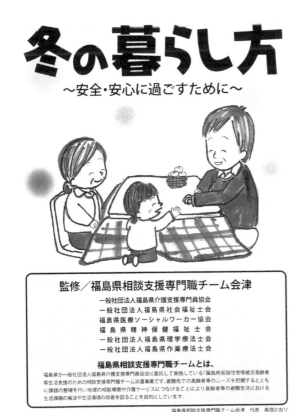

FIGURE 56-2 ■ 'Winter Living' brochure.

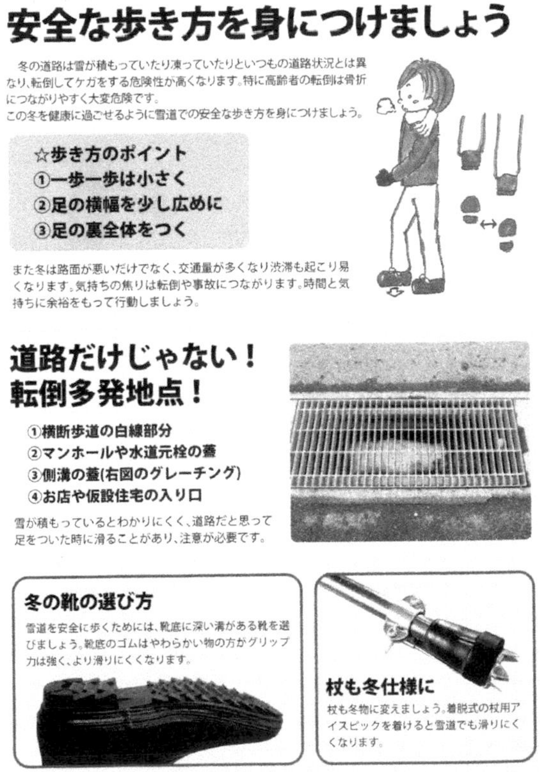

FIGURE 56-3 ■ 'Winter Living' brochure.

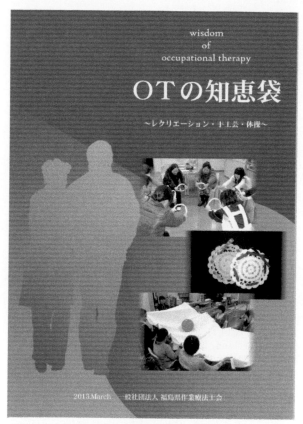

FIGURE 56-4 ■ 'Wisdom of Occupational Therapy' booklet.

Making and Distributing the 'Wisdom of Occupational Therapists' Booklet

It was difficult for the occupational therapist team to visit and support everyone in temporary housing. We created a booklet entitled Wisdom of Occupational Therapy (Figure 56-4), which included various activities: recreation, handcrafts, exercises, etc., to help people make good use of the free time at support centres. We handed it out for free to members of administrative offices who worked in support centres. A local Social Welfare Association picked it up for their public relations magazine as its cover. We distributed it and run workshops about the book. We organized volunteer activities in Fukushima which helped promote the role of occupational therapy. Afterwards, the book was used by many administrative officers and volunteer staff and they performed exercises and activities for evacuees. This book was very popular; 2300 copies were published.

Relation to Developmental Support

There were some reports about increased bone fractures among children experiencing falls. Through the community-based infants' medical examination and in the nursery school, occupational therapists taught the key points for motor and cognitive development to teachers and parents and explained the developmental importance of physical contact for children. We also introduced play for physical balance (Japanese Association of Occupational Therapists, 2014a).

Mental Health

Disorders caused by the considerable stress of the earthquake disaster and an increase in the incidence of depression were reported. Occupational therapists were assigned to the regional care centre for disaster-related mental health and worked on support activities. Some of our colleagues were constantly involved in group work at activity centres. They listened to the voices of both residents and carers in individual and group activities and worked to reduce their stress, anxiety, and feelings of isolation through social interaction and handcrafts. We conducted outreach work to increase evacuees' reassurance through sharing emotions and talking with each other (Japanese Association of Occupational Therapists, 2014a).

CONCLUSION

The consequences of the disaster of the Great East Japan Earthquake remain extensive. In Fukushima prefecture it is hard to erase the effects and harmful stigma resulting from the nuclear accident. The support activities require an extended and sustained effort. We started the support activities by ourselves, that is, there was no clear coordinator or a leader at first. Everyone was affected by the disaster and we started out by seeking to do whatever we could at that time. Depending on each local situation, we developed support activities in cooperation with other types of specialists.

The Japanese Association of Occupational Therapists has a slogan, 'Occupation makes people healthy', and recommends 'meaningful occupation for every person' (Japanese Association of Occupational Therapists, 2014a, 2014b). Most of the evacuees in Fukushima were forced to leave their beloved hometown where the houses are still intact. Furthermore, they were deprived of meaningful occupations, such as jobs and housework. We saw how the evacuees had become unhealthy, both physically and mentally. Daily exercise is recommended to prevent disuse syndrome in general, but it does not seem to make people healthy by itself. We realized again that it is important to keep doing 'meaningful occupations for every person'.

To prepare for the future, it is important to think and act for any disaster, reflecting on the lessons from the Great East Japan Earthquake. The Japanese Association of Occupational Therapists is now preparing support activities as a countermeasure to an anticipated large-scale disaster and has put relevant information on its homepage[1]. It is important to form networks with external organizations depending on the conditions of each country and region, so that there can be preparations in place for a disaster. It might only have a little influence, but the role of occupational therapists could contribute to increasing daily life performance, building a community, and collaborating with various types of professions. In Fukushima, we have managed our daily life and jobs securely and continue to seek new things that we can do in the present, while we advance towards recovery in the future.

Acknowledgements

We want to express our deepest gratitude to Mika Otsuki, who translated this chapter from Japanese. The editors of the book and the authors of this chapter also want to express their gratitude to the Sasakawa Great Britain Foundation. A grant from this foundation made it possible for Dikaios Sakellariou to travel to Japan in July 2015 and work face-to-face with the authors of this chapter.

REFERENCES

Japanese Association of Occupational Therapists Disaster Countermeasure Office. 2014a. The disaster support activity report in the Great East Japan Earthquake disaster. Japanese Association of Occupational Therapists, Tokyo.

Japanese Association of Occupational Therapists, 2014b. Management tool for daily life performance promotion project. <http://www.jaot.or.jp/science/mtdlp.html> (accessed 09.09.14.).

Japan Weather Association, n.d. Overview of the Tohoku-Pacific Ocean Earthquake and Tsunami (the 3rd report). <https://www.jwa.or.jp/news/2011/04/post-000213.html> (accessed 06.01.15.).

Ministry of Internal Affairs and Communications Fire and Disaster Management Agency, 2015. About the Tohoku-Pacific Ocean Earthquake (The Great East Japan Earthquake) in 2011 (the 151th report). <http://www.fdma.go.jp/bn/higaihou_new.html> (accessed 06.01.15.).

Ministry of Land, Infrastructure and Transport Meteorological Agency, 2011a. About an earthquake of the Sanriku offing of 11 March 2011 about 14:46. <http://www.jma.go.jp/jma/press/1103/11b/201103111600.html> (accessed 08.20.14.).

Ministry of Land, Infrastructure and Transport Meteorological Agency, 2011b. About 'Heisei23 (2011) Tohoku district Pacific offing earthquake' (the 15th report). <http://www.jma.go.jp/jma/press/1103/13b/201103131255.html> (accessed 08.20.14.).

Reconstruction Agency, 2015. Transition of the number of evacuees. <http://www.reconstruction.go.jp/topics/main-cat2/sub-cat2-1/hinanshasuu.html> (accessed 06.01.15.).

Yoshikawa, H., 2011. Subete no hito ni yoi sagyo wo *(Better occupational participation for all people)*. In: Japanese Association of Occupational Therapists (Ed.), 'Sagyo' no toraekata to hyokashien gijutsu *(The interpretation of 'occupation' and assessment-support technique)*-Seikatsu koui no jiritsu ni muketa management *(Management toward self-standing daily life performance)*. Ishiyaku Publishers, Inc., Tokyo, p. 24.

[1]http://www.jaot.or.jp/others/saigai.html

57

OCCUPATIONAL THERAPY AT THE TOP OF THE WORLD

ALEXIS DAVIS ■ DEBORAH SIMPSON

This chapter explores an occupational therapy-led global health project called the Ladakh Disability and Rehabilitation Training (LDRT). The aims of this chapter are: (a) to describe the context of the LDRT, (b) to explain the LDRT's development and progress, (c) to review the project's challenges and successes, and (d) to illustrate a partnership model for reapplication in areas where disability services have not been established or are emerging.

The LDRT project is a knowledge exchange partnership between Canada and Ladakh. The LDRT team has included Canadian multidisciplinary rehabilitation professionals and students and Ladakhi community development workers and government health employees. The overall goal of the partnership is to improve the lives of people with disabilities in Ladakh. Since LDRT's inception in 2007, the project has evolved from conducting village-based needs assessments and health-related educational initiatives to supporting service provision in a specialized hospital unit for children who have disabilities.

Ladakh is situated in the Himalayan region of northern India. Impassable by road for most of the year, it has become a popular tourist destination in the summer for sightseers, mountaineers, and anthropologists. Ladakh is often touted as the 'top of the world', and for the Canadian rehabilitation team members this descriptive phrase captures the exhilaration of the project's journey and its rollercoaster ride of successes and challenges.

In 2011, the World Report on Disability (World Health Organization and World Bank) confirmed the dire need for increased rehabilitation services in low- and middle-income regions. LDRT demonstrates that occupational therapy principles are a good foundation for the development of rehabilitation training programmes to address this need.

THE CONTEXT OF THE LADAKH DISABILITY AND REHABILITATION TRAINING

Ladakh, 'land of high passes', in India's northwestern state of Jammu and Kashmir (J & K), is the highest inhabited land and the coldest desert in the world (Hanafi, 2014). Known for its stunning beauty, rich culture, harsh climate, and rugged terrain, Ladakh is nestled between the Himalayas to the south and the Karakoram mountains to the north and is bordered by Pakistan, China, and Tibet. Ladakh is slightly more than 85 000 square kilometres in size (about two-thirds the size of England) and has a population of approximately 275 000. This number is just 2% of J & K's total population despite Ladakh covering two-thirds of its land area (KashmirWatch, 2013; Sikand, 2006). The capital city of Leh is home to half of Ladakh's population, approximately 133 500 people (KashmirWatch, 2013); the other half lives in small, remote villages and survives on subsistence farming. Religion is an important aspect of life in Ladakh; the majority of the population identify as Tibetan Buddhist or Shia Muslim, while a minority are Sunni Muslim or Christian (Bharatonline, n.d.).

There is a strong military presence in Ladakh due to India's border disputes with Pakistan and China (Monasterio, 2000). In 1999, Ladakh garnered international attention as a result of India's armed conflict with Pakistan that was fought in Ladakh's Kargil region. Despite a ceasefire, conflicts occasionally flare up, making Ladakh one of the most volatile regions in the world (North, 2014).

Ladakh's border only opened to tourists in 1974, and in the summer months it has become a popular destination for adventure travellers and Indian tourists who seek respite from the heat. With tourism – now approximately 50% of Ladakh's economy – came an influx of money and exposure to modern habits and behaviours such as the use of technology (Gilman, 1987). Consequently, the people of Ladakh experienced a vast amount of change in a short period of time (Dana, 2007).

Disability in Ladakh

The number of people in Ladakh who have a disability is estimated to be 40 000, based on the global average prevalence rate of 15% (World Health Organization and World Bank, 2011). However, this estimate could be higher as disability statistics are unreliable due to the remoteness of hundreds of Ladakh's villages, the inadequate training that village health workers receive on detecting impairments, and the lack of infrastructure in the healthcare system. Also, having a disability is associated with stigma and shame in Ladakh, which can result in undiagnosed conditions such as hearing loss, cognitive impairments, and mental illness.

Although there is little scholarly literature that connects poverty and disability, McElroy et al. (2011) found that poverty was a major contributing factor to disability in Ladakh. Exclusion of persons with disabilities within valued sectors of Ladakhi society, such as employment, is common and creates a vicious cycle of poverty and disability, as illustrated in Figure 57-1. Nongovernmental organizations (NGOs) in Ladakh, such as HEALTH Inc. (Health, Education & Literacy in the Himalayas) and the People's Action Group for Advocacy and Rights, aim to alleviate this exclusion by promoting awareness of disability issues within the general public and providing opportunities for persons with disabilities to have meaningful roles within their families and communities (Kunzang, 2011).

As recently as 2005, HEALTH Inc. staff reported that community development workers had found children with disabilities hidden away in village homes due to stigma and shame. Since then, due to promotion of disability issues by NGOs, the disability movement has gained strength in Ladakh. Families have started to advocate for services and seek help from doctors and other health professionals, such as audiologists and dentists, for their disabled family members. However, the inaccessibility of schools,

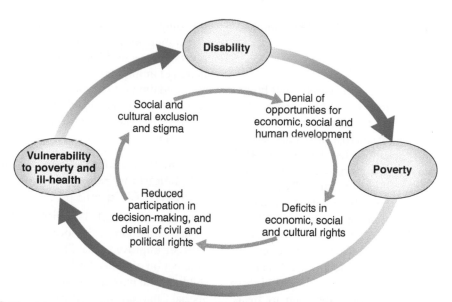

FIGURE 57-1 ■ The vicious cycle of poverty and disability. *Courtesy Department of International Development 2000.*

poor coordination of rehabilitation services, and lack of financial support remain challenges for the provision of services for Ladakhi citizens who have disabilities.

DEVELOPMENT OF THE LADAKH DISABILITY AND REHABILITATION TRAINING PROJECT

In 2005 and 2006, Cynthia Hunt, the founder of HEALTH Inc., brought small groups of Ladakhi community development workers to Vancouver, British Columbia, to learn about rehabilitation services in Canada. The interns' itinerary included a visit to Sunny Hill Health Centre for Children, part of BC Children's Hospital, where occupational therapists oriented them to the centre's rehabilitation services. The occupational therapists and interns found that they had mutual interests and goals, and a partnership was naturally and quickly established. In 2007, the first multidisciplinary team of Canadian rehabilitation professionals travelled to Ladakh to share their knowledge of assessment and treatment approaches with local care providers and to learn directly from the Ladakhi people about the healthcare issues associated with having a disability.

Early Years of the Ladakh Disability and Rehabilitation Training Project

In the 2007 inaugural visit, the tasks of the LDRT team were to meet with key healthcare providers to gather information of the disability services landscape; visit healthcare clinics in remote villages that were identified by the healthcare providers as having a large proportion of children and youth with disabilities; and begin to identify the rehabilitation needs of people with disabilities. Assessment and treatment services were provided by the Canadian LDRT members in partnership with the community development workers. Based on community interest, educational workshops about disability awareness were conducted. From a Canadian perspective, the village health clinics were typically small, ill-supplied, and poorly serviced. Furthermore, the clinic staff had a limited awareness of disability issues due to a lack of training.

In 2008, the LDRT team members returned to the villages to provide follow-up services. In addition, a qualitative research study was conducted. The study explored community readiness for change, and the knowledge, beliefs, attitudes, and practices related to people with disabilities in Ladakh (McElroy et al., 2011). The community development workers were trained in research techniques and participated fully in the research, consistent with the LDRT's foundational value of knowledge exchange.

Mental Health

In 2009, the psychiatrist at Ladakh's government hospital, Sonam-Norboo Memorial (SNMH), asked the Canadian LDRT members to assist with the mental health programme. The psychiatrist shared his view of how mental health problems in Ladakh had increased since 1974 due to the rapid convergence of old and new ideas associated with the influx of tourists. These problems included a rise in alcohol abuse and increased rates of depression and suicide among the region's youth.

The psychiatrist also expressed his concern that religious practices were commonly accepted by the Ladakhi people as the preferred mode of treatment for psychotic illnesses, such as schizophrenia and bipolar disorder, and a pharmacological approach to treatment was typically met with distrust. He hoped that by educating people about the potential benefits of psychiatric medications such as reduced length and severity of disabling symptoms, a major concern in subsistence farming communities, the concurrent use of pharmacology and traditional forms of treatment might become more common. Ladakh has low levels of literacy, and drama is a traditional and effective form of communication. Consequently, the psychiatrist consulted on a theatrical production created by local youth that aimed to heighten awareness of mental illnesses and treatment options. The production travelled to selected remote villages, and the LDRT team accompanied the cast and crew to support the educational component of the initiative by answering questions after the performances.

Another component of the mental health programme was the facilitation of workshops on mental health issues for secondary school students. This initiative provided an opportunity for secondary students to openly discuss issues and trends that might influence their use of substances or contribute to the onset of depression, as well as how to access help if needed.

Lastly, Canadian LDRT team members were invited to participate in an information meeting that brought together traditional healers and local physicians. This gathering allowed the healers – spiritual and allopathic – to share their perspective on the treatment of mental illness. The Canadians described their experience of providing mental health rehabilitation services in cooperation with cultural and spiritual organizations in Vancouver, a multicultural city that has a large population of immigrants and refugees. This exchange laid the foundation for collaborative treatment approaches between traditional and allopathic care providers that could better meet the needs of Ladakh's diverse population.

Current Phase of the Ladakh Disability and Rehabilitation Training – the Paediatric Unit for Special Children

Throughout the LDRT project, the team members brought attention to the local health authority of the need for improved rehabilitation services. This led to the creation of a specifically designed hospital unit for children who have disabilities. The Paediatric Unit for Special Children was established in 2010 with a vision to be a hub for high-quality, comprehensive, and multidisciplinary assessment and treatment services. At the inauguration ceremony (Figure 57-2), high-ranking state government officials, media, armed forces, and local citizens were in attendance and shared in the excitement and pride at the opening of this much-needed service.

With the Paediatric Unit open for patients, the LDRT began to focus on paired training and one-on-one mentoring. For example, the Ladakhi physiotherapist would take the lead in an assessment/treatment

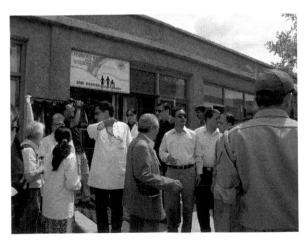

FIGURE 57-2 ■ Inauguration ceremony of the Paediatric Unit for Special Children, Sonam-Norboo Memorial Hospital, 2010.

session providing the Canadian professional with an opportunity to learn about healthcare provision in Ladakh. Coaching and modelling by the Canadian team members allowed the Ladakhi professionals to expand their skills and increase their confidence in several clinical areas, which is particularly important because they work in isolation for much of the year (Wishart, 2014) and opportunities for professional development are limited.

Apart from providing education about clinical services, the Canadian LDRT team members also emphasized the importance of establishing administrative procedures, such as record-keeping – not an inherent aspect of the Ladakhi healthcare system – and communication and follow-up protocols and procedures. Hard data of the Paediatric Unit's activities provides tangible evidence of its unique role in the Ladakhi healthcare system. This validation is important in the continuing need to secure funding. Since the opening of the Paediatric Unit, an annual report has been created with the input of the Ladakhi and Canadian team members that summarizes the goals, achievements, and statistics of the Paediatric Unit throughout the year.

The involvement of the Ladakhi community partners has been a foundation of this phase of the project. From initial meetings about the creation of the unit with healthcare providers and other stakeholders, the Ladakhi LDRT team members have been encouraged to maintain these community connections. The Paediatric Unit has the potential to be a central resource and coordinating body among disability partners in Ladakh as it is government based and supported, and therefore is more sustainable than NGO services.

Future LDRT phases will likely switch from a training focus to more advocacy and lobbying with central government officials. Further research about outreach models for community-based rehabilitation is planned and will be conducted in partnership with the Paediatric Unit staff.

OCCUPATIONAL THERAPY FOUNDATIONS OF THE LADAKH DISABILITY AND REHABILITATION TRAINING

Occupational therapy principles are at the core of the LDRT and have ensured that from its inception the project conceptualized healthcare services from a person, occupation, and environment perspective. This perspective situated the Canadian team's involvement within a holistic view of Ladakh's history and culture, and contributed to team members being consciously aware of their biases and the importance of ethical practice in the field of global health. Occupational therapy competencies have also been integral to project design, such as observation and assessment in real-life environments, a focus on function, community integration, advocacy, and coaching.

Having occupational therapists coordinate the LDRT has been a key factor in the success of the project. Typically, coordinators in Ladakh's healthcare system are physicians, who can be seen as intimidating by other medical staff due to the hierarchy of healthcare services in Ladakh. The occupational therapists were seen as peers, on the same hierarchical level as the Paediatric Unit staff, which was conducive to good communication and joint problem solving. In Canada, occupational therapists often take the lead in interprofessional practice, and this model proved to be equally relevant and effective in Ladakh.

Staffing

Over the years, the Canadian LRDT team members have included representatives from the following professions: occupational therapy, physiotherapy, speech-language pathology, special education, developmental paediatrics, and psychiatry. The staff at the paediatric unit have always been consulted upon as to which professional disciplines would contribute most to their learning. The goal has been to match each Ladakhi staff member with a Canadian counterpart. However, despite occupational therapy training programmes in Delhi and Jammu and recruitment efforts by Ladakh's healthcare authority, to date no occupational therapy positions have been filled in Ladakh. Consequently, the Canadian occupational therapists have been flexible in their mentorship role by working with other professionals, such as maternal-child health workers, to transfer assessment and treatment skills from an occupational therapy lens. In 2013, a newly trained psychologist accepted a posting at the Paediatric Unit and learning assessments became available in the Ladakhi healthcare system for the first time. Hopefully, occupational therapy vacancies will also be filled in the near future.

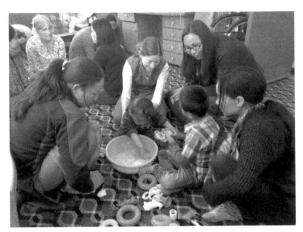

FIGURE 57-3 ■ A busy training session at the Sonam-Norboo Memorial Hospital Paediatric Unit in Leh, 2014.

Interacting with the children and families is a personally fulfilling aspect of this project for the Canadian team members; however, the true work is in empowering the local professionals by supporting their initiatives, setting up systems and protocols, and facilitating new learning. Canadians often take continuing education opportunities and access to the latest research for granted. Sharing these resources with the local professionals in Ladakh (Figure 57-3) is key to the team's role of mentorship (Wishart, 2014).

Student Experiences

Selecting occupational therapy students who have shown interest and engagement in global health is important for the LDRT. Although global heath initiatives offer students the opportunity to combine travel with occupational therapy education, students need to be aware of the challenges inherent in international work prior to applying. To help prepare Canadian occupational therapy students for the contextual factors unique to Ladakh, such as high altitude, rough terrain, lack of modern conveniences, close living quarters, and few therapeutic resources due to remoteness of the region, they participated in several predeparture meetings (McElroy et al., 2011).

Student involvement in the LDRT has had many positive outcomes, such as ensuring that project goals are explicit – a bonus to both students and the Ladakhi partners – and contributing to the lack of hierarchy between the Canadian and Ladakhi team members. The experience of participating in an atypical fieldwork placement presents unique learning opportunities and challenges that can broaden students' understanding of culturally competent healthcare delivery and client-centred practice. These experiences can prepare students for global health work in the future and for clinical practice in their own diverse communities. The presence of students within the LDRT team helps to permeate the culture of shared learning and collaboration among all team members. Quotes from students about their perspectives of involvement in the LDRT project are presented in Boxes 57-1 and 57-2.

Students' evaluations of their LDRT experience indicated that learning about healthcare systems outside of one's home context promoted a deeper understanding of disability perspectives and an awareness of the history of the disability movement. As this information is not necessarily an intrinsic part of occupational therapy curricula, global health placement experiences can fill this gap in education. Several of the students who participated in the LDRT project have become global health clinicians and have completed further education in global health and development.

Students also commented that being immersed in a culture that differs vastly from their own added to their understanding that occupational therapy services need to reflect cultural perspectives on disability. Readiness for treatment has to progress through a natural course of awareness and acceptance in order to lead to sustainable change. As well, the students' experience of client and professional interactions in a context requiring language and cultural interpretation increased their empathy for clients and their families in Canada who have English as a second language and rely on interpreters to understand the healthcare services they are accessing (Wishart, 2014). Furthermore, two Canadian occupational therapy students have conducted evaluative research about the LDRT project by surveying the perspectives of professionals who have been involved in the project since its inception. This research was completed in 2015 and may lead to further studies about perspectives on the LDRT.

CHALLENGES AND SUCCESSES

Challenges

The unique geographical, cultural, and economic characteristics of Ladakh often present a challenge to this knowledge exchange partnership. Although Canada and Ladakh are both mountainous and sparsely populated lands, there is little to compare in terms of social and health infrastructure. Consequently, Canadian LDRT members often questioned if the promotion of disability services and rehabilitation skill training would be relevant to their Ladakhi counterparts. This concern for relevancy was reflected in all aspects of the LDRT programme design.

Development can be a lengthy and arduous process, especially for long-term projects such as the LDRT, that aim for societal and attitudinal change. Often described by LDRT team members as taking two steps forward and one step back, the development of relationships, transfer of knowledge and sequential implementation of services over several years are different kinds of challenges than those faced by short-term aid projects and require ongoing effort and drive to maintain progress.

Another challenge for the LDRT is the change of healthcare administrators in Ladakh every 2 years. This rapid turnover requires that LDRT team members introduce and promote the project, including the SNMH Paediatric Unit, to each new administrator. Also, beyond the human resource challenges already mentioned, there is the constant threat of trained Paediatric Unit staff being reposted to other hospital units. This presents a delicate situation for the Canadian LDRT members who see the value of consistency in the Paediatric Unit staff and want to advocate for their retention, yet do not want to challenge administrative protocols or appear dictatorial. To date, three Paediatric Unit staff members have been in continuous employment over the 5 years of the Paediatric Unit's operation.

Working in Ladakh also requires that the Canadian LDRT members work within the short travel season for village families. Due to hard winter conditions, Ladakh is often isolated from the rest of India for 8 months of the year when its two main access routes become impassable (Monasterio, 2000). Furthermore, during the late summer, families are engaged in harvesting their crops, so the majority of Ladakhi individuals can only access the Paediatric Unit's services in early summer.

Successes

The overarching goal of the LDRT has been to improve the quality of life for people with disabilities in Ladakh. The Canadian team members approached this ambitious task with the underlying values of cultural sensitivity and humility. These values guided the project's inclusion of knowledge acquisition visits to both India and Canada and opened dialogue between Canadian and Ladakhi project members about disability issues, the suitability of Canadian approaches to assessment and treatment in Ladakh, and traditional and newer healthcare practices. Over the several years of the project, the LDRT has progressed gradually and has achieved measurable outcomes. The success of the partnership is expressed in the following statements from members of the Ladakhi team: 'Some NGOs come and do things for us. The Canadian team comes and works with us and teaches us' (Norboo, Paediatric Unit Coordinator). 'It helps when I work with others who increase my understanding, but not do it for me. The Canadian team does that for me. They respect me and work with me. It helps me learn, to do my job' (Dolma, Paediatric Unit Physiotherapist).

Funding

The LDRT is a volunteer-based project with travel expenses for Canadian professionals partially funded by small hospital grants and private donations. The donation of time from the Canadian professionals is an important criterion for engagement in this project. There is no monetary exchange between the Canadian and Ladakhi LDRT members, which helps to enforce the equal partnership between the teams. For example, the new SNMH Paediatric Unit was funded by a one-time grant through the Indian National Rural Health Mission. The Ladakhi healthcare team is responsible for pursuing ongoing funding for Paediatric Unit operations. The Canadian team supports the project in knowledge transfer only, which can be viewed as fiscally responsible development aid in the context of Ladakh (Malhotra, 2000).

Reapplication

The training model that the LDRT has developed over the years was designed for the multifaceted context of Ladakh. This context includes rapid and recent social economic change, a healthcare system with a lack of trained rehabilitation staff, stigma and exclusion of people with disabilities, diverse religious views and traditional beliefs, poverty and illiteracy, and remoteness and isolation in a highly militarized zone. Many elements of the LDRT project may apply to other low- and middle-income regions in the world, where people with disabilities do not have access to the healthcare services that enable them to lead meaningful and productive lives. The World Report on Disability (World Health Organization and World Bank, 2011) provides evidence that rehabilitation services are in dire need in low- and middle-income countries. The LDRT is an example of sustainable rehabilitation services being gradually and methodically developed and executed. Successful strategies included developing trusting relationships with stakeholders over time, being respectful learners of Ladakh's culture, engaging in community life, maintaining an open mind and a watchful eye as to one's biases, and partnering with local partners every step of the way. The foundation of the LDRT project, with its paired-training model, can be an option for further development of rehabilitation services in other global contexts.

CONCLUSIONS

This chapter aimed to explore the diverse context and history of a global health rehabilitation development project in Ladakh, India: the LDRT. The success of the LDRT project is reflected in the development of the healthcare knowledge exchange partnership over several years and in the establishment of a centralized centre of excellence, the SNMH Paediatric Unit. The Paediatric Unit staff are proud of delivering high-quality service for children with disabilities and their families, and value the LDRT partnership. The partnership offers them professional development and the opportunity to train the Canadian team on healthcare provision in a remote, low-resource environment. Lessons learned from the LDRT project, such as the importance of creating paired training opportunities, may be applicable in similar global health situations. Occupational therapy student fieldwork placements and university-supported research partnerships have been successful aspects of the LDRT and are areas for further development.

Global health development work can be challenging and arduous, but also provides tremendous opportunities for learning. Goals include long-term societal and attitudinal changes versus the immediate reduction of threats, which is often the focus of short-term aid projects. Furthermore, the leadership for this development project has been provided by rehabilitation professionals, which has helped steer the training to address the complete picture of life for children with disabilities in a difficult context, rather than focusing on solely one area, such as diagnosis.

Working in a culture other than one's own can challenge belief systems, provide opportunities for mutual learning, and increase cultural awareness (Wishart, 2014). Although it has not been without several 'top of the world' challenges, experiences of the LDRT team in Ladakh have brought both personal and professional learning and fulfilment.

Acknowledgements

We would like to gratefully acknowledge the following people for their assistance with providing content and editing for this chapter: Kate Czapleski, Douglas Herasymuik, Dolma Lhamo, Sonam Norboo, Ross Taylor, and Kathryn Wishart. Our sincere gratitude for support of the LDRT project is given to our families and friends, to the Centre for International Child Health at BC Children's Hospital, Sunny Hill Health Centre for Children, and the Canadian Himalayan Association for Innovation (CHAI).

REFERENCES

Bharatonline.com, n.d. Religions in Leh Ladakh. <http://www.bharatonline.com/kashmir/ladakh/culture/religion.html> (accessed 07.07.15.).

Dana, J.R., 2007. Globalization from below: how Ladakh is responding to globalization with education. <http://www.macalester.edu/educationreform/publicintellectualessay/new%20pies/Dana%20Ladakh%20and%20Education%20PIE.pdf> (accessed 28.09.14.).

Gilman, R., 1987. Ladakh: helping a culture choose its future: an interview with Helena Norberg-Hodge. <http://www.context.org/iclib/ic17/nhodge/> (accessed 12.04.15.).

Hanafi, M.O. 2014. World's Coldest Desert-Ladakh. Pakistan Observer. <http://pakobserver.net/detailnews.asp?id=216290> (accessed 24.09.14.).

KashmirWatch, 2013. J & K census data 2011: Jammu more populated than Srinagar city. <http://kashmirwatch.com/features.php/2013/06/10/j-k-census-data-2011-jammu-more-populated-than-srinagar-city.html> (accessed 04.10.14.).

Kunzang, D., 2011. A journey of a different kind in Ladakh. <http://truthdive.com/2011/02/21/A-journey-of-a-different-kind-in-Ladakh.html> (accessed 24.09.14.).

McElroy, T., Davis, A., Hunt, C., Dadul, J., Stanba, T., Larson, C., 2011. Navigating a way forward: using focused ethnography and community readiness to study disability issues in Ladakh, India. Disabil. Rehabil. 33 (1), 17–27.

Malhotra, K., 2000. NGOs without aid: beyond the global soup kitchen. Third World Q. 21 (4), 655–668.

Monasterio, E., 2000. An experience of psychiatry in Ladakh, India. Australas. Psychiatry 8 (3), 216–219.

North, A., 2014. Siachen dispute: India and Pakistan's glacial fight. <http://www.bbc.com/news/world-asia-india-26967340> (accessed 04.10.14.).

Sikand, Y., 2006. Muslim-Buddhist clashes in Ladakh: the politics behind the 'religious conflict'. <http://www.countercurrents.org/comm-sikand130206.htm> (accessed 28.09.14.).

Wishart, K., 2014. Reflection on an international health project in Leh, Ladakh, India. <http://www.bcaslpa.ca/content/wp-content/uploads/2014/09/Vibrations_September_2014_V1.pdf> (accessed 04.09.14.).

World Health Organization and World Bank, 2011. World report on disability. <http://whqlibdoc.who.int/publications/2011/9789240685215_eng.pdf> (accessed 13.06.11.).

58

REACTIVATING OUR OCCUPATIONAL NATURE FOR SUSTAINABLE OCCUPATIONAL THERAPY

BEN WHITTAKER ▪ GAYNOR SADLO

CHAPTER OUTLINE

Human beings are occupational by nature, evolved with physical, intellectual, social, spiritual, and ultimately creative capacities, as a species that seeks meaning in what we[1] do, born with the capacity to engage in complex, captivating, aesthetic occupations as the essential component of a potentially full, enjoyable, and purposeful life (Ikiugu and Pollard, 2015; Wilcock and Hocking, 2015). How we enact our daily occupations has a powerful impact on our own health and well-being (Clark et al., 2015), but also on that of our world, because there is a symbiotic relationship between human action and the environment in which it takes place (Law et al., 1996).

A very high order of communication (including language) and collaborative skills has become central to our ability to perform occupations of such complexity (Tallis, 2003). Apparently developed from the earlier desire to make tools (using our intelligence to enhance even more our manipulative skills), we thus became 'wired' to connect (Lieberman, 2013) and to care for each other. There is evidence from neuroscience that altruistic behaviour, part of our high social intelligence, is a vital component of our basic occupational nature that has been key to our survival as a species (Wilson, 2015).

Essential to our survival is also care towards our planet. Climate change is the greatest threat to global health in this century (UCL-Lancet Commission, 2009), but we are not acting fast enough to address it (Stern, 2015). In order to sustain the health and well-being of all populations globally, we need to pursue sustainable development (World Health Organization, 2015). This is defined as 'development that meets the needs of the present without compromising the ability

---

[1]When this chapter refers to 'our', 'we' or 'us' this refers to all people as human beings.

of future generations to meet their own needs' (World Commission on Environment and Development, 1987, p. 43). Sustainable development is seen as an altruistic act (Helliwell et al., 2013). This chapter suggests that common negative media messages from advertising and news broadcasts can increase individual anxiety and sense of lack of worth and produce negative feelings about the state of humanity and the wider world. Contemporary culture fosters an increase in materialism and individualism, which can affect health and well-being (Eckersley, 2005), increase narcissism, and reduce empathy (Twenge and Campbell, 2009), and drive climate change through disposable consumerism. In this chapter, the authors propose that we can 'reactivate' our caring, altruistic, occupational nature through doing occupations and live in better harmony with the world.

Sustainable practice is now being advocated within policy documents from governing occupational therapy organizations, such as in Sweden, the UK, and by the World Federation of Occupational Therapists (College of Occupational Therapists, 2013, 2015; Swedish Association of Occupational Therapists, 2012; World Federation of Occupational Therapists, 2012). Occupational therapists need to extend their practice to promote sustainable ways of being at both individual and societal levels, to enable human engagement to promote well-being within a whole-world perspective (Ikiugu, 2008; Whittaker, 2012). Healthier human lifestyles are linked to healthier environments (Goodall, 2007). Occupational therapists can support the 'reactivation' of occupational nature through occupations that are not grounded in consumerism, for example, through the mindful practise of everyday occupations as part of a nurturing self-compassion, community engagement with green spaces and enabling flow experiences through meaningful activity. If we are to change the way we do things (occupational form), then the occupational meaning of these actions must first change.

THE OCCUPATIONAL NATURE OF HUMAN BEINGS

Human nature is occupational in that its hallmark is to engage in, be occupied by, and enjoy a great variety of absorbing, challenging, and highly skilled activities (Hocking, 2013). It is through the experience of participation that occupations acquire meaning, significance, and value to the performer (Kielhofner, 2008). The Person-Environment-Occupation model shows how participation needs to be supported by resources within an environmental context while occupations, in turn, have an impact on those surroundings (Law et al., 1996). Such enquiries are part of occupational science, which has been defined as 'research into the variety of ways in which people are occupied as human beings, and the impact that such engagement has on bodies, selves, communities *and the world*' (Clark and Lawlor, 2008, p. 3, emphasis added).

Our creative productivity and manipulation of the environment owes much to our 'thinking hands' (Pallasmaa, 2009) or their engineered tool equivalents, enacting our intentions (Tallis, 2003) and managing problems presented by different environments (Radman, 2013). We engage in self-care, productive, and enjoyable activities supported by our ability to modify our place, by building protective homes for example, which enhance our survival and pleasure (Wilcock and Hocking, 2015). Occupational scientists Hocking (2013) and Wilcock and Hocking (2015), along with historians, anthropologists, and archeologists, have explored in detail how human societies exponentially developed unique and diverse ways of living over the millennia, tuning with our geographic, climatic, and topographic resources and circumstances (Cochran and Harpending, 2009). The diverse ways we express our occupational nature have forged extraordinary cultural developments (Dutton, 2009). We make deliberate and conscious choices about how we live and act in the world, although hardwired habitual ways of doing can delimit choice (Duhigg, 2013).

Our search for meaning (Hasselkuss, 2011; Ikiugu and Pollard, 2015), need for self-expression, capacity for high skill, and our aesthetic sensibilities foster invention of complex accomplishments, such as the creative arts (Dutton, 2009). Part of our occupational nature is that we seem to have an innate understanding that such profound engagement is essential to health and well-being (Wilcock, 2006); for example, art practices are considered to have a healing function (McNiff, 2004).

The occupational perspective of health (Wilcock and Hocking, 2015) proposes that it is part of human nature to imbibe activities with beliefs, purpose, meaning, and, a sense of belonging (Greenfield, 2002). Basic survival needs, such as feeding, become opportunities to express profound, individual, social, and aesthetic needs; we do not just eat, we *dine* (Jones, 2007; Wrangham, 2010). In Maslow's hierarchy of needs, survival activities (eating, sleeping, mating) are conceptualized as the most basic human requirements, building towards the highest need, self-actualization (Maslow, 1954). Alternatively, an occupational science approach could propose that humans often self-actualize *through* survival activities: by acting out everyday lives in varied, culturally relevant, complex or novel ways. Such combinations form different 'lifestyles', which strongly influence health (Clark et al., 2015). Conversely, when our capacities are compromised through occupational deprivation, alienation, imbalance or injustice (Townsend and Polatajko, 2007), health deteriorates (Wilcock, 2006). Human occupations require high-level capacities indeed, identified in occupational science as encompassing physical, biological, information processing, sociocultural, symbolic, evaluative, and transcendental systems (Clark et al., 1998).

Social neuroscience (Goleman, 2006; Lieberman, 2013; Post, 2005) reveals that occupations depend on our intelligence for the highest levels of interaction, collaboration, and cooperation. A cortical self-awareness network (Andrews-Hamer, 2012; Lou, 2015) computes how we are received; then we modify our behaviour moment by moment to achieve collaborative communication for occupation. Relevant to the need to foster sustainable ways of being, there is growing evidence that the qualities of altruism and empathy are fundamental human traits, contributing to humanitarianism (Decety and Ickes, 2011). 'Doing good' to each other also means 'being good' to ourselves (Keltner et al., 2010) and to the wider natural world. Doing together, and with care and kindness, supports our own health and survival, while connecting us with each other and the biosphere (Ikiugu, 2008; Keltner, 2009; Post, 2005). The authors agree with Einhorn (2005) that human beings are by nature 'good at heart', born to be altruistic and supportive to each other and our world in order to promote survival. Cardiac neurophysiology also reveals that when we enact our capacity for appreciation and love of others, our own health improves (Childre and Martin, 1999)

via reduction of the threat response. The potential for compassion towards our wider world is thus now acknowledged as a research-based aspect of our evolved occupational nature.

There is yet further neurobiological evidence of our occupational nature. Only through activity is capacity built, through neuroplasticity (neurogenesis, synaptogenesis) and increased blood supply (Draganski et al., 2004; Ilg et al., 2008; Nataraja, 2008). A complex occupation (such as playing music) enhances cognition and perception (Kringelbach and Berridge, 2010), builds collaboration, and improves problem solving, memory, vocabulary and numeracy via cognitive reserve (Wan and Schlaug, 2010). Communal activities, such as choirs, significantly improve collective and individual mental health (Baker et al., 2013).

This evidence supports the proposition that human beings are capable of forging positive lives through enriched activities, while being naturally concerned about the welfare of others, and can sense and adjust our ways of doing, to meet different needs. Thus, our complex nature can be a force for good, so that we are caring for our wider environment, using the powers of occupation wisely, while being aware of the impact of our actions to prevent harm (Pierce, 2003).

This section has used an extended overview from occupational science to explore the, often untapped, potential of our occupational nature, which mounting evidence shows to be inherently caring and altruistic, to support survival. With increased global awareness, we also have the potential to extend this energetic power to incorporate the health of our wider environment and the world. However, humans as a species are finding it hard to comprehend and tackle the imminent threat of global climate change (Marshall, 2015).

A CONCERN ABOUT CONTEMPORARY CULTURE

Many problems in the twenty-first century, including individual physical and mental health issues through to global environmental degradation, are (even if inadvertently) caused by how we actually carry out our everyday occupations. We enjoy engagement in occupations without fully considering the cost to our local and global habitats. Anthropogenic climate change is now the most serious crisis of our age; it is described as the biggest global health threat of this century and will affect all populations (World Health Organization, 2008). In the film *The Age of Stupid* (2009), the unnamed archivist looks back from the future at how climate change developed and says:

> *The question I've been asking is: why didn't we save ourselves when we had the chance? Is the answer because on some level we weren't sure if we were worth saving?*

As we live more and more indoors, we increasingly connect with the world through the media, such as watching events through television or the Internet. News updates and product advertising provide messages that can lead to negative feelings that we are not 'worth it' unless we buy the latest thing, which will give us more value and make us feel better. Built-in obsolescence means that products have a limited life span and advertisements repeatedly encourage upgrading to the next new item. Consumer choices can be influenced by social anxiety and envy, which increase as income inequalities widen (Wilkinson and Pickett, 2014). Consumer entitlement can lead to morally irresponsible consumption (McGregor, 2006): for example, 30% of clothes that are bought in the UK are never worn (Dibb et al., 2015). Such disposable consumerism is a key driver of an unsustainable economic model and of climate change (Jackson, 2009).

News is often presented as a summary of all the bad things that have happened that day, highlighting negative images of human activity, the ways we can and do harm each other and the biosphere (World Health Organization, 2005), which can make people feel negatively about the state of the world and humankind. The threat response is also activated by pervasive media stories, such as terrorist acts, coming through all media devices (Stein and Nesse, 2011). Media impact is so complex and indirect that we do not fully understand the mechanisms involved. Negative stories can lead to chronic stress and even depression as the ability to help is thwarted by the distance of the actual event, while discussions about issues can lead people to feeling impotent and unable to change them (Katz and Lazarsfeld, 1955), numbing us to other peoples' pain and suffering (Bushman and Anderson, 2007).

More sustainable forms of being need to be found that are not dependent on consumerism (Wilkinson and Picket, 2014). The things that make us happy are not necessarily consumable 'things', and spending more time focusing on issues of social status may give less time for things which may have broader individual worth and community value, such as close relationships (Lieberman, 2013). The choice of people's occupations and how they do them is influenced by many varied factors, including the effects of illness, poverty, and inequality. These may limit a person's opportunities, work patterns, social networks, leisure pursuits, and the scope of their culture, and environment (Gallagher et al., 2015). These issues relate to occupational injustice.

SUSTAINABILITY AND GLOBAL WELL-BEING

Sustainable development by definition can be seen as an altruistic act, aiming to meet the needs of both current and future generations. The pursuit of sustainable development is a global challenge to all disciplines. World health is arguably inseparable from the global economy, social justice, and the natural environment (Werner, 1998), which matches the three interrelated pillars of sustainable development: economic, social, and environmental. The necessary science, technology, and wisdom exist to forge a more healthy, humane, and sustainable paradigm, and what is required most of all is the political will. The challenges our societies face in pursuing sustainable development will change depending on the broader political and economic pathway taken. Calls have been made to incorporate sustainability and ethics into business models, rather than these being add-ons (Confederation of British Industry, 2009; Worldwatch Institute, 2008). The current political pursuit of ever-increasing economic growth is unsustainable as it does not account for finite environmental resources, which are currently being used up at a greater rate than ever before, and our rapidly expanding global population (Jackson, 2009).

Buying the latest things to try and maintain social status (known colloquially as 'keeping up with the Joneses') can lead to emotional distress, dissatisfaction, and alienation (Carlisle et al., 2009). Economic growth is effective at lifting people out of the worst effects of poverty, such as poor healthcare and education systems, but as countries become richer they pass a threshold beyond which further economic growth appears to produce diminishing returns in levels of well-being. Income inequality significantly correlates to poorer outcomes in measures of physical and mental health, happiness, crime, and addictions, and also notably for both sustainability and ratings of social relations within communities (Wilkinson and Pickett, 2009). It is time to 'shift emphasis from measuring economic production to measuring people's well-being' (Stiglitz et al., 2009, p. 12). Political leaders have recognized the deficiencies of measuring gross domestic product (GDP), and 'beyond GDP' indicators are being explored internationally (Legatum Institute, 2014; Whitby, 2015).

The politics of sustainability and the politics of well-being are considered compatible, interrelated, and mutually dependent (Lucas, 2008), and working towards environmental sustainability can lead to improvements in human well-being (Wilkinson and Pickett, 2014).

Increasing concerns for the environment (and, ultimately, physical limits to resources) have the potential to counter trends towards materialism, individualism and consumerism, and in so doing could also contribute to our health and wellbeing, as individuals and as social beings in a finite but infinitely precious world. (Carlisle et al., 2009, p. 1560)

Occupational therapy's key focus on enabling individual well-being through meaningful activities potentially places the profession at the forefront of providing practical solutions for the current environmental situation (Hudson and Aoyama, 2008). Working with other professions in health, social care, and beyond, occupational therapy can demonstrate the economic, social, and environmental value that our profession can bring.

SUSTAINABLE OCCUPATIONAL THERAPY PRACTICE FOR BOTH THE INDIVIDUAL AND THE WIDER WORLD

Sustainability must become a vital influence on the future of occupational therapy practice globally, extending the borders of present practice in all con-

texts. Ikiugu (2008) has proposed how human beings' occupational capacities could more powerfully serve the world. There have been calls to integrate sustainable development into practice by several occupational therapy organizations (College of Occupational Therapists, 2013, 2015; Swedish Association of Occupational Therapists, 2012; World Federation of Occupational Therapists, 2012) and other theorists (recently Persson and Erlandsson, 2014; Simó Algado and Townsend, 2015; Wagman, 2014). See Box 58-1 for a brief overview of key issues.

BOX 58-1

CONSENSUS STATEMENT ON SUSTAINABILITY IN OCCUPATIONAL THERAPY

Sustainability in occupational therapy engages with environmental, economic, and social issues to address global health and well-being both now and in the future.

Occupational therapists have a particular duty that is rooted in exploring how occupations and activities of daily living impact upon the climate. Occupational therapists can reevaluate practice models and expand clinical reasoning about occupational performance to include global issues, focusing on places, communities and society, as well as individuals and their needs. This is supported by existing concepts, such as occupational ecology, occupational choice, and occupational justice.

Sustainable occupational therapy practice will:
1. Continue to explore the social, economic, environmental, and spiritual determinants of health as part of preventative healthcare approaches.
2. Continue to empower and enable people to take control of their own well-being and their impact on communities.
3. Eliminate wasteful activity.
4. Make use of low-carbon alternatives.

Occupational therapists will share and promote knowledge and research in order to influence health and well-being and commissioning strategies in the future.

Occupational therapists can take a leading role in enabling a shift towards sustainable occupations, including sustainability in activity analysis, supporting public health agendas, utilizing the therapeutic value of natural settings, and nurturing support networks. These are some examples that can improve care for people while reducing economic, social, and environmental costs.

Consensus statement from attendees of 'Saving Resources, Improving Health' networking day at College of Occupational Therapists, London, England, 21 November 2014 (Smyth, 2015).

Whilst occupational therapists are already addressing the first two of the four points regarding sustainable occupational therapy practice mentioned in the Box 58-1, there are compelling reasons to expand occupational therapy to incorporate a global approach to address the second two points (College of Occupational Therapists, 2013). This means incorporating each individual's interdependency with the global ecosystem and to 'think globally, act locally', which could have manifold implications for practice, including gently reframing models and interventions, promoting leadership to develop sustainable healthcare settings, and creating new community opportunities outside of healthcare and social care, where we could use the occupational therapy process to enable people from a 'well population' to live more sustainably (Whittaker, 2012).

Occupational therapists can keep in mind the evidence base outlined above for people's potential as caring, altruistic occupational beings and support them to 'reactivate' this. This can happen through enjoying the sensory experience of doing occupations, which leads us to learn and understand that we are occupational beings and to value the meaning of our occupations (Kielhofner, 2008). Occupational therapists could also foster the development of people's self-compassion, through exploring the three components of kindness for oneself, mindfulness around our shortcomings, and acknowledgement of our common humanity (Neff, 2003). Self-compassion has multiple health benefits, differing from development of self-esteem which can lead to narcissistic traits; self-compassion can instead enhance compassion for others (Germer and Neff, 2013; Neff and Vonk, 2007). It is a process that can support people in reconnecting with themselves and the wider world.

Occupational therapists have always worked with the inherent value of individuals and their power and potential, methods that now need to project to public health and sustainable practice with 'well' populations. The skills of activity analysis and pacing and grading can empower people to engage in more sustainable occupations. There are several ways to foster sustainability locally, socially, and globally. These include doing everyday living and domestic activities with concern for the environment more in mind; reviving engagement in creative activities, including the arts and crafts, leading to flow experiences; and engaging more in community projects, especially in natural environments.

By supporting individuals to carry out everyday tasks with increased consciousness, or awareness, of their effects on the environment, therapists can help people manage the fear and inertia towards the challenge of leading sustainable lives. Mindfulness training – practising doing everyday survival occupations with full focus on the activity – could become a more common approach during therapeutic sessions. Such approaches are evidence-based and bring a return to a focus of finding joy during the everyday (Reid, 2011).

The sustainability of cooking and gardening could be explored by considering their ecological context and mindfully performing them with that focus (Wiseman and Sadlo, 2015). Greater engagement with the growing and cooking of one's own food, sourcing of other ingredients, declining packaging, monitoring water and energy use, composting, recycling, and eating with mindful awareness could improve individual well-being through, for example, deepening occupational meaning and purpose (Sadlo, 2004). Perhaps 51% of global greenhouse gas can be attributed to meat and dairy production (Goodland and Anhang, 2009), while eating less of these can reduce cardiovascular disease and some cancers (International Agency for Research on Cancer, 2015). These and other health cobenefits of a low-carbon lifestyle can be explored with service users (Watts, 2009). Further research needs to focus not only on the experience of occupations but also on an analysis of the occupation itself, regarding sustainability issues and occupational justice (Hocking, 2009). An occupational interpretation of other disciplines' research evidence is also needed. Research and sustainable best practice could be shared among clinicians on networks such as OT Susnet[2] (Centre for Sustainable Healthcare, 2015).

There is rich potential for sustainability in returning to the use of natural, skilled activities as therapeutic media, such as any of the creative arts and crafts.

---

[2]OT Susnet is an online global network for occupational therapists, students, and educators who would like to explore sustainable practice and related resources.

The Arts in Health movement is expanding internationally, and yet such activities are currently often neglected (European Network of Occupational Therapy in Higher Education, 2004). Research shows that occupations that lead to optimal human experiences – a state of flow – activate our natural rewards systems (Reid, 2011; Wright et al., 2007) as rewards for enacting our occupational capacities.

Occupational therapists could deliberately foster and prioritize more connectivity with our environment and each other (Belcham, 2004). Yerxa (2013) encourages therapists to focus on optimizing human flourishing in a way that depends more on realizing our occupational nature than on excessive environmental resources. Messages about health benefits need to promote people's inherent value and potential, to counteract the dominant messages in news and advertising that can lead to stress, inertia, and a sense of lack of worth.

Engaging with the natural environment brings proven health benefits, such as faster patient recovery after surgery (Ulrich, 1984) and improved mood and self-esteem (Barton and Pretty, 2010). Living near to a green space increases opportunities to exercise and improves stress levels (UK National Ecosystem Assessment, 2011). Access to green spaces can be inequitable, but occupational therapists can work to engage in projects on a local level. In the UK's National Health Service (NHS), the NHS Forest aims to increase access to green spaces on or near NHS land and has so far planted nearly 40 000 trees. Occupational therapists are involved in various forest sites working with patients, volunteers, and communities to capitalize on the therapeutic benefits of green spaces (NHS Forest, 2015).

Occupational therapists can promote individual engagement with community projects that encourage sustainable living and can improve individual, social, and global well-being (Griffiths, 2009). Individuals and communities can be encouraged to reconnect with elderly people, who may have used more sustainable living skills in their past, such as making and mending clothes and growing vegetables. They, in turn, may also learn from young people who are being taught about sustainability in school, to bridge the gap in some sustainability skills that have arisen in our society between these generations. Therapists could get involved with

and help raise awareness of projects such as the Transition Network[3] (2015), community allotments, and Repair Cafés[4] (Repair Café Foundation, 2015).

Occupational therapists need to have an awareness of the sustainability of their own clinical practice and also to consider how to work with clients towards more sustainable activities, whilst honouring client-centred practice (Whittaker, 2012). Therapists can become a force within public health policy and practice, seeking work in such departments, or volunteering within communities. By doing so, they could demonstrate and disseminate the evidence that meaningful participation in a range of occupations is as vital an ingredient in the health and satisfaction of persons and communities as are the better-known ones, such as increased exercise and better eating habits. An occupational perspective of health needs to be more widely promoted (Wilcock and Hocking, 2015). The advantages of all the positive cultural, scientific, and technological advances need to be appreciated as they arise, but their use needs to be more conscious, having more awareness for the protection of our planet.

One more aspect of occupational science is relevant here. In order to change how we act in the world (i.e., to change our occupational forms), human beings first need to change the meaning of these actions (Clark et al., 1998). One advantage of contemporary communication systems is that our natural, evolved capacity to empathize with others, to be altruistic, to connect with, and care for those close by, has the potential to expand to a more global perspective (Leith and Whittaker, 2012; Lovelock, 2009). Rapid international communication has increased our awareness and the meaning of the environmental impact of contemporary lifestyles (Lovelock, 2014), while our powerful need to belong (Lieberman, 2013; Wilcock, 2006) can extend to a wider world, through spiritual intelligence (Tolle, 2001; Zohar and Marshall, 2000).

---

[3]The Transition Model is a 12-step process for communities to work together to become more cohesive, resilient and sustainable, eventually reducing reliance on fossil fuels. Transition initiatives (such as Transition towns) follow this process.

[4]Repair Cafés are meetings arranged by local communities, where people bring and mend broken items.

CONCLUSION

The power of occupation to sustain and enhance the quality of human life relates to our distinctive occupational nature, which is now being more fully appreciated and disseminated through occupational science research. Occupations are central to humans living joyful, fulfilling, and meaningful lives, because they characterize our species. Our caring and altruistic occupational nature has enabled us to survive in a great variety of habitats over millennia, and we are rewarded by physical and mental well-being when we engage in collaborative occupations.

However, exponential scientific and technical discoveries combined with the politics of consumerism have led to unsustainable use of fossil fuels and crises in the biosphere, placing unsustainable pressures on the natural world. The pressures of contemporary culture and increased individualism in the twenty-first century can put us under unbearable stress and contribute to a loss of sense of our worth or control. What is needed is a 'reactivation' of our occupational nature, with its naturally positive, altruistic potentials.

Occupational therapists are well placed to use time-proven approaches to encourage human flourishing, through mindful participation in normal, ordinary, everyday activities, through full immersion in creative occupations, and through engagement in communal activities, especially in natural settings. Such engagement can promote feelings of empathy and care for the self and others, because collaboration is an essential component of most occupations. Such activities are seen as pathways to enhanced life satisfaction. Occupations enable us to flourish and express our cultural and creative needs. Occupational therapy practice could more deliberately raise awareness of the need to modify our everyday activities to lessen their effect on the environment. Guidelines formulated by occupational therapy professional organizations highlight the importance of meeting occupational needs with environmentally sustainable practices (World Federation of Occupational Therapists, 2012).

Offering special hope is the recent evidence from neuroscience that suggests that altruism, not selfishness, is a dominant human trait that has supported our survival to date (Wilson, 2015). The global sustainability movement should be supported by this altruism, which favours helping wider communities. Humans need to have the protection of the biosphere more in mind. Occupational therapy can not only support the call that now is the ideal time for our society to move towards sustainable development, but it can also provide a unique perspective to address changes in how we live. As we orchestrate our lives, our natural altruism and highly evolved sense of compassion (Keltner et al., 2010) could hold the key to a more environmental ethic.

Acknowledgement

The authors would like to thank Rebecca Gibbs (Centre for Sustainable Healthcare) for her support in the writing of this chapter.

REFERENCES

Age of Stupid, The, 2009. Directed by Franny Armstrong [Film]. Spanner Films, United Kingdom.

Andrews-Hamer, J.R., 2012. The brain's default network and its adaptive role in internal mentation. Neuroscientist 18, 251–270.

Baker, F.A., Dingle, G.A., Brander, C., Ballantyne, J., 2013. 'To be heard': the social and mental health benefits of choir singing for disadvantaged adults. Psychol Music 41, 405–421.

Barton, J., Pretty, J., 2010. What is the best dose of nature and green exercise for improving mental health? A multi-study analysis. Environ. Sci. Technol. 44 (10), 3947–3955.

Belcham, C., 2004. Spirituality in occupational therapy: theory and practice. Br. J. Occup. Ther. 67 (1), 39–46.

Bushman, B.J., Anderson, C.A., 2007. Measuring the strength of the effect of violent media on aggression. Am. Psychol. 62 (3), 253–254.

Carlisle, S., Henderson, G., Hanlon, P.W., 2009. Wellbeing': a collateral casualty of modernity? Soc. Sci. Med. 69 (10), 1556–1560.

Centre for Sustainable Healthcare, 2015. OT Susnet. <http://networks.sustainablehealthcare.org.uk/network/ot-susnet> (accessed 16.11.15.).

Childre, D., Martin, H., 1999. The Heartmath Solution. Harper, San Francisco.

Clark, F.A., Wood, W., Larson, E.A., 1998. Occupational science: occupational therapy's legacy for the 21st century. In: Neistadt, M.E., Crepeau, E.B. (Eds.), Willard & Spackman's Occupational Therapy, ninth ed. Lippincott, Philadelphia, PA, pp. 13–21.

Clark, F.A., Lawlor, M.C., 2008. The making and mattering of occupational science. In: Crepeau, E.B., Cohn, E.S., Schell, B.A.B. (Eds.), Willard & Spackman's Occupational Therapy, eleventh ed. Lippincott, Philadelphia, PA, pp. 2–14.

Clark, F.A., Blanchard, J., Sleight, A., Cogan, A., Eallonardo, L., Floríndez, L., et al., 2015. Lifestyle Redesign®: The Intervention Tested in the USC Well Elderly Studies, second ed. AOTA Press, Bethesda, MD.

Cochran, G., Harpending, H., 2009. The 10,000 Year Explosion: How Civilization Accelerated Human Evolution. Basic Books, New York.

College of Occupational Therapists, 2013. Essential Briefing: Sustainable Development. COT, London.

College of Occupational Therapists, 2015. Code of Ethics and Professional Conduct. COT, London.

Confederation of British Industry, 2009. Getting Involved: A Guide to Switching Your Employees on to Sustainability. <http://www.cbi.org.uk/media/948812/switching_on_your_employees_to_sustainability.pdf> (accessed 01.07.15.).

Decety, J., Ickes, W. (Eds.), 2011. The Social Neuroscience of Empathy. MIT Press, London.

Dibb, S., Harris, F., Roby, H., Thomas, C., 2015. Sustainable clothing: towards sustainable clothing consumption. <http://www.open.ac.uk/business-school/research/projects/sustainable-clothing> (accessed 03.11.15.).

Draganski, B., Gaser, C., Busch, V., Schuierer, G., Bogdahn, U., May, A., 2004. Neuroplasticity: changes in grey matter induced by training. Nature 427 (6972), 311–312.

Duhigg, C., 2013. The Power of Habit: Why We Do What We Do and How to Change. RH Books, London.

Dutton, D., 2009. The Art Instinct: Beauty, Pleasure and Human Evolution. Bloomsbury Press, London.

Eckersley, R., 2005. Is modern Western culture a health hazard? Int. J. Epidemiol. 35 (2), 252–258.

Einhorn, S., 2005. The Art of Being Kind. Sphere, London.

European Network of Higher Education, 2004. Approaches to Teaching and Learning 'Practical' Occupational Therapy Skills: Sharing Best Practice. ENOTHE, Amsterdam.

Gallagher, M., Muldoon, O.T., Pettigrew, J., 2015. An integrative review of social and occupational factors influencing health and wellbeing. Front. Psychol. 6, 1281. <http://www.ncbi.nlm.nih.gov/pmc/articles/PMC4554961/> (accessed 16.11.15.).

Germer, K.G., Neff, K.D., 2013. Self-compassion in clinical practice. J. Clin. Psychol. 69 (8), 856–867.

Goleman, D., 2006. Social Intelligence: The New Science of Human Relationships. Arrow Books, London.

Goodall, C., 2007. How to Live a Low-Carbon Life. Earthscan, London.

Goodland, R., Anhang, J., 2009. Livestock and climate change: what if the key actors in climate change were pigs, chickens and cows? World Watch Magazine 22 (6), 10–19.

Greenfield, S., 2002. The Private Life of the Brain. Penguin Books, London.

Griffiths, J., 2009. How to take action in the community. In: Griffiths, J., Rao, M., Adshead, F., Thorpe, A. (Eds.), The Health Practitioner's Guide to Climate Change. Earthscan, London, pp. 245–267.

Hasselkuss, B., 2011. The Meaning of Everyday Occupation. Slack, Thorofare, NJ.

Helliwell, J., Layard, R., Sachs, J. (Eds.), 2013. World Happiness Report 2013. United Nations Sustainability Network Development Solutions Network, New York.

Hocking, C., 2009. The challenge of occupation: describing the things people do. J. Occup. Sci. 16 (3), 140–150.

Hocking, C., 2013. Occupation for public health. N. Z. J. Occup. Ther. 60 (1), 33–37.

Hudson, M.J., Aoyama, M., 2008. Occupational therapy and the current ecological crisis. Br. J. Occup. Ther. 71 (12), 545–552.

Ikiugu, M.N., 2008. Occupational Science in the Service of Gaia: An Essay Describing a Possible Contribution of Occupational Scientists to the Solution of Prevailing Global Problems. Baltimore, Publish America.

Ikiugu, M.N., Pollard, N., 2015. Meaningful living across the lifespan: occupational-based intervention strategies for occupational therapists and scientists. Whiting and Birch, London.

Ilg, R., Wohlschläger, A.M., Gaser, C., 2008. Gray matter increase induced by practice correlates with task-specific activation: a combined functional and morphometric magnetic resonance imaging study. J. Neurosci. 28 (16), 4210–4215.

International Agency for Research on Cancer, 2015. Carcinogenicity of consumption of red and processed meat. Lancet Oncol. 16 (16), 1599–1600. Available from: <http://www.thelancet.com/journals/lanonc/article/PIIS1470-2045(15)00444-1/abstract> (accessed 16.11.15.).

Jackson, T., 2009. Prosperity without Growth: Economics for a Finite Planet. Earthscan, London.

Jones, M., 2007. Feast: Why Humans Share Food. Oxford University Press, Oxford.

Katz, E., Lazarsfeld, P., 1955. Personal Influence. Free Press, New York.

Keltner, D., 2009. Born to Be Good: The Science of a Meaningful Life. W.W. Norton & Co., New York.

Keltner, D., March, J., Smith, J.A., 2010. The Compassionate Instinct: The Science of Human Goodness. W.W. Norton & Co., New York.

Kielhofner, G., 2008. The Model of Human Occupation: Theory and Application, fourth ed. Lippincott Williams & Wilkins, Philadelphia.

Kringelbach, M.L., Berridge, K.C., 2010. The functional neuroanatomy of pleasure and happiness. Discov. Med. 9 (49), 579–587.

Law, M., Cooper, B., Strong, S., Stewart, D., Rigby, P., Letts, L., 1996. The Person-Environment-Occupational model: a transactive approach to occupational performance. Can. J. Occup. Ther. 63 (1), 9–23.

Legatum Institute, 2014. Wellbeing and Policy. <http://li.com/docs/default-source/commission-on-wellbeing-and-policy/commission-on-wellbeing-and-policy-report---march-2014-pdf.pdf> (accessed 01.07.15.).

Leith, A., Whittaker, R.H., 2012. Primary Productivity of the Biosphere. Springer-Verlag, Berlin.

Lieberman, M.D., 2013. Social: Why Our Brains Are Wired to Connect. University Press, Oxford.

Lou, H.C., 2015. Editorial: self-awareness – an emerging field in neurology. Acta Paediatr. 104, 121–122.

Lovelock, J., 2009. The Vanishing Face of Gaia: A Final Warning. Allen Lane, London.

Lovelock, J., 2014. A Rough Ride to the Future. Allen Lane, London.

Lucas, C., 2008. The real deal? In: Simms, A., Smith, J. (Eds.), Do Good Lives Have to Cost the Earth? Constable, London, pp. 223–230.

McGregor, S.L.T., 2006. Understanding Consumer Moral Consciousness. Int. J. Consumer Stud. 30 (2), 164–178.

McNiff, S., 2004. Art Heals: How Creativity Cures the Soul. Shambhala, Boston.

Marshall, G., 2015. Don't Even Think About It: Why Our Brains Are Wired to Ignore Climate Change. Bloomsbury, London.

Maslow, A., 1954. Motivation and personality. Harper, New York.

Nataraja, S., 2008. The Blissful Brain: Neuroscience and Proof of the Power of Meditation. Gaia Thinking, London.

Neff, K.D., 2003. Self-compassion: an alternative conceptualization of a healthy attitude toward oneself. Self Identity 2, 85–101.

Neff, K.D., Vonk, R., 2007. Self-compassion versus self-esteem: two different ways of relating to oneself. J. Personal. 77 (1), 23–50.

NHS Forest, 2015. NHS Forest: Growing Forests for Health. Available from: <www.nhsforest.org> (accessed 16.11.15.).

Pallasmaa, J., 2009. The Thinking Hand: Existential and Embodied Wisdom in Architecture. Wiley, Chichester, UK.

Persson, D., Erlandsson, L.-K., 2014. Ecopation: connecting sustainability, glocalisation and well-being. J. Occup. Sci. 21 (1), 12–24.

Pierce, D.E., 2003. Occupation by Design: Building Therapeutic Power. F. A. Davis, Philadelphia.

Post, S.G., 2005. Altruism, happiness, and health: it's good to be good. Int. J. Behav. Med. 12 (2), 66–77.

Radman, Z. (Ed.), 2013. The Hand, an Organ of the Mind. The MIT Press, Cambridge, MA.

Reid, D., 2011. Mindfulness and flow in occupational engagement. Can. J. Occup. Ther. 78 (1), 50–56.

Repair Café Foundation, 2015. About Repair Café. <http://repaircafe.org/en/about/> (accessed 17.11.15.).

Sadlo, G., 2004. Creativity and occupation. In: Molineux, M. (Ed.), Occupation for Occupational Therapists. Blackwell Publishing, Oxford, pp. 90–100.

Simó Algado, S., Townsend, E.A., 2015. Eco-social occupational therapy. Br. J. Occup. Ther. 78 (3), 182–186.

Smyth, G., 2015. Saving resources, improving health. OTnews 23 (1), 30–31.

Stein, D.J., Nesse, R.M., 2011. Threat detection, precautionary responses, and anxiety disorders. Neurosci. Biobehav. Rev. 35, 1075–1079.

Stern, N., 2015. Why Are We Waiting? The Logic, Urgency, and Promise of Tackling Climate Change. MIT Press, London.

Stiglitz, J.E., Sen, A., Fitoussi, J-P., 2009. Report by the Commission on the Measurement of Economic Performance and Social Progress. <www.stiglitz-sen-fitoussi.fr/documents/rapport_anglais.pdf> (accessed 16.11.15.).

Swedish Association of Occupational Therapists, 2012. Occupational Therapy and Sustainable Development – from a Swedish Perspective. SAOT, Nacka, Sweden.

Tallis, R., 2003. The Hand: A Philosophical Inquiry into Human Being. Edinburgh University Press, Edinburgh, UK.

Tolle, E., 2001. The Power of Now: A Guide to Spiritual Enlightenment. Hodder and Stoughton, London.

Townsend, E.A., Polatajko, H.J., 2007. Advancing an occupational therapy vision for health, well-being, and justice through occupation. CAOT Publications, Ottawa, ON.

Transition Network, 2015. Transition Network's Strategy 2014/2017. <https://www.transitionnetwork.org/about/strategy> (accessed 17.11.15.).

Twenge, J.M., Campbell, W.K., 2009. The Narcissism Epidemic: Living in the Age of Entitlement. Free Press, New York.

UCL-Lancet Commission, 2009. Managing the health effects of climate change. Lancet 373 (9676), 1693–1733.

UK National Ecosystem Assessment, 2011. The UK National Ecosystem Assessment: Synthesis of the Key Findings. UNEP World Conservation Monitoring Centre, Cambridge.

Ulrich, R.S., 1984. View through a window may influence recovery from surgery. Science 224 (4647), 420–421.

Wagman, P., 2014. The Model of Human Occupation's Usefulness in Relation to Sustainable Development. Br. J. Occup. Ther. 77 (3), 165–167.

Wan, C.Y., Schlaug, G., 2010. Music making as a tool for promoting brain plasticity across the life span. Neuroscientist 16 (5), 566–577.

Watts, G., 2009. The Health Benefits of Tackling Climate Change: An Executive Summary for The Lancet Series. <http://www.thelancet.com/pb/assets/raw/Lancet/stories/series/health-and-climate-change.pdf> (accessed 16.11.15.).

Werner, D., 1998. Health and Equity: Need for a People's Perspective in the Quest for World Health. Presented at the World Health Organization Conference: 'Primary Health Care 21 – Everybody's Business', Almaty, Kazakhstan, 27–28 November 1998. Available from: <http://www.healthwrights.org/content/articles/healthequity.htm> (accessed 16.11.15.).

Whitby, A., 2015. Measuring the long term. <http://www.futurejustice.org/wp-content/uploads/2015/01/Measuring-the-Long-Term.pdf> (accessed 01.07.15.).

Whittaker, B., 2012. Sustainable global wellbeing: a proposed expansion of the occupational therapy paradigm. Br. J. Occup Ther. 75 (9), 436–439.

Wilcock, A.A., 2006. An Occupational Perspective of Health. Slack, Thorofare, NJ.

Wilcock, A.A., Hocking, C., 2015. An Occupational Perspective of Health, third ed. Slack, Thorofare, NJ.

Wilkinson, R., Pickett, K., 2009. The Spirit Level: Why More Equal Societies Almost Always Do Better. Allen Lane, London.

Wilkinson, R., Pickett, K., 2014. A Convenient Truth: A Better Society for Us And The Planet. The Fabian Society, London.

Wilson, D.S., 2015. Does Altruism Exist? Culture, Genes, and the Welfare of Others. Yale University Press, New Haven, CT.

Wiseman, T., Sadlo, G., 2015. Gardening – an occupation for wellness and recovery. (Chapter in) International Handbook of Occupational Therapy Interventions, second ed. Springer, New York, pp. 797–809.

World Commission on Environment and Development, 1987. Our Common Future: Brundtland Report. Oxford University Press, Oxford. Available from: <http://www.un-documents.net/our-common-future.pdf> (accessed 16.11.15).

World Federation of Occupational Therapists, 2012. Position Statement: Environmental Sustainability, Sustainable Practice within Occupational Therapy. WFOT, Forrestfield, Australia.

World Health Organization, 2005. Ecosystems and Human Wellbeing: Health Synthesis. WHO, Geneva.

World Health Organization, 2008. Protecting Health from Climate Change – World Health Day 2008. WHO, Geneva.

World Health Organization, 2015. Sustainable Development Goals 2030 Agenda for Sustainable Development. WHO, Geneva.

Worldwatch Institute, 2008. State of the World: Innovations for a Sustainable Economy. <http://www.worldwatch.org/files/pdf/State%20of%20the%20World%202008.pdf> (accessed 01.07.15.).

Wrangham, R., 2010. Catching Fire: How Cooking Made Us Human. Profile Books, London.

Wright, J.J., Sadlo, G., Stew, G., 2007. Further Explorations of Flow Process. J. Occup. Sci. 14 (3), 136–144.

Yerxa, E., 2013. The Human Spirit for Occupation. Occupation: Awakening to the Everyday. Keynote Address, University College Cork Occupational Science Conference, September 2013. Available from: <www.oscork2013.com> (accessed 14.12.13.).

Zohar, D., Marshall, I., 2000. SQ Spiritual Intelligence: The Ultimate Intelligence. Bloomsbury, London.

59

ECO-SOCIAL OCCUPATIONAL THERAPY: TOWARDS AN OCCUPATIONAL ECOLOGY

SALVADOR SIMÓ ALGADO ■ MARIA KAPANADZE

CHAPTER OUTLINE

Occupational therapists claim to be experts in appreciating human beings as occupational beings. However, occupational therapists have often neglected key aspects of the environment, such as its political, economic, and ecological conditions. As will be explained in this chapter, the current ecological crisis cannot be ignored by occupational therapists, since human occupation is the dialogue between the person (or community group) and the environment. The ecological crisis is primarily a crisis of scarcity: scarcity of raw materials, energy, land, and environmental space. It is reflected in phenomena such as acid rain, global warming, destruction of the ozone layer, deforestation, desertification, and overpopulation. These realities are endangering the continuation of human life on Earth (Boff, 2000; Latouche, 2009; Lovelock, 1985). This chapter reflects on the impact of ecological factors on health and well-being, as well as the potential role of occupational therapy to confront this ecological crisis. Human occupation has been a key factor in the genesis of the ecological problem and it must be a key factor for its solution, developing an occupational ecology.

Occupational therapists want to promote justice (Simó Algado and Townsend, 2015), through the promotion of economic and social change to ensure that people will have access to meaningful occupations. In order to achieve this goal, occupational therapists need to understand and question critically the current economic system and its consequences on the health, social, and occupational participation of people. The neoliberal economy is the ruling economic system in the major part of the planet and it has a profound impact on the ecology.

The ultimate goal of an eco-social occupational therapy is the cocreation of healthy, inclusive, and sustainable communities where all members can develop their human potential and participate as full citizens through meaningful occupations, satisfying their needs without endangering the next generations' need for survival.

ECOLOGICAL CRISIS

The natural environment can be defined as the set of biotic and abiotic natural beings that surround an organism, population, or human community. As open systems, humans depend on the environment for their survival (García, 2004). Ecology is the study of the interdependence and interaction between living things and their environment. Boff (2000) gives a more holistic view to define ecology as the relationship, interaction, and dialogue of all existing things with each other. Nothing exists outside of this relationship. This is an inclusive definition, which relates nature to society and culture. Boff (2000) says that poverty is the main environmental problem, as it is connected to phenomena such as deforestation, desertification, and overpopulation.

Humans are citizens of a spherical and interconnected world with global problems, such as climate change or poverty, that affect everybody. People need to develop a cosmopolitan citizenship based on the understanding of their interdependence and common destiny (Cortina, 2005).

Despite this reality, in the West one of the *topoi*, or strong beliefs, is in the independence of the human being. It results in a process of severe individualization (Beck and Beck-Gernsheim, 2003) that fragments all community forms and alienates people from the rest of the human beings and the natural environment. Western occupational therapy has been strongly influenced by the reductionistic belief of valuing independence while forgetting the importance of interdependence.

Santos (2005) argues that the Western person considers her/himself separated from the East, the Wilderness, and Nature. The East symbolizes the space of otherness. The Wilderness, represented by the South and indigenous peoples, symbolizes inferiority. Nature symbolizes the exterior space. Animals and the natural environment are considered a pure economic resource to be exploited for human economic production.

A major part of human societies is immersed in a neoliberal economic system based on the idea of unlimited economic growth (Latouche, 2009). Humans need to understand the limits of natural resources. This emphasis on growth is illusory since it ignores the fundamental problem of the law of entropy, that once matter has been transformed into energy the reaction is nonreversible, and therefore at some point the material resources for energy will be used up (García, 2004).

According to Boff (2000), between 1500 and 1850, one species was eliminated every 10 years; between 1850 and 1950, one per year; in 2000, one species per hour. More than 20% of all living species disappeared between 1975 and 2010. The sustainability of the planet, which is the product of billions of years of cosmic activity, is endangered (Boff, 2001). The main issues affecting the global environment are acid rain, global warming, destruction of the ozone layer, deforestation, desertification, and overpopulation.

The ecological footprint is a key concept in understanding the ecological crisis and its origins. It refers to the area per person of biologically productive land required to meet the needs of food, resources, and energy, as well as the area required to absorb the waste produced, adding the environmental impact of human infrastructure. The sustainable ecological footprint per person is 1.8 hectares. At the time of this writing (2015), however, it is estimated that the space consumed per person is 2.2 hectares. From 1970 to 1996, the ecological footprint has increased by 50%. A citizen of the United States consumes 9.6 hectares, a European 4.5, and the ecological footprint of the citizens of rapidly developing countries like India and China is growing (Latouche, 2009). The ecological footprint reflects how current lifestyles are unsustainable.

ECOLOGY, CULTURE, AND SOCIETY

The Report of the Club of Rome on the Limits to Growth (Meadows, 1972) and the Stockholm Conference on Environment were two initial ecological highlights. Lovelock's (1985) Gaia hypothesis described the earth as a living being. In 1983, the United Nations organized a World Commission on Environment and Development, where the famous concept of sustainable development was coined; it refers to a development that meets the needs of the present without compromising the ability of future generations to meet their own needs (WCED, 1998). These pioneering initiatives were followed by the Rio (1992), Johannesburg (2002), and Durban (2011) Earth Summits which have achieved limited results.

Santos (2005) proposes a diatopical hermeneutics, a dialogue between the different cultures, to complete each culture's strong beliefs. Iwama (2006) contrasts the Western worldview based on independence, with an Eastern cosmovision based on the interdependence of human beings, the gods, and nature. My (first author) work with Guatemalan refugee communities (Simó Algado, 1997, 2004) allowed me to delve into the Mayan cosmovision, studying with an Ajgij, a Mayan priest. Their mission is to preserve the balance between man, nature, and god. The Ajgij told me that loss of harmony leads to disease. In Mayan culture, the Earth is our mother; the Earth is a living being. People live on water, wind, fire, and rain. People belong to the Earth. If a person does not respect nature, they will fall sick without hope. When humans are born, they are twinned with an element of nature, called *nagual;* this can be a jaguar or a quetzal, for example, and their fates are linked (Simó Algado and Abregú, 2015). Most indigenous cultures reflect the sacred reality of life. These cultures reflect the idea of connection with the nature: 'I'm all forces and elements with which I am in contact. I am the wind, the trees, the birds, and darkness' (Curtis, 1972, p. 34), 'The sun, the moon, and my trees are symbols of continuity' (Pigem, 1994, p. 48). Societies based on economic values imposed by neoliberal capitalism, appear to have forgotten the sacred character of human life.

The ecological crisis is linked to a cultural crisis. Davis (2001) states that around 300 million people belong to indigenous cultures. There is no stronger evidence for this cultural crisis than the loss of languages. Of the 10 000 which once existed, only 6000 are still spoken today, and only 600 of these are considered stable. From an economic point of view, the loss seems inconsequential. But a language is a reflection of the human spirit, the filter through which the soul of each particular culture relates to the world. At risk is the spiritual, intellectual, and artistic expression of human experience.

Shiva (2006) alerts us to the disappearance of indigenous populations, which is justified through so-called progress. The resulting destruction has a more irreversible character, which is seen in the loss of the cultural mechanisms of indigenous populations, mechanisms that protect both the population itself and its natural environment. When they are gone, who will teach us to walk gently on the earth?

NEOLIBERAL ECONOMIES AND SOCIAL EXCLUSION

The term *neoliberal economy* refers to the resurgence of nineteenth-century ideas associated with laissez-faire economic liberalism. Beginning in the 1970s and 1980s, its advocates supported extensive economic liberalization policies such as privatization, fiscal austerity, deregulation, free trade, and reductions in government spending in order to enhance the role of the private sector in the economy (Duménil and Lévy, 2004). The common features of neoliberal economies are the promotion of consumerism, competition, individualization, hedonism, and the growth of severe economic inequalities.

These inequalities produce significant social discomfort, even in leading economies, through a degradation of middle-class prosperity and an increase in poverty. For example, in 2013 the child poverty rate in Spain was 34%, while the European Union average was 28%. Youth unemployment rate in Spain was 55%, and the European Union average was 28%. This rate of unemployment is combined with a precarious job market in which the numbers of the working poor are growing (people living in poverty although they have a job): Spain 15.7%, European Union average 10.2% (Alternativas Económicas, 2015). European workers are losing their labour rights and are suffering a process of degradation of their working conditions (Beck, 2000). Another important part of the population is considered to be disposable by the system, without any expectation that it can be incorporated in the labour market (Bauman, 2005).

Neoliberal economy is connected to the growing of inequity in remuneration, exemplified by the income divide between the highest and the lowest earners in an organization: the highest earners earn 354 times more than the lowest earnest in the US, 206 in Canada, 147 in Germany, 127 in Spain, and 28 in Poland. Inequality is increasingly affecting all countries around the world. In developed and developing countries alike, the poorest half of the population often controls less than 10% of its wealth. There is growing evidence and recognition of how the powerful and corrosive effects of inequality on economic growth, poverty reduction, social and economic stability, and socially sustainable development inequality can lead to a less stable, less efficient economic system that stifles economic growth and the participation of all members of society in the labour market (Stiglitz, 2012).

In the face of this unsustainable goal, new economic proposals are appearing. Latouche (2009) proposes a serene degrowth (decline), *la décroissance sereine,* based on the commitment to reduce, reevaluate, reconceptualize, relocate, and reuse. Social entrepreneurship promotes enterprises whose main goal is to create meaningful jobs for people solving social and ecological problems through innovation, returning the good to the community rather than operating for profits that only benefit shareholders. In both cases, human occupation linked to productivity is the key factor.

THEORY OF OCCUPATIONAL RENAISSANCE, OCCUPATIONAL ECOLOGY, AND ECO-SOCIAL OCCUPATIONAL THERAPY

Human beings are bio-psycho-social beings with a spiritual essence immersed in a cultural, political, and ecological environment. From an occupational perspective (Wilcock, 2006) health can be defined as: a balance between physical, mental, and social well-being through meaningful occupations that are valued socially and individually; the development of personal potential; opportunities for social participation and cohesion; and social integration, support, justice, in balance with ecology.

The poor attention that occupational therapists have paid to the natural environment is noteworthy, especially when occupation is seen as an expression of the dialogue which takes place between humans and their environment. Occupational therapists have often focused on the physical environment such as architectural barriers to disability but have shown a serious neglect of the political (Pollard et al., 2008) and ecological conditions (Simó Algado, 2012; Thibeault, 2006).

Occupational dysfunction can be due to environmental causes. The United Nations High Commissioner for Refugees (2012) estimates that 24 million people have fled their homes and had to radically change their occupational patterns because of floods, famine, and other environmental disasters. The ecological crisis is worsening; the United Nations High Commissioner for Refugees estimate for 2050 is 150 million environmental migrants, defined as any person who abandons her or his usual territory of residence due to environmental impacts and moves within the same country or crossing borders (Castillo, 2011).

Occupational therapists and occupational scientists have to research the implications of current occupational patterns (productivity, leisure, and self-maintenance), majorly connected with neoliberal economies, for the well-being and occupational participation of people and communities.

Occupational therapists are gradually becoming more aware of the need to develop a profession oriented to human rights (Guajardo and Simó Algado 2010). Freire (2009) invites professionals to denounce the injustices they encounter and to propose possible alternatives to these injustices. Occupational therapists have to be aware and denounce the potential negative effects of the neoliberal economy and then to announce possible alternatives. The theory of occupational renaissance (Simó Algado, 2011) can be helpful in this process (Box 59-1).

Wilcock (2006) argues that human occupation has been a main factor in environmental degradation and must be a force for its restoration. For example, the first author and Abregu (2015) have reflected on the impact of large-scale open cast mining in South America, showing its impact on the ecology, in the well-being, and in people's occupational patterns.

Rozario (1993) argued that occupational therapists need to work to maintain a harmonious relationship between people and the environment, working for sustainability through interaction, occupation, and sociopolitical action. This statement is consistent with the ecological sustainability model of health, understood as promoting healthy relationships between human beings, other living organisms, their ecosystems, habits, and lifestyles (Wilcock, 2006).

Occupational therapists are aware of the therapeutic impact of occupations developed in the natural

THEORY OF OCCUPATIONAL RENAISSANCE

According to Wilcock (2006), a theory is based on the following elements: (a) a basic theory of human nature, (b) a diagnosis of what is wrong, and (c) a prescription on how to improve the situation. Here we outline the theory of occupational *renaissance*. First, the human being is a social and historical being, with a need to experience meaning and the capacity of speech, action, and narrative. Second, the current economic neoliberal system leads to the exclusion of large sectors of the population, the fragmentation of community ties, and the destruction of the biosphere. Third, human occupation can play a key role to improve the situation: occupational therapists have to develop a healthier self-care; give a new meaning to leisure, moving from passive and consumerism-based leisure to a creative leisure; and reconceptualise productivity, which beyond material survival should allow human development, creating healthy, inclusive, and sustainable communities.

The authors would need another chapter to develop this section in depth. Some suggestions are made here.

Self-maintenance: A major part of societies is based on a biomedical model of health. This model predominantly promotes pharmacotherapy, not putting as much emphasis on the prevention of illness or the importance of health promotion. This model also creates new risks; iatrogenic illnesses caused by the health system itself, are the third cause of death in the US after heart disease and cerebrovascular disease, representing 581 926 deaths annually (Null et al., 2011). We need to move to a client-centred model, where the person can take control over his own health based on the promotion of healthier habits.

Productivity: In 2015, young unemployment rate in Spain was 55%, and the European Union average was 28% (Alternativas Económicas, 2015). It is necessary to create meaningful and well-paid jobs that are not contributing to the pollution of the planet. At a macro level, people need to look for alternatives to the neoliberal economy; occupational therapists can contribute to this endeavour from their expert knowledge on occupation.

Leisure: Ninety percent of the teenagers in the US identify shopping as their favourite leisure activity. Most American children spend about 3 hours a day watching TV. Added together, all types of screen time can total 5 to 7 hours a day (Kaneshiro, 2013). It is necessary to explore and develop other leisure patterns not based in mere consumerism. For example, leisure activities connected to the natural environment can be explored, such as trekking or running in nature.

environment or with animals in the well-being of human beings. The first author has worked on projects based on dolphin therapy, gardening/landscaping, and restoration of natural environments (Simó Algado, 2012). His research with mental health survivors has showed how gardening increased the feeling of physical, mental, and social well-being, the sense of meaning and purpose in life, and the feeling of social participation and citizenship (Simó Algado, 2011). Occupational therapists have to carry out research to increase knowledge about the interaction between the natural environment, animals, and people. This is especially important when global developments are leading to the development of more artificial and technological societies that alienate humanity from nature.

Initially, the first author understood occupational ecology as a double reflection-action cycle, which can be understood as the awareness of an ecological crisis that endangers life on earth (reflection cycle); to be followed by taking proactive measures through human occupation, to restore balance to the environment (action cycle). This definition is inspired by Mounier (2002), a philosopher who proposed a revolution based on the cycles of reflection and action. More recently, occupational ecology has been defined as the interdisciplinary work of enabling socioeconomic, cultural, and policy developments to enable economically and environmentally sustainable occupations for all humans, everywhere (Simó Algado and Townsend, 2015).

Occupational ecology is consistent with sustainable development and with the *décroissance sereine* (Latouche, 2009), since human occupation is a medium for recycling, relocating, reducing, and reusing. It resonates with the theory of occupational renaissance (Simó Algado, 2011) as it outlines the negative consequences of the current neoliberal system on wellbeing. Occupational therapists can develop an ecosocial occupational therapy, whose main objective is the cocreation of healthy, inclusive, and sustainable communities through new occupational patterns. The term *cocreation* refers to the common construction process, in partnership with other professionals (ecologists, economists, and anthropologists, among others), and especially with civil society and the public/state and private/market sectors, keeping service users at the heart of all partnerships. Civil society refers to those organizations that do not belong to the state or the market (Barber, 2000), including voluntary or third sector organizations and nongovernmental organizations.

ECO-SOCIAL OCCUPATIONAL THERAPY PROJECTS: FROM THEORY TO PRACTICE

In this section, we present two examples that have been developed by the first author in Spain under the umbrella of a nongovernmental organization called Social, Human, and Ecological Sustainability (SHES)[1]. The aim is to create one integrated project that can confront practical issues of poverty, unemployment, and ecological degradation.

Restoration of Natural Spaces

This project focused on the restoration and reforestation of five protected natural spaces with a high ecological value in the province of Osona, located in northeastern Catalonia in Spain. Creating meaningful and well-paid jobs, particularly where poverty exists, has become an eco-social occupational therapy priority. Under the umbrella of the European Union project *Recover*, 10 jobs in the green economy sector were created between 2009 and 2011 to employ people who have experienced persistent poverty and/or mental health issues.

This project continued with the restoration of El Montseny Natural Park, a protected natural space located near the town of Vic in Catalonia. The local provincial government is funding the project to create jobs for another six persons who have experienced persistent social exclusion. Workers engage in reforestation, building protective fences for the animals, and recovering natural springs.

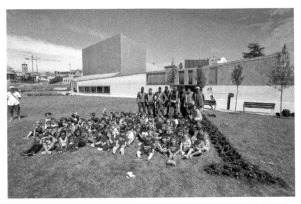

FIGURE 59-1 ■ The Garden of the Arts. *Courtesy of Salvador Simó Algado.*

EcoSPORTech

The project EcoSportech (Simó Algado and San Eugenio, 2013) has created three gardens: the Philosophical garden, where conceptual art is integrated with landscaping; the Identity garden, a combination between landscaping with graffiti and youth art; and the Garden of the Arts. It has also restored the ancient garden of the Cathedral of Vic. These gardens are connected with a riverside forest. The project promotes economic development for the city through tourism. The target population has been 16 young people who have no formal academic qualifications. They have received theoretical and practical training in areas related to landscaping, social entrepreneurship, information and communication technology, and sports in natural environments, among others. These students have received a living grant during this period. The project promotes the use of leisure and sports in the preservation of the natural environment. The faculties of Health Sciences, Economics, and Education at the Universitat de Vic are involved. More than 100 four-year-old children have participated in the flower plantations; 25 local young artists have also collaborated in the creation of a piece of graffiti art covering 400 square metres (Figure 59-1).

CONCLUSION

The human being is part of the whole that we call the universe, a part limited in time and space. He perceives himself, his thoughts and feelings as

---

[1]See first author's portfolio for more projects and related publications (www.salvadorsimo.org).

something separated from the rest, which is a kind of optical delusion of his consciousness. For us this illusion is like a prison that restricts our desires and affections to a handful of people around us. Our task must be to free ourselves from this prison, and we must broaden our circle of compassion to embrace all living creatures and the whole of nature in its beauty.

— *Albert Einstein* (cited in Howard, 2002)

Occupational therapists can no longer ignore the importance of the ecological environment. Occupation is the dialogue between humans and their environment. If humans are to survive, this dialogue should be based on respect: everybody must care for the planet. Human occupation has played a key role in the genesis of the environmental crisis and must play a role in its solution. This crisis is rooted in the neoliberal focus on financial progress and an economic model that seeks unlimited growth in a world with limited resources. It is rooted in a system that puts humans at the service of the economy. Occupational therapists need to explore the effect of neoliberalism on the well-being and social participation of communities, and propose new alternatives based on human occupation.

Understanding the ecological dimension of the environment, occupational therapists will be able to prevent and restore occupational dysfunction caused by environmental conditions. It is a great challenge and opportunity for occupational therapy to become a more relevant profession for society. For example, knowing that the green economy sector is one with a high growth (European Environment Agency, 2013), therapists can use this as an opportunity to enable access into the job market for people excluded from it. For occupational therapists to be able to make a difference, it is necessary to improve their knowledge on areas such as productivity, understanding the possibilities that green economy and social entrepreneurship can offer to the profession.

As Bohm (2001) says, one of the big problems today is that humans tend to be repetitive when they need to be creative. Occupational therapy boasts this creativity: it is time to develop an eco-social occupational therapy that contributes to the cocreation of healthy, inclusive, and sustainable communities. The concept of occupational ecology and the theory of occupational renaissance can help occupational therapists better realise their responsibility to respond to the serious environmental crisis people face, which cannot be separated from the social crisis. The occupational therapists can develop transformative praxis in strategic partnership with all stakeholders.

Occupational therapists have the obligation to sustain the occupational rights of the people of the present and the future, rights which are currently being undermined by a concern with material realities in the present, through the effects of neoliberalism and consumerism. Developing healthier self-care, creative leisure, and new productivity patterns can help ensure the planet's sustainability and, for the people who live on it, personal well-being.

Acknowledgements

The authors wish to thank Nick Pollard and Dikaios Sakellariou for their valuable comments during the revision of this chapter that really have enriched the text.

REFERENCES

Alternativas Económicas, 2015. Gráficos para Comprender la Crsisi y sus Efectos. AE SL, Madrid.

Barber, B., 2000. Un Lugar para Todos. Paidós, Barcelona.

Bauman, Z., 2005. Vidas Desperdiciadas. Paidós, Barcelona.

Beck, U., 2000. Un Nuevo Mundo Feliz. Paidós, Barcelona.

Beck, U., Beck-Gernsheim, E., 2003. La Individualización. Paidós, Barcelona.

Boff, L., 2000. La Dignidad de la Tierra. Ecología, mundialización, espiritualidad. La emergencia de un nuevo paradigma. Trotta, Madrid.

Boff, L., 2001. Ética Planetaria Desde el Gran Sur. Trotta, Madris.

Bohm, D., 2001. Sobre la Creatividad. Kairós, Barcelona.

Castillo, J., 2011. Migraciones Ambientales. Virus Editorial, Barcelona.

Cortina, A., 2005. Ciudadanía. Ciudadanía cosmopolita. Alianza Editorial, Barcelona.

Curtis, E., 1972. The North American Indians. Aperture, Hong Kong.

Davis, W., 2001. Light at the Edge of the World. Douglas McIntyre, Toronto.

Duménil, G., Lévy, D., 2004. Capital Resurgent: Roots of the Neoliberal Revolution. Harvard University Press, Cambridge, MA.

European Environment Agency, 2013. Towards a Green Economy in Europe. EEA, Brussels.

Freire, P., 2009. Pedagogía del Oprimido. Siglo XXI, Madrid.

García, E., 2004. Medio Ambiente y Sociedad: La Civilización Industrial y los Límites del Planeta. Alianza, Madrid.

Guajardo, A., Simó Algado, S., 2010. Hacia una terapia ocupacional basada en los derechos humanos. <http://www.revistatog.com/num12/pdfs/maestros.pdf> (accessed 25.07.12.).

Howard, W., 2002. Mathematical Circles. Mathematical Assocaciont of America, New York.

Iwama, M., 2006. Ubicación en el Contexto: Cultura, Inclusión y Terapia Ocupacional. In: Kronenberg, F., Simó Algado, S., Pollard, N. (Eds.), Terapia Ocupacional sin Fronteras. Aprendiendo del Espíritu de Supervivientes. Editorial Médica Panamericana, Madrid.

Kaneshiro, N., 2013. Screen time and children. <http://www.nlm.nih.gov/medlineplus/ency/patientinstructions/000355.htm> (accessed 15.09.14.).

Latouche, S., 2009. Petit Tractat Sobre el Decreixement Serè. Tres i Quatre, Valencia.

Lovelock, J., 1985. Gaia, una Nueva Visión de la Vida Sobre la Tierra. Orbis, Barcelona.

Meadows, D., 1972. Los Límites del Crecimiento: Informe al Club de Roma. Fondo de Cultura Económica, Ciudad de Méjico.

Mounier, E., 2002. El Personalismo. Antología Esencial. Ediciones Sígueme, Salamanca, Spain.

Null, G., Feldman, M., Rasio, D., Smith, D., 2011. Death by Medicine. Nutrition Institute of America, New York, USA.

Pigem, J., 1994. Nueva Conciencia. Integral, Barcelona.

Pollard, N., Sakellariou, D., Kronenberg, F. (Eds.), 2008. A Political Practice of Occupational Therapy. Elsevier, Oxford.

Rozario, L., 1993. Purpose, place, pride and productivity: the unique personal and societal contribution of occupation and occupational therapy. XVII Australian Occupational Therapy Conference. Darwin, Australia.

Santos, B., 2005. El Milenio Huérfano. Ensayos para una Nueva Cultura Política. Editorial Trotta, Madrid.

Shiva, V., 2006. Manifiesto para una Democracia de la Tierra. Paidós, Barcelona.

Simó Algado, S., 1997. Spirituality in a refugee camp. Can. J. Occup. Ther. 61, 88–94.

Simó Algado, S., 2004. The return of the corn man. In: Kronenberg, F., Simó Algado, S., Pollard, N. (Eds.), Occupational Therapy without Borders: Learning from the Spirit of Survivors. Elsevier, Oxford.

Simó Algado, S., 2011. La palabra y la acción. Lucha contra la pobreza, ciudadanía y salud a partir de nuevas praxis universitarias. Tesis (Doctorado en Educación), Universidad de Vic, Vic, España. Publicado en Tesis en Red. Available from: <http://tdx.cat/bitstream/handle/10803/9325/PALABRAACCION.pdf?sequence=1> (accessed 14.03.13.).

Simó Algado, S., 2012. Terapia Ocupacional eco-social: hacia una ecología ocupacional. Cadernos de terapia ocupacional da UFSCar, São Carlos 20, 7–16. Available from: <http://dx.doi.org/10.4322/cto.2012.001>.

Simó Algado, S., Abregu, M., 2015. Ecología ocupacional: el caso de la megaminería en Argentina. Revista Argentina de Terapia Ocupacional. 1 (1), Dec 2015. Available from: <http://www.revista.terapia-ocupacional.org.ar/descargas/articulo%204%20FF.pdf> (accessed 12.05.16.).

Simó Algado, S., San Eugenio, J., 2013. El proyecto 'Ecosportech' como implicación de la academia con la sociedad en base al 'Problem Based Learning'. Visión, Madrid.

Simó Algado, S., Townsend, E., 2015. Eco-social occupational therapy. Br. J. Occup. Ther. 78 (3), 182–186.

Stiglitz, J., 2012. The Price of Inequality: How Today's Divided Society Endangers Our Future. W.W. Norton & Company, Inc., New York.

Thibeault, R., 2006. Globalization, universities and the future of occupational therapy: dispatches from the majority world. Aust. J. Occup. Ther. 53, 159–165.

United Nations High Commissioner for Refugees, 2012. Format and organizational aspects of the high-level political forum on sustainable development. <http://www.un.org/ga/search/view_doc.asp?symbol=A/67/L.72&Lang=E> (accessed 12.08.13.).

Wilcock, A., 2006. An Occupational Perspective of Health, second ed. Slack Incorporated, Thorofare, NJ.

WCED, 1998. Report of the Report of the World Commission on Environment and Development: Our Common Future. Available at <http://www.un-documents.net/wced-ocf.htm> (accesssed 14.06.14.).

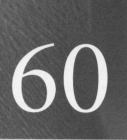

60

VENTURE THINK TANK: THE POLITICS, TECHNOLOGIES, AND OCCUPATIONS OF DISABILITY, AND MECHANICAL VENTILATION

PAMELA BLOCK ■ BROOKE ELLISON ■ MARY SQUILLACE

CHAPTER OUTLINE

The goal of this chapter is to discuss vent-users[1], that is, people who rely on continuous mechanical ventilation for survival. This group is subject to occupational injustice but is not generally discussed in the occupational therapy and occupational science literature. Ventilator technology keeps people alive but does not assure quality of life and meaningful occupation. Cultural perceptions and policies profoundly influence and constrain the occupations of vent-users. This group is cross disability and cross life span and is defined and united, not by their diagnoses, but by the occupations, policies, and support systems that flow from their dependence on ventilator technologies (Divo et al., 2010).

Individuals who comprise this demographic may span a diverse array of medical conditions, including such conditions as spinal cord injury, amyotrophic lateral sclerosis, muscular dystrophy, spinal muscular atrophy, and pulmonary dysfunction (Charlifue et al., 2011; Gelinas et al., 1998). While some of these individuals may have been studied from a disease-specific framework, there is valuable and important information that can be gathered for the vent-users as it cuts across all medical diagnoses. This is a uniquely diagnosis-resistant community, joined entirely by its reliance on their common use of mechanical ventilation technologies. The dependence on a ventilator for their survival unifies vent-users in a particularly interesting way: establishing a community that is especially vulnerable to social challenges but, at the same time, about which very little is known. Questions persist, including exactly who constitutes this population, how similar or dissimilar experiences might be depending

---

[1]For brevity and clarity, we will refer to people who rely on continuous mechanical ventilation as 'vent-users' throughout this chapter.

on demographic characteristics, and what proportion live in their desired social setting. As a result, vent-users have a rich set of experiences that demand greater understanding.

In response to these and other challenges, Pamela Block and Brooke Ellison, along with many university and community partners, including occupational therapist Mary Squillace, have formed the Stony Brook University VENTure Think Tank, an interdisciplinary and community participatory university think thank to encourage policy and technology innovation for people who rely on mechanical ventilation for survival. VENTure is centrally concerned with understanding the experiences of the vent-users and working to better meet their needs. We are interested in uncovering and disentangling the complex factors that contribute to quality of life, an ability to live in the community, and what factors influence how easily this can be done. We are also concerned with what policy intervention strategies ought to be implemented at various societal levels to address these factors in a comprehensive manner. We believe that without gaining firsthand and personal information from ventilator users and their family members, researchers are at risk of misunderstanding the conditions or relying on paternalistic attitudes to attempt to solve the problems faced. We assert that vent-users belong in community contexts and that the perspectives of vent-users and their family members are central to identifying strategies to achieve this. Allies also play an essential role, including both clinicians and disability rights activists who can advocate along with vent-users and families for occupational and social justice, including the cultural and policy shifts needed for lasting beneficial change.

In this chapter, we address two fundamental rights which are often not available for vent-users:

1. **The right to live in the community rather than in institutions.** People on ventilators are routinely forced into institutions due to lack of the human, policy, and technology support networks necessary for people to live safely in the community.
2. **The right to participate in valued occupations.** Even if living in the community, vent-users often face barriers to pursing meaningful activities. It

can be difficult to leave home. Many people are basically shut-in due to lack of human and technological support, appropriate transportation, and other barriers.

Those concerned with the study and practice of occupation can have an important role supporting vent-users in achieving these fundamental rights.

We also need to acknowledge a third area of importance to vent-users: **the right to basic survival.** As New Yorkers, we lived through extended power outages due to Hurricane Irene in 2011 and Super Storm Sandy in 2012. Power outages that might be inconvenient for some, are terrifying and life-threatening for those who rely on mechanical ventilation for survival. The close line between safety and danger experienced by vent-users on a daily basis is especially significant in times of crisis and places without secure power sources. We want to acknowledge the privilege in the US and other countries of the Global North where the (usual) presence of secure power sources allows vent-users to survive. This is not the case everywhere; large disparities of access exist even in the Global North. We wish to work with vent-users and allies on local, regional, national, and international levels to address these disparities and to secure not just survival, but lives well-lived.

OCCUPATIONAL INJUSTICE AND APARTHEID

Wilcock and Townsend (2000) discuss necessities in accomplishing social and occupational justice, such as the political and organizational systems that are based on human, environmental, and economic needs and that are designed to share physical and emotional resources. Although occupational injustice encompasses many levels of deprivation, alienation, and marginalization, occupational apartheid takes these forms of social exclusion to another level that is out of the hands of individuals experiencing the injustice and is 'a systematic segregation of occupational opportunity' (Kronenberg and Pollard, 2005, p. 59; Nilsson and Townsend, 2010). The question remains, how do we correct occupational injustice or apartheid when the source of injustice is beyond the personal control of the parties involved?

The occupational justice framework identifies environments as occupationally just when they contain appropriate resources and supports to enable participation in meaningful occupations (Townsend and Wilcock, 2004; Wolf et al., n.d.). Environments can provide 'affirmation of the individual as a person of worth, a place of belong, and a place to be supported, thereby environment not only influences one's occupational performance, but the meaning of the preferred occupation' (Rebeiro, 2001, p. 83). Occupational deprivation may begin within an immediate environment and spread throughout a community when not addressed. White et al. (2008) discuss the use of the term *occupational deprivation* in relation to those who experience such inequities. Occupational deprivation attracts the attention of social and political powers on a larger scale when people are prevented from engaging in meaningful activities as a result of conditions beyond their control (White et al., 2008). Injustice and deprivation, occupational marginalization, alienation, and occupational imbalance proliferate when systemic structures impose inequities where privileged groups are afforded freedoms to engage in the occupations of everyday life of their choice, while others are discriminated against and left behind (White et al., 2008).

In cases of occupational apartheid, the different life experiences of individuals from different social strata are so severely divided as to result in completely separate social and occupational experiences and opportunities. Such extreme circumstances are a call to action. Change must be made or a downwards spiral of the disregarded will continue or worsen in these communities (Kronenberg and Pollard, 2005). Occupational therapists must take responsibility for clarifying their vision and philosophical goals as well as practices to be available to address moral and political challenges of those in this situation, including vent-users (Kronenberg and Pollard, 2005; Block et al. 2016).

VENT-USERS AND OCCUPATIONAL INJUSTICE

For disabled people, environmental and contextual injustices often lead to access barriers to basic human occupations and to occupational injustices (Block et al. 2016; White et al., 2008). Vent-users experience even greater injustices in getting their occupational needs met, due to systemic and sociocultural discrimination (Ellison and Block, 2014). People on mechanical ventilation desiring to exercise their rights to live within communities, experience a constant battle, or perhaps more accurately a siege, that reveals societal injustices on multiple levels.

As mentioned earlier, ventilator dependence is not, in and of itself, a diagnosis. This group is composed of people of all ages, who experience many different impairments, conditions, or diagnoses. What unifies people in this group is their very intimate and constant reliance on a biomedical technology that both complicates their existence and also makes their existence possible. Similarly, because vent-users come from many different medical diagnoses, there are no data on who these people are, where they are located, what their individual needs and experiences are, or how these needs can best be met. This lack of knowledge about who comprises this population, and the failure to even identify this as a population category, perpetuates the invisibility of vent-users and the neglect of their needs. This erasure, this lack of public acknowledgement of vent-users' existence as a community with shared experiences and needs, can compromise safety and even survival. There are struggles on multiple levels that individuals in this population must face. Vent-users and family members must constantly advocate for healthcare services and the acquisition and maintenance of life-saving technologies that facilitate and monitor breathing (Dupree, 2016; Dybwik et al., 2011). Technological advances can offer an opportunity for occupational change as a step towards addressing occupational justice for vent-users (Dupree, 2016; Ellison and Block, 2014). However, before there can be occupational justice for this group, the struggle must begin from the home and community as we seek change on a society and policy level.

THE PULL OF THE INSTITUTION

In the US, vent-users and their families face enormous pressures in favour of institutionalization, even though hospitals and institutions are neither safe nor appropriate places to live, especially for children and youth. Yet, far more money is available to support people in institutions rather than community settings. Always, but especially during natural disasters, vent-users' lives are threatened by sustained power losses (in homes *and* in institutions). Rather than bringing alternative power sources to the people, the vent-users are told by emergency medical personnel to evacuate to hospitals. This is based on erroneous cultural perceptions that hospitals are safe places for people who use complex medical technologies. Due to policies that require vent-users to swap their equipment for the hospital equipment, they are particularly susceptible to acquiring infections in the hospital setting. It is also extremely expensive for vent-users to use a hospital as if it were a hotel, as they must be housed in critical care units (at tens of thousands of dollars per day), where they are taking beds away from people who might actually need them. This is particularly true in times of emergency, when vent-users are often directed by health professionals and emergency responders to go to hospitals, not for medical reasons, but because the hospital is seen as a stable source of energy to power a ventilator. Additionally, there are strong cultural perceptions that a hospital or nursing home is the most appropriate venue for vent-users to live (Ventusers. org, 2007).

However, this is a fallacy; hospitals are not safe places for people on ventilators and should be avoided except during times of health emergency. Many hospitals lost power in recent environmental crises, and hospitals present many health dangers for people on ventilators. Secondary infections, pneumonia, and other complications are much more common in hospital settings (Ashraf and Ostrosky-Zeichner, 2012; Klompas, 2013; Prospero et al., 2012; Solomkin, 2005). Alternative community-based stable energy sources for ventilator users during times of extended power outage is one example of a policy solution that could be implemented on a large scale and save both money and lives.

PROCEDURAL AND DISTRIBUTED JUSTICE

Impartiality, empowerment, and equality are forms of social justice and are essential components of the moral association between people and the government. Societal equality means opportunities for and access to means and goods (Braveman and Bass-Haugen, 2009; Braveman and Suarez-Balcazar, 2009;

Townsend and Wilcock, 2004). Procedural and distributive justice plays a role in decisions of how resources are equally distributed. Procedural justice theory refers to how the decision-making processes occur between dominant and subordinate social groups, as well as the level of participation on a broader societal level where distributive justice is the method in which social and economic resources are distributed within a society (Braveman and Bass-Haugen, 2009; Braveman and Suarez-Balcazar, 2009). Braveman and Suarez-Balcazar (2009) state:

Distributive and procedural justice plays an important role in the context of human rights. Some societies provide their citizens with opportunities to have access to resources (distributive justice) and opportunities to voice their opinions and make decisions (procedural justice), while at the same time protecting their human rights (intellectual rights, freedom of speech). (p. 14)

People from disability and minority groups have experienced obstacles and barriers in attempts to reach their goals for occupational justice; disabled people are statistically shown to experience a high level of unemployment, thereby limiting access to resources and support for their needs (Balcazar and Hall, 2005). The World Health Organization (2001) discusses inequities as: '(1). Systematic with consistent patterns across a population, (2). Socially produced and thus amenable to change, and (3). Unfair from human rights perspective' (Whitehead and Dahlgren, 2006, p. 8).

TECHNOLOGY AND THE DISABILITY STUDIES FRAMEWORK OF EMPOWERMENT

The Stony Brook University VENTure Think Tank advocates for the removal of barriers that affect community living for vent-users, via technology and policy innovation. This group is highly understudied from an occupational perspective and, as a result, not well understood, in terms of their unique experiences and social challenges. To add to our discussion of occupational justice and apartheid, we add a disability studies framework of empowerment (Block et al., 2006, 2010, 2011). In contrast to a biomedical focus on a physical difference such as an impairment or diagnosis, the disability studies framework of empowerment recognizes shared socioenvironmental experiences and common struggles that cross diagnostic boundaries. In the case of vent-users, ventilation technologies are the dominant common factors. We seek to expand upon existing research in the technologies of disability (Wolbring, 2011, 2012) and develop new critical perspectives of how life-support technology has impacted the lives of disabled people, how disability experience is shaped not just by technology in general, but life-support technology in particular, and how this influences people's sense of self and ways of being in the world.

There have been decades of scholarship on how the interaction between humans and technology has influenced constructions of gender (Haraway, 1985; Harding, 1986; Wajcman, 2009). We seek to extend these theoretical debates to consider how disability and disability experiences are shaped by ventilation technologies. What distinguishes vent-users is not just the focus on the disability/technology relationship, but also the disability/technology/essential-technology triadic relationship. It changes the dynamics, makes certain options more limited, and forces individuals to think very differently about the technology they use. Our approach is translational, moving from disability studies theory to practical community-based strategies for technology development and policy change.

HUMAN RIGHTS ISSUES FOR VENT-USERS

Vent-users experience social challenges that are vast and affect the most fundamental measures of participation. Often the challenges are not related to individual medical needs, but rather to a general lack of social supports that would allow successful life in the community (Ballangrud et al., 2009; Brooks et al., 2002; King, 2012). Vent-using children, commonly living in medical settings, spend prolonged amounts of time in places like intensive care units, with few other alternatives available (Crocket, 2012; Lumeng et al., 2001; Noyes 2000a, 2000b, 2006, 2007). This is the case whether or not there is medical need to be there. There are prevalent and very troubling human rights abuses that can take place against ventilator-dependent children and young adults who live in the hospital (Noyes, 2000b). The abuses that ventilator-users describe include forced hospitalization, the inability to maintain contact with family members, and discrimination in seeking medical care (Noyes, 2000b).

Studies highlight some of the most prevalent barriers that prevent children and young adult vent-users from being discharged from medical settings to the community (Noyes, 2000a; Wallis et al., 2011; Wang, 2004). Among the most significant barriers impeding discharge from a hospital unit are negative attitudes of professionals towards the possibility of discharge; the lack of coordination in funding discharge; poor management both within the health service and in collaborating with other services; complex social issues; housing problems; and a general lack of auditing and outcome measures (Noyes, 2000a). As a result, data indicate that even when focusing exclusively on children and young adults, vent-users experience significant impediments to community living. These impediments are equally, if not more, pronounced for adults (Tsay et al., 2013; Warschausky et al., 2005).

Even if discharge is accomplished, the transition process from hospital to home can often be challenging. Warren and colleagues (2004) discuss the difficulty in creating a strategic discharge plan for ventilator users to leave a hospital setting and enter the community. As the authors note, dependence on a ventilator not only affects the vent-user himself or herself, it affects the entire family and system of support. The establishment of a system of caregivers is essential, as ventilator-users require support and monitoring 24 hours per day. For many vent-users, healthcare needs are maintained by a combination of family members, nurses, and friends who are able to provide such skilled care as suctioning and operating the ventilator. However, such a team of individuals is often extremely difficult to assemble (Warren et al., 2004). This fact significantly diminishes an ability to live in the community or to participate meaningfully in social life.

Vent-users in hospital settings face pronounced difficulty or adverse circumstances, but those who live in the community do as well. Sarvey (2008) addresses some of the challenges that vent-using children who live in the community, as well as their families, experience on a daily basis. These include burdens placed on primary caregivers, usually mothers, who experience significantly increased instances of depression (Sarvey, 2008). Most notably, though, respondents in this qualitative study indicated, as central to their life experiences, perceptions of being different, the inability to be left alone and the desire to be seen as a person. Another study, conducted in Norway, was designed to assess the experiences of community living for 10 ventilator users, including their experiences with caregivers and medical supervision (Ballangrud et al., 2009). This study presented several subthemes implicit in participants' responses, indicating a sense of agency or control in their own situations, and the desire for more competence in personal care providers.

QUALITY OF LIFE FOR VENT-USERS

Though there is great regional variation, the number of ventilator users is growing, as medical technology advances and the population ages (King, 2012). Along with the growing number of ventilator users, there is a growing need to better understand barriers to quality of life that arise, not only for ventilator users living in the institutionalized setting but also for those living in the community. By 'quality of life', we include such aspects of social participation as community living, access to necessary healthcare services, engagement in recreation, safety in one's environment, and ability to secure employment, if desired. While people with disabilities are known to experience disparities in many measures of quality of life, vent-users are especially prone to such occupational and social participation challenges.

The factors that contribute to the decrease in quality of life for vent-users, are disparate and not fully understood. We believe that there are many contributory issues that, separately and together, have a significant effect on whether or not a ventilator-user has the ability to live in the community or to participate in community life. However, to date, there is little information about what these primary factors are, how they affect ventilator users' life experiences, which play the greatest role in population outcomes, and, most importantly, what interventions can be made to promote quality of life. As a result, existing strategies may be ineffective, insufficient, or not applicable to the entire population, thus targeting the wrong areas in the wrong ways. Existing research shows vent-users are in critical need of research on strategies and interventions that would serve to promote quality of life, address community participation, and alleviate some predominant struggles (Charlifue et al., 2011).

CONCLUSION

Irrespective of age or precipitating medical diagnosis, vent-users encounter a set of circumstances that lie at the intersection of health, technology, and society (Crocket, 2012). This group utilizes medical technology in a way unlike nearly any other, with a ventilator serving not only as an essential means of survival but also as the factor that influences social participation (Dybwik et al., 2011; Lindahl, 2011; Lindahl et al., 2003, 2006). Over time, ventilation technology has developed from the early immobile iron lungs to portable units that allow the potential for full engagement in community life, should the social, economic, and policy supports also be present. What are the experiences of this group? What opportunities have been presented to them to increase their quality of life? What do they foresee as the most pressing threats to their survival and what measures can be taken to alleviate these threats? How can members of this group become agents for their own social betterment and what alliances might need to be created in order for this to take place? These are questions that pertain to all vent-users, yet have not been addressed in any comprehensive manner. While advances in medical technology have created a new and diverse group of people, at least in parts of the world where there are secure power sources, little effort has been made to study how their lives have evolved or where society has fallen short in making their lives meaningful.

REFERENCES

Ashraf, M., Ostrosky-Zeichner, L., 2012. Ventilator-associated pneumonia: a review. Hosp. Pract. 40 (1), 93–105. doi:10.3810/hp.2012.02.950.

Balcazar, F.E., Hall, K., 2005. Accessing the world of work: concerns of African Americans with disabilities actively seeking employment. Final report. Disability Research Institute, University of Illinois, Urbana-Champaign.

Ballangrud, R., Bogsti, W.B., Johansson, I.S., 2009. Clients' experiences of living at home with a mechanical ventilator. J. Adv. Nurs. 65 (2), 425–434. doi:10.1111/j.1365-2648.2008.04907.x.

Block, P., Skeels, S., Keys, C.B., 2006. Participatory intervention research with a disability community: a practical guide to practice. Int. J. Disabil. Commun. Rehabil. 5 (1).

Block, P., Vanner, E., Keys, C.B., Rimmer, J., Skeels, S., 2010. Project Shake-It-Up!: a disability studies framework of empowerment for capacity building and health promotion. Disabil. Rehabil. 32 (9), 741–754.

Block, P., Rodriguez, E., Milazzo, M., MacAllister, W., Krupp, L., Nishida, A., et al., 2011. Building pediatric MS community. Res. Soc. Sci. Disabil. 6, 85–112.

Block, P., Kasnitz, D., Nishida, A., Pollard, N., 2016. Occupying Disability: Critical Approaches to Community, Justice and Decolonizing Disability. Springer, Ltd, New York.

Braveman, B., Bass-Haugen, J.D., 2009. Social justice and health disparities: an evolving discourse in occupational therapy research and intervention. Am. J. Occup. Ther. 63 (1), 7–12.

Braveman, B., Suarez-Balcazar, Y., 2009. Social justice and resource utilization in a community based organization: a case illustration of the role of the Occupational Therapist. Am. J. Occup. Ther. 63 (1), 13–23.

Brooks, D., Krip, B., Mangovski-Alzamora, S., Goldstein, R.S., 2002. The effect of postrehabilitation programmes among individuals with chronic obstructive pulmonary disease. Eur. Respir. J. 20, 20–29.

Charlifue, S., Apple, D., Burns, S.P., Chen, D., Cuthbert, J.P., Donovan, W.H., et al., 2011. Mechanical ventilation, health, and quality of life following spinal cord injury. Arch. Phys. Med. Rehabil. 92, 457–463.

Crockett, A., 2012. Technology dependence and children: a review of the evidence. Nurs. Children Young People 24 (1), 32–35.

Divo, M.J., Murray, S., Cortopassi, R., Celli, B.R., 2010. Prolonged mechanical ventilation in Massachusetts: the 2006 prevalence survey. Respir. Care 55 (12), 1693–1698.

Dupree, N., 2016. My World, My Experiences with Occupy Wall Street and How We Can Go Further. In: Occupying Disability: Critical Approaches to Community, Justice and Decolonizing Disability. Springer, Ltd, New York.

Dybwik, K., Nielsen, E.W., Brinchmann, B.S., 2011. Home mechanical ventilation and specialized health care in the community: between a rock and a hard place. BMC Health Serv. Res. 11 (115), 1–8.

Ellison, B., Block, P., 2014. "VENTure Think Tank Seeks Policy and Tech Solutions to Vent User Challenges" Ventilator Assisted Living 28(4):4-6. August 2014. <http://media.wix.com/ugd/fef361_055c4934788a4fd3808993b6ad36d04f.pdf>.

Gelinas, D.F., O'Connor, P., Miller, R.G., 1998. Quality of life for ventilator-dependent ALS patients and their caregivers. J. Neurol. Sci. 160 (Suppl. 1), S134–S136.

Haraway, D., 1985. A Manifesto for Cyborgs: science, technology, and socialist feminism in the 1980s. Social. Rev. 80, 65–108.

Harding, S., 1986. The Science Question in Feminism. Cornell University Press, New York.

King, A.C., 2012. Long-term home mechanical ventilation in the United States. Respir. Care 57 (6), 921–930. doi:10.4187/respcare.01741.

Klompas, M., 2013. Complications of mechanical ventilation – the CDC's new surveillance paradigm. N. Engl. J. Med. 368 (16), 1472–1475.

Kronenberg, F., Pollard, N., 2005. Overcoming occupational apartheid: a preliminary exploration of the political nature of occupational therapy. In: Kronenberg, F., Simo Algado, S., Pollard, N. (Eds.), Occupational Therapy without Borders: Learning from the Spirit of Survivors. Elsevier, Philadelphia, PA, pp. 58–86.

Lindahl, B., 2011. Experiences of exclusion when living on a ventilator: reflections based on the application of Julia Kristeva's philosophy to caring science. Nurs. Philos. 12, 12–21.

Lindahl, B., Sandman, P.O., Rasmussen, B.H., 2003. Meanings of living at home on a ventilator. Nurs. Inq. 10 (1), 19–27.

Lindahl, B., Sandman, P.O., Rasmussen, B.H., 2006. On being dependent on home mechanical ventilation: depictions of patients' experiences over time. Qual. Health Res. 16 (7), 881–901. doi:10.1177/1049732306288578.

Lumeng, J.C., Warschausky, S.A., Nelson, V.S., Augenstein, K., 2001. The quality of life of ventilator-assisted children. Pediatr. Rehabil. 4 (1), 21–27.

Nilsson, I., Townsend, E., 2010. Occupational justice bridging theory and practice. Scand. J. Occup. Ther. 17, 57–63.

Noyes, J., 2000a. Ventilator-dependant children who spend prolonged periods of time in intensive care units when they no longer have a medical need or want to be there. J. Clin. Nurs. 9 (5), 774–783.

Noyes, J., 2000b. Enabling young 'ventilator-dependent' people to express their views and experiences of their care in hospital. J. Adv. Nurs. 31 (5), 1206–1215.

Noyes, J., 2006. Health and quality of life of ventilator-dependent children. J. Adv. Nurs. 56 (4), 392–403. doi:10.1111/j.1365-2648.2006.04014.x.

Noyes, J., 2007. Comparison of ventilator-dependent child reports of health-related quality of life with parent reports and normative populations. J. Adv. Nurs. 58 (1), 1–10. doi:10.1111/j.1365-2648.2006.04191.x.

Noyes, J., Godfrey, C., Beecham, J., 2006. Resource use and service costs for ventilator-dependent children and young people in the UK. Health Soc. Care Commun. 14 (6), 508–522.

Prospero, E., Illuminati, D., Marigliano, A., Pelaia, P., Munch, C., Barbadoro, P., et al., 2012. Learning from Galileo: ventilator-assisted pneumonia surveillance [Letter to the Editor]. Am. J. Respir. Crit. Care Med. 186, 1308–1309.

Rebeiro, K.L., 2001. Enabling occupation: the importance of an affirming environment. Can. J. Occup. Ther. 68 (2), 80–89.

Sarvey, S.I., 2008. Living with a machine: the experience of the child who is ventilator dependent. Issues Ment. Health Nurs. 29 (2), 179–196. doi:10.1080/01612840701792456.

Solomkin, J.S., 2005. Cost-effectiveness issues in ventilator-associated pneumonia. Respir. Care 50 (7), 956–964.

Townsend, A., Wilcock, A.A., 2004. Occupational justice and client-centred practice: A dialogue. Can. J. Occup. Ther. 71 (2), 75–87.

Tsay, S., Mu, P., Lin, S., Wang, K.K., Chen, Y., 2013. The experiences of adult ventilator-dependent patients: a meta-synthesis review. Nurs. Health Sci. 15 (4), 525–533. doi:10.111/nhs.12049.

Ventusers.org., 2007. Take charge, not chances: a portfolio for users of home mechanical ventilation, their caregivers and health professionals. Ventilator-Assisted Living (web newsletter) 21 (4), Available from: <http://www.ventusers.org/edu/valnews/index.html> (accessed 07.06.16.).

Wajcman, J., 2009. Feminist theories of technology. Cambridge J. Econ. 34 (1), 143–152. doi:10.1093/cje/ben057.

Wallis, C., Paton, J.Y., Beaton, S., Jardine, E., 2011. Children on long term ventilatory support: 10 years of progress. Arch. Dis. Child. 96 (11), 998–1002. doi:10.1136/adc.2010.192864.

Wang, K.K., 2004. Technology-dependent children and their families: a review. J. Adv. Nurs. 45 (1), 36–46.

Warren, M.L., Jarrett, C., Senegal, R., Parker, A., Hartgraves, D., 2004. An interdisciplinary approach to transitioning ventilator-dependent patients to home. J. Nurs. Care Qual. 19 (1), 67–73.

Warschausky, S., Dixon, P., Forchheimer, M., Nelson, V.S., Park, C., Gater, D., et al., 2005. Winter. Quality of life in persons with long-term mechanical ventilation or tetraplegic SCI without LTMV. Top. Spinal Cord Injury Rehabil. 10 (3), 94–101.

White, B.P., Arthanat, S., Crepeau, E.B., 2008. Perspectives about occupational justice: can poverty and occupational deprivation influence child development? University Dialogue (Paper 37). Available from: <http://scholars.unh.edu/cgi/viewcontent.cgi?article=1036&context=discovery_ud>.

Whitehead, M., Dahlgren, G., 2006. Concepts and principles for tackling social inequities in health: leveling up (part 1). World Health Organization, Copenhagen.

Wilcock, A., Townsend, E., 2000. Occupational terminology interactive dialogue. J. Occup. Sci. 7 (2), 84–86.

Wolbring, G., 2011. Ableism and energy security and insecurity. Stud. Ethics Law Technol. 5 (1).

Wolbring, G., 2012. Citizenship education through an ability expectation and 'ableism' lens: the challenge of science and technology and disabled people. Educ. Sci. 2 (3), 150–164.

Wolf, L., n.d. Applying an occupational justice framework. Occup. Ther. Now 12 (1), 15–18. Available from: <http://www.caot.ca/otnow/jan10/justice.pdf>.

World Health Organization, 2001. International Classification of Functioning, Disability and Health. WHO, Geneva.

SECTION 6

EDUCATIONAL PRACTICES

61

COMMUNITY ENGAGEMENT IN OCCUPATIONAL THERAPY

MARGARET MCGRATH

CHAPTER OUTLINE

Since its earliest days, occupational therapy practice has had a distinctive social contract. Realizing the link between occupation and health, pioneers in the profession sought to extend access to meaningful occupations for all people (Frank, 1992; Kronenberg and Pollard, 2005; Thibeault, 2002; Townsend, 1993). More recently, interest in issues of occupational justice and occupational participation and engagement reaffirms occupational therapy's commitment to ensure that all people, communities, and populations have the possibility to participate in meaningful occupations of their choice (Fazio, 2008; Whiteford and Townsend, 2011). Advancements in occupational science research have led to acknowledgement that 'occupational therapists have a valuable contribution to make to the prevention of illness for all people not just those who are sick or disabled' (Wilcock, 2006, p. 275).

However, despite recognition of the ethical responsibilities of occupational therapists to respond to the social and political issues that influence possibilities for occupational participation, there continues to be limited scholarship that addresses how occupational therapists promote occupational justice as part of their daily work. In this chapter, I briefly consider the social contract between the profession of occupational therapy and broader society as it relates to occupational justice, and examine the extent to which contemporary practice fulfils this contract. Using the concept of professional citizenship, I explore how occupational therapists might engage in collaborative action with other citizens to address community needs (Box 61-1). I consider the skills needed by occupational therapists to practise in this way and offer some suggestions as to how occupational therapists might attempt to incorporate working for occupational justice into everyday practice.

AN EXTENDED SOCIAL CONTRACT FOR OCCUPATIONAL THERAPY

While occupational therapy has always had a stated aim to promote the occupational well-being of individuals, the introduction of the concept of occupational injustice by Townsend and Wilcock (2004) extended occupational therapy's social contract to include working with those people, organizations, and communities who experience occupational deprivation, alienation, disruption, or imbalance (Box 61-2).

The development of the Participatory Occupational Justice Framework further strengthens professional practice in this area by providing a conceptual tool for occupational therapists to use in doing justice as part of what the authors describe as 'critical occupational therapy' (Whiteford and Townsend, 2011, p. 66) (Box 61-3).

This adoption of a broader remit for occupational therapy practice has also been supported by a number of international standards for human rights including the Convention on the Rights of the Child (United Nations, 1989); the Standard Rules on the Equalisation of Opportunities for Persons with Disabilities (United Nations, 1993); the Convention on the Rights of Persons with Disabilities (United Nations General Assembly, 2007), and position statements published by

BOX 61-3
CRITICAL OCCUPATIONAL
THERAPY

Critical occupational therapy practices are described as
occupational therapy practice guided by a participatory
justice lens that focuses on bringing about change at a
macro level – addressing regulations, policies, economic
factors, and other broad sociopolitical issues that influence how people engage in occupation (Whiteford and
Townsend, 2011).

the World Federation of Occupational Therapists
(WFOT) including Community Based Rehabilitation
(2004); Occupational Science (2006b); Human Rights
(2006a); Diversity and Culture (2010); Environmental
Sustainability Sustainable Practice in Occupational
Therapy (2012); Human Displacement (2014a); and
Occupational Therapy in Disaster, Preparedness, and
Response (2014b). These statements draw attention to
the broader context through which health and occupation are experienced and legitimize occupational
therapy practice that addresses the social, economic,
and political aspects of occupational engagement. Furthermore, the statements from the WFOT clearly set
out the belief that access to meaningful occupation
should be understood as a human right and as such
should be protected and seen as equally important to
other human rights.

OUR PLACE IN THE WORLD: CONCEPTUALIZING OUR OBLIGATIONS IN A RIGHTS-BASED APPROACH TO OCCUPATIONAL PARTICIPATION

So then, in the early stages of the twenty-first century,
there is some evidence that occupational therapists (at
least within their *own* scholarly publications, for as
Pollard and Sakellariou (2014) note, the idea of occupation as a right is not well articulated by professionals
and academics laying claim to it, let alone among a
wider external audience) recognize themselves as
having a social and political role and potential to act
as agents of social transformation (Fazio, 2008; Galheigo, 2011; Whiteford and Townsend, 2011). However,
despite the growth in professional outputs regarding

issues of occupational justice and engagement, concerns continue to be expressed that the profession does
not always meet its obligations to society, particularly
with regard to issues of occupational justice and participation (Galheigo, 2011; Kronenberg et al., 2011).
Within a Western context, the majority of occupational therapists work in clinical settings where interventions are aligned with biomedicine and emphasis
is placed on enabling components of individual occupational performance. Furthermore, such practice is
frequently bounded by organizational demands and
cultures that emphasize 'rapid discharge' and prevent
therapists from addressing wider social, economic,
and political aspects of occupational participation and
engagement (see, e.g., recent explorations of occupational therapy practice in the area of sexuality
(McGrath and Lynch, 2014) and dementia care
(McGrath and O'Callaghan, 2013)). For many occupational therapists, then, the ideals of occupational
justice and critical occupational therapy practice may
appear to be unobtainable and as such may be excluded
from routine practice (McGrath and Lynch, 2014).

Wolf et al. (2010) suggest that addressing issues of
occupational injustice requires occupational therapists
to reframe the way in which they understand and view
issues that prevent occupational engagement. However,
as illustrated in Box 61-4, even when occupational
therapists identify the environmental and systemic
barriers that create occupational injustices, there is no
guarantee that they will feel able to act to enable occupational justice. Given the principle of *ultra posse nemo
obligatur* – that is, the idea that no person can be obligated beyond what he or she is able to do – does it
make sense to expect occupational therapists to grapple
with issues of social transformation? According to a
statement issued by the WFOT (2006a), the profession
is 'committed to advance certain core principles, one
of which is the right of all people – including people
with disabilities – to develop their capacity and power
to construct their own destiny through occupation',
and thus, the response to the question should be a
resounding yes. However, the extent to which this statement reflects the realities and priorities of contemporary occupational therapy practice is unclear, and
terms such as *participation*, *rights*, and *justice* potentially ring hollow if professional practice is not critically questioned and official pronouncements about

BOX 61-4
OCCUPATIONAL JUSTICE AS AN UNOBTAINABLE IDEAL

A community occupational therapist is working with a 75-year-old man who requires an electric bed in order to stay at home. The man asks if it is possible to order a double bed so that he can continue to share his bed with his wife. The occupational therapist knows that the health services will not fund this request and so tells the man that it is not possible and that he will have to be content with sleeping alone for the first time in 50 years. Later, when she discusses the case with her colleagues they all agree that sleeping alone is not desirable, but that nothing can be done because double beds are not considered essential items by the service.

An occupational therapist working with adults with intellectual disability learns that some of the adults would like to go swimming in the local swimming complex. He organizes a group outing to the swimming pool during the public swimming session. When the group arrives, the pool is busy with lots of parents and children. Within 15 minutes the pool empties and the adults with intellectual disabilities are left with no doubt that the other people do not want to share the pool space with them. The occupational therapist feels angry on behalf of the people with intellectual disabilities. He discusses his concerns with his manager, who reminds him that changing public attitudes is not within the scope of his employment. Eventually, he decides that the best solution is to organize future swimming sessions in a pool owned by another organization providing services for people with disabilities. He knows that for the adults with intellectual disabilities this is not the same as going to the local swimming complex but feels unable to tackle the attitudes and actions of the wider community.

occupation gloss over real questions about justice and development. Reflecting on the capacity of professionals to bring about occupational justice, Townsend and Marval (2013) note that at first glance it seems unlikely that professionals can achieve this goal unless they are willing to take a 'radical turn' (p. 222) and use their professional power to challenge prevailing social and political practices which act to marginalize and exclude certain groups from achieving full occupational participation. However, in order to move towards achieving this radical turn in practice, there is a need for therapists to identify and transcend an array of seemingly dichotomous ways of understanding professional obligations.

WAYS OF UNDERSTANDING PROFESSIONAL OBLIGATIONS

Tensions exist between dealing with immediate individual needs and addressing underlying structural causes of inequity. For example, research among occupational therapists working with older people found that issues regarding sexuality were deprioritized by occupational therapists who reported that practice was guided by the need to maintain the individual at home rather than participation in valued occupations (McGrath and Lynch, 2014). There are of course legitimate reasons why occupational therapists might seek to support older people to live at home and as Pollard, Kronenberg and Sakellariou (2009a) point out, occupational therapists must operate in a heteroglossic context navigating through interests of clients, employers, colleagues, and other professionals in order to maintain their position as professionals who can act at all. Furthermore, in an era of increased constraints on public resources, there is inevitably a tension between what is needed and what can be provided. However, by focusing on immediate priorities, occupational therapists are, perhaps unwittingly, reinforcing the notion that therapy practice is essentially focused on the immediate needs of the individual, and that concerns regarding the allocation of resources and prioritization of goals should be left in the public domain to be debated and decided upon by public health specialists and policymakers.

Furthermore, many therapy practices assume that individuals are either a provider of a service or the recipient of a service leading to the development of practice where the professional is the expert on the problems of the consumer-client. Framing occupational therapy in this way influences how we think of ourselves as occupational therapists and excludes not just the idea that our clients are citizens with something to contribute to their communities, but also how we think of ourselves as citizen therapists engaged in partnerships with other citizens to tackle public problems. The growth of the idea of the consumer-client can be linked to the rise in the adoption by many governments of neoliberal principles to reform public sector services (O'Dwyer, 2013). Such principles include adopting the values of the private sector to rationalize the public sector and placing an emphasis on privatization, deregulation, and efficiency (Navarro, 2007). In this approach, the service user is conceptualized as a consumer-client and is assumed to be concerned only with getting the best service for themselves as individuals and is not expected to be concerned with the common good of the community. For Mol (2006), the conceptualization of the service user as a consumer is problematic not least because consumers make different choices to citizens. She argues that consumers choose alone and that the decision as to which is the best treatment, goal, or way of life is a private matter of concern only to the individual. Citizens, on the other hand, make choices with reference to others, they engage in public discussions regarding what is best to be done, and debate with each other in an attempt to reach a collective decision regarding future actions. Research suggests that service users do not always see themselves as consumers but rather feel and act in ways which are guided by their identities as citizens. For example, Johansson (2013) found that among older adults living in Sweden, decisions regarding the use of home modification services were frequently made with reference to fulfilling obligations to the state and to other community members. For participants in the study, such obligations included 'being a good citizen by not causing extensive costs for the society and by finding out about one's own responsibilities to it' (p. 428).

Tensions also exist between personal beliefs and commitments to occupational justice expressed in the form of voluntary works versus accountability for professional obligations that occupational justice demands. Much of the existing work regarding occupational therapy practice in a justice arena has been driven by the personal motivations and choices of individual therapists who have sought opportunities to use their professional skills to enhance occupational participation for marginalized groups (see, e.g., Black, 2011; Simmond, 2005; Simó-Algado and Burgman, 2005). In some ways this is not surprising. After all, many occupational therapists are not employed directly by the client but instead are employees of a state or private health or social care system with its own agenda which often does not extend to issues of justice (Pollard et al., 2009b).

Kivel (2007) suggests that professionals cannot expect to easily combine the role of service provision with that of social transformation and change since paid professionals' jobs and status are dependent upon their ability to maintain the status quo no matter how illogical or unjust that status quo might be. Furthermore, occupational therapists might argue that their relatively low status among healthcare professions limits the extent to which they can act as agents of social transformation (Pollard et al., 2009b). Despite these challenges relying on individual, personal moral commitments to occupational justice cannot be considered an appropriate method of operationalizing the profession's stated commitment to occupational justice. Referring to volunteer work in food poverty, Poppendieck (1998) notes that relying on volunteer practice to address issues of social justice is likely to lead to developments that are 'uneven, unreliable, of unpredictable quantity and erratic quality' (p. 200), and it is likely that the same will apply if occupational justice is seen as an optional endeavour. The need for professional leadership in this area has been acknowledged (Townsend and Marval, 2013; Wolf et al., 2010); however, to date, the profession has failed to hold itself fully accountable for deficits in practice or to acknowledge that the professional obligation to promote occupational justice cannot be met by a small minority of practitioners.

Finally, professional literature focusing on issues of occupational justice may act to limit the scope and the effectiveness of occupational therapists in promoting occupational rights by promoting the view that: (a) occupational justice-based practice is for low-income and low-resource communities, (b) therapists' professional obligations to promote occupational rights and occupational justice can be met through pro bono work, (c) advocating for changes in public policy is the primary means through which therapists can promote justice, and (d) students must develop clinical knowledge and skills before being introduced to occupational justice. The association between occupational justice-based practice and low-income/low-resource communities is based on the assumption that only people living in such communities are likely to experience occupational injustices. Thibeault (2013) has noted that such an assumption undermines the very essence of occupational justice as it leads to skewed perspectives that fail to appreciate the complexity of a community's occupational landscape and can result in damaging outcomes for individuals and communities. Furthermore, such a view may also support the assumption that those therapists who work and live in resource-plentiful communities need not concern themselves with any professional obligation to work to improve the occupational situation of the community.

Situating occupational justice work as pro bono work to be completed outside of therapists' main professional concerns ensures that occupational justice work will continue to remain at the margins of professional practice. While pro bono work is certainly useful, such an approach also encourages occupational therapists to think of working for occupational justice as a personal choice to be taken up by those who have time and capacity for such largesse rather than a professional obligation. Although the Participatory Occupational Justice Framework (Whiteford and Townsend, 2011) highlights the need for therapists to use advocacy skills for sustainability or closure of collaborative partnerships, relying on public advocacy as the sole means to bring about changes in people's occupational situation at best limits the impact of this work and at worst can result in professional elites talking to policy elites while the concerned communities are excluded from the discussions. Such an approach also fails to recognize the knowledge and strengths of the communities involved and increases feelings of disempowerment, passivity, and learned helplessness (Thibeault, 2013).

Galheigo (2011) has highlighted the need for occupational therapy educators to prepare the next generation of occupational therapists to be able to work for social transformation, and there is growing evidence that educators are responding to this need through the development of community-engaged learning opportunities for preprofessional students (McGrath et al., 2014; McMenamin et al., 2014). However, for the most part, community-engaged learning opportunities have been included towards the later stages of the curriculum (McGrath et al., 2014), and the extent to which such experiences have any meaningful impact upon students' future professional practice remains unclear (McMenamin et al., 2014). Van Bruggen (2009) questions if it is sufficient to attempt to 'fit' curricula relating to the social and political aspects of occupation into traditional curricula and proposes that it may be more effective for educators to develop an entirely new curriculum which can incorporate a vision of occupational justice throughout the learning process. Given that the foundations of professional identity are set from the first day of education, it seems reasonable to suggest that opportunities to develop skills in promoting occupational justice should be afforded equal presence in the curriculum as traditional subjects. Such an approach would go some way towards communicating to students that working for occupational justice is both a core part of practice and a professional responsibility.

TAKING UP THE CHALLENGE: PROMOTING OCCUPATIONAL JUSTICE AS A PROFESSIONAL OBLIGATION

How, then, can occupational therapists respond to their professional obligations to support the rights of all people to have opportunities for meaningful occupation? One way to address the gap between what is written about occupational justice and what is done about occupational justice may be for occupational therapists to develop their skills in professional citizenship and the public practice of occupational therapy. Professional citizenship is a term used to describe how professionals might engage in collaborative civic action in communities alongside other community members to address community needs. As described in text Box 61-1, professional citizenship requires occupational therapists to identify and articulate occupational injustices in communities and to use their knowledge and understanding of occupation to collaborate with others to bring about changes and enable occupational justice for all.

The idea of professional citizenship emerges from the work of Doherty (2011) relating to citizen professionals. Doherty (2011) uses the term *citizen professionals* to highlight the role of professionals in developing and enhancing the civic life of communities in addition to their traditional role of providing specialized services to individuals. According to Doherty (2011), citizen professionalism is primarily an issue of identity and involves developing a sense of oneself as a citizen with particular expertise who works with other citizens, each of whom has his or her own expertise, in order to address complex community

BOX 61-5
PUBLIC PRACTICE OF OCCUPATIONAL THERAPY

The concept of public occupational therapy encompasses a variety of connotations and is a political concept. Public occupational therapy is fundamentally political because it is a rationale for collective public action to assure conditions in which people have access to meaningful occupational participation and engagement.

issues. He suggests that citizen professionals have a body of knowledge and a set of skills that enable them to make connections between the personal and public aspects of their professional knowledge and practice. For Doherty (2011), citizen professionalism is enacted by using this professional knowledge and skills to bring together other citizens to generate public conversation and action to address community needs.

Professional citizenship is closely linked to and is supported by the concept of 'public' occupational therapy practice which sets out a clear mandate for collective public action by occupational therapists in order to realize their stated aim of achieving rights to meaningful occupational participation for all (WFOT, 2006a) (Box 61-5).

Situating professional obligations in the context of citizenship requires some discussion about the meaning and use of the concept of citizenship. As Oliver and Heater (1994) note, the language of citizenship is used for a multitude of purposes and in a multitude of contexts including, but not limited to, politics, legislation, philosophy, and academia. Given the diversity of usage, it is not surprising that no one universally accepted definition of citizenship is easily available. At its most basic, definitions of citizenship, irrespective of philosophical or political disposition, are made with reference to three main criteria: (a) legal status, (b) philosophical orientation, and (c) sociopolitical context (Faulks, 2000). Understandings of citizenship drawing from a primarily liberal stance that emphasizes the importance of individually held rights will have a very different approach from a civic republican/communitarian understanding that stresses individuals' commitments and obligations to a wider community (Dwyer, 2010; Heater, 1999).

My conceptualization of citizenship draws from the work of Heater (1999), who identifies three interrelated dimensions of citizenship: status, feelings, and participation. Citizenship status can be understood with reference to Marshall's (1950) understanding of the rights conferred on citizens by the state and the duties owed by these citizens to the state. Depending on the particular state, basic statuses will include a range of civic and political rights while individual citizens may obtain additional status through social, cultural, and economic factors. Feelings about citizenship can refer to identity and civic virtues (moral consciousness). According to Heater (1999), feelings of citizenship generate loyalty among citizens and result in feelings of or duty to responsibilities. Participation refers to citizens' capacity for and attempts to bring about improvements or to counteract deterioration in public life. Motivation for participation comes from feelings of citizenship that generate moral obligations or duty to participate in society and from personal interests to bring about change. In some ways, this conceptualization integrates central aspects of both the liberal and the civic republican tradition and is closely connected to Lister's (1997) assertion that citizenship is both a process and an outcome where one cannot simply be a citizen, but one must also feel and act as a citizen.

LEARNING TO DO 'COLLABORATIVE ACTION'

Developing capacity for professional citizenship among occupational therapists requires that future practitioners are given the opportunity to acquire key skills necessary to engage in collaborative action. These skills include, but are not limited to, (a) understanding formal processes of policy-making and legislature; (b) knowledge and awareness of occupational issues of particular importance in local communities; (c) openness and willingness to work with people of diverse backgrounds and dispositions; (d) grassroots leadership skills including the ability to engage others, the capacity to engender participatory processes, and ability to plan and implement actions for change; and (e) personal belief and commitment to the value of collaborative action.

One method of supporting students to develop such professional citizenship skills is through the use of community engaged learning, an experiential learning approach which facilitates students to work in collaboration with existing community groups to use their disciplinary knowledge to bring about positive change in response to a defined community need. During the period 2006–2014, while working at the National University of Ireland (NUI), Galway, I was responsible for developing such learning opportunities for undergraduate occupational therapy students as part of a wider university commitment to community engagement. Examples of collective actions students engaged in include working with the Going to College Project to support opportunities for people with intellectual disability to participate in higher education (Lyons et al. 2011), developing strategies to support transition of people who experience homelessness from emergency sheltered accommodation to independent living (Connell et al., 2009; Gilligan et al., 2010), and addressing social exclusion of older adults through occupational engagement (Fahy et al., 2010; Gowran et al., 2011) (Box 61-6).

For students, these learning opportunities enabled development of skills in professional citizenship and a renewed sense of commitment to social justice and change, while for community groups, collaborative partnerships with university staff and students enabled real issues of relevance to the community, such as access to health information for older people, opportunities for occupational engagement for men in emergency accommodation for people experiencing homelessness, the inclusion of teenagers with visual impairment and so on to be addressed from an occupational perspective (McMenamin et al., 2011). Fundamentally, these experiences were underpinned by a partnership approach where all stakeholders were assumed to bring knowledge, experience, and personal and professional diversity to address issues of mutual concern. Such an approach is consistent both with a professional orientation towards client-centred practice and a commitment to social justice and transformation.

APPLYING PROFESSIONAL CITIZENSHIP SKILLS IN PRACTICE

There are, of course, challenges in transferring this type of work from the university setting to the wider

---

BOX 61-6
EXAMPLES OF COLLABORATIVE ACTIONS BETWEEN OCCUPATIONAL THERAPY AND THE WIDER COMMUNITY

For adults with intellectual disability, participation in higher education is often limited. At NUI Galway, as part of the Going to College Project, occupational therapy students were asked to work with adults with intellectual disabilities, their parents and caregivers, academic staff, and university management to identify how these adults might be enabled to access the opportunity to attend university. The students' work took place over a period of 1 academic year and involved developing relationships with university management, academic staff, and organizations providing services for people with intellectual disabilities (Lyons et al., 2011). Students investigated potential challenges relating to accessing the university environment, including both physical barriers and attitudinal difficulties. In collaboration with the Going to College Project, the students generated a brief report outlining strategies that needed to be implemented to ensure that adults with intellectual disabilities would be facilitated to participate in university life.

A longstanding partnership between the Discipline of Occupational Therapy at NUI Galway and COPE Galway Senior Services enabled both groups to identify and respond to the needs of older people living in the community. Many of the older people supported by COPE Galway reported that knowing where to get information about health services, social support, and advice regarding welfare entitlements, among other services, was confusing and required a great deal of perseverance and ingenuity on behalf of older adults. Supported by a research grant from the Community Knowledge Initiative at NUI, Galway, the author collaborated with older people, staff at COPE Galway and local healthcare professionals to develop an action research project which sought to build upon older people's existing strengths in health literacy and to raise awareness among healthcare professionals of the need to ensure that information-sharing strategies were adequate and met the needs of the local community (McGrath et al., 2015). Using action research methodology, the collaboration resulted in the development of health and community care information for older adults. Furthermore, the findings were used to inform subsequent discussions with healthcare and social care managers regarding health literacy in the local population.

community, and for occupational therapists who do not have the luxury of supportive employment contexts, it may be difficult to imagine how one can begin to become involved in collaborative actions. In the following paragraph, I attempt to map out a process through which a therapist might become involved in this work. My suggestions draw from the work of Tennyson (2003) in relation to developing partnerships, the Participatory Occupational Justice Framework (Whiteford and Townsend, 2011), and the 3P for political reasoning in occupational therapy described by Pollard, Sakellariou and Kronenberg (2009b). Each of these frameworks highlights a different aspect of collaborative actions that are focused on bringing about social transformations and in combination offers a method of considering both the process (collaboration/ political reasoning) and the intended outcome (occupational justice).

From the outset, the reader should be aware that the linear steps described do not reflect the realities of collaborative practice. Working with individuals and communities to address complex issues with no obvious solution is a complex and messy endeavour. Very often, development of true partnerships occurs over a long period of time and opportunities to engage in processes of transformation appear in an ad hoc manner. Collaborative actions do not always bring about intended results and mostly the change that occurs is small change whose impact may not be as significant as hoped for. For this reason, therapists must be clear about their willingness and ability to commit to collaborative actions and to ensure that actions remain grounded in the needs and desires of communities.

As a point of departure, therapists may wish to reflect on their own personal knowledge and understanding of the formal processes of policy-making and legislation as it occurs in their own communities. Developing the capacity to engage with issues of social justice and social rights requires therapists to understand how such rights are articulated and protected. With this understanding, therapists are in a stronger position to be aware of and contribute to debates concerning issues of particular importance to local communities, such as, for example, access to health services, public transport policies, and environmental protection plans. Therapists must then seek opportunities to engage with other citizens in order to begin to identify possibilities for action and to plan for social transformation and change. Such opportunities frequently present themselves during everyday life and so therapists must be alert to the possibilities for action for occupational justice in all that they do. Through adopting an open attitude towards collaborating with people of diverse backgrounds and perspectives, occupational therapists have the opportunity to share their professional knowledge with others in an attempt to generate sustainable solutions to community challenges. Furthermore, occupational therapists' skills in enabling individuals and communities to bring about change in occupational performance and engagement ensure that they bring a valuable skill set to collective civic actions. However, the extent to which these skills are utilized is largely dependent on professional and personal commitment to social justice and requires ongoing reflection on action and inaction regarding ones' identity as a professional citizen.

CONCLUSION

The profession of occupational therapy sets out an ambitious agenda to enable access to meaningful occupation for all people. However, despite growing professional interest in occupational justice and participation, daily occupational therapy practice often fails to confront issues of occupational injustice. One method of addressing this gap is to consider how the concept of professional citizenship can be used to enable occupational therapists to identify and respond to issues of occupational injustice in collaboration with wider communities. Enacting professional citizenship requires occupational therapists to reflect on and develop their understanding of citizenship and to build collaborative partnerships with other citizens. Through these partnerships, therapists may be enabled to bring an occupational justice lens to bear on community issues and in doing so contribute towards promoting occupational justice.

Acknowledgements

I wish to acknowledge my colleagues at Trinity College Dublin and at the National University of Ireland, Galway, who have previously supported my work in community engagement, including Professor Agnes

Shiel, Dr Lorraine McIlrath, Dr Josephine Boland, Dr Tadhg Stapleton, and Dr Deirdre Connolly. I also acknowledge with much gratitude the vast contribution made by all of my former occupational therapy students, community partners, and colleagues in Ireland, Lebanon, and Singapore who have been involved in this work.

REFERENCES

Black, M., 2011. From kites to kitchens: collaborative community-based occupational therapy with refugee survivors of torture. In: Kronenberg, F., Pollard, N., Sakellariou, D. (Eds.), Occupational Therapy without Borders, vol. 2: Towards an Ecology of Occupation-Based Practices. Churchill Livingstone Elsevier, Edinburgh, pp. 217–227.

Connell, L., Ní Dhufaí-Boltúin, N., Waldron, A., McGrath, M., 2009. Occupational Therapy to promote independent living in the context of a continuing care service for homeless people – a case study. Poster presented at the Campus Engage International Conference 2009 Higher Education and Civic Engagement Partnerships: Create, Challenge, Change, Dublin, Ireland, 4–5th June 2009.

Doherty, W.J., 2011. The Citizen Professional Idea. University of Minnesota Citizen Professional Center, St Paul, MN. Available from: <http://www.cehd.umn.edu/fsos/projects/cpc/idea.asp> (accessed 10.05.14.).

Dwyer, P., 2010. Understanding Social Citizenship: Themes and Perspectives for Policy and Practice. University of Bristol, Policy Press, Bristol, UK.

Fahy, J., O'Grady, N., McGrath, M., Cunningham, T., 2010. Combating Social Exclusion through Empowerment. Paper presented at European Network of Occupational Therapists in Higher Education 16th Annual Meeting. Karolinska Institutet, Stockholm, Sweden, 14–16 October, 2010.

Faulks, K., 2000. Citizenship. Routledge, New York.

Fazio, L.S., 2008. Developing occupation-centred programs for the community, second ed. Prentice Hall, Upper Saddler River, NJ.

Frank, G., 1992. Opening feminist histories of occupational therapy. Am. J. Occup. Ther. 46 (11), 989–999.

Galheigo, S.M., 2011. What needs to be done? Occupational therapy's responsibilities and challenges regarding human rights. Aust. Occup. Ther. J. 58 (1), 60–66.

Gilligan, R., Tolan, S., Gallagher, A., McGrath, M., 2010. Harm reduction and its application to occupational therapy. Paper presented at the Association of Occupational Therapists of Ireland Annual Conference: Occupational Therapists Achieving Goals. Croke Park Conference Centre, Dublin, Ireland. 28–29 May 2010.

Gowran, S., Lynch, E., Cunningham, T., McGrath, M., 2011. Come Dine with Me- promoting social inclusion of older adults through dining clubs. Poster presented at Association of Occupational Therapists of Ireland and College of Occupational Therapists, UK All Ireland Conference: Crossing Borders: Challenges and Opportunities. Promoting Best Practice and Collaboration amongst

Occupational Therapists throughout all Ireland. Dundalk, Ireland. 8–9 April 2011.

Hammell, K., 2009. Sacred texts: a skeptical exploration of the assumptions underpinning theories of occupation. Can. J. Occup. Ther. 76 (1), 6–22.

Heater, D., 1999. What Is Citizenship? Polity Press, Bristol, UK.

Johansson, K., 2013. Have they done what they should? Moral reasoning in the context of translating older persons' everyday problems into eligible needs for home modification services. Med. Anthropol. Q. 27 (3), 414–433.

Kantartzis, S., Molineux, M., 2011. The influences of Western society's construction of a healthy daily life on the conceptualization of occupation. J. Occup. Sci. 18 (1), 62–80.

Kivel, P. (Ed.), 2007. Social service or social change. In: INCITE! Women of Color Against Violence (Ed.), The Revolution Will Not Be Funded beyond the Non-profit Industrial Complex. South End Press Read Write Revolt, Boston, MA, pp. 129–151.

Kronenberg, F., Pollard, N., 2005. Introduction: a beginning ... In: Kronenberg, F., Pollard, N., Sakellariou, D. (Eds.), Occupational Therapy without Borders: Learning from the Spirit of Survivors. Elsevier Churchill Livingstone, Edinburgh, pp. 1–15.

Kronenberg, F., Pollard, N., Ramungondo, E., 2011. Introduction: courage to dance politics. In: Kronenberg, F., Pollard, N., Sakellariou, D. (Eds.), Occupational Therapy Without Borders, vol. 2: Towards Ecology of Occupation-Based Practices. Churchill Livingstone Elsevier, Edinburgh, pp. 1–17.

Lister, R., 1997. Citizenship: Feminist Perspectives. MacMillan Press Ltd, London.

Lyons, A., Campbell, M., O'Brien, M., Killeen, H., McGrath, M., 2011. Exploring Accessibility Issues at NUI, Galway for Students with Intellectual Disabilities. Poster presented at Association of Occupational Therapists of Ireland and College of Occupational Therapists, UK All Ireland Conference: Crossing Borders: Challenges and Opportunities. Promoting Best Practice and Collaboration amongst Occupational Therapists throughout All Ireland. Dundalk, Ireland. 8–9 April 2011.

McGrath, M., Lynch, E., 2014. Occupational therapists' perspectives on addressing sexual concerns of older adults in the context of rehabilitation. Disabil. Rehabil. 36 (8), 651–657.

McGrath, M., O'Callaghan, C., 2013. Occupational therapy and dementia care: a survey of practice in the Republic of Ireland. Aust. Occup. Ther. J. 61 (2), 92–101.

McGrath, M., Moldes, I., Fransen, H., Hofstede-Wessels, S., Lilienberg, K., 2014. Community-university partnerships in occupational therapy education: a preliminary exploration of practice in a European context. Disabil. Rehabil. 36 (4), 344–352.

McGrath, M., Kenny, A., Clancy, K., 2015. An exploration of strategies used by older people to obtain information about health- and social care services in the community. Health Expect. doi:10.1111/hex.12408.

McMenamin, R., McGrath, M., D'Eath, M., 2011. Impacts of service learning on Irish healthcare students, educators, and communities. Nurs. Health Sci. 12 (4), 499–506.

McMenamin, R., McGrath, M., Cantillon, P., MacFarlane, A., 2014. Training socially responsive health care graduates: Is service learning an effective educational approach? Med. Teach. 36 (4), 291–307.

Marshall, T.H., 1950. Citizenship and Social Class and Other Essays. Heinemann, London.

Mol, A., 2006. The Logic of Care Health and the problem of patient choice. Routledge Taylor & Francis Group, New York.

Navarro, V., 2007. Neoliberalism as a class ideology; or, the political causes of the growth of inequalities. Int. J. Health Serv. 37 (1), 47–62.

O'Dwyer, C., 2013. Official conceptualizations of person-centred care: which person counts? J. Aging Stud. 27 (3), 233–242.

Oliver, D., Heater, D., 1994. The Foundations of Citizenship. Harvester Wheatsheaf, New York.

Pollard, N., Sakellariou, D., 2014. The occupational therapist as a political being. Cad. Ter. Ocup. UFSCar 22 (3), 643–652.

Pollard, N., Kronenberg, F., Sakellariou, D., 2009a. Introduction. In: Pollard, N., Kronenberg, F., Sakellariou, D. (Eds.), A Political Practice of Occupational Therapy. Churchill Livingstone Elsevier, Edinburgh, pp. xxi–xxiv.

Pollard, N., Sakellariou, D., Kronenberg, F., 2009b. Political competence in occupational therapy. In: Pollard, N., Kronenberg, F., Sakellariou, D. (Eds.), A Political Practice of Occupational Therapy. Churchill Livingstone Elsevier, Edinburgh, pp. 21–39.

Poppendieck, J., 1998. Sweet Charity ? Emergency Food and the End of Entitlement. Penguin Books, New York.

Reid, L., 2011. Medical professionalism and the social contract. Perspect. Biol. Med. 54 (4), 455–469.

Richardson, H.S., 2006. Rawlsian social-contract theory and the severely disabled. J. Ethics 10 (4), 419–462.

Simmond, M., 2005. Practicing to learn occupational therapy with the children of Viet Nam. In: Kronenberg, F., Simo Algado, S., Pollard, N. (Eds.), Occupational Therapy without Borders: Learning from the Spirit of Survivors. Elsevier Churchill Livingstone, Edinburgh, pp. 277–287.

Simó-Algado, S., Burgman, I., 2005. Occupational therapy intervention with children survivors of war. In: Kronenberg, F., Simo Algado, S., Pollard, N. (Eds.), Occupational Therapy without Borders – Learning from the Spirit of Survivors. Elsevier Churchill Livingstone, Edinburgh, pp. 245–261.

Tennyson, R., 2003. The Partnering Toolbok. The International Business Leaders Forum and the Global Alliance for Improved Nutrition, London.

Thibeault, R., 2002. Muriel Driver Memorial Lecture: In praise of dissidence: Anne Lang-Etienne. Can. J. Occup. Ther. 69 (4), 197–203.

Thibeault, R., 2013. Occupational Justice's Intents and Impacts: From Personal Choices to Community Consequences. In: Cutchin, M.P., Dickie, V.A. (Eds.), Transactional Perspectives on Occupation. Springer, Dordrecht.

Townsend, E.A., 1993. Muriel Driver Memorial Lecture: Occupational Therapy's Social Vision. Can. J. Occup. Ther. 60 (4), 174–184.

Townsend, E.A., Marval, R., 2013. Can professionals actually enable occupational justice? Cad. Ter. Ocup. UFSCar 21 (2), 215–228.

Townsend, E.A., Wilcock, A.A., 2004. Occupational justice and client centred practice: a dialogue in progress. Can. J. Occup. Ther. 71 (1), 75–87.

United Nations, 1989. United Nations Convention on the Rights of the Child (UNCRC). United Nations, Geneva, Switzerland.

United Nations, 1993. The Standard Rules on the Equalization of Opportunities for Persons with Disabilities. United Nations, New York.

United Nations, 2006. Convention on the Rights of Persons with Disabilities. Treaty Series, 2515, 3.

Van Bruggen, H., 2009. Foreword. In: Pollard, N., Kronenberg, F., Sakellariou, D. (Eds.), A Political Practice of Occupational Therapy. Churchill Livingstone Elsevier, Edinburgh, pp. xiii–xvii.

Whiteford, G., Townsend, E.A., 2011. Participatory Occupational Justice Framework (POJF 2010): enabling occupational participation and inclusion. In: Kronenberg, F., Simo Algado, S., Pollard, N. (Eds.), Occupational Therapy without Borders, vol. 2: Towards an Ecology of Occupation-Based Practices. Churchill Livingstone Elsevier, Edinburgh, pp. 65–85.

Wilcock, A.A., 2006. An Occupational Perspective of Health, 2nd ed. Slack, Thorofare, NJ.

Wolf, L., Ripat, J., Davis, E., Becker, P., MacSwiggan, J., 2010. Applying an occupational justice framework. Occup. Ther. Now 12 (1), 15–18.

World Federation of Occupational Therapists, 2004. Position Statement: Community Based Rehabilitation. World Federation of Occupational Therapists, Forrestfield, WA. Available from: <http://www.wfot.org/ResourceCentre.aspx> (accessed 09.12.14.).

World Federation of Occupational Therapists, 2006a. Position Statement: Human Rights. World Federation of Occupational Therapists, Forrestfield, WA. Available from: <http://www.wfot.org/ResourceCentre.aspx> (accessed 09.12.14.).

World Federation of Occupational Therapists, 2006b. Position Statement: Occupational Science. World Federation of Occupational Therapists, Forrestfield, WA. Available from: <http://www.wfot.org/ResourceCentre.aspx> (accessed 09.12.14.).

World Federation of Occupational Therapists, 2010. Position Statement: Diversity and Culture. World Federation of Occupational Therapists, Forrestfield, WA. Available from: <http://www.wfot.org/ResourceCentre.aspx> (accessed 09.12.14.).

World Federation of Occupational Therapists, 2012. Position Statement: Environmental Sustainability Sustainable Practice in Occupational Therapy. World Federation of Occupational Therapists, Forrestfield, WA. Available from: <http://www.wfot.org/ResourceCentre.aspx> (accessed 09.12.14.).

World Federation of Occupational Therapists, 2014a. Position Statement: Human Displacement. World Federation of Occupational Therapists, Forrestfield, WA. Available from: <http://www.wfot.org/ResourceCentre.aspx> (accessed 09.12.14.).

World Federation of Occupational Therapists, 2014b. Position Statement: Occupational Therapy in Disaster, Preparedness and Response. World Federation of Occupational Therapists, Forrestfield, WA. Available from: <http://www.wfot.org/ResourceCentre.aspx> (accessed 09.12.14.).

62

FROM RHETORIC TO REALITY: COMMUNITY DEVELOPMENT IN OCCUPATIONAL THERAPY CURRICULUM

SUSAN GILBERT HUNT ■ BEN SELLAR ■ ANGELA BERNDT ■ EMMA GEORGE ■ KERRY THOMAS ■ KRISTEN MARIE FOLEY

CHAPTER OUTLINE

Occupational therapy educators have a responsibility to prepare graduates for the complexities and possibilities of future practice and as such need to provide opportunities for students to develop tactic knowledge and skills to work with communities in addressing multifaceted issues. This chapter aims to share the learnings of staff in the occupational therapy programme at the University of South Australia that have come from establishing and implementing a curriculum aimed at preparing students to work effectively at a community level. To do this successfully, there is a need for an ethical and robust pedagogy, which focuses on participatory processes rather than premature solutions, and on the importance of holding the space of discomfort as students grapple to understand their potential as occupational therapists. Supporting such a gestalt to occur facilitates a greater appreciation and confidence in the power of occupation, the importance of capacity building, and sustainable outcomes.

'Participatory community practice' (PCP) is an approach to practice that has been a core element of the occupational therapy education programme at the University of South Australia for 20 years (Gilbert Hunt, 2006). PCP is underpinned by a thorough knowledge of primary healthcare and community development principles. Ife (1995) identifies 22 principles that underpin community development work, which is a process of working with people to enable the necessary skill development and mobilization of resources to generate solutions to agreed problems within a community or group.

PCP enables students to partner with community organizations in undertaking projects that address community needs. Moreover, students develop the knowledge and skills to effectively work at the community level from an occupational perspective. This work is often referred to in the literature as a role emerging or 'nontraditional' project placement (Thew et al., 2011), suggesting it sits beyond the border of usual practice. Though we argue that such work is core

561

to occupational therapy practice, when we began this type of placement 20 years ago, it was certainly perceived as challenging tradition.

BACKGROUND

A Challenging Healthcare Climate: Change Catalyst

The catalyst for change and the beginnings of PCP at the University of South Australia was the impact of the 1991 collapse of the South Australian State-controlled bank, which led to a severe economic downturn and the successive conservative governments being committed to reducing state government expenditure and the size of the public service, including health (Newman et al., 2007). This resulted in a freeze on all allied health positions in the health sector and a need for graduating students to consider employment outside of 'traditional' options – that is, community and nongovernment organizations. However, the student group was unclear about how to apply existing occupational therapy knowledge and skills to work in such community contexts.

The previous decade in South Australia had seen a significant increase in the implementation of what is now called the new public health policy (Baum, 2008). The new public health agenda acknowledged the limitations of medical, behavioural, and lifestyle approaches to improving the health status of all people. The Ottawa Charter (World Health Organization (WHO), 1986) clearly outlined the prerequisites for health including peace, shelter, education, food, income, a stable ecosystem, social justice, and equity. Moreover, this perspective acknowledged that health is of concern to all government sectors, and health services needed to shift their focus from hospital-based services to community-based and community-controlled models. This shift in focus resulted in the introduction of the Social Health Strategy (South Australian Health Commission, 1988) and the Primary Health Policy (South Australian Health Commission, 1989) in South Australia and created an environment in which community-focused initiatives flourished with an associated increase in employment opportunities in this area (Baum, 2008).

Concomitantly, there was growing awareness in the literature that a lack of educational focus on public health issues and the skills and competencies needed to work from a primary healthcare perspective was missing in most health professional training (Saunders, 1998), which perpetuated the limitations of responsive healthcare in the field (WHO, 1984). Thus, traction for change came from a very practical imperative, supported by a philosophical rationale for change, which reflected the growing commitment to a public health perspective acknowledging the socioeconomic, ecological, and political contexts that influence health.

Challenging Hegemonic Practice

The move to community development-based student placements was not without its challenges as it questioned the ideological and cultural power of '1000 hours' of occupational therapy-supervised placement identified by the World Federation of Occupational Therapists as the gold standard for practice education. As the organizations we partnered with did not employ occupational therapists, there was not the requirement to have onsite occupational therapy supervision. This was provided at a distance by a university tutor, and some local therapists expressed concerns regarding the adequacy of supervision and the potential for questionable outcomes. As such, PCP was a counterhegemonic process that challenged the status quo regarding placement requirements, contested the legitimacy of placement structures, and provided an alternative option that has proven to be effective (Kronenberg et al., 2011). Initially, local therapists questioned the validity of the learning experience and demarcated the placement as 'other', alternative, or nontraditional. Whilst the placement was acknowledged for the development of student project management and research skills, there were queries as to the core occupational therapy skills development. This stance by local therapists reflected the practice environment of the majority at that time, which involved providing occupational therapy intervention to individuals or small groups in hospitals or health services in the community. However, this issue continues to be discussed in the literature with some authors arguing that such placements provide excellent opportunities for developing the skills needed for future practice and enhanced professional identity (Bosser et al., 1997; Fieldhouse and Fedden, 2009; Thew et al., 2011), whilst others maintain the need for traditional placements to consolidate core practice skills (Kirke et al., 2007).

The need to resist these hegemonic pressures present within the profession necessitated the development of robust and well-scaffolded learning processes that enabled students to critique the rhetoric of the profession's claim of working with communities and envisage the opportunities afforded through community empowerment to enhance community health (Thibeault and Herbert, 1997).

PARTICIPATORY COMMUNITY PRACTICE

The primary focus of the PCP placement is to enhance the ability of communities to take control over issues that influence their own health through empowerment (Williams and Labonte, 2003). It is generally accepted that occupational therapists work to empower individuals, groups, and communities in influencing their health. However, a closer look at key texts highlights an individualistic focus even when encompassing the community. Moreover, dominant practice models in occupational therapy also have a bias towards the individual, which can limit consideration of how to foster interdependence or develop shared visions about collective health and well-being (Hammell, 2009; Thibeault and Herbert, 1997). The lack of clarity around occupation-based models for community development has been identified as a limitation for occupational therapists working with communities (Leclair, 2010). Being able to respond to the emerging gaps in healthcare provision, as well as more deeply analyse how occupation, can be transformative at a community level in creating real and sustainable change to improve health outcomes provides the foundation for teaching and learning processes within and preceding the PCP placement.

Course Structure and Process

Within our 4-year undergraduate programme, PCP is broken into two courses across the third and fourth years of the Occupational Therapy Program. The learning outcomes for both courses are provided in Table 62-1. Table 62-2 provides further details of the activities undertaken and their purpose. In PCP 301, learning is carefully scaffolded to enable students to

---

TABLE 62-1
Learning Outcomes for Participatory Community Practice

PCP 301: Learning Outcomes	PCP 400: Learning Outcomes
1. Apply social health and community development principles to occupational therapy practice with a target community.	1. Demonstrate ability to function as a facilitator rather than assuming an 'expert' position, including effective skills in: working with people rather than for people, listening to and learning from others, awareness of resource options available within the community, and accessing available resources with and on behalf of stakeholders.
2. Effectively undertake a preliminary needs assessment with a target group.	
3. Apply project management skills in the development of a project plan to address a specified issue.	2. Demonstrate the ability to manage and monitor a planned project demonstrating effective skills in: communication and negotiation, participatory techniques, resource management (human and nonhuman), networking, identification of problems and capacity to address these in a politically and socially acceptable manner, and ensuring sustainability.
4. Demonstrate collaborative skills and use of participatory techniques in developing a project plan.	
5. Apply ethical skills to project planning.	
6. Demonstrate capacity for critical reflection through awareness of skills and competencies achieved and those requiring further development.	3. Demonstrate professional conduct and ethical practice.
7. Demonstrate appropriate professional behaviour.	4. Demonstrate ability to evaluate a project including selection and utilization of evaluation methods, use of participatory and capacity-building techniques, and recommendations for the future.
	5. Prepare a comprehensive written project report.
	6. Effectively disseminate project outcomes.

TABLE 62-2
Structure of Participatory Community Practice 301 and 400

PCP 301 (9 Units or ½ Semester Study Load)

Activity	Focus and Purpose
Preclass readings	Curriculum content and priming for learning
13 × 2-hour lectures	Curriculum content and construction of knowledge
7 × 3-hour workshops	Application of knowledge and skill development
Agency visits to learn about the services and potential project ideas	Increased awareness of community-based services and service provision challenges
Online discussion to review information from agency visits and consider project ideas in more depth	Support student in developing their understanding of project processes, challenges, and opportunities
Potential Project Plans – submission of five, based on five specific projects pitched by agencies	Application of knowledge to unique and authentic issues
Allocation of project and project partner	Identification of project and student partner
Partnership contract	Develop skills in effectively working with others
Scoping project parameters with agency and key stakeholders including a brief literature review	Application of skills and knowledge
Project Proposal	

PCP 400 (9 Units or ½ Semester Study Load)

Activity	Focus and Purpose
300 hours placement (4.5 days × 9 weeks)	Effective application of skills and knowledge
Weekly progress reports for tutor and stakeholders	Effective monitoring and evaluation skills
Final Project Report	Effective report-writing skills
Poster and abstract	Effective dissemination skills
Midway and final placement performance review	Feedback on performance led by student
Project management skills review by tutor	Feedback on specific project management skills

develop the skills and confidence to effectively facilitate the 9-week project placement in year 4. Each course constitutes half a semester load of study and is mandatory for all students as part of their 1000 hours of field placement required for World Federation of Occupational Therapists accreditation (WFOT, 2002). Located as it is in the third year, students have already studied core occupational therapy principles and practice as well as preparatory coursework in sociology, occupational science, and primary health.

PCP 301 requires students to increase their understanding and application of primary health, community development, and project management. At the same time, students attend a series of agency visits at which staff and communities pitch potential project ideas. From these visits, students identify their preferred project and are allocated in pairs to projects of best fit to their preferences. The visits also provide an opportunity for students to increase their awareness of the range of agencies providing services beyond the health sector. For the remainder of the course, students collaborate with the agency and community to scope the project, analyse situational factors and produce a comprehensive project proposal that constitutes their final assignment. After the project proposal is reviewed and any amendments undertaken, it becomes a contractual agreement between the agency, university, and students for the implementation of the project and as such it is a professional document, not just an assignment. During this period, students attend weekly workshops with tutors and peers to critique each other's work, identify gaps and limitations in understandings, and promote application of knowledge and processes to fine-tune their proposals.

PCP 400 then requires students to implement their proposals over a 9-week period. Students have one supervisor from the sponsoring agency, often not an occupational therapist, and one university tutor who work as a team to monitor project management performance and scaffold learning. Students are assessed on their individual skills in managing the project process, its complexities and ambiguities. Other assessments include a final project report that is submitted to the agency and made publicly available, as well as an abstract and poster that could be submitted for publication at relevant conferences. Two project examples are provided in Boxes 62-1 and 62-2 to highlight the scope of the projects students undertake.

Tools and Processes Used to Support Student Learning

Despite the course having very specific structures in place, these alone are inadequate to achieve the learning outcomes required of students. Students often come to the course with what we call a 'solution focus'. That is, when they hear community needs they immediately leap to solutions without first examining the issues from multiple perspectives. Many students assume that they will be assessed on the quality of solution that they can imagine for the identified need. This is often learned from previous courses where having 'the right answers' produced better marks. Tutors are required to emphasize and reorient students to the focus on process. That is, we are more interested in how well students can follow a process of information gathering, critical thinking, collaboration, and capacity building with agencies and communities to produce a response from the bottom up. Though not dissimilar to the process of enabling client-centred practice, the diverse and fragmented nature of stakeholders and community contexts forces students to analyse, synthesize, and reconcile a diversity of views and interests that is new, challenging, and at times conflicting. Increasingly, the issues or problems explored in PCP are what have been called 'wicked problems' (Kickbush and Gleicher, 2012) in that they

exceed the capacities of individual sectors, departments or levels and call for multiple perspectives. Such complexity can be overwhelming for students. To enable students to manage these challenges, we provide process-focused tools to unpack the multiplicity of causal factors and perspectives.

One useful tool to help students understand the complexity and underlying causes of the situation associated with the project theme is the why-why diagram. It is a tool they can also use very effectively with key stakeholders. The why-why diagram is based on the work of Kaoru Ishikawa (Ishikawa and Loftus, 1990) and is a structured brainstorm technique to map factors that contribute to a particular situation or issue, an example of which can be seen in Figure 62-1. Concept mapping has been found to be a useful tool in provoking and supporting meaningful student discourse (van Boxtell et al., 2010) and in our experience, assists students to consider underlying assumptions. In PCP, students use the technique to begin to externalize their own perspectives and are encouraged to use it with key stakeholders to develop a deeper, collective, and more layered understanding of the complexity of the presenting issue.

The programme logic model is another tool used to assist students to plan, develop, monitor, and evaluate their project. Programme logic is a diagrammatic representation of the project (see Figure 62-2) depicting the relationship between the overall project aim, project objectives and outcomes, as well as activities and resources (Millar et al., 2001). It is based on change theory and helps students to map their path to long-term outcomes by stating, 'if we do this, then this is likely to occur'. Crucially, this allows for interrogation of underlying assumptions, which is an often forgotten aspect of working with communities (Kaplan and Garrett, 2005).

In most cases, the project ideas pitched by agencies are significantly reframed as students use these tools to delve into the complexities of the issue. However, students can feel uncomfortable challenging the agency interpretations and overwhelmed by a problem that now appears too big or complex to address. As the capacity to resolve complexities and ambiguities is a core aim of the courses, tutors must resist invitations to resolve this discomfort by prematurely foreclosing on the learning potential of student struggles.

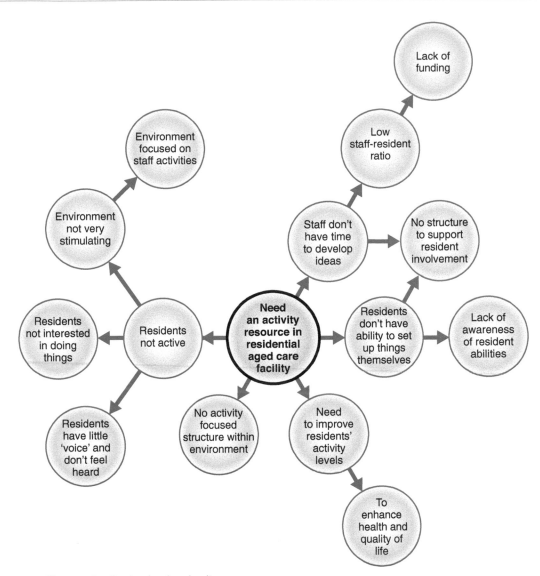

FIGURE 62-1 ■ Example of a simple why-why diagram.

Examples of how this process evolves are evidenced in Table 62-3.

Challenges for Educators

Discomfort is not reserved for students, but is typical for tutors as well because advising students to delve deeper, seek out marginalized voices, and critically engage with power and conflict can produce tensions within the agency. Furthermore, tutors need to manage the tension between prematurely solving student problems and having them flounder. This is an ethical and pedagogical challenge as students learn little without having to solve their own problems, but learn even less when left to their own devices with no guidance at all. As such, maintaining an ethical relationship with communities and a process focus requires that educators attend to the pedagogical problem defining their role: how to enable students to discover problems and solutions with the communities most affected by them? Informed by this problem, tutors approach students with curiosity over the processes and silences in the project.

Text continued on p. 571

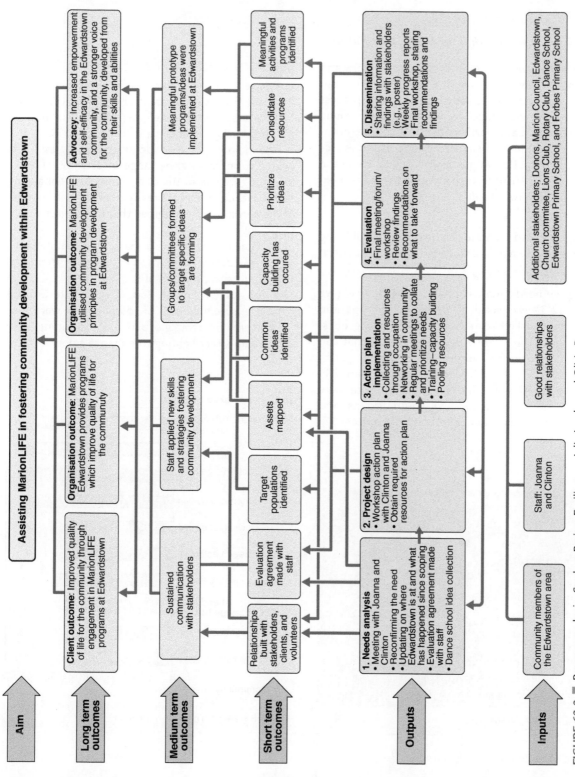

FIGURE 62-2 ■ Programme logic. Student Project Facilitators: Julia Jacobs and Olivia Bowman.

BOX 62-1

Case Study: Our Youth, Our Voice, Our Future

In partnership with the Port Augusta community and headspace, a National Youth Mental Health Foundation initiative, the students facilitated a process that actively encouraged a wide range of young people to share and participate in developing meaningful community engagement opportunities for young people in Port Augusta. Port Augusta is a rural town in South Australia with a population of approximately 15 000 to 20 000.

PROJECT AIM

To promote and increase the health and well-being of young people aged 12 to 25 years in Port Augusta.

NEED IDENTIFICATION AND CONFIRMATION

During the needs analysis phase, a 'needs tree' (see Figure 62-3) was used at multiple locations and people were asked to respond the following question: 'We all think Port Augusta is great. What can we do to make this community better for young people aged 12 to 25 years?' Students had 181 responses to this activity. The collated data were then shared with established youth groups and youth-related events to determine further ideas.

DEVELOPING THE ACTION PLAN

The project action plan was determined by analysing the data from the needs analysis in collaboration with headspace to determine what was feasible within the project timeline.

The majority of needs identified (see Figure 62-4) related to increasing the range of activities suitable for young people in the community and enhancing safety. Headspace was already addressing a number of the needs, so it was agreed that the project would focus on:

- Implementation of a basic car maintenance and safety workshop, as car usage is an important aspect of rural life
- Advocacy role with Port Augusta City Council to ensure the needs of young people were considered in strategic planning, including adequate street lighting to enhance safety

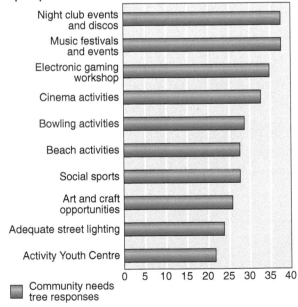

Top 10 prioritized needs

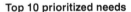

FIGURE 62-4 ■ Top 10 prioritized needs.

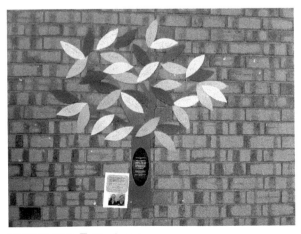

FIGURE 62-3 ■ Needs tree.

BOX 62-1

Case Study: Our Youth, Our Voice, Our Future—cont'd

- Development of a resource folder and associated capacity building of headspace Youth Crew (hYC), an existing working group, to ensure sustainability and continuing development upon conclusion of the project
- Implementation of an outdoor cinema event, with hYC evidencing their event management skill development

IMPLEMENTATION OF ACTION PLAN

In partnership with hYC, the occupational therapy students implemented the project. Informal training and capacity-building opportunities were developed in partnership with hYC members including the establishment of processes for future work. For example, tools to facilitate the effectiveness of future meetings and event planning were trialed, and those proven to be effective were developed into an electronic resource folder for ongoing use.

The basic car maintenance and safety workshop provided an opportunity to evidence the project's responsiveness to community feedback and assisted in the development of trust and rapport. The workshop also allowed young people to develop skills and engage with community members. The workshop involved qualified mechanics from two local providers as well as a community constable (police community support officer). The success of the workshop allowed for further workshops to be scheduled and run in conjunction with the hYC.

The presentation to Port Augusta City Council Strategic Planning Meeting played an important advocacy role. The students provided the Council with a report outlining the project and associated outcomes, and highlighted the importance of a participatory needs analysis in discovering the unmet needs of young people in Port Augusta. Being a formal meeting, meant that the report was formally acknowledged and lodged with the Council.

The Outdoor Cinema Event was undertaken in partnership with headspace Port Augusta and OPAL, a government-funded initiative focused on supporting everyone in the community to eat well and be active. The event attracted over 650 participants. OPAL screened a short film promoting active engagement in outdoor environments highlighting opportunities in the Port Augusta area and also provided free fruit, and headspace Port Augusta had stalls promoting mental health and their services. hYC were closely involved in all aspects of the event to increase their skills and ability to manage future events. Due to the positive response to this event, Port Augusta Council confirmed funding for two further events for 2014.

KEY LESSONS LEARNT

- Tap into existing groups, processes and events, rather than create new or duplicate what exists. This builds on existing strengths within the community, fosters greater community engagement, and promotes capacity building, in keeping with the Ottawa Charter (WHO, 1986).
- Create community ownership and control through partnership and shared decision making. The time and thought involved in determining the project name evidenced the level of ownership as did the time, effort, and pride demonstrated by hYC in promoting and successfully running the various events and activities.
- Engage other local organizations and community members to generate interest, mobilize resources, and actively engage the broader community. Allow community members to be experts of their community and recognize their expertise by involving them, acting on their knowledge, and acknowledging their contribution.

ANNA COOTE AND TAMRA EARDLEY-HARRIS

BOX 62-2

Case Study: MarionLIFE

In partnership with MarionLIFE Community Services and the Edwardstown Community Church, this project sought to foster community development within the Edwardstown community. The project involved a participatory needs analysis to discover the assets and opportunities within to strengthen the sense of community connectedness and support. MarionLIFE is a not-for-profit community organization that provides care and support to vulnerable and at-risk individuals and families. Edwardstown is a suburb of Adelaide located 6 kilometres from the city centre. The Australian Bureau of Statistics (2012) indicates that 27% of Edwardstown residents live alone, which is two times higher than the statistics of the local government area.

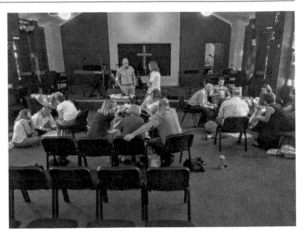

FIGURE 62-5 ■ Capacity-building workshop.

PROJECT AIM

To help facilitate MarionLIFE in fostering community development within Edwardstown.

NEED CONFIRMATION

Although this project was a community needs analysis, there was still a need to define the focus. Data from a Community Development Forum, which included representatives from MarionLIFE, EEC, and local service clubs, indicated a lack of social connectedness in the community and this became the focus of the needs analysis.

PROJECT PLAN

The project plan was to explore ways to facilitate community connectedness and determine community assets that could be mobilized to foster a stronger, thriving community. An asset-based community development (ABCD) approach (Cunningham and Mathie, 2002) was utilized. The capacity and knowledge of key stakeholders within each of the partner organizations around ABCD was built throughout all aspects of the project to facilitate community connectedness, empowerment, and ownership. Some examples of how this was achieved included:

- Inviting key stakeholders to an ABCD training day.
- Using and discussing ABCD at all workshops.
- Supporting and participating in community development forums that involved members of

    local service clubs as well as partner organizations.
- Development of a neighbourhood storybook to showcase positive connection stories.
- Developing capacity of church leaders to ask 'powerful questions' to generate creative insights and promote change (Vogt et al., 2003) (see Figure 62-5).
- Using the *world café* concept (Brown and Isaacs, 2005) with church leaders to engage in the community, using the powerful questioning skills and developing a dialogue about the community's future.

KEY OUTCOMES

The community has expressed the need for a number of large-scale environmental improvements related to parks and upgrading of some council facilities, which were beyond the capacity of MarionLIFE and Edwardstown Community Church. However, the small-scale community and recreation groups, community events, and get-to-know-your-neighbour events were also identified and feasible actions. Developing a thriving and connected community requires ongoing work and capacity building of key stakeholders for it to become sustainable. Therefore, a key outcome was the enhanced capacity of informal community leaders to promote and facilitate meaningful community engagement strategies.

OLIVIA BOWMAN AND JULIA JACOB

TABLE 62-3 Reframing the Issue		
Agency Pitch	**Reframed**	**Project Focus/Objectives**
Need for a report that outlined needs and issues of young people in specific rural area, including demographic trends that could be used to inform service delivery and support funding applications	To focus on community engagement and capacity building of young people in community and connect with the agency	Shifted from a process of finding information to actively involving young people in meaningful and desired activities that increased engagement with agency and facilitated empowerment
Develop an activity resource to help residents of an aged care facility lead a healthier life	Develop a process that enabled residents to facilitate sustainable health-promoting outcomes	Shifted from resources for people to a system including establishment of a residents' committee, staff education, and issue/options tree resource

We might ask whose voice is missing or being invalidated in the process, and why do some voices have more power? We ask students to reflect on why they are being persuaded down one path over another and whose needs that ultimately serves. We examine where alternative perspectives might exist and advise students that we will be suspicious of any project that does not encounter conflict or contest, as this usually testifies to superficial engagement.

In addition to the common problems stated above, educators can also experience additional challenges including:

- Balancing didacticism with scaffolding: some students do not fully comprehend the effects and processes of their project until 7 weeks into their 9-week placement, as outcomes can be slow and hard to see. Forcing this understanding beforehand undermines the learning. However, this does not permit laissez-faire supervision, as learning outcomes are not inevitable and require vigilant and attentive monitoring of student progress, careful self-reflection, and peer support.
- Resisting the desire to 'save' students from distress: for students who perceive learning as a transaction in which technical knowledge is traded, the demand to undertake embodied learning by doing, struggling, and achieving can be distressing. This distress can affect educators, and reflection is required to prevent the desire to 'save' the student.
- Managing conflict between agencies, colleagues, and peers in relation to the way the problem is understood and whose voices should be heard: as

agencies hold a great deal of power over access to communities, students must often advocate for the need to involve people who might otherwise be perceived as peripheral or inexpert. Students can sometimes become unfairly wedged between agency perspectives and course demands for maximal participation, and require support and careful management to achieve a reasonable outcome.

- Determining when to intervene directly with the agency when students are struggling: sometimes student struggles pertain to poor direction or clarity from the agency. It is important to assist students to manage this rather than step in and undermine their role as project managers.

Discomfort, pedagogy, and ethics are all part of the teaching process. Enabling others to define and solve their own problems requires educators to actively resist knowing too soon, which can be uncomfortable. When students bring problems to supervision, educators must establish distance 'from the demand they make upon us to provide answers not questions' (Rabinow and Rose, 2003, p. 21). It can feel vulnerable and fragile to not be in control of the answers, but it is necessary if project outcomes are to be sustainable and students are to build their own capacities. That is, the ethical response to student problems is to teach in a way that subordinates the educators' own certainties and self-assurances to the learning of the student and the interests of the community. This could be described as an ethics of discomfort (Foucault, 1979/2007) and regarded as crucial to effective education.

Connecting With Occupation

There are many disciplines that work from a primary health perspective and apply community development principles to their practice. However, each discipline has a unique lens or focus through which they interpret and act. PCP requires students to use their occupational lens and whilst they may feel comfortable using occupation-based interventions with individuals or in small groups, identifying how to use occupation within a community can be challenging. Tutors play a key role in helping students develop a deeper appreciation and confidence in the power of occupation as a process, a means or an end outcome within projects.

Developing their ability to articulate the rationale behind the use of occupation is part of the process of building rapport and trust with communities and promoting participation and it can be an unexpected learning outcome for many students. It is the students' experience of these moments that delivers the gestalt experience or 'aha' moment of realization, when they become strong advocates of occupation and their profession. Several authors have identified how the autonomous learning and agency of placements, such as this, result in the development of an authentic professional identity in which occupation plays a central role (Bosser et al., 1997; Clarke et al., 2014; Fieldhouse and Fedden, 2009; Thew et al., 2011). Moreover, students need to effectively communicate the purpose of the occupation-based activity across disciplines and agencies, and it has been found to assist in the development of interprofessional skills (Gilbert Hunt, 2007). There is evidence to indicate that collaborative and interprofessional practice such as this is essential for effective community work and allows for a more in-depth appreciation of one's own profession (Gum et al., 2013).

CONCLUSION

PCP is a student project placement experience that seeks to turn the rhetoric of community development into reality. It is a continually evolving and dynamic project, the power and flexibility of which are located in the strong focus on process that allows for and anticipates changing community health contexts and evolving practice needs. It is essential for the profession to have the tools to meet not only the increasing complexity of health issues, including the influences of social determinants, but also the increasing need to work across all sectors and within changes to funding allocations and processes. PCP is at the forefront of building occupational therapy graduate capacity to understand, analyse, and determine how best to address an issue with the resources available and through engaging the strengths and capacity of the community. However, we currently lack extensive research evidence to demonstrate the role of occupation in this process. Moreover, our practice models require further development to extricate the potency of occupation in achieving community outcomes. Turning community development into reality is a challenging undertaking, but it has been made possible by harnessing changing local conditions, changes in global health governance, existing tools and models to scaffold student learning and support for educators to manage the inevitable discomfort of supervision, amid the pressures of health systems and professional values.

REFERENCES

Australian Bureau of Statistics, 2012. 2011 Census of Population and Housing: Basic Community Profile Edwardstown S SC40173 2.3 sq Kms, cat no. 2001.0. ABS, Canberra.

Baum, F., 2008. The new public health: an Australian perspective, third ed. Oxford University Press, South Melbourne, Australia.

Bossers, A., Cook, J., Polatajko, H., Laine, C., 1997. Understanding the role-emerging fieldwork placement. Can. J. Occup. Ther. 64 (1), 70–81.

Brown, J., Isaacs, D., 2005. The World Café community. Berrett-Koehler Publishers Inc, San Francisco, CA.

Clarke, C., Martin, M., Sadlo, G., de-Visser, R., 2014. The development of an authentic professional identity on role-emerging placements. Br. J. Occup. Ther. 77 (5), 222–229.

Cunningham, G., Mathie, A., 2002. Assets-Based Community Development: An Overview. Coady International Institute, Thailand.

Fieldhouse, J., Fedden, T., 2009. Exploring the learning process on a role-emerging practice placement: a qualitative study. Br. J. Occup. Ther. 72 (7), 302–307.

Foucault, M., 2007. For an ethics of discomfort (Hochroth, L., Trans.). In: Lotringer, S. (Ed.), The Politics of Truth. Semiotext(e), Los Angeles, pp. 121–127.

Gilbert Hunt, S., 2006. A practice placement education model based upon a primary health care perspective used in South Australia. Br. J. Occup. Ther. 69 (2), 81–85.

Gilbert Hunt, S., 2007. Participatory community practice: developing interprofessional skills. Focus Health Professionals Educ. 8 (3), 71–78.

Gum, L.F., Richards, J.N., Walters, L., Forgan, J., Lopriore, M., Nobes, C., 2013. Immersing undergraduates into an interprofessional longitudinal rural placement. Rural Remote Health 13 (1), 2271. Available from: <http://www.rrh.org.au> (accessed 25.09.14.).

Hammell, K., 2009. Sacred texts: a sceptical exploration of the assumptions underpinning theories of occupation. Can. J. Occup. Ther. 76 (6), 6–13.

Ife, J., 1995. Community development. Creating community alternatives-vision, analysis and practice. Longman Pty Ltd, South Melbourne, Australia.

Ishikawa, K., Loftus, J.H., 1990. Introduction to Quality Control. 3A Corporation, Tokyo, Japan.

Kaplan, S.A., Garrett, K.E., 2005. The use of logic models by community-based initiatives. Eval. Program Plan. 28 (2), 167–172.

Kickbush, I., Gleicher, D., 2012. Governance for health in the 21st century. World Health Organisation, Copenhagen.

Kirke, P., Layton, N., Sim, J., 2007. Informing fieldwork design: key elements to quality in fieldwork education for undergraduate occupational therapy students. Aust. Occup. Ther. J. 54 (Suppl. 1), 13–22.

Kronenberg, F., Pollard, N., Ramugondo, E., 2011. Introduction: courage to dance politics. In: Kronenberg, F., Pollard, N., Sakellariou, D. (Eds.), Occupational Therapies without Borders, vol. 2. Elsevier, Oxford, pp. 1–16.

Leclair, L.L., 2010. Re-examining concepts of occupation and occupation-based models: occupational therapy and community development. Can. J. Occup. Ther. 77 (1), 15–21.

Millar, A., Simeone, R.S., Carnevale, J.T., 2001. Logic models: a systems tool for performance management. Eval. Program Plan. 24 (1), 73–81.

Newman, L., Biedrzycki, K., Patterson, J., Baum, F., 2007. A rapid appraisal case study of South Australia's social inclusion initiative. A report prepared for the Social Exclusion Knowledge Network of the World Health Organisation's Commission on Social Determinants of Health by the Australian Health Inequities Program (Department of Public Health, Flinders University of South Australia) and the Social Inclusion Unit (Department of the Premier and Cabinet, Government of South Australia), Adelaide, Australia.

Rabinow, P., Rose, N., 2003. The essential Foucault: selections from the essential works of Foucault, 1954–1984. New Press, New York.

Saunders, D., 1998. Executive summary: PHC21 – everybody's business. Primary Health Care Conference, Almaty, Kazakhstan, 27–28 November 1998. World Health Organization, Geneva.

South Australian Health Commission, 1988. A Social Health Strategy for South Australia. South Australian Health Commission, Adelaide.

South Australian Health Commission, 1989. Policy and Primary Health Care. Adelaide, South Australian Health Commission, Adelaide.

Thew, M., Edwards, M., Baptiste, S., Molineux, M. (Eds.), 2011. Role Emerging Occupational Therapy, Maximizing Occupation Focused Practice. Wiley-Blackwell, Chichester, UK, pp. 149–155.

Thibeault, R., Herbert, M., 1997. A congruent model of health promotion in occupational therapy. Occup. Ther. Int. 4 (4), 271–293.

van Boxtell, C., van der Linden, J., Roelofs, E., Erkens, G., 2010. Collaborative concept mapping: provoking and supporting meaningful discourse. Theory Pract. 41 (1), 40–46.

Vogt, E.E., Brown, J., Issaacs, D., 2003. The Art of Powerful Questions: Catalysing Insight, Innovation and Action. Whole System Associated, Mill Valley, CA.

Williams, L., Labonte, R., 2003. Changing health determinants through community action: power, participation and policy. Health Promot. Int. 18 (1), 33–40.

World Federation of Occupational Therapy, 2002. Overview of the WFOT Minimum Standards for the Education of Occupational Therapists 2002, CD ROM. WFOT, Western Australia.

World Health Organization, 1984. The 8th Global Health Promotion Conference. World Health Organization, Geneva.

World Health Organization, 1986. The Ottawa Charter for health promotion. World Health Organization, Geneva.

63

READING, CRITICAL REFLECTION, AND COLLECTIVE KNOWLEDGE CONSTRUCTION AT BIBLIOGRAPHIC ATHENAEUMS

ANDREA FABIANA ALBINO ▪ MARÍA MARCELA BOTTINELLI ▪ FEDERICO JUAN MANUEL ZORZOLI ▪ MARIELA NABERGOI ▪ LILIANA PAGANIZZI ▪ LUIS ERNESTO CHAURA ▪ GUADALUPE DÏAZ USANDIVARAS ▪ NATALIA SPALLATO ▪ ANDREA VERÓNICA MEDINA ▪ MICAELA WALDMAN

CHAPTER OUTLINE

There is a need to create spaces for critical and reflective reading between professionals, teachers, and young graduates of occupational therapy; a need for spaces that could bring together students, teachers, and clinicians with different roles, for example, involvement in community and social health approaches, to generate a space for encounter with each other, so that participants can meet and share. Such a space could also allow the involved actors to build and strengthen bonds and networks. Every year since 2009, Bibliographic Athenaeums have been held in different settings in Argentina (universities, Chairs[1], civic associations, etc.), sharing reading and the spirit of creating a space for exchanging experiences in a horizontal

dialogue between the different actors in occupational therapy. In this chapter, we present Bibliographical Athenaeums and discuss their importance.

HOW DID BIBLIOGRAPHIC ATHENAEUMS BEGIN?

The first Bibliographic Athenaeum was held in 2009 in Buenos Aires as part of the celebrations for the 50th anniversary of occupational therapy in Argentina, following the creation of the National School of Occupational Therapy (ENTO), when occupational therapist Frank Kronenberg was invited to participate in the events, along with other colleagues from various national universities. The first proposal for the Athenaeums was suggested by the previous experiences of those involved in this idea, such as the experience of translating and distributing books and generating reading processes with students, with the aim of

---

[1]Chair (cátedra) denotes a specific subject area and the academics and students involved in it.

meeting authors in a two-way dialogue as an alternative to the one-way conference format[2]. Another relevant experience was the contribution of one member to the translation of some chapters for the Spanish edition of *Occupational Therapy without Borders* in 2006. Other experiences involved participation in personal and virtual meetings and dialogues held at different professional congresses and exchanges between occupational therapy teachers and writers from different countries, together with national processes developing in the profession. All these experiences contributed to the idea of getting to know about, explore, and debate the publication of *Occupational Therapy without Borders* (Kronenberg et al., 2006).

The space for the first of the Athenaeum meetings was made available by the research and education team of the Institute of Rehabilitation Sciences and Movement of the National University of San Martín (ICRM-UNSaM)[3]. Research methodology and statistics students and their teachers from the occupational therapy programme at the University of Buenos Aires also participated. Occupational therapy teaching teams at various universities were invited to address the issues of knowledge production and practices with different social and community perspectives, and to include opportunities for reading and reflection on the different chapters in the book within their classes. This was in preparation for a day event called '*Encuentros de cátedra*' (meetings with the Chair) where the main idea was to share and develop dialogues about these experiences in meetings, held with different invited participants, including one of the editors of the book.

---

[2]That is, Medeiros, M.H., 2003. Occupational Therapy: an epistemological and social approach; Medeiros, M.H., 2008., Terapia Ocupacional. Un enfoque epistemológico y social. Universidad Nacional del Litoral, Santa Fe, Argentina; Nabergoi, M., Benassi, J., Yujnovsky, N. (Trans., Eds.), Colaboration between different chairs of Occupational Therapy Programmes: Metodología de la Investigación (Universidad Nacional de San Martín), Metodología de la Investigación y Estadística (Universidad de Buenos Aires), Práctica Profesional IV y Estética I (Universidad Nacional del Litoral).

[3]Research area of ICRM-UNSaM, Research Proyect R003 'Revisión Histórica de la Creación de la ENTO/UNSAM. Medio Siglo de Crecimiento' and Research Methodology, Final Work Design and Statistics Chairs (Bottinelli – Nabergoi).

WHAT IS A BIBLIOGRAPHIC ATHENAEUM?

The Bibliographic Athenaeum is a pedagogical space that promotes thoughtful and critical reflection on the practices and foundations of occupational therapy and reflective readings of *Occupational Therapy without Borders* and other critical readings in occupational therapy. It brings together students, teachers, occupational therapists, and healthcare professionals with social and community health perspectives, different backgrounds and interests. The focus is in participation in alternative educational practices that allow dialogue and the exchange of ideas, different experiences, and ways of working. Such educational practices can enable training and continuous learning from the horizontal dialogue between different actors and the construction of knowledge with others.

A working group was formed to organize and convene the readings. This group discussed and planned the dynamics of the activity, the number of meetings, their length, the topics covered, suggested which articles, books, and book chapters would be relevant and developed a proposal for a series of three or four meetings.

Each meeting includes the presentation of the theme, a description of the proposed texts for shared reading in small groups (these are formed at the time according to the interest of each participant in the subject), discussion and exchanges on the reading and its connections with the experience of practice in Argentina, with a final closing plenary. These encounters are organized independently from each other, so that participants can attend all of them or go to individual meetings; each is independent in its conception from the rest, since different chapters are worked on in each event. However, there is some focus on cross-cutting themes and the dynamics of the athenaeums allow participants the process of constructing learning throughout the various meetings.

As part of the tools designed to support the process, guiding questions are made available to facilitate the contextualization of chapters and practices. Some of these questions are given below:

• In what context was the chapter written?
• What practices are described and/or proposed?
• What are its actors and/or stakeholders?

- What are the theoretical foundations and concepts that are used?
- How is occupational therapy defined/considered in the chapter?
- What is the role of occupational therapists?
- What aspects caught your attention in the chapter? Why?
- What is the relationship between what you read and professional practices in our country?
- Do you know how similar problems are addressed in our country?
- From your personal/professional perspective, what are the contributions that this chapter gives to your knowledge and perspective on occupational therapy so far? Can you give examples?
- What is new for you? What questions did it open up?

The horizontal form of dialogue and collective contributions promote reflective thinking and the ability to problematize current practices and foundations, as well as allowing dialogue on experiences in different places of the world to be connected with local contexts.

Through these exchanges, participants are enabled to understand different practices, cultural similarities and differences, and reflect on the phenomena of social vulnerability at their own pace. Sharing these different outcomes can extend the horizon and enrich the work of occupational therapy from a perspective that promotes the joint construction of new strategies.

This structure invites participants to meet new people, to discuss and share their interests, which in turn allows the development of new questions and foundations for practice. As there are no set rules, the activities around reading stimulate people to organize the distribution of tasks and functions for the shared lectures in a democratic way, including note-taking, pregroup and postgroup debate, the allocation of work time, the selection of reading spaces, and the group definition of the presentation to others of the thematic and process of the readings, alongside the shared cultural aspects of mate[4] and sharing food. Some of the participants' comments are shared in Box 63-1.

---

[4]Hot-water infusion of yerba mate leaves, characteristic of some countries in Latin America. Culturally, this infusion is for collective consumption and can be used any time of the day.

THE BIBLIOGRAPHIC ATHENAEUM OVER THE YEARS

Over time, through colleagues' regular participation and the maintenance of this activity, the Bibliographic Athenaeum participants have been critically rethinking its content to propose modifications. Thus, every year the Bibliographic Athenaeum develops different approaches to the workshop dynamics, the framework, or the meeting space.

For example, during the last meeting of the first year, a presentation was made about some of the innovative concepts in the profession: occupational apartheid, occupational justice, occupational injustice, and political activities of daily living among others. There was a broad debate on these terms, which included their similarities and differences from our current local context and the potential for their application.

In the following year, one of the meetings took place within the framework of a civil association called Atuel. This organization delivers clinical care approaches for people who face problems with drugs or alcohol, and other social issues. Until then, the athenaeum had been mainly positioned within universities, but now it was taking place in the practice base. As an outcome of some members' involvement in the World Federation of Occupational Therapists Congress in Santiago de Chile in 2010, we discussed the organization of the Second Athenaeum with different representatives of national and Latin American associations, participants and exhibitors at the World Congress, and authors of occupational therapy books. Many of them expressed their desire to participate and understand the working of the athenaeum, but geographic distances, time, and different agendas made it very difficult for them to assist at that time. The possibility of generating audiovisual material was therefore considered. This took the form of sharing some personal experiences, knowledge, and words on what *Occupational Therapy without Borders* meant for each of them and how they came to it. Among those with whom we talked, some authors from different chapters of the book agreed to say a few words to share with participants of the Bibliographic Athenaeums. Elelwani Ramugondo (South Africa) said:

What I appreciate of Occupational Therapy Without Borders *continues to grow, it is not a static*

BOX 63-1

SOME EXAMPLES OF FEEDBACK FROM PARTICIPANTS IN BIBLIOGRAPHIC ATHENAEUMS

'This space offers an alternative position to formal teaching, where the theoretical approach (hard, traditional, institutional) seems to offer fewer opportunities to students than these spaces of reading, discussion, and horizontal exchange.'

'I didn't know about community-based OT intervention, and by participating in the Athenaeum I could think about the profession from another point of view, and it has raised my interest to continue learning more about this proposal.'

'The different chapters have enabled us to open various reflective, critical, and technical theoretical spaces. It has been a pleasure to re-encounter methodologies of group work and the instrumentation or use of activities that are reevaluated and updated in the different experiences presented in the book.'

'The contexts trigger action, or so they should. Activity should be defined from the actors and contexts, not from theory. Activity is not good by itself, it can [either] facilitate or alienate. The experience and activity are not transferable; they are re-signified in different contexts: for example, disabling experience: what dimensions of the context create that experience? It is essential to ensure that the practice of occupational therapy gives power to the people instead of oppressing them. Something in relation to these weaving plots and concepts that are hidden behind the titles.'

'What emerged as topics in several meetings were a focus on the areas of formal education, the dynamics of these spaces and how many visions leave aside places like this, to meet for reading, share, learn and that are very interesting and profitable.'

'This is an initiative to replicate in many places. To reflect on our practices and our fundamentals, and problematize about them is essential. I think this workshop invites us to do so, to question what appears to be evident, natural, obvious.'

'I found the community perspective through the discipline valuable, regardless of the area of professional practice or population with which we work. Not being just a scenario, it becomes a conception of the discipline that involves acting on an ethical basis, beyond merely being a health practice. The ethical basis is a prerequisite for the implementation and development of occupational therapy, and this implies an academic review.'

'I like this space because I [used to] feel stagnant; it has been a long time since I last did anything that has to do with these kinds of exchanges that make me feel enriched. Besides the book and its chapters, I was interested in connecting with colleagues and the proposed revision of the practice of occupational therapy.'

---

destination but the possibilities that open by collective movements…it was only after OT Without Borders and being invited to write in the book that I started gaining confidence over doing what I knew was right and what the people that I worked with confirmed to be the right thing to do in that time.

Alejandro Guajardo (Chile) shared:

I think Occupational Therapy Without Borders is a movement within the Institution of Occupational Therapy which questions its foundations and practices, and I think this is actually what we need to do. It is a movement that also raises a different view of people, of their problems, their relationship to historical contexts, and to their objective, real, material, structural needs. And it also calls for an Occupational Therapy that is creating and reinventing itself in every moment. It is not

about a static and fixed outlook but about an occupational therapy that creates itself from its own daily practices.

Another year, the selection of chapters for reading was organized around different themes suggested by the organization of the book, and the joint reading of the Prologue of the second book, *Occupational Therapy without Borders, Volume 2: Towards an Ecology of Occupation Based Practices* (Kronenberg et al., 2011), was proposed. On another occasion, the spirit of sharing experience through the dynamics of activity was conveyed in a peripatetic proposal of inviting others to generate meetings in their own bases, in their places of practice. Thus, every meeting was held in a different place, including national universities, the Argentina Association of Occupational Therapists, and civil and healthcare associations. We included reading the Preface and Introduction of the book *A Political Practice of Occupational Therapy* (Pollard et al, 2008, not yet translated into Spanish).

In different meetings, we had the opportunity to personally meet colleagues from different parts of our country as well as from other countries, and to share with them the dynamics of the athenaeum; some of them had taken part in the writing of the publications of *Occupational Therapy without Borders*, such as Daniela Albuquerque and Frank Kronenberg, as well as most of the Argentinian coauthors.

During this process, which developed over 6 consecutive years of Bibliographic Athenaeums, new members joined. The group now includes graduates, teachers, scholars, and students with different insertions in the profession. These new members generate other spaces for exchanging of experiences, theory, and practice in a horizontal dialogue between the different actors in addition to the athenaeum. The athenaeum space has also brought together students, academics, professionals in our country and the region (Chile, Peru, and Colombia), delegates from Argentina to the World Federation of Occupational Therapists and the Latin American Confederation of Occupational Therapists (CLATO).

Since 2010, the athenaeum has been replicated in different places. For 3 consecutive years, various faculties at Universidad Nacional del Litoral organized reading meetings, incorporating Bibliographic Athenaeums, with the participation of teachers and students of occupational therapy. We wrote to colleagues in the Universities of Tucuman and Mar del Plata who were interested in replicating the experience as well, and colleagues from neighboring countries (Brazil, Chile, and Uruguay) asked us for advice about the organization. The experience was also held at faculties of different universities and professional practice venues. The first was organized as a preparation for an event called '*Encuentros de cátedra*', organized by the Chair of Research Methodology at the University Buenos Aires. Different actors participated, including some meeting for critical and shared reading with athenaeum dynamics, such as the Chair of Occupational Dynamics in the Community of the National University of San Martín, Occupational Therapy Residency (postgraduate training) of the Government of Buenos Aires City, among others. The athenaeum travelled to different faculties in the different national universities through teachers who, having participated in previous events, wanted to share this experience with their students. Thus, these meetings took place with the support of the chairs of the National University of San Martin, Quilmes National University, and the University of Buenos Aires.

We also proposed to increase the awareness of these experiences through occupational therapy educators, in spaces organized by students, and through participation and presentation at local, regional, national, and international professional and scientific-academic spaces. These activities have had very good reception from participants and we received inquiries about how to replicate these spaces in different contexts.

FINAL COMMENTS

Contemporary ideas in occupational therapy invite the returning to, rebuilding, and invention of concepts and interventions according to the social context in which we live together. *Occupational Therapy without Borders* is a publication that together with other critical readings helps us all learn about experiences from different countries and areas; sharing similar questions drives us to reflect on a widened approach to occupational therapy.

The Bibliographic Athenaeum is an activity that enriches us as participants while allowing the group to multiply, diversify, and weave together our collective knowledge. Through dialogue between the experiences proposed in publications, the knowledge of our own realities, interventions, cultures and the ability to find and create spaces for exchanging views between colleagues, we affirm our desire to build new occupational therapies where we feel represented and included, and where we can be active participants in their construction.

REFERENCES

Kronenberg, F., Pollard, N., Sakellariou, D., (Eds.), 2011. Occupational Therapies without Borders, vol. 2: Towards an Ecology of Occupation-Based Practice. Elsevier, Oxford.

Kronenberg, F., Simo Algado, S., Pollard, N., (Eds.), 2006. Terapia Ocupacional sin Fronteras. Aprendiendo del Espíritu de Supervivientes. Médica Panamericana, Madrid.

Pollard, N., Sakellariou, D., Kronenberg, F. (Eds.), 2008. A Political Practice of Occupational Therapy. Elsevier, Oxford.

64

THE EVOLUTION OF OCCUPATIONAL THERAPY AS A PROFESSION IN THE PEOPLE'S REPUBLIC OF CHINA

KIT SINCLAIR ■ MENGAN CAO

CHAPTER OUTLINE

Occupational therapy is gaining greater recognition in the People's Republic of China, with increased understanding of rehabilitation services. The concepts of rehabilitation now extend far beyond the technical skills of physical medicine, massage, and electrotherapy which have traditionally been considered part of rehabilitation medicine in the People's Republic of China. With the largest population in the world, health issues have become a focus of the government, particularly in relation to its ageing population, the country's industrialization, and rapid economic growth. There has also been an increased social awareness regarding access to health and requirements for quality of care.

The aim of this chapter is to discuss the development of occupational therapy in the People's Republic of China. We will discuss the introduction of rehabilitation and its impact on the development of this new profession. We will also describe the current occupational therapy practice, with reference to the cultural adaptation of internationally held and accepted concepts, using case examples of the role of pioneers in developing occupational therapy within the healthcare system. With awareness of the interdependence of service development and education, we will also discuss the existing education system for occupational therapists, highlighting some of the challenges and opportunities for occupational therapy development.

BEGINNINGS OF REHABILITATION

Since the establishment of the People's Republic of China in 1949, the National Congress has agreed on consecutive 5-year plans to include social and economic initiatives. Each subsequent 5-year plan includes an aspect on healthcare. Starting in the 1950s, for example, Traditional Chinese Medicine precepts were standardized in the People's Republic, including attempts to integrate them with Western notions of anatomy and pathology. Some of the basic principles of Traditional Chinese Medicine include a belief in a balance between movement/activity and rest as key to functional fitness. The traditional approach to functional rehabilitation incorporates Tai Chi (internal martial art form) and Qigong (relaxation and meditation). It incorporates dietary therapy, acupuncture, Tui Na (massage), and Kung Fu (therapeutic exercises). In relation to the health system, which had always had a strong Traditional Chinese Medicine influence, connections with Russia supported the running of three 1-year education programmes (1955–1958) for doctors, introducing physical modalities for rehabilitation into the hospital system including, for example, magnetic therapy and electrotherapy. These doctors from all around China took the ideas home to implement in their own newly developed local hospital departments. Rehabilitation medicine was born and, supported by the government, grew and spread.

CHANGING CONCEPTS OF REHABILITATION

Pufang Deng, son of past Chinese leader Xiaoping Deng, sustained a spinal cord injury during the Cultural Revolution in 1968. He was sent to Canada for rehabilitation in the early 1980s. Experiencing the great benefits of rehabilitation, on his return he led the development of the Chinese Disabled Persons Federation, which became a quasi-governmental organization. This organization started many services for people with disabilities including rural clinics, which opened avenues for modern-day rehabilitation.

Modern rehabilitation medicine subsequently became established in China drawing on Western contemporary methods of assessment and training for function [see Box 64-1 for an overview of the development of rehabilitation medicine and occupational therapy]. Consistent with the time of the introduction/expansion of rehabilitation ideas around the world, Chinese doctors visited Canada and the United States,

---

BOX 64-1
EVOLUTION OF REHABILITATION AND OCCUPATIONAL THERAPY FROM 1983 TO 2016

1983 Chinese Association of Rehabilitation Medicine (CARM) is founded.

1988 Twenty-three colleges offer rehabilitation medicine courses.

1989 WHO/Hong Kong Society for Rehabilitation 11-month course on rehabilitation for clinical doctors.

1995 CARM Committee on Rehabilitation Therapy is established.

2001 Chinese Rehabilitation Research Centre (CRRC) and Capital Medical University 4-year occupational therapy bachelor 2 + 2 programme commences in Beijing.

2005 White Paper by CARM on occupational therapy/physiotherapy education.

2006 Capital Medical University and CRRC's 4-year occupational therapy education programme gain WFOT approval.

2007 Expansion of rehabilitation therapy education to 47 universities in 18 provinces (21 Western-style and 12 Traditional Chinese Medicine).

2009 CARM survey of rehabilitation therapy education programmes.

2010 There are 3288 rehabilitation institutions (general hospitals with rehab department) with 12 523 rehabilitation therapists to serve a population of over 1.2 billion population.

2011 Kunming Medical University (KMU) B.Sc. in Occupational Therapy in Kunming, Yunnan, gains WFOT approval.

2013 Physiotherapy and Occupational Therapy National Education Guidelines published (Li, 2013).

2014 Sichuan University B.Sc. in Occupational Therapy in Chengdu, Sichuan, gains WFOT approval.

2014 Sichuan University commences a master's entry-level occupational therapy course at the Institute of Disaster Management and Reconstruction in Chengdu, in collaboration with Hong Kong Polytechnic University.

2016 Fujian University of Traditional Chinese Medicine B.Sc. in Occupational Therapy and Shanghai University of Traditional Chinese Medicine B.Sc. in Occupational Therapy gain WFOT approval.

and brought Western rehabilitation scholars to China. Specialist courses were run in physiotherapy, occupational therapy, and speech therapy techniques (Zhuo, 2013).

In 1989, the Ministry of Public Health (renamed in 2013 as the National Health and Family Planning Commission of the People's Republic of China) released a policy document on 'Management of hospitals at different levels', instructing every level 3 (higher grade) general hospital at the city and provincial level to set up departments of rehabilitation medicine and offer essential inpatient and outpatient services in rehabilitation to include physiotherapy, occupational therapy, and speech therapy. A room for each service was designated. Level 2 (intermediate) general hospitals had to include at least outpatient rehabilitation medicine. Occupational therapy at the time consisted primarily of activities of daily living training, upper extremity training, and woodwork activities (Hu, 2012).

With a pay-for-service hospital system, the importance and benefits of occupational therapy were gradually recognized with increased patient demand in the late 1990s. The demand was shown by the willingness of patients to pay for the service by cash or through insurance. Some hospitals expanded occupational therapy services as part of physical medicine in such areas as cognitive training for patients with neurological conditions (not covered by insurance), prosthetics and orthotics, and activities of daily living assessment and training.

As the understanding of rehabilitation and specifically of occupational therapy increased globally, professionals in rehabilitation sciences brought more ideas to China, courses were expanded, and continuing education became a way of extending therapists' understanding and skills. A group of dedicated Hong Kong occupational therapists were instrumental in this process by offering workshops and conference/lectures at both hospital and university level through an organization called the Hong Kong Institute of Occupational Therapy.

THE CURRENT OCCUPATIONAL THERAPY SITUATION

Without a national association or separate national occupational therapy registration, it is difficult to esti-

mate the number of practising occupational therapists in the People's Republic of China. In 2014, there was an undocumented estimate of about 1000 occupational therapists. Data from 2009 shows that on average there were only 1.03 rehabilitation therapists per 100 000 people in the country, whereas the international standard on the therapist to client ratio is 50 : 100 000 (Ren et al., 2014). Rehabilitation therapists are trained to cover physiotherapy, occupational therapy, and speech therapy, though they primarily provide physiotherapy.

At the time of this writing (October 2015), the majority of occupational therapists work in hospital settings with adult clients who have major physical dysfunctions, such as stroke, spinal cord injury, or traumatic brain injury. Many occupational therapists understand upper limb function training and activities of daily living training as their main role. Traditionally, clients with mental health issues are not seen by rehabilitation therapists, and mental health was not included in the 2013 national occupational therapy education guidelines (Li, 2013), indicating a lack of readiness for development of that service area. Occupational therapists prefer working in general hospital settings because the bigger hospitals provide a better reputation, better salaries, better promotion opportunities, and better training opportunities. However, public hospitals in the People's Republic of China are partially self-financed, and staff rely on the hospital income for their salary (i.e., working with more clients will increase the bonuses staff receive). In many hospitals, the occupational therapy service has not offered as good financial contribution to the rehabilitation department as other services, such as massage and electrotherapy, creating friction among members. This has a few underlying reasons. One major concern is the physiatrists' lack of initiative to promote occupational therapy to clients and other health professionals, leading to a lack of occupational therapy referrals. Another underlying reason is that some professionals were initially working in other rehabilitation positions before being selected by their directors to act as occupational therapists in the team. Often, these professionals have not received comprehensive occupational therapy training and only have attended intensive short courses. They seem to be satisfied with doing what they are familiar with, which is physiotherapy. There are cases, however, such as the

Guangdong Work Injury Centre, noted below, where occupational therapy services provide the top financial contribution to the centre.

WORK INJURY REHABILITATION – A RECOGNIZED NEED LED TO MAJOR SERVICE DEVELOPMENT

According to national statistics, there are over 1 million people affected by work-related injuries every year in the People's Republic. Work Injury Insurance and policies developed in 2004 have supported the development of this emerging professional area (China.org.cn, 2011).

Work Injury Rehabilitation in Guangdong Province is a good example of the development of an occupational therapy service to meet a specific community need. In Guangdong Province, which has a great number of factories, work injury rehabilitation is provided at a specially designed rehabilitation hospital. In recent years, an average of 150 000 workers have been affected by work injuries each year and 80% of these are reported to be migrant workers from other provinces. In Guangdong, work injury rehabilitation services are categorized into medical rehabilitation, vocational rehabilitation and social rehabilitation, and assistive device provision and training. The major role of the occupational therapists in this area of practice has been physical and vocation rehabilitation. The vocational rehabilitation has developed quickly. For example, in 2006 only 182 people received vocational rehabilitation services, while in 2012 1924 people participated in a vocational rehabilitation programme in Gongdong Work Injury Rehabilitation Center. According to the statistics of this rehabilitation centre, about 80% of the injured workers who participated in vocational rehabilitation programmes returned to work in 2012, but there is still an unmet need for vocational rehabilitation and social rehabilitation (Lu, 2013).

Occupational therapy pioneer Kuicheng Li has worked as an occupational therapist in the work injury rehabilitation field for the last 14 years and is Head of the Occupational Therapy Department at the Guangdong Provincial Work Injury Rehabilitation Hospital. He completed the Diploma in Rehabilitation Medicine in Tianjin Medical University and went on to gain his Bachelor's Degree of Clinical Medicine in Sun Yat-sen University in 2005 and a Master's Degree of Rehabilitation Science at the Hong Kong Polytechnic University in 2009. He worked as a rehabilitation therapist for several years before settling into occupational therapy. This varied background is typical of a number of occupational therapists. He notes that his department has 43 workstations built to simulate environments for various professions, such as drivers, waiters, electricians, and cooks, where patients are given practical training daily to cope with their injuries. Programmes are designed to meet workers' needs. For example, if the patient is a postman, they will add more lifting, pushing, and pulling exercises to his training. Workers often return to companies for trials, with regular evaluations to ensure they are progressing well, while the centre will also carry out home modifications for patients with long-term mobility problems. Patients are followed up every 6 months. Roughly 78% of the department's patients have returned to work in the past 3 years. To replicate this success around the country, rehabilitation staff members now provide technical support and training to over 300 settings in other cities and provinces around the country. Li is involved with research which focuses on specific rehabilitation to meet the growing demand of injured workers, as well as assisting industries to implement safe practice and injury prevention practices.

HOSPITAL-BASED ADULT PHYSICAL REHABILITATION

Occupational therapy pioneer Yanning Yan came to occupational therapy from rehabilitation nursing in 1995. Having studied Japanese, she was able to go to Fukuoka in Japan for 8 months to study and undertake clinical training in occupational therapy. She returned to develop the occupational therapy department in Shijiazhuang, an industrial city in Hebei Province in central China. In 2005, she was elected to the occupational therapy subgroup of the Chinese Association of Rehabilitation Medicine (CARM), the only national group to represent occupational therapists. At the same time, she started teaching occupational therapy at a rehabilitation therapy course in Shijiazhuang. She concentrated on a relatively new practice area for occupational therapy in China, cognitive function, primarily because of the increased number of patients with stroke.

Yan notes that occupational therapy services are changing along with the social changes taking place in the People's Republic of China. In the 1980s, with the breakdown of the iron rice bowl[1] where every member of the agricultural community was guaranteed food, came the decentralization of land use and the development of a market economy under the communist party. The one-child policy implemented in 1980s was also taking effect. People were no longer in a position to stay at home to look after their disabled family members as had been the cultural norm.

Other changes included the increased acceptance of assistive technology. In the past, Yan said, family members were available and expected to provide for the daily needs of ill or disabled members. Economic growth and the availability of affordable assistive technology made this easier. New government policy supported medical and health insurance but imposed limited hospital stay and relevant rehabilitation. People had to go out to work in order to put food on the table and achieve a level of quality of life. Carers were hired to care for family members, both in hospital and at home. She notes that as the population ages, there are more patients with neurological and chronic conditions being treated and a greater need for extended care. Also, with the recent rapid economic growth of the People's Republic of China, accidents resulting from increased high-rise construction and vehicular traffic have created another major patient group.

2008 SICHUAN EARTHQUAKE – A CATASTROPHE BECAME A TIPPING POINT

The 2008 Wenchuan, Sichuan earthquake registered a magnitude of 7.9 and caused the death of more than 70 000 people, leaving 380 000 people injured and about 4.8 million homeless (Wikipedia, n.d.). Money from donations opened many gates for post-disaster rehabilitation and occupational therapy in the area. The Hong Kong Polytechnic University and Sichuan University jointly set up the People's Republic of China's first 'Institute for Disaster Management and

Reconstruction', which was officially launched in 2013. The institute is the first of its kind on 'disaster preparedness, disaster risk reduction and disaster reconstruction' on the Chinese mainland. Not only does it provide training in healthcare, rehabilitation, and disaster management, it also aspires to become a world-class disaster management research centre serving the whole nation, fostering closer collaboration between the Chinese mainland and the global community in the related research area.

Occupational therapy pioneer GuoHui Lin graduated as a Western medicine practitioner in 1985. He attended the World Health Organization course on rehabilitation for medical doctors in Wuhan, Hebei Province, in 1991. In September 2008, he had just completed his MSc in Occupational Therapy at the Hong Kong Polytechnic University, and was sent to the Wenchuan, Sichuan earthquake disaster zone as a member of the Rehabilitation Medicine team of Guangdong Province to support the local healthcare system to deliver occupational therapy services. Occupational therapists were deployed along with the full rehabilitation team to earthquake sites at regular periods after this major disaster. They completed home assessments and made recommendations on home modifications and assistive devices, did follow-up visits, and performed in-home daily living training.

During the visits, he used the translated Canadian Occupational Performance Measure as a client-centred assessment tool (Yun et al., 1995). The successful use of this and other occupational therapy assessment tools in the disaster zone gave him confidence to base his clinic services and teaching on occupation-based, client-centred concepts. By 2014, he was being regularly invited to teach occupational therapy in eight universities. GuoHui Lin is Head of the Medical Administration Department and Department of Rehabilitation Medicine of Guangzhou Rehabilitation Center for People with Disability. With 100 beds in his rehabilitation centre in Guangzhou and a team of three occupational therapists, five physiotherapists, and two speech therapists, about 120 patients are provided rehabilitation services per day. Through his department he provides clinical education for five occupational therapist and rehabilitation therapy education programmes.

---

[1]Iron rice bowl means guaranteed job security.

OCCUPATIONAL THERAPY EDUCATION

As demand for occupational therapy increases, so too does the demand for improved education opportunities for occupational therapy. Because of the variation in training institutes and courses around the country, there was no consistent standard for programme establishment, course objectives, teaching content, and quality of educators, significantly impacting the quality of knowledge and skills of graduates.

Until 2001, rehabilitation therapy was included in the National Full Time Higher Education Plan of the Ministry of Education. Starting from 2011 and following the 12th National 5-Year Plan, the government of the People's Republic, called for 'Rehabilitation for All by 2015' (Central People's Government of the PRC, 2011). Rehabilitation education expanded exponentially to support this demand, growing from only a few programmes in 2002 to over 90 diploma and 160 bachelor's programmes in 2009, focusing on the education of generic rehabilitation therapists (Xu et al., 2014). These courses have been taught in vocational schools, nursing schools, sports universities, and medical colleges/universities. Usually, the diploma is a 3-year course and the bachelor's degree is a 4-year course.

A first rehabilitation therapy textbook based on Japanese textbooks was published in 2003 to provide support for the training of rehabilitation professionals (China Rehabilitation Research Center (CRRC), 2011). From 2001, with the support and cooperation of the Japanese International Cooperation Agency and the Japanese Association of Occupational Therapists, Capital Medical University and the CRRC developed a new approach to teaching allied health professions, using a 2 + 2 format in which all students study core foundation subjects for the first 2 years. During the final 2 years of the bachelor course, students are separated into the two profession-specific streams for physiotherapy and occupational therapy. New Chinese-language textbooks have been developed since then, though mostly edited by rehabilitation doctors.

Occupational therapy pioneer Yue Gu went to Hong Kong from 1986 to 1988 to study occupational therapy, returning to Beijing with a view to further developing occupational therapy. Now, Head of the Department of Occupational Therapy at the CRRC, he supervises 45 members of staff and oversees the student clinical education programme.

This 700-bed, government-owned centre became the first rehabilitation hospital in the People's Republic of China and provides treatment for approximately 300 000 patients a year. Yue Gu notes that involvement of family members is an integral part of rehabilitation and they stay at the hospital with the patient to provide personal care. This is a unique part of the hospital system all over the People's Republic.

CRRC delivered an undergraduate programme for rehabilitation therapists before 2002, when they started a 2 + 2 curriculum together with Capital Medical University, requiring students to complete 2 years generic subjects and then specialize in occupational therapy or physiotherapy in the last 2 years. The Bachelor's of Occupational Therapy programme was approved by the WFOT in 2006. The rehabilitation departments have received very supportive input from the Japanese International Cooperation Agency since 2001, and the CRRC was able to send therapists to Japan to study for their master's degree. Yue Gu has been instrumental in retaining staff and supporting particularly the section of the programme which caters to children with cerebral palsy. In Yue Gu's department, there are now at least 10 master's level-educated occupational therapists and an equal number of physical therapists, providing academic and clinical teaching.

Other universities offering healthcare education have followed in the footsteps of Capital University and actively seek international support to develop occupational therapy courses. Some universities in the People's Republic are moving towards upgrading their present programmes in rehabilitation therapy to an international level by establishing occupational therapy and physical therapy as the framework for the last 2 years of the programme, that is, a 2 + 2 programme. By the year 2014, there were three universities with this course arrangement which gained approval by WFOT. However, there is an urgent demand for qualified educators and appropriate clinical placements and supervision.

In order to make the transition from generic rehabilitation therapy training programmes to profession-specific curricula, a process of professional development was undertaken, involving occupational therapy educators. The 2011 collaborative project group used

BOX 64-2

DEVELOPMENTS RELATED TO OCCUPATIONAL THERAPY EDUCATORS COURSE

- A provincial occupational therapy association was inaugurated on 6 August 2011 in Guangdong Province under the auspices of the CARM.
- A national group, 'Occupational Therapists', was inaugurated in September 2011, under the umbrella of the Rehabilitation Therapy Specialty Committee of the CARM. It was a major step in moving towards a legally recognized occupational therapy association.
- The national occupational therapy curriculum guidelines were completed and published, forming a basis for consistent nationally recognized occupational therapy programmes. Two of the occupational therapy educator participants were involved in the process and development.
- Occupational therapy educators developed a regular Saturday night social networking through QQ (People's Republic of China's favourite free online instant message software). This QQ group had expanded to over 2000 participants by 2014. They pose case studies and questions for discussion. Having this social network available had a solidifying effect on occupational therapy professional development. It created a sense of cohesiveness and community but also a sense of pride, and it raised awareness of the possible future impact of occupational therapy on the health and well-being of the population.

blended (online and classroom) approaches to facilitate change in the curriculum, teaching methods, and clinical practice for a group of 48 occupational therapy educators from over 30 schools throughout the People's Republic (Box 64-2). After 3 years, the programme was taken over by Nanjing Medical University and continues to be run locally. With subsequent years, the first cohort of the programme was engaged as facilitators and teachers, ensuring the sustainability of the programme.

NATIONAL REGISTRATION SYSTEM

In the People's Republic, the National Health and Family Planning Commission is responsible for the registration of health professionals. As of 2014, the national registration identifies rehabilitation thera-

pists as a professional group on the national government registry, but there are no separate registrations for physiotherapists, occupational therapists, and speech therapists. The examination which all therapists must take in order to work in the People's Republic covers physiotherapy, occupational therapy, and speech therapy, meaning that despite learning a specific discipline, to be registered to practice, students must learn a great deal of medical and physiotherapy knowledge. As a result, occupational therapy subjects are usually shortened or taught in an intense way. As most of the occupational therapists' posts available are based primarily in physical rehabilitation settings, graduates need physiologically-based skills to be employable.

In 2009, the Chinese National Government set out a requirement to develop a strong rehabilitation workforce that meets international standards and that is prepared to address the rehabilitation needs of its population. This would specifically require a separation of the disciplines of occupational therapy and physiotherapy.

CHALLENGES AND OPPORTUNITIES FOR THE DEVELOPMENT OF OCCUPATIONAL THERAPY

In order to develop the profession for future sustainability, occupational therapy needs to expand from the present hospital focus into community settings. Professionals need to develop confidence to work with more diverse populations and competencies to move out of hospital practice. The move must be supported by government policy; for instance, there is a need for government to establish policy and licensing so that homes for the elderly which are under the social welfare system can legally hire medical professionals.

Expanding the variety of fields of practice and taking advantage of developing health policy, will push the limits to establish new services. With good standards of healthcare, improving standards of living, and the national government's investment in referral systems nationally, there will be more opportunities and also demands for occupational therapists to extend services into new fields. The involvement of private companies in the provision of healthcare services, might also contribute to the rapid expansion of the role of occupational therapists in the People's Republic.

SUMMARY AND CONCLUSION

There is a need for occupational therapists to establish their services in clinical and community settings. Appropriate outcome measures need to be established in the People's Republic of China to evidence the effectiveness of occupational therapy. Occupational therapists need to see that they have a real impact. They also have to demonstrate effectiveness to other health professionals and the public. There is a need for policy support and organizational support for the profession as it develops. There is also a need for research in occupational therapy to show outcomes and effectiveness.

With this rapidly expanding service development, external support from outside the mainland has been sought. Therapists and educators from Hong Kong and Taiwan, which both have well-developed occupational therapy services, as well as therapists and educators from other countries, such as Japan, have been instrumental in supporting development. As this support is withdrawn, local teachers and therapists need to take up the reins. The pressure on the system and on individuals is tremendous as these pioneers attempt to lead the developments throughout the People's Republic of China. Individual ambitions and needs sometimes overtake altruism. For example, occupational therapists sometimes quit their current position for a higher salary position in more developed provinces; some go overseas to study and decide to stay overseas for better work environment and salary; there is a lack of job satisfaction, heavy workload, and working overtime with the same salary can often be off-putting. Some practising occupational therapists have taken the initiative to invest in their education. The first Master's in Occupational Therapy course in Sichuan University in 2012 attracted many occupational therapy applicants, with some deciding to resign from their current job and pay the full tuition on their own.

In a country with a population of over 1.3 billion people, there is a huge and continuous need for healthcare and rehabilitation. With increased urbanization and the changing needs of an increasingly ageing population, the demand for occupational therapy will escalate. The country's healthcare education system will have to continue to grow in order to accommodate these demands and should be incorporating the People's Republic of China's historical and cultural components. Areas to watch in the future include government policy and related legislation, improving medical and health insurance schemes, raising public awareness of the benefits of occupational therapy, improving registration and licensure, and further developing professional education with well-trained teaching faculty.

REFERENCES

Central People's Government of the People's Republic of China, The (CRRC), 2011. Perspectives of the 12th 5 year plan for people with disabilities. <http://www.gov.cn/jrzg/2011-05/12/content_1862943.htm> (accessed 16.10.14.).

China Rehabilitation Research Centre, 2011. Introduction on School of Rehabilitation Medicine in Capital Medical University. <http://www.crrc.com.cn/html5/jgsz_07.cbs> (accessed 17.10.14.).

China.org.cn, 2011. Injured laborers unaware of free rehab. <http://china.org.cn/china/2011-01/25/content_21813391.htm> (accessed 26.05.15.).

Hu, J., 2012. Development of health and occupational therapy. In: Hu, J. (Ed.), Occupational Therapy. China's Medical Publishing House, Beijing, pp. 65–70.

Li, J.A., 2013. Education Guidelines for Physiotherapy and Occupational Therapy. People's Medical Publishing House, Beijing, p. 180.

Lu, S.W., 2013. Work Rehabilitation *Chinese OT e-newsletter (HKIOT)*. September 2013. Hong Kong Institute of Occupational Therapy, Hong Kong.

Ren, Y.P., Guo, I., Li, Y.Q., Chou, J.H., Lu, Z.Y., Shao, B.H., et al., 2014. Current situation and need on community based rehabilitation resources. Chin. J. Rehabil. Med. 29 (8), 757–759.

Wikipedia, n.d. 2008 Sichuan earthquake. <https://en.wikipedia.org/wiki/2008_Sichuan_earthquake> (accessed 04.07.15.).

Xu, S., Lai, P.F., Lin, X.M., Cheng, H., Wang, Y., Li, J.W., 2014. Current Situation and Future Development of Chinese Higher Education for Rehabilitation Therapy. <http://max.book118.com/html/2014/0516/8281941.shtm> (accessed 02.10.14.).

Yun, X., Packer, T.L., Ouyan, D., Wang, L., Chen, Q., 1995. Application of the Canadian Occupational Performance Measure in patients with different diagnosis: 113 case reports. Chin. J. Rehabil. Theory Pract. 1 (1), 15–19.

Zhuo, D.H., 2013. The chronological track of contemporary development of rehabilitation medicine in China. Chin. J. Rehabil. Med. <www.rehabi.com.cn> doi:10.3969/j.issn.1001-1242.2013.06.00.

65

CHALLENGES IN THE EDUCATION OF OCCUPATIONAL THERAPISTS, DISCUSSED FROM A CRITICAL PERSPECTIVE

MÓNICA PALACIOS TOLVETT ■ MÓNICA DÍAZ LEIVA

Our experiences as occupational therapists in the last decade have been strongly associated with the education of our future colleagues, nourished by the experience we have acquired in practice with vulnerable populations. To systematize this experience of educating occupational therapists from a critical perspective, we need to consider at least two major, interrelated areas: the political and the ethical implications of education.

It is necessary to ask ourselves as the occupational therapist educators, *What is critical?* and *What is critical in the training of occupational therapists?* In turn, this exploration proposes another series of questions: which is the field we are concerned with and what are the relations of power that are established in this; what are the specific conditions of existence in which these relations occur; how can anyone be critical in a non-judgmental way (important, e.g., in the relationship between student and teacher); how can anyone disrupt

the naturalization[1] (Montero, 2004) and the trivialization of relations in the educational process?

The challenge we would like to document and to discuss in this chapter is the experience of a training approach that aims to be critical, of being part of an academic school within a private university context, where education can be seen as a commodity and relationships are determined by the logic of the marketplace.

The education of future colleagues in occupational therapy is a social practice, a transforming human experience, an achievement that constitutes one of the occupations that give meaning to people's lives. As de Sousa Santos (2010) suggests, the emergence of

---

[1]Naturalization is a concept that refers to a psychosocial process where people assume adverse situations as daily and natural ones, so they are able to continue with their lives without bringing them into question. Naturalization is a process that allows people to live in an acritical way (Montero, 2004).

sociology places everybody within the symbolic extension of knowledge, practices, and the possibilities of a future that, on one hand, shows hope and, on the other hand, urges people to turn this hope into reality. This allows students and educators to value the diversity of human experience, whereas an absence of a social perspective would render those experiences invisible. De Sousa Santos (2003, p. 238) explains that hegemonic processes try to disqualify forms of knowledge which counter them by imposing a *rational monoculture* which actively produces the *nonexistence* of knowledges by a process of disqualification, making them 'invisible, unintelligible, or irreversibly discardable'.[2]

We would like to consider, from the beginning, the intuitive and then more conscious attempts to generate a pedagogical area of occupational therapy, from what is becoming identified as a critical occupational therapy. This is an effort to systematize our current practices as educators, not from a neutral or abstract position, but instead from a place which is established in our practices as occupational therapists with social and political commitment. Over time, these practices have been established as exemplifying an occupational therapy approach towards a southern epistemology[3].

In Chile since approximately 2004, several occupational therapists working in academia have begun to reflect on their experiences in community-social practices, primary care, community-mental health, human rights, and more recently in the approaches and models of community-based rehabilitation. This was associated with the creation of occupational therapy schools in private universities and with the opening of schools in other public universities. These developments have been encouraging classrooms to open occupational therapy to diverse fields of activity, such as the vulnerability of the children's and teenager's rights, the intervention with vulnerable communities, inclusion-exclusion, and human rights, among others. These fields bring opportunities to converge different worlds and the possibilities of overcoming disagreements and creating areas of encounter and interaction.

The redirection of the professional gaze towards these diverse fields of activity has also produced tensions within the traditional and established perspectives, approaches, and patterns of occupational therapy. These tensions bring into play contradictory forces that reveal the underlying symbolic powers and material conditions from a critical perspective, where occupational therapists are engaged with vulnerable and often excluded or invisible populations. These critical perspectives imply the need to consider the inclusion of political and ethical reasoning as a part of occupational therapy training.

The experiences of populations whose access to occupation is compromised have been conceptualized as occupational apartheid and occupational injustice (Kronenberg and Pollard, 2007; Townsend and Wilcock, 2004). These terms draw on concepts such as segregation, marginalization, and social exclusion. This glimpse into the social field implies a political stance (without the possibility of neutrality) together with an ethic of human rights.

Now, what is a critical perspective? We, the authors, would like to reflect on this matter from epistemological, ideological, and practical perspectives. Evidence of the critical perspective can be found in the way relations in the educational field are negotiated, involving all actors: students, educators, administrative, and managerial staff.

The challenge of developing a critical perspective is that it generates a lot of questions about our nature as human beings and social actors. The tensions created as we try to gain awareness of our position, our place in society, and to articulate the possibilities these afford us, are very urgent and undeniable. Coming to understand this process is part of developing a critical perspective. During this reflection we have explored several questions that, in this text, we would like to try to discuss.

WHAT IS A CRITICAL PERSPECTIVE?

We understand a critical perspective as an awareness of the conditions of dominance throughout all levels

---

[2]This concept corresponds to de Sousa Santos's explanation of the concealment and invisibility of the knowledges and practices that are excluded from the hegemonic knowledge produced in the West.

[3]For de Sousa Santos, the southern epistemology 'arises from the consideration that the world in which we are in is in the middle of both colonial and capitalist power relations' (Ortega, 2010, p. 177). A southern epistemology proposes a counterhegemonic epistemological construction.

of social existence. This perception enables people to be aware of power relations through each layer of the society and to work for emancipation across them all, from the specifics of interpersonal relations at the micro level, to the macro level in economy and social policy.

A critical gaze has an interest in 'the conversion of reality, not just anything or to merely observe the change, yet the one that being desirable would have the potential to constitute a better world to all' (De la Garza Toledo, 2001, p. 109). However, what does *a better world* refer to? We believe in a world that promotes values of self-determination, justice, solidarity, and humanization of life in several contexts, including the university.

According to Freire (1969), a critical perspective looks at the world through the problematization of reality, from the logic of the question and from seeking to change those realities which alienate human beings and maintain the status quo. Likewise, Foucault (1995) would say that the critical perspective is 'the art of not being governed in a certain way' (p. 5), that is, in certain ways, *for certain purposes*, under certain principles. In this case, critical perspectives concern the art of not being governed by commercial relations of consumption, of the excessive use of technology in daily life, for money, for wages, by the relations of subjugation, among many others.

WHICH IS THE FIELD, AND WHICH RELATIONS OF POWER ARE ESTABLISHED IN IT?

For the purposes of this chapter, our chosen field is the education of occupational therapists. The relationship which occurs through direct contact between educator and learner takes place in an educational arena filled with contradictions. These can be identified through the complex web that comprises the educational process. The idea of education as individual progress or betterment is interwoven with its high economic cost, expressed in a commercialized relationship. The students are established as customers whose demands are based in consumer rights, rather than their rights as human beings. In this context, the educator is the administrator of a specific field or amount of knowledge or even the one who attends to

the customer's needs, providing the necessary supplies, that is, knowledge.

In this field, there are several positions of power – some visible, some hidden and at different levels – since the power is not always vested in the same actor. A first reading would indicate that it is the educator who owns the power, the power of knowledge and the power of evaluation. Nevertheless, when the learners occupy the position of the customer, they hold power over the conditions under which the educational process operates. They may require certain qualities of the product offered, such as particular forms of knowledge or forms of assessment, or exert influence over the conditions in which the knowledge is transferred or distributed.

All of the above, however, become evident when both educator and learner are subject to the power of the educational institution. It is the institution and its surrounding social, political, and legal context which causes and promotes the commodification of education and the power of the knowledge based in a scientific rationality, where both dominant science and employability conditions are important factors. These multiple relations of power are subject to multiple influences, most of them invisible, and obey symbolic forms of oppression where educators and learners occupy the place in the knot of the web; a knot that keeps the web joined, but may also be a place of power, as it may be possible to change the weave of the web or to untie the knots.

About the Critical Perspective in the Educational Field

In the educational field, the critical perspective suggests the creation of a map of relations of power to render visible the concrete conditions of life existence. In our case as educators in private universities, the implications of this critique concern the university, whose aim is to provide professional training, which is understood as another product within the education market.

We aim to analyse the reproduction of the hegemonic system from a critical perspective of pedagogy and propose how to generate a struggle and resistance against this domination. Through this perspective it may be possible to recognize how academic departments replicate the established relations of power, thus legitimizing their organization and structure (Bórquez, 2005). Nevertheless, this educational space also offers the possibility to *disarray* and subvert existing relations of power and produce new ones.

This critical perspective takes the assumption that education is not about instructing in either an impartial or neutral manner; instead, it is about politicizing the educational processes so that learners become themselves educators. This can help learners understand how emancipation in the educational process goes hand in hand with the emancipation of the vulnerable and oppressed populations in society (Bórquez, 2005).

There is an urgent need to generate a resistance to the neoliberalization of education and the reduction of its practices through citizens' education, an education based in dignity and active participation. Such an education can stand against the reproduction of the dominant culture, taking advantage of the gaps and spaces where the domination is not completely imposed, to open up alternative paths, develop countercultures and counterhegemonics (de Sousa Santos, 2010).

For Paulo Freire, 'true education is in Praxis, reflection and in the action of men upon the world to transform it' (Freire, 1969, p. 7). That the words in this dialectical process are understood as action is essential to Freire; words should not be a vehicle of incongruous ideologies, but on the contrary, be the creators of spaces of freedom and credibility in so far as they are embodied in the reality of those who pronounce them (Freire, 1969).

For Freire (1969), to educate from a critical perspective implies doing it from a humanistic conception through which the learner and the educator can lose their fear of freedom, allowing them the possibility of creating an awareness that they are part of a major context beyond the individual state of being (such as a community, district, country, the world, etc.).

There are many complexities in making these principles a reality in contexts such as the one we have already described. The main issues are the invisible restriction on the freedom of the educator and learner placed by the relations of consumption in which both are engaged, and by the illusion of neoliberal freedom, which is in reality an oppressive and very limited form of freedom. For example, in several private universities in Chile, the students are persuaded to choose their representatives[4] with the consent of the university authorities, denying them, however, an autonomous student organization. This also applies to the educators, who are not allowed to establish their own workers' organizations. Therefore, it is necessary to develop strategies of resistance, of openness and of reflection that enable the preservation of awareness and consciousness before the educational process.

About the Relational Conditions in the Educational Field

Within these concrete conditions we can realize positions where educators do not assume the role of alienated workers, learners do not become alienated and socialized towards individualism, the beliefs, values, and laws of neoliberalism, and young people do not develop an *acritical* perspective which is naturalized on superficial and trivialized relationships (Bauman, 2003).

For Bauman (2003), this issue of an *acritical* and alienating environment is understood as a liquid modernity, whereby the dominant power is exercised through the escape from, or evasion of, all responsibility in order to avoid its consequences and commitments. This brings about a dissolution of the social web, of the collective, of social geography, which produces isolated, uprooted, lonely, individual subjects where the power exerted is characterized by its superficiality and its slippery character. According to Bauman (2003), we, educators and students in the classrooms, offices, and hallways of the university, live with the evasion of self-commitment and of other people; with the invisibility of the other and the centrality of hedonism; where we seem to be disaffected in the present and involved in other places, for example, in our social networks and social media. Nevertheless, despite this disaffection, when a deeper relationship between students and educators is established, it is

---

[4]In Chile, private universities have a department of student affairs that regulates the types of student organization. Whenever the students choose their student council, it must be governed by the rules of that department and so students are not free to define their own types of organization.

possible to recognize that students are young people with problems of a different order to those of the educators, yet without references that provide them with support.

This places educators in what we could call a position of *pedagogical perplexity* (Bauman, 2007), that is, working with a reality that from the beginning seems unknown to them, with events that seem to be inexplicable and produce a sense of strangeness. For some teachers the experience is to feel lost and paralysed at first but produces no lasting reaction. In others, the feeling is resolved by recognizing some students as objects or qualifying them negatively, by not recognizing those people who are different in their human dimension, and finally by externalizing the events that occur, becoming *others* themselves through new identifications. From this place, the educator may disengage with the students, with an attitude of rejection, of indifference and acceptance of a perspective of students as simply being 'that is how they are … nothing to do', forgetting that as educators they also coexist in the same reality and ways of being in the world.

The precarious and uncertain economic situation and its consequences for social status should also be recognized by educators. This leads to a tendency for individualism, everyone striving to compete for themselves (both among the educators and among the students), as either could be expelled from the system and become unemployed. This unstable and insecure context incurs a huge cost, in terms of indebted households and learners who must work and pay off expensive loans to be able to afford the education[5] that will enable them to meet the illusion of social improvement.

These economic and material conditions also possess a symbolic element in so far as they are constituted in ways of life and of being in the world, with the effect that education turns out to be just another product in a world of superficial appearances. Becoming a professional has its own status and social

representations and can allow access to goods and services that others are not able to obtain. In particular, becoming an occupational therapist enables access to the world of healthcare, an alignment with the medical profession, and an association with those who help others.

WHAT IS THE CRITICAL PERSPECTIVE IN THE EDUCATION OF OCCUPATIONAL THERAPISTS?

Occupational therapy has been hegemonized from the moment of its origin as a profession supplementary to medicine, through the guiding principles for knowledge requirements established by professional bodies in agreement with state licensing processes, which ultimately shape practice. De Sousa Santos (2010) proposed promoting a southern epistemology in the critical perspective in the education of occupational therapists to enable it to break away from the hegemonic gaze. This is not to ignore the emergence of occupational therapy as a clinical practice, nor its history, but on the contrary, to position the profession in a sociohistorical way as a dynamic discipline with potential for transformation, linked to the areas where change processes are taught and exercised.

Freire (1992) proposes another element to be considered in the education of occupational therapists, that of generating spaces for dialogue. This pedagogical exercise goes beyond revealing a critical perspective of occupational therapy, to a critical perspective that respects and recognizes each learner. Starting from their own life experiences, every student is historicized by considering their social, cultural, economic, and political context to look for diverse paths and learning spaces with a personal meaning. This encourages them to discuss occupational therapy in their own words and allows the establishment of bonds, for both students and educators, which are engaged in transformation.

In the vision of Paulo Freire, the understanding of reality and of the subject within that reality implies overcoming the social relations of domination with the dialectical conjugation between subjectivity and objectivity. This can only happen by not denying human beings access to a process of personal affirmation or the deployment of this affirmation in the

---

[5]In Chile, every year about 130 students enter the department of occupational therapy in which we teach; they study for an average of 6 years. The average monthly salary of a Chilean middle-class family is $600 000 (approximately US$800, and the annual tuition is approximately $3 500 000 (US$5040).

political space. Both are necessary for people to perform their vocation of humanization[6] (Bonnefoy, 2009).

REFLECTIONS ON THE POSSIBLE SOLUTIONS

The challenges of producing a critical perspective are, on one hand, about being conscious of the positions that the educators are dealing with and, on the other hand, about collapsing these positions, in order to search for actions that enable change. Emancipation arises from little acts, small ordinary 'doings', such as finding ways to look at, listen to, and recognize the other's position in a genuine, responsible, and generous way. Then there are challenges of a different order, which are personal, and refer to human relations and how these are recognized in an adverse political, cultural, and economic context.

One of the first actions is to deeply realize both who *we* and the *others* are. This presents us as people with the challenge of implementing a path that allows connection, to think of ourselves as a part of the situation upon which we want to have an impact. Below, we offer some principles to guide pedagogic action from a critical perspective, according to Freire's book *Pedagogy of Indignation* (2012):

1. *Epistemic curiosity*

    This principle could translate into wanting to know more, not taking for granted what learners know about the educational exercise and educators know about the students. Epistemic curiosity does not accept that the truth is unique, generalizable, and immutable or that the truth the teacher holds is superior to that of others. To be led by occupational therapy principles implies the recognition of multiple ways of knowing and doing, deepening the

foundations of knowledge and remaining open to other forms of knowing and doing. The epistemically curious person assumes the attitude of questioner and a state of questioning, in which things are not regarded as obvious.

2. *Positioning oneself in the world from a critical perspective*

    Thinking from a critical perspective is a concrete process. It is historical, which demands that the subjects recognize themselves and assume their historicity, that is, ask what and who will be served by the knowledge or thought that they want to generate.

    Where a pedagogical project involves the commitment and thinking of an educational team, the first thing to do is to take account of self-awareness, to explore the historical position of individuals within the collective and of the collective itself. It is important to know the ideological basis of each member of the educational team, to identify differences and similarities, through spaces of dialogue related to the foundation of the ethical, political, and pedagogical principles.

3. *Think about options for transformation*

    Applying a critical perspective to understanding the world, rather than as an intellectual operation, is a challenge of facing up to the necessity of transforming the world. This requires clarity and rigor, but also a willingness to do so with discipline and not by disciplining, by tearing down the dispensable and trivial logics which are used to maintain social control. The critical perspective Freire (2012) proposes for a pedagogical project should be built upon neither a fatalist determinism nor a naive willfulness.

    Thinking in terms of options for transformation needs to be grounded in possible action, not dreams. Our dreams are not always achieved, are illusory and if we let them guide us, they might lead to frustration. On the contrary, we could make our commitments and principles become a reality with a possible action where little acts, gestures, projects that are materialized in everyday life allow us, the collective, to

---

[6]Freire (1992) proposes that the humanizing vocation implies a responsibility that is acquired in the daily life, where people learn to commit with themselves, the others, with the world, with the transcendental. This commitment leads the person to be related to others and from this place to know the world, deepen and transform it; actions will be acts of love, and therefore of value to the recovery of their humanity.

move forward to possible and necessary changes.

4. *Thinking from a critical perspective*

It is necessary to break down ideologies that block and subjugate learning, through the use of dialogical methodologies which emphasize group and collective reflexivity. It is essential that the learning is developed through the experiences of discovery, of the connection between self and others and not merely by studying concepts.

To generate the conditions for thinking from a critical perspective, it is essential that the educational team is in consonance with this vision, so that there is a matrix that generates a critical pedagogy. For this reason, it is important that a project should be built collaboratively, understood by everyone involved and constantly reflected upon. The motivation of any individual educator is not enough as it cannot allow a deeper change to occur.

5. *A critical perspective needs to be applied to thought and imagination, rather than to contents*

To think from a critical perspective is a complex exercise. Among other things, it introduces the empty word which arises as a slogan, the good *intention* to transform reality rather than a concrete action. Where the critical perspective only relates to intention, it collapses the moment it is put into practice, since it only takes the form of a simplifying and authoritarian shape of complexity but has not been enabled to express itself in daily relations. It is imperative to involve all dimensions of the subject; Freire (2012) proposes a coherent critical perspective of subjectivity between the ideal emancipator and the transformation process.

6. *Reflexivity*

Thinking from a critical perspective demands that one is alert to the risk of naturalizing or taking for granted one's own gaze and converting it into an object of critical reflection. This problem frequently occurs in educational institutions, their pedagogical practices, as well as in the decisions that are made through them. This requires what Freire (2012) calls a self-critical attitude of educators to their own lectures and practices. For Freire (2012), to take a creative approach to the problem of developing one's own way of seeing, thinking, and understanding requires a continuous capability for self-criticism towards one's own comprehensions and practices.

7. *Being critical requires consistency between thinking and acting*

The critical perspective in thinking and subjectivity makes sense in so far as it enables the proper guidance of transformative practices. This is a challenge with a high requirement from Freire (2012) demanding that one acts with good judgement, prudence, responsibility, and commitment.

These principles trace the possible paths by which pedagogical practice can be understood as a dialectic process in the sense of an indissoluble conjunction between practices, knowledges, and new practices. We believe these principles bring us closer to the education of occupational therapists from a critical perspective. Therefore, we can permit ourselves answers to certain questions, presented in Table 65-1.

CONCLUSIONS

In this chapter, we wanted to share our experiences as educators of occupational therapy – experiences which are full of concerns, contradictions, and convergences. Our reflections were guided by a conviction, perhaps a controversial one, that a critical perspective can enable educators to become aware of their own positions, as well as those of others (e.g., learners). To do so, we have proposed a methodology based on experience and not necessarily on evidence, a methodology that places hands and feet in the mud, which walks the streets, forging connections between human beings, while recognizing both the road on which we travel and the living realities that it leads to.

Educators cannot remain passive observers. There is an urgent need to re-create areas where there is dialogue and reflexivity, where the curiosity to know and ask can emerge, and which recognize that each of us is an educator for ourselves and others. As Bauman (2003) points out, we are living in a liquid modernity,

TABLE 65-1	
Queries About Pedagogical Practice in Occupational Therapy	
Queries About Pedagogical Practice in Occupational Therapy	**Possible Answers**
What would be the relation between educators and learners?	Human connection based on recognition and respect. Located in the realities of both the learner and the educator.
How should curriculum content and other academic activities be planned and scheduled?	Oppose self-contained individualism and competition, inviting people to build together. Discuss and agree planning on subjects and other academic activities between educators and learners.
Which methodologies to use?	Methodologies that encourage reflection on experience and discussion with an emphasis on the action and participation. Encourage learners to discover their own ways of thinking and doing.
How should we evaluate?	Challenge ourselves as educators and learners to perform the processes of continuous self-evaluation. Recognize assessment as an essential part of the learning process.
How to qualify?	Understand that the rating is not the assessment, but rather the result of the evaluative process. The qualification is contingent and not the centre of the pedagogical process.
How to transcend practice outside the classroom?	Provide opportunities and practical experiences, which are accompanied by mutual reflection, for example, by participating in collective situations, in research, volunteering and continuing education courses.
How can educators discuss and evaluate what they do?	Strengthen areas that allow the development and transformation of the pedagogical team. Invite educators and learners to evaluate through their real interest by generating significant learning.

which is characterized by a disintegration of the collective and an emergence of individualism. We believe that the educational context must oppose and resist this, through several strategies that encourage thinking from a critical perspective grounded in practice and not merely in academia. Guided by Freire (1969, 1992), all the actors in the process of occupational therapy education need to be enabled to recognize that both small acts and big actions can be emancipatory as long as we recognize the humanity of those who stand beside us.

Acknowledgements

We would like to thank Lorena Guajardo Yevenes for her translation of this chapter.

REFERENCES

Bauman, Z., 2003. Modernidad Líquida. Fondo de Cultura Económica, Buenos Aires.

Bauman, Z., 2007. Los Retos de la Educación en la Modernidad Líquida. Gedisa, Barcelona.

Bonnefoy, M., 2009. El Pensamiento de Paulo Freire y la Intervención Social: ¿Una Relación Anacrónica? CEAAL, Panamá.

Bórquez, R., 2005. Pedagogía Crítica. Ciudad de México, Trillas.

De la Garza Toledo, E., 2001. La Epistemología Crítica y el concepto de Configuración. Revista Mexicana de Sociología 63 (1), 109–127.

de Sousa Santos, B., 2003. The world social forum: toward a counter-hegemonic globalisation (part i). In: Sen, J., Anand, A., Escobar, A., Waterman, P. (Eds.), World Social Forum. Challenging Empires. Viveka Foundation, New Delhi, pp. 235–245.

de Sousa Santos, B., 2010. Descolonizar el Saber, Reinventar el Poder. Trilce, Montevideo.

Foucault, M., 1995. ¿Qué es la Crítica? Crítica y Aufklärung. Daimon-Revista de Filosofía 11, 5–25.

Freire, P., 1969. La Educación como Práctica de la Libertad. Siglo XXI editores, Ciudad de México.

Freire, P., 1992. Pedagogía de la Esperanza. Un Encuentro con la Pedagogía del Oprimido. Siglo XXI Editores, Ciudad de México.

Freire, P., 2012. Pedagogía de la Indignación Cartas Pedagógicas en un Mundo Revuelto. Siglo XXI Editores, Ciudad de México.

Kronenberg, F., Pollard, N., 2007. Superar el apartheid ocupacional: exploración preliminiar de la naturaleza politica de la terpia ocupacional. In: Kronenberg, F., Salvador Simó, S., Pollard, N. (Eds.), Terapia Ocupacional sin Fronteras: Aprendiendo del Espíritu de Supervivientes. Panamericana, España, pp. 55–84.

Montero, M., 2004. Introducción a la Psicología Comunitaria. Desarrollo, Conceptos y Procesos. Paidós, Buenos Aires.

Ortega, J., 2010. Boaventura de Sousa Santos. Epistemología del sur. Revista Mexicana de Sociología 1 (72). sigloXXI Editores, Mexico. <http://www.scielo.org.mx/scielo.php?script=sci> (accessed 06.07.15.).

Townsend, E., Wilcock, A., 2004. Occupational justice and client-centred practice: a dialogue in progress. Can. J. Occup. Ther. 71 (2), 75–87.

66

COLLECTIVE OCCUPATIONS AND SOCIAL TRANSFORMATION: A MAD HOT CURRICULUM

GELYA FRANK

How do we as academics share the emerging global conversation about justice with a wider audience of future occupational therapy practitioners? How can we support the integration of emerging ideas about occupational justice and collective occupations into new forms of occupational therapy practice?

As defined by Ramugondo and Kronenberg (2013, p. 10), collective occupations 'are engaged in by individuals, groups, communities and /or societies in everyday contexts; these may reflect an intention towards social cohesion or dysfunction, and/or advancement of or aversion to a common good' (see also Kantartzis and Molineux, 2014; Peralta-Catipon, 2009). In my own thinking, collective occupations are closely tied to 'occupational reconstructions', a kind of problem solving that becomes evident when people organize themselves to make social change.

Occupational therapy master's students whom I teach from such far-flung developing countries as India, China, Venezuela, and the Philippines tell me that there is typically little or no time in their national curricula to address the perspectives that occupational science offers. In the US, UK, Japan, Singapore, Australia and elsewhere in the so-called developed world, demands for technical proficiency and quality assurance also deflect educators' attention from exploring foundational concerns.

There is no doubt that students must be able to take their place as competent, confident practitioners in healthcare settings. After all, occupational therapy is a paid profession; hospitals and clinics are the settings where most occupational therapists practise. But the vision of occupational science also calls for seeing the world in new ways while using occupation as the lens. It had been anticipated that using an occupational lens to understand human beings and their problems would result in new forms of practice.

Occupational science founder Elizabeth J. Yerxa and colleagues (1990) wrote hopefully: 'The science of occupation could help the profession contribute new knowledge and skills to the eradication of complex problems affecting everyone in society' (p. 3). This work is not yet finished, nor should it ever be considered finished. We should not foreclose on the capacity of occupational science to contribute more to society. Without waiting for gatekeepers to allocate resources to develop a collective occupation approach to practice, educators can begin making use of the digital media and global networks to help to accomplish this goal.

TEACHING ABOUT COLLECTIVE OCCUPATIONS: USING VISUAL MEDIA AND THE INTERNET

This chapter shares a curriculum used with undergraduates in the occupational science minor programme at the Mrs. T. H. Chan Division of Occupational Science & Occupational Therapy at the University of Southern California. The course, Occupational Reconstructions: Collective Occupations and Social Transformations (OT 355), explores real-world examples of collective occupations in diverse social settings used to produce community-level change.

Digital media are key to the curriculum. In an article in the *American Journal of Occupational Therapy*, Doris Pierce (2005) explains in beautiful detail the usefulness of various video methods for occupational therapy and occupational science research. Visual data, Pierce (2005) writes, offer 'great potential for the study of occupation in all its contextual complexity' (p. 9).

Not least, for example, video allows us to immediately experience aspects of the feeling states of others while engaged in occupations. We can see immediately if there is enjoyment or discomfort. We can observe whether participation is tentative or wholehearted. Through interviews, we can gain access to participants' thoughts.

But this, of course, is only one dimension of what we can learn from observing people through the medium of film. We also see and hear where they live, how they live, the problems they face, the resources that may be available and how they typically deal with them. In short, visual media communicates to students differently than textbooks and scholarly articles. It

enables us to teach meaningfully about complex social problems in short, impactful sessions that do not even necessarily require the use of classroom time for viewing media in their entirety.

This chapter discusses three films: *Mad Hot Ballroom* (Agrelo, 2005), *War/Dance* (Fine and Nix, 2006), and *Waste Land* (Walker, 2010). These films are part of an expansive genre of documentaries about ordinary people working together in a focused way, using occupations to introduce desired change into a shared situation. These include:

- *Mad Hot Ballroom:* How to engage boys and girls in New York City schools in activities that promote developmentally appropriate skills and positive self-esteem, while also reducing multicultural and racial tensions. Here, the collective occupation is ballroom dancing.
- *War/Dance:* How to help youth in Northern Uganda to recover from violence that they and their families experienced as victims of the rebel Lord's Resistance Army (LRA), while also regaining pride and respect for their region and tribe. Here, the collective occupation is traditional tribal dance.
- *Waste Land:* How to introduce a different and more empowering perspective of trash pickers in a city dump in Brazil, people whose identity and livelihood depend on a highly marginalized and stigmatized occupation. Here, the collective occupation is a project in which garbage is turned into high art.

These and many similar films are available in DVD and digital formats for purchase, rental, or free streaming on the Internet. The trailers that promote and advertise these films, typically less than 4 minutes long, are also available instantly and without charge to most people with an Internet connection.

Because they tell the story in a highly condensed format, trailers also make a powerful teaching tool. Made by professional filmmakers, trailers function to convey stories and ideas quickly, with great impact, to awaken interest and make students want to know more. But while the films convey a story about social change, our job as educators is to provide students with the needed occupational lens. How can we teach students to view films like *Mad Hot Ballroom, War/*

Dance and *Waste Land* in ways that develop their capacity?

TEACHING STUDENTS TO USE AN OCCUPATIONAL LENS

Students enrolled in Occupational Reconstructions: Collective Occupations and Social Transformations (OT 355) gain an occupational lens on social change. This occurs through use of a one-page worksheet as a learning tool that orients and facilitates analysis, understanding, and comparisons of cases. The learning worksheet helps students to understand each case as an *occupational reconstruction* based on a set of principles or elements.

Occupational reconstructions have been described elsewhere by the author concerning the movements for racial justice in the US and South Africa (Frank and Muriithi, 2015) and work done by nongovernmental organizations in Guatemala after its long civil war ending in 1996 (Frank, 2012). The elements include:

1. *Collective Occupation*
   Occupational reconstructions involve shared actions with a clear purpose. These actions are collective occupations.
2. *Problematic Situations/Problem Solving*
   Occupational reconstructions are a kind of problem solving to make a problematic situation better.
3. *Mind-Body Practices*
   Occupational reconstructions are embodied. Participation and engagement involves mind-body practices, not just ideas or beliefs. They are conscious enactments of change.
4. *Narrative Meanings/Narrative Structures*
   Occupational reconstructions have a narrative meaning in the lives of the participants. Because they involve change in a situation over time, they also have their own narrative structure.
5. *Creative Possibilities*
   Occupational reconstructions open up spaces for doing, being, and becoming. They open possibilities for innovation and creative transformations.

6. *Intrinsic Motivation*
   Occupational reconstructions build upon intrinsic motivations. Participation is voluntary, that is, by choice.
7. *Hopeful Experimentation*
   Occupational reconstructions are hopeful experiments. They necessarily produce some type of change, but only sometimes what was initially intended.

The worksheet uses a grid that directs students to add notes about the content and context of specific scenes and particular moments. The students experience using the worksheet as a game-like challenge at which they become better as they see more examples of collective occupations in films. The worksheet also works as a one-time learning tool, but its repeated use turns the students into highly focused observers, skilled analysts, and knowledgeable commentators.

Let us go right away to the kind of observations, analysis, and commentary that we are seeking to encourage as the outcome of using the worksheet. Through their viewing of *Mad Hot Ballroom* we would like students to be able to use their notes to discuss collective occupational aspects of the ballroom dancing programme in the New York City schools. The description of the film, below, models a coherent understanding of dance as a collective occupation within a specific problematic situation. The discussion is followed by a worksheet based on this example (see Table 66-1).

VIEWING *MAD HOT BALLROOM* WITH AN OCCUPATIONAL LENS

In *Mad Hot Ballroom*, a film released in 2005, the collective occupation introduced into the New York City schools is ballroom dancing. These words float over the opening scene:

> *In 1994 a ballroom dance program was introduced to 5th grades in two New York City public schools. Today 6,000 kids from over 60 schools in Manhattan, Brooklyn, the Bronx and Queens are required to take this 10-week course. In the final citywide competition, only one school's team will be left standing.*

TABLE 66-1			
Visual Analysis Worksheet			

Name: <u>Your Student's Name</u>   Film: <u>*Mad Hot Ballroom (2005)*</u>

Occupational Reconstruction Elements	Example 1	Example 2	Example 3
1. Collective Occupation What is the collective occupation? What is the overall 'doing'? Who is doing it? Why?	*Ballroom dancing*	*Winning the citywide competition*	*Learning specific dances (merengue, foxtrot, swing, etc.)*
2. Problematic Situation What is the shared situation? What problem are the people trying to solve? What is their status and relationship to power?	*Getting preteen boys and girls to get to know and treat each other respectfully*	*Getting students of different economic classes and ethnic backgrounds to work together*	*Reducing tensions and fear of immigrants after the 9/11 attack in New York City*
3. Mind-Body Practices How is change enacted through occupations? How is the 'doing' done? What resources are needed and available?	*Learning skills: steps, rhythmic patterns, motor planning, balance, form, posture, self-awareness, eye contact, attention to partner, coordinated movement*	*Learning to relate and touch respectfully as the children begin their sexual maturation*	*Learning to deal with strong feelings that arise through the 'doing' (anticipation, excitement, criticism, losing, winning)*
4. Narrative Meanings/ Narrative Structures What is the shared story? How are events plotted in time? How do individuals' stories relate to the shared narrative?	*One boy does not speak English yet, but because he's such a good dancer, he is not excluded*	*Excitement builds week by week because the teams have a limited time to prepare for the final competition (the climax)*	*Dominican students in a disadvantaged neighbourhood can be winners*
5. Creative Possibilities What new opportunities become possible? What innovations arise through problem solving?	*Two Muslim boys are not supposed to dance, so instead they become DJs and still participate*	*A boy is able to dance with a much taller partner; a boy competes who is seen as graceful and confident although obviously overweight*	*The Latin music invites appreciation of Dominican culture; conversely, immigrant children come to 'own' the American songbook*
6. Intrinsic Motivation How are people recruited and do they stay? Why do people remain involved despite difficulties and challenges?	*All children in 5th grade take the 10-week course, but they do not have to be on the team that competes*	*A boy walks out of the class and the teacher does not force him to stay*	*Children appear excited and engaged; they show pride in their accomplishments*
7. Hopeful Experimentation What hopes and desires drive participation? What are the stakes? What are the risks? What are the outcomes?	*The kids learn the dances even though they do not know how good they will become*	*They work hard as a team but may not win the competition*	*The school and parents cannot predict which kids will change, but some become better students and attain a better future*

Latin music comes up. The camera pans a street in Washington Heights, a neighbourhood in Upper Manhattan that is home to PS 155. This is one of three schools whose teams will rise to participate in the final citywide competition. The other two schools are located in the higher-income, predominantly white neighbourhood of Tribeca (Lower Manhattan), and the ethnically mixed, middle-class neighbourhood of Bensonhurst (Queens).

The residents of Washington Heights are predominantly American blacks and Spanish-speaking black and brown immigrants from the Dominican Republic. Dominicans are relatively recent migrants to the US and since the 1990s comprise the country's fifth largest Hispanic group after Mexicans, Puerto Ricans, Cubans, and Salvadorans (Nwosa and Batalova, 2014). They make up 2.8% of greater New York City's population.

Students born to parents from the Dominican Republic are at risk. Their parents are more likely than the overall foreign-born population to live in poverty, to have limited English proficiency, and to lack health insurance. Yet, conversely, they are more likely to be US citizens and therefore entitled by law to full participation in US society. In the Washington Heights neighbourhood portrayed in the film, we see the *bodegas* – small grocery stores owned and frequented by Dominicans – that are set in buildings erected before the Second World War. The street is lively, but a burnt-out apartment house with boarded windows marks the environment as poor and disadvantaged.

As the film follows the teams from the three schools, interviews reveal that there is a shared narrative of ongoing competition (see Mattingly, 1998). The teachers at PS 155 would love to win the trophy from the current champion, Bensonhurst. The students are drawn into this story. They become motivated not only to learn the skills associated with ballroom dancing but become identified with their school and team. The competition brings out their willingness to work hard and work together so that their school can win.

By virtue of the competition, the dance programme operates within a powerful, overarching narrative structure. Like all narratives, it has a before-and-after temporal structure. The citywide competition will be a decisive climax to the shared story that marks the part that is 'before' from the part that will be 'after'.

Only one team may take home the challenge trophy. The other teams will have to learn to accept elimination, a lesser victory or defeat. In either case, everyone's lives will have been changed in some way by participating in the shared occupational experience. As the competition approaches, the intensity of practice and emotions rise.

A young teacher of Dominican background at the school in Washington Heights reports to the camera that the programme has resulted in significant changes in students' lives. There is no way to predict which students will be affected or how. The situation of lower-class black and brown students in New York City schools is too often one of occupational alienation. But the programme has helped many in the past to develop confidence, self-esteem, and higher aspirations.

In its mission, the ballroom dancing programme addresses a key situation of physical development and problems of maturation faced by preteens in general. At this crucial stage when their bodies are maturing, the 11-year-old students are given an opportunity to interact with members of the opposite sex in a protected setting with adult instruction. In the same occupational way, however, the programme addresses certain other problematic situations within New York City related to race, class, migration, inclusion, and participation.

In one segment, a school principal notes that ballroom dancing has taken on a new function and meaning, following the 9/11 attacks on the World Trade Center in New York City in 2001. Some students have experienced discrimination and exclusion, particularly those whose families have recently emigrated from Middle East countries. In fact, it is perfectly visible that the programme not only creates new possibilities for gendered interactions, but also opens spaces for shared participation and cooperation among students perceived to be of different ethnicities or races.

Week by week, the students are instructed in the etiquette, protocols, postures, and steps of North American and Latin American dance. They learn the meringue, rumba, tango, foxtrot, and swing. The children's faces and their body language reflect changes, as their practice becomes less self-conscious and more natural. The students learn how to interact and to touch one another in a respectful manner, while developing basic skills such as postural awareness, counting, and rhythmic patterns, motor planning, and coordinated movement.

Mad Hot Ballroom provides the viewer with access to informal, unscripted moments. Seen walking home from school, boys talk to boys (about the girls) and girls talk to girls (about the boys). The excitement is palpable. We glimpse a girl experimenting with makeup in front of a mirror, and boys hanging out around a football table. We see them in a city park, climbing rocks and shooting baskets on the playground. We hear their parents comment on the positive changes they observe in their children.

The final citywide competition is aptly called 'The Colours of the Rainbow'. Members of the team from PS 155 wear sashes indicating that theirs is the 'Indigo Team'. The Indigo Team's performance through the grueling elimination rounds is confident, skillful, and joyful. Their smooth movements thrill parents, teachers, and audience. As cheers rise in the packed arena, the Indigo Team from Washington Heights triumphs over its competitors to take home the citywide trophy. The gleaming trophy is impressive, as tall as the children themselves.

COMPARING PROBLEMATIC SITUATIONS IN *MAD HOT BALLROOM* AND *WAR/DANCE*

War/Dance, a film released 2008, follows three children of the Acholi Tribe living in the Patongo Refugee Camp in northern Uganda. Along with the other students at the Patongo School, Rose, Nancy, and Dominic are learning to perform traditional music and ritual dances of the Acholi people in order to participate in a national music competition in Kampala, the country's capital. Consequently, for the children and also for viewers, anticipating the competition gives *War/Dance* a tightly focused temporal or narrative structure that generates tension and excitement, similar to *Mad Hot Ballroom*.

Rose, Nancy, and Dominic are middle-school-aged children only slightly older than those attending PS 155 in New York City. But the children at the Patongo school are suffering from severe trauma and loss as a result of a war still being waged against the national government by the LRA. Both Rose and Nancy

witnessed the murder and even dismemberment of their parents by the LRA. They were forced to flee and struggled to care for, feed, and find safe hiding places for themselves and their still younger siblings. Dominic was recruited as a child soldier and forced by his LRA captors to commit atrocities, including the murder of an innocent family.

The three children suffer also from the stigma and shame associated with the fact that the rebel LRA leader, Joseph Kony and his followers, are members of the Acholi Tribe. So while the collective occupation is dance, as in the previous film, *Mad Hot Ballroom*, the problematic situation is of a different order, the narrative meanings for the participants are specific to Uganda, and the stakes for the children are much higher. In *Mad Hot Ballroom* the problematic situation concerns: (a) guiding the social and gender development of adolescents, and (b) creating opportunities for positive interactions and identities across race and ethnicity.

In *War/Dance*, however, the problematic situation concerns: (a) healing the psychological, emotional, and behavioural dimensions of war trauma; and (b) achieving social reintegration. Overcoming stigma and shame in order to reenter normal social life as a member of the group is crucial to the children's recovery (Vindevogel et al., 2013). As Rachel Thibeault (2011) explains, selective use of occupations can be used to rebuild lives and societies in postconflict areas such as northern Uganda, beginning with the acute phase of treatment all the way through social reintegration.

Another key difference between *Mad Hot Ballroom* and *War/Dance* concerns mind-body practices. These may appear similar when analysing dancing as an occupation for the individual student (e.g., learning the steps and postures, rhythmic patterns, motor planning). It is also true that we can literally 'read' states and emotions such as intense concentration, excitement, and joy in the faces and bodies of the students in both films. But we can also see important differences in the mind-body practices of dance as an occupation at the collective level.

Acholi dances are public events. The dancers perform in a circle rather than pairing off as couples. This difference in form signals the desired relationship of the individual and society that the dance accomplishes. In Acholi dance, uniformity and precision are key criteria for social proficiency in costume, posture and synchronized movement, as it is not the individual performer who is important but the tribe itself. The Patongo students' most important dance is the Bwola, which is traditionally performed by the Acholi to welcome and entertain the king and his court. Rose says: 'If I made a mistake in Bwola, it would insult my tribe'. The dance itself is with cultural pride and, for the children traumatized by the war, it literally embodies social reintegration.

In each film, the participants themselves want to know what the narrative impact will be of the competition. There is hope and risk: *What will it be like? How will it feel? Will it be good enough? Will good things happen as a result?*

The Patongo School won a prize for their performance of the traditional Bwola dance. But the film reveals that the students are intrinsically motivated regardless of the competition. Nancy says: 'When I dance my problems vanish. The camp is gone. I can feel the wind. I feel the fresh air. I am free and I can feel my home'. Dominic's narrative, which follows immediately, reveals his intrinsic motivation and experience of healing transformation as a participant: 'I feel proud to be an Acholi when I dance. In my heart I am more than a child of war'.

WASTE LAND: PARTICIPATORY ART AND SOCIAL TRANSFORMATION

The documentary film *Waste Land*, released in 2010, also demonstrates the power of the arts as a collective occupation tied to social transformation. While it is important to point out that occupational reconstructions do occur outside of the arts, *Waste Land* exemplifies the contemporary art movement known as 'socially engaged art', 'cooperative art', 'social practice', and 'participatory art' (Finkelpearl, 2013; Thompson, 2012).

Waste Land documents a 2-year participatory social art project conceived and executed by a contemporary artist and his team in collaboration with a small number of *catadores* (trash pickers) who make their living at Jardim Gramacho. A mountain of garbage dumped on marshland outside of Rio de Janeiro, Brazil, for a period of 34 years, Jardim Gramacho was a place of self-employment for 1700 *catadores* who sorted the trash by hand, to sell to recyclers. The dump

was one of the world's largest landfills and continues to emit massive amounts of toxic greenhouse gases after being shut down by the authorities in Rio for environmental reasons, just before receiving delegates for the United Nations Rio+20 conference on sustainable development in 2012.

The film records the situation and occupations of the *catadores,* including their thoughtful and surprisingly diverse narratives about what they do and why. But the film's focus is the transformation that takes place of the image and self-image of the trash pickers themselves through a project designed by renowned contemporary artist Vik Muniz. Born in Brazil but living in New York City, Muniz approached the Garbage Pickers Association of Jardim Gramacho, to gain support for a 2-year project. He recruited seven trash pickers, getting to know them over time, listening to them, meeting their families, filming their lives, and taking portraits of each of them at work. Posed classically and even heroically, the photographs evoked masterpieces of Western art.

The *catadores* were hired as assistants and participated by finding and placing pieces of trash as coloured pixels on the floor of a huge studio. Muniz projected images from a high platform and used a laser pointer to direct the *catadores* to fill in the outlines with different pieces of trash to produce the desired colour or texture. As one student in OT 355 described the collaboration: 'Like an architect Muniz guides the creative process but depends on a team to actualize it'.

Using this technique, the photographs are recreated using garbage to produce textured portraits on a stunning scale. Muniz photographed the massive images made of detritus to floor-to-ceiling *trompe d'oeil* portraits. The panels were exhibited at the Museum of Modern Art in Rio de Janeiro under the provocative exhibit title 'Pictures of Garbage'. The opening was attended by Rio's glitterati as the *catadores*, dressed and coiffed for the event, gave interviews to the filmmakers and the press.

Where is the transformation in this project? Muniz had the pieces shipped to London where they were auctioned off to art patrons to raise USD $50 000. He donated his share of the sales to the Garbage Pickers Association of Jardim Gramacho and continued to collaborate with them. According to art critic

Nato Thompson (2012), Muniz worked with the Association to enact a formal recycling project in Brazil and bring awareness to the dignity of labour by this marginalized sector of society.

A more important result has to do with the role of the contemporary artist to transform perceptions of reality. This is an approach to art anticipated by the philosopher John Dewey, who urged us to understand that art is not about objects, but experience (Dewey, 1934). It is also what Debbie Laliberte Rudman (2014) refers to as a transformative 'occupational imagination'. Transformational perceptions were created not only for the public, but for the *catadores* themselves. Tiao Jose Carlos Dos Santos, the president of the Garbage Pickers Association, exemplifies the awakening of a new self-image when he remarks that as pickers, 'We see only recyclable materials, but what Muniz saw was the potential to be more. 'The moment when one thing turns into another thing is the most beautiful moment of all', Tiao explains. Later, in the film, when he sees his finished portrait, he exclaims: 'Oh, man. That's crazy. . . . I never imagined I could become a work of art'.

CONCLUSION: MORE THAN MEETS THE EYE

The remarks by Tiao, president of the association of the catadores of Gramacho Jardim, carry important messages for occupational therapy educators. His comment, 'The moment when one thing turns into another thing is the most beautiful moment of all', informs us that collective occupations and social transformations are experiential processes. His further comment, 'I never imagined I could become a work of art', reminds us that such processes take place through individuals. The change is always a transaction among individuals and their society (Dickie et al., 2006).

As collective occupations and occupational reconstructions enter the working vocabulary of occupational therapists, lessons from 'naturally occurring' examples such as the three documented can be applied to work with communities. This type of occupational therapy needs to be supported through studies of cases, theory development, curriculum, evaluation research and funded projects. Targeting and preparation for employment opportunities need to be addressed by occupa-

tional therapy associations and occupational therapy professional degree programmes.

Towards this end, we can ask: what if only 5% of the world's 420 000 occupational therapists (www.wfot .org) were better equipped with theories and methods that enabled their legitimacy to work with collective occupations for justice and social change? It is a scenario that could well amplify the ability of occupational therapists to work for occupational justice (Bailliard, 2014; Durocher et al., 2014). Imagine if only 1% of the profession's resources – only 1% of the budget of the American Occupational Therapy Association, for example – were devoted to this goal.

Acknowledgements

The author wishes to thank students at the University of Southern California from 2013 to 2015 who were enrolled in OT 355 for their participation. Contributions by volunteer research assistants Alisa Kim, Katherine Lucas, Danielle Noriega, and Yushi Wang are also gratefully acknowledged.

REFERENCES

Films

Agrelo, Marilyn (Director), 2005. Mad Hot Ballroom. Paramount Classics. (105 min.) Trailer: <https://www.youtube.com/watch?v=-rlJuTC637c> (accessed 14.11.15.).

Fine, Sean, Nix, Andrea (Directors), 2008. War/Dance. Velocity/ThinkFilm. (107 min.) Trailer: <https://www.youtube.com/watch?v=2saj4gJ4Lvw>.

Walker, Lucy. (Director), 2010. Waste Land. Arthouse Films. (99 min.) Trailer: <https://www.youtube.com/watch?v=sNlwh8vT2NU> (accessed 14.11.15.).

Other Sources

Bailliard, A., 2014. Justice, difference, and the capability to function. J. Occup. Sci. 21, 1–4. doi:10.1080/14427591.2014.957886.81.

Dewey, J., 1934. Art as Experience. Putnam, New York.

Dickie, V.A., Cutchin, M.P., Humphry, R., 2006. Occupational as transactional experience: a critique of individualism in occupational science. J. Occup. Sci. 13 (1), 83–93.

Durocher, E., Rappolt, S., Gibson, B.E., 2014. Occupational justice: future directions. J. Occup. Sci. 21 (4), 431–442. doi:10.1080/14427591.2013.775693.

Finkelpearl, T., 2013. What We Made: Conversations on Art and Social Cooperation. Duke University Press, Durham, NC.

Frank, G., 2012. 21st century pragmatism and social justice: problematic situations and occupational reconstruction in post-civil war Guatemala. In: Cutchin, M.P., Dickie, V.A. (Eds.), Rethinking Occupation: Transactional Perspectives on Doing. Springer, Heidelberg, New York and London, pp. 229–243.

Frank, G., Muriithi, B.A.K., 2015. Theorizing social transformation in occupational science: the American civil rights movement and South African struggle against apartheid as 'occupational reconstructions.' South Afr. J. Occup. Ther. 45 (1), 11–19.

Kantartzis, S., Molineux, M., 2014. Occupation to maintain the family as ideology and practice in a Greek town. J. Occup. Sci. 21 (3), 277–295.

Mattingly, C., 1998. Healing Dramas and Clinical Plots: The Narrative Structure of Experience. Cambridge University Press, Cambridge, UK.

Nwosu, C., Batalova, J., 2014. Immigrants from the Dominican Republic in the United States. SPOTLIGHT, 18 July 2014. Migration Policy Institute. <http://www.migrationpolicy.org/article/foreign-born-dominican-republic-united-states#Distribution_by_State_and_Key_Cities> (accessed 01.01.15.).

Peralta-Catipon, T., 2009. Statue square as a liminal sphere: transforming space and place in migrant adaptation. J. Occup. Sci. 16 (1), 32–37. doi:10.1080/14427591.2009.9686639.

Pierce, D., 2005. The usefulness of video methods for occupational therapy and occupational science research. Am. J. Occup. Ther. 59 (1), 9–19. doi:10.5014/ajot.59.1.9.

Ramugondo, E., Kronenberg, F., 2013. Explaining collective occupations from a human relations perspective: bridging the individual-collective dichotomy. J. Occup. Sci. 22 (1), 3–16.

Rudman, D.L., 2014. Embracing and enacting an 'occupational imagination': occupational science as transformative. J. Occup. Sci. 21 (4), 373–388.

Thibeault, R., 2011. Rebuilding lives and societies through occupation in post-conflict areas and highly marginalized settings. In: Kronenberg, F., Pollard, N., Sakellariou, D. (Eds.), Occupational Therapies without Borders, vol. 2. Churchill Livingston, Edinburgh, pp. 155–162.

Thompson, N. (Ed.), 2012. Living as Form: Socially Engaged Art from 1991–2011. MIT Press, Cambridge, MA.

Vindevogel, S., Broekaert, E., Derluyn, I., 2013. 'It helps me transform in my life from the past to the new': the meaning of resources for former child soldiers. J. Interpers. Violence 28, 2413–2436.

Yerxa, E.J., Clark, F., Frank, G., Jackson, J., Parham, D., Pierce, D., et al., 1990. An introduction to occupational science, a foundation for occupational therapy in the 21st century. Occup. Ther. Health Care 6 (4), 1–18.

67

POLITICAL ACTIVITIES IN THE CLASSROOM: ALTHOUGH DIFFICULT, CHANGE IS POSSIBLE

LILIANA PAGANIZZI

The Argentine Republic has 41 million inhabitants in a territory of 3 761 274 km². Forty percent of this population lives in the province of Buenos Aires. The city of Buenos Aires, the capital city of Argentina, is a financial and labour hub and is home to several universities (public and private) and also to the National School of Occupational Therapy (ENTO, for its Spanish acronym). This school not only is the institution where occupational therapy was first taught in Argentina, (1959) but it also contributed to the opening of occupational therapy courses in neighbouring Latin American countries. Currently in Argentina, there are 14 occupational therapy courses of study in 13 universities. Eight of these universities are public and free for all the students, and five of them

are private. According to the Occupational Therapy Human Resources Project (WFOT, 2012), Argentina has a total of 5900 occupational therapists (based on data provided by the Argentine Association of Occupational Therapists).

This chapter refers to the teaching experience at the former ENTO, which is now part of the National University of San Martín, where 100 new students are annually enrolled and which has a total enrollment of 600 students. The position statement of the World Federation of Occupational Therapists (WFOT) on Community-Based Rehabilitation (WFOT, 2004), in which occupational apartheid experiences, occupational injustice, and occupational deprivation are recognized, the Declaration of Human Rights (WFOT, 2006), and the Universal Declaration of Cultural

Diversity (WFOT, 2010) mark a tendency to incorporate political reasoning within the required competences for occupational therapy. Influenced by these developments, and after 50 years of occupational therapy in Latin America, new forms of disciplinary and professional comprehension are becoming evident (Galheigo, 2010; Guajardo, 2011). Teachers are challenged to address the current claims that occupational therapy is transformational (WFOT Congress, 2010).

The purpose of this chapter is to share the teaching experience in an occupational therapy course of study at a public and free university in the city of Buenos Aires, Argentina. The scenario is made up of experiences among students and the author during the teaching of subjects such as: (a) Public Health, (b) Occupational Therapy and Work, (c) Daily Living Occupations, and (d) Professional Practice. Some teachers in occupational therapy, including the author, support a current occupational therapy philosophy based on concepts such as autonomy, participation, empowerment, and citizens' rights which cannot be merely transmitted as theory[1] (ENOTHE, 2013). It is necessary to create conditions so that teachers and students have the opportunity to experience them through an educational practice that generates spaces for participation and dialogue with concepts that are based in the actual lives of the students and teachers. According to Freire's view (Freire, 2011, 2014), education is not just simply developing skills; teaching is a political practice, and learning-teaching methodologies are not neutral since they make power-knowledge relations between teachers and students explicit.

Although we are concerned about content, we will focus here on the manner in which the *objects of study* are posed in the classroom, because learning methodologies imply and construct 'subjectivities' (Quiroga, 2002, p. 3). In this chapter, I use the concept raised by Pollard, Kronenberg, and Sakellariou (2008) of 3P Archaeology (3PA) as a tool for developing political reasoning within the classroom based on its articulating proposal among personal, professional, and political aspects.

ABOUT POLITICS, DAILY LIVING, AND EDUCATION

For Arendt (2007, p. 45), politics can simply be defined as the 'world of relationships'. She raises the concept of humans as naturally social beings, who can be political only in relation to others, so the political character is given by the relation *between* humans. Politics is the manner of relating, that is, the world of relationships.

According to Arendt (Roiz, 2002), political theory originates in the construction of a public space where some people are given the right to talk and be listened to, under equal conditions. In the emergence of the ancient Greek city-state, there existed a decisive division between public and private spheres, between life in the *polis* and in the *family*, between the activities related to the social world and those related to domestic life, which today we can call them activities of daily living. For instance, the right of *isegoría* (Roiz, 2002, p. 4), which concerns the possibility of talking and also of being listened to respectfully, belonged exclusively to the public sphere. Furthermore, Greek philosophers took for granted that the power and violence exercised by the head of the household were justified in the domestic sphere, where humans lived together out of need.

Relationships that were built out of necessities were considered to be a prepolitical phenomenon, particular to domestic organization. Daily chores, such as cooking, laundry care, and home maintenance, essential activities for the living of the individuals and mankind, were, therefore, forcibly mandated to women, children, and slaves.

This conceptualization of activities at home as apolitical and private (with a right of privacy from the social sphere) was maintained in the Western world until the eighteenth century, which is when Arendt places the beginning of the modern age (Álvarez Gardiol, 2005). Where activities of daily living, the household administration, and everything related to the family private sphere are indicated as part of the collective interest, issues such as where to live, how to live, and with whom become a political issue; these

---

[1]For example, learning about citizenship is not the mere acquisition or transfer of knowledge by an individual. It is a process of social participation, which occurs through opportunities for the production or construction of knowledge (ENOTHE, 2013, p. 2).

issues concern another politics, that is, a politics of daily living. So when Kronenberg and Pollard (2007) propose to explore the meanings of politics in relation to occupational therapy, it becomes necessary to distinguish between 'Politics' with capital *P*, that is, politics in the public sphere (state, government or political party's activities) and 'politics' with a small *p*.

To this purpose, Pollard, Kronenberg, and Sakellariou (2008) developed the political activities of daily living reasoning tool and emphasize the need of developing and integrating the political teaching and the political commitment with practice, education, and research in occupational therapy.

EDUCATING IS A POLITICAL PRACTICE

Education is a matter of political interest to any government. During the nineteenth century, the industrial revolution and the growing democracies developed universal education; the introduction of a mandatory and free of charge education was and continues to be the main force in the eradication of illiteracy. In some countries, the expansion of popular education has preceded the industrial advancement, while in others, it has occurred afterwards; but both phenomena have always been closely related to each other (Liu, 1958).

In 1870, the UK established a pattern with Forster's Education Act by guaranteeing basic education for everyone; in France, elementary education was made free in 1881 and mandatory in 1882; the percentage of people unable to read or write rapidly decreased from 16.5% in 1901 to 3.3% in 1946 (Liu, 1958). In 1869, 77% of people were unable to read or write in Argentina, but with the enactment of the law that established the mandatory, free, and nonreligious elementary education and with the construction of schools throughout the country, in less than 15 years the illiteracy rate was reduced to 50% (Torrado, 2003). The Universal Declaration of Human Rights (Paris, 1948), Article 26, established that 'everyone has the right to education. Education shall be free, at least in the elementary and fundamental stages…' but the then illiteracy rate revealed the social inequalities; in India it was 80.7%, in Argentina 13%, and in France 3.3%.

The literacy concept has changed in time and has been defined in several ways. Such concepts account for political and economic emerging circumstances, ever-changing cultural values, and new technological possibilities. Literacy may be defined as the 'use of printed and written information to function in society at large, to meet the personal objectives and to develop the own knowledge and potential' and, in its broadest sense, to reach the necessary capability in the required processes for culturally interpreting significant information (Cabral Perdomo, 2001).

Yet in the twenty-first century, where the literacy rate has considerably increased – 98% in Argentina – it is undeniable that there is an important group of adult people with some difficulties in reading and writing, who, while not being totally illiterate, remain below the school matriculation standard. Limited literacy represents a significant issue of inequality, as it means that those people will often not have access to appropriate or adequate information, for example, regarding their welfare benefits or health.

POLITICS IN EDUCATIONAL PRACTICES

In 1974 in the North of Brazil, Paulo Freire (Brazil, 1921–1997) began his literacy programme for adults, using an informal educational method. He proposed that apart from learning to read and write, education should establish a transformative relationship between the subject and the surrounding world, and he included the concept of politics within educational practice because it involves values, projects, and dreams that reproduce, legitimate, question or transform the power relationships prevailing in society. The social and political context confirmed his proposal: he was sent to prison and was exiled for 16 years, but through this experience, he became the architect of the transformative pedagogy, which currently is known as the pedagogy of autonomy (Freire, 2011, p. 68).

According to Freire (2011), the deepest root of politics in education is based on the *educability* of the human being that is recognized as unfinished. Recognizing this aspect of necessity, of needing others to know how to act and to be in the world, justifies the possibility of education. One of the main questions raised by Freire (2000) refers to knowledge; he argues that knowledge is not transmitted but is constructed or produced, and that both the educator and the learner should perceive and assume themselves as active subjects in the construction process. This proposal is extended to all educational levels, whether formal or informal, from basic education to higher levels.

THE CONTEXT OF EDUCATIONAL PRACTICE: THE 3P ARCHAEOLOGY PROCESS

The everyday shape of education practice is given by its content and form. An enriching educational context is collaborative, in which living human relationships are negotiated and actions are performed in an intellectual and challenging practical environment. Therefore, the creation of such a context is a basic concern for all participants (Ibáñez Herrán, 2004).

According to Morín (1999), it is necessary to develop the natural ability of human intelligence to place information within a context, and at the same time, to teach methods which facilitate the understanding of the mutual relationships and the reciprocal influences between the parts and the whole in a complex world. Educational practices must generate pedagogic activities that enable analysis of the relations between individual daily experiences, the contexts in which they are produced and also the social, cultural, and economic rules of the wider social order (Ibáñez Herrán, 2004).

For the development of this particular competence of understanding the articulation between complex elements, Pollard, Kronenberg, and Sakellariou (2008) developed the 3PA process as a tool for developing political reasoning in occupational therapy. The 3PA process explores values and personal, professional, and political motivations, and even the assumption of an absence of political values and professional practice. It is termed *archaeology* because unraveling the links between these components requires a deep self-questioning investigation of ones' own values.

POLITICAL ACTIVITIES WITHIN THE CLASSROOM

Educational practice requires methods, processes, teaching techniques, and didactic materials which must be consistent with the underlying foundations,

'with the dream where the pedagogic project is impregnated' (Freire, 1993, p. 75). Argumedo (2008) and Argumedo and Rossotti (2012), based on the educational philosophy of Gramsci (Italy, 1891–1937)[2] and Freire (Brazil, 1921–1997), and guided by their own experiences as educators in Argentina, made a list of methodological principles, which are presented below.

Organization

The classroom is mainly organized in what is known as interactive groups (Ferrada, 2010; Ferrada and Flecha, 2008). Although there are narrative or explanatory moments in which the educator expounds on an object of study of a mutually cooperative organization where responsibilities (for teaching and learning) are shared, in general, activities are distributed in small groups.

Participation

Teachers are used to coming into the classroom with a bag full of answers to questions that nobody has asked them. Freire (2011) advises on the need to develop a questioning pedagogy; a questioning enables the opening of a dialogue between persons who are willing to listen to each other, and where news may arise in the chatting context. It is necessary to provide mechanisms that make it possible for participants to have the right of giving and requesting information, of being listened to (the right of *isegoría* mentioned earlier), and being able to intervene in different moments of the learning process. Activities in small groups facilitate participation.

Operativity

Freire (2011) states that the necessary theoretical discourse for a critical reflection has to be so concrete that it merges with practice. The operability principle aims at producing an articulation between practice and theory, that is, learning new concepts and

---

[2]Gramsci opened new roads to political action, and education during the 1930s, a period in the world history characterized by the competition among three models: dictatorship, social organization, and a strong conformism, that ended in the Holocaust during Second World War (Monasta, 2001).

incorporating them to daily living. It, therefore, becomes important to discuss with the students the operability of topics in the group and raise questions such as: what does it serve for an occupational therapist to know the employment or unemployment rates prevailing in the country? Maybe in the future occupational therapists will be able to offer career advice to people, whether disabled or not, guided by the prevailing national context? Knowledge is produced in the articulation spaces created between practice and theory, leading to a close connection between the two.

Significance

Content must be relevant, pertinent, and adequate to the symbolic and material contexts of the students; it must have a meaning and significance for the students. It is necessary to seek and tolerate an unstable balance, between what the group knows – continuity – and what they need to learn – rupture. Teachers should establish a more intimate connection between curriculum and the social world of the students (Freire, 2011).

Globalism and Conceptuality

Globalism assumes that social reality is determined by multiple factors involving different economic, political, and cultural levels operating as influences encompassing the world. Globalism concerns the need to expose the relations between local, national, and worldwide levels and between the past, the present, and the future.

SOME TESTIMONIES OF EDUCATIONAL PRACTICES

Freire (2011) argues that the manner by which knowledge is constructed has received little attention. He invites educators and students to share experiences and encourages a close examination and description of the relationship between the teacher and the students (Freire, 2011). This section outlines some teaching experiences between occupational therapy students and the author during the teaching of subjects such as: (a) Public Health, (b) Vocational Rehabilitation, and (c) Professional Practice (clinical placement) which take place in the seventh and eighth quarters of the

course of study[3]. These courses are coordinated by the author, sometimes there is a paid assistant teacher and, on other occasions, faculty members are assisted by young professional colleagues who work for free.

The students' testimonies are obtained from opinion surveys made in writing and anonymously at the end of each course[4]. We think that this method encourages the students to give their opinion more freely, at least until we are able to incorporate in the classrooms a culture of discussion on various topics, including the teaching methods we use.

Public Health

Topic: Epidemiology and Causes of Death

In Argentina, the current statistics show that the five main causes of death are: (a) heart diseases, (b) malignant tumours, (c) respiratory diseases, (d) cerebrovascular diseases, and (e) accidents (Argentina-Ministerio de Salud, 2014; Barragán, 2007). However, there is a political discussion concerning insecurity, violence, and poverty. The media often emphasize the idea that there is a clear relation between these three elements, while the current (at the time of this writing in October 2015) government under President Cristina Fernandez de Kirchner tries to reverse this concept, which in fact is erroneous.

When dealing with the topic 'causes of death' in the classroom, we began by listening to the students' opinions on this matter. The following question was used to stimulate discussion: which is the main cause of death in Argentina? When the students were asked about the main cause of death in Argentina, the answers were often 'malnutrition' and 'violence', reflecting the discussion in the media. Guided by the class discussion and comments, I proposed that two groups of students were to be in charge of searching epidemiological data. Tools and official sources of data were provided.

In the following class, the groups displayed their search results. Rather than violence or malnutrition,

---

[3]The professional cycle of the course of study comprises thirty-eight theoretical, theoretical-practical, and practical subjects, out of which three are clinical placements. The curriculum is organized in nine quarters (of 16 weeks each) running each year between March and November.

[4]Mainly 23-year-old female students.

chronic noninfectious diseases (cardiovascular, respiratory, and neoplasms) and accidents were the main causes of death in Argentina. Domestic accidents were the main external cause of death in children between 0 and 4 years old, and suicide was the main external cause of death in people between 20 and 24 years old (Argentina-Ministerio de Salud, 2014); this was the same age group as that of most of the students attending the course.

The class discussed the psychosocial character of the causes and the possible role of occupational theory. Safety measures in household daily activities for the care of children and forms of detecting suicidal thoughts often arose as answers. At the end, several students shared experiences about self-harming events of which they became aware in clinical placement and shared testimonies of personal experiences from friends and family.

Topic: Health Determinants and Lifestyles

There is considerable evidence of the correlation between lifestyles and determinants of health. Where the influence of diet in health is addressed, discussion quickly moved to the question of the ignorance of the most economically deprived population groups as a factor in poor nutrition, according to the presentations that are often given in the media and the beliefs of the urban middle class, to which most of the participants in this classroom belonged.

Dialogue and the questions about the students' own lifestyles often revealed that they experienced an urgency and lack of time; the great range of fast and processed food and the cost of food are the determinants of the basic problems. Then, after discussing around the evidence, we saw how malnutrition, poor nutrition, and obesity are, in fact, present in all social sectors (Barragán, 2007).

We also noted that malnutrition is a very serious problem across Latin America[5], and a group of students offered to conduct a search on the topic. Tools and reliable Internet sites were provided and, at the next deadline, they shared their search results with the rest of the class. Other groups suggested searches on

employment, education, housing, or the environment and their relations with health. The finished work was displayed in the classroom and after being discussed, some of this work was recommended as study material.

Achievements and Setbacks

As in every system of relations, there are tensions, conflict situations, and moments of cooperation. Kronenberg and Pollard (2007) explain that conflict and cooperation serve as the engine of all political commitment; they motivate the action and should not be considered as inherently good or bad. Making them explicit is part of the political activities of daily living. Below, I outline some of the main challenges.

Group Size

Since 2005 and until the time of this writing (October 2015), the enrolment in occupational therapy courses has increased considerably. Teachers at some public universities often have class sizes of 70, 80, and up to 100 students. This structure makes it difficult to conduct activities based on dialogue and participation. Whenever possible, academics try to form smaller work groups. With regard to this, one student stated:

> It seemed very useful to me that the class has been split over 2 days to reduce the number of students and, in that way, having more dynamic and participating classes. (Male student, 22 years old)

Another student said:

> I really think that the class increases its potential when everyone participates, but, sometimes people are embarrassed or too shy to participate, one feels more comfortable in small groups. (Female student, 24 years old)

Although teachers and students usually agree on this issue, the current university administrative system will not reconsider the number of hours and teaching positions for the creation of smaller class sizes or for repeating the course in the second term of the year. Having smaller class sizes depends on the educators' willingness to teach and the availability of the

---

[5]Malnutrition, overweight, and obesity affect 23% of adults and 7% of children in preschool age in Latin America (FAO, 2014).

students; if an agreement can be reached, the administration can organize the classes.

Traditional Versus Participatory Methodologies

A participatory educational system does not remove the responsibility of the teacher or the need for rigor in the presentation of the subjects; however, these strategies can occasionally be disruptive to traditional teaching methodologies in which students occupy a spectator role.

While in the opinion of some students, 'the way the module was taught was very good, one gets to incorporate the topics when preparing research assignments, the space for discussion and for listening to our fellow students was very useful, it helps a lot' (female student, 25 years old), others expressed that 'I appreciate the intention of working outside the traditional framework, and although I think it is more useful, I also believe that it is more uncomfortable and less efficient…I do not agree that the student is always called to study and participate' (female student, 25 years old), or 'I am not very participative because I'm afraid of being criticised by the teacher' (female student, 23 years old), or 'the space given for dialogue in group and for discussion is very useful…but the students sometimes do not feel comfortable or confident in doing this because we are not used to it' (female student, 23 years old).

In other opportunities, indeed, teachers are not able to expound or support the intended proposals clearly, or they are not always very supportive.

It is very good that we have to read and that we can discuss the topic in class, but speaking in groups in most of the classes was very tiring for me, and sometimes confusing, I prefer the teacher to teach and the student to participate or ask questions. (Male student, 24 years old)

I dare say that occasionally, we have felt that participations were not well received…as if we failed to live up to the expectations, or as if teachers think that what we say is too elementary. (Female student, 26 years old)

In the dialogue and discussion space during the course, I have dared to give my opinion in group on

certain topics that I would have never imagined, even outside the university. (Female student, 26 years old)

CONCLUSIONS

During the educators' meeting of the 15th WFOT World Congress, taking place for the first time in a Latin American country, Chile, the need to face social issues and maintain a reflexive and critical thought with due respect for diversity, culture, social affairs, and human rights was made clear (WFOT Congress, 2010). The purpose of this chapter has been to share some of the achievements and setbacks of applying this to educational practice.

I have presented some concepts developed from the participatory pedagogies which may enable a classroom discourse on a social and political vision of occupational therapy. My arguments are constructed from within the classroom and across all the subjects comprising the curricula, not just those formerly linked to community practice.

The living thought of Paulo Freire and the 3PA concept as a tool for political and articulating reasoning have resulted in a basic strategy, which supports the methodological principles that guide professional as well as educational practice. This participatory perspective implies the acceptance that nobody has the solution about what, when, or how to teach and evaluate, but alternative solutions may be constructed and improved in time, through agreed and collective dynamics. Such an approach espouses an open, dynamic, and agreeably complex process, like life itself.

Acknowledgements

I wish to thank C.T. Romina Contreras for translating this chapter from Spanish.

REFERENCES

Álvarez Gardiol, A., 2005. Academia Nacional de Derecho y Ciencias Sociales de Córdoba. Argentina. <http://www.acader.unc.edu.ar> (accessed 09.2013.).

Arendt, H., 2007. ¿Qué es política? Ediciones Paidós, Barcelona, p. 45. Available from: <http://www.psikolibro.tk> (accessed 10.10.15.).

Argentina-Ministerio de Salud, 2014. Dirección de Estadísticas e Información de Salud- Serie 5 – Número 55. República Argentina,

Buenos Aires. Available from: <http://www.deis.gov.ar/> (accessed 10.10.15.).

Argumedo, M.A., 2008. Principios metodológicos para una educación emancipatoria. Buenos Aires. Available from: <http://argumedomanuel.wordpress.com/category/metodologia/> (accessed 10.10.15.).

Argumedo, M., Rossotti, A., 2012. Bachilleratos Populares y educación liberadora. VII Jornadas de Sociología de la Universidad Nacional de La Plata. Bs As. Argentina, 'Argentina en el escenario latinoamericano actual: debates desde las ciencias sociales'. Available from: <http://jornadassociologia.fahce.unlp.edu.ar> (accessed 10.10.15.).

Barragán, L., 2007. Fundamentos de la salud pública. La Plata. Available from: <http://sedici.unlp.edu.ar/> (accessed 10.10.15.).

Cabral Perdomo, I., 2001. Alfabetismo Científico y Educación. Campus Central de Veracruz, México. Revista Iberoamericana de Educación: OEI.

ENOTHE, 2013. Ciudadanía: explorando la contribución de Terapia. p. 2. Available from: <www.enothe.eu/activities/.../CITIZENSHIP_STATEMENT_SPANISH.Pdf.2014http://www.rieoei.org/deloslectores/Cabral.PDF> (accessed 10.2014.).

FAO: Organización de las Naciones Unidas para la Alimentación y la Agricultura, 2014. Panorama de la Seguridad Alimentaria y Nutricional en América Latina y el Caribe, 2013. Available from: <http://www.fao.org/docrep/019/i3520s/i3520s.pdf> (accessed 06.2015.).

Ferrada, D., 2010. 'Comunidades de Aprendizaje' y 'Enlazando Mundos': las bases de una pedagogía dialógica que genera igualdad. Revista Eletrônica de Educação. São Carlos, SP: UFSCar, 4: 2, pp. 70–84. Available from: <http://www.reveduc.ufscar.br>.

Ferrada, D., Flecha, R., 2008. El modelo dialógico de la pedagogía: un aporte desde las experiencias de comunidades de aprendizaje. Estudpedagóg 34, 1. Valdivia 2008. Available from: <http://dx.doi.org/10.4067/S0718-07052008000100003> (accessed 10.10.15.).

Freire, P., 1993. Educación y participación comunitaria Extracto-. Nuevas Perspectivas Críticas en Educación, Barcelona, Paidós, p. 75.

Freire, P., 2000. Recopilación de entrevistas a Paulo Freire. Available from: <http://paulofreire19.blogspot.co.uk/2015/08/paulo-freire-recopilacion-de-entrevistas.html> (accessed 15.06.16.).

Freire, P., 2011. Pedagogía da Autonomía. Saberes Necessários á Prática Educativa. Ed 43°, Sao Paulo, Ed Paz e Terra, pp. 45–68.

Freire, P., 2014. Cartas a quien pretende enseñar. Biblioteca Esencial del pensamiento contemporáneo. Ed siglo XXI. Buenos Aires, p. 68.

Galheigo, S., 2010. ¿Qué hay que hacer? Responsabilidades y desafíos de la terapia ocupacional en materia de derechos humanos. Available from: <www.wfot2010.com> (accessed 2014.).

Guajardo, A., 2011. Prólogo. In: Ocupación: sentido, realización y libertad en Diálogos ocupacionales en torno al sujeto, la sociedad y el medio ambiente. Universidad Nacional de Colombia, sede Bogotá. Facultad de Medicina Grupo de Investigación Ocupación y Realización Humana. Claudia Rojas, Colombia.

Ibáñez Herrán, J., 2004. La educación transformadora: concepto, fines y métodos. Available from: <http://www.pangea.org/jei> (accessed 07.2014.).

Kronenberg, F., Pollard, N., 2007. Superar el apartheid ocupacional. In: Kronenberg, F., Simo Algado, S., Pollard, N. (Eds.), Terapia Ocupacional sin Fronteras Aprendiendo del Espíritu de Supervivientes. Médica Panamericana, Madrid.

Liu, B., 1958. Geografía de la ignorancia UNESCO. El Correo 3 (2), 5–6. Available from: <http://unesdoc.unesco.org/images/0007/000781/078161so.pdf> (accessed 10.2014.).

Monasta, A., 2001. Gramsci. ©UNESCO: Oficina Internacional de Educación. <www.ibe.unesco.org/publications/ThinkersPdf/gramscis.pdf> (accessed 10.10.15.).

Morín, E., 1999. Los siete saberes necesarios para la educación del futuro. Organización de las Naciones Unidas para la Educación, la Ciencia y la Cultura. UNESCO, París.

Pollard, N., Sakellariou, D., Kronenberg, F., 2008. A Political Practice of Occupational Therapy. Churchill Livingston, London.

Quiroga, A., 2002. Pichon Riviére y Paulo Freire: El sujeto en el proceso de conocimiento (modelos internos o matrices de aprendizaje). Psicología Social. Ficha 2 p. 3. Available from: <www.psicosocial.geomundos.com> (accessed 10.10.15.).

Roiz, J., 2002. La teoría política de Hannah Arendt (1906–1975). Institut de Ciències Politiqunes i Socials. Universitat Autònoma de Barcelona, Barcelona, p. 4.

Torrado, S., 2003. Historia de la familia moderna (1870–2000). Ed. de la Flor, Buenos Aires.

World Federation of Occupational Therapists (WFOT). 2004. Position Statement on Community-Based Rehabilitation-CBR. Available from: <www.wfot.org> (accessed 10.2011.).

World Federation of Occupational Therapists (WFOT). 2006. Position Statement on Human Rights. Available from: <www.wfot.org> (accessed 02.2012.).

World Federation of Occupational Therapists (WFOT). 2010. Position Statement on Diversity and Culture. Available from: <www.wfot.org> (accessed 02.2012.).

World Federation of Occupational Therapists (WFOT), 2012. Human Resources Project Report. Federación Mundial de Terapeutas Ocupacionales, Western Australia. Available from: <http://www.wfot.org/ResourceCentre.aspx> (accessed 10.2013.).

World Federation of Occupational Therapists Congress, 2010. Informe Día de la Educación. Santiago, Chile. Elab por: Oyarzún, E., Acevedo, C., Olivares Palacios, M., Méndez, P., Comité Día de la Educación. Available at: <www.wfot2010.com> (accessed 11.2012.).

INDEX